Small Animal Internal Medicine
for Veterinary Technicians and Nurses

Editorial offices: 2121 State Avenue, Ames, Iowa 50014-8300, USA
The Atrium, Southern Gate, Chichester, West Sussex, PO19 8SQ, UK
9600 Garsington Road, Oxford, OX4 2DQ, UK

For details of our global editorial offices, for customer services and for information about how to apply for permission to reuse the copyright material in this book please see our website at www.wiley.com/wiley-blackwell.

Library of Congress Cataloging-in-Publication Data

Small animal internal medicine for veterinary technicians and nurses / editor, Linda Merrill.
p. ; cm.
Small animal internal medicine for veterinary technicians and nurses
Includes bibliographical references and index.
ISBN 978-0-8138-2164-1 (pbk. : alk. paper)
1. Cats–Diseases–Handbooks, manuals, etc. 2. Dogs–Diseases–Handbooks, manuals, etc. 3. Animal health technicians–Handbooks, manuals, etc. 4. Veterinary nursing–Handbooks, manuals, etc.
5. Veterinary internal medicine. 6. Veterinary medicine. I. Merrill, Linda (Linda Lee),
1958- II. Title: Small animal internal medicine for veterinary technicians and nurses.
[DNLM: 1. Animal Diseases. 2. Animal Technicians. 3. Internal Medicine–methods. 4. Pets. 5. Veterinary Medicine–methods. SF981]
SF981.S627 2012
636.089–dc23
2011052834

A catalogue record for this book is available from the British Library.

Wiley also publishes its books in a variety of electronic formats. Some content that appears in print may not be available in electronic books.

Set in 10/12 pt Minion Pro by Toppan Best-set Premedia Limited
Printed and bound by CPI Group (UK) Ltd, Croydon, CR0 4YY

Cover images:
Top image: VD radiograph of a 6-month-old puppy with right-sided pneumothorax with secondary lung lobe collapse showing retraction of the peripheral lung margins from the thoracic wall and presence of avascular gas opacity (free air) filling the pleural space and compressing the lung lobes. Image courtesy of Marcella Ridgway
Second image from top: *Histoplasma capsulatum* in a white blood cell in a dog. Image courtesy of Stan Krogman.
Middle image: Image of author Ann Wortinger's cat, Cheyenne, enjoying a garden view during a supervised break from her protective bandage.
Second image from bottom: Focally a myocyte contain onion-cyst (arrow) also note a pyogranuloma (star). Image courtesy of Kuldeep Singh.
Bottom image: Demonstration of the technique to add fenestrations to catheter prior to abdominocentesis. Image courtesy of Diane Greene.
Right hand image: Cody, editor's corgi

Disclaimer

C9780813821641_190924

Dedication

This textbook is dedicated to all those veterinary technicians with a thirst for learning and has been inspired by all the wonderful animals that have touched my life. The idea for this textbook was made into a reality by the combined works of a fantastic group of authors and editors. I hope it inspires you to continue your personal journey in veterinary medicine and provides you with the means to expand your horizons.

I would like to give a special thank you to the veterinary technicians who have helped me along the way and to the veterinary technician specialists of AIMVT and the other academies who continue to motivate me. You are too many to name, but I hope you realize how great you all are. I would also like to express my sincere appreciation to all the knowledgeable veterinarians and colleagues who have taken their time to answer my thousands of questions.

Finally, I wish to acknowledge the love, patience, and support of my husband Jeff.

Linda

Contents

Chapter **4**

The Neurological Examination   99

Chapter **5**

Thrombotic Disorders in Small Animal Medicine   127

Chapter **6**

Respiratory   137

Chapter **7**

Hematology   161

Chapter 8

Gastrointestinal 193

Chapter 9

Liver 263

Chapter 13

Pain and Its Management   433

Chapter 14

Nursing   449

This book is accompanied by a companion website:

www.wiley.com/go/merrill

The website includes:

- More than 400 Multiple-Choice Questions
- Powerpoints of all figures and tables from the book for downloading
- Echocardiography video clips

Contributors

Ale Aguirre, DVM, DACVIM (SAIM), VETMED, Phoenix, Arizona

Constance Barkey, LVT, LMP, LAMP, Seattle Veterinary Associates, Seattle, Washington

Shauna Blois, DVM, DVSc, DACVIM (SAIM), Ontario Veterinary College, University of Guelph, Guelph, Ontario, Canada

Peter J. Bondy, Jr. DVM, MS, DACVIM (SAIM), Central Texas Veterinary Specialty Hospital, Austin and Round Rock, Texas

Kara M. Burns, MS, MEd, LVT, Academy of Veterinary Nutrition Technicians, Inc., Wamego, KS

Rosemary Calderon, LVT, VTS (Oncology), Animal Medical Center, New York, New York

Clay A. Calvert, DVM, DACVIM (SAIM), University of Georgia College of Veterinary Medicine, Athens, Georgia

Marcia Carothers, DVM, DACVIM (SAIM), Akron Veterinary Internal Medical Practice (AVIMP), Norton, Ohio

Anthony P. Carr, Dr. med. vet., DACVIM (SAIM), Western College of Veterinary Medicine, Saskatoon, Canada

Virginia Coyle, DVM, Practice limited to Oncology, Florida Veterinary Specialists, Tampa, Florida

Tanya Crocker, RVT, VTS (SAIM) Canada West Veterinary Specialists, Vancouver, BC, Canada

Tracy Darling, RVT, VTS (SAIM), Anacapa Animal Hospital, Ventura, California

Alice Defarges, DVM, MSc, DACVIM (SAIM), Ontario Veterinary College, University of Guelph, Guelph, Ontario, Canada

Krysta Deitz, DVM, MS, DACVIM (SAIM) Iowa State University, College of Veterinary Medicine, Veterinary Medical Center, Ames, Iowa

Lawren Durocher, DVM, MS, DACVIM (SAIM), Carolina Veterinary Specialists, Winston-Salem, NC

Heather A. Flaherty, DVM, DACVP, Iowa State University, College of Veterinary Medicine, Veterinary Medical Center, Ames, Iowa

Marnin Forman, DVM, DACVIM (SAIM), Cornell University Veterinary Specialists, Stamford, CT

Jennifer Garcia, DVM, DACVIM, JGMedInk, Houston, Texas

Michael Goldstein, DVM, DACVIM (SAIM), Ontario Veterinary College, University of Guelph, Guelph, Ontario, Canada

Diane Green, RVT, VTS (Oncology), Texas A&M University, College of Veterinary Medicine and Biomedical Sciences, Veterinary Medical Teaching Hospital, College Station, Texas

Meri Hall, RVT, RLATG, VTS (SAIM), Colonial Veterinary Hospital, Ithaca, New York

Barry Kipperman, DVM, DACVIM (SAIM), VetCare, Dublin, California

Amy Kubier, DVM, University of Illinois, College of Veterinary Medicine, Veterinary Teaching Hospital, Urbana, Illinois

Katrina Lafferty, BFA, CVT, VTS (Anesthesia), University of Wisconsin, Veterinary Medical Teaching Hospital, Madison, Wisconsin

Ellen I. Lowery, DVM, PhD, Kansas State University (Adjunct), Manhattan, KS

Daniel J. MacArthur, DVM, University of Illinois, College of Veterinary Medicine, Veterinary Teaching Hospital, Urbana, Illinois

Maureen McMichael, DVM, DACVECC, University of Illinois, College of Veterinary Medicine, Veterinary Teaching Hospital, Urbana, Illinois

Linda Merrill, LVT, VTS (SAIM, CP-CF), Seattle Veterinary Associates, Seattle, Washington

Jo Ann Morrison, DVM, MS, DACVIM (SAIM), Iowa State University, College of Veterinary Medicine, Veterinary Medical Center, Ames, Iowa

Jocelyn Mott, DVM, DACVIM (SAIM), Pasadena Veterinary Specialists, South Pasadena, California

Marcella D. Ridgway, VMD, MS, DACVIM (SAIM), University of Illinois, College of Veterinary Medicine, Urbana, Illinois

Beth Rogers, RVT, VTS (ECC, SAIM) Veterinary Specialty and Emergency Center, Overland Park, Kansas

Colleen Ruderman, RVT, VTS (SAIM), Georgia Veterinary Specialists, Atlanta, Georgia

Debra Sauberli, DVM, DACT, University of Illinois, College of Veterinary Medicine, Veterinary Teaching Hospital, Urbana, Illinois

Sallianne Schlacks, DVM, University of Illinois College of Veterinary Medicine, Urbana, Illinois

Thomas Schubert, DVM, DACVIM (Neurology), ABVP (Canine/Feline), University of Florida, College of Veterinary Medicine, Gainesville, Florida

Robin Sereno, BS, CVT, VTS (SAIM) University of Wisconsin, Veterinary Teaching Hospital, Madison, Wisconsin

Elisabeth Snead, DVM, BSc, MSc, DACVIM (SAIM), Western College of Veterinary Medicine, University of Saskatchewan, Saskatoon, Canada

Amy Somrak, MBA, DVM, University of Illinois, College of Veterinary Medicine, Veterinary Teaching Hospital, Urbana, Illinois

Rhonda South-Bodiford, RVT, VTS (SAIM), Animal Emergency Clinic of Conroe, Texas

Rachel Sternberg, DVM, University of Illinois, College of Veterinary Medicine, Veterinary Teaching Hospital, Urbana, Illinois

Allyson Stewart, CVT, VTS (Oncology), The Veterinary Cancer Center, Norwalk, Connecticut

Melissa J. Supernor, AS, BS, CVT, VTS (SAIM), Worcester Technical High School, Worcester, Massachusetts

Justin D. Thomason, DVM, DACVIM (SAIM), University of Georgia College of Veterinary Medicine, Athens, Georgia

William Whitehouse, DVM, University of Illinois, College of Veterinary Medicine, Urbana, Illinois

Ann Wortinger, BIS, LVT, VTS (ECC, SAIM), Sanford-Brown College, Dearborn, Michigan

Kimm Wuestenberg, CVT, VTS (ECC, SAIM), Phoenix, Arizona

Preface

The scope of practice for the veterinary technician is continually evolving. This is especially true as veterinary technicians have progressed to becoming veterinary technician specialists. Lacking formal pathways to specialization, many veterinary technicians are striving to increase knowledge in their area of interest. Some may question why this degree of information is being presented to the technician. It is because I am a firm believer that learning is a lifelong process. Enhancing the technician's knowledge base in internal medicine can lead to improved patient care, increased anticipation of the needs of our patients and of our doctors, and advance our ability to provide clients with timely, accurate information on their pets.

The idea behind this textbook is to provide a resource for the veterinary technician in the area of small animal internal medicine. It is obviously inspired by Drs. Feldman and Ettinger's *Textbook of Veterinary Internal Medicine*, and I hope that it is received as the complement it was intended to be. The definition of internal medicine is extremely broad, and as such, this text cannot possibly encompass all aspects we wished to cover. This textbook is divided into body systems and therefore some overlap of material naturally occurs in this format. I have also included chapters on selected aspects of neurology and cardiology as some of these areas, at times, are intimately related. Some subjects in internal medicine have not been included in this textbook, either due to page constraints or choice. I hope the subjects selected and contained in this text provide the veterinary technician with the information needed, but any suggestions for improving this text are gladly welcomed.

The many individuals that contributed to this book by their selfless devotion of time, experience, and knowledge have been invaluable. The diplomates who contributed to this book, both editors and authors, have demonstrated not only their passion and knowledge but also their support of the profession of veterinary technology and of the specialization of veterinary technicians. The veterinary technician specialists who contributed to this book, both as editors and authors, continually amaze me with their strength, compassion, and thirst for knowledge. A special thank you is owed to all contributors for supporting me in my efforts as a first-time editor.

I would also like to acknowledge the animals in all our lives; they are what keeps us passionate about our work and are why I love working in internal medicine. Thank you to the animals of my childhood who helped guide me to this profession (Pepi, Marmaduke, and Christopher Robin), to the animals that have helped me to learn and grow (Salina and the corgi trio—Wally, Tobin, and Cody), and finally, to the current tribe who continue to amaze me (Sally, the way too smart rescue dog, Audrey, the ex practice cat who is a total purr monster, and Raymond, the adorable but clueless Persian).

Linda Merrill

Chapter 1 Physical Examination

Editor: Peter J. Bondy, Jr.

Author: Marcella D. Ridgway

The initial consultation appointment for the internal medicine patient is vital not only from the standpoint of evaluating the patient's history and performing a complete physical examination but also to establish a positive and effective relationship with the pet owner. In the setting of a specialty referral practice, it is important to recognize that the referring veterinarian (RDVM) is the primary client and should always be included as an essential component of the relationship with the pet owner that has been referred. A solid foundation for this relationship with the RDVM and the pet owner can be established even before the actual appointment. Many specialty referral practices provide a Web site where veterinarians can find referral protocols and pet owners can readily access information about the hospital. This information may include how the patient should be managed before the appointment (e.g., 12-h fast), what to expect during the referral appointment, and some biographical material about the specialist(s) and the veterinary health-care team that will be evaluating the pet. Pamphlets or other written materials provided to the RDVM, which can be given to the pet owner at the time of the referral, are also useful. To nurture good relationships with referring veterinarians, it is particularly important to maintain frequent communications. This can be achieved in several ways: prompt follow-up on cases, participation in local veterinary medical association activities, hosting continuing education programs, distributing newsletters with updates about the specialty practice, arranging for new specialists joining the practice to meet referring veterinarians in person, and, above all, by supporting the relationship of the RDVM and the pet owner through positive communications and by ensuring that the pet owner's visit is otherwise as positive as possible. It can be quite helpful to have short referral forms for the RDVM to fill out online or on paper summarizing the RDVM's impressions about the case, including suspected diagnoses, and results of diagnostic tests that have already been completed. This short, simple form can be tremendously helpful in assuring that the RDVM's reasons for referral are addressed and that miscommunication of such information by the pet owner does not mislead the specialist as to the reason for the visit. The specialist and the RDVM are reliant upon each other to achieve the best care for the pet and the pet owner.

Charting

The SOAP charting system (subjective, objective, assessment, and plan) is the standard approach to formulating the medical record. It is a technique of organizing thoughts so that any person picking up the record will understand what the clinician was and is thinking. The medical record is subpoenable by a court of law, and by law, if it is not written in the record, then it does not exist. Understanding the importance of the medical record is paramount to good medical practice.

S (for subjective) includes the history and other data which cannot be measured in a repeatable manner across different evaluators, such as physical exam findings of patient attitude. This may be recorded and may present documentation in narrative form. Ask targeted questions and document what the owner says, in their own words, without paraphrasing. The O (for objective) includes information that can be graded or otherwise quantified such as body weight and heart rate and also includes laboratory data. The A is the assessment, which is a

Small Animal Internal Medicine for Veterinary Technicians and Nurses, First Edition. Edited by Linda Merrill.

summary and interpretation of the clinical signs and the diagnosis or the differential diagnosis (list of tentative diagnosis). Once the list of differential diagnosis has been established, the clinician forms the plan (P), or how to prove which of the suspect diseases is the actual perpetrator. The plan is divided into three components: the treatment plan (Tx), the diagnostic plan (Dx), and the client education component (CE).

Goals of the consultation appointment

The specific goals of the initial consultation appointment are to

1. build trust with the client and with the pet;
2. establish the client's primary concerns;
3. understand the course of events, diagnostic steps, and treatments prior to referral;
4. carefully evaluate the patient;
5. build a problem list and prioritize problems;
6. consider differentials for each problem on the problem list;
7. establish a diagnostic and/or treatment plan; and
8. communicate patient management plans, associated risks, and costs to the client.

The veterinarian and technician/nurse can consider this list together and determine roles and responsibilities within this framework. These may vary according to the nature of the condition (emergency vs. chronic disease), experience level of the technician(s), or relationships among caregivers.

Build trust with the client and with the patient

Remember this may be the first time that they have come to a specialty hospital. They may have already seen several other veterinarians and it is likely their pet has a serious problem. Recognize that clients are probably distressed by needing to establish yet another new relationship with veterinary caregivers and by the fact that their pet is ill and has a complex disease or an elusive diagnosis that has prompted the referral visit. Working to make the clients feel welcomed and that they are in the hands of capable veterinary professionals is important. This really starts with the receptionist, from the initial phone call to the impression as they walk in the door for the first time. Confidence, consideration, and efficiency on the part of support staff are key in getting consultation visits off to a positive start.

Minimize waiting times—this is a period of uncertainty and discomfort for the client. If they are left with unstructured time to worry about their pet and the visit itself, their anxiety levels may be heightened. Provide something for them to do while waiting; let them know what period of time they can expect to wait and be certain to update them if there will be any delays. Prompt notification of the arrival of the client to the appropriate staff can facilitate the timeliness of the appointment process and can reassure the owner that they are being cared for.

Know the pet and the owner name and greet them both in a welcoming manner. Look the client in the eye, greet them professionally, and introduce yourself by name and position. Invite the client into the exam room, invite them to sit, and ask them to place their pet on the floor or on the table as appropriate. In these initial few minutes, clearly delivered, friendly directions from you will help to build confidence.

Unless this is an emergency, avoid immediately examining the patient. Allow the pet to acclimate to the room while you initiate conversation with the client. Key pieces of information about the patient, such as mentation, respiratory character, ambulation, and vision are often best assessed by a *hands-off* examination, which can be completed at this time.

Establish the *client's* primary concerns

Try to use open-ended questions such as "What made you first take Fluffy to your local veterinarian?" rather than "What seems to be the problem?" In the latter situation, the client is tempted to take on the role of doctor and is likely to paraphrase their RDVM's assessment rather than their own concerns.

Understand the course of events and diagnostic steps prior to referral

Information from the referring veterinarian should be available prior to the consultation, but ask the clients for their own chronological assessment of the course of events. They may admit to seeing another veterinarian or they may add important information omitted from the referred history. It is helpful to work from a history and physical exam checklist to avoid overlooking any details that may eventually prove to be important. After an initial relaxed inquiry of the patient's history, the history form should be checked to ensure that all the details of vaccination, heartworm or retrovirus testing, current medications, previous treatments for the current illness, and prior medical problems have been recorded.

History acquisition

History acquisition may be considered to include two phases. The first phase is acquisition of a *general* history, which covers information that is pertinent to every patient. The second is a *targeted* history, in which information pertinent to specific problems of an individual patient is addressed in greater detail (e.g., more careful questioning about exposure to stagnant water sources in a patient in which leptospirosis is being considered as a differential).

In the general history, it is important to determine the reason for the clients' visit so that their presenting concerns are always addressed even if more significant problems are identified in the referral information or subsequently during the referral visit. Signalment should be determined as a significant factor to be considered in developing appropriate differential diagnoses. Clients should be questioned carefully about preexisting conditions and current medications, keeping in mind that clients may inadvertently omit information about very chronic or common conditions (e.g., osteoarthritis in an older dog) or medication that they give so routinely they may fail to consider it a medication (e.g., heartworm prevention). It is particularly important to determine what treatments, if any, the patient has received for the current illness and what response was noted. Specific information (exact date administered and product used) about vaccinations should be determined as some conditions (e.g., immune-mediated hemolytic anemia, immune-mediated thrombocytopenia, polyneuropathy) have been chronologically associated with vaccination. An accurate travel history helps in assessing the risk of exposure to diseases that are regional in occurrence (e.g., systemic fungal diseases, tick-borne diseases, high altitude disease). Complete information about the patient's diet, including specific types or brands and specific amounts fed, as well as any supplements or treats that the pet receives, should be obtained. It is important to ask open-ended questions that do not "lead" the client into giving a particular answer and to be nonjudgmental when obtaining this information (clients sensing criticism of how they care for their pet may not accurately report historical information) in order to obtain an accurate history.

Evaluate the patient: physical examination

The physical examination begins before ever touching the patient by observing the general demeanor of the animal and how it moves about and interacts with the environment. In fact, hospital receptionists, kennel personnel, and other nontechnical staff can provide important preliminary or monitoring information through their observations and should be advised that their input is welcomed and valuable in providing the best care for patients. This general assessment of patient attitude contributes to the evaluation of vision, mentation, and ambulation. It also allows for a general assessment of the patient's personality, which can lead to an adjustment in technique for aggressive or fearful patients. It is important to know what constitutes a normal physical examination and to recognize breed, age, sex, and species variations. The key to consistent performance of a thorough and useful physical examination is establishing a well-organized and systematic approach that is employed routinely in evaluating patients, whether for their first visit or for reevaluation. This will safeguard against overlooking some physical abnormalities because of distractions or focusing too soon on a particular area of interest suggested by the client or on a preliminary observation of the patient. A logical system is to work from "nose to tail," although with patients of uncertain temperament, delaying examination of the mouth and head until the examiner is better acquainted with the patient may be advantageous. Additionally, postponing the parts of the physical examination that are likely to be objectionable to the patient, such as rectal examination or palpation of a painful limb, until the end of the examination is advisable. Body temperature, respiratory rate, and pulse are best determined when the patient is the most relaxed, which may be early in the exam for some patients, especially cats, and later in the exam for others.

Body temperature is usually determined via rectal thermometer; although otic devices are available, normal ranges have been routinely established for rectal temperature. Respiratory rate can often be determined before beginning a hands-on exam by observation of thoracic wall motion. Heart rate is determined by thoracic auscultation or direct chest wall palpation, and pulse rate may be determined by digital pressure over the femoral artery, or the digital artery. Recording both a heart rate and a pulse rate will determine if a pulse deficit is present.

Head

Starting at the nose, the patient's nose and head should be observed for symmetry and palpated to identify regions of pain, swelling, or muscle wasting. The posture of the head and neck should be observed. Ventroflexion is seen in hypokalemic or thiamine-deficient cats, and patients with neck pain may maintain a lowered straight and rigid posture of the head and neck. Running the hands firmly over the skin of the head can help identify skin lesions; this should be done over all cutaneous surfaces of the patient as part of a complete examination. The nares should be examined for patency (e.g., stenotic nares in brachycephalic dogs and cats), discoloration (e.g., some immune-mediated skin disease, secondary to chronic nasal discharge), swelling of surrounding soft tissues (e.g., chronic rhinitis, fungal rhinitis, atopy), and evidence of discharge. If nasal discharge is present, it should be characterized as to relative volume, unilateral/bilateral and serous/serosanguinous/mucoid/mucopurulent/hemorrhagic as the nature of the discharge may be helpful in distinguishing differentials (e.g., unilateral when associated with unilateral dental disease, hemorrhagic in ehrlichiosis or anticoagulant rodenticide toxicity). Air passage can be confirmed by holding a glass microscope slide under and perpendicular to the nares and watching for fogging of the glass by expired air.

Auscultation of the nose can help localize the source of respiratory noise. Percussion over the nasal sinuses can provide evidence of pain or dullness associated with sinus filling with secretions or tissue. Retropulsion of the globe (gentle pressure on the eyeball through closed eyelids) evaluates for space-occupying lesions affecting the orbit that can be present with some nasal (neoplasia) or paranasal (retrobulbar abscess) diseases. Examination of the oral cavity should be thorough, which may require sedation or general anesthesia in some patients. Oral mucous membrane color should be assessed (pale in patients with anemia or poor perfusion due to dehydration or cardiovascular disease; cyanotic [blue or purple] in patients with reduced oxygen levels in blood supplying the oral cavity). In patients with dark pigmentation of the oral mucous membranes, the conjunctiva and lining of the prepuce or vulva offer alternative sites for observation of mucous membrane color. Capillary refill time (CRT) should be determined by applying digital pressure adequate to blanch the tissue, releasing that pressure and observing the length of time for the mucous membrane color to normalize. CRT reflects perfusion and can be prolonged with dehydration, cardiovascular disease, or other hypotensive conditions.

Teeth should be examined for fractures, discoloration, or disease of the periodontal tissue that may indicate dental disease as a source of nasal or other facial problems or sepsis. Oral tissues should be carefully evaluated for ulceration or erosions (trauma, immune-mediated disease, chemical or electrical burns, renal disease, thromboembolic disease, neoplasia), discoloration (jaundice, petechiation), presence of masses (neoplasia, granuloma), and presence of foreign material. The ability to move the tongue and to swallow should also be assessed. A technique of pressing upward under the external aspect of the intermandibular space allows the examiner to elevate the tongue for examination of the ventral tongue surface and underlying tissues, a potential site for string foreign bodies to lodge. The hard and soft palates should be examined to ensure that they are intact and the palatine tonsils should be checked—normally, the tonsils are contained within the crypts and are not readily visible. The patient should be able to open and close the mouth without discomfort, which might indicate osseous disease, temporomandibular, retrobulbar or pharyngeal disease, or masticatory myositis. It is sometimes difficult to distinguish resistance to opening the mouth due to patient temperament versus actual discomfort.

Eyes

A thorough examination of the eyelids and eyes, including a fundic examination, should be completed in all patients. Structural abnormalities of the eyelids (entropion, ectropion) may cause secondary ocular problems. Eyelid lesions can be seen in immunologic diseases, atopy, hereditary dermal diseases, and infectious diseases (dermatophytes, demodicosis). Unexpected occurrence of conditions like demodicosis in an adult may indicate an underlying immunosuppressive condition (hyperadrenocorticism or use of exogenous corticosteroids). Aberrant growth of eyelashes can cause discomfort and corneal injury. Ocular discharge can be associated with systemic infectious diseases (ehrlichiosis, blastomycosis) as well as local ocular disease. Conjunctival edema may signify conjunctival inflammation or may be associated with generalized peripheral edema due to vasculitis or hypoalbuminemia. In aged or cachectic animals, loss of retrobulbar fat results in a sunken position of the globe, which may then cause accumulation of secretions and possibly irritants, causing tearing or mucoid ocular discharge, which is generally benign. Older animals may have iris atrophy with thinning, defects and irregular edges to the iris that will also cause non-neurological impairment of pupillary light responses. Yellowing of the conjunctiva and sclera occurs in animals with jaundice. Coagulation disorders may manifest as scleral or conjunctival hemorrhages, bleeding into the anterior chamber (hyphema), and iris or retinal lesions. Infiltrative disease (inflammation, neoplasia) may cause lesions of intraocular vascular tissues (iris and retina); retinal granulomatous lesions may be evident in feline infectious peritonitis (FIP), systemic fungal diseases, and lymphoma. Hypertension or other vascular diseases may result in tortuosity of the retinal vessels. The optic nerve should be examined for changes consistent with neuropathy or increased intracranial pressure. Pupillary light responses, corneal reflex, position of the globe and eyelid appearance and response to touch, and ocular response to head motion are part of the cranial nerve evaluation.

Ears

The ears should be palpated for swelling (inflammation, hematoma from trauma, headshaking, or coagulopathy), coolness (poor perfusion), or discomfort (otitis). The ear margin should be examined for alopecia, thickening, or crusting that can be associated with exposure to temperature extremes, excessive UV radiation, and microvascular or dermal disease. Visual and otoscopic inspection of the inner pinna and the external ear canal should be performed to evaluate for inflammation, exudates, foreign materials, or masses. The pinnae may show petechiation and ecchymosis in patients with abnormal platelet numbers or function. Unilateral drooping of an ear may indicate pain or neurological abnormalities. On otoscopic examination, the normal tympanic membrane is a complete thin translucent gray structure with a visible manubrium (opaque bone structure projecting approximately halfway to the center from the periphery). In disease conditions, the tympanic membrane may appear thickened, opaque, discolored, bulging, or perforated.

Neck to thorax

Examination of the cervical region should include general palpation and manipulation to evaluate for pain or masses. In evaluating the neck, the parotid salivary glands should be identified as symmetrical left and right thick disklike structures with their cranial aspect positioned medial and caudal to the mandibular ramus. While these glands may occasionally be diseased (usually unilateral enlargement and discomfort with salivary duct obstruction, uncommon bilateral sialoadenitis in dogs), the usual significance in identifying the salivary glands is to ascertain that they are *not* enlarged lymph nodes. The submandibular lymph nodes are generally much smaller (even when enlarged), spherical, and lie caudal to the parotid glands. Retropharyngeal masses (lymph node, foreign body granuloma, neoplasm) can sometimes be identified on cervical palpation dorsal to the larynx. In dogs with laryngeal paralysis, palpation of the larynx may reveal asymmetry in patients with unilateral dysfunction, and some affected dogs will show noticeable worsening of respiratory noise or dyspnea with laryngeal palpation. Palpation for a thyroid slip is of particular importance in cats, in which hyperthyroidism due to thyroid hyperplasia or adenomas may cause various systemic signs. In dogs with thyroid tumors, the predominant sign is the presence of a cranial to midcervical mass. The trachea should be palpated for structural abnormalities such as dorsoventral flattening in dogs with tracheal collapse. Tracheal palpation may readily elicit a cough (increased tracheal sensitivity) in animals with tracheal inflammation. Caution should be employed in tracheal collapse patients, in which stimulation of a tracheal cough can trigger paroxysmal coughing and exacerbation of tracheal collapse and resulting respiratory distress. Auscultation of the larynx and trachea can aid in localizing a source of respiratory noise and can help differentiate cervical collapse (inspiratory click) from intrathoracic collapse (expiratory click) in patients with tracheal collapse. Auscultation of wheezes in the laryngeal region generally indicated airway narrowing (e.g., laryngeal paralysis, everted laryngeal saccules, laryngeal mass).

A cervical bulge that is most prominent on the left may be evident in patients with megaesophagus. Patients should be checked for abnormal jugular pulses by elevating the nose and observing the jugular groove. Normally, the jugular pulse should not extend more than one-third up the neck. Increased jugular pulses indicate impaired venous drainage into the right heart (e.g., right heart failure, pericardial effusion). This may be difficult to evaluate in obese patients or in those patients with thick or long hair coats. Wetting and flattening the hair with alcohol may aid visualization of the jugular vein. In the distal cervical region, the superficial cervical (prescapular) lymph nodes should be identified and evaluated for size and consistency.

Moving toward the thorax, the axillary lymph nodes can also be evaluated at this point: The axillary nodes are often not identified unless they are enlarged or enveloped in fat and are best identified as movable disk-shaped structures against the ventro-lateral cranial thorax.

In evaluating the thoracic region, the patient's respiratory motions and effort should be examined. Animals with pleural space disease usually take rapid, shallow breaths. Those with upper airway obstruction have a slow, deep respiratory pattern with a prolonged inspiratory phase. Animals with lower airway disease (cats with asthma) may have increased expiratory effort. Animals with pulmonary parenchymal disease and abnormal diffusion of inspired gas from the alveolus to the bloodstream may show increased effort on both inspiration and expiration. With extreme respiratory effort, additional cervical strap muscles are recruited to assist in the expansion of the thoracic cavity, and animals will show drawing back of the commissures of the mouth as a result. As respiratory muscles fail, a paradoxical inward motion of the caudal ribs on inspiration occurs.

Stethoscopes are designed to follow the human ear canal; therefore, for best results, the binaurals (ear pieces) should be placed in the ears facing forward. Both the bell (low frequency sounds) and the diaphragm (high frequency sounds) of the stethoscope are utilized during auscultation. Adequate time should be spent in listening to all lung fields and in a thorough evaluation of heart sounds. Referred respiratory sounds can complicate interpretation of sounds heard on thoracic auscultation. Further evaluation by auscultating the trachea, larynx, and nasal cavity can help delineate the source of the abnormal sounds as their intensity is expected to be greatest over the primary site of disease. Other artifacts that can interfere with auscultation are ambient room noise, purring cats, shivering, and referred upper airway or gastrointestinal noise. Purring cats can be especially problematic. Distracting the cat by the introduction of a new sound, odor, or object may break the purr long enough to adequately assess heart or lung sounds.

Lung auscultation should characterize any abnormal sounds and they should be localized as to the region where they are heard. Breath sounds are best heard in a sternal position: standing, sitting, or laying. To encourage patients to take deep breaths (for best evaluation of lung sounds), temporarily holding off the mouth and nose or covering mouth and nose with an air-inflated bag or exam glove may be effective. In animals that purr, pant, or sniff, holding a cotton swab dampened with alcohol may interrupt the problematic breathing pattern to allow auscultation. The inspiratory phase of respiration is typically louder and longer than the expiratory phase (Table 1.1).

Both sides of the thoracic cavity should be auscultated. In addition, both cranial and caudal, and dorsal and ventral lung sounds should be evaluated. Careful auscultation can reveal reduced or absent lung sounds. If noted, thoracic percussion may aid in further characterization of the pathology. Decreased resonance or dullness may indicate pleural fluid or lung consolidation, and increased resonance may indicate pneumothorax.

Table 1.1 Pulmonary auscultation

Sound	Timing	Location
Bronchial	Normal intense harsh sound heard on both inspiration and expiration	Central chest over caudal trachea/large bronchi
Bronchovesicular	Normal moderate sound heard on full inspiration and short expiration	Bilateral bronchial/hilar region
Vesicular	Normal soft sound heard better on the slightly longer inspiratory phase	Peripheral lung fields
Stertor	Abnormal low pitched snoring sound heard mainly on inspiration; sound radiates	Larynx or trachea
Stridor	Abnormal intense high pitched wheeze heard on inspiration	Larynx or thoracic inlet
Crackles (rales)	Abnormal popping sound heard on inspiration, further classified as either fine or course	Lung fields
Rhonchi (wheezes)	Abnormal high or low pitched musical sounds heard at the end of inspiration/beginning of expiration	Isolated lung fields

Source: Jack CM, Watson, PM. *Veterinary Technician's Daily Reference Guide*, 2nd edition, p. 32. Ames, IA: Blackwell Publishing; 2008.

Auscultation of the heart allows for the assessment of the heart rate, rhythm and murmurs, or other abnormal heart sounds. Cardiac sounds are best heard with the patient's heart in its normal position; therefore, if possible, a standing posture is preferred. Respiratory noise can mask cardiac sounds; this is especially evident in panting dogs. Gently holding the mouth shut and even briefly holding the nostrils closed may facilitate auscultation. A thorough examination includes listening on both the left- and the right-hand sides of the chest from the apex of the heart to the heart base. If an abnormality is heard, the point of maximal intensity (PMI) should be defined. The normal heart rate for dogs varies by size, age, and physical fitness level. Puppies and smaller dogs tend to have faster heart rates than larger or physically fit dogs. Cats have less variability in the normal range.

Accurate cardiac auscultation may be difficult when the patient's heart rate is increased above normal. Allow the patient to acclimate to the environment and to adjust to having the stethoscope in position on the thorax. Simply waiting for a few moments in position to auscultate often allows the nervous animal to calm down enough that the heart rate drops. If the heart rate is elevated because of a cardiac or metabolic abnormality, the rate will remain elevated. Simultaneous auscultation of the heart and palpation of the femoral pulse allows for detection of pulse deficits (auscultated heartbeat without a corresponding pulse). There are four heart sounds that correlate to the closing of the heart valves and to blood flow in the heart. The first heart sound (S_1) is the closing of the atrioventricular (AV) valves (mitral and tricuspid), often referred to as the lub sound. The second heart sound (S_2) is the closing of the semilunar valves (aortic and pulmonary), often referred to as the dub sound. Typically, the third and fourth heart sounds are not heard in a healthy heart. The third heart sound (S_3) is a sound produced at the end of rapid blood filling of the ventricles. The fourth heart sound (S_4) is also a blood flow sound produced by the emptying of the atria and the filling of the ventricles.

Normal dogs may have a sinus arrhythmia (heart rate increases with inspiration and decreases with expiration), while cats do not exhibit this same variation with respiration. Normal sinus arrhythmia should be distinguished from ventricular premature contractions (VPCs), which can sound similar in certain situations. Gallop rhythms may be noted, especially in cats and particularly at higher heart rates. Gallop rhythms are not a true arrhythmia but are actually the auscultation of the third and fourth heart sounds in addition to the first and second heart sounds heard normally. Gallop sounds are low frequency sounds best heard with the bell side of the stethoscope.

Murmurs, which are sounds generated by turbulent blood flow, can be difficult to detect at faster heart rates, especially in cats. For cats, allowing a longer period of time for cardiac auscultation is important for detecting murmurs, and sometimes murmurs can be best identified by auscultation of the parasternal region in feline patients. Murmurs should be classified as to timing, character (pitch, modulation, and quality), intensity, and location (Tables 1.2–1.5).

Table 1.2 Cardiac murmurs—timing

Timing		
Systolic	Heard during systole (ejection)—between S1 and S2	Mitral or tricuspid regurgitation, aortic or pulmonic stenosis, ventricular septal defect (VSD)
Diastolic	Heard during diastole (filling)—start of S2	Uncommon, aortic regurgitation, endocarditis, VSD
Continuous (pansystolic or holosystolic)	Heard throughout the cycle—S1 through S2	PDA

Table 1.3 Cardiac murmurs—character

Character					
Pitch—sound due to velocity					
Pitch	Low	Medium	High		Mixed
Heard best	Bell head	Either head	Diaphragm head		Both heads
Modulation—intensity over time					
Modulation	Plateau	Crescendo–decrescendo			Decrescendo
Sounds like	Machinery	Diamond shape—soft-loud-soft			Loud to soft
Quality—unusual characteristics					
Blowing	Harsh	Rumbling	Honking	Grunting	Musical

Murmurs do not always indicate cardiac disease. Murmurs can arise in patients with changes in blood viscosity due to dehydration or anemia. This is especially true in cats. These innocent murmurs are low intensity murmurs (grade I or II) and are expected to resolve as the inciting condition normalizes (e.g., normal hydration restored).

Abdomen

The abdomen should be observed for distension or asymmetry. Distension can be caused by abdominal masses, organ enlargement (e.g., hepatomegaly or splenomegaly), intestinal gas or accumulation of feces, obesity, gastric distension (e.g., obstruction, GDV, foreign material, food), ascites, free abdominal air, or pregnancy in intact females. Ballottement of the abdomen may allow for the distinction of fluid accumulation (ballottement produces fluid wave) from other causes of distension.

The abdomen should be palpated systematically; working from the cranial to the caudal abdomen is a logical approach, although leaving known or suspected areas of pain until the end of the examination is beneficial to maintain patient comfort and to facilitate palpation. In obese animals, adequate evaluation of the abdomen by palpation may not be feasible, and the evaluation must be made by means of imaging studies. In very fractious or tense animals, starting the abdominal examination by very gently placing the hands on the abdomen and moving them slightly or not at all for a period of time may allow the patient to acclimate to being touched and to relax enough to allow palpation. In small dogs and cats, abdominal palpation may be done using a one-handed technique in which the examiner cups the hand under the abdomen with the fingers directed toward the patient's spine then palpating with the fingers with gentle but steady pressure. Larger patients will require a two-handed approach where the examiner places one hand on each side of the lateral abdomen. In large or deep-chested dogs, abdominal palpation may be facilitated by positioning the patient with the forelimbs elevated to allow abdominal contents situated under the caudal rib cage to shift backward where they are more accessible for palpation.

A large part of successful abdominal palpation is in knowing the normal anatomy and maintaining the confident expectation that identifiable structures will be identified. Only with a few abdominal structures (e.g., the urinary bladder, the kidneys in cats or left kidney in dogs) is the examiner able to grasp and clearly identify the structure in its entirety. Most of the assessment of abdominal organs is made by palpating tissue margins and surfaces (e.g., liver, right kidney) or by feeling structures slip through the fingers or hands as the abdomen is palpated (e.g., intestines, enlarged uterus). In the cranial abdomen, the stomach is usually not palpated unless it is full of food, fluid, or gas. Food or fluid distension of the stomach produces a doughy feel in the left cranial abdomen. The pylorus is sometimes palpable in small lean patients as a firm mass in the mid- to right cranial abdomen. The liver of the cat is not palpable unless it is enlarged. In the dog, the caudal margin of the liver is usually palpable if the fingertips are advanced up under the caudal aspect of the rib cage and drawn caudally. An enlarged liver is easily palpated and rounding of the liver margins may be detectable. The kidneys are located in the right dorsal and left dorsal to mid-abdomen. The left kidney sits more caudal than the right kidney. In the cat, the kidneys are usually readily palpated in the dorsal to mid-abdomen; the right kidney may be partially hidden by the caudal rib cage. The kidneys should be evaluated for size (small in patients with chronic renal disease, large in patients with infiltrative disease, acute renal injury, or portosystemic shunts), shape (irregular with fibrosis or renal cyst formation) and pain (acute renal injury). In the dog, the kidneys are often less identifiable and often only the lateral surfaces or caudal poles can be evaluated. The spleen is not palpable unless enlarged, when it may be palpated caudal to the liver and variably filling the mid-abdomen. The mesenteric lymph nodes, also located in the mid-abdomen, are usually not palpable unless greatly enlarged. In lean small dogs and cats, the normal cecum/cecocolic junction can sometimes be palpated in the mid-abdomen and is an important differential for a mid-abdominal mass. The intestines should be

Table 1.4 Cardiac murmurs—intensity

Intensity—grade	
I/VI	Very soft, faint, or barely audible murmur, localized, only heard after intently listening for a while
II/VI	Low intensity murmur (soft), localized but easily heard
III/VI	Moderate intensity murmur, more than one location, immediately heard
IV/VI	Loud intensity murmur, radiates, no precordial thrill
V/VI	Loud intensity murmur with a palpable precordial thrill
VI/VI	Very loud intensity murmur heard even before the stethoscope touches the chest wall, with an easily palpable precordial thrill

Table 1.5 Cardiac murmurs—location

Location						
Left apex	Heart base	Apex	Left 2–4 intercostal	Left 3–5 intercostal	Left 4–6 intercostal	Right 6–7 intercostal
S1	S2	S3 and S4	Pulmonic valve	Aortic valve	Mitral valve	Tricuspid valve

palpated for any masses (e.g., neoplasia, granuloma, and foreign body), distension (e.g., ileus, mechanical obstruction), presence and character of feces (fluid vs. firm), irregularity (e.g., plication due to intestinal spasm or string foreign body), or changes in wall thickness (generally detected by "slipping" the intestinal loops through the fingertips). The descending colon may be readily palpated as a tubular structure in the caudal dorsal abdomen because of the presence of feces. Feces can be distinguished from a mass by applying gentle pressure, which will cause feces to yield and change shape or location within the colon. The full urinary bladder is easily identified as a somewhat spherical or oblong structure in the caudoventral abdomen. If the bladder is empty, it can often still be identified by allowing tissues in the caudal abdomen to slip through the fingers with a caudal to cranial hand motion, which allows the cranial border of the bladder to be palpated as it slips through the fingers. Wall thickness and irregularities (e.g., neoplasia, polyp) should be noted, and bladder stones will sometimes be palpable. Patients with bladder inflammation may object to palpation because of discomfort and often do not maintain much urine volume in the inflamed bladder, making it more difficult to identify. In male dogs, an enlarged prostate may be identifiable as a structure ventral to the colon and caudal to the urinary bladder on palpation of the caudal abdomen. The prostate should be assessed for irregularities of shape (e.g., prostatic cysts, abscesses, and neoplasia) or pain on palpation (prostatitis). Caution should be exerted when palpating a potentially infected prostate as subsequent development of septicemia may occur. In intact female animals, the uterus is not palpable unless it is enlarged (e.g., pregnancy, pyometra) when it may be identified as a tubular structure extending along the ventral abdomen in a caudal to cranial plane.

The rectal examination allows palpation of some skeletal structures, including examination of the ventral sacral and caudal spine to evaluate for spondylosis, the medial aspect of the left and right ilia laterally and the dorsal pubis ventrally to evaluate for pelvic fractures or narrowing of the pelvic canal. Examination of the soft tissues of the caudal abdomen is also performed. Palpation of the sublumbar lymph nodes evaluates for enlargement due to metastatic neoplasia or, less commonly, severe inflammatory disease. These nodes are dorsal and cranial relative to the examiner. Further examination of the prostate is possible during the rectal examination to evaluate for the size, symmetry, texture of the gland, or any elicited pain. In dogs with significant prostatic enlargement, the prostate may move cranially over the pelvic brim where it is less accessible on rectal palpation. Evaluation of the urethra is possible with ventral palpation to assess for thickening, masses, or urethral calculi. The anal sacs are located caudally, and careful palpation for masses, especially in hypercalcemic patients, along with an assessment for impaction and infection, is recommended. If indicated, the examiner can express an anal sac to collect a sample of secretions as the sacs may become distended with infection or obstruction of the anal sac duct. A sample of feces should be collected at the time of rectal palpation for the determination of fecal consistency and character (e.g., blood, foreign material) and to provide a sample for subsequent fecal analysis if indicated.

The external genitalia should be inspected for evidence of infection, masses, or discharge. The vulva of female patients should be examined for structural abnormalities or perivulvar skin disease. In the male, the prepuce and penis should be examined for inflammation, masses, and discoloration. Male cats with urethral obstruction may have discoloration of the penile tip and palpable "sand" in the urethra that may be extruded with gentle palpation of the penile tip. The testicles of intact males should be palpated for the presence of both testicles in the scrotum and for the identification of masses, swelling, or asymmetry. The ventral abdominal body wall should be palpated for any defects (hernias) especially common at the umbilicus and the inguinal ring. Palpation of the inguinal lymph nodes and evaluation of the mammary chain for masses, swelling, or discharge should be performed.

Musculoskeletal

The examination of the musculoskeletal system begins with a hands-off observation of the patient's posture and ability to move about the exam room, noting any stiffness, lameness, or reluctance to move in a particular direction or to raise the head. For closer examination, running the hands over the trunk and limbs may give a preliminary indication of asymmetry, joint swelling, bony enlargement, or soft tissue swelling or masses and allows for a general assessment of body condition and muscle mass. Deeper palpation and/or manipulation of the spine and limbs may be necessary to detect sources of pain. In patients with lameness, careful examination of the affected limb includes examination of all cutaneous structures including footpads, interdigital spaces, and the nail beds. Deep palpation and manipulation proceeds from the distal to the proximal limb with palpation and manipulation of joints until pain or dysfunction can be localized to direct further diagnostics, such as imaging.

For oncological patients, detailed measurements of any masses and the lymph nodes generally follow a thorough physical exam.

When you think you have finished the physical exam, refer to the checklist on your exam form to ensure that all details are entered.

Build a problem list

The next step in the process is to summarize in point form all of the separate problems ascertained from both the history and the physical examination, always keeping in mind the primary owner concern for which they sought veterinary attention. This is a task typically associated exclusively with the veterinarian, although the team members can certainly help to ascertain that the list is accurate and complete.

Consider differential diagnoses

The clinician will consider all of the possible conditions that could lead to the patient presenting with this combination of problems.

Establish a diagnostic plan

A properly conducted history acquisition and physical examination are critical to the appropriate management of the patient as they form the foundation upon which all diagnostic and treatment decisions will be based. Historical data and results of the physical examination are interpreted and used to help determine what steps need to be taken for further diagnostic testing to identify the underlying cause of clinical abnormalities or for adjustments in therapy in patients with known medical conditions. It is important that history acquisition and physical examination of the referred patient is thorough with careful attention to detail as abnormalities that may provide vital clues to the patient's problem may be quite subtle. A good evaluation of a patient through history acquisition and physical examination includes thorough, accurate record keeping to document findings—multiple individuals should be able to conduct these evaluations and to communicate and record findings in a manner that is consistent, accurate, and understandable to others involved in the patients' care.

Remember, we are not expected to have all the answers at this stage, but rather an organized plan to work through the differentials on our list.

Communicate this plan to the client

One of the best services that can be offered to the patient is to ensure that the owner understands the thought process behind the differential diagnoses and the diagnostic and/or treatment plan. Explain to the clients which laboratory and diagnostic tests are indicated, and what is involved from their pets' perspective. If any shaving of hair is required, obtain permission.

The examination should close with informed consent for any forthcoming diagnostic tests. Provide an accurate estimate of when results should be available and provide the client with a written estimate of costs. Make sure to establish expectations for follow-up communication and to verify preferred contact numbers (Should they call you? What time?).

Referring veterinarians truly appreciate a call or a referral letter at this point in the process to provide an update. Remember, this is their client and their patient that they are entrusting to you. They deserve prompt, professional communication, as well as thanks!

Conclusion

The veterinary technician will be involved in many, but not all, aspects of the consultation and physical examination of the internal medicine patient. Establishing a good rapport with both the client and the patient and the ability to document a complete subjective history are the first steps in the process. The ability to perform a complete physical examination, while not the primary responsibility of the veterinary technician, is very important in accurately monitoring our patient's conditions and response to therapy. The veterinary technician's knowledge of the patient's assessment will help the technician anticipate the needs of the veterinarian and the patient. Finally, knowledge of the treatment and the diagnostic and educational components of the plan will help to ensure the optimal outcome for all involved.

Chapter 2 Endocrinology

Editors: Barry Kipperman and Beth Rogers

SECTION 1 PITUITARY GLAND

The pituitary gland lies ventral to the brain, on midline, outside of the blood–brain barrier. It is a major site of hormone storage, production, and secretion. The pituitary receives vascular and neural input from the hypothalamus. Major hormone products include thyroid-stimulating hormone (TSH), adrenocorticotropic hormone (ACTH), antidiuretic hormone (ADH), and growth hormone (GH). These products have multiple target organs and are responsible for numerous systemic effects. The pituitary may be affected by congenital or acquired disease. It is divided into anterior and posterior portions.

Growth hormone disorders

There are two main clinical diseases associated with GH levels. Growth hormone excess (acromegaly or hypersomatotropism) is most commonly associated with a benign functional tumor of the feline pituitary gland. It is found most often in senior cats (8–14 years) and more often in males. Tumors autonomously secrete GH. Growth hormone is a natural diabetogenic hormone and antagonizes the effects of insulin. The most common clinical presentation of acromegaly is insulin-resistant feline diabetes mellitus (DM).[1,2] In dogs, functional pituitary tumors are less common, and acromegaly is more often associated with natural

Small Animal Internal Medicine for Veterinary Technicians and Nurses, First Edition. Edited by Linda Merrill.
© 2012 John Wiley & Sons, Inc. Published 2012 by John Wiley & Sons, Inc.

estrous cycles or exogenous progesterone therapy. Acromegaly has also been associated with various neoplastic processes (e.g., mammary carcinoma) in the canine.

GH deficiency (hyposomatotropism) is seen most commonly as a congenital lesion, and affected animals are classified as pituitary "dwarfs." German shepherds are overrepresented. It is an autosomal recessive trait.[3,4]

Clinical signs

Acromegaly is most commonly associated with insulin-resistant DM in the feline, and symptoms are consistent with poorly controlled diabetes (polyuria [PU], polydipsia [PD], polyphagia, weight loss, and diabetic neuropathy).[1,2] GH has the effect of promoting linear growth, in conjunction with insulin-like growth factor-1 (IGF-1), and thus other clinical signs may be associated with abnormal growth in an adult animal: increasing body weight, widening interdental spaces, organomegaly, enlarging skull size, and so on.[4] In late-stage disease, cardiomegaly may be noted, which may progress to congestive heart failure (CHF). Azotemia also develops in the late stages of the disease in ~50% of acromegalic cats.

Hyposomatotropism is manifested as poor weight gain, unthrifty body condition, and juvenile hair coat. If GH is the only deficient hormone, affected animals are termed "proportional dwarfs," where body proportions are normal, (but overall size is small)[3,4] (Figure 2.1.1).

If GH deficiency is seen in conjunction with other hormone deficiencies (most commonly TSH), then affected animals are termed "dysproportionate dwarfs." Affected animals typically have larger, wider skulls in comparison to small body size.[4]

Diagnostics

Laboratory

For animals suspected of having acromegaly (insulin resistance, consistent physical exam findings), GH levels can be measured,

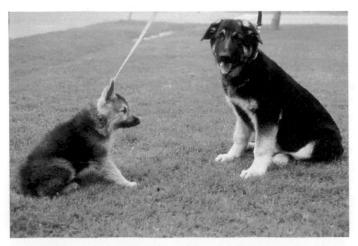

Figure 2.1.1 German shepherd puppy with hyposomatotropism on the left, with normal, unaffected littermate on the right. Photo courtesy of Dr. Jim Noxon.

though normal variation may affect individual results. Serum samples should be collected after a 6- to 12-h fast and sent to the University of Minnesota. One milliliter of serum is needed and samples should be shipped frozen with two ice packs in a Styrofoam container. IGF-1 levels can also be measured and may be considered the preferred diagnostic test. Serum (0.5 mL) should be frozen and sent with an ice pack to Michigan State University. IGF-1 is an indirect measurement of GH excess, and levels are elevated in animals with acromegaly.

For animals suspected of GH deficiency, GH and IGF-1 levels may be measured; however, provocative testing of pituitary GH release is recommended. The xylazine response test is considered the gold standard for diagnosis of GH deficiency. The protocol for the xylazine response test is: 100 pg/kg xylazine intravenously (IV); collect serum samples at baseline (prior to administration), 15, 30, 45, 60 min post.

Biopsy is not applicable for GH disorders. Conditions of GH excess or deficiency are not diagnosed via histopathology.

Imaging

Computed tomography (CT) scan or magnetic resonance imaging (MRI) of the brain can demonstrate pituitary tumors as seen with acromegaly. In cases of hyposomatotropism, additional differential diagnoses for microstature (e.g., portosystemic shunt [PSS]) may be ruled out by other imaging techniques (e.g., abdominal radiographs and ultrasound).

Treatments

Inpatient

For cases of GH excess, radiation therapy (RT) may be considered to reduce the size of the pituitary tumor. Acromegalic feline diabetics that have undergone pituitary radiation have reduced insulin requirements when compared to pretreatment insulin dosages.[1,2] Canine cases of acromegaly due to natural estrous cycles may be treated with ovariohysterectomy. There are generally no requirements for inpatient treatment of hyposomatotropism.

Outpatient

For untreated cases of feline acromegaly associated with DM, increasing doses of insulin are required to control blood glucose levels. Insulin therapy may be combined with oral hypoglycemic agents in an attempt to minimize hyperglycemia.

Animals with hyposomatotropism may be successfully treated with appropriate hormone supplementation. There are currently no commercially available canine or feline GH supplements. Porcine GH is available, with doses for supplementation of 0.1 U (0.05 mg)/kg SQ three times weekly. IGF-1 levels are measured to assess treatment efficacy. Oversupplementation and resultant DM and acromegaly are possible. If other hormone deficiencies (e.g., TSH) are concurrent with GH deficiency, then specific hormone supplementation (e.g., thyroxine [T_4]) is recommended.

Pharmacology

For some cases of acromegaly, therapy may be attempted with GH inhibitors (e.g., octreotide acetate), though therapy is generally expensive and side effects may be significant.

For hyposomatotropism, appropriate hormone replacement therapy may allow a normal life span and quality of life. It is important that all deficient hormones are identified and supplemented accordingly.

Prognosis and survival times

Intact female dogs with acromegaly due to estrous cycling may be cured with ovariohysterectomy. Feline acromegaly due to pituitary tumors cannot be cured, but long-term disease control may be achieved with RT and aggressive glycemic control. Prognosis is often poor despite RT due to the debilitating effects of malnutrition and weight loss that is usually present at the time RT is pursued.

Anesthetic and analgesic considerations

Diabetic felines with acromegaly that are undergoing RT should receive insulin therapy and glucose monitoring as with any anesthetic procedure.

Diabetes insipidus

Clinical signs

There are two main forms of diabetes insipidus (DI), central (brain origin) and nephrogenic (renal origin), and lesions may be congenital or acquired. Most nephrogenic cases are secondary to other diseases (e.g., hyperadrenocorticism [HAC], pyelonephritis, hypercalcemia, and others). Primary nephrogenic and central DI are rare. Abnormalities in the formation (central) or activity (nephrogenic) of ADH, also called arginine vasopressin (AVP), are responsible for the clinical presentation. ADH is responsible for the production of concentrated urine, and in the absence of normal ADH activity, urine remains dilute. The most common clinical signs are severe polyuria and polydipsia (PU/PD), and some cases are severely affected. PD is defined as water consumption in excess of 100 mL/kg/day. PU is defined as urine production >66 mL/kg/day. Animals with congenital disease may present as early as 8–12 weeks of age with complaints of lifelong PU/PD. Acquired diseases may be seen at any time and with any signalment of animal. Other clinical symptoms may be seen and depend on the etiology of the secondary nephrogenic DI, including HAC, pyelonephritis, hypercalcemia, and numerous others.

Diagnostics

DI is a diagnosis of exclusion. As with any diagnosis by exclusion, clients must be prepared for the diagnostics that may be needed to work up the PU/PD patient (Table 2.1.1).

Table 2.1.1   Causes of polyuria, polydipsia, and hyposthenuria

Causes of polyuria and polydipsia	
Definition	Causes of isosthenuria
USG 1.008–1.030	Chronic renal failure
	Diabetes mellitus
	Hyperadrenocorticism
	Hypercalcemia
	Hypoadrenocorticism
	Hypokalemia
	Liver disease
	Pyelonephritis
	Pyometra
Causes of hyposthenuria	
USG < 1.008	Diabetes insipidus
	Hyperadrenocorticism
	Hypercalcemia
	Liver disease
	Pyometra

USG, urine specific gravity.

Laboratory

There are no specific laboratory findings for DI; however, the urinalysis will repeatedly show hyposthenuria (<1.008). Other findings on the urinalysis or the remainder of the minimum database (complete blood count [CBC], serum biochemistry panel) will depend on the specific etiology of the disease. Urinary tract infections are common as a result of poor concentrating ability. Urine cultures are advised.

Water deprivation tests have been used to assess patient ability to concentrate urine in the face of dehydration. These tests are seldom advised as severe dehydration and renal damage can occur. Performing the test properly is extremely labor intensive and requires completely emptying the urinary bladder. Results are often inconclusive. More often, DI is diagnosed after excluding the more common causes of hyposthenuria.

Histopathology is not pursued in the majority of cases. However, if renal biopsy in appropriate cases of nephrogenic DI is considered, precautions should be taken with assessment of coagulation, hydration status, and the determination of blood pressure. Electron microscopy evaluation of renal tissue is recommended for certain disease conditions, and technicians should inquire with the histopathology laboratory for special tissue submission requirements.

Imaging

There are no specific imaging findings in cases of DI. Animals with congenital central disease may show anatomic lesions associated with the pituitary gland on brain CT scan or MRI. There are numerous lesions that may be associated with nephrogenic disease, related to specific etiology. Additional imaging findings may include hepatomegaly with HAC, pyelectasia with pyelonephritis, or sternal lymphadenopathy with hypercalcemia due to lymphoma.

Treatments

Inpatient

Specific inpatient therapy depends upon the underlying etiology for the DI.

Outpatient

Animals may have severe PU/PD, and owners may be tempted to limit access to water. However, client education is crucial as limiting water may lead to severe dehydration and renal insult with possible permanent renal damage. Quality of life may be negatively impacted in animals with severe PU/PD, and realistic discussions regarding prognosis are important. Select cases of central DI may be successfully managed with administration of vasopressin (synthetic ADH). The available form is desmopressin acetate (DDAVP®) as oral, intranasal, and ophthalmic drops. This medication results in increased urine concentration, thus reducing PU/PD.

Prognosis and survival times

The prognosis for animals with congenital lesions is guarded to poor. A few exceptions may be seen in animals that can be managed with vasopressin. In extreme cases of PU/PD, animals may have to urinate every few hours, including overnight. If environmental conditions are favorable (ready access to urinate and free access to water), the short-term prognosis is favorable. Prognosis otherwise depends on the underlying etiology for DI.

Anesthetic and analgesic considerations

Affected animals are at a risk for dehydration and hypotension. Serum electrolytes and blood pressure should be monitored during times of potential water limitation and parenteral fluid administration given in conjunction with anesthetic events. Water restriction prior to anesthesia is contraindicated unless receiving fluid therapy.

SECTION 2 THYROID GLANDS

The thyroid glands are two reddish-brown glands (also called lobes) located in the neck on either side of the trachea, just below the cricoid cartilage, from approximately the fifth to the sixth rings of the trachea. The microscopic structure consists of thyroid epithelial cells that synthesize the thyroid hormones (arranged in spheres called thyroid follicles) and parafollicular or C cells, which secrete calcitonin. The two principal thyroid hormones are thyroxine (T4) and triiodothyronine (T3), both of which are basically two tyrosines linked together with iodine. The thyroid glands are ductless glands that serve only an endocrine function. The thyroid is the only endocrine gland in the body that can be palpated.

Canine hypothyroidism

Hypothyroidism is a disorder that results from inadequate production of T_4 and T_3. It is relatively common in dogs but is rarely seen in cats.

Primary hypothyroidism accounts for more than 95% of cases and develops as a result of progressive destruction of the thyroid gland.[1] Frequently, this occurs either from an immune-mediated process called lymphocytic thyroiditis in which thyroid tissue is destroyed and replaced by fibrous connective tissue[2] or by idiopathic atrophy in which the thyroid tissue atrophies and is replaced by adipose tissue.[1] Less common causes of primary hypothyroidism include follicular cell hyperplasia and infiltrative neoplasia.[3]

Secondary hypothyroidism is rare but may be caused by pituitary malformation or neoplasia.[2]

Hypothyroidism can arise at any age and in any breed. Most commonly affected breeds include Golden retrievers, Doberman pinschers, Irish setters, Great Danes, Airedale terriers, Old English sheepdogs, dachshunds, miniature schnauzers, cocker spaniels, poodles, and boxers.[4] There is no apparent gender predisposition[1]; however, spayed females and neutered males are at increased risk for developing hypothyroidism compared with sexually intact animals.[5]

Clinical signs

Thyroid hormone is required for normal cellular metabolic functions; deficiencies can affect the metabolic function of almost all organ systems.[1] The extensive list of clinical manifestations associated with hypothyroidism is further testimony to the systemic impact that thyroid hormone, or the lack thereof, can have on the entire body.

Signs are often nonspecific and gradual in onset,[3] with the most common being lethargy, weight gain, and alopecia. Owners may attribute many of these signs to aging or overfeeding (Table 2.2.1).

Diagnosis

Prior to any diagnostic testing, it is important to take into consideration any concurrent medical therapies the patient may be receiving. Common drugs including (but not limited to) glucocorticoids, phenobarbital, sulfa antibiotics, furosemide, some nonsteroidal anti-inflammatory drugs (NSAIDs), clomipramine, and radiocontrast agents have been reported to alter thyroid concentrations,[2,6] thereby making diagnostic interpretation that much more difficult.

Another factor that should be considered is that of concurrent illness causing a reduction in thyroid hormone levels. This phe-

Table 2.2.1 Clinical manifestations of canine hypothyroidism

Metabolic	Cardiovascular
Lethargy	Bradycardia
Mental dullness	Cardiac arrhythmias
Unexplained weight gain	
Cold intolerance	Ocular
	Corneal lipid deposits
Dermatologic	Keratoconjunctivitis sicca
Alopecia	Corneal ulceration
Seborrhea sicca, oleosa, or dermatitis	Uveitis
Dry, brittle hair coat	Gastrointestinal
Changes in hair coat color	Diarrhea
Pyoderma	Constipation
Hyperpigmentation	Hematologic
Otitis externa	Anemia
Myxedema	Hyperlipidemia
	Coagulopathy
Neuromuscular	
Weakness	Reproductive
Ataxia	Female cycle abnormalities
Vestibular signs	Testicular atrophy
Facial nerve paralysis	Hypo/azoospermia
Seizures	

Source: Feldman EC, Nelson RW. Hypothyroidism/the thyroid gland. In: *Canine and Feline Endocrinology and Reproduction*, 3rd edition. St. Louis, MO: Saunders Elsevier; 2004, 86+, print.

Table 2.2.2 Factors causing low T_4 values in euthyroid animals

Factor	Example
Concurrent drug therapy	Prednisone, phenobarbital
Nonthyroidal illness	Hyperadrenocorticism
Naturally occurring different reference ranges for specific breeds	Greyhounds, whippets, basenjis, sled dogs
Hourly fluctuations	Circadian cycle changes
Fasting over 48 h	Anorexia
Age	An older dog is more likely to have lower TT_4 values than a younger dog
Ambient temperature	Car ride on a hot summer day
Stress	Visit to the veterinary hospital

Sources: Wilford C, DVM (Veterinary News columnist for the *AKC Gazette*). The enigmatic nature of hypothyroidism makes it difficult to distinguish from other diseases. *AKC Gazette* November, 1995; pp. 67–71; Neiger R, Prof. Dr. med. vet., PhD, DACVIM, DECVIM–CA. Canine hypothyroidism. In: *50° Congresso Nazionale Multisala SCIVAC*, Rimini, Italy. Giessen, Germany: Small Animal Clinic, Justus-Liebig University; 2005.

Urinalysis is often normal in dogs with primary hypothyroidism; however, in dogs with lymphocytic thyroiditis, immune complex glomerulonephritis may result in proteinuria. PU, hyposthenuria, and urinary tract infections are not typical of hypothyroidism.[1]

Endocrine testing

Total T_4 values will fall below normal reference range in most hypothyroid dogs; however, because this test is highly sensitive but not as *specific*, it is recommended that a free T_4 by equilibrium dialysis (fT_4 [ED]) and a TSH level be evaluated. A decreased fT_4 (ED) and an increased TSH in a dog with typical hypothyroid signs is highly suggestive of a true hypothyroid condition. It should be emphasized that measuring fT_4 (ED) is considered more accurate than radioimmunoassay (RIA) and should be specifically requested when submitting samples for testing.

Certain dog breeds such as greyhounds, whippets, basenjis, and conditioned sled dogs have been shown to have T_4 concentrations lower than established reference ranges of most other dogs. A diagnosis of hypothyroidism can therefore be difficult in these breeds and further diagnostic testing is recommended.[5,7,8]

Due to highly variable T_3 concentrations in both hypothyroid and euthyroid dogs, this test is of little value in the diagnosis of canine hypothyroidism.

The TSH stimulation test has been reported as highly accurate in diagnosing hypothyroidism in dogs; however, cost and availability of TSH has limited its use in veterinary medicine.

Dogs demonstrating abnormalities in other parameters of testing should be further evaluated for other conditions that may have overlapping diagnostic findings and clinical signs such as HAC or other nonthyroidal illnesses (Table 2.2.2).

nomenon, known as nonthyroidal illness or euthyroid sick syndrome, can be brought on by conditions such as HAC, renal disease, hepatic disease, heart failure, severe infections, and diabetic ketoacidosis (DKA). It is thought to be a physiological adaptation of the body in an attempt to decrease cellular metabolism[1] and to conserve energy. In general, the relative reduction in basal T_4 levels correlates with the severity of clinical illness.

For dogs demonstrating signs typical of hypothyroidism, a minimum database including a CBC, a chemistry profile with electrolytes, urinalysis, and total T_4 (TT_4) is recommended for the initial diagnostic workup.

Abnormal findings in the CBC that may be consistent with hypothyroidism are a mild, normocytic, normochromic, nonregenerative anemia, as well as leukocytosis, which could be a result of any skin infections that are present.[1]

Common abnormalities found in the serum chemistry profile are hypercholesterolemia and/or hypertriglyceridemia despite the collection of fasted samples. This may be due to the body's diminished capability to degrade lipids in its hypothyroid state.[1]

Treatments

The treatment of choice for hypothyroid dogs with clinical signs is supplementation of a name brand synthetic levothyroxine sodium product that is approved for use in dogs. Initial standard doses are 0.02 mg/kg (0.1 mg/10 lb) twice daily, up to a maximum of 0.8 mg twice daily.[9] Animal origin and generic synthetic thyroid supplements have historically been criticized for either having variable bioavailability or the potential of having variable, and sometimes considerably less, hormone than what is stated on the label.[1,2]

It is recommended that a T_4 level be reevaluated 4–8 weeks after starting replacement therapy or after any changes in dose or supplement brand. Dosage should then be adjusted according to test results as well as clinical response. If the patient responds well to therapy, once-daily therapy can be tried; however, some patients will require continued twice-daily therapy.[4] In dogs, peak plasma concentrations after oral dosing reportedly occur 4–12 h after administration, and the serum half-life is approximately 12–16 h.[5] Ideally, blood samples should be drawn immediately before the next dose is due (trough level) and then 4–6 h post pill (peak level). Once a consistent therapeutic dose has been achieved, routine monitoring may only require testing of peak T_4 levels every 6–12 months.

Clinical improvement should be observed within 4–6 weeks of initiation of therapy, although improvement in mental alertness and activity level may be seen in as little as 1–2 weeks.[4] Dermatologic and reproductive abnormalities may take several months to completely resolve.[5] If resolution of symptoms is not noted within this time frame, the diagnosis of hypothyroidism should be questioned.

Prognosis and survival times

With proper diagnosis, therapy, and monitoring, the prognosis for canine hypothyroidism is excellent and life expectancy is normal.[4]

Feline hyperthyroidism

Hyperthyroidism (thyrotoxicosis) is a multisystemic disorder that results from the excessive production and secretion of T_4 and T_3. Overall, it is the most common endocrine disorder of cats[10]; it is typically only diagnosed in middle age to older cats with a median age of 13 years. Feline hyperthyroidism has no gender predisposition, and with the possible exception of the Siamese and the Himalayan having fewer reported incidences than other breeds, there does not appear to be a significant breed predisposition.[11]

Fortunately, 97–99% of cases are histologically characterized as benign adenomatous hyperplasia, adenomas, or multinodular adenomas.[12] The remaining 1–3% of hyperthyroid cats, however, have malignant thyroid carcinomas.[11] Furthermore, over 70% of hyperthyroid cats are found to have bilateral involvement with the majority of cats having asymmetrical disease.[11]

At this point, the etiology of hyperthyroidism in cats is unknown; however, studies suggest that diet, environment, and genetics may all play a role in the development of the disease.[13]

Table 2.2.3 Common signs associated with feline hyperthyroidism

Weight loss
Polyphagia
Tachycardia
Heart murmurs
Palpable thyroid
Increased ALT/SAP
Polydipsia
Polyuria
Vomiting
Diarrhea
Unkempt appearance of skin and hair coat
Behavioral changes (i.e., increased vocalization, restlessness, irritability)

Clinical signs

Clinical signs of feline hyperthyroidism may vary depending on the severity of the disease, the duration of occurrence, and individual eccentricities (Table 2.2.3). Two of the most common signs that are reported, and are oftentimes the most distinguishing feature of feline hyperthyroidism, are those of unintended weight loss (in 92% of hyperthyroid cats) coupled with polyphagia (in 61% of hyperthyroid cats).[11] As it pertains to hyperthyroidism, this paradox is believed to be the result of the hypermetabolic state that is produced when chronically elevated levels of circulating thyroid hormone are present. Simply put, despite their increased drive to do so, most cats with significant hyperthyroidism often cannot consume enough food to compensate for the speed in which their bodies are burning energy, sometimes to the point of cachexia. A smaller subset of hyperthyroid cats, however, becomes anorexic as the disease progresses, thereby accelerating their rate of weight loss. This condition is referred to as apathetic hyperthyroidism and is seen in approximately 14% of hyperthyroid cats.[11]

Gastrointestinal (GI) signs of the disease may include vomiting, caused by stimulation of the chemoreceptor trigger zone (CRTZ), as well as rapid ingestion of large volumes of food, and diarrhea, which may be caused by a decrease in GI transit times and subsequent malabsorption.[11,14]

PU/PD is another clinical feature that has been reported to occur in 47%[11] of hyperthyroid cats and may be a result of increased renal perfusion (which subsequently reduces renal medullary solute concentration),[15] the diuretic effects of T_4, an associated renal insufficiency, or compulsive PD.[16]

Other common signs include hyperactivity and behavioral changes such as increased vocalization, irritability, or increased socialization. These may be attributable to either an increased stimulation of the sympathetic nervous system or a result of the cat's heightened drive to seek out food or water.

Diagnostics

Although some diagnoses are incidental findings following routine lab work, hyperthyroidism is more often diagnosed by linking history and clinical signs with one or more of the following: physical examination, abnormal laboratory findings, and thyroid scintigraphy.

Physical examination of hyperthyroid cats often identifies tachycardia (with heart rates often >220 beats/min), systolic heart murmurs, cardiac arrhythmias, weight loss, muscle wasting, and a poor hair coat.

In addition, a palpable thyroid nodule, which is sometimes referred to as a thyroid slip or goiter, may also be present. The term "thyroid slip" indicates that one or both of the glands are enlarged. Initially, the glands are pushed ventral (down) during palpation and then "slip" back up into position. The classic method to palpate the glands is to place the thumb and the index finger on either side of the trachea. With the cat in a sitting position and the legs held still, the neck is extended and the examiner gently sweeps their digits from the cat's larynx to the thoracic inlet, feeling for any lumps running under the digits. In the alternate technique, the examiner is positioned behind the cat, which is either standing or in sternal recumbency. The cat's head is elevated and turned 45° to the right or left, and the examiner places his or her index finger in the groove formed by the larynx and moves it downward toward the thoracic inlet.

One of the most common abnormalities that may be observed on routine lab work of hyperthyroid cats is mild to moderate elevations in liver enzymes, specifically in the alanine aminotransferase (ALT) and serum alkaline phosphatase (SAP) measurements. Suggested explanations for such abnormalities have included malnutrition, CHF, infections, hepatic anoxia, and direct toxic effects of thyroid hormones on the liver.[10]

Erythrocytosis, neutrophilia, and lymphocytosis are also frequently observed.

Elevated total T_4 (TT_4) serum concentrations are typically the most reliable test in confirming the disease. However, because of naturally occurring thyroid hormone fluctuations, as well as the potential suppressive effects of nonthyroidal illness, hyperthyroidism cannot be ruled out based on one normal TT_4 value; this is particularly true when clinical signs and physical examination suggest otherwise. In instances where the TT_4 value is within the normal reference range but hyperthyroidism is still suspected, a TT_4 should be repeated along with fT_4 (ED). Occasionally, true hyperthyroid cats will have a normal or high normal TT_4 but have an elevated free T_4. Because the free T_4 is less affected by nonthyroidal illness than TT_4, it is considered a more sensitive test; therefore, when elevated, it may lend supportive evidence of the disease. Free T_4 should not, however, be used as an initial screening tool because it is a less specific test than the TT_4. In other words, when used alone, it has a higher incidence of false positives.[11]

Other thyroid function tests such as the T_3 suppression test and the thyrotropin-releasing hormone (TRH) stimulation test have been described as potential aids in diagnosing mildly hyperthyroid cats with vague or borderline resting serum T_4 concentrations.[11] However, when considering that these tests may be difficult to interpret, expensive, or more labor intensive to perform in comparison with total and free T_4 assays, they should be reserved for occasions when repeated traditional testing proves nondiagnostic.[10,17]

The TSH response test is not recommended as it may be difficult to differentiate mildly hyperthyroid versus euthyroid results.

Furthermore, in cats with clearly elevated TT_4 values, the TSH response test offers no additional diagnostic information.[11]

Additional diagnostics

A thyroid scan, by means of scintigraphy, is considered both a highly sensitive and specific method of diagnosing feline hyperthyroidism.

Because thyroid scintigraphy allows the direct visualization of the functional adenomatous thyroid tissue responsible for the development of hyperthyroidism,[18] cats diagnosed with the disease based on clinical signs and laboratory findings alone should have scintigraphy performed to definitively confirm the diagnosis, as well as to determine the location of the abnormal tissue. This is especially important for cats scheduled to undergo irreversible treatments for hyperthyroidism such as surgical thyroidectomy or radioactive iodine.

Thyroid scans are performed by first injecting an intravenous radionuclide that is actively concentrated by thyroid tissue. Although iodine-131 (^{131}I) and iodine-123 (^{123}I) could also be utilized, technetium-99m as pertechnetate ($^{99m}TcO_4^-$) is the most commonly used compound because it is readily available, relatively inexpensive, has a rapid uptake of as little as 20 min, and has a short half-life of 6 h.

Once an appropriate uptake time has lapsed, the cat is imaged by a gamma camera, which will detect and display areas where gamma-emitting radionuclides are concentrated in various degrees. Pertechnetate concentrates primarily in the thyroid tissue, salivary glands, and gastric mucosa. A 1:1 uptake ratio of salivary glands to thyroid lobes is the standard for a normal study, whereas the radioactive uptake of the thyroid lobe(s) must be greater than that of the salivary glands to confirm a diagnosis of hyperthyroidism[11] (Figures 2.2.1 and 2.2.2).

Considering that a high percentage of hyperthyroid cats have clinical evidence of heart disease, cardiac screening is also advisable. At a minimum, this should include thoracic radiographs; however, an electrocardiogram (ECG) evaluation and echocardiography may also be warranted to further identify the type and severity of the heart disease present. Thyrotoxicosis causes cardiac hypertrophy related to a hypermetabolic state, peripheral vasodilation, and increased demands for cardiac output. In addition, increased sympathetic activity and thyroid hormone levels may stimulate myocardial hypertrophy. In chronic cases of hyperthyroidism, the left ventricle (LV) becomes thickened. Concurrent systemic hypertension probably contributes to this in many cases. Hypertension in these cats can be multifactorial: from high cardiac output, aortic stiffness in cats with aortoannular ectasia, or related to concurrent renal disease. In advanced hyperthyroidism, there will be sufficient cardiac dysfunction and

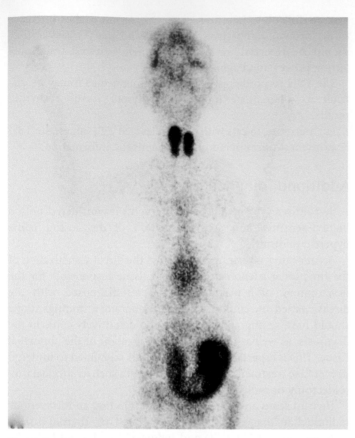

Figure 2.2.1 Thyroid scintigraphy performed on a hyperthyroid cat illustrating an increased uptake of $^{99m}TcO_4^-$ by functional adenomatous thyroid tissue. The figure demonstrates bilateral disease.

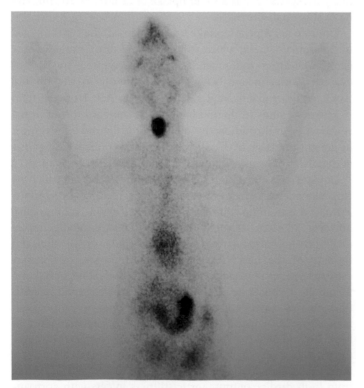

Figure 2.2.2 Thyroid scintigraphy performed on a hyperthyroid cat illustrating an increased uptake of $^{99m}TcO_4^-$ by functional adenomatous thyroid tissue. The figure demonstrates unilateral disease.

fluid retention to cause more generalized cardiomegaly or even CHF. Echocardiography will reveal bi-atrial dilatation with normal or reduced LV ejection fraction.[19]

Because of the high incidence of systemic hypertension in hyperthyroid cats, measurement of systolic, and if possible diastolic, blood pressure as well as an ophthalmic examination should be performed on all hyperthyroid cats. Consequences of uncontrolled hypertension include retinopathy, progressive renal disease, and central nervous system (CNS) hemorrhage.[20]

Fortunately, hypertension associated with this disease results in less end-organ consequences compared to the hypertension associated with chronic renal failure.

Concurrent disease

As hyperthyroidism is typically a disease of middle age to older cats, it is important to recognize the increased likelihood of existing concurrent disease. Furthermore, as the differentials for hyperthyroidism oftentimes overlap with those of other illnesses such as primary GI, renal, hepatic, or cardiac disease, it is strongly recommended for the overall well-being of the patient to identify and address, when possible, any concurrent illnesses while considering therapy options for hyperthyroidism.

Treatments

Failure to institute some kind of therapy for hyperthyroidism will result in an insidious progression of emaciation, severe metabolic and cardiac dysfunction, and, ultimately, death. However, because of the benign nature of the thyroid lesions, the disease carries a favorable prognosis with effective therapy. Standard options for treating hyperthyroid cats consist of one or a combination of the following methods: medical management, surgical thyroidectomy, radioiodine therapy, and iodine-restricted diets.

Medical management

In the United States, medical management of feline hyperthyroidism is most commonly achieved with the use of methimazole (trade names Tapazole® or Felimazole®). Elsewhere, carbimazole, a prodrug to methimazole, may be used with similar effects. Antithyroid drugs such as methimazole and carbimazole inhibit synthesis of thyroid hormones; they are not, however, cytotoxic. Therefore, thyroid nodules may continue to grow, necessitating the need for dose adjustments over time. In humans, the plasma half-life of methimazole is reported as anywhere from 4 to 14h; however, the biological effects of the drug appear to exceed its plasma half-life.[11] In cats, once- to thrice-daily administration of antithyroid drugs has been described with most cats requiring lifelong twice-daily dosing to achieve stable euthyroidism.

Although many cats will respond well to daily methimazole treatments for the remainder of their lives, others experience some form of adverse reaction such as inappetence, vomiting, lethargy, and dermatologic or hematologic disturbances. In these cats, alternative methods in treating their disease may be required.

Regardless of the long-term means of hyperthyroid treatment, an initial short-term trial period of methimazole is recommended to assess the possibility of occult renal disease before a permanent resolution is sought. Once a euthyroid state has been achieved through administration of either oral or transdermal methimazole, serum chemistry and urinalyses should be repeated to determine if renal function remains normal in the face of the reduction in renal perfusion induced by the euthyroid state.

Methimazole administration may also be a helpful tool in preparing a cat for eventual surgical thyroidectomy as it can halt or reverse significant weight loss, as well as decrease cardiac and metabolic complications,[10] thereby making the patient a better surgical candidate. It is recommended that methimazole be administered for 6–12 weeks prior to surgery, until the cat is medically and clinically euthyroid.[11]

Surgical thyroidectomy

Although radioiodine therapy appears to be the safest, most effective,[21] and preferred method of treatment by both veterinary surgeons and internal medicine specialists alike, surgical thyroidectomy may be an option for hyperthyroid cats that have been determined to have minimal anesthetic risks *and* do not have access to, or funding for, radioiodine therapy.

It should be noted, however, that a significant number of cats have been found to have ectopic hyperplastic thyroid tissue located in their thoracic inlet or anterior mediastinum.[12] It is therefore advisable that nuclear scintigraphy be utilized to identify ectopic tissue and to alter treatment plans if necessary. Should surgery proceed without identification of the ectopic tissue via scintigraphy, the hyperthyroid condition will often persist despite removal of a coexisting hyperfunctional cervical thyroid gland. In addition, surgical thyroidectomy can carry detrimental risks. Damage to, or the inadvertent removal of, adjacent parathyroid glands or their blood supply may result in postoperative hypoparathyroidism and subsequent hypocalcemia. Postoperative hypoparathyroidism is rarely a permanent occurrence; however, because calcium regulation is vital to proper electrical conduction of the nervous and muscular systems, serum calcium levels should be evaluated daily for up to 7 days and patients should be closely observed for the onset of hypocalcemic signs.[11] Other potential complications include laryngeal paralysis as a result of damage to the recurrent laryngeal nerve, Horner's syndrome, and permanent hypothyroidism. Although some cats undergoing bilateral total thyroidectomies will retain and grow enough accessory thyroid tissue to remain clinically euthyroid, others will demonstrate manifestations of hypothyroidism and therefore will require long-term thyroid supplementation and subsequent dose monitoring postoperatively.

As described earlier, due to the high incidence of cardiovascular and metabolic disturbances and the debilitated condition of untreated hyperthyroid cats, they often are poor anesthetic candidates. Therefore, every effort should be made to stabilize hyperthyroid patients prior to anesthetic events. This may be achieved by initiating methimazole administration several weeks to months prior to the event or, at minimum, by formulating an anesthetic plan that incorporates careful selection of nonadrenergic stimulating drugs and close monitoring.

Finally, it should be reiterated that although surgical thyroidectomy may be convenient and readily accessible, due to a significantly increased risk of life-threatening complications when compared to radioiodine therapy, it is rarely advised.

Radioiodine therapy

Radioiodine therapy has been shown to provide a simple, safe, and effective means of treating feline hyperthyroidism.[22] [131]I is the therapeutic radionuclide of choice[11] as it has a >95% success rate in destroying hyperfunctional thyroid tissue, regardless of where it resides, with a single dose. [131]I can be given IV, subcutaneously (SC), or orally; however, because oral administration may increase the risk of radiation exposure to veterinary personnel, it is most often given IV or SC. After administration, up to 60% of ^{131}I is trapped or concentrated in the thyroid gland where it selectively destroys hyperfunctional tissue by emitting both gamma rays and beta particles. Eighty percent of the tissue destruction is caused by the beta particles; however, because they only travel a maximum of 2 mm into the tissue, adjacent hypoplastic thyroid tissue, parathyroid glands, and other cervical structures are usually spared. [131]I not trapped in the thyroid gland is excreted primarily in the urine and, to a lesser degree, in the feces.[22] The half-life of ^{131}I is 8.1 days and requires patients to be hospitalized while radiation levels decrease. Duration of hospitalization is usually between 3 days and 2 weeks depending on the dose used and the state or local radiation regulations.[10,23]

In order to reduce human exposure to radioactivity still present in the cat at the time of discharge, owners should be advised to abide by the following instructions for 1–3 weeks after the cat is discharged from the hospital:

Keep the cat indoors.

Minimize close contact with the cat.

Eliminate all contact with the cat and its waste products for all children and pregnant women.

Dispose of all waste products and litter according to state and local radioactive waste disposal regulations.

Although most cats will have normal thyroid function within 1 month of ^{131}I treatment, postprocedure rechecks are recommended at 1, 3, and 6 months to assess thyroid levels, serum chemistry profiles, and the overall health status of the cat.

Adverse reactions to ^{131}I are rare; however, the disadvantages to ^{131}I treatment are a higher upfront cost of treatment, the limited availability of facilities that are equipped and licensed to offer the procedure, and quarantine requirements after administration.

Treatment with iodine-restricted diets

Most recently, a fourth option for the treatment of feline hyperthyroidism has emerged by way of dietary iodine restriction. Although correlating studies were performed on a relatively small number of test subjects, abstracts published in the *Journal of Veterinary Internal Medicine* demonstrated that hyperthyroid cats fed a diet with iodine levels ≤0.32 parts per million dry matter basis maintained normal T_4 concentrations.[24]

The factors to consider if dietary management is elected are the following:

- Cats on an iodine-restricted diet need to be fed that diet exclusively, as even small volumes of erroneous food items can cause unacceptable elevations in thyroid levels.

- Rechecks including a physical exam, T_4, CBC, serum chemistry profile, and urinalysis should be conducted indefinitely at a minimum of 6-month intervals.

- Excluding those that have experienced adverse reactions, cats receiving antithyroid medication should be down-titrated off medication over a period of several weeks while transitioning to the iodine-restricted diet.

Prognosis and survival times

Prognosis and survival times for cats with hyperthyroidism are highly variable depending on the age of the cat, concurrent illnesses, and method of treatment. As previously stated, hyperthyroidism is a systemic disease that eventually leads to death if untreated.

Excluding cats classified as having renal disease prior to treatment, one study found that the average survival time for hyperthyroid cats treated with methimazole alone was 2 years, with a range of 1.0–3.9 years, whereas cats treated with ^{131}I alone averaged 4-year survival times with a range of 3.0–4.8 years.[25]

Although few statistical evaluations of prognosis and long-term survival times of hyperthyroid cats undergoing surgical thyroidectomy with or without pretreatment with methimazole have been published, most literature agrees that the presurgical health status of the patient, the location of the tumor(s), the skill of the surgeon and the anesthetist, and perioperative monitoring and care are all very important factors in determining outcome. In one study, the recurrence rate of hyperthyroidism postoperatively was reported as low. Of those that did recur, most were cases that had presurgical scintigraphic evidence of ectopic hyperplastic thyroid tissue.[26]

Conclusion

Hyperthyroidism, the most common endocrine disorder of cats, is frequently encountered by the veterinary technician. As such, a thorough understanding of this disease process is necessary. This knowledge should also include a complete understanding of the diagnostic testing and treatment options. Because radioiodine therapy is the superior method for treating most hyperthyroid cats, licensed facilities offering this treatment are becoming more common and accessible in the United States. As such, the veterinary technician should be comfortable in providing client education for this treatment option.

The role of the veterinary technician

As with many aspects of veterinary medicine, the role of the veterinary technician in the care of hyperthyroid cats can be quite extensive. Client knowledge regarding hyperthyroidism can range from pet owners who just thought their cat was "getting old" and are completely unaware that such a disease exists to clients armed with reams of information gleaned from the internet. It has been well documented that hyperthyroid cats that have been identified and treated effectively often have favorable outcomes. Therefore, if hyperthyroidism is suspected or diagnosed, technicians can go a long way in providing in-depth information to the client about the many facets of the disease and how it relates to their cat so that they can make an informed decision about treatment options.

Likewise, technicians play a vital role in the treatment of hyperthyroid cats through their involvement with diagnostic testing, assisting in therapeutic procedures, such as surgery or radioactive iodine, and providing at-home client education.

Canine thyroid tumors

Thyroid tumors account for 1–2% of all canine neoplasms.[27,28] Of these, 70–100% are malignant, with 30–60% of dogs having metastasis at the time of diagnosis.[27,28] Boxers, beagles, and golden retrievers are overrepresented.[27,28] Tumors typically affect middle-aged to older dogs, with an average age of 10 years, with no sex predilection.[28]

Clinical signs

The most common reason for presentation to the veterinarian is palpation of a ventral neck mass by the owner.[28] The mass may be large and may extend to the thoracic inlet. Other clinical signs include trouble swallowing, regurgitation, tachypnea, dyspnea, loud breathing, coughing, and bark change.[28,29] Nonspecific signs such as lethargy, weight loss, and decreased appetite can occur.[29] Clinical signs due to hyperthyroidism can occur as 10% of thyroid tumors are functional. Functional canine thyroid tumors are almost always malignant carcinomas. Clinical signs associated with hyperthyroidism include weight loss, PD, PU, polyphagia, hyperactivity, diarrhea, and vomiting. Thyroid tumors can be clinically silent if benign, small, noninvasive, and nonfunctional. Thyroid masses of this nature are often found incidentally on necropsy due to their silent nature.[28,29]

Diagnostics

Diagnostic testing is used both to definitively diagnose the tumor and to clinically stage the tumor.

Physical exam

The only physical exam finding may be a mass in the ventral cervical region.[27,28] Other causes of cervical swellings include abscess, salivary mucocele, granuloma, and cellulitis. Other physical exam abnormalities can be seen with large, invasive tumors and are similar to what the owner notes at home as described in the previous section. The neck should be palpated very carefully to determine the size and extent of the mass, as well as if the mass is freely movable. An immovable mass implies local invasion and should raise suspicion for a malignant thyroid tumor. Mandibular lymph nodes should be carefully palpated and may be enlarged due to tumor spread. Physical exam findings associated with hyperthyroidism can be seen with functional thyroid tumors, as described above, and may include tachycardia and heart murmur.[29]

Laboratory testing

A CBC, serum biochemistry profile, and urinalysis should be performed to assess for concurrent conditions. There are no specific findings on these tests to indicate a malignant tumor. Rarely, hypercalcemia has been reported as a paraneoplastic syndrome. Urinalysis is usually unremarkable.[29]

A basal T_4 level, and potentially a TSH concentration, should be obtained in any dog suspected of having a thyroid tumor. Thyroid tumors can destroy the thyroid gland leading to hypothyroidism. In addition, 10% of dogs with malignant thyroid tumors have hyperthyroidism due to a functional tumor.[29]

Imaging

As a part of staging the tumor, and prior to making a treatment plan, thoracic radiographs (three views) should always be performed to evaluate for metastatic disease.

Cervical radiographs can be performed to evaluate for displacement of neck structures. Ultrasound of the neck is used to determine mass origin, invasiveness, vascularity, and whether the tumor is unilateral or bilateral.[29,30]

Abdominal radiographs and ultrasound can also be performed to look for metastasis to the abdominal organs, such as the liver. This is also useful as the geriatric dog may have other disorders that may influence decisions regarding therapy.

CT or MRI of the cervical region can help determine the invasiveness of the tumor. They are especially recommended if surgical excision or RT is being considered (Figure 2.2.3).

Other diagnostic tests

A cardiac workup is recommended if murmurs or arrhythmias are detected. This can occur in dogs with hyperthyroidism.

As radiolabeled pertechnetate is trapped by any cells that trap iodine, thyroid scintigraphy can be used to locate ectopic thyroid tissue and to determine extent of invasion or lymph node metastasis. It is not useful for pulmonary metastasis.[31] This can also be used to determine if the tumor can be treated with [131]I (see the section "Treatment").

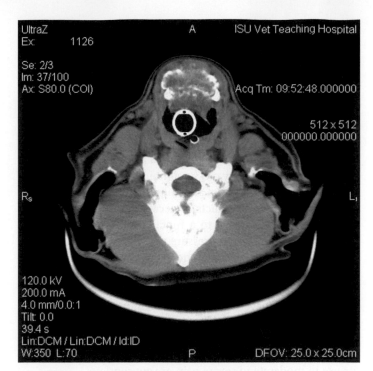

Figure 2.2.3 CT scan of invasive thyroid tumor.

Fine needle aspiration and biopsy

Thyroid tumors are typically vascular tumors that hemorrhage when aspirated or biopsied. Fine needle aspiration using a 21- to 23-gauge needle with ultrasound guidance is recommended.[30] This can help differentiate thyroid tumors from other masses, such as abscesses, cysts, salivary mucoceles, other tumors (sarcomas or mast cell tumors), or lymph nodes. Be prepared for postsampling hemorrhage. Firm pressure should be applied to the site with special attention to keep the airway open. Pressure should be continued until sure of the clotting status of the biopsy site. Frequent checks of the area should continue throughout the day. If fine needle aspiration and cytology does not yield a diagnosis of thyroid malignancy, then biopsy of the mass should be considered. Incisional biopsy of masses that are fixed to the underlying or adjacent tissue may be considered for definitive diagnosis. If the tumor is freely movable and nonfixed to adjacent and underlying tissues, surgical excision is recommended.[29]

Treatment

Treatment options include surgical excision, radiotherapy, radioiodide therapy (^{131}I), chemotherapy, or a combination of these. The type of treatment chosen depends on the size of the tumor, invasiveness, metastasis, and availability of treatment modalities.

Surgical excision

Surgical excision is especially recommended for smaller, mobile masses. Dogs with freely movable thyroid carcinomas without evidence of metastasis have a median survival time (MST) of greater than 36 months.[32] Surgery is not recommended when the tumor invades adjacent structures (vasculature, recurrent laryngeal nerves, parathyroid glands, larynx, or trachea). Tumors that are bilateral and fixed are difficult to resect without significant morbidity, including laryngeal paralysis and hemorrhage.[33] It is estimated that only 25–50% of thyroid carcinomas are resectable at the time of diagnosis.[32,34] MST with surgery is 6–12 months if the tumor is invasive.[32,34]

Anesthetic and analgesic considerations

Blood loss during surgery can be significant due to the vascularity of the tumor. The surgeon and anesthetist should be prepared to administer blood products if necessary. Additionally, dogs with hyperthyroidism due to a functional tumor should have their heart rate and blood pressure monitored closely. Animals with large tumors are placed in dorsal recumbency for imaging, RT, and surgery. Care should be taken to protect the airway as tracheal compression by the tumor can occur in this position.

Patients may have significant discomfort, especially if not treated, as the tumor increases in size. Client education on recognizing the signs of discomfort along with strong patient advocacy will ensure adequate pain management. Analgesics intended for use in moderate to severe pain are appropriate.

Radiation therapy

RT is indicated when complete surgical excision of the tumor is not possible due to invasion of adjacent structures. Dogs treated with RT have an MST of 24.5 months.[35] RT may be attempted when there is incomplete surgical excision. Palliative RT has also been used as the sole therapy to reduce tumor size or to decrease tumor growth.[36] Palliation is indicated for pain relief or relief of other complications due to the tumor. The option for palliative radiotherapy should be reserved for dogs that are not good candidates for surgery or a full course of radiation (e.g., the dog has metastasis to the chest but is experiencing discomfort from a large thyroid carcinoma).[37] Acute side effects of RT include skin desquamation, hair loss, and mucositis within the treatment field. Side effects usually develop during or shortly after treatment and are generally reversible and are treated with symptomatic care (pain management and soft, highly palatable foods). Permanent alopecia and skin pigmentation are common after treatment.[37]

Radioiodide 131 (^{131}I)

^{131}I can be used as an adjunct to surgery, with an MST of 34 months; when used alone, MST is 30 months. In contrast, dogs that did not receive any treatment at all had an MST of 3 months.[30] ^{131}I therapy is recommended when surgery alone is not likely to be curative due to metastatic disease or local invasion, or when surgery has been attempted but complete surgical excision has not been achieved.[30] Another study showed similar results, and reported MSTs similar to RT.[38] Three dogs (out of 39, or 8%) died of radioiodine-associated myelosuppression in this study.[38] Dogs should undergo thyroid scintigraphy with pertechnetate prior to ^{131}I treatment. ^{131}I should be considered in most dogs that accumulate pertechnetate in

an abnormal pattern on thyroid scintigraphy regardless of T_4 measurement.[38]

Chemotherapy

Cisplatin or doxorubicin chemotherapy can be used with response rates of 40–50%.[39,40] Chemotherapy should be recommended following surgery or RT in dogs at high risk for developing metastasis (large, fixed, bilateral tumors).[33] Anecdotally, Palladia® (toceranib phosphate) or metronomic chemotherapy protocols may be of benefit in some cases. Anti-inflammatory steroid therapy may be helpful in decreasing inflammation and edema associated with the tumor.

Prognosis

The prognosis of dogs with thyroid carcinomas is considered good to excellent following curative intent treatment. See "Treatment" section for prognosis with specific treatments. The MST for untreated dogs is only 3 months.[30] The risk of metastasis increases when there is >20 cm³ tumor volume[41] or when the tumor is bilateral.[42] When tumor volume is greater than 100 cm³, metastatic potential approaches 100%.[41]

Client education

Clients should receive instruction on home care including the importance of using a harness instead of a neck leash/collar, exercise restriction to avoid hypoxic situations, and keeping the pet cool on warm days to prevent overheating.

Client education should also include information on quality of life in the terminal phase of the disease process. These pets have the potential for death from slow asphyxiation and owners may need instruction on humane care.

SECTION 3 PARATHYROID GLANDS

The two parathyroid glands lie in close approximation to the thyroid gland on either side of the cervical trachea. They release parathyroid hormone (PTH) with the primary goal of maintaining normal blood calcium levels. In a normal animal, hypocalcemia stimulates the release of PTH and hypercalcemia will reduce the amount of PTH released from the parathyroid glands, allowing blood calcium levels to return to normal range. The three main actions of PTH are the conversion of vitamin D to its active form (vitamin D_3), which increases absorption of calcium from the GI tract, renal conservation of calcium, and calcium release from bony stores. The net effect of PTH is to increase blood calcium levels back to normal range.

Hypoparathyroidism

Hypoparathyroidism is characterized by the loss of functional parathyroid tissue. The naturally occurring disease (primary hypoparathyroidism) is immune mediated in origin and is more common in the dog. The toy poodle is overrepresented. Iatrogenic hypoparathyroidism may be seen secondary to inadvertent parathyroid removal or damage (as in surgical therapy for feline hyperthyroidism) or as a temporary or permanent result of therapy for primary hyperparathyroidism.

Clinical signs

The clinical signs of hypoparathyroidism are due to hypocalcemia. As blood ionized calcium levels fall, animals present with primarily neuromuscular symptoms. Clinical signs include weakness, lethargy, and muscle fasciculations, which can become severe enough to resemble tonic clonic seizure activity. Animals that present with severe fasciculations or seizures may also be febrile. However, the fever is most commonly due to the increased muscle activity and is self-limiting with appropriate therapy for hypocalcemia. Facial pruritus, which may be severe, is another manifestation of hypocalcemia. Clinical signs may appear acutely, so additional neurological differentials (e.g., distemper, rabies) should be considered.

Diagnostics

Calcium levels are measured in animals with consistent clinical signs. Ionized calcium levels are recommended, as total calcium levels do not accurately represent the levels of the ionized form and may be affected by serum albumin levels. Severe hypocalcemia may be life threatening, so once hypocalcemia is documented, supportive measures should be immediately instituted. Once animals are stable and additional diagnostic testing is pursued, PTH levels should be measured in animals suspected of having hypoparathyroidism. The diagnosis is made by demonstrating decreased PTH levels concurrent with hypocalcemia.

In the majority of cases, there is no reason to consider parathyroid gland biopsy.

Imaging

There are no diagnostic imaging procedures that are specific to hypoparathyroidism.

Treatments

Inpatient treatment

Inpatient treatment centers on identification of the hypocalcemic state and emergency stabilization of the patient. Calcium may be administered via slow intravenous injection, but this therapy may result in significant cardiac arrhythmias. Therefore, concurrent, continuous ECG monitoring is recommended. Once calcium levels have stabilized, additional calcium may be administered via constant rate infusion (CRI), subcutaneous injection, and oral therapy. Protocols for subcutaneous injections are available but are controversial. Severe cutaneous lesions have been reported as a result of subcutaneous calcium administration. Calcium chloride is highly irritating to tissues and calcium gluconate has been associated with calcinosis cutis and skin necro-

sis. Rectal temperatures should be monitored in febrile animals. External cooling measures are rarely necessary. When animals are stable and eating, oral supplementation with calcium and vitamin D_3 (in the form of calcitriol) may be initiated.

Outpatient treatment

In the immediate period, animals may require therapy with both oral calcium and calcitriol. Once calcium levels have stabilized, animals may be able to be maintained on single-agent calcitriol therapy. Additional therapy is not indicated in uncomplicated cases of primary hypoparathyroidism. In the absence of clinical signs, recheck examinations are recommended every 6 months. These examinations should, at a minimum, include recent history, physical examination, body weight and body condition score, and blood ionized calcium levels.

Pharmacology

Oral or parenteral forms of PTH are not available, so therapy consists of supplementation with calcium and vitamin D_3. Vitamin D_3 is necessary for absorption of calcium from the GI tract.

Prognosis and survival times

With accurate diagnosis and committed owners, prognosis for primary hypoparathyroidism is good to excellent. Animals may be expected to have normal survival times with successful therapy.

Nutritional considerations

Animals with hypoparathyroidism do not require special diets or dietary supplements. An age-appropriate and nutritionally complete diet is required.

Client education

Client education is imperative with hypoparathyroidism. Clients need to be made aware of signs of hypocalcemia, including weakness, lethargy, muscle fasciculations, and facial pruritus. It must be stressed that signs may be noted at any time and that emergency intervention may need to be pursued. Clients must also be aware that monitoring of blood calcium levels, on a routine basis or in an emergency situation, requires measurement of ionized calcium, as opposed to total calcium. Clients should identify veterinary practices that can provide in-house and accurate ionized calcium measurements. Clients must also be aware of signs of hypercalcemia (PU/PD). Oversupplementation with calcitriol may lead to clinical hypercalcemia, and if signs are noted, then dosing adjustments may be necessary.

Hyperparathyroidism

Hyperparathyroidism is characterized by an abnormal increase in the amount of functional parathyroid tissue. This can be a primary disease (more common in the dog) or can occur secondary to renal disease (renal secondary hyperparathyroidism). Naturally occurring primary hyperparathyroidism is most commonly a benign condition and keeshonds are overrepresented.

Clinical signs

Clinical signs of hyperparathyroidism are due to hypercalcemia. The predominant clinical signs are PU/PD. If signs are chronic, weight loss and lethargy may also be reported.

Diagnostics

The most significant finding on laboratory testing is hypercalcemia. The total calcium on serum chemistry is elevated and, in most cases, ionized calcium will also be increased. Hypercalcemia may be severe. Phosphate levels are normal to low; this is in contrast to other causes of hypercalcemia (chronic renal failure [CRF]) in which phosphate levels are elevated. Diagnosis is usually suspected by excluding the more common causes of hypercalcemia (e.g., LSA, anal sac tumors, renal failure). PU/PD may contribute to evidence of dehydration, including elevated blood urea nitrogen, hematocrit, and albumin. Urine specific gravity may be in the isosthenuric range, even in the face of dehydration. Assays for PTH are definitive, documenting either normal or elevated values, consistent with autonomous hypersecretion of PTH.

Imaging

Cervical ultrasound is a recommended imaging modality for primary hyperparathyroidism. Animals may require sedation for maintaining dorsal recumbency and cervical extension, allowing for improved imaging of the cervical region. Cervical ultrasound aids in the diagnosis and in the therapeutic approach to primary hyperparathyroidism, especially when a solitary parathyroid nodule is identified. This assists in planning for surgical or percutaneous approaches. Diffuse, bilateral enlargement of the parathyroid gland is more consistent with renal secondary hyperparathyroidism.

Biopsy

In the majority of cases, biopsy of the parathyroid tissue is performed at the time of surgical parathyroidectomy. Tissue should be submitted for histopathologic examination to ensure hyperparathyroidism is a benign condition. Malignant parathyroid disease is rare, but when present, metastatic disease may be seen.

Treatments

Inpatient treatments

Inpatient treatment centers on maintenance of ionized blood calcium levels. Animals with primary hyperparathyroidism may present with dangerously elevated blood calcium levels. Therapy for hypercalcemia consists of intravenous fluid support with a balanced crystalloid solution (0.9% NaCl), diuretic therapy once volume status has been normalized, and potentially, corticoster-

oids to promote calciuriesis. Animals with primary hyperparathyroidism should be medically managed to minimize anesthetic risks and reduce complications of parathyroidectomy. Certain protocols call for preoperative therapy with calcium and vitamin D_3 for 24–72h to help prevent life-threatening postoperative hypocalcemia. Definitive treatment for primary hyperparathyroidism may consist of surgical parathyroidectomy or percutaneous ablation techniques. In either scenario, postoperative monitoring of ionized calcium levels is imperative. Depending on the levels of preoperative hypercalcemia, postoperative *ionized* calcium levels may need to be assessed from every 4 to 12h. Animals also require close monitoring for signs of hypocalcemia (lethargy, weakness, muscle fasciculations, facial pruritus). Emergency measures for hypocalcemia may be indicated and may require intravenous calcium supplementation. Continuous ECG monitoring is a necessary component of intravenous calcium therapy.

Anesthetic and analgesic considerations

Anesthetic considerations concentrate on repeated measurement of ionized calcium levels and appropriate supplementation of calcium.

Outpatient treatments

Long-term supplemental therapy is not required for most cases of primary hyperparathyroidism. In cases of subtotal parathyroidectomy for primary hyperparathyroidism, short-term therapy for hypocalcemia may be indicated. However, once PTH and calcium levels have equilibrated, long-term supplemental therapy is not required in most cases. Renal secondary hyperparathyroidism is a medically managed condition and parathyroidectomy is not considered a part of therapy. PTH levels may be controlled with therapy for renal disease and, in appropriate cases, with calcitriol therapy. See Chapter 10 for more information.

Pharmacology

In animals with primary hyperparathyroidism, the ability to respond to hypocalcemia is diminished as PTH would normally be downregulated in response to hypercalcemia. Therefore, in light of autonomously functioning parathyroid tissue, the compensatory mechanisms that would be in place for hypocalcemia are downregulated. Thus, the animal's ability to compensate for hypocalcemia (brought on by surgical parathyroidectomy or percutaneous parathyroid ablation), by increasing PTH levels and resorbing calcium in various sites, is insufficient. Postprocedural ionized calcium concentration may significantly decrease and can reach life-threatening levels. Therefore, close monitoring of ionized calcium and appropriate parenteral supplementation is critical.

Prognosis and survival times

Prognosis for long-term survival is good to excellent with successful therapy and appropriate and intensive perioperative monitoring and therapy. In cases with malignant disease, the prognosis is worse and animals may succumb to metastatic disease.

Nutritional considerations

As with any critical animal, nutritional needs, calculated by basal energy requirement (BER), should be assessed for every patient. There are no specific short- or long-term nutritional requirements for patients with primary hyperparathyroidism. Nutritional considerations are more important for cases of renal secondary hyperparathyroidism.

SECTION 4 ADRENAL GLANDS

The adrenal glands consist of an outer cortex and an inner medulla.[1] There are three layers, or zones, which make up the cortex. The outer most layer is the zona glomerulosa (ZG), which produces aldosterone. Aldosterone's main function is to increase sodium absorbtion and potassium excretion.[2] The middle layer, the zona fasciculata (ZF), and the inner most layer, the zona reticularis (ZR), function as a unit.[2] Together they are responsible for the production of cortisol and androgens.[2] Cortisol has a multitude of effects on many body systems including hepatic glucose production, protein and fat catabolism, as well as maintaining normal blood pressure.[2]The destruction of the three layers leads to inadequate secretion of both mineralocorticoids (primarily aldosterone) and glucocorticoids (primarily cortisol).[1,2]

Hypoadrenocorticism: Addison's disease

Hypoadrenocorticism, also known as Addison's disease, is characterized by glucocorticoid or mineralocorticoid deficiency that results from a failure of the cortex of the adrenal glands. The most common cause of hypoadrenocorticism in dogs is immune-mediated adrenalitis, also called primary hypoadrenocorticism. Less common causes of primary hypoadrenocorticism can include granulomatous destruction and hemorrhagic infarction of the adrenal gland, amyloidosis, necrosis, and metastatic neoplasia.[2] Deficiency of ACTH or secondary hypoadrenocorticism can occur with destructive or neoplastic lesions of the hypothalamus or pituitary gland, postoperative hypophysectomy, or can be idiopathic.[2]

Hypoadrenocorticism has been documented to be inherited in a variety of breeds including standard poodles, Portuguese water dogs, and Nova Scotia duck tolling retrievers.[2] While any dog can be affected, it appears there is a predisposition for young to middle-aged female dogs.[2]

Clinical signs

Clinical signs associated with hypoadrenocorticism are nonspecific and can involve many different body systems. Waxing and waning lethargy, vomiting, diarrhea, and dehydration are the most common clinical signs on presentation.[2] Other clinical signs can include PU/PD, muscle tremors, abdominal pain, shock, and collapse.[2]Since some of these animals have a painful abdomen, care should be used when picking up these animals.

Classically, dogs presented for an Addisonian crisis are lethargic, dehydrated, and are hyponatremic and hyperkalemic due to the lack of aldosterone.[3]

Diagnostic testing

In 95% of dogs with hypoadrenocorticism, the sodium : potassium ratio is less than 27:1.[3] Nonregenerative anemia (21–25%) and lack of a stress leukogram (92%), (neutrophilia [32%], lymphopenia [10–13%], and eosinopenia [10–20%]) may be present.[1,2] A serum biochemistry panel may reveal prerenal azotemia due to hypovolemia in up to 95% of dogs with primary hypoadrenocorticism.[1] Other significant clinicopathologic abnormalities can include hypoglycemia, increased liver enzymes, hypercalcemia, hypoalbuminemia, and hyperphosphatemia.[3] A urine specific gravity of <1.030 is noted in 60–88% of Addisonian dogs.[1]

Imaging

Thoracic radiographs can reveal microcardia, reduced caudal vena cava size, and pulmonary vasculature related to hypovolemia. Radiographs may reveal a megaesophagus (0.9%).[2] Abdominal radiographs are often performed to rule out a GI foreign body. An abdominal ultrasound may reveal a significantly smaller adrenal gland size on ultrasound compared to normal dogs.[1]

The nickname of this disease is "The Great Pretender" or "The Great Masquerader" because the clinical signs and test results can resemble those in patients with renal failure, infectious enteritis, and GI obstruction, to name a few. The veterinary team must have a high index of suspicion for Addison's disease to pursue this diagnostic route. Measurement of the basal cortisol concentration can be helpful in ruling out hypoadrenocorticism. A basal cortisol concentration of greater then 2 μg/dL (55.2 mmol/L) in dogs (not on any medications) has a high negative predictive value, meaning that these dogs are unlikely to have hypoadrenocorticism.[4] The gold standard for diagnosis of hypoadrenocorticism is the ACTH stimulation test to document a decreased functional adrenal reserve.[4] Blood samples for measurements of serum cortisol concentrations are collected prior to and 1 h after administration of synthetic ACTH (Cortrosyn®).[2] Confirmation of hypoadrenocorticism is made if both the pre- and post-ACTH cortisol concentrations are less than 2 μg/dL (27.6 mmol/L).[4] Endogenous ACTH concentrations and plasma aldosterone concentrations can be measured to support a diagnosis of hypoadrenocorticism but are limited by their availability.

Treatment and pharmacology

The treatment for hypoadrenocorticism can be divided into acute and maintenance therapy.

Acute

An acute Addisonian crisis represents a true medical emergency that requires prompt intervention. The goals of emergency therapy include correction of hypovolemia, electrolyte abnormalities, and metabolic acidosis.[2] Shock rate (90 mL/kg) administration of 0.9% sodium chloride intravenous fluid should be initiated immediately upon presentation. If possible, an ACTH stimulation test should be performed and the dog should be administered a dose of dexamethasone (0.25–1.0 mg/kg IV). This medication can be started prior to the ACTH stimulation as it does not interfere with the test unlike prednisone, but if possible, it is best to wait until after the second sample has been drawn. Blood pressure, electrocardiography, serum electrolytes, and acid–base status should be monitored.

Maintenance

Once stabilized and a diagnosis of hypoadrenocorticism has been established, maintenance therapy should be initiated. Prednisone (0.1–0.22 mg/kg/day) is the standard of care for glucocorticoid replacement.[2] The dose should be doubled under any stressful circumstances. Mineralocorticoid supplementation can be achieved with desoxycorticosterone pivilate (DOCP, Percorten') or fludrocortisone (Florinef®). Both drugs can provide good control. Fludrocortisone offers both mineralocorticoid and glucocorticoid supplementation, whereas DOCP is only a mineralocorticoid. Fludrocortisone may be more attractive for owners because of the low cost of the medication. However, most dogs require an increased dose of fludrocortisone to control the mineralocorticoid deficiency, which may induce PU/PD (secondary to glucocorticoid activity). For this reason, the clinician may have to replace the fludrocortisone with the DOCP after several weeks. Most dogs receiving DOCP require prednisone (0.1 mg/kg/day) to control glucocorticoid deficiency.

Anesthetic and analgesic considerations

Prior to anesthesia, the Addisonian patient should be stabilized and all electrolyte disturbances should be resolved. It has been previously recommended that animals with adrenal insufficiency requiring general anesthesia should be treated with intravenous dexamethasone at 2–4 mg/kg at the time of premedication.[5] Treatment should be administered immediately prior to surgery and continues until the patients have recovered from surgery and are eating and drinking well on their own.

Nutritional considerations

Animals with hypoadrenocorticism should be fed a well-balanced diet. No special diets are recommended unless there is a concurrent disease that requires a specific diet.

Prognosis

Once recognized and treated, dogs with hypoadrenocorticism have an excellent prognosis. Clinical improvement is spectacular, usually within 12–24 h. The MST was 4.7 years in one study of 205 dogs with hypoadrenocorticism.[2] Due to the vague clinical signs, hypoadrenocorticism should be considered in any dog suffering from nonspecific clinical signs.

Client education

Client education is pivotal to ensure successful treatment and to avoid potential life-threatening effects secondary to the therapy itself. Rapid recognition of clinical signs associated with hypoadrenocorticism can possibly prevent acute decompensation and the need for emergency treatment. Addison's disease requires lifelong therapy with regular monitoring of serum electrolytes and adrenal functioning. Routine contact with the client provides a noninvasive method for monitoring the patient's response to treatment.

Hyperadrenocorticism: Cushing's disease

HAC, also known as Cushing's disease or Cushing's syndrome, is the result of hypersecretion of cortisol by a functional adrenal tumor (FAT) (15–20% of cases) or secondary to increases in ACTH from a pituitary tumor (80–85%).[6] Iatrogenic HAC can occur secondary to the administration of glucocorticoid medications. In normal dogs, the pituitary gland secretes ACTH, which stimulates the adrenal glands to release cortisol. The presence of cortisol exerts a negative feedback on the pituitary gland (Figure 2.4.1).

In dogs with pituitary-dependent hyperadrenocorticism (PDH), this feedback loop is disrupted by the tumor and ACTH is released despite high plasma cortisol concentrations.

In dogs with FAT, excessive amounts of glucocorticoids are released, exerting a negative feedback on the pituitary gland, resulting in low concentrations of ACTH and atrophy of the contralateral (normal) adrenal gland (Figure 2.4.2).

Spontaneous HAC occurs more frequently in middle-aged to older dogs (mean age at diagnosis is 11 years) and is less commonly recognized in dogs less then 6 years of age.[6] All breeds can be affected with HAC, but dachshunds, various terrier breeds, poodles, and boxers appear to be overrepresented.[6] While no sex predilection is evident in dogs with PDH, 60–65% of dogs with HAC secondary to an adrenal tumor are female.[6] HAC is one of the most commonly diagnosed endocrine disorders in dogs; it is very rare in cats with only 70 cases reported in the veterinary literature.[7]

Clinical signs

The clinical signs and laboratory changes are the result of glucocorticoid excess. Dogs with HAC are presented to the veterinarian for PU, PD (>90%), and polyphagia.[8] A complete history can help to discriminate a "healthy appetite" from polyphagia. Other commonly reported clinical signs include weight gain, weakness, "pot-bellied" appearance, excessive panting, and truncal, bilaterally symmetrical hair loss.[6] Less common clinical signs include calcinosis cutis and facial paralysis[6] (Figure 2.4.3).

The same clinical signs are recognized in cats with HAC, as well as excessively fragile skin.[6]

Diagnostic testing

Excessive secretion of glucocorticoids typically results in a "stress leukogram" characterized by lymphopenia, eosinopenia, neu-

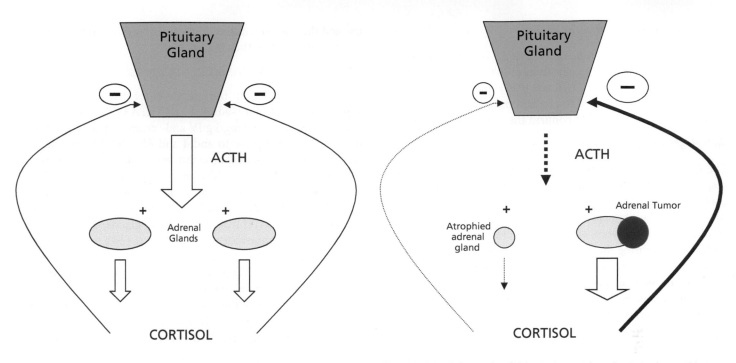

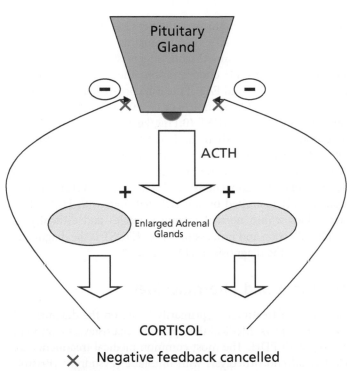

Negative feedback cancelled

Pituitary adenoma

Figure 2.4.1 A schematic of the pituitary–adrenal axis in normal dogs and a schematic of dogs with pituitary-dependent hyperadrenocorticism.

Figure 2.4.2 Schematic of the pituitary–adrenal axis in dogs with adrenal tumor.

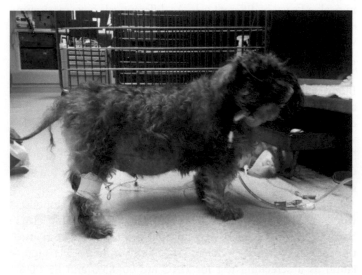

Figure 2.4.3 Dog exhibiting the typical clinical signs of "pot-bellied" appearance and truncal, bilaterally symmetrical hair loss associated with HAC.

trophilia, and monocytosis.[8] These changes are nonspecific and can occur in any sick dog.[7] An increase in alkaline phosphatase (ALP) activity is noted in 85–90% of dogs with HAC.[6] It is not uncommon for dogs with HAC to have a mild fasting hyperglycemia, but overt DM occurs in only 5–10% of dogs with HAC,[6] whereas 80% of cats affected by Cushing's disease have concurrent DM.[9]

The urinalysis reveals a specific gravity of less then 1.020 in the majority of the patients, glucosuria (5–10%), and proteinuria (46%).[6] Due to the immunosuppressive effects of high cortisol concentrations, 40–50% of dogs with HAC have a urinary tract infection. However, only a few develop clinical signs related to the lower urinary tract disease.[6]

Endocrine testing

In conjunction with clinical suspicion, endocrine testing plays an important role in the diagnosis of HAC.

Urine cortisol:creatinine ratio

The urine cortisol:creatinine ratio (UCCR) is a rapid, noninvasive screening test with high sensitivity (100%) but low specificity (22%).[10] Thus, a normal UC:CR test (<10) rules out HAC, but a high UCCR cannot be used to confirm the diagnosis of HAC.[10] Further tests are required to confirm the diagnosis of HAC.

ACTH stimulation test

The ACTH stimulation test is used to evaluate the adrenal gland's response to exogenous administration of ACTH and is most useful in differentiating spontaneous HAC from iatrogenic HAC. The test can be performed using an aqueous porcine gel or a synthetic ACTH. Every effort should be made to minimize patient stress during the testing period. Also, these patients may bruise easily, so care must be taken with venipuncture. Icterus and lipemia may adversely affect the results, so fasting blood draws are recommended. Samples should be centrifuged and refrigerated within 1 h of draw.

ACTH gel protocol

Blood samples for serum cortisol are obtained prior to, as well as 1 and/or 2 h after, intramuscular (IM) injection (2.2 U/kg) of ACTH gel.[6] A 1- and/or 2-h sample is recommended due to the variability in peak efficacy of different gels. As different gels have maximum effects at 60 min and others at 120 min, collection of both samples will ensure a most accurate representation of the adrenal axis.

Synthetic ACTH protocol

Blood samples are collected prior to and 1 h after intravenous administration of synthetic ACTH (Cortrosyn). Previously, the dose of Cortrosyn was one vial (250 mcg) per patient.[6] Recently, with supply and cost issues, the dose has been amended to 5 mcg/kg with a maximum dose of 250 mcg administered IV. Once reconstituted, the remaining solution may be frozen and stored for up to 6 months.

Dogs with spontaneous HAC have an exaggerated response, whereas those with hypoadrenocorticism or iatrogenic HAC have diminished response or normal-to-diminished response, respectively.[9] The sensitivity and specificity of the ACTH stimulation as a screening test for HAC are 60–85% and 85–90%, respectively[11] (see Table 2.4.1). In cats, the ACTH stimulation test and the low dose dexamethasone suppression test (LDDST) are less reliable than they are in dogs.[6]

Low-dose dexamethasone suppression test

The LDDST evaluates the negative feedback loop of the hypothalamic–pituitary–adrenal axis (HPAA). Dexamethasone is administered at 0.01 mg/kg IV and serum cortisol concentrations are collected prior to and 4 and 8 h after administration. As with the ACTH stimulation test, every effort should be made to minimize patient stress. This includes postponing other diagnostic testing, such as ultrasound, during the testing period. In normal dogs, the administration of dexamethasone suppresses the secretion of ACTH from the pituitary glands, decreasing the cortisol concentration to less than 1.4 μg/dL (38.6 nmol/L) at 8 h. The administration of dexamethasone has a minimal effect on dogs with PDH or FATs and the blood cortisol concentrations remain elevated (equal to or greater than 1.4 μg/dL [38.6 nmol/L]) at 8 h. The sensitivity of the LDDST is 90–95% in dogs with PDH and approximately 100% in those with FATs. However, as other diseases can affect the HPAA, the specificity is low (40–50%).[11]

Differentiating PDH and FAT

Once HAC has been confirmed, the next step is to differentiate between PDH and FATs. Discriminating tests include the LDDST, High dose dexamethasone suppression tests (HDDSTs) and endogenous ACTH concentration. The LDDST can aid in differentiating PDH and FAT if the 4-h cortisol concentration is less than 1.4 μg/dL (38.6 nmol/L) or is <50% of the basal cortisol concentration.[6] The HDDST (0.1 mg/kg IV) may identify 15% more dogs with PDH than the LDDST.[6] Additional testing to differentiate between the two diseases can include an abdominal ultrasound to screen for the presence of an adrenal tumor and measurement of endogenous ACTH levels. However, endogenous ACTH is limited by the fact that dogs with HAC often have values within normal reference ranges and difficulty in sample collection and processing.[6] The HDDST is the diagnostic test used for the diagnosis of HAC in cats.[6]

Treatment and pharmacology

The choice of treatment is primarily based on the diagnosis of PDH versus FATs. Medical therapy is the mainstay of treatment for dogs with PDH. The most common medical treatments are selective adrenocorticolysis with mitotane (Lysodren® [Bristol-Myers Squibb], Op'-DDD) or by selectively inhibiting the synthesis of adrenal cortex hormones with trilostane (Vetoryl®). Mitotane treatment is usually given at high doses (30–50 mg/kg/day) during the induction phase (usually 4–5 days) until the dog has a decrease in appetite or water intake. The owner is contacted daily to ensure compliance. If a dog with HAC is being treated with mitotane, an ACTH stimulation test is performed at the time the owner detects the change in water intake or appetite. The goal of the induction phase is to achieve a basal cortisol of 1–4 μg/dL (or 25–125 mmol/L) and a post-ACTH stimulation cortisol of <4 μg/dL or <125 nmol/L.[6] Once this is achieved, mitotane is continued at a dosage of 50 mg/kg/week.[6] Adverse

Table 2.4.1 Sensitivity and specificity of endocrine screening tests in dogs for the diagnosis of hyperadrenocorticism

Test	Sensitivity (%)	Specificity (%)
Basal cortisol	100	78.2
UC:CR	100	20
ACTH stimulation	60–85	85–90
LDDST	90–95	40–50

Source: Modified from Nelson RW, Feldman EC. Chapter 6: canine hyperadrenocorticism. In: *Endocrinology and Reproduction.* Philadelphia, PA: Elsevier Science 2004.

side effects of mitotane can include lethargy, ataxia, weakness, vomiting, diarrhea, and complete adrenocorticalysis and iatrogenic hypoadrenocorticism. To prevent a relapse of HAC and deleterious side effects of the treatment, ACTH stimulation tests should be repeated after 3, 6, and every 6 months thereafter.[6] Dogs treated with trilostane should be monitored with an ACTH stimulation at 10 days and 1, 3, and every 3 months thereafter.[6] The ACTH stimulation must be performed 4- to 6-h after trilostane administration. No significant difference in survival time has been documented with either protocol, but the high proportion of side effects and relapses associated with the use of mitotane has led to the increased use of trilostane among veterinarians.[12] Other less commonly utilized therapies for PDH include ketoconazole, selegiline hydrochloride (l-deprenyl), hypophysectomy, and RT.[13] Periodic monitoring throughout the life of the HAC patient is indicated. The typical monitoring program is for an ACTH stimulation test assay, initially every 3 months and then increasing to every 6 months. One cost-saving measure is to only submit the postsample for analysis as the presample level is typically not needed for monitoring purposes.

A unilateral adrenalectomy is the treatment of choice for FATs. However, a small percentage of patients will have inoperable tumors. In these instances, adrenocorticolysis and necrosis of the ZF and ZR with mitotane are recommended. Trilostane has been reported to improve quality of life but has little effect on tumor size.[6,13] The treatment of HAC in cats is more difficult compared with dogs.[6] Unlike dogs, the medical treatment is often not successful in cats, and adrenalectomy is often the treatment of choice.[6]

Anesthetic and analgesic consideration

If possible, it is recommended to stabilize a patient with HAC prior to anesthesia. Dogs with HAC may have a steroid hepatopathy and, as such, an opioid premedication, induction with propofol and inhalant anesthesia for maintenance, is often the protocol of choice.[5]

Nutritional considerations

Up to 50% of dogs with HAC can have mild to moderate serum cholesterol and triglyceride concentrations; therefore, mild fat restriction is recommended.[14] Diet recommendations are often based on concurrent comorbidities, including DM, that have specific dietary requirements.

Prognosis

The MST for animals treated with trilostane was 662 days (range 8–1971), and for mitotane, it was 708 days (range 33–1399).[12] In the study of 148 dogs with HAC, multivariable analysis revealed that only age at the time of diagnosis was negatively associated with overall survival.[12]

Client education

Client education is important to ensure the goals of treatment, the risks of therapy, and the frequency of monitoring are understood. The goals of treatment are to improve the animal's quality of life while minimizing the side effects of the disease. Treatment of PDH should only be pursued if the patient's quality of life is detrimentally affected by the disease. Testing and treatment of HAC requires a significant commitment in time and expense on the part of the owner, lifelong medication, and periodic blood testing.

A client questionnaire that addresses the clinical signs of HAC can be helpful in a monitoring program. The questionnaire should inquire about appetite, water consumption, urination habits, current dose and frequency of medications, when the last dose was administered, supply of medication (are refills needed), and any other changes to behavior or health.

The educated veterinary technician plays a very important role in the successful management of the HAC patient.

Pheochromocytoma

A pheochromocytoma is a neuroendocrine tumor of the sympathetic nervous system capable of secreting catecholamines. The neoplasm usually arises from chromaffin cells of the adrenal medulla (most common) but can also arise from extramedullary chromaffin cells in sympathetic ganglia in other parts of the body (rare). Clinical signs associated with this tumor either result from the sporadic and unpredictable secretion of catecholamines (e.g., epinephrine, norepinephrine, and dopamine) or relate to the space occupying nature and locally invasive and metastatic behavior of the tumor. A pheochromocytoma is an example of an APUDoma type of tumor because it is capable of amine precursor uptake and decarboxylation.

Usually, the tumor is solitary, slow growing, and highly vascular. The size of the tumor can range from 0.5 to >10.0 cm in diameter. In rare cases, bilateral adrenal pheochromocytomas or an adrenal pheochromocytoma with a contralateral adrenocortical tumor has been reported. These tumors are always considered malignant; in one study, 40% of dogs had evidence of local extension/invasion by the tumor. In another study, 30% of the dogs had evidence of distant metastasis at the time of necropsy. Common sites of metastasis include the liver, lung, regional lymph nodes, spleen, heart, kidney, bone, pancreas, CNS, and spinal cord.

Catecholamine secretion by a pheochromocytoma may be stimulated by blood flow, direct pressure, or various chemicals and drugs; secretion is not neurally mediated. Catecholamines exert their physiological effects via interaction with α- and β-adrenergic receptors. Elevated plasma catecholamine concentrations stimulate predominately α_1-adrenergic receptors, resulting in arteriolar vasoconstriction and hypertension, mydriasis, increased tone on all smooth muscle sphincters, stimulation of hepatic gluconeogenesis, and glycogenolysis.

Pheochromocytomas are identified most commonly in older dogs (mean age 11 years of age, range 1–18 years of age). Rare cases in cats have also been reported (mean age 14.5 years). No sex or breed predilection exists.

Clinical symptoms

The clinical signs are often vague and intermittent. A hypertensive crisis, manifesting as intermittent collapse and generalized weakness, is the most common presentation. Other clinical signs may include intermittent excessive panting, agitation, a "pounding" heart, syncope, PU, PD, lethargy, vomiting, inappetence, and anxiety. Less common clinical manifestations include cutaneous flushing, sudden blindness from systemic hypertension, signs associated with spontaneous hemorrhage (weakness, epistaxis, neurological signs), and, rarely, sudden death from a massive sustained release of catecholamines by the tumor. In cats, PU, PD, lethargy, and anorexia are the most common clinical signs seen.

A positive correlation may exist between the size of the tumor and the presence and severity of clinical signs with small tumors (<1.5 cm in diameter) resulting in minimal findings, while larger tumors (>2.0 cm in diameter) tend to be associated with severe clinical signs and potentially a worse prognosis. In cats, PU, PD, lethargy, and anorexia are the most common clinical signs seen.

Findings on physical examination are variable. The tumor size, its secretory activity, and existence of other concurrent problems will impact the physical findings. Typically, the physical exam is unremarkable, but findings attributable to excessive catecholamine release can involve the respiratory (increased bronchovesicular or alveolar sounds, crackles), cardiovascular (tachycardia, cardiac arrhythmias, weak femoral pulses, pale mucus membranes), and musculoskeletal systems (weakness, muscle atrophy). Mydriasis, retinal hemorrhage, retinal detachment, blindness, and epistaxis may develop secondary to systemic hypertension. Neurological signs that may be attributed to pheochromocytomas include systemic hypertension and CNS hemorrhage or metastasis, which may lead to seizures, head tilt, nystagmus, and strabismus. A palpable abdominal mass is rarely appreciated but ascites, peripheral edema of the hind limbs, and abdominal pain may be appreciated if the tumor has invaded or is obstructing the caudal vena cava.

Diagnostics

Diagnosis of a pheochromocytoma requires a high index of suspicion as signs are usually episodic and vague. Pheochromocytoma are often not suspected until an adrenal mass is found using ultrasound or at necropsy.

Results of routine blood work are rarely helpful; anemia, erythrocytosis, thrombocytopenia, elevated liver enzymes, hypercholesterolemia, azotemia, isosthenuria, and proteinuria may be seen.

Arterial blood pressure measurement is indicated if a pheochromocytoma is suspected: Multiple measurements should be taken and averaged. The prevalence of hypertension (sustained systolic pressure >160 mmHg, sustained diastolic pressure >100 bpm) in dogs with a pheochromocytoma varies from 25% to 86% in different retrospective studies. Failure to document hypertension in a dog with appropriate clinical signs does not rule out a pheochromocytoma.

Imaging

Survey radiographs may show evidence of a perirenal mass, but radiographs are far less sensitive than ultrasound or CT for iden-

tification of an adrenal mass. About 10% of pheochromocytomas show evidence of mineralization.

Specialized radiographic studies including a pneumoperitoneogram (room air insufflated into the abdominal cavity), excretory urography, venography, and arteriography can be used to help visualize the tumor and to assess vascular and renal displacement or invasion by the tumor. These modalities are somewhat outdated in light of the availability and superiority of CT.

Thoracic radiographs are important as part of the clinical staging; approximately 10% of dogs have evidence of pulmonary metastasis at the time of initial diagnosis. Evidence of pulmonary congestion or edema secondary to systemic hypertension may also be seen.

Abdominal ultrasound performed by a skilled operator accustomed to locating and assessing adrenal glands plays a critical role in the diagnosis and is the most reliable screening test readily available in private practice. Ultrasound is also helpful for detecting intra-abdominal metastasis and, to a limited degree, for assessing local invasion into blood vessels or the kidney by the tumor. The most common finding is adrenomegaly with a normal-sized contralateral adrenal gland.

Advanced imaging with CT or MRI of the abdomen is also excellent for tumor detection and is more sensitive than ultrasound for the detection of metastases, local invasion of the kidney, epaxial muscles, and adjacent vessels. Advanced imaging should be strongly recommended prior to surgery for the purposes of surgical planning.

Endocrine testing

Rule-out of an adrenocortical tumor using an ACTH stimulation test or preferably an LDDST should be performed as an adrenocortical tumor can cause clinical signs that are similar to a pheochromocytoma.

Hormone assays

Measurement of increased serum and urine catecholamines and urinary metabolites of catecholamines is often confirmatory in humans with a suspected pheochromocytoma; however, because of limited availability, lack of established reference ranges, expense, the inconvenience of 24-h urine collection, and the requirement to freeze the urine quickly after collection, this is infrequently used to help confirm the diagnosis in cats and dogs.

Differential diagnoses

The differential diagnoses for an adrenal mass include a nonfunctional adrenal mass (incidentaloma) or an adrenocortical tumor that is functional (cortisol-secreting) or nonfunctional. The differential diagnoses for intermittent systemic hypertension include renal disease, essential or primary hypertension, HAC, primary hyperaldosteronism, hyper- or hypothyroidism, DM, obesity, liver disease, and tumors that result in inappropriate ADH secretion.

Treatment

A period of medical therapy to control the effects of excessive adrenergic stimulation followed by surgical resection, when possible, is the treatment of choice. The chance of cure is enhanced if the dog does not have significant concurrent disease, metastasis of the tumor, or evidence of local tissue invasion. If a tumor thrombus is identified, evaluation by a skilled surgeon is indicated as surgical resection (adrenalectomy plus venotomy) may still be possible.

Outpatient preoperative medical therapy prior to adrenalectomy is recommended in order to control blood pressure, expand the extracellular fluid (ECF) volume, and hopefully limit or reduce hypertensive episodes intraoperatively. For 1–3 weeks prior to adrenalectomy, an α-antagonist medication is administered. The drug of choice is phenoxybenzamine, a nonselective, long-acting, noncompetitive α$_1$-antagonist. The initial dose for phenoxybenzamine is 0.5 mg/kg q 12 h, and this should be gradually increased every 4–5 days until either a maximum dose of 2.0–2.5 mg/kg q 12 h has been achieved or there are clinical signs of either hypotension (e.g., lethargy, weakness, or syncope) or adverse effects of the drug (e.g., vomiting). This medication is continued until the day of surgery. Prazosin, a selective, competitive α$_1$-antagonist, can be used as an alternative.

β-Adrenergic blocking drugs (e.g., propranolol) may be used to control arrhythmias but only after α$_1$-adrenergic blockade has been initiated. This is a challenging surgery and all cases that are candidates for adrenalectomy should be referred to a facility with 24-h intensive care and with a board certified anesthesiologist and surgeon on staff. Postoperative complications are common and include hypertension, cardiac arrhythmias, respiratory distress, and hemorrhage. Most patients become normotensive within 24–48 h of surgery. If the blood pressure fails to return to normal or intermittent hypertension continues after adrenalectomy, undetected metastasis should be suspected.

Other treatment options are limited; however, RT can be attempted on inoperable tumors.

For nonresectable tumors or for patients with widespread metastasis at the time of initial diagnosis, palliative management with phenoxybenzamine is indicated. Alpha-methyltyrosine, a drug that inhibits the rate-limiting enzyme involved in catecholamine synthesis by decreasing the production and secretion of catecholamines from the tumor, has been used as an adjunct treatment to an α$_1$-antagonist.

Anesthetic and analgesic considerations

Anesthetic induction and intraoperative tumor manipulation can be associated with life-threatening intraoperative complications. Anesthetic drug selection to help limit the potentiation of catecholamine-induced hypertension and arrhythmias during induction and intraoperatively is very important. Also, excellent communication between the surgeon and anesthesiologist combined with continuous monitoring of the patient's direct arterial blood pressure and ECG during the entire anesthetic period and for the first 24 h postoperatively are important. This allows for rapid recognition of hypertensive crises and cardiac arrhythmias and immediate intervention. Phentolamine (a short-acting, competitive α-adrenergic antagonist) may be administered as a bolus or by a CRI to treat intraoperative hypertension. If this is insufficient to control intraoperative hypertension or tachyarrhythmias, esmolol, a short-acting α1-adrenergic antagonist, can be used. Intraoperative hypotension after tumor removal is managed by decreasing the dose of or discontinuing phentolamine, by the administration of a short-acting α-adrenergic agonist such as phenylephrine, and by the administration of colloid and crystalloid fluids to expand the ECF volume.

Analgesia postoperatively should be provided. Repeated doses of a short-acting opioid analgesic would be appropriate.

Prognosis

Prognosis is dependent on a number of factors including the size of the mass, the existence of metastasis or local invasion at the time of diagnosis, the ability to control perioperative complications, and the presence and nature of concurrent disease.

Surgically resectable tumors carry a guarded to good prognosis. If patients survive beyond the immediate postoperative period, extended survival times of 18 months to 2 years are possible.

SECTION 5 PANCREAS

Feline diabetes mellitus

DM is the second most common endocrinopathy in cats and affects approximately 1 in 50 to 1 in 400, depending on the population studied.[1] DM is a disease that results in persistent hyperglycemia. Traditionally, the classification of DM in cats has been extrapolated from the model used in human medicine. The Committee on the Diagnosis and Classification of Diabetes Mellitus of the American Diabetes Association has abandoned the long-used terms *insulin-dependent diabetes mellitus* (IDDM) and *non-insulin-dependent diabetes mellitus* (NIDDM) because they were based on treatment rather than on etiology and were therefore regarded as more confusing than helpful. The vast majority of human cases falls into two broad categories now called *type 1* and *type 2 DM*. Unlike diabetic dogs, type 1 DM seems to be rare in cats.[2–4]

Antibodies against beta cells and insulin have not been demonstrated in cats, and lymphocytic infiltration, as a marker of immune-mediated destruction, has only been described in a small number of diabetic cats.[5,6] It is assumed that approximately 80% of diabetic cats suffer from a type 2-like DM,[3] although there is little data to support this. It is a clinical estimate only because differentiation of the two types of DM is clinically very challenging in cats. Nevertheless, most endocrinologists would agree that a type 2-like DM is the most frequent form in cats. Similar to human type 2 DM, feline type 2 DM is a heterogeneous disease attributable to a combination of impaired insulin action in liver, muscle, and adipose tissue (insulin resistance) and β-cell failure. Environmental as well as genetic factors are thought to play a role in the development of both defects. Genetic factors have not been characterized in the cat. The only evidence for their existence comes from studies in Australia and in the United Kingdom, in which the frequency of DM was shown to be about four times higher in Burmese cats than in domestic cats.[7,8] Management of diabetic cats depends on the stage of β-cell failure. In most cats, diabetes is usually not diagnosed until relatively late in the disease process when extensive β-cell function has been lost. Diagnosis is typically made once blood concentration is above the renal threshold (e.g., 180–216 mg/dL [10–12 mmol/L]) and signs of polyuria, polydypsia, and weight loss are apparent.[1]

DM etiology in cats

The cause of beta-cell degeneration is not known. Other diabetic cats have a reduction in the number of pancreatic islets and/or insulin-containing beta cells on immunohistochemical evaluation, suggesting additional mechanisms may be involved in the physiopathology of DM in cats. Although lymphoplasmocytic infiltration of islets, in conjunction with islet amyloidosis and vacuolation, has been described in diabetic cats, this histological finding is very uncommon. Beta cell and insulin autoantibodies have not been identified in newly diagnosed diabetic cats, and the role of genetics remains undetermined. Non-insulin-dependent (NIDDM) type 2 diabetes may be identified in as many as 50–70% of newly diagnosed diabetic cats. The majority of owned cats in developed countries that develop diabetes likely have type 2 diabetes, which is characterized by a relative lack of insulin secretion and insulin resistance. In type 2 diabetes, beta cells are damaged by chronically high blood glucose concentrations (BGCs) suppressing insulin secretions; this is called glucotoxicity. Other specific types of DM or secondary DM may occur in 10–20% of diabetic cats. Pancreatic lesions are frequently identified by ultrasonography or histological examination of islets.[9] However, the changes are often mild and are therefore probably not involved in the initiation of diabetes. Severe pancreatitis may be the triggering factor for diabetes and DKA. In general, it is difficult to know which of the two diseases (DM or pancreatitis) is the cause and which is the effect. Glucocorticoids and GH have strong diabetogenic actions because approximately 80% of cats with hypercortisolism and presumably 100% of cats with hypersomatotropism are diabetic. Gestational diabetes is very unlikely in cats.

Based on data in other species, BGC below the renal threshold but persistently above normal (e.g., 180–216 mg/dL [10–12 mmol/L]) are likely associated with adverse effects such as glucotoxic damage to beta cells and in cats should be considered as diabetes.[1] A small percentage of diabetic cats have other specific types of diabetes resulting from β-cell destruction associated with pancreatitis and neoplasia, or have marked insulin resistance from excess GH or corticosteroids. Cats may have IDDM or NIDDM at the time diabetes is diagnosed. Cats with NIDDM may progress to IDDM with time. Cats with apparent IDDM may revert to a non-insulin-requiring state after initiation of treatment, and cats may flip back and forth between IDDM and NIDDM as severity of insulin resistance and impairment of beta-cell function waxes and wanes.[2,3,10]

Signalment and physical examination of cats with DM

Although DM may be diagnosed in cats of any age, most of the cats are 9 years old at the time of diagnosis (mean 10). DM can occur in either gender; however, higher incidences have been reported in neutered male cats.[11] Burmese cats seem to be overrepresented.[12]

Major risk factors for the development of DM in cats are increasing age, male gender, being neutered, physical inactivity, glucocorticoid and progestin administration, and obesity.[2,3,12–14]

The majority of the cats are presented for PU, PD, polyphagia, and weight loss. Potential complications of unregulated DM in cats include hypertension (with or without secondary chronic renal failure), hepatic lipidosis, DKA, and the development of a plantigrade posture as a result of peripheral neuropathy. The predisposing factors are obesity, steroid or megestrol acetate treatment, Cushing's disease, and acromegaly.[2]

The nonketotic diabetic cat may not have any classic clinical physical examination findings, although many cats are obese.

Diagnosis of DM

Diagnosis is based on persistent hyperglycemia and glucosuria. Transient stress-induced hyperglycemia is common in cats and can cause the BGC to increase higher than 300 mg/dL. Glucosuria usually does not develop in cats with transient hyperglycemia but can be present if stress is prolonged (i.e., hours).[2]

If further diagnostics are needed to discriminate stress hyperglycemia from true hyperglycemia, a serum fructosamine concentration can be measured. Fructosamine is a glycated protein complex found in blood. It results from an irreversible, nonenzymatic, insulin-independent binding of glucose to serum proteins. The fructosamine level reflects the mean BGC over the circulating life span of the protein (2–3 weeks) so it is not affected by acute transient increases in BGC. Documenting an increase in serum fructosamine concentration in the upper range of normal confirms the persistent hyperglycemia.[15] The minimal laboratory evaluation in any diabetic cat should include a biochemistry profile, a serum T_4 concentration, a urinalysis, and urine culture to rule out chronic renal failure, hyperthyroidism, and urinary tract infection.[2,3,16]

Treatment of DM

The most important goal of therapy is to resolve the clinical signs while avoiding clinical hypoglycemia, which can be life threatening. The best way to resolve clinical signs is to achieve diabetic remission. Glycemic control can be maintained in some cats with dietary changes, oral hypoglycemiant drugs, control of concurrent diseases, discontinuation of insulin antagonist drugs, or a combination of these modalities,[2] while some cats will require insulin therapy in order to achieve glycemic control.

Dietary changes

The primary goal of dietary therapy is to minimize the impact of a meal on postprandial BGC. Current recommendations include diets with high protein and low carbohydrate content and diets containing high fiber and moderate carbohydrate content.[2] Reducing the carbohydrate content of the diet decreases the demand on beta cells to secrete insulin. Cats in diabetic remission likely have reduced β-cell mass, and, from the limited testing reported, approximately 50% have impaired glucose intolerance. It is vital that these cats be fed diets that spare β-cell function. Feeding a low carbohydrate diet once diabetic remission is achieved will likely prolong remission.[1] Diet modifications may need to be introduced gradually in order to enhance patient compliance.

Oral hypoglycemiant drugs

Acarbose reduces postprandial BGCs by decreasing intestinal glucose absorption (alpha-glucosidase inhibition). However, changing to an ultra-low carbohydrate diet has a greater glucose-lowering effect than administering acarbose. If a cat needs reduced-protein diet (high carbohydrate) for control of azotemia, it might be beneficial to add acarbose at 12–25 mg/cat twice daily at the time of eating.[1]

Sulfonylureas (glipizide, glyburide) are the most commonly used oral hypoglycemic drugs for the treatment of DM in cats. They stimulate insulin secretions by pancreatic cells. Clinical response to these medications in diabetic cats has been variable, ranging from excellent (i.e., BGC lower than 200 mg/dL ≈ 11 mmol/L) to partial response (i.e., clinical improvement but failure to resolve hyperglycemia) to no response.[2,3] These oral hypoglycemiants should not be offered as first-line treatment because of the poorer control of BGC. However, these drugs may be utilized in select cases of owner compliance or owner need.

Control of concurrent disease

Any inflammatory, infectious, neoplastic, and endocrine disorder can cause insulin resistance, as well as obesity and drugs such as glucocorticoids and progestagens (steroid hormones). There are currently no published prospective or retrospective studies specifically evaluating the causes of insulin resistance in cats. However, insulin resistance is most commonly caused by severe obesity, chronic renal failure, chronic pancreatitis, stomatitis/oral infections, HAC, and hypersomatotropism (acromegaly). Hyperthyroidism is often mentioned as a cause of insulin resistance; however, in our cats, the coexistence of the two diseases is extremely rare. In some cases, the cause of insulin resistance is easy to identify (e.g., obesity, infections, chronic renal failure), and in others, a thorough workup is required.

The diseases that have the potential to cause the most severe insulin resistance are HAC and hypersomatotropism (acromegaly), although insulin resistance may also be mild or variable.[11] Approximately 80% of cats with HAC and nearly all cats with hypersomatotropism will develop DM.[11] Hypersomatotropism in cats is caused by a GH-producing tumor (usually an adenoma)

Table 2.5.1 Causes of insulin resistance in cats

Causes
Drug administration (progestagens/corticosteroids)
Infection (urinary tract/oral cavity/sepsis/bronchopneumonia)
Hyperthyroidism
Acromegaly
Pancreatic disease (pancreatitis, tumor)
Renal disease
Hepatic disease
Cardiac insufficiency
Hyperlipidemia
Neoplasia
Severe obesity
Exocrine pancreatic insufficiency
Hyperadrenocorticism
Pheochromocytoma

Source: Modified from Scott-Montcrieff JC. Insulin resistance in cats. *Vet Clinics of North America, Small Animal Practice* 2010;40(2):241–257.

in the pars distalis of the pituitary gland. The catabolic effects of GH are mainly due to insulin antagonism and are the reason for the DM (Table 2.5.1).

Discontinuation of insulin antagonist drugs

Exogenous glucocorticoids and progestagens such as megestrol acetate cause insulin resistance.[3] Administration of these drugs has been identified as an important precipitating factor for DM in cats.[9] The use of these drugs in a diagnosed diabetic cat should be avoided. If the patient absolutely requires these drugs for concurrent diseases, it is recommended to taper the dose of the drug to the minimum that will control the disease process[3] or to use an alternative drug that is not an insulin antagonist (e.g., such as inhalants steroids for asthma: Fluticasone®).

Objectives of insulin therapy

1. Reversion of a transient diabetic cat to a subclinical diabetic if possible

2. Elimination of owner-observed signs (e.g., polyphagia, polydypsia, and weight loss) leading to normal appetite, normal water consumption, and a stable (if normal weight) or increased body weight (if body condition score was <5/9).

3. Improved quality of life and normalization of body weight and activity

4. Prevention of diabetic complications (hypoglycemia, weakness, chronic infections, neuropathy)

Insulin therapy

Insulin therapy is the mainstay of therapy in diabetic cats. Veterinary insulin preparations available for maintenance treatment of

DM in cats include porcine lente insulin (Caninsulin®/Vetsulin® at 40 U/mL by Intervet Inc.), and protamine zinc insulin (PZI) (Insuvet® at 100 U/mL by Schering-Plough and PZI Vet® at 40 U/mL by IDEXX Pharmaceuticals). Human insulin preparations include neutral protamine Hagedorn (NPH), glargine, and detemir. Human lente and ultralente preparations have been removed from the market in most countries.[9,17,18] The availability of insulin products is rapidly changing; every effort has been made to provide a current list at the time of publication.

Diabetic cats are totally unpredictable in their glycemic response to exogenous insulin. There is no single type of insulin that will effectively control glycemia in all diabetic cats, even with twice-daily administration.

Current recommendations regarding the initial insulin of choice for treating diabetic cats are based on personal experiences and vary between clinicians. Some clinicians prefer PZI or glargine insulin, whereas others use lente or NPH as the initial insulin. It is important to remember that the response to insulin is always unpredictable and that individual cats respond individually to any or all insulin preparation. For this reason, it is important to be conservative when selecting initial insulin doses, either at the start of therapy or when switching a cat from one type of insulin to another.

Although porcine lente and NPH insulin are consistently and rapidly absorbed following subcutaneous administration in cats, the duration of effect of porcine lente, and especially NPH, can be considerably shorter than 12 h. These intermediate duration insulins can result in inadequate control of glycemia despite twice-a-day administration. Although these insulins may be adequate in some cats, they usually produce too short a duration of action for optimal blood glucose control in cats. This commonly leads to poor glycemic control and/or induction of the Somogyi phenomenon. It must be remembered, however, that the response to porcine lente or NPH insulin is variable. There may be cats in which these intermediate-acting insulin preparations have a longer action, making one of them suitable for twice-a-day dosing.

In general, long-acting insulin preparations, such as PZI or insulin glargine, have worked the best in diabetic cats. Currently, the author's preference for the initial treatment of newly diagnosed DM in cats is glargine administration twice a day.

Insulin glargine (Lantus® by Sanofi Aventis Pharmaceuticals) is a long-acting, slow-onset, minimal curve insulin analogue in cats. It forms some precipitates at the site of injection from which small amounts of insulin glargine are slowly released. In general, the duration of effect of insulin glargine appears quite variable, with the glucose nadir occurring as soon as 4–6 h and as late as 18–22 h after administration. As with other insulin preparations, the glycemic response to glargine is always unpredictable, and each cat treated with this insulin must be carefully monitored and evaluated to determine the cat's response.

Glargine has been successfully used in cats with a starting dose of 0.25–0.5 U/kg BID. The initial starting dose should not exceed 3 U/cat BID. It is strongly recommended that glargine be administered BID to maximize glycemic control and diabetic remission. The dose should not be increased during the first week of treatment. Typically, once the cat has been on insulin glargine for 7–10 days, the glucose curve will flatten out. The flattening of the curve is the result of the long duration of action and the slower absorption rate of glargine. This may lead to an overlap of efficacy occurring with the BID injections. In some cats, the dose may have to be lowered at this point of therapy. It is important that the dose of insulin is not increased during this time without adequate monitoring. Increased insulin administration coupled with the overlap of efficacy may result in clinical hypoglycemia. It is recommended that close monitoring and adjustment of dose is continued throughout the first month of treatment because some cats will achieve diabetic remission within this time.

The response of diabetic cats to detemir insulin (Levemir®) appears to be very similar to glargine, but the pharmacokinetics have not yet been studied in cats and there is no published information on its use.

Most insulins are available as 100 U/mL (U-100) preparations (NPH, lente, insulin glargine). Low dose U-100 (0.3–0.5) syringes should be routinely utilized for cats. Note that insulin glargine cannot be diluted as dilution alters the pH and, hence, absorption characteristic. In general, using low dose syringes to improve dosing accuracy is preferable to diluting any insulin preparation. Label directions state insulin glargine does not require refrigeration but that it has a shelf life of 28 days maximum once opened. Glargine is commonly being used for 3–6 months with refrigeration in veterinary medicine. Note that Caninsulin and PZI are available only in concentrations of 40 U/mL, and it is strongly recommended that U40 insulin syringes are utilized in order to reduce the chance of dosage miscalculation.

Glargine is the longest-acting commercially available insulin for treatment of DM in humans and is currently a popular initial choice by veterinarians for diabetic cats.[17,18] In a trial of 24 cats, 8/8 newly diagnosed diabetic cats treated with glargine and ultralow carbohydrate diet achieved remission compared to 3/8 for PZI and 2/8 for porcine lente. However, lower remission rates occur in long-term diabetic cats changed to glargine therapy. Diabetic remission is unlikely in cats that have been diabetic for more than 2 years. For this reason, if a cat has been well controlled with a different insulin, it is not recommended to change to glargine (Tables 2.5.2 and 2.5.3).

During the first 24 h of therapy, perform spot blood glucose measurement to check for evidence of hypoglycemia (every 3–4 h for initial 18 h). Whenever insulin therapy is initiated or changed, the cat should be allowed to "equilibrate" at home for 3–6 days before response to insulin therapy is assessed.

At each recheck, remember that the goals of therapy are resolution of clinical signs and avoidance of hypoglycemia. Therefore, the owner's assessment of thirst and urine production, and accurate weight measurement are very important. A blood glucose curve (a series of timed measurement of blood glucose, such as every 2 h for 12 h) is recommended every 10–14 days until an appropriate insulin dose is achieved and thereafter as necessary for monitoring (usually every 2–4 months).

Cats are more prone than dogs to develop the Somogyi phenomenon (hypoglycemia-induced glucose counter-regulation), even at conservative doses of insulin. The Somogyi phenomenon

Table 2.5.2 Parameters for changing insulin dosage and frequency based on blood glucose measurements when using lente or NPH insulin in cats

Blood glucose variable	Recommendations
Initial therapy	
If blood glucose ≥360 mg/dL (>20 mmol/L)	Use of an initial dose of 0.5 U/kg of lean body weight BID
If blood glucose ≤360 mg/dL (<20 mmol/L)	Use of an initial dose of 0.25 U/kg of lean body weight BID
Nadir response	
If nadir blood glucose concentration is <54 mg/dL (<3 mmol/L)	Dose should be reduced by 50%
If nadir blood glucose is 54–90 mg/mL (3–5 mmol/L)	Dose should be reduced by 1 U if poor control of clinical signs of DM, otherwise no change in dose
=If nadir blood glucose concentration is 91–180 mg/dL (6–9 mmol/L)	Dose should remain the same
If nadir blood glucose concentration is >180 mg/dL (>10 mmol/L)	Dose should be increased by 1 U
If nadir blood glucose concentration occurs at 8 h or later	Once-daily administration may be used, although BID administration at a reduced dose is preferred
Baseline response	
If blood glucose returns to baseline within 8 h Or if nadir blood glucose concentration occurs within 3 h of insulin administration	Change to longer-acting insulin (e.g., glargine, detemir, or PZI)

Source: Modified from Rand J, Marshall R. Management of feline diabetes mellitus: part I. Which insulin do I choose and how do I adjust the dose? ACVIM 2009 Proceedings, Quebec, Canada, June 3–6.

occurs in response to impending hypoglycemia (<65 mg/dL). The cat's low blood glucose level stimulates the release of catecholamines, glucagon, glucocorticoids, and GH, which causes a rapid release of glucose in the blood. If only a spot check blood glucose level is performed at the time of hyperglycemia, the insulin dose might be further increased in response to the perceived hyperglycemia. This will exacerbate the hypoglycemia. For this reason, the use of glucose curves to assess the status, especially in cats, on high doses of insulin is recommended.

In general, BGC following glargine administration does not change as quickly as with shorter-acting insulin; therefore, monitoring every 4 h is usually adequate. The critical time points to monitor are the BGC just before each injection (preinsulin morning and evening).

Serum fructosamine concentration may be used every 3–4 months in lieu of serial glucose profiles as long as history, clinical signs, and random blood glucose measurements also suggest good glycemic control.

An alternative to hospital generated blood glucose curves is to have the client perform the blood glucose curve at home using the marginal ear vein prick technique in cats (the ear or lip prick technique in dogs) and a portable home blood glucose monitoring device that allows the client to touch the drop of blood on the ear with the end of the glucose test strip.[19,20] The advantages of the at-home method include minimizing patient transport, decreasing stress to the cat, and less cost to the client. Disadvantages include uncertain reliability of the glucose values and inability to monitor body weight.

Which glucometer?

The choice of glucometer is important because an accurate assessment of blood glucose levels is needed to determine if the goal of normoglycemia has been achieved. To avoid clinical hypoglycemia or unnecessarily high BGC, it is important to recognize and understand whether the meter is calibrated for human or cat blood. Meters calibrated for human diabetic patients that report glucose concentrations for whole blood (not plasma equivalent) read cat's blood glucose on average 1.5–2.0 mmol/L lower than actual BGCs. All the reputable companies such as Abbott, Bayer, and Roche make precise meters that have close correlation ($r \geq 0.90$) with feline BGC measured by a serum chemistry analyzer. This means that the results they provide are very repeatable. You should recommend a glucometer that is user-friendly, requires a microquantity of blood, and utilizes readily available test strips. AlphaTRAK® glucometer (Abbott) has met all of these criteria and is highly recommended.

Table 2.5.3 Parameters for changing insulin dosage and frequency based on blood glucose measurements when using glargine insulin in cats

Blood glucose variable		Recommendations
Initial therapy		
If blood glucose ≥360 mg/dL (>20 mmol/L)		Use of an initial dose of 0.5 U/kg of ideal body weight BID
If blood glucose ≤360 mg/dL (<20 mmol/L)		Use of an initial dose of 0.25 U/kg of ideal body weight BID
Note: Do not increase the dose in the first week unless minimum response to insulin occurs, but decrease if necessary. Monitor response to therapy for first 3 days. If no monitoring occurs during the first week, begin with 1 U/cat BID		
Preinsulin blood glucose level and nadir response		
Preinsulin level	Nadir response	Recommendations
If preinsulin blood glucose concentration is >216 mg/dL (>12 mmol/L) provided nadir is not in hypoglycemic range	Or if nadir blood glucose concentration is >180 mg/dL (>10 mmol/L)	Increase by 0.25–1.0 U
If preinsulin blood glucose concentration is 180–216 mg/dL (10–12 mmol/L)	Or if nadir blood glucose concentration is 90–160 mg/dL (5–9 mmol/L)	Same dose
If preinsulin blood glucose concentration is 198–252 mg/dL (11–14 mmol/L)	Or if nadir glucose is 54–72 mg/dL (3–4 mmol/L)	Use nadir glucose, water consumption, urine glucose, and next preinsulin glucose concentration to determine if insulin dose should be decreased or maintained
If preinsulin blood glucose concentration is <180 mg/dL (<10 mmol/L)	Or if nadir blood glucose is <54 mg/dL (<3 mmol/L)	Dose should be reduced by 0.5–1.0 U or if total dose is 0.5–1.0 U SID, stop insulin and check for diabetic remission
Note: If clinical signs of hypoglycemia are observed		Reduce by 50%

Source: Modified from Rand J, Marshall R. Management of feline diabetes mellitus: part I. Which insulin do I choose and how do I adjust the dose? ACVIM 2009 Proceedings Quebec Canada June 3-6 .

Continuous glucose monitoring system

A continuous glucose monitoring system (CGMS) has recently been introduced in veterinary medicine as a method for monitoring glucose concentrations in dogs and cats. The technology of the CGMS is designed to measure subcutaneous interstitial fluid (ISF) rather than BGCs.[21] The subcutaneous ISF is ideal for glucose concentration measurements because it is easily and safely accessed, has rapid equilibration with the blood, and has good correlation with BGC. The CGMS measures ISF glucose with a small, flexible sensor inserted through the skin into the subcutaneous space, secured to the skin, and attached to a recording device. The ISF glucose is recorded and stored every 5 min. After the CGMS is removed, the data are downloaded to a computer for analysis. The CGMS avoids several limitations of the traditional blood glucose curves including intermittent assessment of BGC, hospitalization, patient restraint, and repeated phlebotomy. For this reason, the CGMS is usually used in referral centers to monitor patients with DKA while avoiding multiple phlebotomies or placement of a central venous catheter. The wireless, real-time CGMS allows the monitor to be attached to the outside of the patient's cage where readings can easily be recorded, thereby minimizing patient stress.

Education of clients and the role of the veterinary technician

At the time of discharge of the newly diagnosed diabetic, the clients should go back home with a form that reminds them of:

- all of the steps of the subcutaneous injection technique for the insulin and the necessity of changing injection sites at each administration;

- the specific recommendations on how to store the insulin (e.g., write the date of expiration on the vial and do not shake the vial);

- the description of the clinical signs of hypoglycemia and what to do in case it happens; and

- the specific recommendations regarding the dose of insulin to administer ("do not give any if no appetite," "assume that you have given the insulin if you do not remember").

The education of the client is a key role in the success of the treatment, thereby improving the quality of life and the life expectancy of the patient, their pet.

Remission or not?

Determining if diabetic remission is present is very important as it is strongly recommended that insulin therapy not be withdrawn prematurely. Cats with almost normal β-cell function can tolerate 0.5–1.0 U of insulin SID or BID and rarely develop clinical hypoglycemia. If insulin therapy is stopped prematurely and hyperglycemia recurs, the reinstituted insulin therapy can take weeks or months to achieve the same level of glycemic control as was previously obtained. It is not recommended that insulin therapy be stopped within a minimum of 2 weeks of initiating treatment in order to facilitate β-cell recovery from glucotoxicity. Instead, the insulin dose should be decreased gradually based on dosing guidelines.

Once the preinsulin BGC is ≤10 mmol/L and the total dose of insulin is decreased to 0.5–1.0 U BID, the dosing frequency should be reduced to SID. If after 1-week preinsulin BGC is still ≤10 mmol/L and the nadir BGC is in the normal range (preferably determined at home) of 4–7 mmol/L, insulin therapy may be discontinued and the BGC should be monitored during the first day. If BGC rises above 10 mmol/L within 12–24 h, immediately reinstitute insulin at 1 U SID and wait for a minimum of 2 weeks before again trying to discontinue insulin. If BGC is ≤10 mmol/L, continue to withhold insulin, checking BGC every 3–7 days for several weeks. Owners should monitor for the clinical signs consistent with a relapse such as increased water consumption, increased appetite, and/or weight loss.

Does the type of insulin influence the remission rate?

Based on the studies available, the remission rate depends on multiple factors such as the quality of glucose monitoring (intensity, home-generated glucose curve), the diet, the control of the underlying disease(s), and risk factors (obesity, physical inactivity). The long-acting insulins are more likely to induce remission than the intermediate-acting insulins because they control the glucose level fluctuations more tightly and are more likely to resolve glucose toxicity. Because nearly all the studies reporting remissions with insulin types other than porcine insulin zinc suspension (Vetsulin) also included other diabetes management strategies (e.g., dietary control) in their design, simple comparison of the remission rates can be misleading.

In one study of newly diagnosed diabetic cats, eight of eight cats became insulin independent when treated with twice-a-day insulin glargine and an ultralow carbohydrate diet.[22]

This remission rate was higher than the remission rate for cats treated with protamine zinc and PZI (three of eight) and lente (two of eight) in the same study. The duration of illness before inclusion in the study was not mentioned and the allocation into treatment groups was not random. Also, treatment protocols were not identical between groups. Lower remission rates were reported in another study in which the goal of treatment was to achieve euglycemia.[23]

In this study, 84% of cats that were started on a treatment protocol (insulin glargine and intensive home monitoring of blood glucose) within 6 months of diagnosis achieved remission, while only 35% of cats that were started on the protocol after more than 6 months from diagnosis achieved remission. These remission rates are similar to the results of another study in which cats treated with various insulin formulations other than insulin glargine (mostly PZI) had 68% remission rate when fed a low carbohydrate diet.[24]

Diabetes had been diagnosed recently (within 45 days) in only 11 of 31 cats in this study, but there were no differences in remission rates between those cats and others that had been diabetic for more than 45 days.

In a small clinical study in cats, once-a-day insulin glargine was compared with twice-a-day lente in cats fed an ultralow carbohydrate diet.[18] In that study, both treatment groups experienced improvement in serum fructosamine concentrations and 16-h blood glucose curves were improved. Four of the thirteen cats experienced remission of diabetes (one in the insulin glargine-treated group).

Taken together, these studies suggest that a low carbohydrate diet in combination with glargine or any other insulin formulation is clinically useful in treating diabetes in cats. In newly diagnosed diabetic cats, treatment with glargine might be more likely to achieve remission.

The wide range of remission rates reported in the literature with insulin glargine treatment reinforces the influence of multiple factors in achieving remission.

If a patient has been treated for more than 6 months for DM, it is very unlikely that this patient will go into remission. For this reason, we do not recommend changing such patients to another type of insulin if well controlled.

Outcome and prognosis

The majority of the cats will go into remission within 3 months on insulin glargine therapy. If insulin therapy is discontinued, it is recommended to continue feeding the diabetic with a specific diet.[2]

The mean survival time in diabetic cats is 3 years from the time of diagnosis. However, this survival time is skewed because cats are usually 8–12 years old at the time of diagnosis. Concurrent diseases (e.g., ketoacidosis, pancreatitis, renal failure) increase the mortality rate during the first 6 months. Overall, the prognosis of diabetic cats depends on the cooperativeness of the cat, the compliance of the owners, and the regularity of the recheck by the veterinarian.

Canine diabetes mellitus

DM is a common endocrinopathy in dogs with a prevalence of 0.005–1.5%. Affected dogs are usually 7 years of age or older.[25] Females are at an increased risk for diabetes. Genetics play a role as some breeds have either an increased or decreased risk of developing diabetes. Australian terriers, standard and miniature schnauzers, Samoyeds, fox terriers, keeshonds, bichon frises, Finnish spitzes, cairn terriers, miniature and toy poodles, and Siberian huskies are breeds at increased risk of diabetes,[26] whereas German shepherds, golden retrievers, and American pit bull terriers are at low risk.[25]

Anatomy and physiology

The pancreas consists of two lobes that lie in the cranial abdominal cavity. The right pancreatic lobe is closely associated with the duodenum, whereas the left limb extends behind the stomach toward the spleen. The endocrine pancreas is composed of tissue called islets of Langerhans. The islets of Langerhans are composed of alpha, beta, F, and delta cells. Each cell secretes a different hormone—alpha cells secrete glucagon in response to low blood glucose levels, which stimulates the liver to convert stored glycogen into glucose. Beta cells secrete insulin in response to high blood glucose levels, which stimulates cells to take up glucose from the bloodstream and store it as glycogen in the liver and muscles. Thus, the alpha cells, by secreting glucagon, and the beta cells, by secreting insulin, are opposite hormones of the feedback system that regulates blood glucose levels. The delta cells secrete somatostatin (SST) (GH-inhibiting hormone) and F cells secrete pancreatic polypeptide (PP). When each different cell line is stimulated, it secretes its hormone directly into the bloodstream.

In normal animals, after a meal, insulin secretion is dramatically increased in response to increasing BGCs.

Insulin has several metabolic effects: carbohydrate metabolism, suppressing hepatic glucose production, promoting glucose uptake by the liver and then storage as glycogen, and stimulating glucose uptake into the peripheral tissue. Insulin also decreases the breakdown of fat and prevents the formation of ketones.

When insulin deficiency occurs, glucose production by the liver is not suppressed and there is a resultant decreased glucose uptake in the peripheral tissues. The result is hyperglycemia. As the BGC continues to increase, it eventually exceeds the renal threshold (approximately 180–200 mg/dL in dogs and >300 mg/dL in cats).[27] Glucosuria results in an osmotic diuresis and PU with compensatory PD. Protein catabolism and muscle wasting also occur. Glucosuria results in loss of calories, and weight loss and polyphagia ensue.[28]

Classification of canine diabetes mellitus

The most common form of diabetes in dogs is type 1, which is characterized by pancreatic beta-cell deficiency or destruction resulting in an absolute insulin deficiency. Thus, dogs with type 1 diabetes lose the ability to secrete insulin. The cause of the beta-cell deficiency is unknown, but it is thought that more than one mechanism is responsible. In approximately 50% of diabetic dogs, immune-mediated destruction of pancreatic beta cells is speculated to occur based on the presence of inflammatory cell infiltration of pancreatic islets[30] and circulating antibodies against beta cells in newly diagnosed diabetic dogs.[31] This form of type 1 canine diabetes most closely resembles latent autoimmune diabetes of adults (LADA). LADA occurs in middle-aged to older humans typified by gradual beta-cell destruction over months to years resulting in absolute insulin deficiency and is not associated with obesity.[31] Similarly, canine diabetes typically affects dogs over 7 years of age with a slow onset of weeks to months and evidence of immune-mediated destruction of beta cells.

Damage from pancreatitis is another mechanism of beta-cell destruction that occurs in approximately 30% of diabetic dogs. A congenital form of type 1 canine diabetes with pancreatic islet hypoplasia or aplasia has also been reported. Breeds affected with familial diabetes are keeshonds, golden retrievers, Samoyeds, and miniature poodles.[25]

Some dogs develop a form of diabetes with a relative insulin deficiency. In other words, the dogs are still producing insulin, but it is an inadequate amount because its function is being antagonized by other hormones or medications. Endocrinopathies such as HAC and acromegaly can cause insulin resistance. Insulin resistance can also occur in intact female dogs during diestrus or during pregnancy. The latter is known as gestational diabetes. Dogs receiving glucocorticoids or synthetic progestagens can also become insulin resistant. The diabetes may or may not be reversible once the underlying disease is treated or the antagonistic drug is discontinued. However, with chronic hyperglycemia that persists for 2 weeks or more, the resulting glucose toxicity can cause loss of beta cells and permanent DM.

Clinical signs

PU, PD, polyphagia, and weight loss are the classic signs of DM. A dog that has been housebroken for years may suddenly begin having urinary accidents in the house. Less frequently, diabetic dogs present for lethargy, weakness, decreased vision, or even blindness. Dogs in DKA can be very ill systemically and present with vomiting, dehydration, and anorexia.[31]

Diagnostic testing

Persistent hyperglycemia with glucosuria in a dog with PU/PD, polyphagia, and/or weight loss is consistent with DM. The diagnosis can be easily achieved with a glucometer and a urine dipstick. However, further biochemical testing to assess the dog's overall health and to evaluate for concurrent diseases is recommended in all newly diagnosed diabetics. A minimum database is a complete blood cell count (CBC), chemistry panel, urinalysis, and urine culture. In a diabetic patient with subnormal appetite, thoracic radiographs and abdominal ultrasound are also strongly advised.

Complete blood cell counts are often normal but may show a stress leukogram or an inflammatory neutrophilia. A left shifted neutrophilia with or without toxic change is often an indication of concurrent inflammatory or infectious disease. Chemistry panels reveal hyperglycemia with or without additional abnormalities. Elevated liver enzymes, ALP, and ALT are common, along with hypercholesterolemia and hypertriglyceridemia.[31] Urinalyses reveals glucosuria with or without proteinuria, bacteriuria, pyuria, and/or ketonuria. Diabetic dogs have an increased incidence of urinary tract infections due their depressed immune system and ready supply of glucose in the urine. Inactive urinary sediment does not rule out the presence of a concurrent urinary tract infection. Thus, all urine samples should be cultured.

HAC, pancreatitis, and hypothyroidism are a few of the concurrent diseases that may be present in a diabetic dog. If concurrent pancreatitis is suspected, it can be investigated with canine pancreas-specific lipase. However, adrenal and thyroid testing should be delayed until the diabetes has been initially treated. The uncontrolled diabetes may influence the test results and may interfere with their interpretations.

Imaging

Imaging can be useful to uncover concurrent diseases in the diabetic dog. Therefore, thoracic radiographs and abdominal ultrasound may be indicated to complete the initial workup. However, imaging is not necessary for the diagnosis of uncomplicated DM. The most common finding on abdominal radiographs is hepatomegaly. Abdominal ultrasound is useful to identify pancreatitis, neoplasia, hepatic abscesses, and/or adrenomegaly. Hyperechoic hepatic parenchyma is the most frequent ultrasound abnormality.

Pharmacology

All dogs with naturally occurring DM require lifelong insulin therapy. The goals of insulin therapy are to ameliorate clinical signs and to prevent insulin-induced hypoglycemia. Currently, the best insulin options for dogs with uncomplicated DM include Vetsulin (porcine insulin zinc suspension) and human recombinant NPH (also known as Humulin-N*) insulin administered twice daily. Both insulins are intermediate in the duration of action. NPH insulin is synthetic human recombinant insulin and differs from canine insulin by one amino acid. Vetsulin is porcine insulin and has the identical amino acid sequence to canine insulin.

Insulin is available in two concentrations—U-100 (100 U/mL) and U-40 (40 U/mL). Each concentration requires its own type of syringe. Vetsulin is U-40 insulin and requires U-40 syringes for its administration. U-100 NPH insulin requires U-100 syringes. It is possible to overdose or underdose a patient if the wrong concentration type of syringe is used with the opposite insulin. Insulin syringes also are available in 30- and 100-U sizes to facilitate all dosages.

Vetsulin is the first Food and Drug Administration (FDA)-approved insulin for dogs. However, currently, there are availability issues with Vetsulin in the United States. The availability of insulin products is rapidly changing; every effort has been made to provide a current list at the time of publication.

Client education and the role of the veterinary technician

Client education on the administration and handling of insulin is critical. A veterinary technician can have a crucial role in facilitating a clear and informative diabetic discharge for newly diagnosed dogs. Clients should be instructed on how to gently mix insulin by rolling the bottle between their hands prior to withdrawing the injection. Insulin has a crystalline structure and shaking the mixture will break down the medication. For this reason, the shelf life of insulin, once opened, is usually rated at 3 months. Clients need to be instructed to change bottles of insulin even if there is still insulin left in the bottle. The insulin should also be warmed to room temperature prior to administration. Clients should practice withdrawing the correct dosage with an insulin syringe from a bottle of saline. This should be practiced until the veterinary technician is satisfied that the client is consistently drawing the correct dose. The veterinary technician can then instruct the client on the administration of the insulin injection. Sometimes, to better facilitate the client's understanding, a small patch of hair can be shaved where the injection will be given. The injection should be given at a 45° angle to the skin. Administration sites should be rotated along the lateral thorax and abdomen. The client should practice administering several saline injections to their pet in front of the veterinary technician. In some cases, multiple sessions may be needed to achieve the goal of ensuring that all family members who will be administering insulin can do so correctly.

Some veterinarians will work with select patients and clients to obtain blood glucose samplings in the home environment. This method of monitoring diabetes is less costly, less stressful to the patient than spending a day in the hospital, and may yield more accurate data. The technician may be asked in these situations to guide apprehensive clients in how best to obtain the blood samples. New on the market are continuous glucose monitoring systems that are attached to our patients, allowing us to bypass frequent patient venipuncture.

It is advised to have a specific form clients can complete when leaving pets for diabetes evaluation. The technician should ensure the form is completed by the client. Pertinent information should include

What is the pet's water consumption compared to last time? Is it increased or decreased?

How much is the pet urinating compared to last time? Is it increased or decreased?

What is the present dose of insulin? How often is it given? When was the last dose given?

What is the current diet? How much are you feeding? How often? When was the last time it was fed? Did it eat? How much?

Are insulin refills needed? When was the last time the bottle was replaced?

Are there any other problems or concerns?

What are your goals for today's visit?

Anesthetic and analgesic considerations

A normal meal and the regular dose and type of insulin are given the night before an anesthetic procedure. Food is withheld after 10 p.m. the night before and the morning of surgery. On the morning of surgery, 0.25–0.5 of the regular dose of insulin is given dependent on the blood glucose level, the time of surgery, and the glycemic control of patient. Blood glucose levels need to be monitored preoperatively and approximately every 30 min perioperatively. Blood glucose concentrations are maintained between 150 and 250 mg/dL during surgery with either dextrose infusions and/or regular insulin. Diabetic patients are encouraged to eat as soon as possible after surgery and a subnormal dose of insulin is reinitiated that evening once the patient is eating.

Nutritional considerations

Diets should be complete and balanced, palatable, and should not contain simple sugars.[31] Diabetic dogs are typically fed twice a day at the time of each insulin injection. Each meal should be equal in size and consistency. Some diabetic dogs will show improved glycemic control with high fiber diets. In diabetic dogs with concurrent diseases, dietary therapy is aimed at the most serious disease and that takes precedence over the DM in regard to nutrition.

Canine diabetic ketoacidosis

Diabetic ketoacidosis is a complication of decompensated DM. Although this section is written for canine diabetic ketoacidosis, this information (except dosage information) is generally applicable to feline diabetic ketoacidosis. DKA is associated with significant morbidity and mortality rates in dogs. DKA occurred in 65% of newly diagnosed diabetic dogs and approximately 70% of DKA dogs had other concurrent diseases at the same time in one study.[32] DKA is characterized by hyperglycemia, glucosuria, ketonemia and/or ketonuria, and metabolic acidosis.

Anatomy and physiology

When a combination of insulin deficiency and excessive counter-regulatory hormones such as glucagon, cortisol, GH, and epinephrine occurs, hyperglycemia and the generation of ketone bodies are the end result. Concurrent diseases and/or stress can contribute to an increase in counter-regulatory hormones. The hyperglycemia is due to increased hepatic glucose production and decreased glucose uptake by peripheral tissues. Increased lipolysis secondary to insulin deficiency and increased counter-regulatory hormones favors ketogenesis. The ketone bodies cause vomiting and also contribute to osmotic diuresis, dehydration, metabolic acidosis, and the resulting peripheral vasodilatation.

Clinical signs

The most common clinical signs of DKA are depression, anorexia, and vomiting.[28] The spectrum of severity of clinical signs can be quite varied. Some dogs with DKA will present recumbent, severely dehydrated, and weak, while others will still be eating with polyuria and polydipsia as the only clinical signs. Clinical presentation also depends on the concurrent diseases. A DKA dog with pancreatitis may be vomiting, whereas another patient with pneumonia may be predominantly coughing.

Diagnostic testing

Dogs with DKA require a more thorough workup than healthy diabetics to uncover concurrent diseases and to assess the current health status. A minimum database should include a complete blood cell count (CBC), chemistry panel, urinalysis, urine culture, canine pancreas-specific lipase, blood gas, thoracic and abdominal radiographs, and abdominal ultrasound.

Complete blood cell counts may be normal or may show a stress leukogram or an inflammatory neutrophilia. A left shifted neutrophilia with or without toxic change is often an indication of concurrent inflammatory or infectious disease.

Chemistry panels often reveal marked hyperglycemia. Elevated liver enzymes, ALP and ALT are common abnormalities, along with hypercholesterolemia and hypertriglyceridemia.[29] Electrolyte and acid–base abnormalities are very common. Potassium may be normal, elevated, or low, although there is often a total body potassium deficit due to GI losses (vomiting, diarrhea) and osmotic diuresis.[33] Hyponatremia, hypochloremia, hypocalcemia, and hypomagnesemia frequently occur as well.[34] Azotemia may be present, signaling dehydration or renal failure. Patients with DKA may be hyperosmolar due to the hyperglycemia. There is often an increase in anion gap due to ketone bodies (beta hydroxybutyric acid and acetoacetic acid) and/or lactic acidosis. A blood gas analysis often reveals a metabolic acidosis. The ketone bodies overwhelm the body's buffering capabilities and a metabolic acidosis ensues. Electrolytes need to be monitored closely with treatment (every 4–6 h) as hypokalemia and hypophosphatemia commonly occur.[33,35]

Urinalysis reveals glucosuria, with or without proteinuria, and ketonuria. The nitroprusside reagent detects acetone and acetoacetate but not beta hydroxybutyrate. Thus, a urine dipstick that is negative for ketones does not rule out the possibility of ketoacidosis.[33] All urine samples should be cultured as infection is a common cause of DKA.

Imaging

Imaging is critical to help identify any concurrent diseases that may have resulted in a DKA crisis. Thoracic radiographs and abdominal ultrasound can be used to help identify the most commonly associated diseases with DKA—acute pancreatitis, urinary tract infection, HAC, neoplasia, pneumonia, pyelonephritis, and chronic renal disease.[34]

Pharmacology

The goals of treatment of DKA are to restore hydration and electrolyte imbalances, to diminish ketogenesis, and to correct acid–base imbalances. A central line may be helpful, particularly in small patients to prevent repeated venipunctures for blood monitoring and to measure central venous pressures (CVPs). A peripheral intravenous catheter can also be placed for intravenous fluids and insulin therapy. Intravenous fluid therapy should be initiated for 1–2 h prior to beginning insulin therapy in dehydrated patients.[33,35] Isotonic fluids are recommended for initial fluid therapy and 0.9% sodium chloride is often the first choice.

Potassium chloride supplementation is recommended, dependent on serum potassium levels. Iatrogenic potassium depletion occurs as a result of fluid and insulin therapy and is a common cause of morbidity in patients treated for DKA. The amount of supplementation may need to be increased once insulin therapy is started since potassium will move intracellular. Phosphorus should also be supplemented in initial fluids (usually as potassium phosphate) if warranted by serum phosphorus levels. Serum phosphorus levels should also be reevaluated shortly after insulin and fluid therapy are initiated as additional phosphorus supplementation may be needed.

Regular crystalline insulin is administered to dogs with DKA due to its rapid onset and short duration of effect. There are two main protocols by which insulin is administered.

Constant rate infusion

A low dose CRI of regular insulin has been proposed as the treatment of choice, but definitive studies are not available. This protocol decreases blood glucose levels slowly to reduce the risk of neurological signs, hypoglycemia, and electrolyte abnormalities. Blood glucoses are monitored every 1–2 h, and based on the result, the insulin CRI rate is increased or decreased and fluid composition may be changed to maintain blood glucose levels within a certain range.[35] When preparing the CRI of insulin, it is important to remember that insulin binds to the plastic tubing in the intravenous set. Thus, with a 250-mL bag of fluids spiked with regular insulin, 50 mL of fluid must be run through the line and discarded before it is hooked up to a patient.

Intermittent injections

Another protocol is IM injections of regular insulin for DKA dogs. An IM injection of insulin is given hourly until blood glucose levels reach approximately 250 mg/dL. Then the insulin injections are switched to subcutaneous injections every 6 h. Regular insulin therapy is usually continued until the dog is eating and drinking, and then longer-acting insulin can be initiated.[36]

Anesthetic and analgesic consideration

DKA dogs are typically metabolically unstable patients. They may also have some cardiovascular compromise. Thus, DKA dogs are usually very poor anesthetic candidates. Anesthesia should be delayed until the DKA has been stabilized if possible. The only exception to this is if the DKA is caused by high progesterone levels in a female intact patient wherein ovariohysterectomy would be a necessary part of treatment.

Nutritional considerations

DKA dogs often present anorexic and vomiting. If the dog has concurrent pancreatitis, oral food may need to be withheld for a period of time. In these cases, parenteral nutrition may be necessary. Other DKA dogs may have significant renal impairment or other disease processes that require special nutritional therapy. If there are no concurrent diseases requiring nutritional therapy, DKA dogs should be fed diets that are complete and balanced, palatable, and do not contain simple sugars.[29]

Client education

Owners of dogs with DKA should be informed regarding the following:

1) Prognosis for resolving DKA is guarded, even with intensive care.

2) All dogs with DKA will require lifelong insulin treatment and periodic checkups in order to maintain an acceptable quality of life.

3) All dogs with diabetes will lose their vision from cataracts.

4) Most dogs with diabetes can maintain a good quality of life for many years with the above measures.

5) Dogs with diabetes are predisposed to pancreatitis; diet should be consistent.

Testing and intensive care for DKA should never be pursued without informed consent as above.

Insulinomas

Etiology

Tumors arising from the beta cells of the pancreatic islets can secrete insulin in excessive quantities. Clinical signs are related to hypoglycemia induced by this relatively autonomous hypersecretion. Insulinomas are uncommon in dogs and are very rare in cats.

Pathophysiology

Glucose homeostasis

Ingested carbohydrates, fats, and proteins provide a source of energy for cell metabolism for periods of 4–8 h. Beyond this time period, the body is dependent principally on glucose production by the liver (Figure 2.5.1).

Initially, glucose is provided by hepatic breakdown of stored glycogen (glycogenolysis). Once glycogen is depleted, the main source of glucose arises from the production of glucose from fatty acids, amino acids (supplied by muscle), lactate (supplied by blood via glycolysis), and glycerol (supplied by fat).[37,38]

The pancreatic beta cells are responsible for regulating blood glucose concentrations (BGC). When blood glucose exceeds the normal range (>110 mg/dL), insulin is secreted and blood glucose is reduced into the normal range (70–110 mg/dL) via cell utilization and suppression of hepatic glucose production. When blood glucose levels are <60 mg/dL, insulin synthesis and secretion is inhibited.

Response to hypoglycemia

The CNS, especially the cerebral cortex, is dependent on normal BGCs to maintain normal function. For this reason, in normal individuals, mechanisms are in place to counteract any declines in blood glucose levels (Table 2.5.4).

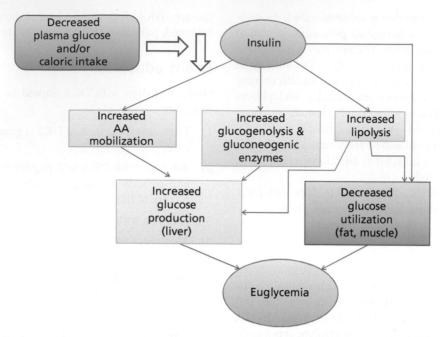

Figure 2.5.1 Hormonal and substrate changes by which euglycemia is maintained (and hypoglycemia is prevented) in normal subjects during a fast. The fall in the plasma insulin concentration is the key hormonal change resulting in increased glucose production and decreased glucose utilization. The decline in the plasma insulin concentration is, in turn, a result of a small decrease in the plasma glucose level (5–10 mg/dL) and/or a decrease in caloric intake. AA, amino acid.

Source: Feldman EC, Nelson RW. *Canine and Feline Endocrinology and Reproduction*, 3rd edition. St. Louis, MO: Saunders Elsevier; 2004.

Table 2.5.4 Hormonal response to hypoglycemia

Hormone	Response
Insulin	Decreased secretion
Glucagon	Increased secretion
Catecholamines	Increased secretion
ACTH, cortisol, growth hormone	Increased secretion

Source: Feldman EC, Nelson RW. Beta-cell neoplasia: insulinoma. In: *Canine and Feline Endocrinology and Reproduction*, 3rd edition, p. 618. St. Louis, MO: Elsevier Science; 2004.

Hypoglycemia leads to rapid secretion of counter-regulatory hormones, which restore an adequate supply of glucose to maintain cerebral function, and suppression of insulin secretion.

Increases in plasma glucagon, epinephrine, and norepinephrine occur acutely, and increases in GH and cortisol occur later. Glucagon is believed to be the primary mediator of the body's response to hypoglycemia; this hormone is secreted by the alpha cells of the pancreas into the portal circulation and results in glycogenolysis and gluconeogenesis within minutes.[39,40]

The adrenal gland also plays a major role in recovery from hypoglycemia. Epinephrine stimulates hepatic glycogenolysis and gluconeogenesis and inhibits glucose utilization by the skeletal muscle.[41]

Pathophysiology in dogs with beta-cell tumors

In dogs with insulinomas, autonomous secretion of insulin by tumor cells results in increased utilization of glucose and hypoglycemia. Normal glucose homeostasis is disturbed with the result being reduced blood glucose (due to exaggerated tissue consumption of glucose) and interference with hepatic production of glucose.

Clinical signs

Insulinomas typically occur in older dogs; there is no apparent breed predisposition. Clinical signs are often insidious and are attributed to old age. The most common signs include seizures, weakness/ataxia, tremors, and behavior changes (Table 2.5.5).

Symptoms often resolve after a few minutes, presumably due to the actions of counter-regulatory hormones. Signs may be precipitated by exercise and excitement, as activity calls for increased glucose utilization by muscles.

Causes of clinical signs

As carbohydrate/energy reserves in the CNS are limited, proper tissue function relies on a steady supply of glucose. In mammals, the cerebral cortex is the first region to be affected. Although the entrance of glucose into brain cells is not dependent on, or regulated by, the level of insulin, hypoxia of brain cells still occurs due to hypoglycemia. The presence or absence of clinical signs is dependent on the duration and degree of

Table 2.5.5 Clinical signs of insulin-secreting tumors in dogs

Sign	Percentage (%)
Seizures	56
Weakness	47
Collapse	30
Ataxia	19
Muscle tremors	18
Hind end weakness	16
Behavior changes	12

Source: Feldman EC, Nelson RW. Beta-cell neoplasia: insulinoma. In: *Canine and Feline Endocrinology and Reproduction*, 3rd edition, p. 621. St. Louis, MO: Elsevier Science; 2004.

Table 2.5.6 Causes of hypoglycemia

Insulin-secreting tumor

Paraneoplastic

Hypoadrenocorticism

Hepatic failure–PSS, acquired

Toxic–xylitol

Sepsis

Toy breed/fasting puppy

Sampling artifact

hypoglycemia and on the success of the counter-regulatory hormones in combating hypoglycemia.

Lab abnormalities

The only consistent biochemical abnormality is the presence of mild to marked hypoglycemia. In most dogs with insulinomas, blood glucose is <60 mg/dL. If other abnormalities are noted, they are usually associated with other concurrent conditions (Table 2.5.6).

As artifact can be a potential cause of an expensive diagnostic evaluation for hypoglycemia, veterinary professionals handling laboratory samples must be aware of this in order to minimize its occurrence. Delay in the separation of cells from serum results in the utilization of glucose by red blood cells (RBCs) and a reduction in the glucose concentration reported. This occurs most commonly when whole blood sits overnight without being centrifuged and separated prior to lab pickup. Placing samples in serum-separator tubes and spinning the sample within an hour after collection minimize this artifact.

Glucose values measured using whole blood portable glucose meters designed for humans often can result in values 10–50 mg/dL lower than actual glucose values, resulting in an artifactual diagnosis of hypoglycemia.

Diagnostic imaging

Insulinomas are usually small (<3 cm) nodules within the pancreas and are seldom recognized on survey radiographs. Pulmonary metastases occur late in the course of disease, so thoracic radiographs are often unremarkable. Abdominal ultrasonography is often viewed as a definitive diagnostic aid for insulin-secreting tumors. While identification of masses/nodules in the region of the pancreas is supportive of the existence of an insulinoma, failure to identify the lesion in the pancreas is common and should not be interpreted as evidence that excludes insulinoma from consideration. CT may be a more sensitive means of detecting the primary tumor and metastases, but studies have not evaluated this modality as a diagnostic tool for insulinoma.

Diagnostic approach

The causes of hypoglycemia can be narrowed based on a brief history, patient signalment, and known breed predispositions to portosystemic shunts. In puppies, young dogs, and toy breeds, hypoglycemia, PSS, and Addison's disease would be the most likely causes. In a geriatric dog, sepsis, insulinoma, and paraneoplastic causes are the most common etiologies. A dog with Addison's disease would usually have electrolyte abnormalities and azotemia with hypoglycemia. Insulinoma should be suspected in any geriatric dog presenting with appropriate clinical signs and hypoglycemia as the only lab abnormality in the absence of artifact.

The diagnosis of insulin-secreting tumor can only be confirmed by evaluating concurrent serum insulin and glucose concentrations. In a normal dog, hypoglycemia suppresses insulin secretion; in dogs with insulinoma, this suppressive effect is minimized due to the semiautonomous release of insulin by the tumor. Serum should be obtained when blood glucose is <60 mg/dL, for insulin/glucose evaluations. If blood glucose is higher than 60 mg/dL, fasting serial samples should be obtained to determine the degree of glucose decline. If human-specific portable glucose meters are used to evaluate blood glucose, hypoglycemia should be <50 mg/dL prior to serum submission as these meters run erroneously low.

One of the most common obstacles in confirming a diagnosis of insulinoma is premature administration of dextrose. Administration of dextrose to hypoglycemic patients will elevate serum glucose and insulin levels, thereby interfering with blood testing relied upon to accrue a diagnosis. Furthermore, in most cases, hypoglycemic signs may resolve with cage rest. As it is very difficult to withdraw therapeutic dextrose once it has been initiated, every effort should be made to ensure that the pretreatment serum has been collected and that the sample is handled properly to avoid artifact. Attempts to improve/resolve hypoglycemia can be initiated after these samples have been obtained.

Past literature has discussed insulin/glucose ratios be used to gauge confidence in the diagnosis.[42] In this author's experience, one to two appropriately obtained serum samples are all that is needed to accrue a diagnosis. If insulin levels are elevated in the face of hypoglycemia, this confirms a diagnosis of insulin-secreting tumor. A common misconception in interpretation occurs if/when insulin concentrations are not elevated but are within the normal range. This should be viewed as an abnormal finding, as serum insulin levels should be nonexistent in patients with severe hypoglycemia. Thus, normal insulin levels in a patient with severe hypoglycemia are consistent with a diagnosis of insulinoma.

Client education and the role of the veterinary technician

Although the veterinary team is usually able to achieve a tentative diagnosis quickly and alleviate clinical signs in the hospital, providing useful information to the client is extremely valuable if the veterinary team is to act on decisions based on informed consent. Pivotal data relayed should include the following:

a) Dogs manifesting signs of hypoglycemia are not in pain.
b) This disease cannot be cured and is considered terminal.
c) Symptoms can often be managed and diminished for periods of months-years with inexpensive measures at home. Medications may have side effects.
d) Signs of hypoglycemia (which may include seizures) will recur in all patients.

An exhaustive workup for a dog with insulinoma should not be completed until the client has been apprised of the key data points above.

Treatment

Acute/hospitalized patient

A common misconception in managing hypoglycemic patients with suspected insulinoma is that restoring euglycemia should be an immediate goal of therapy.

The goal of in-hospital care is to

a) perform appropriate testing to achieve a tentative diagnosis,
b) establish whether surgery is to be performed, and
c) minimize clinical signs related to hypoglycemia.

The latter goal is generally achieved with intravenous dextrose supplementation. Although no particular protocol has been proven to be most effective, most endocrinologists believe that IV fluids supplemented with 50% dextrose to a 2.5–5.0% solution achieve resolution of signs in most cases. Frequent or rapid boluses of dextrose have the potential to create a rebound hypoglycemia due to stimulation of the tumor and release of insulin.[43] In some patients, signs persist despite these measures; in refractory cases, glucagon can be considered as a CRI at 5–10 ng/kg/min.[44]

Is surgery reasonable?

Resection of the pancreatic tumor is considered the most definitive treatment for dogs with insulinoma. In most cases, surgical removal can improve response to chronic medical management, and thereby prolong survival times.[45] In rare cases,

excision can be curative. Despite these data, pancreatectomy may be declined due to the age of the patient, operative and postoperative risks, high rate of metastases and rare surgical cures, cost of surgery and aftercare, and the good success rates of medical management.

If surgery is declined, medical treatment is advised to palliate clinical signs (see chronic management). It should be reinforced that signs are expected to recur in the future and that metastases will occur or progress with time. As many dogs have very good quality of life for months-years without surgery, euthanasia is seldom advised if surgery is not elected.

Pancreatectomy

The goal of surgery is to debulk as much cancer burden as possible and to minimize preventable postoperative complications. Euthanasia is not advised even in the face of a perceived high burden of metastases due to the frequency of benign hepatic nodules in geriatric dogs and the positive response to medical management.

Preoperative administration of glucose as a 5% solution is continued as during the acute period of stabilization and especially during the period of fasting prior to surgery. A glucose >40 mg/dL is ideal. Placement of a central venous catheter prior to the procedure is advised to allow for frequent intraoperative and postsurgical glucose monitoring.

Insulinomas can occur within any portion of the pancreas, with no predilections for a particular lobe. It is believed that tumors associated with the body of the pancreas are associated with much higher risks of pancreatitis after surgery, and excision in these circumstances must be weighed against these risks.[46]

Postoperative care

Postoperative complications are common and include the following.

Pancreatitis

This can be a devastating complication for the postsurgical patient as it delays the ability to feed the patient and is associated with fatal outcomes in select instances. Aggressive intravenous fluid therapy is advised (dextrose initiates a polyuric state) and food is often withheld for 24–48 h after pancreatic surgery to minimize the incidence of this complication.

Diabetes mellitus

This is a rare complication of aggressive resection of a large portion of the pancreas in which atrophy of remaining normal islet cells results in insufficient insulin secretion. Insulin therapy is only advised after a few days of persistent hyperglycemia and glucosuria. In treated cases, hypoglycemia recurs due to tumor regrowth and insulin is discontinued.

Hypoglycemia

Hypoglycemia may persist after surgery due to incomplete tumor resection or due to persistence of functional metastases.

Chronic medical management

Lifelong medical management is advised only if surgery has been declined or when clinical signs recur after surgery due to tumor recurrence and/or metastases. The goals of treatment are to reduce the frequency and severity of clinical signs and to avoid hospitalization if at all possible. Euglycemia may never be achieved.

a) *Frequent Feedings.* It is believed that provision of a constant source of calories for the elevated blood levels of insulin to act on will minimize hypoglycemic symptoms. Feeding three to six meals per day is advised.

b) *Minimize Exercise and Excitement.* Exercise and excitement increase glucose utilization and inhibit hepatic release of glucose.[47]

c) *Glucocorticoids.* These drugs are advised when the above measures no longer control clinical signs adequately. Steroids are insulin antagonists and stimulate hepatic glycogenolysis. Prednisone is started at 0.5 mg/kg/day divided BID, and the dose is increased as needed based on recurrence of symptoms. The limiting factor in dosing is the typical side effects of PU/PD, lethargy, and panting.

d) *Diazoxide.* This is a diuretic that inhibits insulin secretion and tissue utilization of glucose, and stimulates hepatic gluconeogenesis. The drug is expensive, and GI side effects are common. Initial dosage is 10 mg/kg/day divided BID. Giving the drug with food may diminish side effects.

e) *SST.* Octreotide acetate (Novartis Pharmaceuticals, East Hanover, NJ) is an analogue of SST that inhibits synthesis of insulin by beta cells in the pancreas. Doses of 10–50 μg SC BID-TID have been reported.[12]

Monitoring of the insulinoma patient

As a general rule, it is not advised to perform random rechecks of blood glucose in patients with insulinoma as at-home therapy is palliative and changes in therapy are based on clinical signs only. It is advised, however, to check blood glucose levels once the owner reports recurrence of symptoms. It is possible that, with the increased use of at-home glucose monitoring, future guidelines may change.

What to advise for episodes at home

It is generally advised for owners to always have honey, Karo˙ syrup or some form of sugar solution available at home. If the animal is actively seizuring, advise rubbing the solution on the gums (counsel properly so the owner does not get bitten). If the animal is weak or ataxic and is alert enough to eat, offer a small meal.

Prognosis: biological behavior of insulinoma

All beta-cell carcinomas are considered malignant, and most dogs have cancer spread at the time of diagnosis. Most common sites of metastases are the liver, peripancreatic omentum, and lymph nodes. Despite the extent of malignancy, many dogs can maintain prolonged (months-years) symptom-free periods with medical and/or surgical management. The owner's willingness to accept the potential for recurrent episodes and to comply with chronic medical management plays a large role in decision making and patient survival times.

Glucagonoma

Glucagonoma is a very rare malignant endocrine tumor of the alpha cells of the pancreatic islet of Langerhans. No feline glucagonoma cases have been reported. This tumor has been associated with an erosive, crusting skin rash called necrolytic migratory erythema (NME) in people and superficial necrolytic dermatitis (SND) in dogs. Other terms for the skin condition seen with a glucagonoma in dogs include diabetic dermatopathy, metabolic epidermal necrosis, and glucagonoma syndrome. The term diabetic dermatopathy was coined because some canine and human patients with this tumor develop concurrent DM.

Signalment

No breed or sex predilection exists. Middle-aged to older dogs are more commonly affected.

Clinical symptoms

The presenting complaint for most dogs with this condition is an erosive and crusting dermatitis. The footpads or other pressure points are most often the first skin areas affected. Often these animals have concurrent footpad pain and pruritis. Interdigital erythema, crusting, and fissuring of the footpads is typical (Figure 2.5.2).

The skin signs may wax and wane and may also involve other areas that experience increased trauma—distal limbs, muzzle, elbows, hocks, and mucocutaneous areas of the face. Weight loss and PU/PD are other common complaints. Catabolic effects of glucagon may contribute to weight loss.

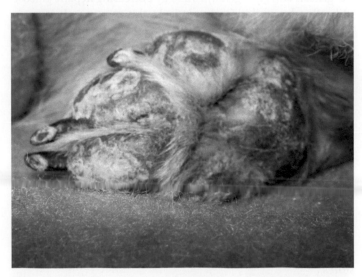

Figure 2.5.2 Footpad of a dog with superficial necrolytic dermatitis.

Pathogenesis of skin lesions

Hyperglucagonemia from autonomous secretion by the tumor is thought to play an important role in the development of the skin lesions; however, the pathogenesis for the skin condition is not well understood and other metabolic and nutritional abnormalities including zinc deficiency, liver dysfunction, hypoalbuminemia, and deficiencies in essential fatty acids and amino acids also likely play a role. In addition, this skin rash is not considered pathognomonic for a glucagonoma.

Association with liver disease

In dogs, a distinctive chronic liver disease is actually a more common cause of this skin condition than a pancreatic glucagonoma and would be a major differential diagnosis in suspected cases of a glucagonoma. The hepatopathy linked to SND can be primary or secondary. Secondary hepatopathy cases have been linked to ingestion of mycotoxins and to chronic treatment with certain anticonvulsants including phenobarbital, primidone, or phenytoin administration. Hepatocutaneous syndrome is another term coined to link the signs of the skin rash with the severe liver disease that occurs in most of the canine cases of SND. See Chapter 9 for more information. A potential case of an extrapancreatic tumor-secreting glucagon has also been reported in a dog, and a pseudoglucagonoma syndrome, in which NME occurs in the absence of a pancreatic tumor, has been reported in association with a number of other conditions in people including cirrhosis, celiac sprue, pancreatitis, malignancies (other than pancreatic), hepatitis, inflammatory bowel disease, generalized malabsorption syndromes, and specific nutritional deficiencies (i.e., zinc and essential fatty acids).

Association with diabetes mellitus

DM with expected weight loss is also a common finding in canine and human patients with glucagonomas. Hyperglucagonemia leads to hyperglycemia by stimulating hepatic gluconeogenesis and glycogenolysis and by decreasing hepatic glucose utilization by inhibiting glycolysis. In this capacity, glucagon is a potent anti-insulinogenic hormone. The insulin resistance that results may lead to signs of DM (PU/PD). Some dogs with hyperglucagonemia associated with liver disease or from a glucagonoma also have concurrent pancreatitis, which can further impair insulin secretion and contribute to the onset of signs of DM. In adipose tissue, hyperglucagonemia activates hormone-sensitive lipase and increases the free fatty acid delivery to the liver, which promotes ketogenesis. At the same time, hyperglucagonemia inhibits hepatic lipoprotein production. Enhanced breakdown of muscle protein is promoted resulting in increased release of the amino acids alanine and glutamine for hepatic gluconeogenesis. Ultimately, hyperglucagonemia reduces plasma amino acid concentrations due to enhanced essential amino acid catabolism. As a consequence of persistent hyperglucagonemia, DM develops at the expense of tissue, muscle, and fat glycogen stores.

Laboratory findings

Normocytic, normochromic, nonregenerative anemia may be seen secondary to chronic disease. Elevated liver enzymes are typical in dogs with glucagon-secreting tumors. If these are associated with elevated bile acid levels, then a primary or secondary hepatopathy should be suspected. If serum bile acids are normal, then primary glucagonoma is most probable.

Hypoalbuminemia, low urea, and hypoaminoacidemia may be seen in these patients due to advanced muscle catabolism. Hypoaminoacidemia is very common with glucagonoma cases, and in affected dogs, serum amino acids are reduced by more than 50%. The molar ratio of branched-chain amino acids to aromatic amino acids is also commonly decreased. Serum amino acids can be measured through only a few laboratories (e.g., University of California, Davis). Hyperglycemia with glucosuria is expected if the patient has concurrent DM. Elevations in amylase and lipase may occur with concurrent pancreatitis.

An elevated serum glucagon concentration may be seen, but this has not been documented in all reported canine cases; the reference range has not been established, but values <200 pmol/L are considered normal. This assay is not commonly performed and has limited availability.

Diagnosis

Histopathology

Skin biopsies are the gold standard for the diagnosis of superficial necrolytic dermatitis. Multiple punch biopsies from the edges of early lesions should be submitted. With early or acute lesions, diffuse parakeratotic hyperkeratosis with vacuolation of keratinocytes, no edema, and minimal dermal changes are seen. Biopsies of more chronic lesions show epidermal edema, marked parakeratotic hyperkeratosis, epidermal hyperplasia, and surface crusting, resulting in the classic red, white, and blue layering with standard histopathologic staining.

Differential diagnoses for the skin lesions seen with a glucagonoma include autoimmune skin disorders (e.g., pemphigus foliaceus, toxic epidermal necrolysis, erythema multiforme), nutritional causes (e.g., zinc responsive dermatosis), infectious causes (e.g., dermatophytosis, bacterial pyoderma), parasitic causes (e.g., demodicosis), and neoplastic causes (e.g., epitheliotropic lymphoma). Definitive diagnosis requires immunohistochemical staining of the excised pancreatic mass or biopsy for glucagon.

Laboratory testing

Serum glucagon concentration has been elevated in most but not all of the canine cases with a confirmed glucagonoma.

A complete plasma amino acid profile should be done to confirm hypoaminoacidemia in suspected cases of SND as amino acid supplementation is often provided as part of the therapy. Monitoring of the serum amino acid profile with therapy may also be warranted.

Imaging

Abdominal ultrasound should be done both to look for a pancreatic tumor and for possible metastasis to other abdominal organs such as the liver. Abdominal ultrasound is also important to rule out a pseudoglucagonoma syndrome due to a hepatopathy. In cases of SND caused by a hepatopathy, the characteristic hepatic ultrasonographic appearance is a honeycomb or Swiss cheese appearance.

Because pancreatic islet tumors are often not visible with ultrasound, failure to visualize a tumor does not rule out a glucagonoma even if cutaneous signs of SND are present. CT and MRI of the abdomen with contrast are both more sensitive imaging modalities for the detection of pancreatic islet tumors in dogs. Indium-111-labeled somatostatin/octreotide acetate scintigraphy can also be used to detect these tumors in some cases or to corroborate CT findings and identify metastatic disease. Although not commonly available in veterinary medicine at this time, endoscopic ultrasound is a very sensitive method for detection of pancreatic islet tumors in people.

Treatment

Complete surgical resection of the pancreatic tumor is the treatment of choice and can be curative for cases of SND induced by a glucagonoma. Any suspicious areas in the liver seen at the time of surgery should be biopsied as should local lymph nodes to evaluate for possible metastasis. Surgical excision of pancreatic tumors is associated with a high risk of postoperative pancreatitis; this can be severe and in rare cases fatal.

Chemotherapy (dacarbazine, streptozotocin combined with 5-fluorouracil) for glucagonomas has had limited palliative success in people with unresectable or metastatic tumors.

Parenteral (Aminosyn*) or oral (ProMod*) amino acid solutions or total parenteral nutrition (TPN) along with a high quality protein diet are used to help resolve the rash signs. Zinc and essential fatty acid supplementation are often used supportively for the skin lesions. Hydrotherapy and topical glucocorticoids may also be indicated along with treatment of a secondary bacterial or fungal pyoderma.

The administration of octreotide acetate, a synthetic SST analogue that binds with high affinity to somatostatin receptors (SSTRs) and inhibits the release of several GI hormones including glucagon, has been used to treat glucagonemia in humans and appears to be effective in cases where surgery is not an option (e.g., patients with widespread disseminated metastatic disease). Few reports are available in dogs, but in one case, SC administered octreotide acetate did resolve cutaneous signs and improve quality of life for the dog in the short term. The drug is expensive and anorexia is the major adverse effect.

Hepatic arterial chemoembolization for the treatment of hepatic metastasis of pancreatic tumors has been reported in dogs and is a palliative option.

Insulin therapy for patients with concurrent DM will be required.

Prognosis

The prognosis for a pancreatic glucagonoma in dogs is considered guarded to poor because in most cases, the diagnosis is made late in the course when the tumor has already metastasized. If caught early, complete surgical excision may be possible.

SECTION 6 MISCELLANEOUS HORMONES, GLANDS, AND DISEASE

Calcitriol

Calcitriol, otherwise known as bioactive vitamin D, or 1,25 dihydroxycholecalciferol $(1,25(OH)2D_3)$, is a steroid hormone that plays an important role in regulating the concentrations of calcium and phosphorous in the blood and in the mineralization of bone.

Pathophysiology of calcitriol

Production of bioactive vitamin D is a multistep process involving sequential hydroxylation of the initial precursor, vitamin D_3. In dogs and cats, vitamin D_3 is exclusively obtained from the diet since they are not capable of synthesizing it in their skin. Vitamin D_3 is first hydroxylated to form vitamin D_2 within the liver. Vitamin D_2 is then released into the bloodstream and is transported to the kidney. In the kidney, vitamin D_2 is hydroxylated again, inside the proximal renal tubule cells, by the enzyme 1α-hydroxylase to form bioactive vitamin D. Only the final product in vitamin D synthesis, calcitriol or 1,25 dihydroxycholecalciferol, is biologically active; the earlier precursor molecules are not biologically active.

Three major mechanisms contribute to the regulation of active vitamin D production. The first mechanism involves regulation by a multifactorial classic endocrine negative feedback system. Low calcium, phosphorus, calcitriol, or elevated PTH increases 1α-hydroxylase activity; the reverse conditions decrease the activity of 1α-hydroxylase. Feedback regulation by calcitriol limits its circulating concentration and prevents excessive synthesis.

The second major regulatory mechanism is accomplished intracellularly within virtually all target cells. This involves the production of an enzyme (24-hydroxylase) that catalyzes a series of oxidation reactions leading to inactivation of calcitriol. This enzyme is regulated in a reciprocal manner to 1α-hydroxylase. Its activity and expression are increased by high serum phosphorus and calcitriol concentrations and reduced by elevations in PTH.

The third major regulatory mechanism is the binding of calcitriol (99%) to protein (making it inactive). Carrier proteins help to act as a buffer guarding against vitamin D intoxication.

Biological actions of vitamin D: Calcium and phosphorus homeostasis

The vitamin D endocrine system is an essential component of the complex interactions involving the kidney, bone, parathyroid gland, and intestine that maintain extracellular calcium and phosphorus levels within very narrow limits. Such tight control of calcium and phosphorus concentrations in the body is vital for normal cellular physiology and skeletal integrity. Vitamin D acts in concert with PTH produced by the parathyroid glands to tightly regulate these minerals in the body. The main site of action of vitamin D is the GI tract where it stimulates active absorption of Ca^{2+} as well as stimulating absorption of phosphorus and magnesium by enterocytes.

Vitamin D is essential for the development and maintenance of a mineralized skeleton. Vitamin D deficiency results in rickets (softening of bones) in young growing animals and osteomalacia in adults.

The vitamin D endocrine system is a potent modulator of parathyroid function. Vitamin D is important for determining the parathyroid gland responsiveness to calcium. As expected, prolonged calcitriol deficiency (as occurs in chronic kidney disease [CKD]) leads to markedly reduced parathyroid receptors and calcium receptor levels, thereby requiring higher serum calcium or 1,25(OH)2D3 doses to suppress PTH synthesis or to arrest growth. The administration of 1,25(OH)2D3 in patients with CKD inhibits PTH synthesis and parathyroid cell growth and has been utilized for the treatment of secondary hyperparathyroidism from CKD. Calcitriol also potentiates the effect of PTH on bone.

Through all these effects, but especially through its action on the intestine, vitamin D ensures that the blood levels of calcium and phosphorus are sufficient for the normal mineralization of type I collagen in the skeleton.

Other nonclassic biological actions of vitamin D

Vitamin D is being increasingly recognized for its role in modulating cell growth and differentiation in a diverse array of tissues. Vitamin D has been shown to have potent antiproliferative, prodifferentiative, and immunomodulatory activities. These functions have suggested a possible role for vitamin D in preventing cancers and in the modulation of the immune system.

Clinical disease states and applications involving vitamin D

Deficiency of vitamin D in young animals leads to rickets, a devastating skeletal disease characterized by undermineralized bones. In adult animals, vitamin D deficiency leads to osteomalacia. Nutritional rickets results from a dietary deficiency of vitamin D or phosphorus; this is very rare in humans, but cases have been reported in young cats and dogs fed with a nutritionally incomplete and unbalanced diet. Other forms of rickets seen in people (type I and II, nutritional rickets, and X-linked hypophosphatemic rickets) that are caused by mutations in genes involved in vitamin D synthesis or that affect the sensitivity of vitamin D receptors, have also been described in cats and dogs.

In adult animals, CKD can result in acquired vitamin D deficiency due to the reduction in the kidney's ability to produce bioactive vitamin D. The resulting deficiency is an important factor promoting the development of renal secondary hyperparathyroidism in CKD because one of calcitriol's important functions is to modulate PTH activity. With renal secondary hyperparathyroidism, increased secretion of PTH occurs due to ionized hypocalcemia. Renal secondary hyperparathyroidism is very common in cats with CKD. Renal osteodystrophy may result from renal secondary hyperparathyroidism. This is usually a subclinical syndrome in adult dogs with CKD; however, in young animals with CKD and in rare cases in older animals with CKD, it will manifest clinically as skeletal abnormalities such as bone pain, pathologic fractures, loose teeth, and rubber jaw syndrome.

PTH has been recognized as a uremic toxin, and supplementing cats and dogs with calcitriol has been advocated by some veterinary nephrologists in order to ameliorate the adverse effects of excessive PTH production in CKD patients. At this time, current evidence does not support the use of calcitriol in cats with CKD but does support its use in dogs.

Hypervitaminosis D toxicity

Vitamin D toxicity is usually the result of overdosing on vitamin D supplements or of exposure to toxins such as rat bait that contain high concentrations of vitamin D. Certainly, vitamin D supplements are a valuable treatment for individuals with vitamin D deficiency or hypocalcemia from hypoparathyroidism, but overzealous supplementation over a period of weeks or months can be severely toxic to humans and animals. Excessive dietary supplementation of vitamin D by uninformed owners or inadvertent oversupplementation of feedstuffs from problems with ration formulations can also lead to severe hypercalcemia, renal failure, and possibly death.

Hypervitaminosis D toxicity from cholecalciferol containing rodenticides (Quintox˚, True Grit Rampage˚, and Ortho Mouse & Rat-B-Gone˚) can result in hypercalcemia as soon as 12–18 h post ingestion. Other causes of hypervitaminosis D toxicity have also been reported in dogs consuming vitamin D containing psoriasis medications (Davionex, Dovenex, and Psorcutan).

If toxicity or deficiency of vitamin D are suspected, then measurement of vitamin D metabolites, 25-hydroxycholecalciferol (calcidiol) and 1,25 dihydroxycholecalciferol (calcitriol), is indicated. A competitive protein binding assay that is not species specific is available for the measurement of vitamin D. To avoid handling errors, protect the frozen serum from light.

Erythropoietin

Erythropoietin (EPO) is a glycoprotein hormone that regulates RBC production (erythropoiesis); it is produced by peritubular interstitial cells in the kidneys in the adult animal and in hepatocytes in the fetus. Small amounts of extrarenal EPO are also produced by the liver in humans and potentially in other species.

Pathophysiology of erythropoietin

EPO binds to an erythroid progenitor cell surface receptor to regulate bone marrow erythroid cell proliferation, differentiation, and survival. The highest number of EPO receptors is located on the colony-forming unit-erythroid (CFU-E) cells, which are considered the primary target cells for EPO. When EPO binds to the receptors on the colony-forming unit (CFU) progenitor cells the end result is to rescue these progenitor cells from undergoing apoptosis (programmed cell death). This leads to an increase in the number of progenitor cells that survive to differentiate into mature RBCs that can be released from the bone marrow.

EPO is not the only growth factor involved in erythropoiesis. Other growth factors that act synergistically with EPO in this role include granulocyte colony-stimulating factor (G-CSF), interleukin (IL)-6, stem cell factor (SCF), IL-1, IL-3, IL-4, IL-9, IL-11, granulocyte-macrophage (GM)-CSF, and IGF-1.

Ubiquitous EPO receptor expression in nonerythroid cells has been associated with the discovery of diverse biological functions for EPO in nonhematopoietic tissues. During development, EPO-EpoR signaling is required not only for fetal liver erythropoiesis but also for embryonic angiogenesis and brain development. A series of recent studies suggest that endogenous EPO-EpoR signaling contributes to wound healing responses, physiological and pathological angiogenesis, and the body's innate response to injury in the brain and heart. EPO and its novel derivatives have emerged as major tissue-protective cytokines. Other effects of EPO include a hematocrit-independent vasoconstriction-dependent hypertension, increased endothelin production, upregulation of tissue renin, change in vascular tissue prostaglandin production, stimulation of angiogenesis, and stimulation of endothelial and vascular smooth muscle cell proliferation.

Erythropoietin secretion

The intrarenal physiology and pharmacology of EPO production is highly complex. To maintain a stable hemoglobin (Hb) concentration, the erythroid precursor cell compartment (or erythron) must be able to respond promptly and appropriately to increased oxygen demands caused by acute (e.g., blood loss) or chronic (e.g., infection) conditions. The primary means by which the body regulates RBC production in response to such demands is through a feedback loop regulated by tissue oxygen levels. Tissue hypoxia prompts renal tubular epithelial cells to secrete EPO, while an increase in tissue oxygenation causes a decrease in EPO secretion to basal levels. A certain basal level of EPO is necessary for a normal rate of erythropoiesis, but when there is a decrease in the number of RBCs (e.g., after hemorrhage or with hemolytic anemia) leading to hypoxia, renal peritubular cells detect this and increase their secretion of EPO. The concentration of EPO will vary with the degree of hypoxia or severity of the anemia. The degree of oxygenation and the number of RBCs in circulation act as a feedback mechanism to either increase or decrease EPO secretion in response to increased red cell production. This process helps to ensure that there is a normal red cell circulating mass to prevent hypoxia while preventing overproduction of RBCs, which could lead to a dangerous increase in blood viscosity. Other factors that increase secretion of EPO include other hormones such as androgens, T_4, GH, prolactin, ACTH, and adrenocortical steroids. Products released from premature RBC destruction (hemolysates) have also been shown to enhance EPO secretion. Drugs that cause marked vasoconstriction and result in renal hypoxia can also stimulate EPO production. Adenosine and estrogens are factors other than polycythemia that decrease EPO secretion by the kidneys.

Clinical disease states and therapeutic uses

Following the cloning of the EPO gene and the characterization of the selective hematopoietic action of EPO on erythroid CFU cells, recombinant EPO forms (epoetin-alfa, epoetin-beta, and the long-acting analogue darbepoetin-alfa) were produced for therapeutic use. Today, these products are widely used in people for the treatment of anemia in patients with CKD, aplastic anemia, and chemotherapy-induced anemia. Human recombinant erythropoietin (rHuEPO; Epogen®, Amgen, Thousand Oaks, CA) and darbepoetin (Aranesp®, Amgen, Thousand Oaks, CA) have also been used in dogs and cats to treat the anemia of advanced CKD and chemotherapy-induced anemia.

The principal cause for the anemia associated with advanced chronic renal failure is erythroid hypoplasia in the bone marrow secondary to inadequate renal production of EPO. Hormone replacement therapy using recombinant human EPO has been shown to be effective in correcting anemia of CKD in dogs. Uncontrolled clinical trials in cats with CKD have also shown that treatment of anemia of CKD results in improvement in appetite and improved quality of life. Unfortunately, the development of antibodies directed against rHuEPO has limited the usefulness of rHuEPO in some dogs and cats with CKD. The development of anti-EPO antibodies may result in failure of drug efficacy, progressive anemia in spite of therapy, and the need for blood transfusion. This has led to the recommendation to withhold the use of rHuEPO until the patient's packed cell volume is less than 20% and clinical signs are seen attributable to the anemia. The serious nature of these complications requires a thorough discussion with the pet owner so that risks and benefits of therapy can be weighed prior to proceeding with therapy.

Darbepoetin, when compared with rHuEPO, has a longer plasma half-life, so it requires less frequent dosing and has been reported to be just as effective at maintaining Hb levels in human patients with CKD as rHuEPO. Although unproven, darbepoietin alpha may be less immunogenic in dogs and in cats than EPO. However, studies on the clinical effectiveness and safety of this product in dogs and cats with CKD have not been published, and evidence regarding its effectiveness and recommendations for its use in dogs and in cats with CKD is limited to expert opinion. Usage of rHuEPO or darbepoetin requires an express consent form as these are not approved for use in dogs and cats. Nevertheless, rHuEPO has been in use since approximately

1990, and nephrologists have been using darbepoetin for the past few years on clinical patients.

Recombinant forms of both canine and feline EPO have been synthesized and have been shown to be effective and safe when used to treat the anemia of CKD in dogs and in cats, respectively. The immunogenicity problems observed with rHuEPO administration to dogs were not observed with the use of this canine recombinant EPO. Recombinant canine and feline EPO are not, however, currently available commercially.

Regardless of the underlying disease process for which human or species-specific recombinant EPO is being administered, iron supplementation is typically necessary in order to prevent the development of iron deficiency due to the increased rate of erythropoiesis.

Systemic hypertension is a recognized complication of EPO therapy in human beings receiving rHuEPO.

Measurement of plasma EPO

Various methods are available for the measurement of EPO in plasma and serum; however, in clinical medicine, immunoassays are the most commonly used. The concentration of EPO in the sample is expressed in international units per liter and is determined by calibration against a reference standard. The availability of this test is variable at the time of print; check with your reference laboratory. When serum EPO is measured, 5 mL of blood should be collected into tubes containing no additive; once clotted, the samples should be centrifuged immediately and the serum separated and stored in a plastic vial at 2–8°C for up to 24 h. For longer storage, up to 18 months, serum or plasma can be frozen at −20°C. Samples with gross hemolysis or lipemia are unsuitable for analysis. A same-day Hb or hematocrit measurement from the patient along with other relevant clinical information should be provided to the laboratory to aid with accurate interpretation of the serum EPO concentration. Sex and age do not affect serum EPO levels in healthy cats and dogs.

The primary indications for the measurement of serum or plasma EPO is as a diagnostic tool to differentiate between the two major causes for absolute polycythemia—primary polycythemia (polycythemia vera [PCV]) and secondary polycythemia. See Chapter 7 for more information on polycythemia.

Abuse potential

The use of rHuEPO and darbepoetin to enhance athletic performance is officially banned by most sports-governing bodies because the resulting excessive erythrocytosis can lead to increased thrombogenicity and can cause deep vein, coronary, and cerebral thromboses. Veterinarians need to be aware of the abuse potential for recombinant EPO if this drug is not carefully prescribed.

Gastrin

Gastrin is a GI hormone that is produced by G cells located primarily in the antral portion of the stomach. Smaller numbers of gastrin-secreting cells are also located in the pancreas, proximal duodenum, various parts of the CNS (pituitary gland, the hypothalamus, and the medulla oblongata) as well as in the vagus and sciatic nerves.

Pathophysiology of gastrin

Gastrin has many functions, but its two major effects on the GI tract are stimulation of gastric acid secretion by parietal cells and promotion of gastric mucosal growth.

Gastrin receptors are found on parietal cells, and binding of gastrin, along with binding of the other two major ligands that promote gastric acid secretion (histamine and acetylcholine), is required for maximal gastric acid secretion by parietal cells. Histamine produced by neighboring histamine-secreting enterchromaffin-like cells and acetylcholine released from post-ganglionic parasympathetic neurons bind to H2 and M3 receptors, respectively, located on parietal cells. Binding of gastrin to cholecystokinin (CCK)-2 receptors on enterchromaffin-like cells stimulates histamine release, and histamine then is free to bind to H2 receptors on parietal cells to promote gastric acid secretion.

Gastrin has also been shown to stimulate many aspects of gastric mucosal development and growth. Gastrin has trophic actions on the gastric mucosa by stimulating the production of members of the epidermal growth factor family, which in turn stimulate growth and hypertrophy of surface epithelial cells in the stomach and intestine.

Gastrin is secreted in response to chemical (e.g., elevated pH and protein) and mechanical (e.g., stomach distension) stimuli that act directly on the G cell and/or indirectly via adjacent neuroendocrine cells and neurons. The primary stimulus for secretion of gastrin by gastric G cells is the presence of certain foodstuffs (especially peptides, certain amino acids and calcium) in the gastric lumen. Secretion of gastrin is inhibited when the gastric luminal pH becomes too acidic (pH < 3) through a classic negative feedback loop. Circulating gastrin in the blood is inactivated by the kidney, liver, and small intestine.

Disease states that involve excessive gastrin secretion

Excessive secretion of gastrin, also referred to as hypergastrinemia, is a well-recognized cause of a rare but severe disease known as Zollinger–Ellison syndrome, which has been reported in dogs, cats, and human beings. The hallmark of this disorder is gastric and duodenal ulceration resulting from excessive and unregulated secretion of gastric acid. Most commonly, this is the result of a gastrin-secreting tumor (gastrinoma) arising in either the pancreas or the duodenum.

A gastrinoma tumor is an example of an APUDoma-type GI tumor. While a gastrinoma is the most serious and potentially life-threatening cause for hypergastrinemia, other causes for elevations in serum gastrin include collection of a postprandial blood sample, renal failure, gastric obstruction, pyloric stenosis, gastric dilatation and volvulus, atrophic gastritis, prior small intestinal resection leading to short bowel syndrome, and administration of certain antacid drugs (H2 blockers, proton pump inhibitors). Because the liver is responsible for the breakdown of gastrin, diffuse and severe liver disease can also lead to hypergastrinemia due to the resulting prolonged half-life of the hormone.

Gastrinoma

A gastrinoma is a rare, malignant, neuroendocrine tumor arising from either delta islet pancreatic cells or from G cells within the duodenum. In dogs and in cats, the majority of reported cases have had a pancreatic mass.

In 1955, Zollinger and Ellison were the first to describe a triad of gastric acid hypersecretion, a non-beta-cell pancreatic islet cell tumor, and GI ulceration that has come to be called the Zollinger–Ellison syndrome. As in dogs, gastrinomas in people resulting in clinical symptoms compatible with the Zollinger–Ellison syndrome can arise from either the pancreas or an extrapancreatic (renal, duodenum) site. In people, duodenal gastrinomas are the most common form of this tumor. Rare cases of gastrinomas arising within a lymph node or the kidney have also been reported in people.

Signalment

Most dogs diagnosed with gastrinoma are middle-aged (mean 8.2 years; range 3.5–12.0 years of age). Only a few feline cases have been reported; affected cats were middle-aged (mean age 10–12 years). No breed predilection for this tumor exists.

Clinical signs

Clinical signs seen with gastrinoma result from an excessive secretion of gastrin by the tumor, which leads to gastric acid hypersecretion, gastric mucosal hypertrophy, GI ulceration, melena, and malassimilation secondary to digestive enzyme inactivation and bile salt precipitation.

The most common clinical signs are vomiting and weight loss. Other signs include depression, lethargy, anorexia, hematemesis, hematochezia, melena, and abdominal pain. Collapse and signs of shock have been reported with acute perforation of a gastric ulcer leading to peritonitis. Physical examination findings may vary from being unremarkable to findings compatible with shock. Pale mucus membranes, tachycardia, abdominal pain, emaciation, and fever are other signs that have been reported. In one feline case, an abdominal mass was palpated, but generally, these tumors are too small to be detected on physical examination.

Laboratory findings

Anemia (regenerative or nonregenerative), secondary to GI bleeding, may be seen on the CBC. In addition, neutrophilia may be seen due to the inflammation associated with GI ulceration. Findings on a serum biochemistry profile can include panhypoproteinemia compatible with GI hemorrhage, electrolyte abnormalities (hypokalemia, hypochloridemia) secondary to vomiting, and elevations in liver enzymes from inflammatory disease or from tumor metastasis. Hyperbilirubinemia, from compression of the bile duct by the pancreatic or duodenal mass, has also been reported. A metabolic alkalosis, with or without aciduria, may occur if the tumor causes an upper GI obstruction.

Imaging

Abdominal radiographs are usually unremarkable; however, a perforating ulcer and subsequent peritonitis may result in loss of serosal detail and free abdominal air. A radiographic upper GI contrast study may reveal gastric wall thickening and gastroduodenal ulceration. Abdominal ultrasound may reveal a thickened gastric wall or pylorus, evidence of metastatic disease to the liver, spleen, regional lymph nodes, and other organs, and in rare cases, the primary tumor in the pancreas or duodenum may be visualized. Failure to detect a pancreatic or duodenal tumor using ultrasound does not rule out a gastrinoma. CT or MRI with intravenous contrast administration should be performed if a gastrinoma is suspected as these imaging modalities have a higher sensitivity than ultrasound for the detection of pancreatic tumors and metastases.

Thoracic radiographs with three views to check for evidence of pulmonary metastasis are indicated but rarely will show evidence of visible metastasis.

Upper GI endoscopy may show evidence of rugal and pyloric antrum hypertrophy, gastric or duodenal ulceration and hemorrhage, and possibly, evidence of reflux esophagitis (erythema, erosions, and ulceration). Endoscopic ultrasound, which is currently not readily available in veterinary medicine, is highly useful for localizing these tumors within the pancreas and duodenum in humans.

Diagnosis

Most commonly, the diagnosis of a gastrinoma is made based on the presence of elevated levels of serum gastrin in a fasted patient (fasting hypergastrinemia), detection of a pancreatic mass using imaging, signs consistent with gastroduodenal ulceration, and subsequent confirmation using immunohistochemistry to stain for gastrin in the excised tumor.

An elevated fasting serum gastrin concentration is expected, but in some dogs with confirmed gastrinomas, gastrin levels have been low or normal. Other causes for elevated gastrin levels need to be ruled out or considered, including collection of a postprandial blood sample, renal failure, gastric obstruction, pyloric stenosis, gastric dilatation and volvulus, atrophic gastritis, prior small intestinal resection leading to short bowel syndrome, hepatic disease, and administration of certain antacid drugs (H2 blockers, proton pump inhibitors).

Provocative testing involves the measurement of gastrin levels before and after administration of secretin or calcium to stimulate gastrin secretion. This test is performed in people with suspected gastrinomas but has not been widely adopted for domestic animals. Provocative testing by injecting secretin or calcium into an artery supplying the viscera can be combined with hepatic venous sampling to help locate some tumors that are not visible with advanced imaging and that are not visible at the time of surgery.

Scintigraphy using [111]iridium-octreotide acetate or pentetreoctide (SST analogue) to bind to receptors expressed on gastrinomas has facilitated localization of tumors and metastatic lesions in people. Such diagnostic techniques are not widely used in veterinary medicine at the current time.

Definitive confirmation relies on immunohistochemical staining of surgical biopsies for gastrin.

Differential diagnoses for GI ulceration include drug administration (NSAIDs, steroids), ingestion of toxic chemical irritants, stress associated with shock, sepsis, multiple organ dysfunction syndrome (MODS), strenuous exercise, neurological disease (head trauma, intervertebral disk disease), metabolic disease (liver, kidney, pancreatitis, hypoadrenocorticism), inflammatory bowel disease or GI neoplasia, systemic mastocytosis, other APUDoms, and GI motility disorders.

Treatment

The treatment of choice for a gastrinoma involves surgical excision; however, the cure rate with surgery is low because the metastatic rate in dogs, as in people, is high at the time of initial diagnosis. In addition to excision of the primary tumor, surgery may also permit resection of deep or perforated ulcers and visible metastatic lesions.

Chemoembolization, hepatic transplantation, radiofrequency ablation, and hepatic cryosurgery are other treatment modalities used in people to relieve symptoms and to reduce tumor burdens. Tumor-targeted radioactive treatment, also called receptor-mediated radiotherapy, using a radionucleotide-labeled somatostatin analogue is an option in the selected group of patients with tumors that have a strong uptake of [^{111}In]pentaoctreotide (OctreoScan) documented with scintigraphy.

For nonresectable tumors, a combination of medical management plus or minus surgical debulking of the tumor is the best option.

Medical management involves the use of antacids, gastroprotectants, and possibly, other adjunctive therapies (chemotherapy and octreotide acetate) to reduce the hypersecretion of gastric acid, reduce the clinical effects of gastric hyperacidity, and/or inhibit hormonal secretion from the tumor itself. The infiltrative nature of the tumor and high metastatic rate makes medical management the only tenable option in the majority of our patients where diagnosis is often made late in the clinical course of the disease.

Reducing hypersecretion of gastric acid can be accomplished using H2 blockers to prevent histamine-mediated parietal cell gastric acid secretion or by the administration of more potent proton pump inhibitors. The use of proton pump inhibitors has largely replaced the use of H2 blockers for the treatment of a gastrinoma. Proton pump blockers available include omeprazole, lansoprazole, and pantoprazole. For patients with bleeding ulcers, sucralfate and or misoprostol can also be administered to promote healing.

Long-acting SST analogues such as octreotide acetate have also been effective for controlling symptoms in dogs and in people with metastatic disease. These drugs reduce gastric hyperacidity by directly inhibiting tumor cell secretion of gastrin and indirectly by binding to high affinity SST receptors on gastric parietal cells. Addition of alpha interferon to the somatostatin analogue has been shown in one human study to be beneficial. The use of these drugs in nonfunctioning gastrinomas is controversial.

A range of different chemotherapeutic agents have also been used to treat metastatic disease with limited short-term survival benefit. Streptozotocin as a sole agent or in combination with 5-flurouracil, dacarbazine, and epirubicin has been shown to be effective for palliative therapy for metastatic disease in people.

Prognosis

Long-term prognosis for dogs diagnosed with a gastrinoma at the current time is grave with survival times following diagnosis ranging from 1 to 18 months in one study ($n = 4$). The primary determinants of long-term survival in people are tumor size at diagnosis and liver metastasis.

The kinins

The kininogen–kallikrein–kinin (KKK) system, is a complex multiprotein system that is a metabolic cascade that, when activated, triggers the release of vasoactive polypeptides called kinins. The kinins that are produced by the activation of the KKK system participate in the acute phase inflammatory response and in the intrinsic coagulation system. In addition, there is mounting evidence that the KKK system is also involved in the regulation of blood pressure and plays a role in renal and cardiac function.

Pathophysiology of kinins

There are two main pathways by which kinins are generated. The plasma KKK system, by far the more complex, initiates activation of the intrinsic coagulation pathway and is involved in the acute inflammatory response through the activation of complement. The second and simpler tissue KKK system generates kinin through the action of tissue kallikrein. Each of these enzyme systems may play different roles in the body.

The plasma KKK system, also called the contact system of plasma, consists of three serine proenzymes (coagulation factor XII or Hageman factor, factor XI, and prekallikrein) and the kinin precursor high molecular weight kininogen (HMWK). The contact of plasma with a negatively charged surface leads to the binding and autoactivation of factor XII. Factor XII activation is not only a first step in the initiation of the intrinsic clotting cascade and the generation of kinins but it also leads to the activation of the complement pathway.

Tissue kallikrein is widely distributed (kidney, blood vessels, CNS, pancreas, gut, salivary and sweat glands, spleen, adrenal, and neutrophils) and this wide distribution suggests a paracrine (local) function. The regulatory mechanism of tissue kallikrein remains partly unknown.

Almost all cells express kinin receptors, such as the vascular endothelium, primary sensory afferent neurons, vascular and nonvascular smooth muscle, epithelial cells, and perhaps some types of leukocytes. Receptor stimulation causes increased vascular permeability, relaxation of venular smooth muscle, hypotension, contraction of intestinal smooth muscle, contraction of the smooth muscle in the airways (increasing airway resistance), stimulation of sensory neurons (pain), alteration of ion secretion by epithelial cells, production of nitric oxide (vasodilator), release of cytokines by leukocytes, and release of eicosanoids from various cell types. The various pharmacological effects derive from the presence of these receptors on various cell types.

Circulating levels of kinin peptides are typically very low in health. Tissue levels of kinin peptides are higher than circulating levels, consistent with tissues being the main site of formation of kinin peptides. Very high levels of kinin peptides are measured during acute inflammation particularly during episodes of acute allergic reactions resulting in angioedema.

Clinical disease states and applications

Research has helped shed light on the role of the KKK system. Recent findings suggest a possible role in blood pressure regulation.

Inhibition of angiotensin-converting enzymes (ACEs) with ACE inhibitors, which are commonly used drugs in dogs and in cats with cardiac or renal diseases, leads to a decrease in angiotensin II (a vasoconstrictor) but also to an increase in kinin end products (bradykinin) due to decreased degradation. This explains why some patients on angiotensin-converting enzyme inhibitors (ACEIs) develop a dry cough, and some react with angioedema, a dangerous swelling of the head and neck region. Contact activation of the plasma KKK system with dialyzer membranes may also account for why some canine and feline patients have an anaphylactic reaction during hemodialysis. It has also been hypothesized that many of the beneficial effects of ACE inhibitors may be due to their influence on the KKK system. This includes their effects when used for the treatment of arterial hypertension, ventricular remodeling (after myocardial infarction), and possibly, for diabetic nephropathy.

Although the pathophysiology of sepsis remains largely unknown, experimental and clinical data point to a role of kinins in inducing sepsis through the activation of the complement cascade, consumption of contact activating factors in the intrinsic coagulation pathway, and by promoting vasodilation and increased vascular permeability. All of these mechanisms can contribute to hypotension, edema, and disseminated intravascular coagulation (DIC) with shock. A significant increase of plasma bradykinin was also measured in patients suffering from *Staphylococcus aureus* sepsis. These observations could open a new area for the clinical application of B2R antagonists (receptor antagonists for the end products of the KKK system).

Melatonin

The pineal gland is located near the center of the brain between the two thalamic bodies, in the space between the two cerebral hemispheres on the roof of the third ventricle. There are two types of cells within the pineal gland: pinealocytes and glial cells. The main function of the pineal gland is the production of the hormone melatonin, which is synthesized and secreted by the pinealocytes.

Pathophysiology of melatonin

The synthesis and secretion of melatonin by the pineal gland is synchronized to diurnal circadian rhythms (the dark–light cycle). During the daytime when it is light, synthesis and secretion are decreased such that serum concentrations are undetectable. At night when it is dark, synthesis and secretion increase dramatically. The pineal gland is unique in this way, as it is the only endocrine gland to have its secretion directly tied to information received from the retina.

Information from retinal photoreceptors is transmitted to higher brain centers in the hypothalamus and from there to the pineal gland via the superior cervical ganglia and postganglionic adrenergic sympathetic neurons. Changes in the levels of noradrenaline (NA) ensure proper translation of the light information (via the circadian clock) into melatonin synthesis by the pineal gland.

The overall amount of melatonin that is secreted over a 24-h period is determined by the length of the photoperiod. Other factors besides the photoperiod that may influence pineal gland secretion of melatonin include ambient temperature and dietary factors, such as the availability of tryptophan, folate, and vitamin B_6.

Melatonin is synthesized from a dietary amino acid precursor, L-tryptophan. The rate of melatonin formation depends on the activity of two enzymes: serotonin N-acetyltransferase (AANAT) and, to a lesser extent, tryptophan hydroxylase (TPH), which controls the availability of serotonin, an important intermediate within the pathway. The expression of these two rate-limiting enzymes in melatonin secretion fluctuates in a clock-driven circadian rhythm, with high concentrations occurring during the night and low to negligible concentrations occurring in the daylight. Once synthesized, melatonin is not stored within the pineal gland but is released directly into the cerebrospinal fluid (CSF) and blood to exert its biological actions by binding to melatonin receptors in various tissues.

There are two major classes of melatonin membrane-bound receptors (ML1 and ML2 receptors) that belong to a superfamily of G protein-coupled receptors. The different classes of melatonin receptors are differentially expressed in different tissues; this varied distribution is important in implementing the various biological effects of melatonin. The highest density of melatonin receptors has been found in the hypothalamus, the anterior pituitary, and the retina. Receptors are also found in several other areas of the brain (cerebral cortex, thalamus, hippocampus, and cerebellum) and in several peripheral tissues, including the adrenal gland, arteries and heart, lung, liver, kidney, small intestine, skin, and on T and B lymphocytes.

More than 90% of circulating melatonin is deactivated by the liver and a very small amount is excreted unchanged in the urine.

Functions of melatonin

With its secretion being tied to a circadian rhythm, melatonin has been implicated in the regulation of various neural and endocrine processes that are cued by the daily change in the photoperiod. This includes regulation of the seasonal effects on reproduction, body weight, pelage (coat growth and color) in some species, appetite, and activity and hibernation. Melatonin has also been shown to be important in the neuroendocrine control of puberty in animals and has been implicated in playing an important role in the modulation of retinal function.

Reproduction

Melatonin is considered an antigonadotropic hormone; by inhibiting the release of gonadotropin-releasing hormone (GnRH) from the hypothalamus, it inhibits the release of the gonadotropic hormones (luteinizing hormone and follicle-stimulating hormone) from the anterior pituitary gland. In some wild and domestic species, these hormonal effects play an essential role in determining the timing of the breeding season.

In some species, melatonin secretion, influenced by seasonal variations, determines the timing of puberty, provided that a sufficient degree of physical maturity has been reached.

Miscellaneous effects

There is evidence that melatonin may influence circadian aspects of glucose homeostasis, the immune system, and cardiovascular function. Melatonin receptors are expressed in several skin cells (including normal and malignant keratinocytes, melanocytes, and fibroblasts), and it has been experimentally implicated in skin functions such as hair growth cycling and fur pigmentation. Melatonin is able to suppress ultraviolet (UV)-induced damage to skin cells and shows strong antioxidant activity in UV-exposed cells. It is believed to play a role in the development of cancer of melanocytes (melanoma).

Clinical disease states and applications

Reproduction in domestic ruminants and the desired winter fur coat of animals farmed for their fur such as mink, arctic foxes, and cashmere goats can be manipulated by photoperiod and melatonin implant administration. Due to melatonin's effect on the fur coat and the skin, it has been used with variable success to treat a variety of dermatologic problems in dogs including canine acanthosis nigricans, canine recurrent flank alopecia, canine pattern baldness, sex hormone-responsive alopecia, and alopecia X in Pomeranians and in artic dog breeds.

Melatonin has also been recommended for the treatment of atypical HAC. Melatonin is particularly recommended for the treatment of mild cases because it is cheap, has few side effects compared to other treatments for adrenal disease, and is readily available through health food stores. While typical HAC results from excess production of cortisol, atypical HAC, alopecia X, and sex hormone-responsive alopecia refer to HAC caused by increased levels of intermediate adrenal steroids. It is now recognized that other steroids besides cortisol have a negative feedback effect on the hypothalamic–pituitary axis, and steroid profiling in dogs and cats has led to the realization that HAC can be due to primary adrenal tumors that secrete other steroids besides cortisol.

In vitro cell culture studies have shown that both 21-hydroxylase and aromatase enzymes, two enzymes in the steroid synthesis pathway, are inhibited by melatonin. Inhibition of the 21-hydroxylase enzyme should lower cortisol production and secretion, and inhibition of the aromatase enzyme should lower estradiol production and secretion by adrenal cortical cells. In dogs with adrenal disease treated with melatonin, cortisol levels are consistently reduced, and estradiol levels are variably reduced when extended adrenal steroid panel values after treatment are compared to pretreatment values.

Treatment of cases of mild adrenal disease, particularly cases where sex steroids are increased, is often initiated with melatonin alone or melatonin with phytoestrogens. If clinical response over time is less than desired, then the addition of a maintenance dose of mitotane can be added to the treatment regimen.

Although there is no scientific data from clinical trials to support its use, melatonin has also been used as a sedative and anxiolytic for the treatment of behavioral problems in dogs such as separation anxiety and anxiety associated with thunderstorms or fireworks. It has also been used in the management of idiopathic epilepsy to reduce the risk of epileptic seizures at night. Finally, melatonin has also been used for the treatment of canine cognitive dysfunction. It is used for its sedative effects, to treat restlessness associated with this condition, and to improve the quality of sleep.

Formulations of melatonin

The use of melatonin in dogs must be considered experimental at this time. There is no information on possible harmful long-term side effects in dogs or in any other species. Melatonin is easily synthesized and is available as tablets or capsules and as a constant-release SC implant. However, because melatonin is classified as a nutriceutical, not a drug, there is a lack of standardization in existing products. This means that there may be variable drug content within and between preparations, as well as variable absorption and bioavailability between products.

For oral dosing, typically a dose of 3 mg is given q 12 h for dogs <15 kg and a dose of 6 mg is given q 12 h for dogs >15 kg. Regular melatonin is typically used, rather than rapid release or extended-release products. Subcutaneous melatonin implants are available for dogs in 8, 12 and 18 mg doses. The effects of these implants last 3–4 months. Unfortunately, some dogs have experienced sterile abscesses or granulomas at the site of implantation.

At least 4 months must be allowed to determine if there is any response to treatment with melatonin, and the response time is variable between dogs. Response to treatment is monitored by improvement in clinical signs, by improvement in serum biochemical abnormalities, or by repeat of steroid profiles.

Natriuretic peptides

Atrial natriuretic peptides (ANP) belong to a family of structurally related peptide hormones that inhibit tubular reabsorption of sodium ions in the glomerulus. Natriuretic peptides also include brain natriuretic peptide (BNP) and C-type natriuretic peptide (CNP). ANP is synthesized mainly by cells in the cardiac atria and BNP is synthesized mainly by cells of the cardiac ventricles and atria, but both can be produced by cells of other tissues (including the brain, pituitary gland, lung, and kidney). Both ANP and BNP are released as hormones into the bloodstream and they have paracrine (local) effects. CNP is produced by the vascular endothelium of many organs and appears to exert exclusively autocrine (self-stimulation) and paracrine effects within the vasculature. Through the production of ANP and BNP, the heart is recognized as an important endocrine organ that plays a role in the regulation of blood pressure, blood volume, and electrolyte balance.

Pathophysiology of natriuretic peptides

The primary stimulus for ANP release is stretch of the cardiac atria in response to expansion of the intravascular volume. Secretion of ANP is also stimulated in response to some vasoactive substances (e.g., angiotensin II, catecholamines, endothelin-1, and vasopressin). Secretion of ANP is inhibited by nitric oxide and by intravascular volume depletion (e.g., dehydration, hemorrhage) and hypotension. Stretch of the cardiac atria and ventricles with intravascular volume expansion is the primary stimulus for the release of BNP, but angiotensin II, hypoxia, α1-adrenoceptor agonists, endothelin-1, transforming growth factor-β, and vasopressin can also stimulate release.

Functions of natriuretic peptides

ANP and BNP possess diuretic, natriuretic, and hypotensive activity. They promote vasodilation and counteract the vasoconstrictive and sodium-retaining effects of the renin–angiotensin–aldosterone system (RAAS). ANP, BNP, and CNP also inhibit the release and actions of vasopressin (ADH) and the secretion and actions of renin and aldosterone.

ANP has direct tubular actions that include inhibition of angiotensin II-stimulated sodium and water transport in the proximal convoluted tubules, which leads to a decrease in sodium reabsorption by the renal tubules. This is a dose-dependent effect and is a major aspect of the natriuretic and diuretic effects of ANP. With more chronic stimulation, ANP decreases blood pressure through another mechanism (involving a decrease in intravascular volume) resulting from increased permeability of the endothelium to water and macromolecules. ANP also induces dilation of arteries and veins in an endothelium-independent manner.

There is a large body of evidence supporting the fact that ANP and BNP have important autocrine/paracrine roles within the heart itself. These local actions may be particularly prominent in disease states and may involve cytoprotective actions in response to myocardial ischemia, possible vasodilator actions in the coronary vasculature, inhibitory effects on cardiac myocyte hypertrophy, and suppression of fibroblast proliferation.

The expression of ANP and BNP is increased in cardiac hypertrophy, dilation, and heart failure in response to atrial or ventricular wall stress. Systemic hypertension, which induces left ventricular hypertrophy, is also associated with increased plasma concentrations of ANP and BNP.

Clinical disease states and applications of natriuretic peptide measurement

The ELISA assays currently available for measurement of BNP measure the circulating concentrations of the N-terminal portion (N-terminal prohormone of atrial natriuretic peptide [NT-proANP] and N-terminal prohormone of brain natriuretic peptide [NT-proBNP]) of the protein (inactive prohormone fragments) rather than the biologically active peptide. This is because the N-terminal portion is less rapidly eliminated or degraded and reaches a higher concentration than the active portion (C-ANP and C-BNP).

In humans, the measurement of natriuretic peptide (NP) in blood has been shown to serve as a biomarker for underlying cardiac disease and is used in the diagnosis of CHF, differentiation of cardiac disease from respiratory disease, and to provide information regarding the risk of morbidity and mortality with cardiac diseases. In addition, NP has been used therapeutically for the treatment of patients in acute CHF.

The plasma half-lives of ANP, BNP, and CNP are similar at approximately 1–2 min. The assay used for measuring or detecting canine and feline ANPs in tissues is a human assay: The high level of homology between human, canine, and feline ANPs allows accurate measurement of circulating feline and canine ANPs using antibodies directed against the human peptide. This is not the case for BNP. A species-specific BNP assay must be used to measure circulating BNP in cats and dogs. Currently, BNP assays are available for the detection of C-BNP and NT-proBNP in humans, and, in general, the diagnostic utilities of the tests are similar. In dogs and cats, a commercial test is available to detect NT-proBNP, for which recent clinical data are available.

The strongest indication for BNP or NT-proBNP testing is to help rule out or confirm a diagnosis of volume overload due to CHF in dogs and cats. The test has little diagnostic value in patients already having clear evidence of heart failure based on conventional diagnostic tests but has proven to be useful for differentiating whether symptoms in a patient are due to cardiac or respiratory disease when conventional diagnostics are inconclusive. This is especially important in geriatric small breed dogs that commonly suffer from both cardiac diseases (e.g., mitral valve endocardiosis) and airway diseases (e.g., chronic bronchitis or tracheal or bronchial airway collapse). It is also useful for cats that present with signs of respiratory distress, when it cannot be determined from the history, physical examination, or radiographs whether dyspnea is from respiratory or cardiac disease.

Two veterinary studies have evaluated the use of the NT-proBNP assay in evaluating the presence of early heart failure in dogs with respiratory signs. The results of these studies closely mimic those in humans, wherein the likelihood of heart failure is very high when the NT-proBNP concentration is high but very low when the NT-proBNP concentration is low. In the first study, 46 dogs with respiratory distress or coughing were examined and the results showed that the median NT-proBNP concentration was significantly higher in dogs with heart failure than in dogs with respiratory diseases such as chronic bronchitis, infection, or neoplasia. In the second study, NT-proBNP concentration >1158 pmol/L was found to differentiate dogs with CHF from dogs with respiratory disease with a relatively high accuracy of 83.6%.

Three feline studies have investigated the utility of natriuretic peptides to distinguish cardiac from noncardiac causes of respiratory distress in cats, when the compromised state of cats with severe respiratory distress often limits other diagnostic testings (e.g., radiography and echocardiography). The studies have included cats with a wide range of causes for heart and respiratory disease, and results from all three studies suggest that circulating NT-proBNP concentrations can be used to reliably discriminate cats with CHF (caused by different types of cardiomyopathy) from those with primary respiratory disease as the cause of respiratory distress.

Another possible indication for measurement of serum NT-proBNP is the identification of patients with asymptomatic or occult cardiomyopathies or the identification of feline patients with hypertension. However, to date, the few studies done suggest that BNP or NT-proBNP only have a limited role in the detection of occult cardiomyopathy in dogs and cats. Because NT-proBNP testing reveals information specific to a single time point and a normal value does not exclude the possibility of disease in the future, this test is not considered a good screening test.

Measurement of NT-proBNP in one study has shown promise as a diagnostic marker for systemic hypertension in cats. The use of this test was able to distinguish hypertensive from normotensive cats with a sensitivity of 80% and a specificity of 93% using a cutoff value of greater than or equal to 203 pmol/L. This could be very useful for detecting clinically significant hypertension in cats where assessment of blood pressure measurements is difficult to interpret due to a "white coat effect" possibly causing transient hypertension. Coexistence of other comorbidities, such as severe CKD and myocardial disease, will need to be ruled out in order to accurately interpret the finding of an elevated NT-proBNP in any cat where this test is done to screen for hypertension.

Another indication for BNP or NT-proBNP testing has been for the assessment of a patient's risk of morbidity and mortality related to cardiac disease. In people, practice guidelines indicate that either one-time or serial testing can be used to assess a patient's risk for death or to track a patient's clinical status with the risk of death increasing by 35% for every 100-ng/L increase in BNP level above the reference range. A final indication for BNP

or NT-proBNP testing is to help guide therapy. Only time will tell whether NP concentrations in dogs or cats are useful in assessing the risk of morbidity and mortality or in guiding therapy.

Practicalities and limitations of BNP and NT-proBNP testing

Limitations for BNP and NT-proBNP testing include the existence of concurrent diseases that can affect results (e.g., renal disease and systemic hypertension) and issues with stability following collection. BNP and NT-proBNP are both partially excreted by the kidney so circulating levels can be elevated in cats and dogs with renal disease and decreased glomerular filtration rate. In two separate veterinary studies, a significantly higher mean NT-proBNP concentration was documented in azotemic dogs when compared with healthy control dogs. Renal disease can therefore influence concentrations of ANP and BNP in cats and dogs.

Hypertension could affect plasma NP concentrations because of its effects on atrial stretch. Plasma NT-proBNP concentrations are significantly higher in cats with hypertensive CKD compared with normal cats and those with normotensive CKD. Furthermore, in cats where treatment with the vasodilator amlodipine resulted in normalization of blood pressure, a significant reduction in plasma NT-proBNP concentration was seen. These results show that hypertension does influence NT-proBNP concentrations in cats.

In humans, circulating NP concentrations are also influenced by obesity, pulmonary hypertension, pulmonary embolism, sepsis, hyperthyroidism, and age. The influences of these factors on feline and canine NP concentrations have not yet been definitively established.

The administration of medications that have the potential to alter volume status (i.e., diuretics) must also be accounted for when interpreting results of BNP and NT-proBNP testing. It has also been shown that there is a high degree of weekly variability with respect to NT-proBNP concentrations. As such, NT-proBNP values must be carefully interpreted in the light of each patient's complete clinical picture.

It is important to realize that sample handling and assay performance can affect results. It is likely these factors (variation in sample handling, storage conditions, shipping conditions, and potential variation in NP concentration between plasma or serum samples) have played a role in the conflicting results seen in feline and canine studies evaluating the diagnostic utility of these assays for detection of occult cardiomyopathies. The half-life of canine BNP is very short (approximately 90 s), and although NT-proBNP is thought to be more stable, sample collection, handling, and shipping protocols can affect results. The *ex vivo* stability of canine NT-proBNP is highly time and temperature dependent. Canine and feline NT-proBNP samples should be collected into ethylenediaminetetraacetic acid (EDTA) lavender top tubes, spun immediately, and samples should either be transported to an external laboratory frozen or in manufacturer-supplied pink top tubes that contain a protease inhibitor. At present, no patient side test currently exists.

Currently, there are several available canine- and feline-specific NT-proBNP ELISA assays. Since the introduction of this test, the assay for canine NT-proBNP has also undergone several changes, and differences in assay performance as well as sample handling have likely contributed to important differences in the reference ranges and diagnostic cutoff points reported in different clinical studies.

Therapeutic uses of natriuretic peptides

While no studies have been done in veterinary patients to assess the therapeutic use of natriuretic peptides, there are data from human studies. In CHF, both the RAAS and the natriuretic peptide systems are activated, and as heart failure worsens, the activities of both systems increase. However, there is a relative imbalance between these two systems with the net effect favoring vasoconstriction as well as fluid and sodium retention, especially in the later stages of heart disease.

Given the diuretic, natriuretic, and vasodilating activities of ANP, shortly after its discovery cardiologists hypothesized that ANP might be useful for the treatment of CHF. In Japan, recombinant ANP (carperitide) is licensed for intravenous administration in patients with CHF and is used to treat acute crises. In clinical trials, transient low dose ANP infusion has been shown to improve the long-term prognosis in patients with acutely decompensated heart failure (ADHF). Inhibition of the RAAS and the antioxidant effect of low dose infusion of ANP are the mechanisms believed to be responsible for the long-term beneficial effect.

The renal-protective effect of ANP infusion has been demonstrated in human patients during cardiac bypass surgery and in patients receiving potentially nephrotoxic intravenous contrast reagents for cardiac catheterization.

In addition to the administration of synthetic natriuretic peptides, the development of neutral endopeptidase inhibitors and NPR antagonists has also facilitated the investigation of the physiological and pathophysiological effects of natriuretic peptides. Administration of drugs that inhibit neutral endopeptidase has been shown to reduce blood pressure in dogs with hypertension secondary to experimentally induced renal disease. Their administration may be useful for inducing diuresis for the treatment of patients that were inadvertently overhydrated and are in danger of developing life-threatening pulmonary edema.

Renin

Renin is the initial hormone released in the cascade referred to as the renin–angiotension–aldosterone system (RAAS). The RAAS plays a vital role in regulating salt, blood volume, and systemic vascular resistance, which together influence cardiac output and arterial pressure.

Pathophysiology of renin

Renin is a proteolytic enzyme that is secreted exclusively by the juxtaglomerular cells located in the walls of renal afferent arterioles in the kidneys. It is synthesized as an inactive zymogen called prorenin, and the juxtaglomerular cells are capable of secreting both renin and prorenin.

Release

Renin's release is stimulated by sympathetic nerve activation (acting via β_1-adrenoceptors), renal artery hypotension (caused by systemic hypotension or renal artery stenosis), or decreased sodium delivery to the distal tubules of the kidney. Inhibition of renin secretion by juxtaglomerular cells is regulated by a negative feedback loop with angiotensin II, high blood pressure, high plasma sodium, and volume overload all inhibiting renin secretion.

Action

In addition to renin, the other two important hormones involved in the RAAS system are angiotensin II and aldosterone. When renin is released into the blood, it acts upon a circulating substrate, angiotensinogen, which undergoes proteolytic cleavage to form angiotensin I in the liver. Vascular endothelium, particularly in the lungs, has an enzyme, ACE, which cleaves off two amino acids from angiotensin I to form the enzyme angiotensin II. Angiotensin II has several very important functions: It constricts resistance vessels, thereby increasing systemic vascular resistance and increasing the systemic arterial pressure. Angiotensin II also acts on the adrenal cortex to promote the release of aldosterone, which in turn acts on the kidneys to increase sodium and water retention in addition to promoting urinary excretion of potassium and protons. Angiotensin II also stimulates the release of vasopressin (ADH) from the posterior pituitary, which increases fluid retention by the kidneys; and finally, angiotensin II stimulates thirst centers within the brain and facilitates the release of norepinephrine from sympathetic nerve endings and inhibits norepinephrine reuptake by nerve endings, thereby enhancing sympathetic adrenergic function.

The renin–angiotensin–aldosterone pathway is regulated not only by the mechanisms that stimulate renin release, but it is also modulated by natriuretic peptides (ANP and BNP) released by the heart. These natriuretic peptides act as an important counter-regulatory system (Figure 2.6.1).

Clinical disease states and applications

Therapeutic manipulation of the RAAS pathway is very important in treating patients with hypertension, heart failure, and renal disease (especially suspected cases of glomerulonephritis). ACE inhibitors, angiotensin II and aldosterone receptors blockers, for example, are used to decrease arterial pressure, ventricular afterload, blood volume, and hence, ventricular preload, as well as inhibit and reverse cardiac and vascular hypertrophy for patients with cardiac disease. ACE inhibitors have also been shown to have renoprotective effects in the treatment of glomerulonephritis, and in some species, they are beneficial for slowing the progression of CKD.

Measurement of plasma renin

Measurement of plasma renin activity (PRA), along with, possibly, measurement of other hormones such as aldosterone,

Renin–angiotensin–aldosterone system

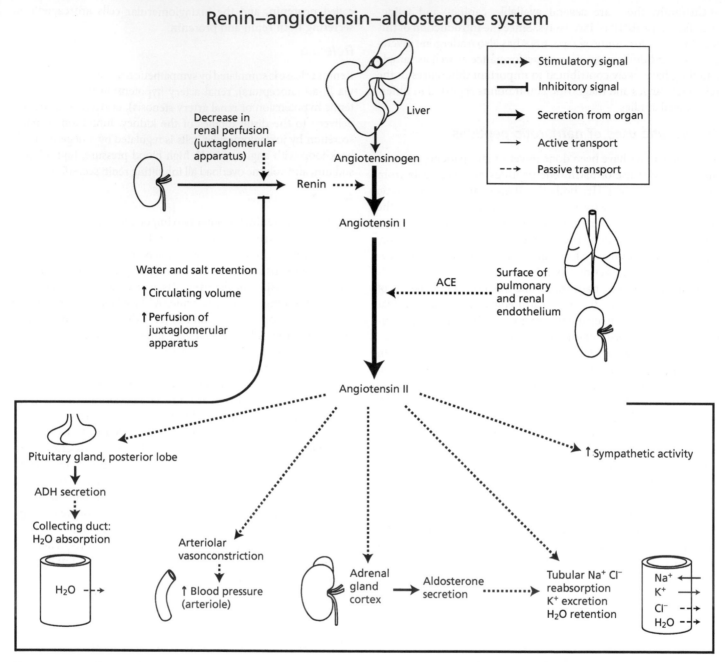

Figure 2.6.1   Pathways of the rennin–angiotensin–aldosterone system (RAAS). Illustration by Juliane Deubner, medical illustrator, Western College of Veterinary Medicine.

catecholamines, and glucocorticoids in dogs and cats may be indicated in patients with systemic hypertension where conventional diagnostics (imaging, serum biochemistry profile, other endocrine testing) have failed to reveal an underlying cause. Measurement of plasma renin or PRA can also be useful for cases of suspected hypoadrenocorticism, especially if a selective deficiency of only mineralocorticoids is suspected. Most cases of primary hypoadrenocorticism (Addison's disease) result from an immune-mediated attack of the adrenal cortex and result in a deficiency of both glucocorticoids and mineralocorticoids. The diagnosis is usually made by measuring the plasma cortisol con-

centration before and after stimulation with ACTH. An alternative approach for diagnosing primary hypocortisolism and hypoaldosteronism in cases of suspected primary hypoadrenocorticism is to determine changes in the interrelationships of relevant endogenous hormones. This dual assessment is particularly relevant when an isolated hormone deficiency is suspected. The occurrence of isolated glucocorticoid deficiency and isolated mineralocorticoid deficiency in dogs has been reported. In one study where PRA and aldosterone concentrations were measured along with plasma cortisol and ACTH concentrations in dogs with primary hypoadrenocorticism and were compared to concentrations in healthy dogs, there was an overlap in the plasma concentrations of cortisol, ACTH, and aldosterone and PRA between the two groups. However, when the ratio of cortisol : ACTH and aldosterone : renin activity was compared between groups, there was no overlap. From these observations, measurement of these endogenous variables (in one blood sample) with calculation of the two independent ratios allows the specific diagnoses of primary hypocortisolism and primary hypoaldosteronism in dogs with primary hypoadrenocorticism and could be used as an alternative to ACTH stimulation testing, which only evaluates for hypocortisolemia.

Measurements in patients with unexplained persistent hypokalemia, patients with renal tumors associated with hypertension, and patients with adrenal tumors suspected to be secreting aldosterone are other indications for measuring plasma rennin or PRA. With primary hyperaldosteronism caused by an adrenal tumor-secreting aldosterone, plasma aldosterone concentrations will be high in the face of normal or low PRA. With renal tumors secreting renin causing hypertension both plasma renin and aldosterone should be elevated.

The most common methods for measuring plasma renin are the PRA assay and the renin immunoassay. In most current renin assays, enzymatic activity is what is measured, and protocols for this assay vary among laboratories. As for most laboratory variables, reference intervals for PRA should be generated by each laboratory. Concentrations could be altered by therapies including potassium supplementation, fluid therapy, and ACE inhibitors.

Somatostatin

SST was first discovered as a hormone secreted by the hypothalamus and was named for its ability to inhibit the release of GH from the anterior pituitary gland. However, it is now known that SST is produced by a wide variety of cell types throughout the body and that SST actually is a family of peptide hormones of variable length that regulate the endocrine system and affect neurotransmission and cell proliferation. SSTs can be thought of as inhibitory hormones based on their ability to suppress two key cellular processes: secretion and cell proliferation. Other names for STT produced by the hypothalamus include growth hormone release-inhibiting factor (GHIH) or somatotropin release-inhibiting factor (SRIF).

Pathophysiology of somatostatins

SSTs are produced by a variety of different cell types including other neuroendocrine cells widely distributed throughout the CNS and the peripheral nervous system, as well as in the pancreas and gut.

Secretion of SST is under the influence of a broad array of secretagogues (substance which causes another substance to be secreted) ranging from ions and nutrients to neuropeptides, neurotransmitters, classical hormones, growth factors, and cytokines.

SST acts by both endocrine and paracrine pathways to affect its target cells. The majority of SST in the blood appears to come from the pancreas and the GI tract. In most other organs, SST is secreted only locally and acts in a paracrine manner. The specificity of endogenous SST derives from the fact that it is produced mainly at local sites of action and that following release is rapidly inactivated by peptidases in the tissue and blood, thereby minimizing unwanted systemic effects.

SST acts through high affinity plasma membrane receptors (termed SSTRs). To date, five receptors for SST have been identified, and these all share common signaling pathways.

Function of somatostatin

Role in the regulation of growth hormone secretion

In the hypothalamus, SST is produced in neuroendocrine cells and is transported to the anterior pituitary gland by the hypothalamic-hypophyseal portal circulation where SST inhibits the secretion of GH from somatotrope cells. The SST neurons in the hypothalamus secrete SST in response to high circulating concentrations of GH or somatomedins to mediate negative feedback effects on GH release. Low circulating concentrations of these hormones inhibit the release of SST. In addition to inhibition of GH release by the pituitary, SST secreted from the hypothalamus also inhibits the release of TSH by the pituitary gland and so plays a limited role in thyroid hormone regulation.

Role in the regulation of gastrointestinal tract hormone secretion

Within the GI tract, SST is secreted by scattered delta cells in the GI epithelium and by neurons in the submucosa that are part of the enteric nervous system. SST in the GI tract has been shown to inhibit the secretion of virtually every GI hormone that has been tested, including gastrin, CCK, secretin, motilin, gastric inhibitory polypeptide (GIP), enteroglucagon, and vasoactive intestinal peptide (VIP). Through such actions, SST has a generalized inhibitory effect on gut exocrine secretion (gastric acid, pepsin, bile, colonic fluid). It suppresses motor activity generally as well, through inhibition of gastric emptying, gallbladder contraction, and small intestinal segmentation. Collectively, these activities seem to have the overall effect of decreasing the rate of nutrient absorption.

Role in the regulation of pancreatic enzyme and hormone secretion

SST is produced by delta pancreatic islet cells, which lie in close proximity to other islets cells that secrete insulin, glucagon, and pancreatic PP. SST in the pancreas acts primarily in a a paracrine manner inhibiting the secretion of insulin and glucagon. In this capacity, SST is important in the regulation of intermediary energy metabolism.

SST also inhibits secretions from the exocrine portion of the pancreas by inhibiting CCK-stimulated enzyme secretion and secretin-stimulated bicarbonate secretion.

Role in the regulation of neurotransmission

SST-positive neurons and fibers are abundantly distributed throughout the CNS and the peripheral nervous system with the notable exception of the cerebellum. SST is often referred to as having neuromodulatory activity within the nervous system and appears to have a variety of complex effects on neural transmission including having a role as a neurotransmitter. In this capacity, it has effects on cognitive, locomotor, sensory, and autonomic functions. It inhibits the release of dopamine from the midbrain and of norepinephrine, TRH, corticotrophin-releasing hormone (CRH), and endogenous SST from the hypothalamus.

Antiproliferative actions of somatostatin

In addition to its antisecretory effects, SST inhibits the release of constitutively secreted proteins such as growth factors and cytokines by unknown mechanisms. In contrast to the antisecretory properties of SST, its antiproliferative effects were relatively late in being recognized and came about largely through the use of long-acting analogues such as octreotide acetate in the early 1980s for the treatment of hormone hypersecretion from pancreatic, intestinal, and pituitary tumors. It was noted that SST not only blocked hormone hypersecretion from these tumors but also caused variable tumor shrinkage through an additional antiproliferative effect. The antiproliferative effects of SST have since been demonstrated in normal dividing cells (e.g., intestinal mucosal cells, activated lymphocytes, and inflammatory cells), as well as *in vivo* in solid tumors.

Miscellaneous functions of somatostatin

Many tumor cells have also been shown to produce SST in small amounts, and SST has been implicated as playing a role in the pathophysiology of several disease states including cancer, inflammation, DM, epilepsy, Alzheimer's disease, Huntington's disease, and AIDS.

Somatostatinoma: A rare neuroendocrine tumor

Somatostatinoma is a very rare neuroendocrine tumor comprising <1% of all gastroenteropancreatic endocrine neoplasms in people. Only a few have been reported in dogs. Most somatostatinomas derive from the SST-producing delta cells of the pancreas or the neuroendocrine cells of the digestive tract. Most somatostatinomas are carcinomas and have typically already metastasized by the time they are detected. Common sites of metastasis include the regional lymph nodes or the liver.

Since the clinical symptoms are often variable and nonspecific, a great many somatostatinomas are "incidentalomas" found during surgery for other disorders (e.g., cholelithiasis) or during GI imaging studies. Pathological examination of the surgical biopsies with immunohistochemical staining for SST provides the definitive diagnosis.

Treatment for a somatostatinoma largely depends on the site and size of the tumor and on the extent of the disease at the time of diagnosis. Surgical resection is the treatment of choice when

feasible. In cases of locally advanced disease or widespread metastases, tumor debulking, chemoembolization of the primary tumor and of hepatic metastases, chemotherapy, SSTR-analogues (octreotide acetate), and interferon-alpha can be used to control the clinical symptoms.

Pharmacological uses of somatostatin

Scintigraphy using [111]iridium-octreotide acetate or pentetreotide (SST analogue) that bind to receptors expressed on gastrinomas has facilitated the localization of tumors (gastrinoma, insulinomas, VIPomas) and metastatic lesions in people and, in rare cases, in dogs. Such diagnostic techniques are not widely used in veterinary medicine at the current time.

SST and its synthetic analogues are used clinically to treat a variety of pancreatic, pituitary, and GI neoplasms in people (e.g., insulinoma, somatotropinoma, gastrinoma, acromegaly). The first clinically useful synthetic analogue that was produced was octreotide acetate.

In veterinary patients, SST analogues have been used in the treatment of gastrinomas, carcinoid tumors, and insulinomas. Octreotide acetate (a long-acting synthetic analogue of SST that suppresses pituitary release of GH), although effective for the treatment of acromegaly in people, has not been reported effective in most cats with this condition.

Other rare neuroendocrine tumors

Neuroendocrine tumors are rare neoplasms that arise from the neuroendocrine cell system and have widely divergent clinical presentations. These tumors can be divided into two main groups: carcinoids and endocrine pancreatic tumors. These tumors are classified as functional if they are associated with a clinical syndrome related to hormone production or as nonfunctional if they are not associated with clinical symptoms of hormone release. Functioning islet tumors are further designated according to the main hormone produced and the related clinical syndrome, for example, insulinomas, gastrinomas, VIPomas, glucagonomas, and somatostatinomas. Nonfunctional islet tumors include tumors that make pancreatic PP, chromogranin A, peptide YY (PYY), and neurotensin but do not have signs associated with the hormone release. In addition to whether they are functional or not, carcinoid tumors are also further designated by their location (e.g., lung, gastric, duodenal, pancreatic, colonic, and rectal).

Pathogenesis

Neuroendocrine tumors are sometimes referred to as APUDomas (amine precursor uptake and decarboxylation), which indicates that the tumor cell types have the ability to accumulate amine precursors 3,4-dihydroxyphenylalanine (DOPA or 5-hydroxytryptophan [5-HTP]) and can decarboxylate them to produce biogenic amines (catecholamines or serotonin). In addition, many of these tumors also secrete one or more peptide hormones (i.e., VIPomas that secrete VIP, gastrinomas that secrete gastrin) that can be responsible for the clinical signs seen.

The term APUDoma was first coined in 1974 to signify that these tumor cells were of neural crest origin and had migrated during their embryonal development into other tissues such as the intestinal tract, pancreas, lung, and several endocrine glands. The term APUDoma has largely been abandoned in human medicine, but since it provides a convenient framework for explaining the multipotential capacity of these cells to produce various hormones and amines, it is still in use in veterinary medicine.

Clinical signs

The most common clinical syndrome associated with a neuroendocrine tumor in veterinary patients is a hypoglycemic syndrome related to insulin oversecretion by a pancreatic islet beta-cell tumor (insulinoma). In people, insulinomas are also one of the two most common types of neuroendocrine tumors; the other most common type of neuroendocrine tumor in people is a gastrinoma, which causes the Zollinger–Ellison syndrome. Gastrinomas are also reported in dogs and cats but are comparatively rare. Another type of functional neuroendocrine tumor that has been reported in dogs and in people is the glucagonoma syndrome. This syndrome is characterized by a skin rash referred to as NME in people and SND in dogs. All of the clinical signs seen are related to oversecretion of glucagon by this tumor. Please see their respective sections in this text.

Carcinoid tumors, secreting a variety of peptide hormones including SST, pancreatic PP, and 5-hydroxytryptamine (serotonin), have also been reported in dogs and in cats. These tumors have been documented in a variety of anatomical locations, including the stomach, liver, gallbladder, intestine, and lung. In humans, carcinoid neuroendocrine tumors are associated with the release of physiologically active substances, including 5-hydroxytryptamine (serotonin), 5-HTP, histamine, bradykinins, tachykinins, and prostaglandins, which cause the unique paraneoplastic carcinoid syndrome. Symptoms of paraneoplastic carcinoid syndrome vary widely depending on the vasoactive substance released but can include cutaneous flushing, diarrhea, endocardial plaque formation leading to right heart failure, and, in severe cases, can potentially cause a life-threatening syndrome with extensive cutaneous flushing combined with hypotension and severe frequent diarrhea manifesting as a "carcinoid crisis." One case of paroxysmal ventricular tachycardia and gastric ulceration in a boxer dog with an ileocecal carcinoid tumor has been reported with full clinical remission following surgical excision of the mass. In addition, syndromes of gallbladder dysfunction with GI hemorrhage and cholestasis associated with biliary carcinoids have been reported. However, in most carcinoid tumors in dogs and in cats, clinical signs mainly relate to GI signs (e.g., chronic vomiting and diarrhea) caused by obstruction or metastatic spread.

A VIPoma tumor is another type of neuroendocrine tumor that oversecretes vasoactive intestinal protein (VIP) causing a syndrome accompanied by extensive diarrhea, hypokalemia, and achlorhydria (decreased gastric acid production). This syndrome is referred to in people as the Verner–Morrison syndrome. Cutaneous flushing may occur due to vasodilatory effects. VIPoma tumors have not been reported in cats or in dogs; however, in people, these tumors are typically located in the pancreas and occasionally arise in other locations (e.g., lung or sympathetic ganglia).

Diagnosis

Diagnosis of neuroendocrine tumors is based on histopathologic diagnosis and immunohistochemistry for chromogranin A, synaptophysin, and other hormones (e.g., gastrin, glucagon, and insulin).

Pathology

Although there is a histological resemblance, carcinoid tumors must be differentiated from mast cell tumors or undifferentiated epithelial neoplasia by using a combination of routine hematoxylin and eosin (H&E) staining, special silver stains, immunohistochemistry with antibodies against chromogranin A, synaptophysin and other peptide hormones, and electron microscopy.

Laboratory testing

Depending on clinical symptoms, the measurement of other peptide hormones (e.g., gastrin and insulin) in plasma may also be indicated to establish a definitive diagnosis. In human medicine, chromogranin A is also measured in the plasma when screening for a neuroendocrine tumor, but this has not been reported in veterinary patients. Measurement of urinary hydroxyindolacetic acid (5-HIAA), a serotonin metabolite, is also important in the diagnosis of certain carcinoid tumors in people; this has not been done for veterinary patients to date.

Imaging

Localization of neuroendocrine tumors relies on imaging with CT, MRI, and ultrasound in veterinary patients. Adjunct imaging with SSTR scintigraphy and endoscopic ultrasonography are also commonly used in people; neither of these imaging modalities is commonly available for veterinary patients; however, because SST scintigraphy has been helpful in the localization of insulinomas in dogs, it is reasonable to believe it would also be useful for the diagnosis of other neuroendocrine tumors. SST scintigraphy is useful because almost 80% of neuroendocrine GI tumors in people express the SSTR subtype 2 and will bind 111-indium-radiolabeled octreotate acetate. Radionucleotide scanning can be used not only for diagnostic purposes but also for staging to detect metastatic disease and also for indicating sensitivity to treatment with SST analogues. Similarly, positron emission tomography (PET) using nC-labeled 5-HTP and L-dopa has also been shown to be effective in localizing carcinoids and endocrine pancreatic tumors as small as 0.5 mm in people. This imaging technique also provides information about the metabolism of the tumors because 5-HTP is a precursor of serotonin synthesis.

Treatment

Surgery remains the cornerstone of treatment for neuroendocrine GI tumors, although cure is often not possible. While aggressive debulking operations can be helpful in people with metastatic disease for improving patient quality of life and for facilitating medical treatment, too few cases in veterinary medicine are reported to really assess the surgical success rate. Other means of tumor reduction used in people include liver transplantation and arterial embolization. Arterial embolization has been used for hepatic metastatic disease in veterinary patients.

Medical treatments for neuroendocrine tumors include chemotherapy and biotherapy using SST analogues and alpha interferons. Chemotherapy, in particular the combination of streptozotocin with 5-FU or doxorubicin, is still considered the first-line treatment for most endocrine pancreatic tumors in people, while SST analogues and alpha interferons are considered first-line for some carcinoids. Long-term remission (>18 months) with carboplatin chemotherapy has been seen in one dog with a jejunal carcinoid tumor following surgical excision. Too few cases have been reported on to adequately assess the efficacy of chemotherapy in veterinary patients. SST analogues, particularly octreotide acetate, are commonly used today in people to control hormonally related symptoms. In addition to suppressing hormone secretion by these tumors, SST analogues have also been shown to be inhibitors of tumor growth. Tumor-targeted radioactive treatment with indium-labeled octreotide acetate, similar to use of radioactive iodine for the treatment of hyperthyroidism in cats, has been used for local therapy for neuroendocrine tumors in people and in the future may be an option in veterinary patients. Chemotherapy and biotherapy are combined in many human patients, and while medical treatment is palliative and not curative, disease symptoms can be controlled for extended periods of time in some patients.

In general, external radiation therapy has not been successful in the treatment of metastatic neuroendocrine tumors but has been used for the treatment of symptomatic bone, skin, and brain metastases in people with these tumors and could be considered for palliative care in veterinary patients.

Prognosis

Because the clinical manifestations of many neuroendocrine tumors are not specific and they are typically small in size, early diagnosis can be difficult. These tumors tend to be malignant and, in most cases, they are not diagnosed early enough for a surgical cure to be possible. Hence, palliative medical treatment is often the only viable option.

Bibliography

Section 1

1. Hurty CA, Flatland B. Feline acromegaly: a review of the syndrome. *Journal of the American Animal Hospital Association* 2005;41:292–297.

2. Niessen SJM, Petrie G, Gaudiano F, Khalid M, Smyth JBA, Mahoney P, Church DB. Feline acromegaly: an underdiagnosed endocrinopathy? *Journal of veterinary internal medicine/American College of Veterinary Internal Medicine* 2007;21:899–905.

3. Kooistra HS, Voorhout G, Mol JA, Rijnberk A. Combined pituitary hormone deficiency in German shepherd dogs with dwarfism. *Domestic Animal Endocrinology* 2000;19:177–190.

4. Donaldson D, Billson FM, Scase TJ, et al. Congenital hyposomatotropism in a domestic shorthair cat presenting with congenital corneal oedema. *Journal of Small Animal Practice* 2008;49: 306–309.

5. Ramsey IK, Dennis R, Herrtage ME. Concurrent central diabetes insipidus and panhypopituitarism in a German Shepherd dog. *Journal of Small Animal Practice* 1999;40:271–274.

6. Schwedes CS. Transient diabetes insipidus in a dog with acromegaly. *Journal of Small Animal Practice* 1999;40:392–396.

7. Rossi TA, Ross LA. Diabetes insipidus. *Compendium of Contin Educ Vet* 2008;Jan;30(1):43–52.

Section 2

1. Feldman EC, Nelson RW. Hypothyroidism/the thyroid gland. In: *Canine and Feline Endocrinology and Reproduction*, 3rd edition, eds. EC Feldman, RW Nelson, pp. 86–151. St. Louis, MO: Elsevier Saunders; 2004.

2. Scott-Moncrieff J, Catharine R, Guptill-Yoran L. Hypothyroidism/endocrine disorders. In: *Textbook of Veterinary Internal Medicine*. Comp., 6th edition, Vol. 2, eds. SJ Ettinger, EC Feldman, pp. 1535–1544. St. Louis, MO: Elsevier Saunders; 2005.

3. Cote E. Hypothyroidism/diseases and disorders. In: *Clinical Veterinary Advisor*, 1st edition, ed. E Cote, pp. 575–577. St. Louis, MO: Mosby Elsevier; 2007.

4. Tilley LP, Smith FWK, Jr. Hypothyroidism. In: *The 5 Minute Veterinary Consult: Canine and Feline*, 3rd edition, eds. DB Troy, MJ Hauber, KM Ruppert, pp. 686–689. Baltimore, MD: Lippincott Williams & Wilkins; 2004.

5. Scott-Moncrieff J, Catharine R. Hypothyroidism/endocrine and metabolic diseases. In: *Kirk's Current Veterinary Therapy*, 14th edition, eds. JD Bonagura, DC Twedt, pp. 185–191. St. Louis, MO: Elsevier Saunders; 2009.

6. Gulikers KP, Panciera DL. Influence of various medications on canine thyroid function. *Compendium on Continuing Education for the Practicing Veterinarian* 2002; 24(7):511–523.

7. Daminet S. Canine hypothyroidism: update on diagnosis and treatment. Proceedings of the World Small Animal Veterinary Association World Congress 2010, Geneva, Switzerland. http://www.VIN.com (accessed December 2010).

8. Evason MD, Carr AP, Taylor SM, Waldner CL. Alterations in thyroid hormone concentrations in healthy sled dogs before and after athletic conditioning. *American Journal of Veterinary Research* 2004;65(3):333–337.

9. Plumb DC. Levothyroxine sodium. In: *Veterinary Drug Handbook Pocket Edition*, 5th edition, ed. DC Plumb, p. 457–460. Ames, IA: Blackwell; 2005.

10. Mooney CT. Hyperthyroidism. In: *Textbook of Veterinary Internal Medicine: Diseases of the Dog and Cat*, 6th edition, Vol. 2, eds. SJ Ettinger, EC Feldman, pp. 1544–1560. St. Louis, MO: Elsevier Saunders; 2005.

11. Feldman EC, Nelson RW. Feline hyperthyroidism (thyrotoxicosis). In: *Canine and Feline Endocrinology and Reproduction*, 3rd edition,

eds. EC Feldman, RW Nelson, pp. 152–218. St. Louis, MO: Saunders; 2004.

12. Harvey A, Hibbert A, Barrett E, Day M, Quiggin A, Brannan R, Caney S. Scintigraphic findings in 120 hyperthyroid cats. *Journal of Feline Medicine and Surgery* 2009;11(2):96–106.

13. Kass PH, Peterson ME, Levy J, James K, Becker DV, Cowgill LD. Evaluation of environmental, nutritional, and host factors in cats with hyperthyroidism. *Journal of Veterinary Internal Medicine* 1999;13(4):323–329.

14. Greco DS. Feline thyroid disorders. *The NAVTA Journal* Fall 2008;62:59–63.

15. Thyroid tumors. VSSO—Veterinary Society of Surgical Oncology. http://www.vsso.org/Thyroid_Tumors_-_Feline.html (accessed August 29, 2010).

16. Gunn-Moore D. Feline endocrinopathies. *Veterinary Clinics of North America: Small Animal Practice* 2005;35(1):171–210.

17. Mooney CT. Feline hyperthyroidism. Diagnostics and therapeutics. *Veterinary Clinics of North America: Small Animal Practice* 2001;31:963.

18. Broome MR. Thyroid scintigraphy in hyperthyroidism. *Clinical Techniques in Small Animal Practice* 2006;21(1):10. Print.

19. Bonagura JD. Feline cardiovascular diseases. Proceedings of the Atlantic Coast Veterinary Conference, Atlantic City, October 5–11, 2007.

20. Panciera DL. Cardiovascular complications of thyroid disease. In: *Kirk's Current Veterinary Therapy XIII: Small Animal Practice*, ed. JD Bonagura, pp. 716–719. Philadelphia, PA: W.B. Saunders; 1999.

21. Bruyette DS. The options for treating feline hyperthyroidism. *Veterinary Medicine* 2004;99(11):964–972.

22. Peterson ME. Radioiodine for feline hyperthyroidism. In: *Kirk's Current Veterinary Therapy XIV*, eds. JD Bonagura, DC Twedt, pp. 180–184. St. Louis, MO: Elsevier Saunders; 2009.

23. Peterson ME. Hyperthyroidism. In: *Textbook of Veterinary Internal Medicine: Diseases of the Dog and Cat*, 5th edition, Vol. 2, eds. SJ Ettinger, EC Feldman, pp. 1400–1419. Philadelphia, PA: W.B. Saunders; 2000.

24. Yu S, Wedekind KJ, Burris PA, Forrester DS, Locniskar MF. Controlled level of dietary iodine normalizes serum total thyroxine in cats with naturally occuring hyperthyroidism. *Journal of Veterinary Internal Medicine* 2011;25:683–684. Print.

25. Milner RJ, Channell CD, Levy JK, Schaer M. Survival times of cats with hyperthyroidism treated with iodine 131, methimazole, or both: 167 cases (1996–2003). *Journal of the American Veterinary Medical Association* 2006;228:559–563.

26. Nann EC, Kirpensteijn J, Kooistra HS, Peeters ME. Results of thyroidectomy in 101 cats with hyperthyroidism. *Veterinary Surgery* 2006;35:287–293.

27. Birchard SJ, Roesel OF. Neoplasia of the thyroid gland in the dog: a retrospective study of 16 cases. *Journal of the American Animal Hospital Association* 1981;17(3):369–372.

28. Harari J, Patterson JS, Rosenthal RC. Clinical and pathologic features of thyroid tumors in 26 dogs. *Journal of the American Veterinary Medical Association* 1986;188(10):1160–1164.

29. Feldman EC, Nelson RW. Canine thyroid tumors and canine hyperthyroidism. In: *Canine and Feline Endocrinology and Reproduction*, 3rd edition, eds. EC Feldman, RW Nelson, pp. 219–249. St. Louis, MO: Saunders; 2004.

30. Worth AJ, Zuber RM, Hocking M. Radioiodide (^{131}I) therapy for the treatment of canine thyroid carcinoma. *Australian Veterinary Journal* 2005;83(4):208–214.

31. Marks SL, Koblik PD, Hornof WJ, et al. 99mTc-pertechnetate imaging of thyroid tumors in dogs: 29 cases (1980–1992). *Journal of the American Veterinary Medical Association* 1994;204(5):756–760.

32. Klein MK, Powers BE, Withrow SJ, et al. Treatment of thyroid carcinoma in dogs by surgical resection alone: 20 cases (1981–1989). *Journal of the American Veterinary Medical Association* 1995;206(7):1007–1009.

33. Bailey DB, Page RL. Tumors of the endocrine system. In: *Small Animal Clinical Oncology*, 4th edition, eds. SJ Withrow, DM Vail, pp. 583–609. St. Louis, MO: Saunders; 2007.

34. Carver JR, Kapatkin A, Patnaik A. A comparison of medullary thyroid carcinoma and thyroid adenocarcinoma in dogs: a retrospective study of 38 cases. *Veterinary Surgery* 1995;24(4):315–319.

35. Pack LA, Roberts RE, Dawson SD, et al. Definitive radiation therapy for infiltrative thyroid carcinoma in dogs. *Veterinary Radiology & Ultrasound* 2001;42(5):471–474.

36. Brearley ML, Hayes AM, Murphy S. Hypofractionated radiation therapy for invasive thyroid carcinoma in dogs: a retrospective analysis of survival. *Journal of Small Animal Practice* 1999;40(5):206–210.

37. Mayer MN, MacDonald VS. External beam radiation therapy for thyroid cancer in the dog. *The Canadian Veterinary Journal. La Revue Veterinaire Canadienne* 1997;48(7):761–763.

38. Turrel JM, McEntee MC, Burke BP, et al. Sodium iodide I 131 treatment of dogs with nonresectable thyroid tumors: 39 cases (1990–2003). *Journal of the American Veterinary Medical Association* 2006;229(4):542–548.

39. Fineman LS, Hamilton TA, De Gortari A, et al. Cisplatin chemotherapy for treatment of thyroid carcinoma in dogs: 13 cases. *Journal of the American Animal Hospital Association* 1998;34(2):109–112.

40. Jeglum KA, Whereat A. Chemotherapy of canine thyroid carcinoma. *Compendium on Continuing Education for the Practicing Veterinarian* 1983;5(2):96–98.

41. Leav I, Schiller AL, Rihnberk A, et al. Adenomas and carcinomas of the canine and feline thyroid. *American Journal of Pathology* 1976;83(1):61–122.

42. Theon AP, Marks SL, Feldman ES, et al. Prognostic factors and patterns of treatment failure in dogs with unresectable differentiated thyroid carcinomas treated with megavoltage radiation. *Journal of the American Veterinary Medical Association* 2000;216(11):1775–1779.

43. Wisner ER, Nyland TG. Ultrasonography of the thyroid and parathyroid glands. *Veterinary Clinics of North America: Small Animal Practice* 1998;28(4):973–991.

Section 3

1. Henderson AK, Mahony O. Hypoparathyroidism: pathophysiology and diagnosis. *Compendium* 2005;27(4, April):270–278.

2. Henderson AK, Mahony O. Hypoparathyroidism: treatment. *Compendium* 2005;27(4, April):280–287.

3. Feldman EC, Hoar B, Pollard R, Nelson RW. Pretreatment clinical and laboratory findings in dogs with primary hyperparathyroidism: 210 cases (1987–2004). *Journal of the American Veterinary Medical Association* 2005;227(5):756–761.

4. Pollard RE, Nelson RW, Hornof WJ, Feldman EC. Percutaneous ultrasonographically guided radiofrequency heat ablation for treatment of primary hyperparathyroidism in dogs. *Journal of the American Veterinary Medical Association* 2001;218(7):1106–1110.

Section 4

1. Klein SC, Peterson ME. Canine hypoadrenocorticism: part I. *The Canadian Veterinary Journal. La Revue Veterinaire Canadienne* 2010;51:63–69.

2. Scott-Moncrieff JC. Hypoadrenocorticism. In: *Textbook of Veterinary Internal Medicine*, eds. SJ Ettinger, EC Feldman, pp. 294, 1847–1857. St. Louis, MO: Saunders; 2010.

3. Adler JA, Drobatz KJ, Hess RS. Abnormalities of serum electrolyte concentrations in dogs with hypoadrenocorticism. *Journal of Veterinary Internal Medicine/American College of Veterinary Internal Medicine* 2007;232:413–416.

4. Lennon EM, Boyle TE, Grace R, et al. Use of basal serum or plasma cortisol concentrations to rule out a diagnosis of hypoadrenocorticism in dogs: 123 cases (2000–2005). *The Journal of the American Medical Association* 2007;231:413–416.

5. Robertson SA. Endocrine system. In: *Textbook of Small Animal Surgery*, ed. D Slatter, pp. 187, 2589–2590. Philiedlphia, PA: Saunders; 2003.

6. Melian C, Perez-Alenza M, Peterson M. Hyperadrenocorticism in dogs. In: *Textbook of Veterinary Internal Medicine*, eds. SJ Ettinger, EC Feldman, pp. 292, 1816–1840. St. Louis, MO: Saunders; 2010.

7. Gunn-Moore D. Feline endocrinopathies. *Veterinary Clinics of North America: Small Animal* 2005;35:171–210..

8. Behrend EN, Kemppainen RJ. Diagnosis of canine hyperadrenocorticism. *Veterinary Clinics of North America. Small Animal Practice* 2001;31(5):985–1003.

9. Kooistra H, Galac S. Recent advances in the diagnosis of Cushing's syndrome in dogs. *Veterinary Clinics of North America. Small Animal Practice* 2010;40:259–267.

10. Feldman EC, Mack RE. Urine cortisol : creatinine ratio as a screening test for hyperadrenocorticism in dogs. *Journal of the American Veterinary Medical Association* 1992;200:1637.

11. Feldman EC, Nelson RW. Hyperadrenocorticism (Cushing's syndrome). In: *Canine and Feline Endocrinology and Reproduction*, 2nd edition, eds. EC Feldman, RW Nelson, pp. 187–265. Philadelphia, PA: Saunders; 1996.

12. Clemente M, Andres PJD, Arenas C, et al. Comparison of non-selective adrenocorticolysis with mitotane or trilostane for the treatment of dogs with pituitary-dependent hyperadrenocorticism. *The Veterinary Record* 2007;161:805–809.

13. Brown C, Graves T. Hyperadrenocorticism: treating dogs. *Compendium on Continuing Education for the Practicing Veterinarian* 2007;29:137–145.

14. Zicker SC, Ford RB, Nelson RW, Kirk CA. Endocrine and lipid disorders. In: *Small Animal Clinical Nutrition*, 4th edition, eds. MS Hand, CD Thatcher, RL Remillard, P Roudebush, pp. 850–885. Topeka, KS: Mark Morris Institute; 2000.

15. Maher ER, McNeil EA. Pheochromocytoma in dogs and cats. *Veterinary Clinics of North America. Small Animal Practice* 1997; 27:359–380.

16. Feldman EC, Nelson RW. Pheochromocytoma and multiple endocrine neoplasia. In: *Canine and Feline Endocrinology and Reproduction*, 3rd edition, eds. EC Feldman, RW Nelson, pp. 440–463. St. Louis, MO: Elsevier Saunders; 2004.

17. Bouayad H, Feeney DA, Caywood DD, et al. Pheochromocytoma in dogs; 13 cases (1980–1985). *Journal of the American Veterinary Medical Association* 1987;191:1610.

18. Barthez PY, Marks SL, Woo J, et al. Pheochromocytoma in dogs: 61 cases (1984–1995). *Journal of Veterinary Internal Medicine/ American College of Veterinary Internal Medicine* 1997;11:272.

19. Herrera MA, Mehl ML, Kass OH, et al. Predictive factors and the effect of phenoxybenzamine on outcome in dogs undergoing adrenalectomy for pheochromocytoma. *Journal of Veterinary Internal Medicine/American College of Veterinary Internal Medicine* 2008;22:1333–1339.

20. Kook PH, Boretti FS, Hersberger M, et al. Urinary catecholamine and metanephrine to creatinine ratios in healthy dogs at home and in a hospital environment and in 2 dogs with pheochromocytoma. *Journal of Veterinary Internal Medicine/American College of Veterinary Internal Medicine* 2007;21:388.

Section 5

1. Rand. JS. Feline diabetes mellitus. In: *Current Veterinary Therapy XIV*, eds. JD Bonagura, DC Twedt, pp. 199–204. St. Louis, MO: Saunders Elsevier; 2009.

2. Feldman EC, Nelson RW. Feline diabetes mellitus. In: *Canine and Feline Endocrinology and Reproduction*, 3rd edition, eds. EC Feldman, RW Nelson, pp. 539–579. St. Louis, MO: Saunders; 2004.

3. Scott-Montcrieff C. Insulin resistance in cats. *Veterinary Clinics of North America. Small Animal Practice* 2010;40(2):241–258.

4. Hoenig M Comparative aspects of diabetes mellitus in dogs and cats. *Molecular and Cellular Endocrinology* 2002;197(1–2):221–229.

5. Hall DG, Kelley LC, Gray ML, Glaus TM. Lymphocytic inflammation of pancreatic islets in a diabetic cat. *Journal of Veterinary Diagnostic Investigation* 1997;9:98–100.

6. Hoenig M, Reusch C, Peterson ME. Beta cell and insulin antibodies in treated and untreated diabetic cats. *Veterinary Immunology and Immunopathology* 2000;77:93–102.

7. Rand JS, Baral RM, Catt MJ, Farrow HA. Prevalence of feline diabetes mellitus in a feline private practice. *Journal of Veterinary Internal Medicine/American College of Veterinary Internal Medicine (Abstract)* 2003;17:433–434.

8. Lederer R, Rand JS, Jonsson NN, et al. Frequency of feline diabetes mellitus and breed predisposition in domestic cats in Australia. *Veterinary Journal (London, England: 1997)* 2009;179:254–258.

9. Goossens MM, Nelson RW, Feldman EC, Griffey SM. Response to insulin treatment and survival in 104 cats with diabetes mellitus (1985–1995). *Journal of Veterinary Internal Medicine/American College of Veterinary Internal Medicine* 1998;12:1–6.

10. O'Brien TD. Pathogenesis of feline diabetes mellitus. *Molecular and Cellular Endocrinology* 2002;197:213–219.

11. Reush C. Feline diabetes mellitus. In: *Textbook of Veterinary Internal Medicine*, 7th edition, eds. SJ Ettinger, EC Feldman, pp. 1796–1816. Philadelphia, PA: Saunders; 2010.

12. Rand JS, Bobbermein LM, Hendrikz JK. Overrepresentation of Burmese cats with diabetes mellitus. *Australian Veterinary Journal* 1997;75:402–405.

13. Prahl A, Guptill L, Glickman NW, et al. Time trends and risk factors for diabetes mellitus in cats presented to veterinary teaching hospitals. *Journal of Feline Medicine and Surgery* 2007; 9:351–358.

14. McCann TM, Simpson KE, Shaw DJ, et al. Feline diabetes mellitus in the UK: the prevalence within an insured cat population and a questionnaire-based putative risk factor analysis. *Journal of Feline Medicine and Surgery* 2007;9:289–299.

15. Crenshaw KL, Peterson ME, Heeb LA, et al. Serum fructosamine concentration as an index of glycemia in cats with diabetes mellitus and stress hyperglycemia. *Journal of Veterinary Internal Medicine/American College of Veterinary Internal Medicine* 1996; 10:360–364.

16. Bailiff NL, Nelson RW, Feldman EC, et al. Frequency and risk factors for urinary tract infection in cats with diabetes mellitus. *Journal of Veterinary Internal Medicine/American College of Veterinary Internal Medicine* 2006;20:850–855.

17. Marshall RD, Rand JS. Treatment with glargine results in higher remission rates than lente or protamine zinc insulins in newly diagnosed diabetic cats. *Journal of Veterinary Internal Medicine/American College of Veterinary Internal Medicine (Abstract)* 2005; 19:425.

18. Weaver KE, Rozanski EA, Mahony OM, et al. Use of glargine and lente insulins in cats with diabetes mellitus. *Journal of Veterinary Internal Medicine/American College of Veterinary Internal Medicine* 2006;20:234–238.

19. Wess G, Reusch C. Capillary blood sampling from the ear of dogs and cats and use of portable meters to measure glucose concentration. *Journal of Small Animal Practice* 2000;41:60–66.

20. Reusch CE, Kley S, Casella M. Home monitoring of the diabetic cat. *Journal of Feline Medicine and Surgery* 2006;8:119–127.

21. Wiedmeyer CE, DeClue AE. Continuous glucose monitoring in dogs and Cats. *Journal of Veterinary Internal Medicine/American College of Veterinary Internal Medicine* 2008;22:2–8.

22. Marshall RD, Rand JS, Morton JM. Treatment of newly diagnosed diabetic cats with glargine insulin improves glycaemic control and results in higher probability of remission than protamine zinc and lente insulins. *Journal of Feline Medicine and Surgery* 2009; 11:683–691.

23. Roomp K, Rand J. Intensive blood glucose control is safe and effective in diabetic cats using home monitoring and treatment with glargine. *Journal of Feline Medicine and Surgery* 2009;11: 668–682.

24. Bennett N, Greco DS, Peterson ME, et al. Comparison of a low carbohydrate-low fiber diet and a moderate carbohydrate-high fiber diet in the management of feline diabetes mellitus. *Journal of Feline Medicine and Surgery* 2006;8:73–84.

25. Hess RS, Kass PH, Ward CR. Breed distribution of dogs with diabetes mellitus admitted to a tertiary care facility. *Journal of American Veterinary Medical Association* 2000;216:1414–1417.

26. Guptill L, Glickman L, Glickman N. Time trends and risk factors for diabetes mellitus in dogs: analysis of veterinary medical database records (1970–19999). *The Veterinary Journal* 2003;165: 240–247.

27. Nelson RW. Disorders of glucose metabolism in the dog—1: diabetes mellitus. *Veterinary Medicine* 1985;1:27–36.

28. Greco DS. Diagnosis of diabetes mellitus in cats and dogs. *Veterinary Clinics of North America. Small Animal Practice* 2001; 31(5):845–853.

29. Rucinsky R, Cook A, Haley S, et al. AAHA diabetes management guidelines for dogs and cats. *Journal of the American Animal Hospital Association* 2010;46:215–224.

30. Fleeman LM, Rand JS. Management of canine diabetes. *Veterinary Clinics of North America. Small Animal Practice* 2001;31(5):855–879.

31. Rand JS, Fleeman LM, Farrow HA, et al. Canine and feline diabetes mellitus: nature or nurture? *The Journal of Nutrition* 2004;Aug;134(8 Suppl):2072s–2080s.

32. Hume DZ, Drobatz KJ, Hess RS. Outcome of dogs with diabetic ketoacidosis: 127 dogs (1993–2003). *Journal of Veterinary Internal Medicine/American College of Veterinary Internal Medicine* 2006; 20:547–555.

33. Connally HE. Critical care monitoring considerations for the diabetic patient. *Clinical Techniques in Small Animal Practice* 2002; 17(2):73–79.

34. O'Brien MA. Diabetic emergencies in small animals. *Veterinary Clinics of North America. Small Animal Practice* 2010;40:317–333.

35. Boysen SR. Fluid and electrolyte therapy in endocrine disorders; diabetes mellitus and hypoadrenocorticism. *Veterinary Clinics of North America. Small Animal Practice* 2008;38:699–717.

36. Rothman DL, Magnusson I, Katz LD, et al. Quantitation of hepatic glycogenolysis and gluconeogenesis in fasting humans with C13 NMR. *Science* 1991;254:573.

37. Karam JH. Hypoglycemic disorders. In: *Basic and Clinical Endocrinology*, 6th edition, eds. FS Greenspan, DG Gardner, p. 699. New York, NY: Lange Medical Books/McGraw Hill; 2001.

38. Cryer PE, Gerich JE. Glucose counterregulation, hypoglycemia and intensive insulin therapy in diabetes mellitus. *The New England Journal of Medicine* 1985;313:232.

39. Cryer PE, Polonsky KS. Glucose homeostasis and hypoglycemia. In: *Williams Textbook of Endocrinology*, 9th edition, eds. JD Wilson, DW Foster, HM Kronenberg, PR Larsen, p. 939. Philadelphia, PA: W.B. Saunders; 1998.

40. Cryer PE. Catecholamines, pheochromocytoma and diabetes. *Diabetes Reviews* 1993;1:309.

41. Feldman EC. Diseases of the endocrine pancreas. In: *Textbook of Veterinary Internal Medicine*, ed. SJ Ettinger, pp. 1615–1649. Philadelphia, PA: W.B. Saunders; 1983.

42. Feldman EC, Nelson RW. Beta-cell neoplasia; insulinoma. In: *Canine and Feline Endocrinology and Reproduction*, 3rd edition, eds. EC Feldman, RW Nelson, p. 638. St. Louis, MO: W.B. Saunders; 2004.

43. Fischer JR, Smith SA, Harkin KR. Glucagon Constant-Rate Infusion: a novel strategy for the management of hyperinsulinemic-hypoglycemic crisis in the dog. *Journal of the American Animal Hospital Association* 2000;36:27–32.

44. Tobin RL, Nelson RW, Lucroy MD, et al. Outcome of surgical versus medical treatment of dogs with beta-cell neoplasia; 39 cases.(1990–1997). *Journal of the American Veterinary Medical Association* 1999;215:226.

45. Feldman EC, Nelson RW. Beta-cell neoplasia; insulinoma. In: *Canine and Feline Endocrinology and Reproduction*, 3rd edition, eds. EC Feldman, RW Nelson, p. 635. St. Louis, MO: W.B. Saunders; 2004.

46. Feldman EC, Nelson RW. Beta-cell neoplasia; insulinoma. In: *Canine and Feline Endocrinology and Reproduction*, 3rd edition, eds. EC Feldman, RW Nelson, p. 622. St. Louis, MO: W.B. Saunders; 2004.

47. Feldman EC, Nelson RW. Beta-cell neoplasia; insulinoma. In: *Canine and Feline Endocrinology and Reproduction*, 3rd edition, eds. EC Feldman, RW Nelson, p. 640. St. Louis, MO: W.B. Saunders; 2004.

48. Mizuno T, Hiraoka H, Yoshioka C, et al. Superficial necrolytic dermatitis associated with extrapancreatic glucagonoma in a dog. *Veterinary Dermatology* 2009;20:72–79.

49. Oberkirchner U, Linder KE, Zadrozny L, Olivry T. Successful treatment of canine necrolytic migratory erythema (superficial necrolytic dermatitis) due to metastatic glucagonoma with Octreotide. *Veterinary Dermatology* 2010;Oct;21(5):510–516. Epub ahead of print.

50. Lurye JC, Behrend EN. Endocrine tumors. *Veterinary Clinics of North America. Small Animal Practice* 2001;31:1083–1110, ix–x. Review.

51. Allenspach K, Arnold P, Glaus T, et al. Glucagon-producing neuroendocrine tumour associated with hypoaminoacidaemia and skin lesions. *Journal of Small Animal Practice* 2000;41:402–406.

52. Langer NB, Jergens AE, Miles KG. Canine glucagonoma. *Compendium on Continuing Education for the Practicing Veterinarian* 2003;25:56–63.

53. Tierney EP, Badger J. Etiology and pathogenesis of necrolytic migratory erythema: review of the literature. *MedGenMed* 2004;6:4.

54. van Beek AP, de Haas ER, van Vloten WA, et al. The glucagonoma syndrome and necrolytic migratory erythema: a clinical review. *European Journal of Endocrinology/European Federation of Endocrine Societies* 2004;151:531–537.

Section 6

1. Dusso AS, Brown AJ, Slatopolsky E. Vitamin D. *American Journal of Physiology. Renal Physiology* 2005;289:F8–28. Review.

2. LeVine DN, Zhou Y, Ghiloni RJ, et al. Hereditary 1,25-dihydroxyvitamin D-resistant rickets in a Pomeranian dog caused by a novel mutation in the vitamin D receptor gene. *Journal of Veterinary Internal Medicine/American College of Veterinary Internal Medicine* 2009;23:1278–1283.

3. Taylor MB, Geiger DA, Saker KE, Larson MM. Diffuse osteopenia and myelopathy in a puppy fed a diet composed of an organic premix and raw ground beef. *Journal of the American Veterinary Medical Association* 2009;234:1041–1048.

4. McMillan CJ, Griffon DJ, Marks SL, Mauldin GE. Dietary-related skeletal changes in a Shetland sheepdog puppy. *Journal of the American Animal Hospital Association* 2006;42:57–64.

5. Malik R, Laing C, Davis PE, et al. Rickets in a litter of racing greyhounds. *Journal of Small Animal Practice* 1997;38:109–114.

6. Lourens DC. Nutritional or secondary hyperparathyroidism in a German shepherd litter. *Journal of the South African Veterinary Association* 1980;51:121–123.

7. Sarkiala EM, Dambach D, Harvey CE. Jaw lesions resulting from renal hyperparathyroidism in a young dog—a case report. *Journal of Veterinary Dentistry* 1994;11:121–124.

8. Carmichael DT, Williams CA, Aller MS. Renal dysplasia with secondary hyperparathyroidism and loose teeth in a young dog. *Journal of Veterinary Dentistry* 1995;12:143–146.

9. Geisen V, Weber K, Hartmann K. Vitamin D-dependent hereditary rickets type I in a cat. *Journal of Veterinary Internal Medicine/American College of Veterinary Internal Medicine* 2009;23:196–199.

10. Tanner E, Langley-Hobbs SJ. Vitamin D-dependent rickets type 2 with characteristic radiographic changes in a 4-month-old kitten. *Journal of Feline Medicine and Surgery* 2005;7:307–311.

11. Godfrey DR, Anderson RM, Barber PJ, Hewison M. Vitamin D-dependent rickets type II in a cat. *Journal of Small Animal Practice* 2005;46:440–444.

12. Schreiner CA, Nagode LA. Vitamin D-dependent rickets type 2 in a four-month-old cat. *Journal of the American Veterinary Medical Association* 2003;222:337–339, 315–316.

13. Gnudi G, Bertoni G, Luppi A, Cantoni AM. Unusual hyperparathyroidism in a cat. *Veterinary Radiology & Ultrasound: The Official Journal of the American College of Veterinary Radiology and the International Veterinary Radiology Association* 2001;42:250–253.

14. Henik RA, Forrest LJ, Friedman AL. Rickets caused by excessive renal phosphate loss and apparent abnormal vitamin D metabolism in a cat. *Journal of the American Veterinary Medical Association* 1999;215:1644–1649, 1620–1621.

15. Randolph JF, Scarlett JM, Stokol T, et al. Expression, bioactivity, and clinical assessment of recombinant feline erythropoietin. *American Journal of Veterinary Research* 2004;65:1355–1366.

16. Roudebush P, Polzin DJ, Adams LG, et al. An evidence-based review of therapies for canine chronic kidney disease. *Journal of Small Animal Practice* 2010;51:244–252.

17. Roudebush P, Polzin DJ, Ross SJ, et al. Therapies for feline chronic kidney disease. What is the evidence? *Journal of Feline Medicine and Surgery* 2009;11:195–210.

18. Randolph JE, Scarlett J, Stokol T, MacLeod JN. Clinical efficacy and safety of recombinant canine erythropoietin in dogs with anemia of chronic renal failure and dogs with recombinant human erythropoietin-induced red cell aplasia. *Journal of Veterinary Internal Medicine/American College of Veterinary Internal Medicine* 2004;18:81–91.

19. Cowgill LD, James KM, Levy JK, et al. Use of recombinant human erythropoietin for management of anemia in dogs and cats with renal failure. *Journal of the American Veterinary Medical Association* 1998;212:521–528.

20. Cowgill LD. *Erythropoietin-replacement therapy*. Personal communication on American College of Veterinary Internal Medicine listserve. http://www.acvim.org (accessed September 1, 2009).

21. Arcasoy MO. Non-erythroid effects of erythropoietin. *Haematologica* 2010;95:1803–1805.

22. Fisher JW. Erythropoietin: physiology and pharmacology update. *Experimental Biology and Medicine* 2003;228:1–14.

23. Marsden JT. Erythropoietin—measurement and clinical applications. *Annals of Clinical Biochemistry* 2006;43:97–104.

24. Hughes SM. Canine gastrinoma: a case study and literature review of therapeutic options. *New Zealand Veterinary Journal* 2006;54:242–247.

25. Brooks D, Watson GL. Omeprazole in a dog with gastrinoma. *Journal of Veterinary Internal Medicine/American College of Veterinary Internal Medicine* 1997;11:379–381.

26. Green RA, Gartrell CL. Gastrinoma: a retrospective study of four cases (1985–1995). *Journal of the American Animal Hospital Association* 1997;33:524–527.

27. Simpson KW. Gastrinoma in dogs. In: *Kirk's Current Veterinary Therapy XIV*, eds. JD Bonagura, DC Twedt, pp. 617–621. St. Louis, MO: Saunders; 2009.

28. Katkoori D, Samavedi S, Jorda M, et al. A rare case of renal gastrinoma. *The Scientific World Journal* 2009;9:501–504.

29. Oberg K, Jelic S, ESMO Guidelines Working Group. Neuroendocrine gastroenteropancreatic tumors: ESMO clinical recommendation for diagnosis, treatment and follow-up. *Annals of Oncology: Official Journal of the European Society for Medical Oncology/ESMO* 2009;20:150–153.

30. Shaw DH. Gastrinoma (Zollinger–Ellison syndrome) in the dog and cat. *The Canadian Veterinary Journal. La Revue Veterinaire Canadienne* 1988;29:448–452.

31. Diroff JS, Sanders NA, McDonough SP, Holt DE. Gastrin-secreting neoplasia in a cat. *Journal of Veterinary Internal Medicine/American College of Veterinary Internal Medicine* 2006;20:1245–1247.

32. Moreau ME, Garbacki N, Molinaro G, et al. The kallikrein-kinin system: current and future pharmacological targets. *Journal of Pharmacological Sciences* 2005;99:6–38.

33. Campbell DJ. Towards understanding the kallikrein-kinin system: insights from measurement of kinin peptides. *Brazilian Journal of Medical and Biological Research* 2000;33:665–677.

34. Zawilska JB, Skene DJ, Arendt J. Physiology and pharmacology of melatonin in relation to biological rhythms. *Pharmacological Reports: PR* 2009;61:383–410.

35. Diaz SF, Torres SM, Nogueira SA, et al. The impact of body site, topical melatonin and brushing on hair regrowth after clipping

normal Siberian husky dogs. *Veterinary Dermatology* 2006;17(1): 45–50.

36. Frank LA, Hnilica KA, Oliver JW. Adrenal steroid hormone concentrations in dogs with hair cycle arrest (Alopecia X) before and during treatment with melatonin and mitotane. *Veterinary Dermatology* 2004;15(5):278–284.

37. Frank LA, Donnell RL, Kania SA. Oestrogen receptor evaluation in Pomeranian dogs with hair cycle arrest (alopecia X) on melatonin supplementation. *Veterinary Dermatology* 2006;17(4): 252–258.

38. Baxter GF. The natriuretic peptides. *Basic Research in Cardiology* 2004;99:71–75. Epub January 23, 2004. Review.

39. Saito Y. Roles of atrial natriuretic peptide and its therapeutic use. *Journal of Cardiology* 2010;56:262–270. Epub September 29, 2010.

40. Connolly DJ. Natriuretic peptides: the feline experience. *Veterinary Clinics of North America. Small Animal Practice* 2010;40:59–70. Epub May 14, 2010. Review.

41. Zimmering TM, Hungerbühler S, Meneses F, et al. Evaluation of the association between plasma concentration of N-terminal proatrial natriuretic peptide and outcome in cats with cardiomyopathy. *Journal of the American Veterinary Medical Association* 2010;237:665–672.

42. Sisson D. B-type natriuretic peptides. *Journal of Veterinary Cardiology* 2009;11 Suppl 1:S5–S7. Epub April 24, 2009.

43. Hsu A, Kittleson MD, Paling A. Investigation into the use of plasma NT-proBNP concentration to screen for feline hypertrophic cardiomyopathy. *Journal of Veterinary Cardiology* 2009;11 Suppl 1:S63–S70. Epub April 22, 2009.

44. Oyama MA, Singletary GE. The use of NT-proBNP assay in the management of canine patients with heart disease. *Veterinary Clinics of North America. Small Animal Practice* 2010;40:545–558.

45. Sisson DD. Neuroendocrine evaluation of cardiac disease. *Veterinary Clinics of North America. Small Animal Practice* 2004; 34:1105–1126. Review.

46. Fox FP, Oyama MA, Reynolds C, et al. Utility of plasma N-terminal pro-brain natriuretic peptide (NT-proBNP) to distinguish between congestive heart failure and non-cardiac causes of acute dyspnea in cats. *Journal of Veterinary Cardiology* 2009;11 Suppl 1:S51–S62, 20.

47. Zimmering TM, Meneses F, Nolte IJ, et al. Measurement of N-terminal proatrial natriuretic peptide in plasma of cats with and without cardiomyopathy. *American Journal of Veterinary Research* 2009;70:216–222.

48. Lobetti RG. Hyperreninaemic hypoaldosteronism in a dog. *Journal of the South African Veterinary Association* 1998;69:33–35.

49. Javadi S, Galac S, Boer P, et al. Aldosterone-to-renin and cortisol-to-adrenocorticotropic hormone ratios in healthy dogs and dogs with primary hypoadrenocorticism. *Journal of Veterinary Internal Medicine/American College of Veterinary Internal Medicine* 2006; 20:556–561.

50. Mazza A, Zamboni S, Armigliato M, et al. Endocrine arterial hypertension: diagnostic approach in clinical practice. *Minerva Endocrinologica* 2008;33:127–146. Epub February 15, 2008.

51. Della Bruna R, Kurtz A, Schricker K. Regulation of renin synthesis in the juxtaglomerular cells. *Current Opinion in Nephrology and Hypertension* 1996;5:16–19.

52. Patel YC. Somatostatin and its receptor family. *Frontiers in Neuroendocrinology* 1999;20:157–198. Review.

53. Hoenerhoff M, Kiupel M. Concurrent gastrinoma and somatostatinoma in a 10-year-old Portuguese water dog. *Journal of Comparative Pathology* 2004;130:313–318.

54. Nesi G, Marcucci T, Rubio CA, et al. Somatostatinoma: clinicopathological features of three cases and literature reviewed. *Journal of Gastroenterology and Hepatology* 2008;23:521–526.

55. Peterson ME. Acromegaly in cats: are we only diagnosing the tip of the iceberg? *Journal of Veterinary Internal Medicine/American College of Veterinary Internal Medicine* 2007;21:889–891.

56. Norman EJ, Mooney CT. Diagnosis and management of diabetes mellitus in five cats with somatotrophic abnormalities. *Journal of Feline Medicine and Surgery* 2000;2:183–190.

57. Niessen SJ. Feline acromegaly: an essential differential diagnosis for the difficult diabetic. *Journal of Feline Medicine and Surgery* 2010;12:15–23.

58. Tappin S, Brown P, Ferasin L. An intestinal neuroendocrine tumor associated with paroxysmal ventricular tachycardia and melaena in a 10-year-old boxer. *Journal of Small Animal Practice* 2008;49: 33–37.

59. Lippo NJ, Williams JE, Brawer RS, Sobel KE. Acute hemophilia and hemocholecyst in 2 dogs with gallbladder carcinoma. *Journal of Veterinary Internal Medicine/American College of Veterinary Internal Medicine* 2008;22:1249–1252.

60. Oberg KE. Gastrointestinal neuroendocrine tumors. *Annals of Oncology: Official Journal of the European Society for Medical Oncology/ESMO* 2010;21 Suppl 7:vii72–vii80.

61. Oberg KE. Neuroendocrine gastrointestinal tumors. *Annals of Oncology: Official Journal of the European Society for Medical Oncology/ESMO* 1996;7:453–463.

62. Morrell CN, Volk MV, Mankowski JL. A carcinoid tumor in the gallbladder of a dog. *Veterinary Pathology* 2002;39:756–758.

63. Sako T, Uchida E, Okamoto M, et al. Immunohistochemical evaluation of a malignant intestinal carcinoid in a dog. *Veterinary Pathology* 2003;40:212–215.

64. Spugnini EP, Gargiulo M, Assin R, et al. Adjuvant carboplatin for the treatment of intestinal carcinoid in a dog. *In Vivo* 2008;22: 759–761.

65. Rossmeisl JH, Jr., Forrester SD, Robertson JL, Cook WT. Chronic vomiting associated with a gastric carcinoid in a cat. *Journal of the American Animal Hospital Association* 2002;38:61–66.

66. Garden OA, Reubi JC, Dykes NL, et al. Somatostatin receptor imaging in vivo by planar scintigraphy facilitates the diagnosis of canine insulinomas. *Journal of Veterinary Internal Medicine/ American College of Veterinary Internal Medicine* 2005;19:168–176.

Suggested reading

1. Connolly DJ, Magalhaes RJ, Syme HM, et al. Circulating natriuretic peptides in cats with heart disease. *Journal of Veterinary Internal Medicine/American College of Veterinary Internal Medicine* 2008;22:96–105.

Chapter 3 Musculoskeletal

Editor: Colleen Ruderman

SECTION 1 ANATOMY AND PHYSIOLOGY

The skeletal system

Introduction

The skeletal system is the support structure for the body. It functions as the framework as well as the area where blood cell formation occurs. Bone is the second hardest substance in the body, the hardest living tissue, and is capable of repair after injury. While the main function of the skeletal system is support, it also serves to protect internal organs and makes movement possible by allowing skeletal muscle to attach via tendons to move joints. Bone is the main storage area for calcium and other minerals. The skeletal system can be divided into two distinct areas based on function. The axial skeleton's principal function is support and includes the skull, vertebrae, sternum, and ribs. It is typically more rigid than the appendicular skeleton, which is responsible for movement and includes the pelvic girdle and limbs.

Bone growth

Bones begin as cartilage during the fetal stages of development and become hardened bone by endochondral ossification as the body develops after birth. Osteoclasts are the cells that make bone by secreting a material called the matrix, which will then harden by a process called ossification. Calcium and phosphorus will enter the matrix during ossification. During this process, osteoclasts will become trapped within the bone and mature into osteocytes (bone cells). The areas of hardened matrix that contain the osteocytes are lacunae. Osteocytes obtain their blood supply through canaliculi, which are channels within the bone that allow nutrients and communication between cells. Osteoclasts are the sculptors of the skeletal system and are also a part of the

Small Animal Internal Medicine for Veterinary Technicians and Nurses, First Edition. Edited by Linda Merrill.
© 2012 John Wiley & Sons, Inc. Published 2012 by John Wiley & Sons, Inc.

mononuclear phagocytic system (MPS), breaking down skeletal tissue during remodeling and injury. Heteroplastic ossification is a similar process that occurs in tissue other than bone, such as the os penis. Intramembranous ossification is bone formation without the intervention of cartilage, such as the bones of the skull, face, and mandible.

Bone repair

Bone repair begins with a bridging callus formation by the periosteum at the location of the injury, hemorrhage, or clot formation. When complete, this will form the external callus and will be followed by the formation of an internal callus by the endosteum and will be composed of spongy bone or cartilage. Once the internal and external callus formation is complete, the ossification process will begin. Any nonfunctioning bone located within the callus is removed by osteoclasts and replaced with matrix by osteoblasts. Once ossification is complete with the formation of compact bone, any area of the callus that is no longer needed is reabsorbed.

Types of bones

Each bone in the body can contain several types of material. Cancellous bone (spongy bone) is named for its sponge-like appearance. Cancellous bone is made up of spicules, and located in the space between the spicules (also called trabeculae) is the marrow. As well as the housing for marrow, cancellous bone also functions to absorb shock and to lighten the overall weight of bone. Bone marrow is hematopoietic tissue (blood cell forming). It is in larger quantities in younger animals and lessens as the body ages. Older animals contain stores of red marrow mainly within the long bones and pelvis. These are also the main areas used for bone marrow collection procedures. Yellow bone marrow can be considered old red marrow and is primarily adipose connective tissue. This type of marrow cannot produce any cell lines; however, it can be converted to red marrow during a disease process that requires the increased production of blood cells. Compact bone is a heavy and dense material that comprises the outside layer of most bones within the skeletal system. Within compact bone is the Haversian system, which is a series of canals that house blood vessels, lymph vessels, and nerves that supply the bone. This is also the area where calcium is stored. Cancellous bone, red and yellow marrow, and compact bone make up the bones of the skeletal system, which are further defined by their shape and include long, short, flat, irregular, and sesamoid bones.

Long bones serve as a prime area for collection of bone marrow and, for this reason, are important to internal medicine and are the best example to describe the anatomy of bone. Long bones develop starting at the diaphysis, or primary growth center, which is the shaft of the long bone. As development progresses, secondary growth centers called epiphyses (proximal and distal) are created. These are located at the ends of long bones. Epiphyseal plates (growth plates) are located between the diaphysis and epiphysis and are where bone growth occurs during development after birth. These plates are further broken

down into zones of reserve cartilage (newest), proliferation, hypertrophy, and calcified matrix (oldest). Where the epiphysis and diaphysis join is the metaphysis. Within the bone is a medullary cavity that contains the yellow marrow. The medullary cavity is lined by the endosteum and its structure is formed from compact bone. Cancellous bone is located on the ends of the medullary cavity within the epiphysis and is the location for the red marrow. The outermost surface of the bone is called the periosteum. Located at the most distal and proximal ends of the bone are cartilages. Where there is cartilage, there is no periosteum (Figure 3.1.1).

The short bones consist of a core of cancellous bone surrounded by compact bone. Examples of short bones include the phalanges, carpus, and tarsus. Flat bones are made of a thin layer of cancellous bone surrounded by flat layers of compact bone on

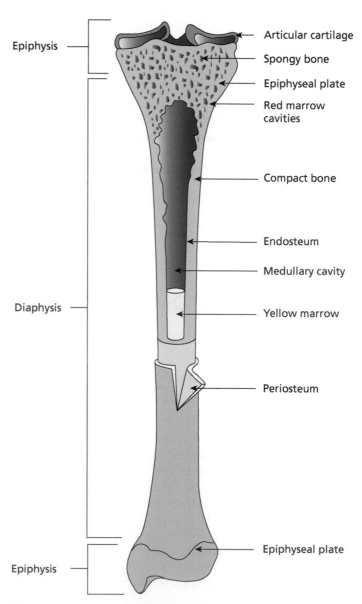

Figure 3.1.1   Structure of a long bone (tibia).

Source: Used with permission, Colville T, Bassert JM. *Clinical Anatomy and Physiology for Veterinary Technicians*, 2nd edition. St. Louis, MO: Mosby Elsevier; 2008.

either side, creating a flat structure (ribs, skull, and scapula). Irregular bones can share characteristics from long, short, and flat bones. Examples of irregular bones are the sesamoid bones located within tendons and include the patella, which is the largest sesamoid bone in the body. Splanchnic or visceral bone is bone that forms within organs, such as the os penis.

A part of most bones are projections and grooves that serve a variety of functions. Articular projections are located where bone meets bone to form a joint and are covered in a layer of articular cartilage. Nonarticular projections are areas located on bones and function as a location for tendons to attach. Nonarticular depressions called fossae and holes called foramina are located on bones where vessels or nerves must cross or in areas where large bones are located and weight must be reduced, such as the obturator foramen of the pelvis.

Joints

Joints serve as the junctions between bones. There are several types, each with its own level of flexibility. The fibrous joints (synarthroses) are immovable joints, such as the sutures of the skull. Cartilaginous joints (amphiarthroses) are slightly movable and include the intervertebral disks and mandibular symphysis. Synovial joints are the most flexible, and most appropriate for internal medicine uses as these are joints where synovial fluid samples are obtained from. Synovial joints allow for flexion, extension, adduction, abduction, rotation, and circumduction of appendages.

Several components are involved in the structure of synovial joints. The joint capsule is made of fibrous connective tissue lined with the synovial membrane and makes up the joint cavity. The joint cavity is the space filled by synovia (joint fluid), which is what is sampled during arthrocentesis. Articular cartilage covers the surface of the bone and functions to absorb shock and provides for the smooth movement between two bones. Articular cartilage is hyaline and covers the surface of bones. Its main function is to reduce friction and wear within the joint and to absorb shock. Matrix secreting cells called chondrocytes are embedded in the cartilage. Because there is no blood supply within the cartilage, it obtains its nutrients from the synovial fluid within the joint, as well as from small vessels located within a thin membrane surrounding the cartilage. Ligaments are the bands of tissue between two bones that function to stabilize the joint.

There are many types of synovial joints within the body and are named for the movement they provide for. Ginglymus (hinge type) for flexion/extension, arthrodial (gliding/rocking) for flexion/extension and minimal abduction/adduction, trochoid (rotating/pivoting) for rotation only, and spheroidal (ball and socket), which allow for flexion/extension, abduction/adduction, and rotation/circumduction and is the most versatile joint in the body.

The muscular system

Introduction

There are three types of muscles within the body and they are defined by their cellular structure, which is further dictated by function. The skeletal muscle is responsible for controlled and conscious movement, which is stimulated by the nervous system. Smooth and cardiac muscles are not under conscious control and do not require stimulation from the nervous system to carry out their function. The muscles in the body can be further broken down into two categories. Voluntary muscles move on conscious command such as the skeletal muscles. Involuntary muscles move with nonconscious control and include smooth and cardiac muscles.

Skeletal muscle

Most skeletal muscles extend from one bone, across a joint, to another bone. The origin is the muscle attachment to the more stationary bone, and the insertion is the attachment to the more movable bone (ex. biceps brachii extends from its origin on the scapula to its insertion to the radius). The movement of the skeletal muscle is a result of contraction. Most skeletal muscles are paired for positive and negative resistance. Agonist muscles work with antagonist muscles in opposition (ex biceps/triceps). Synergist muscles work together to achieve the same movement. Fixator muscles work to stabilize joints.

The skeletal muscle is made of bundles of cells, or fibers, creating striated (striped) tissue. Muscles are composed of layers of connective tissue that encompasses muscle cells/fibers into bundles, or groups. Surrounding each muscle fiber is connective tissue called endomysium. The end point of these connective tissues is what makes up the tendons and aponeuroses that connect the muscle to the bone, or to another muscle.

The muscle cells, or fibers, that comprise the bundles, also called the muscle belly, have a fibrous cell membrane called the sarcolemma. Within each muscle fiber are multiple nuclei surrounded by myofibrils, which are made up of actin and myosin filaments, sarcoplasmic reticulum, and transverse tubules. Actin and myosin are the layered protein myofilaments of muscle fibers that move against each other to create contraction. The layers of actin and myosin are called sarcomeres. Muscle cells also contain a neuromuscular junction where nerve fibers connect into muscle fibers. The small space between the nerve fiber terminal branch and muscle fiber is a synaptic space, or gap, between the nerve ending and the sarcolemma. Synaptic vesicles are located in this space and contain acetylcholine, a neurotransmitter. When stimulated, the nerve will release acetylcholine that will bind to receptors located on the sarcolemma. These receptors will trigger a reaction that will travel the length of the sarcolemma and through the transverse tubules into the muscle fiber. The acetylcholine receptors (AChRs) also allow for sodium transfer that will result in the depolarization of the muscle and subsequent contraction. The sarcoplasmic reticulum will receive the impulse and release stored calcium into the myofibrils, which use adenosine triphosphate (ATP) for energy to perform the contraction via the movement of the sarcomeres. Once the depolarization of the muscle is complete, the myofibrils will use ATP and active transport to release the calcium back into the sarcoplasmic reticulum. As the calcium leaves the myofibrils, relaxation takes place.

Cardiac muscle

Cardiac muscle is an involuntary, striated muscle located only within the heart. Cardiac muscle cells contain a single nucleus and are smaller than skeletal muscle fibers. The cells link together by intercalated disks to form the muscles of the heart. The intercalated disks allow for the transmission of impulses between cells. This allows for the cells of the atria and ventricles to function as a syncytium or a single cell. The sinoatrial (SA) node will stimulate the cardiac muscle cells to contract at a specific pace that is dictated by the body's perfusion needs.

Smooth muscle

The smooth muscle is involuntary, nonstriated muscle, and comprises visceral structures associated with the digestive, urogenital, respiratory, and vascular systems. The smooth muscle is regulated by the autonomic nervous system and contracts without external stimulation. The smooth muscle cell structure of actin and myosin is arranged in a cross pattern that allows for significant elasticity. This provides for expansion when needed, such as in the stomach, bladder, and uterus. Smooth muscle cells are spindle shaped with a single nucleus.

SECTION 2 SELECTED DIAGNOSTICS IN MUSCULOSKELETAL DISEASE

Arthrocentesis

Arthrocentesis is a relatively simple procedure to either collect a sample of joint fluid for analysis (diagnostic) or to drain joint fluid and/or to inject medication (therapeutic). This section will discuss diagnostic arthrocentesis only, commonly called a joint tap.

Indications and contraindications

Arthrocentesis may be indicated to aid in the diagnosis of joint diseases and synovial effusions (inflammatory, noninflammatory, and infectious), to measure the response to therapy, and, in addition, to aid in the diagnosis of certain diseases. Arthrocentesis is typically performed by a clinician; however, if state law allows, it may be performed by a credentialed veterinary technician.

Arthrocentesis may be contraindicated in patients with coagulopathy, and alternate site selection is indicated if the skin or surrounding tissues are infected.

Site selection

There are multiple site options available for the collection of synovial fluid. Typically, the site of lameness and/or joint swelling is used for sampling. If indicated, multiple sites may be used and either submitted separately or the samples may be pooled

for testing. The most common sites for collection of synovial fluid are the radiocarpal and intracarpal, tarsal, and stifle joints.

Materials

1. Clippers
2. Surgical scrub/alcohol
3. Sterile gloves
4. 22- to 25-g needles, 1.0- to 1.5-in. length
5. 3- to 6-cc syringes
6. Slides
7. Culturette
8. EDTA and plain Vacutainer

Patient preparation and restraint

Sedation is recommended since arthrocentesis is an uncomfortable and sometimes painful procedure. The sample quality can be greatly affected by excessive movement of the patient (blood contamination from trauma). In severely painful or fractious animals, general anesthesia may be needed; however, this is not common. Local anesthetics are not recommended as they add extra fluid to the sample area and can contribute to contamination. Once the site(s) for arthrocentesis is chosen, the area is shaved and surgically prepared.

Technique

Using aseptic technique, the gloved hand will palpate for anatomical landmarks. This can be aided by the flexion and extension of the joint. With the joint in the flexed position (to allow an opening into the joint capsule), the needle with the syringe attached is inserted into the joint capsule. Once the needle has reached the joint space, the syringe is gently aspirated. In small patients, it is typical for only a minimal amount of synovial fluid to be obtained (0.01–1.0 mL); however, if significant inflammation or infection is present, large amounts of fluid can be obtained. Once the sample is collected, prior to removal of the needle, negative pressure is released in order to minimize contamination from hemorrhage or the surrounding tissues. If blood contamination occurs, reaspiration or relocation to a different joint is recommended. It is important to note that joint disease can cause a hemorrhagic effusion within the joint capsule itself. Samples with blood contamination may still be submitted for culture; however, clean samples are recommended for fluid analysis, cell counts, and cytology. Typical synovial fluid in animals is minimal in volume, clear to straw colored, and does not clot. If clots are noted within the sample, hemorrhage should be suspected, either caused by underlying disease or by blood contamination during collection.

Synovial fluid analysis

Volume, color, turbidity, and viscosity should be noted during collection. Normal volume should be between 0.01 and 1.0 mL, which varies with the joint used for collection as well as the size of the patient. Clinical experience can help determine if abnormal volumes are collected.

The color of joint fluid should be clear to straw colored. Abnormal samples can appear green yellow with mild to marked turbidity. Synovial fluid is highly viscous and can be checked by using the "strand" method. To perform this check, a small drop of synovial fluid is placed on the thumb. Press the thumb and forefinger together and then spread them apart. A strand of the sample material will extend across the gap. It is important to note that if this test is performed after the sample is added to EDTA, the viscosity can be falsely decreased due to the breakdown of hyaluronic acid that occurs in EDTA.

Sample submission is greatly determined by the volume of fluid obtained during arthrocentesis. If a significant amount of joint fluid is obtained, the sample may be placed into an anticoagulant, such as EDTA, and submitted for cell counts and cytology. If viscosity testing (e.g., mucin clot test) is needed and sample size is sufficient, a small amount of fluid should be placed into heparin, which does not affect viscosity. A small sample is also placed on a culturette or in a plain Vacutainer to submit for culture and sensitivity, as well as mycoplasma culture if indicated. If multiple sites are used, pooling of samples for culture/cytology can be performed. If only a small amount of synovial fluid is obtained, the sample is placed directly onto slides for squash preparation and submission for cytology.

Muscle biopsy

Muscle biopsies are performed when a myopathy of skeletal muscle, or an infectious disease affected muscle (e.g., hepatozoonosis), is suspected. Muscle biopsies are not commonly performed as less invasive testing methods are available (e.g., serum antibody testing, serum creatine phosphokinase (CPK) levels, and electrophysiology/myelography). It should be noted that electrophysiological testing is more valuable in the diagnosis of peripheral neuropathies than in that of myopathies. Within internal medicine, a muscle biopsy is most commonly performed to aid in the diagnosis of masticatory muscle myositis (MMM). The 2M antibody titer commonly performed can have a false-negative result due to low circulating numbers of the 2M antibody. This is uncommon occurrence, but in these circumstances, a muscle biopsy may be helpful in the diagnostic process.

Site selection

Most often, the muscle belly affected by the disease is biopsied. The site may be identified by pain response, muscle atrophy, or muscle hypertrophy.

When a muscle biopsy site is selected, electrophysiological testing should be avoided in the muscle belly that is to be biopsied. This testing can cause inadvertent changes and can affect the diagnosis. Single biopsies are common; however, biopsies of multiple muscle biopsies increase the chance of obtaining a diagnostic sample.

Patient and sample care

The procedure is surgical in nature and performed under general anesthesia. Typically, a 4- to 5-mm-wide, 2-cm-long section of a muscle belly is removed. The biopsy is then divided into two equal sections. One section is fixed in formalin for histopathology. The other portion of the biopsy should be refrigerated in a gauze sponge and submitted for histochemical staining that cannot be performed on formalin-fixed tissue.

Following the muscle biopsy monitoring of the surgical site for hemorrhage or signs of infection is recommended. In addition, adequate analgesia should be provided for a minimum of 2–3 days post biopsy depending on the patients needs.

SECTION 3 DISEASES OF THE MUSCULOSKELETAL SYSTEM

There are several diseases that affect the musculoskeletal system. This chapter will discuss joint disease (inflammatory, noninflammatory, and infectious), neuromuscular disease, and neoplastic disease.

Inflammatory joint disease

Infectious arthritis

Infectious arthritis is a form of inflammatory joint disease. Due to certain anatomical structures within the joint, as well as the blood supply within the bone itself, several pathogens are able to affect the joints of small animals. Most often, this occurs as a result of previous damage to joint structure from injury, congenital deformity, degenerative joint disease (DJD), or surgery. Older, large breed dogs are more susceptible to infectious arthritis. Most often, it is only one to two joints that are affected, whereas systemic infections typically affect most or all joints. Pain on palpation, in addition to swelling of the outlaying areas, is a common physical examination finding. Infectious arthritis can have several causes (bacterial, fungal, protozoal, and viral), which have been attributed to several disease processes including urinary tract, skin, and prostatic infections, as well as cardiac disease and myocarditis. Infectious arthritis is uncommon in cats. More information on specific infectious diseases can be found in Chapter 11.

Bacterial arthritis

Bacterial arthritis can be blood-borne (hematogenous) or local. Common causes for blood-borne bacterial arthritis include genitourinary tract, skin, oral, and respiratory infections. Most often, blood-borne bacterial arthritis is seen with juvenile cellulitis, also called sterile granulomatous dermatitis and lymphadenitis or puppy strangles. Septicemia with progression into the joint cavity as a result of pyelonephritis, cystitis, and prostatitis has also been noted. Bacterial arthritis can affect proximal joints as well as intervertebral disks. Local causes for bacterial arthritis are most often a result of surgical contamination, nonsterile arthrocentesis, and wounds. Common organisms for bacterial arthritis include *Streptococcus canis*, methicillin-resistant *Staphylococcus aureus* (MRSA), *Pasteurella* sp., *Brucella* spp., and *Salmonella* spp.

Clinical symptoms of bacterial arthritis include weight-bearing and non-weight-bearing lameness, fever, swelling and redness of the joint and surrounding tissue, nonhealing wounds, and draining tracts. Imaging results that are often noted with bacterial arthritis are thick synovial membranes, distended joint capsule, displacement of fiscal planes, widening of the joint space, destruction of the synovial membrane, and osteomyelitis. The diagnosis of bacterial arthritis is made by collection and culture of the synovial fluid. Concurrent cultures of blood and urine can also be performed. It has been reported that 50% of dogs with infectious arthritis have bacteria that reach the bloodstream as a result of concurrent urinary tract infection.[1]

Treatment of bacterial arthritis is composed of general supportive care and antibiotic therapy based on culture results. If blood and/or urine cultures are positive for bacterial growth, it is often considered the primary cause for the bacterial arthritis. Local infusions of antibiotics can be used in addition to systemic bactericidal medications.

L-form bacterial arthritis is a disease that affects cats. L-form bacteria are cell wall deficient and are similar to mycoplasma. L-form bacteria cause subcutaneous draining wounds and are most often attributed to bite wounds. For this reason, they are often located in the distal portion of the limbs and invade the joint cavity via the bloodstream. Culture of synovial fluid in these cases is often negative; however, treatment with tetracycline antibiotics is often successful. Mycoplasma arthritis is rare and typically associated with immune compromise and localization of mycoplasma to other areas (mostly respiratory).

Viral arthritis

Viral arthritis is not common in small animals; however, there are reports of a limping syndrome in cats with concurrent calicivirus infection, as well as following the use of live feline calicivirus vaccine.[1] Effusive forms of feline infectious peritonitis have been associated with potential viral arthritis in cats. Live vaccination has also been shown to cause limping in Weimaraners.[1] Distemper virus may affect the joints of dogs and may possibly lead to rheumatoid conditions later in life.

Fungal arthritis

Fungal arthritis is rare in small animals and is most often secondary to systemic fungal disease such as coccidioidomycosis, blastomycosis, histoplasmosis, and cryptococcosis. Fungal culture on synovial fluid is the diagnostic test of choice in the face of systemic fungal infections with acute arthritis symptoms.

Protozoal arthritis

Protozoal arthritis is not common in North America. *Leishmania donovani* is the organism associated with this disease and affects Mediterranean dogs and foxhounds in New York (see Chapter 11). It is transmitted via bloodsucking sand flies (*Phle-*

botomus spp.). Dogs will typically show signs of polyarthropathy. Arthrocentesis will yield a macrophage-filled synovial fluid with *Leishmania* bodies.

The treatment of all forms of infectious arthritis should include proper sterility to guard against nosocomial infections, primarily during arthrocentesis. In addition, when dealing with potentially zoonotic organisms, the use of personal protection equipment (PPE), adequate disinfection, and proper isolation procedures is necessary.

Tick-related joint disease

Tick-borne diseases can cause a form of infectious arthritis typically affecting the joints of dogs. Tick-borne diseases can affect cats; however, they are not associated with joint-related disease.

Lyme disease

Lyme disease, or Lyme borreliosis, is associated with a spirochete bacterial arthritis. *Borrelia burgdorferi* is a spirochete bacterium that is transmitted by ticks. These bacteria can become systemic and have been found in the synovial fluid and central nervous system of dogs. The vector associated with this disease is *Ixodes* spp. The musculoskeletal symptoms of Lyme disease are most often joint related in the limb closest to the tick bite. Acute polyarthritis and shifting leg lameness are the most common clinical signs and can become chronic intermittent. Other symptoms include joint swelling and effusion, fever, and lymphadenopathy. General laboratory findings are often normal; however, other forms of Lyme disease can result in abnormal biochemical and complete blood count (CBC) findings. Radiographs of the limbs will typically reveal soft tissue swelling and nonerosive arthritis.

Several diagnostic tests exist for Lyme disease; further discussion is found in Chapter 11. Most often, suppurative inflammation is noted on joint fluid cytology. Cultures of the synovial fluid are typically not performed due to the difficulty in isolating the bacteria from joint fluid.

The treatment for arthritis associated with Lyme disease is multifocal. Non-steroidal anti-inflammatory medications, in addition to opioids, are typically used to manage pain. Anti-inflammatory doses of glucocorticoids may also be used; however, it is often contraindicated due to their immunosuppressive properties. See Chapter 11 for more information.

Rickettsial/ehrlichial arthritis

Rickettsial and ehrlichial arthritis are other forms of vector-borne bacterial infections that can have joint-related symptoms. The most common rickettsial disease is Rocky Mountain spotted fever (RMSF), which is caused by *Rickettsia rickettsii* and an intracellular bacterium that is transmitted by *Dermacentor* spp. (deer ticks). RMSF can cause severe vasculitis and associated polyarthritis. The clinical symptoms are often joint, muscle, and neurological pain, as well as a stiff gait caused by generalized inflammation, lymphadenopathy, and fever.

Ehrlichial infections are transmitted by the *Rhipicephalus* spp. (brown dog) tick and cause a nonerosive polyarthritis. Different types of *Ehrlichia* are associated with more severe forms of arthritis (*Ehrlichia ewingi* and *Ehrlichia equi*) and are considered to be the granulocytic forms. However, cross reactivity in diagnostic testing will not differentiate between various types of ehrlichial disease. The clinical symptoms are similar to RMSF and include muscle stiffness, lameness, polyarthritis, lymphadenopathy, fever, and stilted gait.

Canine granulocytotropic anaplasmosis (*Anaplasma phagocytophilum*) is a previous member of the *Ehrlichia* genus and is also an obligate intracellular organism that causes musculoskeletal pain, stiffness, and lameness. It is transmitted by the *Ixodes* spp. tick and is diagnostically and clinically similar to ehrlichiosis.

Diagnostic testing for rickettsial and ehrlichial arthritis is needed to distinguish it from other forms of polyarthritis. Clinical history is needed to determine exposure to ticks as well as general laboratory abnormalities such as thrombocytopenia. The granulocytic forms of *Ehrlichia* can be seen on blood film evaluation; however, polymerase chain reaction (PCR), ELISA, and titers are the diagnostic tests of choice. The treatment for rickettsial and ehrlichial infections include tetracycline antibiotic therapy, supportive care, analgesia, vector control, and client education.

Any form of infectious arthritis can be difficult to treat. Treatment duration can vary depending on the organism in question, with weeks to months being typical. It is important to educate clients not only on treatment duration but also on the amount of time typically needed to see improvement. Proper compliance is needed for successful recoveries, and maintaining communications with veterinary professionals during the course of treatment can be helpful in determining if complications, relapse, or adverse effects from medications occur. During the recovery period, exercise should be restricted so as not to cause further pain/inflammation of the joints. In addition, climate control can be helpful as temperature extremes can increase pain and inflammation in the joints. Working dogs should be placed on hiatus until cleared from a veterinarian and gradually reintroduced to their working environment while monitoring for recurrence of symptoms. Some permanent damage can result from infectious forms of arthritis, and intermittent to persistent lameness may require treatment with physical therapy or medication.

Frequent rechecks are needed to properly evaluate the patient's recovery, which may include repeat antigen testing, radiographs, and blood work. It is helpful to develop a recheck schedule; this can increase client compliance and improve patient outcome. Developing a schedule of fees for these rechecks can also provide an opportunity for budgeting the long-term costs of patient care.

Noninfectious arthritis/immune-mediated arthropathies

Immune-mediated polyarthropathy

Immune-mediated polyarthropathy (IMPA), also known as idiopathic nonerosive, noninfectious arthritis, is the most common immune-mediated joint disease in dogs. It is less common in cats but has been reported. IMPA is one of the leading causes of cases

that present with fever of unknown origin.[2] It can affect single joints; however, the polyarticular form is most common. IMPA is divided into four types. Type I is idiopathic, or immune related, and is the most common form. Type II is associated with infection; type III is associated with gastrointestinal (GI) or hepatic disease, and type IV is associated with neoplastic causes.

The clinical symptoms and history of IMPA patients are a cyclic fever that is unresponsive to antibiotics; lethargy, stiff gait, lameness, spinal pain, and immobility being the most common signs.[2] Generalized muscle atrophy, joint swelling, lymphadenopathy, and anorexia are other possible clinical symptoms. IMPA most often affects medium to large dogs 1–6 years of age, and pure breeds are overrepresented (Labrador retrievers, German shepherds).

CBC will often show signs of general inflammation with neutrophilia and leukocytosis. The serum biochemistry panel is typically normal. Some liver enzyme elevation can be seen if glucocorticoid therapy has been started prior to diagnosis. Radiographs of affected limbs will show soft tissue swelling. Arthrocentesis is the diagnostic test of choice, and fluid analysis and cytology will be consistent with a sterile inflammation. The treatment for IMPA is supportive and immunosuppressive. Single immunosuppressive therapy with glucocorticoids is typical; however, multidrug therapy with additional immunosuppressives such as azathioprine, cyclosporine, and leflunomide may be needed. Approximately 30–50% of dogs with IMPA will suffer relapse.[1]

As with any immune disease, client compliance is imperative for successful treatment. Most immune-mediated arthropathies require treatment for 3–6 months. The most common medication prescribed is prednisone, and adverse effects can be pronounced in some patients. These include polyuria, polydypsia, polyphagia, panting, abdominal distension, and poor hair coat or growth. For some clients, the side effects of prednisone can significantly affect the quality of life at home and may lead to poor compliance. Rapid tapering of prednisone can increase the chance of relapse and a strict medication schedule should be discussed in detail. Clients should be made aware that patients requiring long-term treatment with immunosuppressive medications are prone to resistant infections and poor wound healing. Injuries should be monitored closely and examined if infection is suspected. In addition, periodic urine testing can be helpful in detecting subclinical urinary tract infections. Patients requiring treatment with more than one immunosuppressive medication often require longer treatment periods than with prednisone alone. Recheck and fee schedules can provide additional information that can increase client compliance and can aid in patient recovery.

Canine rheumatoid arthritis

Canine rheumatoid arthritis (RA) is a type I noninfectious inflammatory joint disease that affects small, toy breeds ranging from 8 months to 8 years of age. The clinical symptoms include shifting leg lameness and swelling, most often affecting the carpal/tarsal joints, but it can affect any joint including vertebral articulations. Other symptoms are fever, lethargy, anorexia, and lymphadenopathy.

A CBC will show evidence of generalized inflammation with leukocytosis and neutrophilia. Radiographic abnormalities are typically loss of bone density at the joint, soft tissue swelling, luxations/subluxations, and narrowing or widening of the joint spaces. There is no specific rheumatoid factor testing in dogs due to lack of sensitivity; however, antinuclear antibodies (ANAs) can occasionally be detected in canine RA. Arthrocentesis will yield an inflammatory fluid analysis with an elevated white blood cell count. IgG containing mononuclear cells within the synovial fluid is the defining test resulting in a diagnosis of canine RA.

The treatment for canine RA consists of supportive care and lifelong immunosuppressive doses of corticosteroids. Most often, a combination of multiple immunosuppressive medications is needed for the resolution of the clinical symptoms of canine RA.

Joint laxity and physical deformity is common due to the erosive nature of RA. While patients undergoing treatment for RA may have minimal pain, they often require extensive care at home as a result of decreased mobility. Carts or wheelchairs are available, which can aid mobility and decrease the extensive nature of home care. The mobility of dogs with erosive arthritis varies between cases, and larger dogs often carry a poorer prognosis as a result of the increased care needed at home.

For patients with significantly decreased mobility, providing adequate bedding and cushioning is imperative to prevent decubital ulcers or bed sores. Since these patients are immunosuppressed, infection of decubital ulcers can be common and prevention is often the best treatment. Decubital ulcers should be cultured, if possible, to identify any potential resistant infections that may require more extensive treatment. In addition, physical therapy can help increase muscle strength, which will in turn aid mobility.

Frequent monitoring of CBC, biochemistry panels, and urinalysis is required for patients undergoing lifelong immunosuppression to detect any potential adverse effects of medication such as liver or kidney damage, or subclinical urinary tract infections.

Drug related

In a similar fashion as immune-mediated hemolytic anemia (IMHA), some medications can incite an immune response that affects the joints of dogs. These medications include sulfonamides, penicillin, erythromycin, lincomycin, and cephalosporins. Drug-related antibody complexes are deposited throughout the body and cause the immune response. The clinical symptoms are similar to IMPA but can also include hemorrhagic rashes and acute vasculitis. Symptoms will typically present themselves 10–21 days following the start of the medication. Treatment consisting of general supportive care and discontinuation of implicated medication most often yields a quick resolution; however, some patients will require some immunosuppression medications.

For patients with drug-induced IMPA, a list of medications to avoid can be given to the client and will be helpful in preventing relapse.

Systemic lupus erythematosus

Systemic lupus erythematosus (SLE) is an immune disorder in both dogs and cats. While it can be seen in mixed breeds, the highest incidence of SLE is in purebred animals.[1] Most often, the clinical symptoms are dermatology related; however, some patients will experience SLE-related polyarthritis. The diagnosis of SLE is typically made by performing an ANA test and the exclusion of underlying causes. The treatment for SLE-related polyarthritis is single or combination immunosuppressive therapy.

Enteropathic polyarthritis

There is a rare occurrence of polyarthropathy that has been linked to chronic GI or hepatic disease. The clinical symptoms are similar to most joint disease with swelling, fever, and shifting leg lameness being the most common. The treatment is aimed at the underlying disease process and pain control. Most often, immunosuppressive therapy is initiated if indicated for the underlying GI or hepatic disease.

Noninflammatory joint disease

Degenerative joint disease/osteoarthritis

DJD is the most common joint disease in small animals and the most common cause for chronic pain. DJD can be divided into primary and secondary forms of osteoarthritis (OA). Primary OA is idiopathic, and secondary OA is the most common form in small animals. With secondary OA, changes occur within the joint as a result of abnormal force on normal joints, or normal force on abnormal joints. This excessive or abnormal force will lead to synovitis and cartilage loss. With OA, there is a possible overproduction of destructive and proinflammatory substances by the chondrocytes (cells of the cartilage), which leads to this progressive breakdown of the cartilage.

Any canine or feline breeds can be affected by DJD; however, overweight animals are at risk as a result of the excessive force that occurs on all joints. Other predisposing factors of DJD include misalignment, excessive activity (working dogs), joint injury, preexisting arthritis, and hip dysplasia. Secondary DJD is most often seen in large breed dogs; however, intervertebral disk disease (IVDD) is a form of DJD that commonly occurs in small/short-legged breeds of dogs. The most common factor leading to DJD in large dogs is hip dysplasia. Hip dysplasia is the result of a shallow acetabulum that results in significant coxofemoral joint laxity and flattening of the femoral head, and is most often attributed to developmental, environmental, and hereditary causes. The occurrence of DJD in cats is mostly associated with age and typically affects the front limbs.

The clinical symptoms of DJD (primary or secondary) of dogs and cats are progressive. Early symptoms encompass reluctance to perform normal activity, lameness/stiff gait after activity or periods of rest, and during cold or damp weather. As the damage to joint cartilage increases, symptoms will progress to include abnormal gait, vocalization, pain, decreased range of motion (ROM), crepitus, and change in personality.

The diagnostic used for DJD is typically radiographic but can be aided by palpation of the joints during a musculoskeletal examination. Depending on the level of pain in the patient, sedation may be required for the proper manipulation of limbs during the radiographic process. Images of joints will typically reveal evidence of bone remodeling and narrowing of the joint space. If arthrocentesis is performed, it will yield normal to increased amounts of fluid, often after periods of activity, and cytology will demonstrate a sterile synovitis.

The treatment of DJD requires significant client education as the goal is aimed at the improvement of the quality of life. Owners of young animals should be educated to know that some causes of DJD, such as obesity and excessive activity, can be prevented by proper nutrition and appropriate exercise and rest. In addition to medical therapy, many treatments that aid in the reduction of pain caused by DJD/OA and the subsequent improvement of the quality of life occur in the home. They include weight reduction, physical therapy, and controlled or limited exercise.

There are several medical therapies available for the improvement of the quality of life for animals with DJD. The most common is the use of non-steroidal anti-inflammatory medications such as deracoxib, meloxicam, carprofen, and firocoxib. The side effects of NSAIDs include impaired renal/liver function as well as GI upset and may not be appropriate for all patients. Glycosaminoglycans such as Adequan® and Hyalovet® are intra-articular and intramuscular injections of compounds derived from bovine cartilage that have been shown to reduce the degenerative changes that are seen with DJD. Glucosamine and chondroitin are supplements used for their possible effect on cartilage metabolism and breakdown and typically have a cumulative effect. The most common veterinary supplements of glucosamine and chondroitin are Cosequin® and Dasuquin®. Because of their cumulative effect, several weeks of treatment are required before improvement may be noted. A multifocal medical approach is often the most successful.

There are surgical treatment options for some forms of DJD. The most common is for arthritis associated with hip dysplasia and includes total hip replacement or femoral head osteotomy. Other joints may be most benefited by arthrodesis.

Stem cell therapy, also called autologous adipose-derived mesenchymal stem cell (AD-MSC) therapy, is an emerging field of treatment for some types of DJD/OA. A surgical harvest of adipose tissue from the patient is performed. This sample is submitted to the laboratory, which forms a pellet of regenerative cells including fibroblasts, parricides, endothelial cells, and AD-MSCs. The pellet is then administered as an intra-articular injection. Clinical studies[3,4] have shown significant improvement in the coxofemoral and elbow joints in dogs with DJD/OA.

Neuromuscular diseases

Myasthenia gravis

Myasthenia gravis is a neuromuscular transmission disease caused by a reduction in the numbers of AChRs on muscle cell membranes and affects both dogs and cats. Both congenital and acquired forms exist. Acquired myasthenia gravis is the most common form seen in small animals. It is a result of the production of antibodies against the AChRs that block neuromuscular transmission. The blockage can occur as a result of complement or by accelerated normal destruction. Several disorders associated with myasthenia gravis are thymomas and paraneoplastic disorders, drug-associated disorders (methimazole in cats), third-degree heart block, hypothyroidism, and concurrent immune-related problems (IMHA, IMPA, hypoadrenocorticism). For more information, please refer to Chapter 4.

Myasthenia gravis affects dogs and cats 2–3 years of age and older than 8–9 years of age. Breed dispositions for myasthenia gravis include German shepherds, Labrador retrievers, Akitas, terriers, and Abyssinian and Somali cats. The clinical signs are skeletal muscle weakness, exercise intolerance, worsening of symptoms with exercise and improvement with rest, regurgitation of food, dysphagia, and dyspnea associated most often with aspiration pneumonia.

There are focal, generalized, and acute fulminant generalized forms of myasthenia gravis. Focal myasthenia is associated most often with the cranial nerves, and symptoms include change in voice, regurgitation, dysphagia, and facial, pharyngeal, laryngeal, and esophageal dysfunction. Generalized myasthenia is a chronic disease and, most often, patients present with dyspnea as a result of aspiration pneumonia that occurs with megaesophagus. Approximately 80–90% of generalized myasthenia patients have megaesophagus.[3,5] Dogs with generalized myasthenia gravis may also present with symptoms consistent with laryngeal paralysis. Acute fulminant generalized myasthenia gravis is severe. Patients will typically present in a nonambulatory fashion with tetraparesis and dyspnea. This form is fatal as respiratory arrest occurs as a result of poorly functioning intercostal muscles and aspiration pneumonia.

Routine serum biochemistry panels are often normal; CBCs can be normal or may show evidence of infection with leukocytosis; and thyroxin levels are often low as a result of concurrent hypothyroidism or euthyroid sick syndrome. Thoracic radiographs can reveal megaesophagus, aspiration pneumonia, mediastinal masses, or other evidence of metastasis.

There are several specific tests available to help diagnose myasthenia gravis. An AChR autoantibody test is commonly performed. This test detects specific antibodies against the AChRs. False negatives can occur in approximately 2% of patients with generalized myasthenia gravis[3] and is thought to be a result of low numbers of circulating acetylcholine antibodies in the serum.[5] False-positive results with this test are rare. It is important to note that AChR antibody testing should be performed prior to the use of corticosteroids, which may lower antibody concentrations.[3] Another useful test is the edrophonium (Tensilon®) response test. Edrophonium is an indirect acting cholinergic/anticholinesterase drug that, when administered intravenously (dog: 0.1–0.2 mg/kg, cat: 0.25–0.5 mg/kg), can cause a myasthenic patient to have short-lived markedly increased muscle strength. Edrophonium overdose or use in nonmyasthenic animals will cause hypersalivation, vomiting, and diarrhea and can be treated with 0.02–0.04 mg/kg of atropine. Pretreatment with atropine is recommended in cats as they are predisposed to hypersensitivity to edrophonium. A similar test can be performed with neostigmine (20 μg/kg IV or 40 μg/kg IM); however, there is limited specificity and sensitivity with this test. Electromyelograms can also detect delayed neuromuscular transmission and can aid in the diagnosis of myasthenia gravis. Histopathologic evaluation of muscle biopsies can show decreased numbers of AChRs. A presumptive diagnosis of myasthenia gravis can be obtained by noting a decreased response to repetitive stimuli under anesthesia.

The treatment for myasthenia is medical and supportive. Medical treatments include anticholinesterase agents that prolong the activity of acetylcholine and increase the reaction at the neuromuscular junction. Pyridostigmine bromide (Mestinon®) at 1–3 mg/kg orally every 8–12 h is the maintenance treatment of choice. It can be given as a constant rate infusion at 0.01–0.03 mg/kg/h. Injectable neostigmine at 0.04 mg/kg given IM every 6 h can be used if megaesophagus prevents the use of oral medications. Oral neostigmine bromide can be given at a dose of 2 mg/kg/day. In addition to anticholinesterase drugs, the avoidance of medications that reduce neuromuscular transmission (magnesium, phenothiazine, aminoglycosides, ampicillin, and antiarrhythmic drugs) is highly recommended. Constant monitoring of clinical symptoms and the response to treatment is indicated as a spontaneous remission is possible. Adverse side effects of anticholinesterase treatment include bradycardia, hypotension, heart block, diarrhea, vomiting, increased GI activity and GI rupture. The use of corticosteroids may also be helpful in long-term, mild cases but is not recommended until a positive response to anticholinesterase treatment is seen. This is due to the initial weakness and immunosuppression that can be seen with myasthenia gravis. Treatment should also include the removal or treatment of concurrent thymoma or neoplastic syndromes that may be causing myasthenic symptoms.

The supportive treatment for myasthenia gravis can be extensive due to the common finding of megaesophagus and concurrent aspiration pneumonia. Supportive care for myasthenics with megaesophagus includes specific feeding instructions and can require significant time to perfect as the specifics can vary from patient to patient. Upright, gravity feeding is the most common. Patients are fed varying consistencies of food from gruel to meatballs in an upright position and are then held upright for 5–10 min following feeding to ensure gravity has pulled the food from the nonfunctioning esophagus into the stomach. Gastrostomy tubes can help with feedings; however, they do not prevent the possibility of aspiration pneumonia. Extensive supportive care for patients with aspiration pneumonia is required, with fluid therapy, antibiotics, and oxygen supplementation often needed. Nutritional support with partial parenteral and total parenteral nutrition can be helpful in speeding recovery. A significant amount of education should be made so the owners may be able to tell the difference between regurgitation and vomiting, as well as the symptoms for aspiration pneumonia.

The congenital form is a defect in the number of AChRs and no production of AChR antibodies. It is typically diagnosed by Tensilon testing and muscle biopsy showing a decreased number of AChRs. The breeds associated with this disease include Jack Russell and fox terriers, English springer spaniels, miniature dachshunds, Siamese cats, and domestic shorthair cats. Clinical symptoms are typically noted at a very young age and do not typically include megaesophagus. The treatment is similar to acquired myasthenia gravis; however, it is generally unsuccessful and most perish within the first year of life.[4]

Inflammatory myopathies

Muscle disease caused by inflammation can occur in dogs and cats and are either immune related (idiopathic), or associated with other diseases such as parasite, viral, protozoal, and fungal infections (secondary). Clinical symptoms of inflammatory myopathies are associated with the muscle groups affected and can often be systemic.

Masticatory muscle myositis

MMM is a canine idiopathic inflammatory myopathy that affects the masticatory muscles, specifically the 2M myosin fibers located only in the masticatory muscles (digastricus, temporalis, masseter, and pterygoid). MMM mostly affects large breed dogs (German shepherds, Labrador retrievers, Doberman pinschers, golden retrievers) with a median age of 3 years[4]; however, any breed can be susceptible.

The clinical symptoms associated with MMM include acute or chronic bilateral hypertrophy of the temporal and masseter muscles. This can progress to atrophy and fibrosis of these muscles. Fever, jaw pain, and trismus (inability to open the jaw normally) with the associated signs of dysphagia and hypersalivation are also common. Ocular muscles may be involved in approximately 44% of the cases.[4] As a result, exophthalmos and conjunctivitis may be noted and blindness, as a result of optic nerve compression, can occur. Poor body condition scores as a result of inadequate nutrition from dysphagia may be noted.

Routine blood work is typically nonspecific; however, common findings include evidence of inflammation on CBC and elevated creatine kinase (CK) on serum biochemical analysis. CK is a muscle enzyme involved in energy storage and increases are seen with muscle necrosis as a result of inflammation. CK results on serum biochemical analysis can be affected by poor blood collection and hyperbilirubinemia, so high quality blood collection is imperative. CK levels may be decreased in late/chronic disease states. Urinalysis results may reveal proteinuria. Testing for tick-borne diseases may be indicated to rule out secondary causes for inflammatory myopathy. Imaging results can aid in diagnosis as well. If CK results are low, MRI may be helpful by showing inflammatory lesions in the masticatory muscles and may help by revealing the optimum locations for muscle biopsy. Thoracic radiographs may show mediastinal masses (thymoma) or other tumor metastases associated with paraneoplastic issues that may be related to secondary causes for MMM.

Diagnostic procedures include electromyography (EMG), where abnormal spontaneous activity can be found in the acute stages of MMM, and decreased activity is noted in later stages. However, EMG findings may be nonspecific as it is unable to distinguish between myopathies and neuropathies. Muscle biopsies may be helpful in revealing necrosis and/or phagocytosis of the 2M fibers. Biopsy may also help with prognosis as it can give an indication as to the duration and severity of the illness. Higher levels of fibrosis are associated with a poorer prognosis and increased loss of function of the masticatory muscles. The gold standard for the diagnosis of MMM is a 2M antibody test. This test measures the presence of antibodies against the 2M fibers in the serum. It is 100% specific and 85–95% sensitive.[6] It is important to note that the results can be affected by corticosteroid treatment for 7–10 days prior to collection.[4]

The treatment for idiopathic MMM involves immunosuppression, most often with corticosteroid administration. The dose is tapered over a 4- to 6-month period based on clinical symptoms and CK levels. It is important to educate clients on the clinical symptoms so that close home monitoring is accurate. Multidrug immunosuppressive therapy is needed in more severe cases or in patients that cannot tolerate long-term prednisone. Nutritional interventions may also be needed as many cases have significant jaw pain and/or lock jaw, preventing them from chewing properly. Experimentation with food consistency may be needed. Many patients have less pain and an easier time eating with gruel consistency food in the early stages of treatment. Once a response to immunosuppression is seen, most patients can slowly transition back to their normal consistency of food. In severe cases where symptoms are slow to resolve, esophageal or gastrostomy feeding tubes may be needed. Since many patients do not have a full range of jaw motion, close monitoring for vomiting and aspiration pneumonia should be performed. Physical therapy can also hasten some recovery. Toys, massage, and ROM exercise, patient willing, have been shown to help; however, no forcible retraction of the jaw should be attempted.

Polymyositis

Polymyositis is an idiopathic inflammatory myopathy that is similar to MMM. Unlike MMM, there are no circulating 2M antibodies, so it typically affects large muscle groups rather than local disease. It can have clinical findings similar to MMM with lock jaw, temporalis muscle wasting, as well as ocular signs noted. Polymyositis is also associated with lupus patients.

Most often, large breed dogs are affected, and there is no known breed disposition in cats. The clinical symptoms include fever, pain, cervical ventroflexion, dysphagia, change in voice, and muscle weakness, stiffness, and atrophy. Megaesophagus, regurgitation, and aspiration pneumonia are also common findings. Focal muscle groups can be affected, but most often, systemic skeletal muscles are involved.

As with most inflammatory myopathies, serum biochemical analysis often shows elevated CK values and CBC results will be consistent with generalized inflammation. Infectious disease testing for secondary causes of inflammatory myopathy should be performed as well. Diagnostic testing is similar to MMM and

includes EMG and muscle biopsy. Muscle biopsy will show inflammation with evidence of necrosis and/or regeneration. Treatment of polymyositis is immunosuppression, supportive and nutritional care, and monitoring for complications such as aspiration pneumonia.

For patients with megaesophagus, at-home care can be difficult, and experimentation with food consistencies can be helpful in determining what works best for each patient. Meatballs or small boluses of food will do better for some, while gruel will do better for others. Gravity is the key in aiding digestion as the esophagus lacks the contractility to move food into the stomach. Feeding and watering from an elevated position, as well as allowing the animal to remain elevated for 10–15 min following feeding, will allow the food to pass from the esophagus into the stomach. Larger dogs may be fed with their front end on the stairs or a counter, while smaller- to medium-sized dogs can be held or may use a Bailey chair. Bailey chairs may be constructed or purchased and can help decrease the stress and time it takes to feed a patient with megaesophagus. See Figure 4.4 (Chapter 4, "Neurology").

Clients should also be instructed to monitor closely for evidence of aspiration pneumonia, which is a common complication in patients with megaesophagus. If food or vomitus is regurgitated and aspirated, the patient may exhibit cough, rattles, or difficulty in breathing and may require medical intervention.

Hepatozoonosis

Hepatozoonosis is a protozoal vector-borne disease that primarily affects dogs. *Hepatozoon americanum* infection is associated with muscle and bone infection. Cats are susceptible; however, it is rare, has different clinical symptoms, and is typically associated with other hepatozoonosis species. Following ingestion, sporozoites travel through the gut to the striated muscle, the skeletal muscle, muscle fibers, and the cardiac muscle. Once it has reached the target organs, it forms an "onion skin" cyst. The cysts will rupture at various times, creating inflammation and creating a pyogranuloma at the site of the cyst. The pyogranulomas that form in muscle tissue surrounding long bones can cause periostial pain and proliferation. Information on hepatozoonosis, diagnosis, and treatment can also be found in Chapter 11.

Hepatozoonosis cases are most often seen in the warmer months when exposure to ticks is highest; however, symptoms can be seen year round due to the waxing and waning nature of this disease. The clinical symptoms are the result of the pyogranulomatous inflammation and include fever, cachexia, muscle atrophy, weakness or stiffness, hyperesthesia, ocular discharge, and possible keratoconjunctivitis sicca (KCS). Pain may be generalized or may be localized to joints, lumbar, and cervical regions. As a result, neck guarding and gait abnormalities may be noted.

Radiographs may show periosteal proliferation of the long bones, most commonly a result of inflammation in skeletal muscle surrounding the diaphysis. This finding is most common in younger dogs with hepatozoonosis.[7] Bone scintigraphy has also shown early bilateral bone lesions and may be helpful for early *H. americanum* bone detection.

Neoplasia

Osteosarcoma

Osteosarcoma (OSA) is the most common primary bone tumor in dogs and causes bone lysis, bone production, or both. OSA accounts for 85% of skeletal malignancies.[8,9] Breed dispositions include rottweilers, St. Bernards, Great Danes, Doberman pinschers, German shepherds, and golden retrievers. It is relatively uncommon in small breed dogs and more common in intact animals. OSA affecting the appendicular skeleton is found in the majority of patients accounting for up to 75% of OSA cases.[8,9] The primary location for the tumor is in the metaphyseal area of the long bones; however, it can also be found in the mandible/maxillary, spine, cranium, ribs, and nasal passages. The front limbs are most often affected at the distal radius and proximal humerus.[8,9] OSA can also affect the spleen, liver, mammary tissue, testicles, and kidneys. It is uncommon for OSA to cross joint spaces (joint spaces cause bone confinement); however, metastasis will occur through soft tissue contact and the lungs are the most frequent site of metastasis.

The clinical symptoms of appendicular OSA are localized swelling, pain, and acute or chronic lameness. Axial skeletal symptoms vary and are dependent on the area affected. Localized swelling is the most common general symptom of axial skeletal OSA. Maxillary and mandibular OSAs may cause dysphagia and pain upon opening/closing of the jaw. Facial, nasal, or cranial OSA may cause exophthalmos, facial deformity, and nasal and ocular discharge. Spinal OSA is associated with spinal pain and swelling, paraparesis, and ataxia. OSA of the ribs can be seen and most often causes pain, occasionally resulting in dyspnea.

CBCs may show evidence of inflammation and serum biochemical analysis may have elevated alkaline phosphate results, but it is not uncommon for general blood work to be normal. Radiographs of the affected area will often show lysis and other osteogenic changes, periosteal proliferation around the lesion, and soft tissue swelling, and it is possible to see pathological fractures. A biopsy of the lesion is needed to differentiate between OSA and other diseases or neoplastic processes.

Following the diagnosis of OSA, staging is required for adequate prognosis due to its high rate of metastasis. Stage 1 comprises local lesions with no metastasis; stage 2 is high grade lesions with no metastasis; and stage 3 is OSA lesions with metastasis. Staging typically includes fine needle aspirate and/or biopsy of regional lymph nodes, three-view thoracic radiographs, abdominal ultrasound, and a thorough orthopedic examination for pain and other possible sites of OSA. Bone survey radiographs, computed tomography (CT), and MRI may be helpful in determining the presence of early lung lesions or other soft tissue involvement.

The treatment of canine OSA is focused on pain control and the extension of a good quality of life. With appendicular OSA, amputation is the standard surgical treatment. Most dogs will do well with the absence of a limb; however, overweight dogs, dogs with preexisting degenerative joints, or dogs with neurological disease will often have a quick progression of postsurgical problems. The amputation of a thoracic limb most often will include the scapula, and the pelvic limb amputations will involve coxofemoral disarticulation for distal femoral lesions, and en bloc acetabulectomy or subtotal hemipelvectomy for proximal femoral lesions. Limb-sparing surgery with allograft or steel implants is a possible option for dogs with preexisting conditions that indicate the possibility of postoperative complications. Good candidates for limb-sparing surgery include patients whose lesions were detected early and those patients whose lesions are confined to the limb. Most often, this will be lesions of the distal radius/ulna and lesions where the majority (50%) of the remaining bone is intact. Limb-sparing surgery does have a high rate of complications, including local infection, graft infection and rejection, and recurrence of local disease. Postoperative care for limb-sparing surgery includes exercise to minimize swelling of the distal limb and to prevent flexure contracture of the digits.

Adequate pain control with epidurals, opioid injections, and constant rate infusions are extremely important for postoperative amputations. Most dogs will be able to ambulate without assistance in 12–24 h. The technician should assist and encourage movement during the recovery period. Extra care should be taken to prevent further injury to the other limbs. Detailed client education on home care should be performed including encouragement to exercise with restrictions for confinement when not monitored, avoidance of stairs, and leash walking only. Infection, air embolism (as a result of minute amounts of air left inside the body following closure of the incision), hemorrhage, and recurrence of disease at the surgery site are the most common complications.

Following surgery, chemotherapy may be used to control metastasis. The mean survival time for most OSA patients with amputation and chemotherapy is 12 months.[10] Technicians should be aware of specific chemotherapy administration protocols, side effects, handling guidelines, and elimination times. Technicians should educate clients on the side effects of the treatments and the care the patients will need at home. The most commonly used chemotherapy agents for OSA are cisplatin, carboplatin, and doxorubicin. Cisplatin is nephrotoxic and is given with saline diuresis at a dose of $70\,mg/m^2$ intravenously every 3 weeks. This medication is fatal in feline patients. Carboplatin is less nephrotoxic than cisplatin; however, side effects include myelosupression and severe GI upset. Carboplatin is typically given at a dose of $300\,mg/m^2$ intravenously every 3 weeks in dogs and $240–260\,mg/m^2$ intravenously every 3 weeks in feline patients. Doxorubicin is an anthtracycline chemotherapy agent with possible myocardial toxicity typically seen with cumulative doses of $>180\,mg/m^2$. Myelosuppression, GI upset, hypersensitivity/allergic reaction during administration, nephrotoxicity (in cats), and perivascular damage with extravasation can also be seen. The dose is typically $30\,mg/m^2$ intravenously every 3 weeks in patients weighing more than 10 kg, and

1 mg/kg intravenously in patients weighing less than 10 kg. Radiation therapy may also be used for palliative purposes and can relieve pain in some cases. It is most useful when surgery is not an option or is refused. The side effects of radiation therapy are most often a moist desquamation, alopecia, depigmentation, and pathological fracture. See the section on radiation therapy in this chapter for more information.

As previously stated, control of pain is an integral part in the treatment of OSA. Pain can be relieved by amputation; however, patients not undergoing surgery or patients with advanced disease require significant analgesia. A multidrug approach is commonly used with non-steroidal anti-inflammatory medications and opiates such as tramadol, gabapentin, and amantadine. Glucocorticoids can also be used to decrease inflammation and are often helpful in patients with pulmonary metastasis, but cannot be used concurrently with NSAIDs. Analgesia should be started immediately following the diagnosis of OSA. A better quality of life can be maintained with preventative or proactive pain control.

OSA is an aggressive tumor where metastasis is likely and, as noted earlier, is most often pulmonary related. If only amputation is performed, 90% of dogs will die of metastatic disease within 1 year of diagnosis,[9] and most within 3–4 months.[8] Mandibular OSA, however, does have a higher survival rate with just mandibulectomy. Feline OSA is rare but can occur, most often in the pelvic limbs. Unlike canine OSA, amputation may be curative in cats.

Chondrosarcoma

Chondrosarcoma (CSA) is the second most common primary bone tumor in dogs. Golden retrievers are most likely to be afflicted by CSA. CSA will most often occur in the flat bones (including the nasal cavity and ribs) but will occasionally occur in the long bones. CSA can also be found in soft tissue including mammary tissue, heart valves, aorta, larynx, trachea, lung, and omentum. Unlike OSA, CSA is slow to metastasize and prognosis is based on the location of the tumor. The treatment for CSA is surgical resection of the area, if possible, which can be curative. No known chemotherapeutic treatments for CSA exist. The clinical symptoms of CSA comprise pain and localized swelling. A diagnosis is based on histopathologic findings.

Rhabdomyosarcoma

Rhabdomyosarcoma (RSA) is a malignant tumor of striated muscle cells (soft tissue sarcoma) that occurs in young dogs and has been reported in dogs as young as 4 months.[11] RSA is relatively uncommon and carries a moderate risk for metastasis. Common areas of metastasis are the lungs, liver, spleen, kidney, and adrenal glands. RSA can appear as soft or firm, slow growing, locally invasive, and nonpainful tumors. Rapid increases in size can be seen with internal hemorrhage or necrosis of the mass. Symptoms can vary with location, and intra-abdominal RSA can cause vomiting, diarrhea, melena, weight loss, and anorexia.

RSA can also be found in the bladder and may cause hematuria, dysuria, and stranguria.

The diagnosis of RSA is made from biopsy, and the biopsy procedure is based on location. A fine needle aspirate may be attempted but may not be diagnostic due to poor cell exfoliation with RSA. Other diagnostics such as CT and radiographs of the site may be needed to prepare for surgical biopsy and/or removal. Staging of RSA, as with most neoplasia, is recommended and should include routine serum biochemical analysis and thoracic radiographs.

The treatment of choice for RSA is surgical resection; however, recurrence is common at the surgery site. Wide surgical margins (3 cm is typical) are recommended to ensure adequate margins are obtained.[11] The resection of any tissues adhered to the tumor, including bone, is recommended. Postsurgical chemotherapy for sarcoma can be administered; however, sarcomas have a poor response to chemotherapy. Radiation therapy can also be used; however, poor response has been noted with larger-sized tumors. Most often, the vincristine, adriamycin/doxorubicin, and cyclophosphamide (VAC) protocol is used for the treatment of sarcomas. Vincristine (0.5–0.7 mg/m2 IV) is an antitubulin agent and its side effects are myelosupression, perivascular damage with extravasation, peripheral neuropathy, and GI upset; in cats, constipation can also be seen. Cyclophosphamide is typically bone marrow toxic and can cause GI upset. A sterile hemorrhagic cystitis may occur as a side effect of the inflammatory effects of the metabolites of the drug on the lining of the bladder. For this reason, it is advised to encourage water intake, to provide ready access to water, and to encourage frequent urination in patients on this medication. The dose for cyclophosphamide varies, and it comes in oral and intravenous formulations.

Other neoplasia

Fibrosarcoma (FSA) of the bone in dogs has no specific chemotherapy or radiation protocols. The recommendation for bone FSA is surgical resection. FSA carries a poor prognosis. Metastasis is common with FSA and commonly affects the heart, pericardium, skin, and other bones before spreading to lung tissue.

Hemangiosarcoma (HSA) can also rarely occur as a bone tumor. It carries a similar presentation to most bone neoplasia and will appear as lysis on radiographs. HSA of the bone carries a poor prognosis with <10% surviving 1 year[9] after surgical resection and VAC protocol.

SECTION 4 GENERAL MUSCULOSKELETAL EXAMINATION

A thorough musculoskeletal examination performed by the technician can provide the clinician additional information that may help localize potential musculoskeletal disease and aid in the creation of a diagnostic plan. The most important part of any examination includes a complete history including signalment, current medications, preexisting conditions, as well as the current complaint or presenting problems. When performing a musculoskeletal examination, which can be lengthy, it is important to take a systematic approach. Maintaining a consistent systematic approach for each patient will ensure that little to no information is missed during a musculoskeletal examination.

The beginning of a thorough muscular examination should begin with gross observation of the patient, starting in the front (facing the patient), continuing to the rear, moving to the right and left flanks, and continuing down the limbs, including the joints and toes. During the entire examination, it is important to take note of any swelling, muscle atrophy, or asymmetry in the body, as these are often indications of disease or injury.

Gross observation at the front of the patient should involve noting the head position, any displacement of the ears, tilting of the head left or right, or any severe angling above or below the shoulders. When observing the placement of the head, also noting the patient's mental status can be helpful. Following the length of the spine and moving toward the rear of the patient, observe any obvious hunched posture or sagging of the spine. From the rear, evaluate the patient's distribution of weight between the limbs or any obvious lameness. A limb with atrophy or injury can cause an uneven distribution of weight and can help localize a potential area of injury or disease. Moving to the right and left flanks of the animal, observe the length of all four limbs and lift the paws and evaluate each one. Patients with some musculoskeletal disease can drag the limbs, leaving scuffed or broken nails, as well as minor abrasions.

Following general gross observation, the next portion of the musculoskeletal examination should involve palpation of musculature and bone. As with any assessment with the potential for pain, it is recommended to have proper restraint in place before the start of the examination. Begin the palpation with the muscles of the head and jaw; move down the spine all the way to the sacrum. Then, palpate down each limb; gentle pressure should be placed with the tips of the fingers noting atrophy, asymmetry, or swelling. For finding asymmetry, it is helpful to palpate the left and right portions of the body at the same time. Atrophy can be an indicator of poor usage due to chronic injury or disease (e.g., MMM). Swelling or heat can be an indication of acute muscle injury or tearing. During palpation, masses or areas of abnormal tissue may also be noted and mapped. Bone and muscle palpation can be performed simultaneously using a similar technique. Gentle pressure with the thumb or the fingertips should be used to palpate the bones of each limb, noting any areas of pain, swelling, or abnormal bony protrusions. It is important to avoid palpation of obvious fractures or areas of significant pain without proper restraint and/or analgesia for the patient.

Evaluation of the joints should include flexion and extension to find any areas of crepitus, joint effusion, or heat/inflammation. Mobility of the joint should be assessed as any decrease in flexion/extension can indicate disease or injury. Similarly, an increase in joint laxity can also be an indicator of injury or disease (e.g. RA). When assessing the joint, placing a thumb or fingertip on the area of the joint that will open with flexion/extension and applying gentle pressure during joint movement can help assess for effusion or swelling. Care should be taken to avoid hyperextension or overflexing of the joint, specifically in cases where joint disease is expected as this can cause further injury and pain to the patient. In some patients, it may be helpful to have them held in lateral recumbency during this portion of the examination. The spine should also be included in this evaluation. Palpation of the spine should include musculature as well as the spinus processes. Firm pressure should be placed on each spinus process and the surrounding muscle while noting the patient's reaction, specifically looking for tensing, splinting, or movement away from the area of palpation, indicating an area of potential disease or injury.

Assessment of the patient's gait should be performed by watching as the patient is walked and trotted. Observation from the front, sides, and rear of the patient during movement should be performed. During this portion of the examination, specific symptoms to monitor for include bunny hopping, limping, lameness, stilted or stiff gait, decreased joint movement, abnormal movement of the limbs either away or into the body, as well as any inability to lift a limb from the floor, or dragging of the toes. Assessment of gait is difficult in feline patients but can be performed by monitoring them inside a closed exam room. For feline patients that are reluctant to move even in an enclosed room, patient history and the clients' observations about their behavior at home is key.

Specific palpation of the pelvic joints looking for Ortolani's sign, in addition to diagnostic radiographic procedures, can help diagnose hip dysplasia. To perform this palpation, the animal should be placed in lateral recumbency. With the animal in lateral recumbency, the stifle is held and the hip is flexed and extended several times with a hand, stethoscope, or ear placed over the coxofemoral joint during evaluation to check for crepitus. While the joint is adducted, pressure is applied to the proximal area of the joint. In a patient with hip dysplasia, subluxations will occur during the adduction, and the proximal pressure applied during abduction of the stifle will create a thudding noise. This noise is Ortolani's sign indicating likely hip dysplasia. Barden's technique is a specific subluxation of the coxofemoral joint in puppies to evaluate them for potential hip dysplasia. This is a painful procedure and should be performed under anesthesia or sedation. Because this type of evaluation for hip dysplasia is subjective and inconsistent, it is not often performed; a definitive diagnosis is made radiographically.

SECTION 5 MUSCULOSKELETAL THERAPY

Veterinary rehabilitation therapy

Veterinary rehabilitation therapy (also called veterinary physical therapy) is the use of noninvasive therapies for the rehabilitation of animals following physical trauma, surgery, or prolonged illness. Animal rehabilitation therapy employs many different modalities, both manual and mechanical, to produce the desired effect. The goal of therapy is to reduce pain, to enhance recovery following surgery or injury, and to maintain function and mobility of joints and muscles in animals. These goals are accomplished through strength building exercises, proprioceptive retraining, therapeutic stretches, joint mobilization, and controlled physical exercise. Conditions frequently benefiting from rehabilitation techniques include musculoskeletal imbalances, tendon and ligament injuries and contractures, chronic inflammatory disease, and degenerative conditions producing pain. Utilizing various modalities, rehabilitation therapists can increase circulation, reduce swelling and edema, promote tissue healing with reduced scarring and adhesions, as well as reduce pain. Physical rehabilitation therapies can be utilized in both the acute and the chronic stages of healing, with attention to the appropriate treatment being utilized at the optimal time. Contraindications for veterinary rehabilitation include animals suffering from elevated temperatures (febrile), systemic disease, gross fracture, infected or bleeding wounds, tumors not determined to be benign, or recent surgical incisions. Each therapeutic regimen is specifically designed by the referring veterinarian or rehabilitation specialist to meet each patient's treatment goals.

The traditional approach to pain management has been through the use of pharmaceuticals even though veterinary physiotherapy has long been recognized for its focus on pain reduction. More recently, the use of rehabilitation therapy modalities for the treatment of acute and chronic pain has increasingly been utilized. The complimentary use of rehabilitation therapy modalities with the concurrent use of medication has highlighted the synergistic effects of both.

There are many different physical rehabilitation modalities. These include manual therapies and those provided by means of mechanical equipment. Manual therapies are generally identified as those provided directly by the therapist via the use of the hands. Examples of manual therapies are application of heat and/ or cold therapy, joint mobilization and stretching, therapeutic ROM exercises, massage, and hydrotherapy. Machine directed therapies include therapeutic ultrasound, neuromuscular electrical stimulation, transcutaneous electrical neuromuscular stimulation (TENS), and low level laser therapy. Orthotics and prosthetics may also be prescribed for rehabilitative purposes. This chapter will discuss some of these modalities while encouraging the interested reader to continue their education in physical rehabilitation therapy. Postgraduate programs for licensed veterinary technicians are available. Technicians interested in pursuing certification should seek an accredited program recognized by the American Veterinary Medical Association (AVMA) and the state of intended practice.[1]

Cryotherapy and thermotherapy

Cryotherapy

Cryotherapy involves the utilization of various forms of cold to slow or reduce the inflammatory process, absorb heat, reduce muscle spasm, decrease pain, and induce localized vasoconstric-

tion. This localized vasoconstriction slows bleeding and decreases the accumulation of edema that is caused by lymphatic and venous drainage into the injured area. The application of cold therapy also aids in slowing the inflammatory process by slowing local metabolism and decreasing enzyme activity, thereby affecting the inflammatory process at the cellular level. Cryotherapy decreases muscular activity and slows nerve conduction, which in turn reduces muscle spasms and decreases pain (by numbing the area). Following cryotherapy, the body will rebound with vasodilation, causing a flush of nutrients to the affected tissues.

Cold or cryotherapy is especially useful during the first phase of the inflammatory process referred to as the acute stage, typically defined as the first 24–72 h after injury, when other treatments would be contraindicated. Cryotherapy can also be used as an adjunct therapy during chronic phases of inflammation such as in patients with OA.

Cryotherapy is achieved by the use of cold packs, cold wraps, cold whirlpools, or by ice massage. Cold packs can be as simple as a ziplock bag filled with ice and water. Cold packs should never be applied directly to the skin and never on wet hair; always use a protective cloth to prevent frostbite. Commercial flexible ice packs are preferred as they can be easily molded to the area receiving treatment. To make your own flexible ice pack, mix one part isopropyl alcohol to three parts water; place in a ziplock freezer bag; remove most of the air, and seal. Double bag the ice pack in case of leakage and place it in the freezer. If the pack is not slushy enough, add more water; if it is too solid, add more alcohol. The addition of food coloring or dye can help to distinguish the ice pack in the freezer. If ice packs are reused, always disinfect the outer surface between uses. Ice packs should be used for no longer than 8–10 min at a time. The use of alarm timers and continuous local tissue monitoring is strongly recommended. Cryotherapy may be repeated every 2–3 h until the desired effect is reached or as directed by the veterinarian or rehabilitation specialist.[2]

Ice massage is frequently utilized by human physical therapists to reduce pain in a localized area. This method also has applications in veterinary medicine. If prescribed, one method of ice massage is to freeze a small amount of water in a small paper or Styrofoam cup. Once it is frozen, peel off the sides of the cup to expose a small amount of ice all around and use the remaining portion of the cup to hold the ice. Place the ice directly onto the area to be treated; keep the ice constantly moving in circular motions to ice massage the area. Do not hold the ice in one area for any longer than 1 min to avoid causing frostbite. The total time for ice massage should not exceed 10 min.

Cryotherapy is contraindicated in areas of reduced circulation as further vasoconstriction can lead to tissue hypoxemia, damage, and necrosis. It should also be used judiciously in patients with subnormal temperatures to avoid exacerbating preexisting hypothermia. Close monitoring of nonambulatory patients is indicated since they lack the ability to move away from the cold source; ice packs should not be left with unattended patients. Patients with peripheral neuropathies should be treated as nonambulatory patients and should be closely monitored.

Thermotherapy

Thermotherapy is the utilization of superficial heat therapy. Heat therapy is generally utilized during the second phase (subacute stage) of the inflammatory process, typically defined as after the first 72 h following injury, overuse, or surgery. Heat therapy can also be used in chronic conditions and as an aid to warming muscles before the prescribed exercise.

The physiological effects of thermotherapy include increased extensibility of connective tissue, decreased joint stiffness, increased cellular metabolism, reduced muscle spasm, analgesia, and increased lymphatic and venous drainage. Thermotherapy causes an increase in local metabolism and the vasodilation provides enhanced circulation to the tissue; both of these mechanisms aid in the healing process.

Heat therapy is achieved by the use of hot packs (dry and moist), infrared heat lamps, and hydrotherapy. Dry hot packs include rice bags, hot water bottles, fluid bags, therapeutic clay packs, and heating pads. Moist hot packs include warm wash cloths and moist heating pads. Infrared heat lamps, more commonly used with exotic companion animals, can also provide an external heat source, although this type of warming provides heat to a much broader area. Regardless of the heat source, extreme care needs to be used to avoid thermal injury to the patient. Hot packs should never be applied directly to the skin; always use a protective cloth to prevent burns. Heat, as a therapy, differs from rewarming techniques typically used in veterinary medicine. The temperature should be very warm to the touch but never hot. The length of time for thermotherapy is quite variable, depending on the injury or condition. Thermotherapy is often applied for short periods of time (15–20 min) prior to joint mobilization therapy. The use of alarm timers is strongly recommended. Heat therapy may be repeated as directed, typically every 6–8 h. For chronic conditions, where heating of the deep layers of the muscles is desired, therapy can be of longer duration (hours).

The contraindications for thermotherapy are similar to those of cryotherapy and include close monitoring of nonambulatory patients since they lack the ability to move away from the heat source. Patients with peripheral neuropathies should be treated as nonambulatory patients and should be closely monitored. It should also be used judiciously in patients with above-normal temperatures to avoid exacerbating preexisting hyperthermia. Additionally, since heat is a vasodilator, thermotherapy should be used with caution in areas of bruising, infection, thrombosis, or other vascular diseases.

Joint mobilization, stretching, and therapeutic exercise

Range of motion

In ROM, the exercises or movements can be divided into three categories: *passive range of motion (PROM)*, *active-assisted range of motion (AAROM)*, or *active range of motion (AROM)*.

ROM means the movement of a joint through its entire range, from fully flexed to fully extended, with care not to hyperextend or to overflex the joint. This is important to help maintain or improve the motion of the joints, maintain or strengthen the muscles, improve circulation, and reduce pain after an injury or illness. Measuring the ROM of a joint helps to understand how much joint mobility is present and to monitor the response to therapy. Flexing and extending the joint helps maintain the nutrition and health of the joint tissues through the movement of joint fluid throughout the joint capsule.

During ROM exercises, the therapist should be in a comfortable position and should use proper body mechanics to avoid personal injury as well as to provide effective treatment to the patient. The patient should be placed in lateral recumbency with the affected limb up. The joints proximal and distal to the affected joint should be supported to avoid excessive stress and pressure on adjacent structures. ROM exercises should only be performed by skilled therapists certified in exercise therapy.

The process begins by slowly and gently flexing the joint. Be careful to avoid any painful areas, such as incisions or wounds. The other joints of the limb should be maintained in a neutral position (relaxed, not flexed or extended). Slowly continue to flex the joint until the patient shows any initial signs of discomfort, such as tensing of the limb, moving, vocalizing, turning toward the therapist, or trying to get away. During ROM exercises, avoid any undue discomfort or pain in the patient. Continue these techniques for 15–20 repetitions, two to four times daily until the ROM returns to normal. Continually monitor the patient for discomfort throughout the exercise period and alter the technique accordingly. It is very important during ROM therapy to maintain the normal ROM in the other joints of the affected limb by exercising the entire limb. Once normal, the frequency and duration of physical therapy exercises can be gradually decreased.

Passive range of motion (PROM)

In PROM exercises, the therapist provides the guiding force to produce joint movement. PROM can be used to evaluate as well as to improve the available range of extension and flexion available at a specific joint. The exercises are performed without muscle contraction by the patient.

Passive flexion and extension can be performed in conjunction with each other to improve the joint's ROM. PROM exercise goals are to maintain and improve joint function while not exceeding ROM limits, thereby causing pain or injury to the patient. The tissues that limit PROM exercises may be normal or diseased and may include the joint capsule, the soft tissue surrounding the joint, muscles, ligaments, tendons, fasciae, and skin.

Surgical incisions may result in adhesions and fibrosis between skin, subcutaneous tissues, fasciae, muscles, or bone, limiting the ability of tissues to glide over one another. Muscle, tendon, and ligament tissue may also be relatively shortened as a result of spasm or contracture. Any restriction of these tissues may result in resistance to movement and pain.

PROM is appropriate for many different patients, such as those who are unable to move a joint on their own or if active motion across a joint may be injurious to the patient. PROM is used sometimes in anxious patients to relax them. Common indications for PROM exercises are, immediately following surgery, before weight-bearing exercises, to aid in the prevention of ligament and tendon contracture and soft tissue adaptive shortening, to reduce pain, to enhance blood and lymphatic flow, to maintain muscular flexibility, and to improve synovial fluid production and diffusion.

PROM can also be used in the prevention of joint contracture during healing and recovery in paralyzed or recumbent patients. These exercises can be performed many times a day depending on the severity of the disease under the supervision of the veterinarian. Despite aggressive efforts, the patient may not regain normal functional neuromuscular control and the joint can still undergo some degree of contracture.

PROM exercises are limited in that they will not prevent atrophy of the muscles, increase strength, improve endurance, or be as effective in improving vascular and lymphatic flow as will more active therapeutic techniques eliciting active muscle contraction. For this reason, it is typically not the sole modality used in a physical therapy program.

Proper technique in PROM is important. The treatment should be administered to the patient in a quiet, comfortable, and relaxed atmosphere away from all distractions, such as loud noises, other pets, or people not participating directly in the therapy. It is especially important to be gentle, not creating any pain or discomfort. If the patient is painful before treatment, is resistant to treatment, or is overly anxious, a muzzle or other restraint tool should be used for initial treatment. As the patient starts to relax, the muzzle or other restraint tool can be removed. The concurrent use of pain medication administered prior to therapy can reduce pain and anxiety in the patient, although the use of pain medication may mask the response to treatment and increase the risk of injury.

Active range of motion

There are two types of AROM—active-assisted (therapist assists the movement) ROM and active (patient performs the prescribed movement without assistance) ROM. Both AROM and AAROM can be used simultaneously to produce the desired result.

AROM is defined as the ability of a patient to voluntarily move a limb through a ROM. AROM exercises may be initiated to encourage voluntary joint movement through a more complete ROM than the PROM exercises could achieve.

AROM exercises are achieved by active muscle contraction. Coordination between muscle groups is necessary in AROM because the therapist no longer assists the patient to perform the exercise. AROM exercises may be performed during a regular gait cycle, such as walking or trotting. Since normal joint ROM is somewhat limited during exercises such as walking or trotting, the patient may benefit by performing other activities that encourage a more complete ROM. Special conditions designed to increase joint flexibility and to more completely elicit full ROM include swimming, climbing the stairs, treadmill use, crawling through tunnels, negotiating cavalletti rails, and walking in water, tall grass, snow, or sand. Be creative, there are many other activities that can be employed, depending on the patient's condition and restrictions. Each of these activities possesses different advantages and disadvantages; therefore, it is advisable to consult a certified veterinary rehabilitation therapist to design an appropriate regimen. It is important to determine the patient's needs and what benefits could be expected from a particular exercise.

As the patient's joint flexion and extension improves, it is important to continue the PROM exercises and to add muscle stretching exercises to achieve the most complete ROM possible. Emphasis should be placed on encouraging the patient to regain complete use of the limb.

Greater strength is necessary during some ROM exercises, so it is important to transition between AAROM and AROM. AROM exercises may be the prelude to other strengthening activities. Also, owners may be taught to perform exercises at home to augment their pet's rapid recovery.

Active-assisted range of motion

During AAROM exercises, the patient is assisted by the therapist to achieve a normal ROM when the prime muscle mover is weak or injured. The physical therapist guides the joint movement, and some degree of the patient's muscle activity assists with the joint motion. In the animal patient, the amount of muscle activity provided by the patient is difficult to control. This makes it difficult to avoid muscle activation in patients that are not paralyzed; therefore, most of the ROM exercises involve some degree of AAROM.

AAROM exercises are most useful in those patients that are weak or those recovering from lower motor neuron conditions. The assisted range of motion is usually performed in lateral recumbency. Other exercises may be performed using a sling, where the therapist assists limb movement and joint ROM during ambulation. Another form of AAROM exercises can be performed while swimming, where the patient may have limited ability to ambulate. The water buoyancy helps support the weight of the patient while the therapist concentrates on assisting the limb through the normal ROM.

AAROM can also be used to combat the negative effects of immobilization on the limbs. Any degree of active muscle contraction will aid in strengthening the musculoskeletal system. In addition, AAROM can facilitate neuromuscular reeducation, proprioceptive retraining, and postural realignment.

Precautions and contraindications

Any form of ROM is contraindicated when the motion may result in further injury or instability, such as unstable fractures near joints, unstable ligaments, or tendon injuries.

It is important that communication lines between the veterinarian and the therapist remain open to ensure that the appropriate ROM exercises are performed and the limits of the patient are not exceeded.

In most cases, PROM done early in the disease or injury process will have beneficial effects, as long as the therapist stays within a reasonable ROM for the patient and for the condition being treated. The therapist should only perform the appropriate exercises at a reasonable speed that is not painful or detrimental to the patient.

Massage therapy

Therapeutic massage is the manual manipulation of muscle and connective tissues. The physiological effects of therapeutic massage include improved circulation, enhanced tissue healing, pain relief, reduced swelling and edema, reduced muscle spasms, realignment of muscle fibers, improved ROM, reduced adhesions, lengthening of contracted tissue, drainage of lymph tissues, and relief of anxiety and stress. Massage therapy has been shown to increase the endogenous production of chemical compounds such as endorphins that help to decrease pain. Conditions that most frequently benefit from veterinary massage include chronic inflammatory conditions, ligament and muscle injuries, postsurgical and recovering trauma patients, patients recovering from orthopedic surgery, and long-term medical conditions.

There are many different types of manual therapy techniques used in therapeutic massage. Each stroke has its own specific application and benefit. Techniques can be applied with varying amounts of firmness and for varied durations. Instruction on the proper application of strokes, the direction, the indications, and the contraindications is essential. Veterinary massage therapy strokes are adapted from Swedish massage techniques developed for use by human massage therapists. Traditional strokes used to treat animal patients include effleurage (gliding), petrissage (kneading), pin and stretch, lymphatic draining, wringing, cross-fiber friction, tapotement (percussive), coupage (cupping), skin rolling, deep tissue and myofascial release. Massage therapists typically include hydrotherapy, stretching regimens, ROM exercises, muscle strengthening, as well as cranial sacral techniques, laser, cold and thermal therapies.

Contraindications of therapeutic massage are similar to physical rehabilitation therapies and include elevated temperature, active infection, systemic disease, fractures, active bleeding, or patients on medications that would prematurely be released into the system through increased circulation.

Veterinary massage therapy should only be undertaken by a person trained in both veterinary medicine and massage therapy.

Hydrotherapy

Hydrotherapy, also known as aquatic therapy, is defined as the therapeutic treatment of disease or injury with the use of water, as in baths, pools, and underwater treadmills. Hydrotherapy can be used to improve cardiovascular conditioning, to support postsurgical rehabilitation, to provide superficial massage therapy, and can also be used as part of a program for wellness, weight loss, conditioning, and for recreation.

The principal benefit of hydrotherapy is the minimization of gravitational forces on the joints during exercise, thereby reducing pain and accelerating the healing process. Consequently, water exercises can be initiated earlier in the rehabilitative process with little or no risk of reinjury.[2] Older animals are capable of effectively exercising in water without the undue stress to their musculoskeletal systems they might experience on land. These benefits are directly associated with the physical properties of water as described below.

The most common forms of hydrotherapy in physical rehabilitation are the use of pools and underwater treadmills. The advantage of the underwater treadmill is that it provides a stable surface allowing the patient to walk comfortably while being partially supported by the water. This circumvents the panic sometimes experienced by animals when they are unable to touch the bottom of a traditional swimming pool. Underwater treadmills also provide a more controlled environment for a specific rehabilitation program. The speed, resistance, and water depth are all controlled, which allows for individualization of the rehabilitation program. To illustrate, filling the treadmill up to the height of the shoulders effectively diminishes the patient's weight by 38%, providing maximum joint support while still encouraging weight-bearing exercise. In contrast, swimming in deeper water allows the animal to use several muscles simultaneously with increased stretch of the muscle fiber but without bearing weight. Underwater treadmills provide low impact cardiovascular exercise that is well suited to older arthritic dogs. This modality is often utilized in programs designed for weight loss and cardiovascular fitness.

Rehabilitative swim therapy should only be performed when the rehabilitation therapist is in the pool with the patient. This allows the therapist to control intensity and effectiveness of exercise. Pool therapy is typically used later in the rehabilitation process in order to increase conditioning. A gradual, stepwise approach to rehabilitation will decrease the possibility of other injuries and facilitate a slow increase in the patient's exercise endurance level.

Principles and properties of water

To understand the benefits of hydrotherapy, a basic understanding of the principles and properties of water is needed. Hydrotherapy makes use of the properties of water—thermal conductivity, relative density and buoyancy, hydrostatic pressure, viscosity and cohesion, turbulence, resistance, and surface tension. These properties act together to help strengthen the animal, to improve cardiovascular fitness, and to increase blood flow, which aids in the healing process. Each of the properties has its own advantages.

Thermal

The thermal properties of water allow it to conduct heat efficiently. Heated water allows for superficial warming of the involved limbs, which in turn will increase circulation and help to decrease pain and to relax the muscles (especially the skeletal muscles) in order to increase flexibility.

Buoyancy

When a body is immersed in water, it is subjected to two forces—gravity and buoyancy. Buoyancy is defined as the upward thrust of water acting on a body that creates an apparent decrease in the weight of a body while immersed.[3] Buoyancy counteracts the force of gravity subjected on the pet's body as it is submerged in the water. Buoyancy, by minimizing the amount of weight the patient bears on its muscles and joints, decreases pain and allows for modified ambulation (or swimming). For neurological patients whose balance is compromised, buoyancy helps the body regain its vertical position, thereby allowing the patient to exercise in an upright position.

Hydrostatic pressure

While the patient is submersed, pressure is exerted by the water on the body; this is called hydrostatic pressure. Hydrostatic pressure is defined as the pressure exerted by a fluid at equilibrium at a given point within the fluid due to the force of gravity.[3] Hydrostatic pressure provides constant pressure to a limb or body immersed in water. Lung volumes are also affected by these pressures; as a result, patients with respiratory compromise or disease must be monitored closely.

Hydrostatic pressure is directly proportional to the depth of the part that is immersed. This sustained pressure opposes the tendency of blood and/or edema to pool in the dependent portions of the body and therefore aids in the reduction of fluid accumulation. This reduction in edema is helped by a general increase in circulation as a result of the prescribed exercises and may decrease pain during exercise. Hydrostatic pressure may also decrease muscular pain, particularly muscle spasms, by inhibiting sensory receptors through sustained pressure. This, in turn, acts to decrease an animal's pain perception, thereby allowing the patient to comfortably complete the prescribed exercise.

Cohesion and viscosity

Viscosity is a measure of the frictional resistance caused by cohesive or attractive forces between the molecules of a liquid. The viscosity (or resistance to fluid flow) is greater in water than in air, making it harder to move through the water. The water provides increased resistance to help strengthen muscles and to improve cardiovascular fitness. Viscosity is important in aquatic therapy for additional reasons: It may increase sensory awareness in animals with poor balance, assist in the stabilization of joints, and help prevent falling by increasing the time span for patients to react. The increased reaction time may also help to reduce anxiety in the patient.

Turbulence

When a body moves through water, turbulence is created, causing even greater resistance. Most therapy pools and underwater treadmills are equipped with a water jet system. This provides a variable velocity of water, which allows the therapist to increase or decrease resistance based on the patient's needs and the rehabilitation program. The turbulence also provides superficial massage to the submerged area.

Surface tension is the force of attraction between surface molecules of a fluid. Surface tension is not a factor if the moving body part is completely submerged in water. It becomes a sig-nificant factor when a limb breaks the surface of the water. Therapeutically, if a patient is extremely weak, movements may be performed more easily in the water just beneath the surface rather than at or on the surface.

Therapeutic benefits

There are numerous benefits to the use of aquatic therapy. Exercising in water is effective for improving strength, muscular endurance, ROM, agility, and psychological well-being, all while minimizing pain. Other benefits for aquatic therapy include increased circulation to muscles, increased joint flexibility, improved cardiorespiratory endurance, and decreased stress on healing tissue.

The type of aquatic therapy will depend on the specific rehabilitation needs of the individual.

Conditions benefiting from hydrotherapy/aquatic therapy

There are many different conditions that benefit from aquatic therapy. Specific conditions include postoperative fractures, cruciate stabilization, neurological conditions, tendinitis, conditioning, and other disorders in which a patient is reluctant to use extremities or there is a lack of strength, ROM, proprioceptive awareness, or weight-bearing ability.

Contraindications and precautions

Some patients have a fear of water or are reluctant to swim. This is important to consider before prescribing any of these aquatic therapies. Panic or significant anxiety in the patient may cause injury to himself/herself or the therapist. The patient should be introduced slowly to therapy to reduce any anxiety. It is imperative that the patient be monitored throughout therapy and never left unattended while in the water.

Postoperative patients may need to wait until incisions or wounds are completely healed before starting therapy to minimize the risk of infection. There may be instances where therapy needs to commence prior to the removal of sutures or wound closure. Water therapies in this case will be under the direct supervision of the veterinarian. Special consideration will need to be given in protecting the surgery or trauma site.

It is also important to consider the patient's overall health and medical history. The cardiovascular health and fitness level of the patient must be considered. The patient may be unable to swim more than a few minutes before becoming fatigued. Swimming the patient several times a day for 2–5 min may help improve the patient's strength, ROM, and overall cardiovascular function. As the patient responds, the length of the sessions or the resistance may be increased to make the therapy more beneficial to that patient.

Conclusion

Veterinary rehabilitation therapies complement traditional veterinary treatments in various ways and are becoming increasingly accepted. Rehabilitative techniques can aid in the reduction of pain, help to restore function, accelerate the healing process, and retain movement, thereby increasing the quality of life of our patients. This text is provided as an introduction and only specifically trained veterinary personnel should perform rehabilitation therapy.

Palliative radiation therapy

Radiation therapy involves the use of high energy beams of radiation to destroy cells by damaging their DNA. The total dose of radiation is usually fractionated, meaning that the total dose is given over a number of treatments. Fractionated dosing is performed to allow normal cells to repair and repopulate so they can tolerate high doses of radiation. Cancer cells do not typically repair as quickly as normal cells. The dose of radiation (measured in gray [Gy]) used to treat a tumor depends on the type of tumor being treated and the goals of the treatment.

Goals of radiation therapy

Radiation is used for definitive, adjuvant, or palliative therapy. The goals of treatment depend on the type of tumor, the tumor location, and the overall health of the patient.

Definitive therapy involves treating patients daily for 3–4 weeks. They receive a small dose of radiation, typically 2–4 Gy, for each treatment. The goal of this treatment is to deliver the highest dose of radiation to the tumor while minimizing damage to surrounding tissues.

Adjuvant therapy is when radiation is used in combination with other modalities such as chemotherapy or surgery.

With palliative radiation therapy, the goal of treatment is to try to alleviate pain or to relieve symptoms caused by the tumor while limiting the side effects caused by the radiation. Pain relief is achieved by reducing tumor size or by killing other cells such as cytokines and inflammatory cells.[12] This typically involves between one and six treatments. Palliative therapy can be used to treat a variety of tumors.

Concerns that a client may have can affect which protocol is chosen. These concerns can be due to financial constraint, worries over anesthetic complications, or fear of potential side effects.

Bone tumors

Osteosarcoma (OSA)

The most common bone tumor in dogs is OSA. About 75% of OSAs occur in the appendicular skeleton. Axial tumors have been reported in the mandible, maxilla, spine, cranium, ribs, nasal cavity or sinuses, and pelvis.[12] Typically with OSA, radiation is performed in a palliative setting. When treating these patients it is important to monitor pain. Over 70% of dogs exhibit significant pain relief from the radiation treatment.[12]

Chondrosarcoma (CSA)

CSA is the second most common bone tumor in dogs. This tumor can occur in the nasal cavity, ribs, long bones, pelvis, vertebrae, facial bones, digits, os penis, and extraskeletal sites.[12] The nasal cavity is the most common location, and therefore

surgery is usually not feasible. Radiation treatment for this tumor can be either palliative or definitive based on the aggressiveness of the tumor.

Rare bone tumors

Hemangiosarcoma (HSA) is a rare bone tumor. Less than 5% of bone tumor cases are HSAs.[12] Due to the high metastatic rate of has, the patient should be fully staged prior to treatment or therapy (e.g., thoracic radiographs, abdominal ultrasound). Fibrosarcomas (FSAs) are another rare bone tumor that account for less than 5% of cases.[12] This tumor also can have a high rate of metastasis, so staging is recommended. Multilobular osteochondrosarcoma is another uncommon tumor. These tumors are usually found in the skull and are locally aggressive tumors that can recur following surgical excision and have the potential to metastasize.[12] It is difficult to define a treatment course with the tumors mentioned above since they are rare and the prognosis is not known. FSAs and multilobular osteochondrosarcoma radiation therapy can either be palliative or definitive depending on how aggressive the tumor is and how aggressive an owner wants to be.

Feline bone tumors

Bone tumors in cats are rare. OSAs are the most common type. These can occur in the appendicular or axial skeleton. FSA is the second most common bone tumor, while CSAs and HSAs are very rare.[12] With little information on these tumors, the treatment course depends on how aggressive the owner wants to be.

Radiation side effects

Side effects from radiation are dependent on the dose a patient receives and the location treated. With palliative treatment, even though the dosage increases with each treatment, the overall dose is far less than a definitive protocol. The goal of palliative radiation therapy is to minimize radiation side effects while maximizing effectiveness for these patients. The majority of these patients have a guarded prognosis and the expectant life span is typically 6 months or less. The main focus for these patients is pain control and maintaining an acceptable quality of life. There are a variety of different medications that can be used to help control pain, and client communication is essential in finding the right drug or combination of drugs. It is also important for clients to be aware that often the entire course of the radiation treatments will need to be completed before a favorable response may be seen.

Patients receiving definitive therapy typically get treated 5 days a week for approximately 1 month. The location of the radiation and the dose will determine the type of side effects a patient will develop. If the skin is involved in treatment, then radiation dermatitis will occur, as well as side effects including severe erythema, moist desquamation, and ulceration. These side effects can cause significant pain (Figure 3.5.1).

If footpads are treated, the pads typically slough, making it very painful to walk. Antibiotics, pain medications, ointments (silver sulfadiazine), and glucocorticoids can be used to mediate

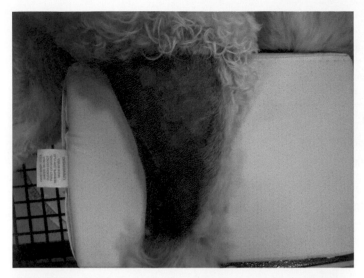

Figure 3.5.1 Dermatitis of the hind leg following radiation therapy.

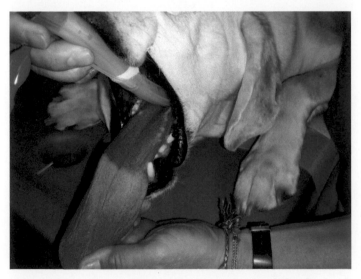

Figure 3.5.2 Oral mucositis on the tongue following radiation therapy.

these side effects. It is important to monitor the patient's comfort level and to emphasize to owners that their pet must not be allowed to traumatize their radiation site. An Elizabethan collar is recommended when the patient is not being directly supervised.

With radiation of the nasal cavity, the mouth and eyes are often involved, resulting in moderate to severe mucositis and ulceration. Side effects will occur in any part of the oral cavity that is treated. Monitoring patients for discomfort and decreased appetite is extremely important. Again, antibiotics, pain medications, and glucocorticoids can be used. Oral anesthetic rinses that contain lidocaine can be prescribed if the oral cavity is affected (Figure 3.5.2).

If an eye is treated, it is important to keep it well lubricated using topical antibiotics and lubricating ointments. It is also important to prevent patients from rubbing or scratching at their face; therefore, the use of an Elizabethan collar is recommended.

Side effects in cats are typically much less severe than those in dogs. Skin can get dry, flaky and itchy, so it is important to prevent patients from licking or scratching. An Elizabethan collar or a loose-fitting baby T-shirt may be helpful.

While these side effects can be painful, they usually persist for a few weeks post radiation. It is important to speak with owners and to monitor the comfort level throughout the treatment protocol. While radiation therapy personnel see these types of side effects often, pet owners generally have no experience with radiation and its effects, so client communication about potential side effects and what to monitor for is extremely important. It is also important to note that patients are different in terms of how they will respond and how much supportive care they may need. Veterinary technicians need to be strong advocates for their patients to ensure their treatment is as comfortable as possible.

SECTION 6 MUSCULOSKELETAL NUTRITION

Chemical energy is stored in the high energy phosphate bonds found in ATP; this provides the sole source of energy for muscle contraction. ATP is also vital for relaxation and maintenance of the ion gradients found in the muscles. Approximately one-third of the basal energy requirements for dogs and cats are used to maintain the electron concentration gradients across cellular membranes.[1]

There are both anaerobic and aerobic pathways for energy production in muscles. Which pathway is utilized is dependent on the duration and intensity of the activity and on the condition and nutritional status of the animal.[1] For short bursts of activity of low intensity exercise, glucose is the preferred energy source. Glucose can be stored endogenously as muscle glycogen, exogenously as hepatic glycogen, and very small amounts as free glucose in the bloodstream. For high-intensity or long-duration activity, fatty acids are the preferred energy source. These are stored in the adipose tissues and within the muscle cells. Amino acids are not used as a primary energy source for exercise. When protein is used for energy, it is produced primary from the branched-chain amino acids—leucine, isoleucine, and valine. The primary use of protein in the diet is structural and functional, with the amount being required dependent on the frequency and duration of exercise.[1]

The intensity and duration of exercise dictates which metabolic pathway is used and which substrates are utilized. When the anaerobic pathway is utilized, lactic acid is one of the major by-products. This is a strong acid within the body and is oxidized for energy by the muscle or converted back to glucose through the Cori cycle. The aerobic pathway produces primarily carbon dioxide (CO_2) and water. Carbon dioxide acts as a weak acid and causes significantly fewer changes to plasma or tissue pH.[1]

If the animal is engaging in a high intensity exercise, anaerobic metabolic pathways will be providing the majority of the energy used for muscle activity. With endurance exercise, aerobic pathways are used, with glucose and glycogen being the primary

Table 3.6.1 Comparison of energy sources during exercise

Nutrient	Sprint	Intermediate	Intermediate	Endurance
		Low frequency/ moderate duration	High frequency and duration	
Water	Unlimited	Unlimited	Unlimited	Unlimited
Energy density	3.5–4.0 kcal ME/g DM	4.0–5.0 kcal ME/g DM	4.5–5.5 kcal ME/g DM	>6.0 kcal ME/g DM
Fat	20–24% ME	30–55% ME	45–65% ME	>75% ME
Unsaturated	–	>60%	>60%	–
Carbohydrate (digestible)	50–60% NFE	20–50% NFE	15–30% NFE	<10% NFE
Protein	20–25%	20–25%	18–25%	18–22%
Digestibility	>80%	>80%	>80%	>80%

Source: Toll PW, Gillette RL, Hand MS. Feeding working and sporting dogs. In: *Small Animal Clinical Nutrition*, 5th edition, eds. MS Hand, CD Thatcher, RL Remillard, P Roudebush, BJ Nototny, pp. 326–345. Topeka, KS: Mark Morris Institute; 2010.
ME, metabolizable energy; DM, dry matter; NFE, nitrogen-free extract.

energy sources. For intermediate exercise, a combination of both pathways can be utilized[1] (Table 3.6.1).

Nutrients

Water

Water is undeniably the most important nutrient in the body even though it contributes no calories, vitamins, or minerals to the animal. It is the primary solvent found in the body, as well as the primary transport medium used in the intracellular, transcellular, and extracellular spaces. Hydration status is the single most important determinant in exercise endurance.[1]

Animals should have access to clean, fresh water at all times during exercise. This is even more important when ambient temperatures are elevated, as dogs use respiration as their primary means of cooling.[1]

Energy is produced through the metabolism of fats, proteins, and digestible carbohydrates. These nutrients alone provide the calories to run the machine.

Fats

Increasing the fat content of a diet is the only practical means of increasing the caloric density of a diet. Fats provide 8.5 kcal/g, while carbohydrates and proteins provide only 3.5 kcal/g. Increasing the fat content of a diet also tends to enhance the palatability, improving the chance that an animal will consume a greater amount of the desired food.[1]

Dogs rely more heavily on free fatty acids for energy generation at all levels of exercise intensities than do people. Because of this, dogs are able to tolerate much higher levels of dietary fat if the increase is introduced gradually and an adequate intake of nonfat nutrients is maintained.[1]

On a dry matter (DM) basis, approximately 2% of the diet should be composed of the essential fatty acids. The remainder can be composed of either plant or animal fats, in either saturated or unsaturated forms. High levels of unsaturated fatty acids may increase oxidative damage to cellular membrane lipids, causing damage to cell membrane functions.[1] Total fat intake should be 20–24% of the metabolizable energy (ME).

Working or sporting dogs should not be fed high fat meals immediately before or during intense exercise as digestion and assimilation of fats is slower than either proteins or carbohydrates diverting blood from the muscles to the intestines.[1]

Carbohydrates

Dogs and cats have no dietary requirements for carbohydrates if enough gluconeogenic precursors are available. The exceptions to this would be during gestation and neonatal development. Even though there is no requirement for carbohydrates per se, dogs and cats are still able to digest and utilize carbohydrates, freeing up fats and proteins for uses other than energy generation. Dogs are indeed much more efficient at this than are cats, but cats, too, can use carbohydrates for energy.[1]

The rate of glycogen use and energy production is dependent on the concentration of glycogen found in the muscle. Increased levels of muscle glycogen can be achieved through a combination of dietary adjustments and training. Glycogen loading is probably not as beneficial for canine endurance athletes as would feeding a higher fat food on a regular basis. Athletes who require short bursts of energy, such as sprint racers, may benefit more from carbohydrate loading, but the benefits have not been conclusively established.[1]

Carbohydrates are found in many forms, ranging from highly digestible to nondigestible for dogs and cats. Increasing the digestibility of the carbohydrates in the diet can help to decrease fecal water loss, flatulence, and fecal bulk and weight in the colon.[1]

Digestibility should be at least 85% as some fiber is required for normal colon function. For sprint athletes, carbohydrate levels ~50–70% ME are recommended. Intermediate athletes, dependent on intensity and duration of exercise, can tolerate levels of 15–50% ME. Endurance athletes should receive no more than 15% carbohydrates in their diets.[1]

Protein

The primary use of proteins is for structural, biochemical, and energy requirements. Cats are more efficient at using protein for energy than dogs. Cats have the protein requirements for muscle and cell repair, plus their energy requirements, thereby increasing their overall protein requirements.

Working animals have increased protein requirements that vary based on the frequency and duration of exercise. This is due to increased synthesis of structural and functional proteins, increased enzyme and transport proteins being used in energy production pathways, and increased blood volume.[1]

Amino acids may provide 5–15% of the energy used during exercise; this is primary through the use of the branched-chain amino acids—leucine, isoleucine, and valine. Compared to glucose and fatty acids, branched-chain amino acids provide very little fuel to the body. This comes at the expense of functional tissue because if you are using amino acids for energy, you have less available for tissue repair, thereby sacrificing your functional tissue to provide energy.[1] The disadvantage for athletes relying on proteins for energy is that there are no protein stores in the body (all protein is functional), making protein an inefficient source of energy, unlike fats or carbohydrates.

All proteins found in the body, other than small amounts found in the amino acid pools in individual cells, are either functional or structural. Increasing the protein in a diet is not an advantage to the animal either as any protein consumed in excess of that required is deaminated. This process produces keto acids that are either oxidized for energy directly or converted to fatty acids and/or glucose and stored in the adipose tissue or muscle and liver as glycogen.[1] High protein diets are expensive for the owner, and the added protein (above the required amounts) is unnecessary to the diet, being quickly converted into fats or carbohydrates, providing no benefit to the animal.

Proteins, like carbohydrates, also have varying degrees of digestibility, with muscle and organ meat having the highest digestibility and hair and connective tissue having the lowest digestibility. Feeding proteins of low digestibility not only slows down the process of the animal receiving the nutrients that they require but also increases the fecal bulk—providing unnecessary additional fecal weight to the animal athlete.[1]

It is recommended that protein digestibility should be at least 80%.[1] The only way to assess the digestibility of a food is through the use of feeding trials.

Antioxidants

With exercise, the innate antioxidant capabilities are often overwhelmed, leading to increased oxidative stress. This oxidative stress may contribute to and/or exacerbate a wide variety of degenerative diseases.[1] The more often this occurs, the more significant the potential damage. Oxidative stress can be mitigated to a degree through training. By increasing endurance through training, the cells become more efficient at energy utilization, decreasing the production of oxidative by-products, decreasing the need for endogenous antioxidants.

High levels of an individual antioxidant can be counterproductive as well, as many antioxidants at high levels become pro-oxidants. Ensuring balanced levels of antioxidants is best, so that they may act synergistically to the benefit of the athlete.[1]

Vitamin E

Vitamin E or the mixed tocopherols are the primary lipid-soluble antioxidant found in plasma, tissues, and red blood cells. They are also one of the most effective antioxidants for polyunsaturated fatty acid oxidation. The minimum level of vitamin E for performance is 500 IU/kg of DM in the food (not kilogram of body weight).[1]

Vitamin C

Vitamin C is the most powerful reducing agent available to the cell and is an important co-oxidant with vitamin E. Dogs and cats are able to synthesize normal amounts of vitamin C required for maintenance and are able to rapidly absorb supplemental vitamin C from the GI tract. Recommended levels are 150–250 IU/kg DM of food.[1]

Selenium

Selenium is found in the antioxidant glutathione peroxidase. It is responsible for protecting tissues against oxidative stress by catalyzing the reduction of peroxides and organic hydroperoxides. This has a sparing effect on vitamin E. Recommended levels are 0.5–1.3 mg/kg DM in food.[1]

Energy and growth

Excessive amounts of food (energy) intake and or calcium during early growth contributes to the development of hip and elbow dysplasia as well as ostochondrosis.[2] In young growing animals, excess energy, either through feeding adlib and not controlling the energy provided or feeding energy dense foods, does not cause a substantial increase in fat deposits. Instead, excess food energy causes an increased rate of growth. This rapid growth rate decreases the time period that animal has for growth, causing increased weight to be placed on an immature skeleton and support system.[2]

Skeletal problems are associated more with the increased body weight rather than with the protein content found in the diets.

Dogs who received less food during growth, maintaining a body condition score only slightly lower than ideal, had a slower growth rate and a longer growing period but no substantial change in their overall adult size.[2] OA in multiple joints, such as elbows, hips, and shoulders, is seen more frequently in overweight dogs as opposed to slim dogs. Remember, overweight is defined as only 15% over ideal, with obesity being 30% over the ideal weight.

Calcium

During the active growth phase, calcium requirements are dependent on the stage of growth (i.e., the age of the puppy) and the growth rate (i.e., expected adult size and weight).[2] High levels of calcium decrease osteoclastic activity. Osteoclasts are the cells that replace bone-removing old cells so that the osteoblasts can make new cells. Excessive calcium also disturbs the endochondral ossification process (when the growth plate stops growing). Additionally, puppies younger than 6 months of age are unable to protect themselves from excess calcium intake as well as older animals. In older animals, GI absorption of calcium decreases as the dietary level increases.[2]

A chronically high calcium intake will cause chronic hypercalcitoninism, preventing calcium release from the skeleton by decreasing bone-resorbing osteoclastic activity. Absorbed calcium levels in the diet are a better determinant for the occurrence of skeletal abnormalities when compared with the calcium/phosphorus ratio.[2]

Osteoarthritis

OA is the largest orthopedic problem found in companion animals and is the main orthopedic cause of euthanasia. The age of occurrence is dependent on breed and adult size but can range from 3.5 to 9.3 years. Overloading the joint(s), either through obesity or overuse, is the primary cause for the development of OA.[2]

Chondroprotectants

Chondroprotectants work primarily by enhancing the metabolism of chondrocytes and synoviocytes, inhibiting degrading enzymes and inflammatory mediators, as well as decreasing thrombi formation in local blood vessels.[2]

The protectants we see most commonly include glucosamine and chondroitin—both glycoaminoglycans, eicosapentaenoic acid (EPA) and docosahexaenoic acid (DHA)—omega-3 fatty acids, vitamin E, vitamin C, lutein and polyphenols—all antioxidants and green lipped mussel extract, which contains anti-inflammatory agents, as well as glucosamine and chrondroitin.[2]

Glucosamine and chrondroitin are both precursors to the glucoaminoglycans (GAGs). GAGs are mucosaccharides consisting of long, unbranched chains of polysaccharides, composed of repeating disaccharide units of hexoses (a type of sugar). GAGs stimulate synthesis of prostaglandins and collagen. By increasing the amounts found in the body, increased levels can be found in the arthritic joints, helping to decrease inflammation and providing additional cushioning to the joint.[2]

While all causes of OA cannot be prevented, by keeping our growing dogs leaner, we can significantly decrease the incidence in older animals.

In older animals, additional comfort can be found by decreasing their weight in order to decrease the load on the damaged joints. Also, maintaining consistent exercise will help to maintain mobility and muscle strength in the damaged area.

Body condition scoring

Body condition scoring (BCS) is a subjective assessment of an animal's body fat and to a lesser extent protein stores.[1] The scoring system takes into account the animal's frame size independent of its weight. In animals, the subcutaneous fat adheres more to muscle than to skin, making skinfold thickness a questionable means for determining body fat in cats and dogs.[3]

There are two main scoring systems: the five-point scale and the nine-point scale. Both systems use defined criteria to help make the subjective process of body evaluation more objective, but all subjectivity cannot be removed when assigning a score to an animal. For this reason, it is important that the same person assign the score each time the animal is evaluated. The five-point scale scores the animals to the nearest half score, and the nine-point scale scores to the nearest whole score.[1]

Studies have shown that body fat increases 5–7% for each whole increment increase using a nine-point scale with mid-range-scoring animals (4/9–5/9) having 15–20% of their body mass as fat.[3] When trying to detect small changes in body fat, the use of BCS scores would probably not be your best choice, but for monitoring and routine care, it is quick, easy, and painless (Table 3.6.2).

Body condition score uses

A body condition score should be recorded with the weight each time an animal is examined. Body weight alone does not indicate how appropriate the weight is for the individual animal. The BCS puts in perspective what an individual animal should weigh.[1]

Table 3.6.2 Excess weight estimate using a five-point scale

Body condition score	Excess weight (%)
3.0 (ideal body score)	0
3.5	10
4.0 (overweight)	20
4.5	30
5.0 (obese)	40

Source: German A, Martin L. Feline obesity: epidemiology, pathophysiology and management. In: *Encyclopedia of Feline Clinical Nutrition*, eds. P Pibot, V Biourge, D Elliott, p. 46. Aimargues, France: Aniwa SAS; 2008.

In general, dogs and cats with an optimal body condition have

- normal body contours and silhouettes,
- bony prominences that are easily palpated but are not seen or felt above the skin surface, and
- intra-abdominal fat that is insufficient to obscure or interfere with abdominal palpation.

Normal BCSs are 3/5 or 4-5/9, when scores are below 2/5 or 3/9 or above 4/5 or 7/9 than action should be taken to bring the animal into a more normal BCS[1] (Table 3.6.3 and Figures 3.6.1 and 3.6.2).

Just because an animal scores a 5/5 or a 9/9 does not mean that this is the maximum size or weight that this animal can attain. In fact, animals can be scored as a 5/5+ or 9/9+ if morbid obesity is present. There is no "maximum" amount of body fat compatible with life.[1]

Using BCS is an effective means of monitoring an animal's condition as well as its weight and is something that can be easily learned by most pet owners and done at home. This should be instituted early on in the client/patient/veterinary team relationship so that we can prevent obesity and all of the associated problems.

Muscle condition scoring

Muscle condition scoring differs from BCS by looking at the muscle mass of the animal, not at the fat layer. This is helpful in animals where significant muscle wasting has occurred but not a loss of subcutaneous fat.

With acute metabolic challenges, the body's preferred fuel is protein, not fat, so muscle will be used preferentially over stored fat for energy. This could be seen in animals suffering from an acute illness as seen with infectious diseases, a chronic illness such as cancer, or a muscle wasting disease such as Cushing's disease.[4]

Overcoat syndrome can be seen when the animal being examined has more fat than muscle, making a muscle condition score of 1 or 2 seem normal by providing artificial bulk to the muscle where none actually exists. Upon palpation, some areas of the body may feel normal, but on continued interrogation, marked muscle wasting can be felt over the bony prominences. This syndrome should be considered when the physical examination and the history do not correlate. Palpation will help to define if overcoat syndrome is present.[5]

The primary areas to check for muscle condition would be the scapula, the occipital crest of the skull, and the wings of the ilium[5,6] (Table 3.6.4).

Table 3.6.3 Five-point body condition score

BCS	What you see	What you feel
1/5 emaciated	Obvious ribs, pelvic bones, and spine; no body fat or muscle mass	Bones with little covering of muscle
2/5 thin	Ribs and pelvic bones, but less prominent; tips of spine, an "hourglass" waist (looking from above), a tucked-up abdomen (looking from side)	Ribs and other bones with no palpable fat, but some muscle is present
3/5 moderate	Less prominent hourglass and abdominal tuck	Ribs without excess fat covering
4/5 stout	General fleshy appearance, hourglass, and abdominal tuck hard to see	Ribs, with difficulty
5/5 obese	Sagging abdomen, large deposits of fat over chest, abdomen, and pelvis	Nothing, except general flesh

Source: Case L, Carey D, Hirakawa D, Daristotle L. Obesity. In: *Canine and Feline Nutrition*, 2nd edition, p. 315. St. Louis, MO: Mosby; 2000.

Table 3.6.4 Muscle condition scoring system

Score	Condition	Muscle mass	What you see
0	Severe muscle wasting	Pronounced decreased muscle mass palpable over the scapula, skull, or wings of ilia	Bony prominences highly visible from a distance
1	Moderate muscle wasting	Clearly discernible decreased muscle mass palpable over the scapula, skull, or wings of ilia	Bony prominences visible from a distance
2	Mild muscle wasting	Slight but discernible decreased muscle mass palpable over the scapula, skull, or wings of ilia	Bony prominences slightly visible from a distance
3	Normal muscle mass	Normal amounts of muscle palpable over the scapula, skull, or wings of ilia	No visible bony prominences when viewed from a distance

Sources: Buffington CA, Holloway C, Abood SA. Nutritional assessment. In *Manual of Veterinary Dietetics*, pp. 4–5. St. Louis, MO: Saunders; 2004b; and Michel KE, Sorenmo KU. Nutritional status of cats with cancer: nutritional evaluation and recommendations. In: *Encyclopedia of Feline Clinical Nutrition*, eds. P Pibot, V Biourge, D Elliott, pp. 389–400. Aimargues, France: Aniwa SAS; 2008.

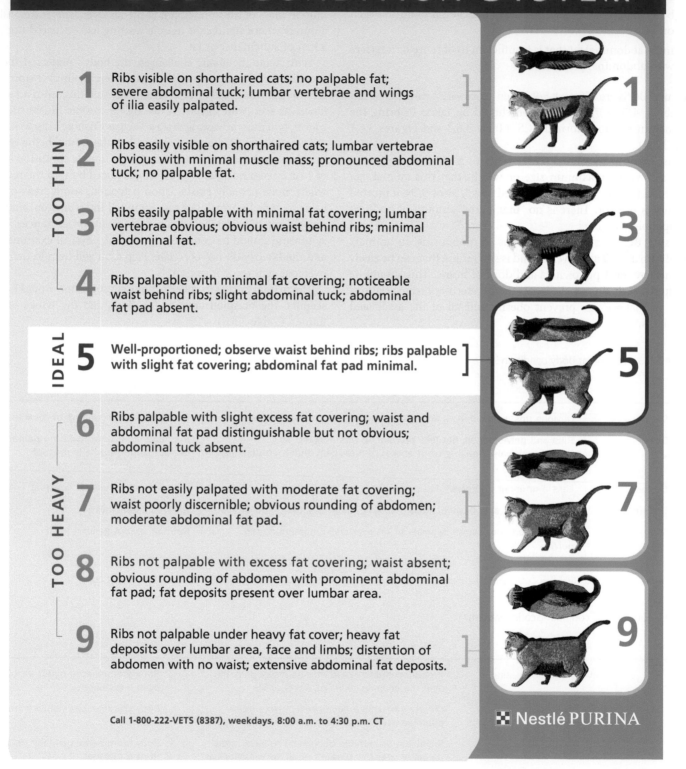

Nestlé PURINA

BODY CONDITION SYSTEM

TOO THIN

1 Ribs visible on shorthaired cats; no palpable fat; severe abdominal tuck; lumbar vertebrae and wings of ilia easily palpated.

2 Ribs easily visible on shorthaired cats; lumbar vertebrae obvious with minimal muscle mass; pronounced abdominal tuck; no palpable fat.

3 Ribs easily palpable with minimal fat covering; lumbar vertebrae obvious; obvious waist behind ribs; minimal abdominal fat.

4 Ribs palpable with minimal fat covering; noticeable waist behind ribs; slight abdominal tuck; abdominal fat pad absent.

IDEAL

5 Well-proportioned; observe waist behind ribs; ribs palpable with slight fat covering; abdominal fat pad minimal.

TOO HEAVY

6 Ribs palpable with slight excess fat covering; waist and abdominal fat pad distinguishable but not obvious; abdominal tuck absent.

7 Ribs not easily palpated with moderate fat covering; waist poorly discernible; obvious rounding of abdomen; moderate abdominal fat pad.

8 Ribs not palpable with excess fat covering; waist absent; obvious rounding of abdomen with prominent abdominal fat pad; fat deposits present over lumbar area.

9 Ribs not palpable under heavy fat cover; heavy fat deposits over lumbar area, face and limbs; distention of abdomen with no waist; extensive abdominal fat deposits.

Call 1-800-222-VETS (8387), weekdays, 8:00 a.m. to 4:30 p.m. CT

Nestlé PURINA

Figure 3.6.1 Nine-point feline body conditioning score card.

Nestlé PURINA
BODY CONDITION SYSTEM

TOO THIN

1 Ribs, lumbar vertebrae, pelvic bones and all bony prominences evident from a distance. No discernible body fat. Obvious loss of muscle mass.

2 Ribs, lumbar vertebrae and pelvic bones easily visible. No palpable fat. Some evidence of other bony prominence. Minimal loss of muscle mass.

3 Ribs easily palpated and may be visible with no palpable fat. Tops of lumbar vertebrae visible. Pelvic bones becoming prominent. Obvious waist and abdominal tuck.

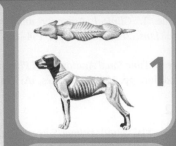

IDEAL

4 Ribs easily palpable, with minimal fat covering. Waist easily noted, viewed from above. Abdominal tuck evident.

5 Ribs palpable without excess fat covering. Waist observed behind ribs when viewed from above. Abdomen tucked up when viewed from side.

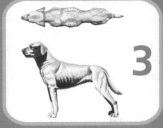

TOO HEAVY

6 Ribs palpable with slight excess fat covering. Waist is discernible viewed from above but is not prominent. Abdominal tuck apparent.

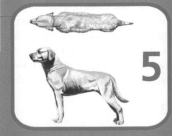

7 Ribs palpable with difficulty; heavy fat cover. Noticeable fat deposits over lumbar area and base of tail. Waist absent or barely visible. Abdominal tuck may be present.

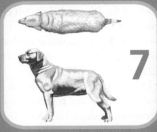

8 Ribs not palpable under very heavy fat cover, or palpable only with significant pressure. Heavy fat deposits over lumbar area and base of tail. Waist absent. No abdominal tuck. Obvious abdominal distention may be present.

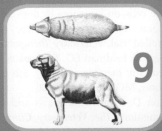

9 Massive fat deposits over thorax, spine and base of tail. Waist and abdominal tuck absent. Fat deposits on neck and limbs. Obvious abdominal distention.

The **BODY CONDITION SYSTEM** was developed at the Nestlé Purina Pet Care Center and has been validated as documented in the following publications:

Mawby D, Bartges JW, Moyers T, et. al. *Comparison of body fat estimates by dual-energy x-ray absorptiometry and deuterium oxide dilution in client owned dogs. Compendium 2001; 23 (9A): 70*

Laflamme DP. *Development and Validation of a Body Condition Score System for Dogs. Canine Practice July/August 1997; 22:10-15*

Kealy, et. al. *Effects of Diet Restriction on Life Span and Age-Related Changes in Dogs. JAVMA 2002; 220:1315-1320*

Call 1-800-222-VETS (8387), weekdays, 8:00 a.m. to 4:30 p.m. CT

Nestlé PURINA

Figure 3.6.2 Nine-point canine body conditioning score card.

Source: Nestle Purina.

Bibliography

Section 1

1. Colville T. *Clinical Anatomy and Physiology for Veterinary Technicians*, 2nd edition, pp. 154–204. St. Louis, MO: Mosby; 2008.
2. Reece W. *Functional Anatomy and Physiology of Domestic Animals*, 4th edition, pp. 179–223. Ames, IA: Wiley-Blackwell; 2009.

Section 2

1. Fossum TW. *Small Animal Surgery*, 3rd edition, pp. 1144–1146. St. Louis, MO: Mosby; 2007.
2. Ettinger SJ. *Textbook of Veterinary Internal Medicine*, 5th edition, Vols. 1–2, pp. 79, 1865, 1879. St. Louis, MO: Saunders; 2000.
3. Pratt PW. *Laboratory Procedures for Veterinary Technicians*, 3rd edition, p. 580. Philadelphia, PA: Mosby; 1997.
4. Hendrix CM. *Laboratory Procedures for Veterinary Techncians*, 5th edition, pp. 323–325. Philadelphia, PA: Mosby-Elsevier; 2007.
5. Cowell RL. *Diagnostic Cytology and Hematology of the Dog and Cat*, 2nd edition, pp. 104–118. St. Louis, MO: Mosby; 1999.
6. McCurnin DM. *Clinical Textbook for Veterinary Technicians*, 6th edition, p. 105. St. Louis, MO: Elsevier-Saunders; 2006.
7. Ettinger SJ. *Textbook of Veterinary Internal Medicine*, 5th edition, Vol. 1, pp. 685–686. St. Louis, MO: Saunders; 2000.
8. Melmed C. Masticatory muscle myositis: Pathogenesis, diagnosis, and treatment. *Compendium* 2004;26(8):590–605.

Section 3

1. Ettinger SJ, Feldman EC. *Textbook of Veterinary Internal Medicine (Diseases of the Dog and Cat)*, 5th edition, Vol. 2, pp. 1867–1886. St. Louis, MO: Saunders; 2000.
2. Clements D. Type I immune mediated polyarthritis in dogs—39 cases. *Journal of the American Veterinary Medical Association* 2004;224(8):1323–1327.
3. Black LL. Effect of intra-articular inj. of autologous adipose-derived mesenchymal stem and regenerative cells on clinical signs of OA of the elbow joint in dogs. *Veterinary Therapeutics* 2008;9(3):192–200.
4. Black LL. Effect of adipose-derived mesenchymal stem and regenerative cells on lameness in dogs with chronic OA of the coxofemoral joints: a randomized, double-blinded, multicenter controlled trial. *Veterinary Therapeutics* 2007;8(4):272–284.
5. Ettinger SJ, Feldman EC. *Textbook of Veterinary Internal Medicine (Diseases of the Dog and Cat)*, 5th edition, Vol. 2, pp. 675–676. St. Louis, MO: Saunders; 2000.
6. Shelton D. Myasthenia gravis and disorders of neuromuscular transmission. *The Veterinary Clinics of North America. Small Animal Practice* 2002;32(1):189–206.
7. Podell M. Inflammatory myopathies. *The Veterinary Clinics of North America. Small Animal Practice* 2002;32(1):147–167.
8. Green CE. *Infectious Diseases of the Dog and Cat*, 3rd edition, pp. 195–197, 203–216, 232–241, 417–435, 705–711. St. Louis, MO: Saunders; 2006.
9. Potter T. *Hepatozoon americanum*: an emerging disease in the south-central/southeastern United States. *Journal of Veterinary Emergency and Critical Care* 2010;20(1):70–76.
10. Withrow S. *Small Animal Clinical Oncology*, 3rd edition, pp. 283–289, 378–386. Philadelphia, PA: Saunders; 2001.
11. Ettinger SJ, Feldman EC. *Textbook of Veterinary Internal Medicine (Diseases of the Dog and Cat)*, 5th edition, Vol. 2, pp. 536–538. St. Louis, MO: Saunders; 2000.
12. Melmed C. Masticatory muscle myositis: pathogenesis, diagnosis, and treatment. *Compendium* 2004;26:590–605.
13. Medici E. American canine hepatozoonosis. *Compendium* 2008;30(11):E1–E9.
14. Sessions J. Canine appendicular osteosarcoma: curative-intent treatment. *Compendium* 2004;26(3):186–196.

Section 4

1. Piermattei D. *Handbook of Small Animal Orthopedics and Fracture Repair*, 4th edition, pp. 3–15, 478–480. St. Louis, MO: Saunders; 2006.
2. Bloomberg M. *Canine Sports Medicine and Surgery*, pp. 20–27. St. Louis, MO: Saunders; 1998.
3. Wheeler S. *Small Animal Spinal Disorders, Diagnosis and Surgery*, pp. 21–30. Edinburgh, NY: Elsevier; 1994.

Section 5

1. McGowan C, Goff L, Stubbs N (eds.). *Animal Physiotherapy, Assessment, Treatment, and Rehabilitation of Animals*. Oxford, UK: Blackwell Publishing; 2007.
2. Rivera PL. Canine rehabilitation therapies I and II. *Proceedings of the 79th Annual Western Veterinary Conference, February 18–22, 2007, Las Vegas, NV*; p. 11.
3. *Webster's Dictionary*, 2nd edition, p. 1074; 1982.
4. Hellyer P, Rodan I, Brunt J, et al. AAHA/AAFP pain management guidelines for dogs and cats. *Journal American Animal Hospital* 2007;43:235–248.
5. Millis DL, Levine D, Taylor RA. *Canine Rehabilitation and Physical Therapy*. St. Louis, MO: Saunders/Elsevier; 2004.
6. Williams J (ed.). *The Complete Textbook of Animal Health and Welfare*. St. Louis, MO: Elsevier/Sanders; 2009.
7. Jack CM, Watson PM. *Veterinary Technician Daily Reference Guide, Canine and Feline*, 2nd edition. Ames, IA: Blackwell Publishing; 2008.
8. Kahn CM (ed.). *The Merck/Merial Manual for Pet Health, Home Edition*. New Jersey, NJ: Merck and Company; 2007.
9. Cote E (ed.). *Clinical Veterinary Advisor—Dogs and Cats*. St. Louis, MO: Mosby/Elsevier; 2007.
10. Gaynor JS, Muir WW. *Handbook of Veterinary Pain Management*, 2nd edition, Chapter 27, pp. 513–515. St. Louis, MO: Mosby Elsevier; 2009.
11. Bassert JM, McCurnin DM. *McCurnin's Clinical Textbook for the Veterinary Technician*, 7th edition, pp. 791–802. St. Louis, MO: Saunders Elsevier; 2010.
12. Withrow SJ, Vail DM. *Small Animal Clinical Oncology*, 4th edition, St Louis MO, Saunders Elsevier, 2007.

Section 6

1. Toll PW, Gillette RL, Hand MS. Feeding working and sporting dogs. In: *Small Animal Clinical Nutrition*, 5th edition, eds. MS Hand, CD Thatcher, RL Remillard, P Roudebush, BJ Nototny, pp. 326–345. Topeka, KS: Mark Morris Institute; 2010.
2. Hazewinkel H, Mott J. Main nutritional imbalances implicated in osteoarticular diseases. In: *Encyclopedia of Canine Clinical*

Nutrition, eds. P Pibot, V Biourge, D Elliott, pp. 316–338. Aimargues, France: Aniwa SAS; 2006.

3. Burkholder WJ. 2000. Precision and practicality of methods assessing body composition of dogs and cats. In: *Nutrition Forum Proceedings*, pp. 1–9. St. Louis, MO: Ralston Purina.

4. Buffington CA, Holloway C, Abood SA (eds.). Clinical dietetics. In: *Manual of Veterinary Dietetics*, p. 60. St. Louis, MO: Saunders; 2004.

5. Buffington CA, Holloway C, Abood SA (eds.). Nutritional assessment. In: *Manual of Veterinary Dietetics*, pp. 4–5. St. Louis, MO: Saunders; 2004.

6. Michel KE, Sorenmo KU. Nutritional status of cats with cancer: nutritional evaluation and recommendations. In: *Encyclopedia of Feline Clinical Nutrition*, eds. P Pibot, V Biourge, D Elliott, pp. 389–400. Aimargues, France: Aniwa SAS; 2008.

Chapter 4 The Neurological Examination

Author: Thomas Schubert

Clinical signs and the relevant anatomy

When evaluating the neurological patient, the clinician systematically reviews each anatomical section of the nervous system. Understanding neuroanatomy is essential to the goal of the neurological examination, that goal being to *place the lesion*.

Brain

The brain is divided into five main parts: telencephalon, diencephalon, mesencephalon, metencephalon, and myelencephalon.

Telencephalon

The telencephalon, otherwise considered the forebrain, is further divided into four lobes, each with a specific function. The four lobes are the frontal, parietal, temporal, and the occipital lobes.

Because the frontal lobe deals with motor function, an abnormality in it often presents as compulsive pacing, circling, or partial or generalized seizures.

The parietal lobe is the brain's area for interpretation of the physical environment and interpretation of the body's position in space. Lesions in the parietal lobe result in proprioceptive deficits.

Difficult to evaluate in the veterinary patient, the temporal lobe is associated with hearing. The temporal lobe has a propensity toward generating seizures.

The occipital lobe interprets visual input and a lesion in it may result in visual field deficits as evaluated by the menace reflex.

Menace deficits may also arise from lesions in the optic nerve or cerebellum.

Brain stem

The remainder of the brain is collectively referred to as the brain stem. The most rostral part of the brain stem is the diencephalons, which is made up of the epithalamus, the thalamus, and the hypothalamus. Caudal to the diencephalon is the mesencephalon (midbrain); next is the metencephalon (pons and cerebellum), and finally, the myelencephalon, which is the medulla oblongata. The diencephalon is adjacent to and part of the forebrain. It consists of the epithalamus (pineal body), the thalamus, the hypothalamus, the pituitary gland, and a few other structures. The mesencephalon is considered the midbrain. The metencephalon and the myelencephalon are considered the hindbrain. The hindbrain consists of the pons and cerebellum (metencephalon), and the medulla oblongonta (myelencephalon). What assists the clinician in lesion placement throughout the brain stem is the association of the 12 cranial nerves with their respective areas of the brain stem.

Cranial nerves

Anatomists have logically placed the 12 cranial nerves starting with I, olfactory, the most rostral, to XII, hypoglossal, the most caudal.

Loss of the sense of smell, cranial nerve 1 (CN I), is rare. CN I may be tested by offering the blindfolded patient some food. Alcohol or other mucosal irritating compounds should be

Small Animal Internal Medicine for Veterinary Technicians and Nurses, First Edition. Edited by Linda Merrill.
© 2012 John Wiley & Sons, Inc. Published 2012 by John Wiley & Sons, Inc.

avoided. Cranial nerve 2 (CN II), the optic, is evaluated in conjunction with CN VII, the facial. A menacing gesture is made toward the eye and there should be a reflexive blink. If the patient has a facial paralysis (CN VII), then the reflex will be incomplete. Cotton balls may be tossed toward or into the peripheral area of the patient's visual field to assess vision.

A distinction must be made between a peripheral and a central blindness. A central blindness may be the result of a lesion in the occipital lobe where a peripheral blindness will be associated with lesions of the retina, optic nerve, or chiasm. A method of differentiating is with the pupillary light reflex (PLR). Shining a light into the eye stimulates the retina. Electrical impulses are sent via the optic nerve through the optic chiasm and along the optic tract to the pretectal motor nucleus in the mesencephalon. Crossing to the opposite side of the mesencephalon, the impulse synapses on the parasympathetic nucleus of the oculomotor nucleus. The oculomotor nerve then acts to constrict the pupil. A lesion in the pathway of the PLR can result in blindness and a loss of the PLR (Figure 4.1).

CN III, IV, and VI all work in conjunction to move the eye, and deficits in any of these may result in a strabismus.

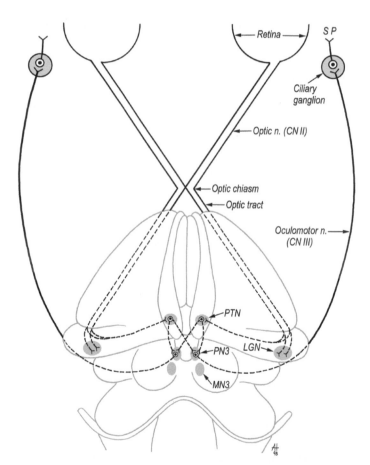

Figure 4.1 Neuroanatomic pathways for vision and pupillary constriction. LGN, lateral geniculate nucleus; PTN, pretectal nucleus; PN3, parasympathetic nucleus of cranial nerve III; MN3, motor nucleus of cranial nerve III; SP, sphincter papillae muscle.

Source: Illustration by Hoffman A; reprinted with permission from Dewey CW. *A Practical Guide to Canine and Feline Neurology*, 2nd edition, figure 2.8, p. 24. Ames, IA: Wiley; 2008.

A CN III palsy results in a ventral lateral deviation, CN IV a lateral rotation of the dorsal aspect of the eye, and a CN VI a medial deviation. CN VI is also responsible for the retraction of the globe into the orbital socket. A light touch of the cornea (sensory CN V) will result in the patient reflexively pulling the eye into the socket. Abnormalities of CN IV and VI are very rare.

CN V is called trigeminal because of its three branches: the mandibular (motor to muscles of mastication and sensory to the lower half of the face), the maxillary (sensory to the upper lateral half of the face), and the ophthalmic (sensory to the medial portion of the face and top of the head).

The patient is evaluated for muscle symmetry and atrophy of the muscles of mastication; the mandible is assessed for muscle tone and sensation. The palpebral reflex is used to evaluate the maxillary and the ophthalmic branches. Touching both the medial (ophthalmic) and the lateral (maxillary) canthi of the eye should cause the patient to reflexively blink. Unless there is a CN VII (facial) deficit, the patient should feel the touch (CN V) then blink (CN VII). CN V may also be evaluated by lightly touching the mucosa of the nares; normal patients should pull their heads away. This is a cerebral response to a noxious stimulus.

CN VII (facial) controls the muscles of facial expression. Parasympathetic fibers travel with CN VII to control tear formation so a facial paralysis may result in an inability to close the eye and an inability to produce enough tears.

CN VIII (vestibular/cochlear) has two parts: the vestibular for balance and the cochlear for hearing. There may be a dysfunction of either one or both.

The cochlear is tested with the crude test of clapping hands or banging two dog food bowls together. This test will not define that portion of the population with a unilateral deafness (25% of Dalmatian puppies may have congenital unilateral deafness). Brainstem auditory evoked response (BAER)/brainstem auditory evoked potential (BAEP) testing is an objective way to evaluate hearing. Using the same electrodiagnostic equipment as is used for electromyography (EMG) and nerve conduction velocities (NCVs) the actual electrical impulse of hearing is measured as it travels up the cochlear nerve (see BAER testing in "Diagnostic Testing").

The vestibular portion of CN VIII is commonly affected by disease. The patient may present with a head tilt, leaning to one side, rolling, and variations of nystagmus.

In the normal patient, a movement of the head will elicit the normal oculocephalic reflex. In the oculocephalic reflex, the eyes will fix on one point as the head turns, then after the eyes reach the limit of their sideway glance, they will quickly move to a point in the direction of head movement. This ratcheting movement (nystagmus) is controlled by CN VIII (vestibular) inputting head movement information into the medial longitudinal fasciculus where the information is relayed to the nuclei of CN III, IV, and VI. They in turn move the eyes appropriately. If the information being given to III, IV, and VI is erroneous because of a diseased vestibular system, the eyes will be moving spontaneously without head movement. There are different types of nystagmus: horizontal, rotatory, vertical, and pendulous. Nystagmus is always characterized by its type and the direction of the fast phase of the eye movement. Pendulous nystagmus is a nystagmus with the speed in both directions being the same, like the pendulum of a clock. Pendulous nystagmus is normal in certain breeds of cats (e.g., Burmese and Siamese) and should not be considered a sign of pathology.

CN IX (glossopharyngeal) is sensory to the pharynx and caudal third of the tongue. It also innervates the muscles of the pharyngeal and palatine structures. The stimulus of a finger in the back of the throat or a gentle squeeze of the larynx should result in the patient swallowing.

CN X (vagus) controls the laryngeal and vocalization function. The parasympathetic fibers of the vagus control the heart and the thoracic and abdominal viscera. Difficulty eating, changes in the voice (bark), stridulous breathing, and megaesophagus may all be signs of vagal dysfunction.

CN XI (spinal accessory) is motor to the trapezius and other muscles of the neck. Abnormalities of this nerve are exceedingly rare.

CN XII (hypoglossal) controls the tongue. Early signs of dysfunction may be rippling fasciculations of the surface on the affected side of the tongue. At first, the tongue deviates away from the affected side due to lack of opposing tone, then with chronicity, it will contract and pull toward the affected side. Abnormalities of the hypoglossal nerve are rare.

Abnormalities in the cerebellum are most evident when there is movement since the cerebellum's main purpose is to coordinate movement. The patient may have a generalized ataxia and hypermetria in the gait, yet strength is preserved. They stand with a broad base and will have an intention tremor of the head. An intention tremor is only evident when the patient intends to do something, such as lap water or eat. Some cerebellar patients may have anisocoria and some may have a menace reflex deficit since the pathway for the menace reflex courses through the cerebellum.

Spinal cord

Caudal to the foramen magnum, the spinal cord begins. For lesion placement purposes, the spinal cord is divided into sections C1–C5, C6–T2, T3–L3, L4–S2, and coccygeal. The logic behind this division is based on the function of the upper motor neuron (UMN) and the lower motor neuron (LMN). This concept of UMN and LMN is essential to the understanding of neuroanatomy and the neurological exam.

Within the cerebral cortex (telencephalon) is the UMN. The simple way to think of this is that the UMN, in order to command motor movement, transmits an electrical impulse (action potential) down the axon to synapse on the LMN. The LMN may be in the facial nucleus of the brain stem if the patient wishes to blink the eye, or the LMN may be in the cervical or lumbar intumescences if the patient wishes to curl a toe or lift a leg. The intumescences are the enlarged areas of the spinal cord, C6–T2 and L4–S2. These areas are enlarged because of all the interconnections of UMN to multiple LMNs.

The general influence of the UMN is not only the initiation of motor movement but also the overall one of calming. If the con-

nection to the UMN is lost, there is a release of the calming influence on the LMN and the reflex arc, resulting in exaggerated reflexes.

As part of the neurological exam, we will "tap tendons"; this is a myotatic reflex. What is happening is that by tapping a tendon, we quickly cause the muscle to stretch; intrafusal fibers in the muscle sense this stretch and send a signal to the spinal cord notifying the cord of this unexpected lengthening of the muscle. The spinal cord (not the brain), in response to this unexpected stretch, sends a signal to the extrafusal fibers in the muscle to increase muscle tone. This increased tone results in the resultant "jerk" after the tendon has been tapped. Generally, the jerk is mild and only acts to prevent overstretching of the muscle and maintains the status quo. If the "calming" effect of the UMN has been removed because of pathology in the central nervous system (CNS) rostral to the reflex arc, then the reflex will appear more brisk or exaggerated. Segmental reflexes are those that we test that show the integrity of the reflex arc, for example, the knee jerk. Segmental reflexes of the limbs are in the sections of the spinal cord C6–T2 and L4–S2. They go no farther than from the limb to the cord then back to the limb.

If the lesion is in the reflex arc, then the reflex will be depressed or nonexistent. That is why one of the cardinal rules states, "If the reflex is depressed or absent, then you must *place the lesion in the reflex arc!*"

Postural responses go from the limb to the brain then back to the limb. Postural responses differ from segmental reflexes in that the response is initiated from the brain. This necessitates that sensation from the periphery, whether it be nociception or joint position sense, be interpreted by the brain (parietal lobe), then a motor movement (frontal lobe) is initiated with the result of returning the limb to its normal position or away from the pain.

C1–C5

Lesions in the C1–C5 region of the spinal cord may present with exaggerated (UMN) reflexes in all the limbs because the LMN for the limbs has been released from the calming effect of the UMN. These animals may also present with a weakness or paralysis in all four limbs (quadriparesis/quadriplegia) or only on one side (hemiparesis/hemiplegia), loss of postural responses in all four limbs or only on one side, urinary incontinence, cervical pain, and in some severe cases, loss or difficulty in respiration.

C6–T2

Lesions in the C6–T2 area should give LMN signs in the forelimbs and UMN signs in the rear; however, up to 30% of lesions here will not result in depressed or absent reflexes in the forelimbs. This fact illustrates one of the idiosyncrasies of neurology; there are always exceptions to the rule and always the possibility of shades of gray. A lesion in the C6–T2 area may also present with weakness in all four limbs (which may be asymmetrical), depressed postural responses in all four limbs, urinary incontinence, Horner's syndrome, and a possible loss of the panniculus/lateral cutaneous trunci reflex bilaterally or unilaterally.

T3–L3

The T3–L3 area is the most common for spinal neurological lesion placement. These patients will have normal forelimbs (Schiff–Sherrington is the exception); they may have weakness or paralysis in the rear limbs (paraparesis/paraplegia), normal to brisk segmental reflexes in the rear limbs, postural response deficits in the rear limbs, increased focal sensitivity at the level of the lesion, possible urinary incontinence, and a possible disruption of the panniculus/lateral cutaneous trunci reflex. Disruption of the panniculus, when present, is an invaluable aid in localizing spinal lesions. Cutaneous sensation enters the cord via the dorsal nerve root and travels rostral to the upper thoracic area where it connects with the LMN for the lateral cutaneous trunci muscle. Exiting with the T2 nerve root, it makes the cutaneous trunci muscle flinch, functionally to perhaps chase flies off the back. If the impulse is blocked anywhere along this path, then the reflex muscle flinch is arrested. Once the examiner ascends to above the blockage/lesion, the reflex is once again completed.

The Schiff–Sherrington posture is an exception to this rule since a severe lesion in the T3–L3 area may disrupt a spinal tract that ascends the cord from border cells in the lumbar intumescence. This tract has an inhibitory effect on the extensors of the front limbs. If this inhibition is removed because of interruption of the spinal tract, then when the front limbs are at rest, they remain in extension.

L4–S2

Lesions in the L4–S2 region may cause flaccid weakness or paralysis in the pelvic limbs, a flaccid weakness or paralysis of the tail, postural response deficits in the rear limbs, urinary/fecal incontinence, depressed or absent anal reflex, and possible focal pain. Absent or depressed reflexes and flaccid or limp muscle tone are LMN signs.

Diffuse or multifocal locations may be encountered. The most common would be a diffuse LMN disease. These are most characteristically a toxin (botulism, tick, or coral snake) or immune mediated (polyradiculoneuritis, fulminating myasthenia gravis [MG]). The patient will have LMN signs in more than one limb or the signs may be progressing from the rear to the thoracic limb. The presence of LMN signs in both the pelvic and thoracic limbs can only be explained by a diffuse or multifocal lesion.

After placing the lesion, the clinician will formulate a list of possible suspect diseases based on signalment, history, and the lesion location.

Seizures

When we speak of seizures, we must have a basic understanding of the nomenclature. Epilepsy is commonly thought of as a disease; however, the word epilepsy only means recurring seizures. There are different types of epilepsy; true epilepsy is defined as recurrent seizures over a long period of time of a nonprogressive nature. True epilepsy may be inherited, acquired, or idiopathic. Symptomatic epilepsy is a seizure disorder of a progressive nature. The patient has the symptoms of epilepsy; however, they are the result of an intracranial disorder, for example, brain tumor. A third classification is reactive epilepsy; the patient is having seizures as a reaction to something elsewhere in the body, such as liver disease, low blood sugar, or intoxication. No longer are the terms grand mal or petit mal used to describe the seizure. Instead, we use grades of severity. Simple partial or a focal seizure is where there is no impairment of consciousness and possibly only a minor twitch in one muscle group. Complex partial seizures are where there are serial movements with some impairment of consciousness. The severe generalized seizure is the most common and troublesome form of seizure. Other less observed forms of generalized seizures are classified as absence and myoclonic seizures. Absence seizures are a very short (seconds) loss of cerebral function without motor involvement, and myoclonic seizures consist of one large muscular jerk without loss of cerebral function.

Generalized seizures account for about 60% of all seizures in cats and 80% of those seen in dogs. Typically, the seizure has four phases: prodromal, aura, ictus (active seizure), and postictal. In humans, the prodromal and aura are more well-defined since the patients can describe the sensations that they experience in those minutes to seconds just before the seizure. Many clients will describe how they know their dog is about to have a seizure because the animal will seek them out. For this to happen, the dog must be experiencing a prodrome or aura. The duration of the actual ictus is variable but is typically between 30 s and 1.5 min. For the clinician, the postictal period is a critical length of time to define since the patient with active intracranial disease (symptomatic epilepsy) will have a protracted postictal period or possibly never return to normal between seizures. Most patients have a normal interictal period (i.e., period between seizures) with some demonstrating distinct calendar rhythms. Status epilepticus is a seizure that persists for a sufficient length of time or is repeated frequently enough that recovery between attacks does not occur. Status epilepticus is a true medical emergency. This is not to be confused with cluster seizures, which are multiple seizures spaced over a day or two.

Diagnostic approach

The diagnostic approach to seizures starts with the signalment since true epilepsy usually begins at 6 months to 5 years of age. Certain breeds are more commonly afflicted: Tervuren, beagle, German shepherd, keeshonden, collie, golden retriever, Irish setter, Saint Bernard, cocker spaniel, and miniature poodle. There appears to be no gender preference.

In taking the history, there are specific questions to ask the client—previous illnesses, family history, vaccination status, describe what the seizure looks like, symmetry of the seizure, frequency, duration, when was the first seizure, are they becoming more frequent, time of day, length of seizure, and the length of each phase of the seizure.

The physical examination should not be overlooked for its importance; for example, an ophthalmoscopic exam may show the chorioretinitis of distemper or feline infectious peritonitis (FIP) (feline coronavirus). Similarly, cardiac auscultation is important since syncope may be confused with a seizure. The seizure patient may have a normal neurological exam or the clinical signs may localize to the cerebrum.

Minimum database should include a complete blood count (CBC), serum chemistries (fasting blood glucose if possible), urinalysis, thoracic radiographs, and abdominal ultrasound. Choice of additional diagnostics such as bile acids, tick titers, and fungal titers may change with initial blood values and geographical location.

Cerebrospinal fluid (CSF) analysis is required to rule out CNS inflammatory disease, and advanced imaging with MRI or computed tomography (CT) is invaluable for further defining intracranial disease.

Treatment

The decision to initiate anticonvulsant therapy is based on many variables. Most veterinary neurologists start anticonvulsants if there is more than one seizure a month. However, other variables may be included, including concerns of the owner (e.g., time commitment, ability to medicate), seizure frequency, character of the seizures, and monitoring costs. It is essential for the owner to know that 20–30% of animals may not be controlled despite medical therapy. Selection of an anticonvulsant may be based on a clinician's personal preference. With canine patients, the author starts with phenobarbital then bromide, saving the tertiary anticonvulsants (levetiracetam [Keppra®], zonisamide, felbamate) until later.

Monitoring of drug levels is only a guide; the patient will tell if the medication is working. See the pharmacology section for more information on anticonvulsants.

Home seizure therapy may help clients from having to run to the emergency clinic every time there is a seizure. Injectable diazepam may be administered rectally with the aid of a plastic teat cannula or other similar device. A dose of 1 mg/kg of rectally administered diazepam is almost as effective as if given IV. Another at-home technique is vagal stimulation achieved by pressing on the eyeballs. This may have some effect in preempting the seizure if done in the prodromal period.

One study in the early 1990s with only 11 patients showed that acupuncture, straight needle, or gold bead implant had a benefit in 50% of the patients by reducing either seizure frequency or severity.

Status epilepticus

Status epilepticus, or repeated seizure activity without intermission, is a medical emergency. It can lead to hyperthermia, hypoxia, and acidosis. Sixty percent of epileptics will experience status epilepticus at some time. Increased body weight has been shown to predispose epileptic patients to having status. Where epilepsy will not normally shorten life span, an episode of status epilepticus may.

Treatment of status epilepticus entails all of the following to take place almost simultaneously: Establish an IV and start crystalloids, obtain blood samples (especially for glucose), take a history to define if there has been exposure to toxins, and do a physical exam. Body temperature is most important! Seizure activity readily makes the body temperature go up. Often these patients are hyperthermic and are in need of immediate cooling. If hypoglycemia is suspected, administer 2–4 mL/kg of 50% glucose that has been diluted 1:2 with sterile water intravenously. Diazepam is the drug of choice to arrest seizures. It is generally dosed between 0.5 and 1.0 mg/kg IV. If there is no response to diazepam, proceed to propofol. Both diazepam and propofol may be used as a constant rate infusion (CRI). The use of propofol will necessitate intratracheal intubation and constant monitoring. Oxygen is supplied at the same time. You now have a critical care patient that may not be left when the clock hits five and everyone wants to head home! Phenobarbital is not used to stop status. Some clinics may still be using pentobarbital; however, its cost has risen so dramatically as to make its use prohibitive. If toxicity is suspected, now is the time to perform gastric lavage with copious amounts of warm saline or water followed by the instillation of activated charcoal. If there is a response to diazepam, then seizure control may be continued with phenobarbital loading. Give phenobarbital q 6 h at a dose of 2–4 mg/kg IV for 48 h. This protocol may be abbreviated if the patient is having good seizure control. Loading with bromide rectally is another alternative.

If 24-h care is not available at your clinic, then the client should be advised to transfer the patient to a 24-h care facility where the patient may be monitored throughout the night. If the client declines this level of care, then make a note of this in the medical record. Seizure patients should not be left in the hospital unattended.

Encephalopathies

Storage diseases

Storage diseases are rare and generally inherited by an autosomal recessive mechanism. The signalment is typically a young animal with a slowly progressive loss of function. The compound that is to be metabolically transformed in a stepwise fashion accumulates because these animals are missing an enzymatic step in cellular metabolism. The storage of this compound leads to disruption of the cell function. Some diseases have forebrain signs (e.g., dementia, wandering, and behavior changes), while others have signs referable to the cerebellum (e.g., hypermetria, ataxia, and broad-based stance).

Some storage diseases have had their exact genetic defect identified and have the ability to be diagnosed by genetic testing (see http://www.CanineGeneticDiseases.net to find a list of breed-dependent tests).

Hydrocephalus

Hydrocephalus is a developmental malformation that is common in certain small, toy, and brachiocephalic breeds (e.g., the Chihuahua, toy poodle, and pug). Congenital stenosis or blockage of the normal circulatory paths for CSF (as may be acquired from trauma, tumor, or infection) results in disruption of the ependymal lining of the ventricles with fluid migration into the brain parenchyma. This leads to progressive parenchyma loss with expansion of the ventricles. In the very young animal where there has not been closure of the cranial bone sutures, this

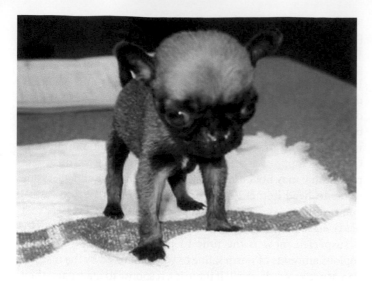

Figure 4.2 Chihuahua with hydrocephalus and the "setting sun sign."

internal pressure causes a large dome-shaped cranium often with bilateral ventrolateral strabismus or "setting sun sign" (i.e., eyes directed downward and outward) (Figure 4.2).

Plain radiographs may demonstrate a lack of detail within the cranial vault; however, CT or MRI is the desired imaging modality.

Medical treatment involves carbonic anhydrase inhibitors, proton pump inhibitors, and steroids. These are palliative at best. Surgical intervention is with shunt placement. A shunt is placed into one lateral ventricle after making a small burr hole in the skull. From there, a tube is placed under the skin to the dorsum of the neck where a one-way valve is placed; from this valve, the subcutaneous tube is directed to the abdominal cavity where the fluid is allowed to be absorbed. This shunt apparatus has a complication rate of approximately 25% due to blockage, kinking, infection, and breakage.

Caudal occipital malformation syndrome

Caudal occipital malformation syndrome (COMS) has become a very common problem in the Cavalier King Charles spaniel; however, other breeds have been shown to have COMS (e.g., toy poodle, Maltese, Yorkshire terrier, pug, and Pekingese). With COMS, there is less room in the caudal fossa because of a congenital malformation of the occipital bone. This lack of space results in the cerebellum being partially forced out the foramen magnum, altering normal CSF flow. The abnormal flow causes changes in pressure gradients with the result being the formation of syrinxes within the spinal cord. Because these syrinxes impinge or destroy the dorsal horn of the spinal cord, the animal often presents with pain as a primary clinical sign. This pain may be a paresthesia around the neck and shoulder region causing the patient to scratch at the area. The pain caused by COMS may also be much more severe. If the syrinx is large and is affecting the LMN, there may also be torticollis, muscle atrophy in the thoracic limb, and paresis in the pelvic limb. Most patients present between 3 and 6 years of age. Diagnosis is made with

MRI of the caudal fossa and cervical spine. Syrinxes may be throughout the cord; however, the most common site is the rostral cervical spinal cord.

Treatment may be medical or surgical. Medical treatment typically includes pain relief, reduction of CSF, and steroids. Drugs used to relieve pain include gabapentin, tramadol, and non-steroidal anti-inflammatory drugs (NSAIDs). Drugs used to reduce CSF are acetazolamide (Diamox®) or, anecdotally, omeprazole (Prilosec®). The steroid typically used is prednisone. Success with medication will depend on the severity of clinical signs. Surgical therapy involves removing part of the occipital bone (foramen magnum decompression), thereby relieving the compression of the cerebellum. With the restoration of normal fluid flow, the clinical signs ameliorate; however, the syrinxes do not go away. Postoperative scarring has been the major complication. Up to 47% of animals treated with the older surgical techniques require a second surgery. With newer surgical techniques, the success rate is closer to 80%.

Hepatic encephalopathy

An important function of the liver is to act as a filter of potential toxins emanating from the gut. If there is a vascular shunt (i.e., a virtual bypass), toxins have direct access to the systemic circulation. With congenital shunts, the circulatory system bypasses the liver. Acquired shunts are caused by severe liver damage through infection or other insult. Any shunt can lead to encephalopathy. The congenital form is overrepresented in Old English sheepdogs, Yorkshire terriers, Australian cattle dogs, Maltese, and miniature and toy breeds.

The clinical signs of encephalopathy include depression, behavior abnormalities, pacing, head pressing, and rarely, seizures. These signs may wax and wane with the animal's appetite.

Typically, the changes on the minimum database include decreased blood urea nitrogen (BUN), albumin, cholesterol and glucose levels, and a mild microcytic, nonregenerative anemia. Urate crystals in the urine may also raise suspicion. The diagnosis of hepatic encephalopathy requires specific liver function tests, most commonly, blood ammonia and pre- and postprandial bile acid levels, both of which should be elevated.

Abdominal radiography may show microhepatica. Definitive diagnosis is typically made by means of abdominal ultrasound (80–90% sensitivity); however, other imaging modalities may be indicated to diagnose the shunt (e.g., scintigraphy or portal, arterial, CT or MR angiography). Liver biopsy may be required if portal vein hypoplasia with microvascular disease is suspected.

Medical management may be indicated prior to surgery and in case of microvascular disease, where surgery is not feasible. Management includes fluid therapy to correct and maintain hydration status, any electrolyte abnormalities, glucose levels, and metabolic acidosis. Initially, the animal may be NPO, and when feeding is reinstituted, a low protein diet (e.g., Hill's k/d) is usually prescribed. Antibiotics to decrease bacterial translocation numbers and therefore ammonia production, such as metronidazole and ampicillin, are indicated. Medication to control seizures and to treat gastric bleeding or ulcers and/or diuretics may be needed. Lactulose, administered either orally or rectally, has many benefits. Lactulose lowers the pH in the gut (thus trapping ammonia as nonabsorbable ammonium), changes the colonic flora, accelerates gut transport time, and may have an antiendotoxin effect. With medical therapy alone, survival prognosis ranges from 2 to 5 years. If there is a solitary shunt, then following stabilization, surgical ligation is the treatment of choice.

Cerebral neoplasia

Cerebral neoplasia occurs with a frequency of 14.5 in 100,000 canines and 3.5 in 100,000 felines.

Signalment may be any breed of dog or cat, but generally, they are middle-aged or older. In dogs, the median age is 9 years, and in cats, it is over 10 years of age. Dogs present with seizures as the most common clinical sign, while cats typically present for behavior abnormalities. There is no specific history associated with cerebral neoplasia; the onset of seizures may be sudden or it may present as a slow, insidious progression of neurological dysfunction.

There are many tumor types associated with cerebral neoplasia. The basic delineation is between primary versus secondary neoplasia. Primary tumors are derived from neuroepithelial tissue (e.g., astrocytoma, oligodendroglioma, glioblastoma, choroid plexus papilloma, meningeal, or meningioma). Secondary tumors originate from other tissues, for example, lymphoid (lymphoma), vascular (hemangiosarcoma), nerve sheath (neurofibroma), and metastatic tumors. In dogs and cats, the most common cerebral neoplasia is meningioma. Cats may have multiple meningiomas at one time, giving a neurological exam typical of multifocal disease. Staging of the patient to rule out secondary tumors is a necessity. The minimum database should include a CBC, serum chemistries, and chest and abdominal ultrasound. Skull radiographs are rarely diagnostic, while CSF's main benefit is in ruling out inflammatory disease. The prime modality for diagnosis is MRI due to the superiority of soft tissue detail with MRI over CT.

Once a definitive diagnosis of a brain tumor has been established, options for treatment may be divided into palliative or definitive. Palliative therapy typically includes steroids and seizure control. Steroids reduce the permeability of the tumor capillaries, reduce the tumor blood supply, and may reduce the tumor blood volume by up to 21% in the first 24 h. However, steroids also have many deleterious effects (see "Pharmacology" section). Seizure control is generally through the use of phenobarbital or newer anticonvulsants.

The choice for surgery depends on the species, the location of the tumor, and accessibility. Once accessed, meningiomas in cats tend to easily peel out, while the character of a meningioma in the dog is much more invasive and nonresectable.

With radiation therapy, either palliative or definitive, the patient receives small fractionated doses repeatedly over multiple weeks until an accumulated dose is achieved. If available, stereotactic radiation surgery (i.e., Gamma Knife) utilizes special computerized targeting of the tumor based on combined CT and MRI images to deliver a single high dose of radiation.

Table 4.1 Canine meningioma survival times based on modality

Modality	Average survival time
Steroids	1–2 months
Radiation	250–322 days
Surgery alone	5–7 months
Surgery and radiation	15 months

Chemotherapy is not considered very effective in the treatment of cerebral neoplasm. The blood–brain barrier (BBB) isolates the brain from the systemic circulation, making it difficult for large nonlipophilic drugs to penetrate. In a published study, BCNU (Carmustine®), at 50mg/m^2 every 6 weeks, had a survival time of 6–17 months no matter what kind of mass was being treated. Small numbers in this report give marginal validity to the data.

The prognosis for patients with cerebral neoplasia is dependent on tumor type, location, and species. While the invasive astrocytoma may have a survival time after diagnosis in dogs of only 1–4 months, canine meningioma survival time can be up to 15 months (Table 4.1).

In felines with operable meningiomas, 71% were alive 6 months postoperative, 66% at 1 year, and 50% at 2 years.

Inflammatory/infectious etiologies: encephalitis

Bacterial

The patient with inflammatory brain disease may present with a spectrum of possible clinical signs ranging from focal signs of unilateral cranial nerve loss to a diffuse encephalopathy. Many of the clinical signs are nonspecific (e.g., mental dullness, ataxia, and cervical hyperesthesia) and may be confused with cervical disease, while "brain pain," as evidenced when the clinician squeezes on the head and the patient exhibits pain, may be seen with any form of intracranial disease.

Bacterial infections of the brain are not common. Bacterial organisms generally gain access to the CNS via the bloodstream. The changes in the CBC expected with a systemic infection are normally not seen with infections of the CNS. *Staphylococcus*, *Streptococcus*, and *Escherichia coli* are those organisms most often isolated, but culturing of the CSF is rarely definitive. When possible, antibiotic selection should be based on culture results. However, in the absence of a definitive culture, Gram staining may suffice. Gram-negative organisms should be treated with enrofloxacin or with third-generation cephalosporin. If no organisms are seen, yet the cytology of the CSF is indicative of bacterial infection, high intravenous doses of ampicillin (which will cross the inflamed BBB) may be started.

The prognosis for bacterial meningoencephalitis is guarded.

Rickettsial

Rickettsial infections in the dog may cause neurological dysfunction. Rocky Mountain spotted fever and ehrlichiosis (*Rickettsia rickettsii* and *Ehrlichia canis*) are intracellular parasites that may cause vasculitis and hemorrhage within the CNS.

The history of tick exposure in the patient presenting with an acute onset of encephalopathy and systemic signs of illness warrants the evaluation of titers to Rocky Mountain spotted fever and ehrlichiosis. A single high serum titer combined with clinical signs is indicative of infection, while paired serum titers with an evident rise over 2 weeks' time is definitive. The Snap 3DX Test® (heartworm, *E. canis*, Lyme) is a good screening test. Doxycycline is the treatment of choice. More information may be found in Chapter 11.

Viral

The most commonly encountered viral meningoencephalitis in the dog is distemper. Despite the widespread use of vaccines, this virus is still a major cause of encephalitis. Young animals with absent or incomplete vaccine history, animals coming from shelters, or nutritionally/immunologically compromised individuals are all at high risk. The paramyxovirus of distemper has two infective phases. The animal may have a history of upper respiratory infection that has resolved and is now presenting as a patient with CNS signs. Chief among the clinical signs may be myoclonus, a rhythmic muscular jerk normally about the head and neck. The patient may also present with posterior paresis or "chewing gum" seizures. Distemper has a predilection for the pontine-medullary angle of the brain stem often giving cranial nerve signs in conjunction with seizures. The fundic exam may reveal chorioretinitis. Titers of serum and CSF (both IgG and IgM) may be indicated to definitively diagnose distemper. There is no treatment for distemper other than supportive and nursing care. Some patients may mount a competent immune response and survive, often to be left with a residual myoclonus.

In cats, the most common CNS viral disease is feline coronavirus (FIP), which may cause a multifocal encephalopathy in the noneffusive (dry) form. The diagnosis of CNS FIP is based upon clinical signs, physical examination findings (chorioretinitis), compatible serum chemistries (elevated immunoglobulin), susceptible age group (young or old), and titers. MRI may also be of value in that periventricular enhancement has been equated to FIP meningoencephalitis. The only confirmatory test is tissue biopsy. The prognosis for the cat with CNS FIP is poor, with most progressing and dying over a few weeks. There is no effective treatment. Steroids may be used to ameliorate clinical signs, but they do not arrest disease progression.

Fungal

Fungal meningoencephalitis may be caused by a number of fungi, most of which are geographically specific. *Cryptococcus* is the most common isolate in dogs and cats and is typically found in young to middle-aged animals. Often there is an intrusion from an external infection, and if a demonstrable source of fungal infection is found in the encephalopathic patient, then it should be presumed to be the cause (e.g., as in a cat with nasal *Cryptococcus* infection breaking through the cribriform plate).

A fungal encephalitis may have the organism demonstrable in the CSF, while viral or bacterial encephalitis is much less likely to have the organism visible.

Testing the CSF or serum for antibodies to the varied fungi is readily available. Latex agglutination testing for *Cryptococcus* is very sensitive and specific. The most basic of screening tests should not be overlooked since often *Aspergillosis* has been identified in the urine.

Treatment for CNS fungal disease is rarely rewarding with the exception of *Cryptococcus*. The BBB is a hindrance to penetration of many antifungals; however, fluconazole does penetrate well and should be the drug of choice. If there is a favorable response to treatment, the patient may need treatment for an extremely extended period, often for the rest of its life.

Protozoan

Protozoal agents are not common causes of meningoencephalomyelitis but must still be on the potential list of suspects. *Neospora caninum* and *Toxoplasma gondii* are similar in their pathophysiology. *Neospora* was mistaken for *Toxoplasma* until refinement of diagnostic capabilities proved the difference in the 1980s. Infective routes are transplacental, the ingestion of fecally shed oocysts, or the ingestion of intermediate hosts harboring the tachyzoite or bradyzoite stage of the protozoa. Young animals may be more susceptible to infection. Diagnosis by serology is with either a rising paired IgG titer or a positive IgM titer with a negative IgG, indicative of active infection.

The organism is rarely seen in CSF or muscle biopsy despite the fact that the cysts may cause a myopathy. The CSF of an active intracranial infection should have a mixed cell pleocytosis with an elevation of protein; these findings, compatible with many diseases of the brain, are not definitive for protozoal infection. The diagnosis may also be supported by a response to treatment. Clindamycin or trimethoprim–sulfa is commonly used for treating protozoan infections.

Granulomatous meningoencephalomyelitis

Granulomatous meningoencephalomyelitis (GME) is an inflammatory disease of unknown etiology that may occur at a rate of 1% of all neurological diseases. There are three forms of GME: disseminated, focal, and ocular. Previous names for GME have been reticulosis, reticulitis, inflammatory reticulosis, and neoplastic reticulosis. Pathology is limited to the CNS. Inflammatory cells may produce granulomas, and these granulomas may compress or invade nearby structures, giving the symptoms of a focal lesion. Thirty-five percent of GME is the focal form with lesions usually in the brain stem, especially the pontine-medullary area, but it may be in the cervical region. Sixty percent of GME is the disseminated form. These lesions may be throughout the CNS but primarily in the white matter. The predilection is for brain stem and cerebral hemispheres. Five percent of GME cases are the ocular form with lesions in the retina, optic disk, and optic nerve. The common presentation of this form is known as optic neuritis. The etiology of GME remains unknown, but a short illness is often a precipitating factor. There is an acute onset with rapid decline in condition. The clinical course is generally 3–8 weeks. Diagnosis is based on clinical signs and history. Most conclusive is the CSF results, a pleocytosis of 50–900 nucleated cells with a predominance of mononuclear cells and occasional neutrophils. CSF protein ranges from 40 to 400 mg/dL. The definitive diagnosis of GME is with brain biopsy, and it is because of this rarely used diagnostic that many inflammatory diseases of the CNS have been lumped together as GME. There is a trend toward using the newer nomenclature, meningoencephalitis of unknown etiology (MUE). With or without the definitive diagnosis treatment is the same for these encephalitidies, steroids (prednisone) as the first drug then when prednisone is no longer effective switching to cytosine arabinoside (Cytarabine/Cytosar®), which has given longer survival times than prednisone alone. Prognosis is poor, depending on the form of MUE it may be a few weeks to 12 months before euthanasia due to a lack of response to therapy. A recent publication had a survival time averaging 1800 days when the second therapeutic agent was azathioprine; however, there was no histological confirmation of the disease type. Cytosine is dosed at 50 mg/m^2 given twice a day for 2 days in a row every 3–4 weeks. Cyclosporin at 3–10 mg/kg bid PO has also been advocated. Cyclosporin inhibits cytokines that modulate macrophages and monocytes. Another treatment is with mycophenolate mofetil (CellCept®) at 20 mg/kg PO. Mycophenolate's main side effect is gastrointestinal upset. Once the patient is showing improvement, the dose may be halved.

Breed-specific inflammatory disease has been recognized. In the pug and Maltese, it is necrotizing meningoencephalitis (NME), and in the Yorkshire terrier, necrotizing leukoencephalitis (NLE). As the name necrotizing implies, these forms of encephalitis are more severe with seizure activity more prevalent. The course of the disease is more rapid with survival times often less than 2 weeks.

Other breeds of dogs have been reported to fall subject to NME and NLE, these being typically young, small breed animals. Differentiating NME and NLE from GME antemortem is difficult; however, MRI lesion distribution to either gray or white matter may aid in diagnosis.

NME and NLE are resistant to successful treatment.

Meningitis

More commonly seen in veterinary practice is sterile meningitis (steroid-responsive meningitis). These are usually young dogs (less than 2 years) that present with severe neck pain and fever. There may be a peripheral neutrophilia on the CBC. As a breed, boxers seem to be predisposed. CSF analysis will have a neutrophilic pleocytosis and high protein levels. Treatment is with immunosuppressive doses of steroids (prednisone) with an excellent prognosis.

Necrotizing vasculitis is a severe sterile meningitis/vasculitis seen in Bernese mountain dogs, beagles (beagle pain syndrome) and German shorthaired pointers. Signs are as in the above steroid-responsive meningitis; however, the response to therapy and prognosis is not as good.

Cranial nerve syndromes

From an evolutionary aspect, it was necessary for the body to be able to right itself before it was even able to stand; hence, the vestibular component of the brain is contained within the oldest parts of the CNS. Although the cerebral cortex receives balance projections via the medial geniculate body, the cortex does not maintain balance; balance is maintained by the rhombencephalon/hindbrain. The neurons of the vestibular ganglion receive impulses from five sites: the crista of the ampulla of each of the three semicircular canals and the macula of the utricle and macula of the saccule. The crista records the movement of the head, while the macula records the position of the head. These neurons synapse in the vestibular nuclei (there are four main vestibular nuclei) in the medulla (Figure 4.3).

Neurons from the vestibular nuclei ascend ipsilaterally, while others decussate then ascend. They project to the medial geniculate body and, on the way, give off multiple branches to the nuclei of CN III, IV, and VI, thereby giving a strong influence to eye movement. The ascending tracts are predominantly in the medial longitudinal fasciculus. There are also numerous projections into the ascending and descending reticular formations. Some of these descending reticular projections are involved in the vomiting and cardiovascular reactions which may occur in vestibular disturbances. Clinical signs may be used to define a central versus a peripheral vestibular lesion (Table 4.2).

Idiopathic vestibular syndrome

Idiopathic vestibular syndrome is also known as senile vestibular syndrome. The signalment is an older dog (mean of 12.5 years of age) with an acute onset of unilateral peripheral vestibular symptoms, head tilt, rolling/leaning, unilateral ventral strabismus, and nystagmus. Diagnosis is by ruling out other causes of the vestibular syndrome (e.g., otitis media, otitis interna, and trauma). A minimum database should include a CBC and serum chemistries. The treatment is palliative therapy, usually with meclizine at 25 mg PO daily; steroids are not indicated. Protective cage padding and tranquilizers may be needed if the patient is attempting to ambulate and causing self-trauma. In the older debilitated patient, fluid support may be needed. These patients may be unable to stand, and close attention to hygiene may be needed to avoid urine scald and fecal soiling.

Improvement comes in stages; nystagmus, and with it the vertigo, is the first clinical sign to wane, typically within the first 48 h. The patient may be left with a permanent, slight head tilt.

Otitis media-interna

Otitis media-interna patients present with similar clinical signs as peripheral vestibular syndrome (e.g., head tilt, nystagmus, leaning or falling against walls, ataxia, and occasionally vomiting). If severe, Horner's syndrome may also be present. The route of infection is usually by ascending the eustachian tube to the middle ear with secondary inflammation affecting the endolymph of the semicircular canals, utricle, and saccule. Penetration of the tympanic membrane with intrusion from the

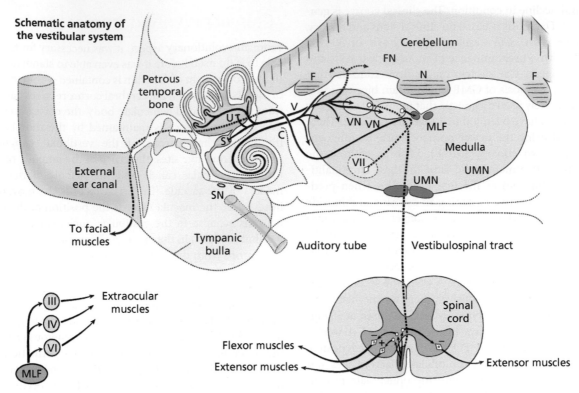

Figure 4.3 Schematic anatomy of the vestibular system. III, oculomotor nucleus; IV, trochlear nucleus; VI, abducent nucleus; VII, facial nucleus; C, cranial nerve VIII—cochlear portion; V, cranial nerve VIII—vestibular portion; F, flocculus; FN, fastigial nucleus; MLF, medial longitudinal fasciculus; N, nodulus; S, saccule; SN, sympathetic neurons; U, utricle; UMN, upper motor neuron; VN, vestibular nucleus.

Source: Reprinted with permission from de Lahunta A, Glass E. *Veterinary Neuroanatomy and Clinical Neurology*, 3rd edition. St. Louis, MO: Elsevier; 2009.

Table 4.2 Central versus peripheral based on clinical symptoms

Clinical symptoms	Central	Peripheral
Loss of balance	Yes	Yes
Head tilt	Yes	Yes
Falling/rolling	Yes, greater tendency	Yes
Nystagmus	Yes	Yes
Horizontal	Yes	Yes
Rotatory	Yes	Yes
Vertical	Yes	No
Positional	Yes	No
Strabismus (ventral)	Yes	Yes
Cranial nerve deficits	Possible V, VI, VII	Possible VII
Horner's syndrome	No	Possible
Cerebellar signs	Possible	No
Mental depression	Possible	No
Hemiparesis, ipsilateral conscious proprioception (CP) deficits	Possible	No

external ear may also be a source of infection. Common bacterial organisms are *Staphylococcus*, *Streptococcus*, and *Pseudomonas*. Diagnosis may be aided by visualization of a cloudy or darkened bulging tympanic membrane.

Skull radiographs, if taken, should include an open mouth view; however, only 70% of the cases will have radiographic changes. CT or MRI is very useful since it provides much better visualization of soft tissue and fluids. The treatment of otitis depends upon the severity. Patients presented for the first time typically require cleaning of the external ear canal (be sure to avoid oily compounds and medications) and treatment with 4–6 weeks of antibiotics (first choice is enrofloxacin; second choice is cephalosporins). For chronic cases, additional diagnostics may be required including skull radiographs and myringotomy to obtain a culture and sensitivity from the middle ear. While still anesthetized, a deep ear flush and cleaning should be performed. For the extremely chronic case with radiographic changes of the bullae, a bulla osteotomy or total ear ablation may be required. In all cases, a residual head tilt may persist.

Central vestibular

The major differences between central vestibular disease and peripheral vestibular disease are a greater tendency to roll, the possibility of vertical nystagmus, or a nystagmus that changes with head position; in addition, there may be cerebellar signs, depression, loss of proprioception on the ipsilateral side and other cranial nerves involved. Etiologies may vary and include distemper (predilection for cerebellar peduncles), GME, and, to a lesser extent, neoplasia (neurofibroma). The diagnosis of central vestibular disease necessitates CSF analysis and special imaging with CT or MRI. A paradoxical head tilt may be seen with lesions in or about the cerebellar peduncles or the flocculonodular lobe of the cerebellum.

Hypothyroidism has been proven as a cause of central vestibular disease; a recent article described adult canines, predominantly Labradors, presenting with an acute onset of central vestibular syndrome. MRI demonstrated lesions compatible with vascular infarct. All the patients improved with thyroid supplementation. It was presumed that the elevated triglycerides caused cerebrovascular disease. Thyroid screening should be a part of any vestibular patient's database.

Idiopathic trigeminal paralysis

The patient with idiopathic trigeminal paralysis presents for an acute onset of a nonpainful inability to close the jaw. In addition, these patients may have drooling and difficulty eating. The signalment has golden retrievers overrepresented. Pathology demonstrates nonsuppurative neuritis of the motor branches of CN V, while the sensory branches do not seem to be affected. The diagnosis is one of rule-outs. In one study of 29 dogs, 26 were idiopathic, 1 had lymphosarcoma, 1 had *Neospora*, and 1 had a severe polyneuritis of unknown etiology. Usually, no treatment is needed; however, the patient may need to be hand-fed. Steroids make no difference in the prognosis, which is generally good with function returning in 2–3 weeks.

Unilateral trigeminal paralysis

Unilateral trigeminal paralysis is an uncommon condition that may be preceded by facial pruritis on the affected side. Neoplasia is the most common cause since the trigeminal nerve is a common site for nerve root tumors. Diagnosis requires advanced imaging with MRI.

Masticatory muscle myositis

Masticatory muscle myositis (MMM) is an autoimmune focal myositis that targets the muscles of mastication because of their unique type IIM muscle fibers. It may present as an acute onset or it may be chronic in nature. The acute cases present with temporalis and masseter pain and a desire to not open the jaw due to pain. These muscles may be swollen and painful. The chronic cases are usually presented because of a change in the shape of the dogs' head. Signalment is usually large dog breeds; Cavaliers are an exception. With an average age on presentation of 3 years, there is no gender predilection. Diagnosis is based on physical findings, elevation of serum creatine kinase, abnormal EMG, and serology for type IIM muscle antibody titer. This titer is the gold standard and is 100% specific and 85–90% sensitive. If caught early, the treatment is aggressive use of immunosuppressive doses of steroids. More information can be found in Chapter 3.

Idiopathic facial paralysis

Idiopathic facial paralysis is an acute onset of a nonpainful paralysis of the facial nerve in mature canines. At first, there is a lip droop on the affected side of the face and then with time (weeks), the resultant muscle contraction produces a deviation of the nose toward the affected side. Pathology is an active degeneration of myelinated fibers, not an inflammatory response (Bell's palsy in humans is an active inflammation). Diagnosis is based on history, physical and neurological exams, minimum database (facial paralysis has been linked with hypothyroidism), EMG, skull radiographs, CT, and MRI. If no etiology is defined, treatment is conservative care (with ophthalmic ointments) to prevent corneal damage since the patient cannot blink. Steroids are not indicated. The prognosis is guarded for the full return of function.

Spinal diseases

Quadriparesis and quadriplegia are common problems in all animals. An animal who has neurological disease affecting all four limbs and who has been determined to have a lesion below the foramen magnum (i.e., spinal cord or peripheral disease) has four possible anatomic locations for the disease process:

1) If there is UMN dysfunction in all four legs, the lesion is most likely in the cervical spinal cord between C1 and C5.

2) If there is LMN dysfunction in the thoracic limbs and UMN dysfunction in the pelvic limbs, the lesion is severe and involves spinal cord segments C6–T2.

3) If there is UMN dysfunction in the rear legs and "root signature" (lameness due to nerve root involvement) in the forelegs, the lesion is mild and affecting spinal cord segments C6–T2.

4) If there is LMN dysfunction in all four limbs, the lesion is a diffuse LMN disease.

In developing the differential diagnosis for quadriparesis, the basic mechanisms of disease must be considered along with the signalment and history. Congenital diseases are often diagnosed in the cervical spinal column of dogs. These include agenesis of the dens (with resultant atlantoaxial subluxation), blocked vertebra, multiple cartilaginous exostoses, leukoencephalomyelopathy of rottweilers, and hereditary ataxia of Jack Russell and smooth-haired fox terriers. In older animals, degenerative intervertebral disk (IVD) disease, inflammatory meningomyelitis, and neoplasia are the most common. If the signs are symmetrical, nutritional, metabolic, and toxic diseases must be considered. Asymmetrical diseases can be separated into their most likely causes: discospondylitis, meningomyelitis, IVD disease, vascular fibrocartilaginous embolization (FCE), and neoplasia.

Like the rest of the nervous system, the neurological examination is the single most important diagnostic method to localize diseases of the cervical spine. The ancillary diagnostic tests for spinal cord disease are similar regardless of the cause and may include the minimum database, spinal radiographs, EMG, CSF tap and analysis, CT, myelography, and MRI. In older patients, routine chest and abdominal radiographs and abdominal ultrasound may assist in the diagnostic process and in determining the prognosis, especially when metastatic neoplasia is in the differential.

Spinal radiographs may demonstrate signs of degenerative disk disease, congenital malformation, spinal arthritis, or discospondylitis, the later disease being one of the few disease diagnoses that may be made on plain spinal radiographs. In acute diseases, the EMG may not help identify denervation until 5–7 days have passed, but in chronic diseases, the EMG may help to localize the disease process so that radiographs can concentrate on the appropriate area. The CSF tap can help determine the presence of inflammation or infection in cases of cervical disease. The problem of inflammatory myelitis is increasing, making CSF collection and analysis critical in assessing cervical neurological disease. Even when other neurological conditions are identified, myelitis may also be present. Unfortunately, many patients are treated with corticosteroids before being adequately evaluated for cervical disease. The CSF analysis performed in the face of steroids may be erroneous, and as such, surgical intervention may be performed to only later discover the cause of neck pain was inflammatory meningomyelitis. Spinal CT myelography can help to contrast the spinal cord when looking for mass lesions and can be an extremely valuable diagnostic aid in determining the need for surgical intervention and which surgical approach is best. MRI is important in assessing neoplastic disease processes including nerve root tumors. The sequence of diagnostic tests logically follows the pattern of minimum database, EMG, spinal radiographs, CSF tap, and CT myelography and/or MRI.

Meningomyelitis

It is almost impossible to see animals with neck pain and not be suspicious of meningomyelitis. For this reason, even with clinical signs of early degenerative disk disease, surgery should not be considered without ruling out meningitis. In the face of meningomyelitis, myelography can exacerbate the clinical signs and is therefore generally contraindicated in meningomyelitis.

The clinical signs of meningomyelitis are generally neck pain and asymmetrical neurological deficits. The deficits depend upon the pathways that are involved in the disease process. The signs are usually progressive but may develop acutely. In dogs and cats, causes of meningomyelitis in order of likelihood are viral, inflammatory, protozoal, fungal, rickettsial, and bacterial diseases. The viral disease most commonly seen in dogs is canine distemper (even in vaccinated dogs), while in cats feline leukemia virus (FeLV), FIP, and feline immunodeficiency virus (FIV) are the most common viral infections. *Toxoplasmosis* can occur in both dogs and cats, while dogs also may develop *N. caninum* infections. *Aspergillosis* is common in dogs, while *cryptococcosis* is more common in cats. Cats do not appear to have rickettsial diseases, but dogs have been shown to develop meningomyelitis from both ehrlichiosis and Rocky Mountain spotted fever. Titers for these agents should be performed on the serum and/or CSF when presented with meningomyelitis.

Steroid-responsive meningomyelitis probably represents a form of vasculitis which results in inflammation of the CNS. Conventional therapy consists of prednisone at 2–4 mg/kg/day in divided doses. Once the signs resolve (usually within 72 h), the dosage is reduced. Therapy may last for months. Conventional therapy with corticosteroids may not always resolve this condition; it may only suppress the signs of the disease. Also see the section "Meningitis."

Discospondylitis

Discospondylitis represents an infection of the vertebrae and intervertebral space. It may be secondary to a migrating foreign body, but often no specific source of the infection is found. It is thought that in most cases of discospondylitis, there is a hematogenous spread of the infection which isolates into a small area of necrosis in the disk space or adjacent bone. These small necrotic areas of the vertebra are in locations where there is microtrauma of the spinal column. This occurs in areas where one segment of the spine is affixed to another more ridged area (e.g., lumbar spine to pelvis or cervical spine to thoracic rib cage). One possible source of infection is infectious agents entering through inflamed tissues that are associated with periodontal disease.

In cases where there is persistent or intermittent fever, bacterial cultures are indicated. Blood cultures may provide information about the infection approximately 70% of the time; urine culture may yield the organism approximately 45% of the time.

The primary clinical sign in patients with discospondylitis is pain at the site of infection. In severe cases, quadriparesis and anorexia may be present. The diagnosis is confirmed by routine spinal radiographs showing characteristic lysis and sclerosis of the adjacent end plates of the vertebrae. This is one of the few neurological conditions where the diagnosis can be made with routine radiographs. Since the radiographic changes may not occur until 2–3 weeks from the start of clinical signs, repeat radiographic examination is indicated when discospondylitis is high on the differential list. The CBC may reflect changes consistent with infection (including neutrophilia) or may be normal. The most common bacterial causative agents are *Staphylococcus*, *Streptococcus*, and *Corynebacterium* or, if fungal, *Aspergillus*. The treatment and prognosis vary depending upon the causative organism. Discospondylitis secondary to bacteria can be treated using a combination of sulfa drugs (sulfadimethoxine, 15 mg/kg every 12 h) and either cephalosporin (22 mg/kg every 8–12 h) or enrofloxacin (5.0–7.5 mg/kg every 12 h). The infection must be treated for a minimum of 6–8 weeks. Radiographic repair usually lags behind remission of the infection; however, continuing therapy beyond the time of radiographic quiescence is the best policy. Rarely will the infection result in bony compression or instability requiring surgical intervention. Most often, spinal cord compression is the result of soft tissue inflammation, which subsides quickly with appropriate antibiotic therapy.

Cervical vertebral malformation complex (wobbler disease)

Cervical vertebral malformation (CVM) or wobbler disease occurs in young and old animals. In young animals, it appears to be secondary to inherited malformation and malarticulation of the cervical vertebrae, which is accentuated by high protein diets. In older animals, it appears to be secondary to chronic degenerative disk disease. Although other large breeds can be affected, it is said to be a disease of young Great Danes and old Doberman pinschers.

The onset of clinical signs can be acute or slow and insidious. Patients with wobbler disease have evidence of ataxia in all four limbs with the pelvic limbs being more affected with both conscious and unconscious proprioceptive dysfunction. These patients have a wide-based stance in the rear legs, and the forelegs may show a stiff and stilted gait (two-engine gait). The diagnosis can be suspicioned from survey radiographs of the neck, looking for narrowed IVD spaces and sclerosis of the facets. The diagnosis is confirmed with myelography or MRI. The treatment of CVM is surgery, but in cases where surgery is not possible (e.g., other medical complications, poor anesthesia candidate), medical management with prednisone and diazepam may provide temporary relief. There are several surgical techniques available to treat wobbler disease including dorsal laminectomy, ventral slot, and ventral slot with distraction. In cases of multiple lesions, dorsal laminectomy is the method of choice. This technique has risks and its success rate is the lowest of the methods for correcting CVM, but in qualified hands, it is still a good technique. The overall success rate is around 75% with 20–25% morbidity and 5–10% mortality. Ventral slot is excellent for IVD protrusion but increases compression from ligamentous hypertrophy. A number of techniques have been described to perform a ventral slot and to maintain distraction across the IVD space. Following surgery, the patient should be kept quiet for 30 days. After the first month, the activity level is gradually returned to normal. Depending upon the severity of the initial damage, most patients will improve, reaching 80% of their recovery in the first 3 months. There is a potential for the "domino" effect whereby the IVD on either side of the surgery site will develop problems in 6 months to 2 years following the initial correction.

As an alternative to surgery, in one group of 104 dogs where medical management was compared to surgery, the resulting mean survival times were not statistically different. Medical management alone is a viable option.

Acute and chronic paraparesis and paraplegia

Paraparesis or paraplegia unaccompanied by signs of additional CNS disturbance suggests that the disease is located caudal to T2. If the rear limb reflexes are intact, the lesion is between T3 and L3. If the rear limb reflexes are diminished to absent, the lesion is between L4 and S2. This can be refined further in that lesions between L4 and L5 result in loss of femoral nerve function manifested as a decrease in the patellar tendon reflex and inability to support weight in the rear legs. Lesions between L6 and S2 result in sciatic nerve dysfunction, reducing rear leg withdrawal, cranial tibialis muscle, gastrocnemius muscle, and sciatic nerve reflexes.

The differential diagnosis of paraparesis and paraplegia includes a number of congenital diseases such as vertebral mal-

formations, various spinal cord malformations, multiple cartilaginous exostoses, and breed-specific disorders. Other disorders are similar to those that affect the cervical spinal cord including meningomyelitis, degenerative disk disease, spinal cord trauma, FCE, and neoplasia. In some breeds, the differential also includes degenerative myelopathy (DM).

The neurological assessment for patients with rear leg problems can help to confirm that the disease is neurological in nature and is not an orthopedic or systemic illness. Reproducible deficits in proprioception usually are indicative of neurological disease whether the deficit is knuckling, stumbling, falling, conscious proprioceptive deficits, or the dysmetria of unconscious proprioceptive dysfunction. When determining whether rear leg lameness is secondary to orthopedic or neurological disease, an examination of proprioceptive function can help to make the differentiation.

Unlike cervical disease, there are several neurological tests that can assist in lesion localization with thoracolumbar (TL) disease. If the lesion is between T3 and L3, Schiff–Sherrington syndrome may be seen. Also, between T3 and L4, the panniculus response may be elicited, where superficial stimulation of the skin over the back results in the stimulation of intraspinal pain pathways with the resultant contraction of the cutaneous trunci muscle. Due to the overlap of sensory dermatomes, the panniculus response will be absent one to two segments caudal to the lesion. Hyperpathia on deep palpation will be present at the cranial edge of the lesion and hyperesthesia will be evident on pinprick of the skin at the cranial and caudal edges of the lesion. By locating hyperpathia and hyperesthesia and by demonstrating the loss of the panniculus response one to two segments caudally, the lesion is localized.

The ancillary diagnostic tests for TL spinal disease are identical to those for cervical disease with the exception that lumbar CSF should be obtained in most instances since the flow of CSF is from cranial to caudal. Lumbar CSF more accurately represents changes within the TL spinal column.

Thoracolumbar intervertebral disk disease

IVD disease can occur as a protrusion of the intervertebral disk (Hansen's type II IVD) with the dorsal annulus still covering the disk material or as an extrusion of the nucleus pulposus into the neural canal (Hansen's type I IVD). Type II is most common in nonchondrodystrophic animals (straight-legged dogs) and occurs as a result of age-related changes in the IVD. As animals age, the water content of the disk diminishes and the collagen content increases; this results in a decrease in elasticity, leading to degeneration of the annulus fibrosis and protrusion of the disk. Depending upon the location, this can result in spinal cord or nerve root compression and in the development of neurological signs. The onset of clinical signs from type II IVD increases with age peaking around 8–10 years. This type of IVD protrusion is uncommon before 5–6 years of age.

Chondrodystrophic breeds of dogs are prone to the development of type I herniation early in life. In these breeds (including dachshunds, beagles, Pekingese, miniature poodles, cocker spaniels, Pomeranians, and basset hounds), there is a metaplasia of the nucleus pulposus whereby the normal collagen fibers of the nucleus are replaced by hyaline fibers. The hyaline fibers are less elastic than collagen fibers, leading to degeneration of the annulus fibrosis. The hyaline fibers calcify, creating further inelasticity. Due to the fact that the annulus fibrosis is thinnest dorsally under the spinal cord, the least line of resistance for the degeneration and breakdown of the annulus is toward the spinal cord. Ultimately, the annulus ruptures, allowing the extrusion of the degenerative nucleus into the neural canal compressing the spinal cord. Not only does the IVD material compress the spinal cord but the degenerative material is irritative in nature. The presence of the extruded material in the epidural space causes inflammation, furthering the swelling associated with the herniation.

Almost all chondrodystrophic dogs will show some degree of IVD degeneration within a year of age. Usually, the age of onset is between 2 and 3 years with the peak incidence being between 4 and 6 years of age. IVD herniation is less common in the upper thoracic region due to the intercapital ligament, which connects the rib heads and reinforces the dorsal annulus in that area. Of the remaining spinal column regions, 20% of IVD herniations occur in the cervical region (C2–C7) with 80% of these at C2–C3. In the TL spinal column, 80% of the IVD herniations occur, with 67–75% of these occurring at T12–13 or T13–L1. The incidence rapidly dissipates cranially and caudally from the TL junction. The incidence between T1 and T9 is less than 0.5%. From L4, caudally each disk has an incidence of around 2.5%.

In addition to location, the dynamic factor dictates the severity of clinical signs. The dynamic factor states the amount of traumatic force imparted by a small amount of material traveling rapidly is greater than a larger amount going slow. In the worst case scenario, this means that the time for intervention is also quite short. In most cases of IVD disease, definitive treatment must be started within 24 h in order to achieve the greatest success. The specific therapy is dependent on the grade of spinal injury.

Grade 1. The patients' only clinical sign is pain. This is the earliest stage of the disease; at grade one only the meninges are involved and only the meninges, not the spinal cord, have pain nerve endings. There is no compression of the cord.

Grade 2. The patient is paretic (weak and ataxic) but still walking. The compressive nature of the protruding disk is starting to affect the outer white matter of the cord. These white matter tracts carry proprioceptive information within large, very sensitive fibers that are very susceptible to compression.

Grade 3. The patient is no longer walking but still has voluntary control of urination and, if supported, will have very weak voluntary motor movements. The patients may act uncomfortable and may whine to go out or drag themselves to the door to urinate. Once outside, they can voluntarily initiate urination. The cord compression is now affecting the motor fiber tracts found deeper in the cord parenchyma.

Grade 4. The patient is not walking, has no voluntary motor movement even with support, no control of urination, but does retain the ability to sense deep pain.

Grade 5. The patient is paralyzed and has no sensation of deep pain below the level of the lesion. Deep pain is evaluated by seeing the patient not only pull the limb back when the toe is pinched but also turn and look at the limb and or try to bite (i.e., there must be cerebral recognition). Once deep pain is lost, the cord has suffered such compressive forces as to render ineffective those very small nonmyelinated type C fibers that are most resistant to crush.

The grade of injury will determine the treatment plan. Grade 1 requires strict confinement and the use of an NSAID to relieve discomfort. Strict confinement (crate or cage) for 3 weeks is absolutely indicated. Grade 1 patients generally will have 100% recovery in 3 weeks. These patients are treated as outpatients unless there is a question as to the possible progression of signs, in which case it is advisable to hospitalize and perform serial neurological exams. Keep in mind that steroid use has been repeatedly shown to cause complications, create polypharmacy, and increase the cost of hospital stays. In fact, in one study of dachshunds given steroids for CNS injury, their neurological status was better than the nonsteroid group 24 h post-op, but there was no difference in neurological status at the time of suture removal.

Grade 2 is treated as grade 1, with absolute confinement if the process is not progressing. This therapy gives a prognosis of 84% recovery within 6 weeks. Steroids may be used with caution at a one-time dose only if the patient is seen within 8 h of the initial insult; otherwise, steroids should be avoided. Polyethylene glycol (PEG), a 30% solution given IV at 2.2 mL/kg twice over 24 h may be used. PEG has not yet been shown to be of an absolute benefit; however, a multicenter study is currently underway to document its benefit. If it has been longer than 72 h since injury, the benefit of PEG is questionable. In those patients presented as grade 2 and having decompressive surgery versus conservative care only, the recovery rate improves to 95% and the recovery time is shortened to less than 2 weeks; however, cost versus benefit is to be weighed.

Grade 3 is the same as grade 2. The recovery percentages and time to recovery are the same as for grade 2; however, if cost is not an issue, surgery would be advised because of the extra nursing care required to maintain a nonambulatory patient over a 6-week rehabilitation time versus less than the 2-week expected postsurgery.

Grade 4 should have immediate decompressive surgery; however, even at this grade, conservative care will result in an ambulatory patient 81% of the time. Recovery time without surgery may take 9–12 weeks, while recovery time with surgery will be approximately 1–4 weeks. For some clients, conservative care is still a viable option.

Grade 5 should have immediate decompressive surgery. Conservative care gives only a 7% chance of recovery, while surgery within the first 24 h will increase that percentage to 64%. After 24 h, the chance of recovery drops to 50% and continues to drop after that. The longer the compressive force stays on the cord, the more permanent the deficit.

Fibrocartilaginous embolization

Even though animals do not suffer from the same degree of vascular disease as human beings, infarction of the spinal cord with fibrocartilaginous material is not uncommon. It occurs in any breed of dog but is most common in large breeds such as Great Danes, Labrador retrievers, and German shepherds; it is also the most common myelopathy of schnauzers. Both arteries and veins can be affected, and it is believed that herniation of the nucleus pulposus takes place either into the vertebral body or the venous sinuses within the spinal column. Since the vertebral body represents a vascular space communicating with the spinal venous system, the material gains access to the spinal veins. These spinal veins do not have valves, thus allowing the fibrocartilaginous material to flow up and down the spinal column. Exactly how this material causes the infarct remains the subject of multiple theories, but pathologically, a pattern of infarction usually affecting a single quadrant of the spinal cord is seen, although initial signs may indicate more spinal pathways involved from concurrent inflammation and spinal cord swelling. The infarction can occur anywhere along the spinal cord, but the cervical and lower lumbar spinal cord segments appear to be most frequently involved.

The presence of spinal cord infarction should be suspected whenever a patient presents with an acute onset of paresis or paralysis that is markedly asymmetrical, and there is no evidence of hyperpathia. Vascular disease is generally acute, nonprogressive, and nonpainful (the spinal cord contains pain pathways but no pain receptors so disease within the spinal cord without meningeal involvement is usually not painful). CSF analysis may demonstrate an increase in protein, which is nonspecific. Spinal radiographs do not demonstrate the disease and myelography will be normal or demonstrate mild intramedullary swelling. MRI will have evidence of hyperintensity in the cord parenchyma on T2 weighted images. The treatment of spinal cord infarction is as for acute spinal cord injury. If the patient is seen within the first 8 h post insult, then methylprednisolone at 15 mg/kg may be given. Many cases will improve dramatically within the first week. PEG 30% solution at 2.2 mL/kg IV repeated within 24 h may help. The benefit of PEG after 72 h of insult is not known.

Degenerative myelopathy of German shepherds

DM has a typical age of onset between 5 and 14 years. In addition to German shepherds, a few cases have been reported in other large breeds of dogs: boxer, ridgeback, Belgium shepherd, Old English sheepdog, Rhodesian ridgeback, Weimaraner, and Great Pyrenees. There is a genetic predisposition in German shepherds and corgis. DM in the corgi has a later age of onset, approximately 12 years, and it may not be the same mechanism as the German shepherd dog. Diagnosis of DM is made by a history of progressive spinal ataxia and weakness that may have a waxing and waning course or may be steadily progressive. This is supported by the neurological findings of a diffuse TL spinal cord dysfunction. Clinical pathologic examinations are generally normal except for an elevated CSF protein in the lumbar cistern. The EMG reveals no lower motor unit disease. Spinal cord evoked potentials show changes compatible with loss of white matter in the cord. Radiographs of the spinal column including myelography and MRI are normal (other than old age changes) in uncomplicated DM.

DM is a diagnosis of exclusion. Once suspect diseases have been excluded and with the added benefit of a positive genetic test showing predisposition to DM, the clinician may, with some certainty, say that the patient has DM.

Treatment for DM is severely lacking of any proven modalities. Antioxidants, nutraceuticals, and experimental medications have all gone without validation. The one modality that has proven to help patients maintain mobility (as it has also been shown in people with multiple sclerosis) is exercise. Daily walking or swimming slows the decline of the patient. In the German shepherd, duration from onset until euthanasia is 6 months to a year.

There is genetic testing available for both the German shepherd and the corgi at the University of Missouri. Contact University of Missouri via their Web site at http://www.caninegeneticdiseases.net/DM/testDM.htm or through the Orthopedic Foundation for Animals at http://www.offa.org.

Neuromuscular diseases

Myasthenia gravis

Myasthenia gravis (MG) may be the congenital form (as is seen in springer spaniels, Jack Russell terriers, Samoyeds, smooth-haired fox terriers, and miniature dachshunds), or it may be the acquired form. The acquired form is immune mediated; antibodies are produced that target the acetylcholine receptor in the neuromuscular junction. The loss of receptors results in an interruption of transmission across the synaptic cleft with a resultant muscle weakness, typically worsening with exercise. This weakness may present as focal, generalized, or the most severe acute fulminating form. More information can be found in Chapter 3.

The myasthenic may have a normal neurological exam until the patient is exercised when the weakness then becomes evident. A megaesophagus with regurgitation is a common presenting clinical sign. For this reason, the minimum database should include thoracic radiographs, which may demonstrate the megaesophagus and, in a small percentage of patients, a concurrent thymoma.

A diagnostic challenge test may be performed with edrophonium chloride (Tensilon®). Edrophonium temporarily binds to acetylcholinesterase, thus slowing its ability to hydrolyze acetylcholine. This allows more acetylcholine to remain in the synaptic cleft longer, thereby improving muscle strength. If edrophonium availability is an issue, neostigmine 0.05 mg/kg IM may be used as a challenge. If the clinical signs resolve in 15–20 min, then a presumptive diagnosis of myasthenia is made. Atropine should always be available in the event of a cholinergic crisis (vomiting, diarrhea, excessive salivation, lacrimation, and bronchospasm). The gold standard to diagnose the acquired form of myasthenia

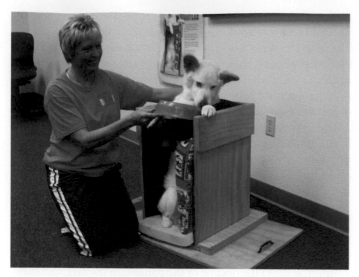

Figure 4.4 Roxie in her "Bailey chair."

is serologic testing for the circulating antibodies to the Ach receptor. This test is readily available through most labs. The patient must have been off of steroids for at least 2 weeks for this test to be valid.

Long-acting anticholinesterase drugs, such as pyridostigmine (Mestinon®) will help to control the muscular weakness, but the megaesophagus rarely resolves. The possibility of aspiration pneumonia gives most myasthenics a poor prognosis.

The Bailey chair is one way of maintaining an upright position, thus assisting eating in the myasthenic suffering from the complication of megaesophagus (Figure 4.4). See Chapter 8 for more information on feeding patients with megaesophagus.

Diagnostic testing

Cerebrospinal fluid collection and analysis

CSF is produced within the ventricular system of the brain by the choroid plexus and circulates through the ventricles and the subarachnoid spaces of the brain and spinal cord. This fluid is in such close proximity to the CNS that it often gives us important insights into the disease processes that can affect the CNS.

The indications for CSF collection are seizures, other encephalopathies, myelopathies not diagnosed by noncontrast radiography or MRI, prior to myelography, meningiopathies, and radiculopathies such as polyradiculitis (coonhound paralysis). The contraindications to CSF collection are elevated intracranial pressure and anesthetic risk.

Cerebellomedullary cistern CSF collection

The cerebellomedullary cistern is the site used for CSF collection when the patient's clinical signs suggest cranial or cervical disease. Because of the proximity of important neural structures to the cerebellomedullary cistern, inadvertent penetration of these structures is possible. The most common structures to be injured are the cerebellum, the brain stem, or the cervical spinal cord. Iatrogenic injury produces a vestibular syndrome, usually

transient, that is apparent upon recovery from anesthesia. A rare injury with more serious consequences is the induction of apnea. The emergency treatment for injury-induced apnea is mannitol and ventilator support, but even these measures may not save the life of the patient. The client should always be counseled on the potential adverse effects from CSF collection prior to the procedure.

The materials needed for a CSF tap are a styleted spinal needle (22 ga., 1.5–3.5 in. long) for dogs or a 22 gauge nonstyleted needle for toy dogs and cats, syringe, sterile gloves, drape, and sterile test tubes or syringes with stoppers for CSF. For this procedure, the patient must be completely immobilized under general anesthesia and in right lateral recumbency for a right-handed collector. Adequate airway patency must be guaranteed because the patient's neck is flexed to open up the joint space. The hair is clipped from the occipital protuberance to the lateral tips of the wings of the atlas. A surgical prep is performed within the triangle formed by the landmarks.

This is a sterile procedure and as such the needle is handled as in any surgical procedure. The puncture is made with the needle placed in the caudal center of the three landmarks aiming toward the patients' larynx. The needle is advanced slowly and, as each facial layer (approximately 4 to 5) is crossed, there will be a barely perceptible pop or change in resistance. After each of these layers is crossed, the stylet should be removed and a few seconds allowed to pass to see if CSF flows into the hub of the needle. If no CSF flows into the hub, the stylet is replaced and the needle is advanced farther. For cats and tiny dogs, a regular 22 gauge needle is used and the needle is slowly advanced while the clinician watches the hub for CSF. If at any time pure blood is encountered, the needle is withdrawn and the tap reattempted with a new clean needle. Often the first drip of CSF may have a bloody tinge to it; this is allowed to drip and clear; uncontaminated CSF may then follow. A guideline for the amount of CSF to be collected is 1 mL/10 lb of body weight.

Lumbar puncture CSF collection

In animals with disease in the thoracic or lumbar area, lumbar puncture is the preferred site for collection because of the close proximity to the affected area. In animals that may have difficulty with general anesthesia, the lumbar tap may be done under a local anesthetic and a tranquilizer or heavy sedation.

The needed materials are the same as for above. The position of the patient is in lateral recumbency but which side down depends on the comfort of the clinician. The preferred space for lumbar collection is the interarcuate space of L5–6. The wings of the ileum are used as landmarks and are palpated, and then the interarcuate depression between L7 and the sacrum is identified. From this site, the dorsal processes are identified and counted rostrally to the space of L5–6. The hair is clipped and a surgical prep is performed over the landmarks.

For needle placement, there are two different approaches; the first is to enter the skin over the dorsal spinous process of L6. The needle slides alongside the process in a rostral direction until it penetrates the interarcuate space and through the interarcuate ligament. As the needle goes through the dura or contacts the cauda equina, there may be a twitch to a rear limb (this causes no serious damage to the nerve). CSF may flow at this time; if not, the needle may be advanced to the floor of the canal, then the needle is retracted slightly and the stylet removed. A few seconds are allowed to pass while the hub of the needle is observed for the flow of CSF. The second technique is to direct the needle perpendicular to the spinal canal going down parallel to the rostral edge of the dorsal process of L6 or L5. Penetration is the same with the same consequences. Once there is flow of CSF, it is allowed to drip into a sterile test tube. Expect the amount of CSF removed to be less than that obtainable from the cisternal site because of the smaller subarachnoid site.

Laboratory analysis of CSF

There are many tests that may be run on CSF, but only the most common will be outlined here. Immediately upon retrieval, the fluid should be grossly observed for color and clarity. Normal CSF should have all the appearance of water, clear and colorless; to facilitate observation of the fluid, the tube can be held against a clean white sheet of paper. Any change in color or clarity should be noted.

Evaluation of cellularity is the most important aspect of any CSF collection, and this may be done easily using a standard hemocytometer. Undiluted CSF is placed on one side of the hemocytometer counting chamber, while on the other side the CSF is mixed with diluting fluid. On the undiluted side, the number of cells in five large squares is counted then multiplied by 2 to give the total cell count per microliter (Figure 4.5).

On the other side, the diluting fluid lyses red blood cells (RBCs) and stains the nucleated cells, thus facilitating their enumeration. The lysing fluid is a mixture of 0.2-g crystal or methyl violet dissolved in 10 mL glacial acetic acid, which is then expanded to 100 mL with distilled water. Use this to dilute the CSF at a 1:10 ratio (1 part diluting fluid, 10 parts CSF). Five squares of the hemocytometer are counted then multiplied by 2.2 for the total nucleated cell count. One may substitute dilute white vinegar with Quick-Dip™ thiazine dye solution added for the lysing solution (Figure 4.6).

The total nucleated cell count in cats is under five per microliter and under eight per microliter in dogs. Because of the caudal flow of CSF in the spinal canal, the cell count will be higher from lumbar punctures. Cell counts should be performed immediately because the cells will start to disintegrate within 30 min. One storage technique is to add 10% by volume of the patient's serum to the sample; hetastarch is another option added in a 50:50 ratio. This has been shown to maintain cell count and morphology for 24–48 h, allowing extra time for transport to an outside lab. If serum is used, then the protein determination will be greatly affected and the lab must be made aware of its presence.

There are correction factors for bloody or otherwise contaminated taps, 1 white blood cell (WBC) for every 500 RBC per microliter in dogs, 1 WBC/100 RBCs in cats. The differential cell count may be done by multiple techniques: cytocentrifuge, microfiltration, and sedimentation. In the general practice setting, sedimentation is very simple and requires no special

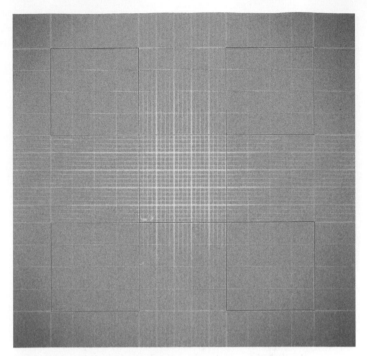

Figure 4.5 Hemocytometer with five squares to be counted. Courtesy of Dr. Mark Dunbar.

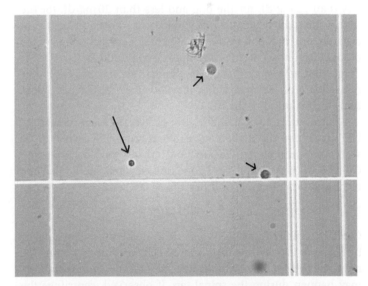

Figure 4.6 Close-up of hemocytometer showing nucleated cells after red cells have been lysed. Courtesy of Dr. Mark Dunbar.

equipment. A simple technique to make a sedimentation slide is to cut a test tube to be open at both ends and then affix the outside of the tube to a glass slide with paraffin. One milliliter of CSF is placed within the tube and allowed to sit for 20 min. After 20 min, carefully pipette off the supernate; the test tube is broken away from the slide, and the remaining fluid is allowed to air dry. Once dry, the paraffin is scraped away and the slide is stained with Quick-Dip (Figure 4.7).

For total CSF protein determination, the refractive index of the fluid is a general guide; the normal range is 1.3348–1.3350.

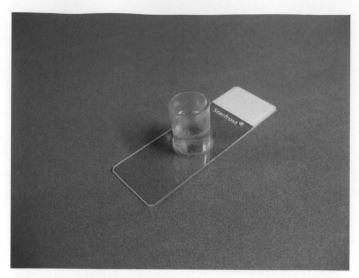

Figure 4.7 Sedimentation chamber.

The protein content of urine test strips may also be used; however, these will only provide a rough estimate. For the specific milligram per deciliter of protein, the sample must be sent to a commercial lab. The protein content of the sample will be stable and allows for the delay in evaluation. Normal cisternal protein is less than 25 mg/dL for the dog and less than 20 mg/dL for the cat. In the lumbar tap, the protein content may be twice that of cisternal and may still be normal. There is a correction factor for bloody taps; it is 1 mg/dL protein for every 1000 RBC.

IgG and IgM levels for specific diseases are normally very low or nonexistent; if elevated, they may indicate intrathecal production or disruption of the BBB.

Albuminocytological dissociation is defined as an increase of CSF protein without the concurrent elevation of cells. This is seen in immunologic diseases and spinal cord compression. Culture and sensitivity is not done routinely but should be done if the cell type suggests or if organisms are seen.

CSF findings in response to disease

CSF is normally translucent and clear. If the fluid is opaque or turbid, it is usually due to increased cells or protein. A pink or red tinge to the CSF may indicate fresh blood contamination, as may happen during the spinal tap. If observed, centrifuge the sample; the color should clear but remember the cellularity evaluation must be performed before centrifugation. A yellowish color (xanthochromia) is due to bilirubin from previous hemorrhage or may be seen as a result of severe icterus.

An increased cell count (pleocytosis) is typically due to inflammation secondary to infection, trauma, or immune-mediated causes. Cellularity will have two qualities: suppurative (the majority of the cells are polymorphonuclear) and nonsuppurative (where the majority of cells are mononuclear). Nonsuppurative is indicative of viral infections, CNS tumors, and some immune-mediated inflammations.

Increased protein is nonspecific and can be seen in many different disease processes either from disruption of the BBB or from intrathecal production. Specific titers may be run on the

CSF for specific diseases, for example, distemper, Lyme, toxoplasmosis, and equine protozoal myelitis (EPM). Vaccination may affect the titers so the clinician must be aware of recent or past vaccination history. In some cases, Western blot (WB) analysis may differentiate between vaccine induced and natural exposure titers.

Imaging

Radiology

Skull radiographs necessitate general anesthesia in order to achieve diagnostic quality images. The standard views are both left and right laterals, dorsoventral, open mouth, and oblique. The open mouth view is best for evaluating the tympanic bullae. Much information can still be gained by standard radiology, but older techniques are now being replaced with the superior images produced by CT and MRI.

For good quality spinal radiographs, anesthesia or sedation is recommended. The most common reasons for poor quality films are rotation, very low milliamperage (mA) for lumbar spinal films, and a lack of collimation allowing for more scatter radiation. However, with good quality plain radiographs, there is a 50% chance of correctly diagnosing TL intervertebral disk disease. Plain radiographs may also be diagnostic for some spinal abnormalities, for example, atlantoaxial subluxation, dens aplasia, spinabifida, hemi- and wedge vertebra, and discospondylitis.

Myelography

Myelography utilizes an iodinated contrast agent to diagnose spinal disorders. The myelography contrast agent used is iohexol, available in 20-mL single-use bottles with differing concentrations of iodine. The standard dosage of 240 mg/mL iohexol is 0.3 mL/kg if administered near the lesion and 0.45 mL/kg if distant from the lesion. Given as a very slow injection into the subarachnoid space, the newer contrast agents have less risk of adverse effects than the early agents. However, myelography may exacerbate underlying pathology and may result in the barely ambulatory patient becoming nonambulatory. There is also a risk of postmyelography seizures (21% may have seizures), and is dependent on the weight of the patient, hydration status, and injection site.

CT

CT (*Tome* = Latin for part, area, segment) is the combination of computers and X-rays. The same basic radiographic principles apply. CT slices the patient in "axial" slices, hence the term computerized axial tomography (CAT). Older scanners would take one slice at a time; in newer scanners, the patient slides through the portal while a continuous spiral image is generated, providing much faster scanning times. The contrast of the image is adjusted by the computer in Hounsfield units or CT units where +1000 = densest bone, 0 = water, and −1000 = air. The computer may manipulate the "central window" to enhance certain areas, for example, bone window. CT is primarily for bone and has limitations with size of detail especially in the caudal fossa where thick bone causes "beam hardening," a streak artifact that hinders detail. CT uses an iodinated contrast agent to which 5% of patients may be sensitive and run the risk of anaphylaxis.

CT benefits are low cost, fast scan times (3–5 min), and may be used post myelogram. CT drawbacks are lack of good soft tissue detail, the need for sedation, and artifacts.

MRI

MRI utilizes different physics from traditional radiology by using a strong magnetic field to cause a uniform alignment of hydrogen protons. Once aligned, the protons are bombarded with a radiofrequency pulse of energy that sends the protons spinning. Once the pulse is stopped, the protons start to relax to their original position. Differing proton relaxation times emit different radiofrequencies, and it is these differences that are interpreted and presented as an image. The image may be interpreted many ways; however, the most common images are T1 weighted and T2 weighted. By varying the pulse frequencies, you produce different images. T1 has fat as white and fluid as dark, T2 has the fat and fluid/edema as white. The contrast agent for MRI is an inert element, gadolinium, to which it is extremely rare to have any patient reactions. Gadolinium enhances the relaxation time of the protons. Where CT is superior for evaluating bone and lung, MRI is far superior for evaluating soft tissue.

Electrodiagnostics

Electromyography

EMG utilizes electrodes placed within the muscle to demonstrate and characterize the electrical activity (potentials) in the muscle. These potentials are amplified, displayed, and recorded for the patients' record. Each type of potential has a characteristic sound. While normal muscle is electrically silent at rest, diseased or denervated muscle is not. By evaluating specific muscles that are a part of the motor unit, the clinician may localize the lesion. The motor unit is composed of the LMN in the ventral horn of the spinal cord, the nerve root, the peripheral nerve, the neuromuscular junction, and a number of muscle fibers. Motor neurons may innervate a varied number of muscle fibers. EMG is best done under general anesthesia. When utilizing this test, there is a time delay after injury; it will be 5–7 days post injury before abnormalities develop in the EMG.

Normal EMG has an audible insertion potential followed by silence. The abnormal EMG may have elongated insertion activity, positive sharp waves, fibrillation potentials, bizarre high frequency waves, myotonic-like potentials, and myotonic (dive bomber) potentials. None of these abnormalities are pathognomonic for any one particular disease; however, their presence is indicative of pathology in the motor unit.

Repetitive nerve stimulation

Repetitive nerve stimulation (stimulating a peripheral nerve at five times per second) is used as an aid to diagnose MG. With MG, there is a fatigue of the nerve transmission across the synaptic cleft and the repetition of stimulation results in a sequen-

tially smaller motor unit action potential (MUAP). This is termed a decremental response.

Nerve conduction velocities

By stimulating a nerve at three separate locations, measuring the distance traveled, and then dividing by time, the actual conduction velocity of the nerve is determined. This diagnostic test may be performed on motor or sensory nerves. The speed of conduction is primarily dependent upon fiber diameter. Normal nerve velocities range from 50 to 90 m/s, but it is dependent on age and temperature. Animals greater than 10 years of age decline 10% in speed each year. Long anesthetic times with cold extremities will also slow NCVs. Slow NCVs may indicate nerve compression or loss of myelin. A complete block of conduction is an indication of nerve severance.

The size or amplitude of the motor unit action potential (MUAP) is also an indicator of disease. If there is loss of nerve fiber or loss of muscle fibers, then the number of muscle fibers brought into action with each impulse will be less, giving smaller amplitude to the MUAP.

Other EMG evaluations are F waves (evaluate ventral nerve roots), H waves (dorsal nerve roots) and somatosensory evoked potentials. F waves are generated when a nerve is stimulated and electrical activity flows in both orthodromic and antidromic directions. The antidromic activity excites the ventral horn LMN eliciting a smaller orthodromic depolarization. This smaller depolarization is the F wave. Stimulating nerves in the limbs elicits potentials that may be recorded as they proceed cranially in the spinal cord; these are somatosensory evoked potentials.

Sensory nerve conduction velocity (SNCV) is the stimulation of peripheral sensory nerves which can produce a measurable potential. When this potential reaches the ventral horn cell via the dorsal root, it produces a small waveform in the peripheral motor nerve called the H wave. The speed at which the nerve transmits is determined by physically measuring the distance traveled divided by the time taken.

Brainstem auditory evoked responses

In BAER testing, an audible click is delivered to the external ear and the resultant eighth cranial nerve transmission is picked up by electrodes placed at the base of the ear and at the top of the head. Because of the small amplitude of this potential and the interference of background noise, the signal must be averaged by a computer that time locks the stimulus to a specific time when the computer "listens" for the action potential. The computer takes the raw data and averages the signal, thereby accentuating the one repeating action potential (Figure 4.8).

The generators of the different peaks are theorized to be (1) the cochlear nerve, (2) the cochlear nuclei in the medulla, (3) the dorsal nucleus of the trapezoid, (4) rostral pons and lateral lemniscus, and (5) the caudal colliculus. Both amplitudes and latencies between peaks may be evaluated. BAER testing is used frequently to evaluate hearing in puppies at the age of 6 weeks or older as normal hearing patterns should be in place by 30–40 days of age.

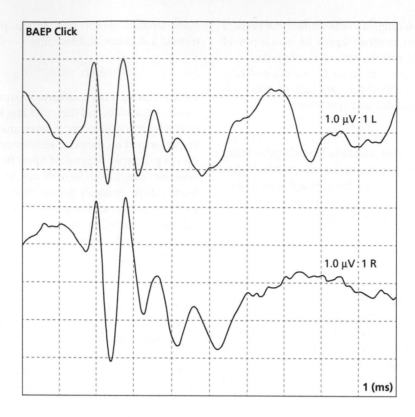

Trace Name	Side	Stime Type	Stmr Type	Intensity L/R (db)	Threshold L/R (db)	Mask (db)	Polarity	PW (µs)	AvgCnt	Reject (%)	RepRate	Gain (µV/div)	Hicut (Hz)
1.0 µV : 1 L	Left	Click	Phones	70/Off	0/0	Diff 30	Alt	100	300	24.2	11.10	1.00	3000.00
1.0 µV : 1 R	Right	Click	Phones	Off/70	0/0	Diff 30	Alt	100	300	5.7	11.10	1.00	3000.00

Figure 4.8 A brainstem auditory evoked potential recording of the right and left ear with typical peaks.

Congenital deafness is associated with a lack of melanocytes. Normally, precursors of melanocytes migrate from the neural crest to the ear and other parts of the body. The lack of melanocytes in the ear is associated with a degeneration of the organ of Corti and its associated hair cells. Twenty-five percent of Dalmatians may have congenital deafness in one ear and 7% in both ears.

Electroencephalography

Electroencephalography (EEG), while widely used in the past, has fallen out of favor. Electrodes are placed in a standard montage on the scalp of an awake but calm animal. Subcutaneous injections of lidocaine must be used to null out muscle electrical artifacts. Restraint is a major problem, promoting some neurologists to advocate using anesthesia or sedation for the study. With the standard EEG montage, the electrodes present the sum of all electrical activity in the surface 3 mm of the cortex. EEG characteristics of normal animals will vary with the patient's different states of arousal or sleep. The EEG is interpreted on the basis of background rhythms (frequency and amplitude), transient events (sleep spindles), and generalized and focal characteristics (spike wave complexes).

Nerve and muscle biopsy

For the definitive diagnosis of many neuropathies and myopathies, biopsy is needed. The biopsy allows for a direct evaluation of most motor unit components. The techniques are not complicated and may be performed by any veterinarian.

For nerve biopsy, a mixed motor and sensory nerve is most representative. One that is easily accessed is the common peroneal. With the patient under a general anesthetic and in lateral recumbency, a surgical prep is done on the lateral aspect of the stifle. If EMG testing has been performed on the patient, choose the opposite side for tissue sampling, thereby avoiding any needle trauma artifact.

A skin incision is made and with strict adherence to hemostasis, the common peroneal is isolated as it crosses the head of the gastrocnemius muscle. Using fine scissors (iris scissors), a longitudinal segment of the nerve is removed. The common peroneal is well suited for this since it is flat and the separate fascicles are easily identified. The segment removed is usually 30% of the nerve width and up to 5 cm long (2 cm being sufficient).

Half of the nerve biopsy is then pinned to a wooden tongue depressor and fixed in 10% formalin or 2.5% glutaraldehyde. The other half is placed in a small airtight container with saline-moistened gauze (the muscle biopsy will also be placed in the container).

Closure of the site is routine, but care should be taken to avoid placing absorbable suture in close proximity to the harvest site so as to prevent an inflammatory response with possible scarring (which can entrap the nerve). Other nerves commonly biopsied are the ulnar, caudal cutaneous antebrachial, superficial radial, and buccal branches of the facial.

The muscle biopsy is easily performed at the same time via the same site as the nerve biopsy. After harvesting the segment of the common peroneal nerve, the fascia overlying the cranial tibialis muscle is incised and a piece of the muscle approximately 1.5 cm long by 1 cm wide by 1 cm deep is removed. The muscle is pinned to a small piece of tongue depressor and placed with the nerve biopsy in an airtight container with saline-moistened gauze. The muscle is *not* placed in formalin. This entire package is shipped chilled (not frozen) overnight to the diagnostic laboratory. Delivery should not be delayed so always perform biopsy procedures early in the week allowing ample time for the lab to receive the samples well before Friday. It is always a good idea to contact the lab ahead of time for exact procedures and to answer any questions.

In the United States, contact

Dr. Diane Shelton

Comparative Neuromuscular Laboratory

Basic Science Building, Room 2095

University of California, San Diego

La Jolla, CA 92093-0612

858-534-1537

http://vetneuromuscular.ucsd.edu/

E-mail: musclelab@ucd.edu

or in the United Kingdom, contact

Dr. Caroline Hahn

Neuromuscular Disease Laboratory

Royal (Dick) School of Veterinary Studies

Easter Bush Veterinary Centre

Midlothian

EH25 9RG

44 (0)131 650-6403

http://www.neurolab.vet.ed.ac.uk/

E-mail: vetneurolab@ed.ac.uk

Pharmacology

Anticonvulsants

Phenobarbital

Phenobarbital is one of the first choice anticonvulsants for use in dogs and it is the first choice in cats. First discovered in 1912 in Germany, the First World War delayed its debut in the United States. Phenobarbital's effect is to potentiate the effects of gamma-aminobutyric acid (GABA) on the chloride channel, thus allowing influx of more chloride into the neuron; this hyperpolarizes and stabilizes the neuron. Due to a half-life of approximately 70 h, it will take about 2 weeks to reach steady state; however, a beneficial effect will be noted long before that. Adverse effects seen most commonly are sedation, polydipsia/polyuria, and polyphagia. While on phenobarbital, the patient will have some expected alterations in their thyroid levels; T4 may be reduced by 50%, free T4 a 50% reduction, thyroid-stimulating hormone (TSH) a 50% increase, while total T3 will have minimal reduction. Liver enzymes will also be affected; alanine aminotransferase (ALT) may triple, alkaline phosphatase (ALP) may increase sevenfold, gamma-glutamyl transferase (GGT) has minor changes, albumin is unchanged, and cholesterol may increase by 50%. If the liver is evaluated histopathologically, there are few if any pathological changes observable.

Bromide

Bromide is available in two compounds, potassium bromide (KBr) and sodium bromide (NaBr). The bioavailability of bromide is different in each compound. KBr has 67% bromide available to the patient and NaBr has 78% bromide available. Bromide is eliminated through the kidneys and has no effect on the liver. The half-life of bromide in the canine is 21 days; in cats, it is 12 days. Analytical grade KBr mixed with distilled water to give 250 mg/mL (60 g KBr in 8 oz of H_2O) has been used in the past. However, if compounded in-house, there may be liability questions; the use of a compounding pharmacy is recommended. When using bromide, the goal is to obtain therapeutic blood levels of at least 1 mg/mL. Bromide is a salt, so side effects are a salty taste, possible pancreatitis, megaesophagus, and skin eruptions. In the diagnostic laboratory, bromide will falsely elevate chloride determination since most analytical machines "see" bromide as chloride.

Bromide loading may be accomplished either orally via the stomach tube or rectally via enema at 400–600 mg/kg bid for 2 days.

Bromide may be used in the cat; however, the most troublesome adverse effect is an asthmatic-like condition presenting as a cough shortly after initiating the bromide therapy. This complication necessitates discontinuation of the bromide.

Diazepam

Diazepam is not used as a maintenance anticonvulsant in dogs due to its short half-life; however, the half-life of diazepam in cats is approximately 15–20 h. Diazepam at 0.5–2.0 mg/kg divided t.i.d. may be used in cats as a maintenance therapy, but up to 20% of cats do not respond. When starting diazepam therapy in cats, it is advisable to check liver enzymes over the first few days as a fatal hepatic necrosis has developed in some cats with maintenance diazepam therapy.

For both dogs and cats, an alternative or home therapy that may be of benefit in seizure control is rectal diazepam. Injectable diazepam is inserted into the rectum with the aid of a teat cannula or other similar device. Rectally administered; diazepam will achieve blood levels in 15–20 min. This therapy has been used since the early 1990s for breakthrough seizure control to lessen emergency room visits. It is very useful for those patients suffering from cluster seizures. Diazepam reacts with plastic and should not be stored in syringes.

Levetiracetam (Keppra®)

An anticonvulsant used in dogs in combination with phenobarbital and/or bromide, levetiracetam is usually well tolerated. It is not substantially metabolized by the liver. In cats, levetiracetam at 20 mg/kg bid as a single drug or in combination with phenobarbital at a reduced dose of 10 mg/kg bid has recently been published to be efficacious.

Zonisamide

Zonisamide is a sulfonamide-derived antiepileptic first approved in 2000. It has a long half-life in dogs (15 h), which allows for bid dosing at 5–10 mg/kg. There is minimal hepatic metabolism with 80% excreted unchanged in the urine. It appears to be very safe in dogs; adverse effects may be transient sedation, ataxia, and inappetence. One study showed 58% of poorly responding epileptics having good control when zonisamide was added to the regime. Since it is costly, it may be used as a tertiary drug.

Drugs for CNS trauma

Steroids are not used in the treatment of head trauma. In spinal trauma, Solumedrol® (prednisolone sodium succinate) may be given if the patient is seen within the first 8 h post injury. There is extensive documentation noting the deleterious effects of steroids, and the frequency and severity of these deleterious effects outweigh the minimal benefit. Steroids do have their use in the treatment of inflammatory brain disease and in the palliative treatment of CNS neoplasia. The veterinary staff must be aware of and diligent in the prevention of steroid-induced delayed healing, gluconeogenesis and its effect on potentiating diabetes, immunosuppression, gastric irritation, pancreatitis, and muscular weakness.

Polyethylene glycol (PEG) is classed as a surfactant that is known to seal defects in cell membranes, specifically axons. Early work shows benefit from administering 2.2 mL/kg IV of a 30% solution of PEG. PEG is given within 72 h of CNS trauma and repeated within the following 24 h. A large multicenter study is now underway to confirm or deny PEG's clinical effect.

Mannitol is an osmotic diuretic that in the brain has the benefit of causing a reflex vasoconstriction, a decrease in blood viscosity, and scavenging of oxygen-derived free radicals. Dosage is 0.5–1.0 g/kg IV given slowly; its effect is reached in 20 min and is repeatable every 6–8 h. CRIs of mannitol may be used; however, some report a better response if used as repeat boluses.

Assisting maintaining urination pharmacologically

See the section "Urinary Control" on diazepam, phenoxybenzamine, prazosin, bethanechol, and propranolol.

Anesthetic and analgesic considerations

The neurological patient is evaluated as any other patient as it concerns anesthesia. Certain presenting issues may necessitate immediate use of anesthesia and may not allow the clinician the luxury of complete patient evaluation prior to anesthesia, for example, the spinal patient in need of immediate decompression or the head trauma with depressed skull fractures. The most high risk anesthesia patients are those with intracranial disease, and anesthetic agents that may increase intracranial pressure or increase cerebral metabolism demands are to be avoided (e.g., ketamine and xylazine). Barbiturates, propofol, and etomidate do not affect cerebral blood flow or increase cerebral metabolic demand and, as such, would be better choices for induction or short procedures. Both isoflurane and sevoflurane increase cerebral blood flow and should be used with caution in patients with head trauma or increased intracranial pressure; however, they are the most readily available and are widely used.

Neurosurgery will cause pain. Since many of our patients may not overtly demonstrate pain, we must be alert to the clinical signs of pain. These may include tenseness, mydriasis, increased blood pressure, vocalizing, biting, lethargy, and withdrawal. One should always strive to preempt pain; anticipating the pain associated with neurological procedures and responding with the appropriate preanesthetic or intra-anesthetic drugs are not only beneficial for the patient but will reduce the overall use of pain medications. The use of an acute pain scale (e.g., Melbourne, Colorado, or Glasgow University's pain scales) may provide an objective idea of the patient's level of pain. See Chapter 13 for more information.

Fentanyl transdermal patches allow a slow release of an opioid (narcotic) that works in the periphery and the dorsal gray column. For these patches to be effective, they must be placed 8–12 h before the anticipated pain.

Butorphanol (Torbugesic®) is a synthetic opiate that is about five times more potent than morphine (morphine is the standard to which narcotics are compared). Butorphanol's main drawback is that it needs repeating every 2–4 h.

Buprenorphine is a synthetic partial opiate that is 30 times more potent than morphine. It has a longer-acting effect than butorphanol, allowing dosing every 6–12 h.

Hydromorphone is a semisynthetic opiate that on a weight basis is five times more potent than morphine. Hydromorphone needs repeating every 2–6 h.

Methadone is a synthetic opioid that is approximately 1.5 times more potent than morphine. Needing to be repeated every 2–4 h, methadone's main benefit is fewer side effects than morphine.

Tramadol is a synthetic opiate that may be given twice to three times a day. It is most frequently used postoperatively as an oral medication for pain control and in those patients suffering from neuropathic pain. It works well when combined with a NSAID.

All of the opiates must be used with caution in head trauma patients or those with potential elevation of intracranial pressure or intracranial disease because the opiates cause respiratory and mental depression. This may be contributory to the patient's clinical signs, making patient monitoring more difficult.

Analgesia may also be achieved through the use of NSAIDS. There are currently many available (e.g., carprofen, deracoxib, etodolac, ketoprofen, and meloxicam). NSAIDs affect cyclooxygenase, lipooxygenase, prostaglandins, and leukotrienes, and each patient may have a varied response to each medication, often necessitating trial and error to find the optimum drug.

Acepromazine and diazepam do not have analgesic effects but go more to the mental state of the patient with diazepam being a good anxiolytic. Diazepam also has the benefit of relieving muscle spasm, another source of pain. The avoidance of acepromazine in veterinary seizure medicine is more of an anachronism. Some researchers have reported that acepromazine has anticonvulsant activity.

Nursing considerations

Nutritional support

Nutritional support for the postoperative neurological patient should consist of a high quality diet. Depending on the condition of the patient, this may be a maintenance diet, a higher calorie critical care diet, or a gastrointestinal diet may be indicated for patients on high dose corticosteroids.

As with any critically ill animal, ensure that adequate amounts of food are being consumed. For the oral route to be used, 85% of the resting energy requirements (RERs) needs to be consumed daily. If this amount is not being consumed, additional assistance in supplying calories needs to be pursued. On average, no animal should go longer than 3 days without adequate nutritional support.

Partial parenteral nutrition can be used to help supplement oral intake as can tube feeding. Because nerves and the brain have a preferential requirement for glucose, ensuring that neurological patients are receiving adequate nutrition is very important for the prevention of muscle catabolism and the breakdown of fat by the body for energy use.

As many of these animals may have difficulty prehending, swallowing, or protecting their airways, special care needs to be taken when feeding orally. If indicated, consideration should be given to the placement and use of a feeding tube.

Vitamins, minerals, and antioxidants

All American Association of Feed Control Officials (AAFCO) certified therapeutic and maintenance diets are complete and balanced and already contain the required amount of vitamins needed for maintenance. Depending on any metabolic challenges the animal may face, additional amounts of specific vitamins and minerals, over maintenance may be required. For B complex, a multicomplex compound will work. The B vitamins are water-soluble vitamins, so any excess consumed above maintenance is excreted in the urine. Brewer's yeast is another good source of B complex, and the flakes are palatable and may be sprinkled directly onto the diet. Vitamin C is a water-soluble vitamin with antioxidant actions; if supplementation is needed, it can be given at a dose of 250–500 mg/day. Each animal's tolerance to vitamin C is defined by its intestine. Excess amounts may cause diarrhea and flatulence. Vitamin E is a fat-soluble vitamin that has strong antioxidant actions and can be given at a dose 400 IU per day for dogs. Do not exceed this dose in cats (since it is fat soluble, storage is in the liver) as excess amounts may cause hepatic lipidosis. Vitamin E can also act as a pro-oxidant when consumed in excess, causing an increase in oxidative damage.

Selenium is a mineral with antioxidant properties. It works synergistically with vitamin E, providing increased antioxidant protection and allowing a lower dose of vitamin E to be taken. The dosage is 100 mcg/day.

L-Carnitine is a nonessential amino acid in dogs and is conditionally essential in cats. It is not inexpensive but generics are available. L-Carnitine helps to improve the utilization of oxygen at the cellular level and may be beneficial for any patient with nerve problems and especially those with myopathies. Dosage is 50 mg/kg PO bid.

Coenzyme Q, also known as ubiquinone, is a fat-soluble antioxidant used in the mitochondrial respiratory chain to control the flow of electrons within the cell. By controlling the flow of electrons, it helps increase the rate of ATP synthesis. Dosage is 1–2 mg/kg daily.

Nursing care

Postural support is especially important in the paralyzed patient; every attempt should be made to maintain the patient in sternal recumbency. Getting the nonambulatory patient up and walking not only helps prevent atelectasis, but it helps their attitude. Sling walking is relatively easy to perform; slings may be made of simple PVC piping from the hardware store and a sturdy cloth or canvas. Turning every 4 h helps to prevent atelectasis; in addition, coupage of the thorax will help to prevent and/or treat atelectasis.

Prolonged recumbency promotes pressure sores over bony prominences; soft dry surfaces and frequent turning are a must for prevention. To prevent formation of pressure sores, which may lead to decubital ulcers, egg crate foam, padded doughnuts, trampolines, fleece bedding and baby powders may be used. Medical management of decubital ulcers includes topical antibiotic creams, enzymatic debriding agents, and astringents such as Tanni-Gel.

Urinary control

Urinary control is important to aid in the prevention of retention cystitis and urine scald. Pharmacologically, diazepam, phenoxybenzamine, and prazosin are used in patients with UMN bladder disorders because they will help relax the spastic paralysis of the urethra and sphincter muscles. Diazepam will affect the striated muscle while phenoxybenzamine and prazosin (being alpha-adrenergic antagonists) will relax the smooth muscle. In the cat, propranolol may be of a greater benefit since the feline urethra has beta-adrenergic fibers and a beta blocker will help to relax these fibers.

In patients with LMN bladder disorders where there is a flaccid urethral sphincter, bethanechol may be used to promote bladder contraction.

The overall goal of urinary control is to keep the bladder as empty as possible, and as such, both the UMN and LMN bladder will often require manual expression at least three times a day. Catheters may be used, but repeated catheterization may cause trauma or introduce infection.

Postoperative rehabilitation therapy

Postoperative care of the neurological patient is divided into three main periods: the immediate, the early, and the late period. In this manner, the patient is slowly returned to full function.

The immediate post-op period consists of pain control, cryotherapy, and passive range of motion exercises. Pain control may be of varied modalities; please see the previous section on analgesia. Cryotherapy or cold therapy induces vasoconstriction, helps muscles relax, and decreases nerve conduction. Superficial cryotherapy only penetrates 1–4 cm and needs to be repeated two to four times daily for 10–15 min. Passive range of motion exercise requires no effort from the patient. Each joint in the limb should be flexed and extended for 10–15 cycles two to three times a day. Please see rehabilitation therapy in Chapter 14 for more information.

In the early period, thermotherapy, massage, therapeutic ultrasound, and neuromuscular electrical stimulators are utilized. Thermotherapy or heat therapy is for use after acute inflammation has subsided. Hot packs or damp hand towels heated in the microwave are applied for 10–20 min two to three times a day. If electrical heating pads are to be used, great caution must be exercised to avoid thermal injury. Heat therapy is optimally applied before massage therapy. Massage is used to break down adhesions of the muscles and to promote circulation. Many clients enjoy performing this therapy for their pets. Massage may be performed once or twice a day for 20 min. Therapeutic ultrasound uses sound energy converted to heat as a form of thermotherapy. Low frequencies are utilized for deep tissue penetration. Typically, therapeutic ultrasound is performed for 5 min once a day. Clients should be told in advance that the site must be shaved in order to provide ultrasound therapy. Neuromuscular electrical stimulation or transcutaneous electrical neuromuscular stimulation (TENS) units help to maintain muscle mass and to decrease edema. The hair must be shaved for good contact; the therapy is applied for 12 s on then 25 s off for 30 min once a day.

The late period is when exercise is started. This exercise regime may be active, active assisted, or active resistive in nature. Examples of active assisted movement are towel walking, Swedish exercise ball, wheelbarrow, dancing, trampoline, using a syringe cap taped to the bottom of the good paw to entice the patient to be weight bearing on the injured paw, sled pulling, and hydrotherapy. More information can be found in the rehabilitative section of Chapter 14.

For patients who have permanently lost function in the rear limbs or until function of the rear legs returns in surgical/medical patients, there are walkers/wheelchairs for dogs and cats. One Web site is that of K9 Carts', http://www.k9carts.com, or they can be reached via e-mail at wheels@k9carts.com.

Low level light therapy

LLLT is the use of laser light of a specific wavelength. The mitochondria are the power-producing organelle of the cell, an increase of function here benefits the entire cell. LLLT is theorized to boost mitochondrial respiration. LLLT has shown benefit in nerve grafts, spinal cord injury, and disk disease.

In one study, using LLLT postoperatively for hemilaminectomy, patients returned to walking status in half the time compared to those not receiving the treatment. LLLT is now being tried in patients with head trauma.

Neurological glossary

Anisocoria. Inequality of the pupil size

Ataxia. Incoordination, when walking the patient deviates from a straight line, the axis

Atrophy. Wasting away or reduction in size

BAER/BAEP. Brainstem auditory evoked response/brainstem auditory evoked potentials

BBB. Blood–brain barrier

Cauda Equina. The accumulation of nerve roots in the lumbosacral and coccygeal area

COMS. Caudal occipital malformation syndrome

Clonus. A rapid tensing and relaxing repeatedly, often seen with release of inhibition of the lower motor neuron

Consensual. The reaction of the opposite pupil when a light is shone in one pupil

Contralateral. Situated on or pertaining to the opposite side

Craniectomy. The removal of part of the skull

Craniotomy. Surgical opening of part of the skull

CVM. Cervical vertebral malformation

Decussate. To cross in the form of an X

Dermatome. That area of the skin supplied by one nerve

Disk Disease. Clinical syndrome of a disk protrusion or extrusion

Disk Extrusion. Rupture of the annulus fibrosus with extrusion of the disk material into the spinal canal

Disk Protrusion. A bulging of the annulus into the spinal canal without the extrusion of disk material

Diskospondylitis. An infection of the intervertebral disk with involvement of the juxtaposed vertebral end plates

DM. Degenerative myelopathy

Dysmetria. Disturbance in the control in the range of muscular movement

Dysphonia. Any impairment of voice (bark/meow)

EEG. Electroencephalography

Embolus. A clot or other plug brought by the blood from another vessel causing an obstruction

EPM. Equine protozoal myelitis

Falx. Used in context of the cranial fault, the falx is the sickle-shaped fold of dura mater that extends ventrally to separate the two cerebral hemispheres

FCE. Fibrocartilaginous embolization

Fenestration. The act of making a defect (window) in the annulus of the disk so as to remove the nucleus pulposus

Flaccid. Weak, lax, or soft

Fucosidosis. A storage disease resulting from an enzyme deficiency resulting in the accumulation of fructose-containing glycolipids in the cell

Gangliosidosis. A storage disease resulting from a deficiency of various hydrolases; storage substrates accumulate these being gangliosides and glycolipid metabolites

Globoid Leukodystrophy. A storage disease resulting from an enzyme deficiency; also known as "Krabbe disease." The storage substrate is glucocerebroside.

GME. Granulomatous meningoencephalomyelitis

Hemilaminectomy. A surgery where one-half of the lamina is removed to expose the spinal cord

Hemiparesis. Weakness affecting one-half of the body

Hemiplegia. Paralysis of one-half of the body

Hemivertebra. A developmental anomaly manifested by a vertebral body with incomplete development of one-half

Hepatic Encephalopathy. Malfunction of the brain secondary to disease of the liver. This malfunction is most often associated with congenital vascular shunts; however, encephalopathy may be seen with infections and toxins

Hydrocephalus. Abnormally large accumulation of fluid within the ventricles of the brain

Hypalgesia. Reduced sensation to painful stimuli

Hyperalgesia. Increased sensitivity to painful stimuli

Hypermetria. Overreaching or excessive range of movement

Hypertonus. Excessive tone or tension

Hypomyelinogenesis. A deficiency of myelin secondary to a lack of normal production/development

Hypoplasia. Defective or incomplete development

Idiopathic. Of unknown cause

Incontinence. Bowels and bladder may be emptied involuntarily

Incoordination. A lack of normal adjustment of muscular motions

Infarction. An area of tissue loss secondary to obstruction of the vascular supply

Intention Tremor. Usually about the head, a tremor that is evident when the patient initiates a voluntary movement

Ipsilateral. Pertaining to the same side of the body

Ischemia. Deficiency of blood in a part due to lack of circulation or blockage

Kyphosis. Abnormal dorsal arching to the spine

Labyrinthitis. Inflammation of the labyrinth of the inner ear, otitis interna

Laminectomy. Surgical removal of the lamina (roof) of the spinal canal

Leukodystrophy. Disturbance or malformation of the white matter of the central nervous system

Lissencephaly. Malformation of the brain where the normal sulci are missing resulting in a smooth appearance to the surface

LLLT. Low level light therapy

Lordosis. An abnormal ventral curvature to the spine, swayback

LMN. Lower motor neuron; neurons whose cell bodies lie within the brain stem or spinal cord and whose axons leave the central nervous system to activate muscles in the periphery

Luxation. Dislocation with major displacement

Malacia. Pathological softening

Mannosidosis. A disease resulting from an enzyme deficiency. The storage substrate is a mannose rice material, including oligosaccharides

Meningitis. Inflammation of the meninges

Meningocele. A herniation of the meninges from the skull or spinal column

Meningomyelocele. A herniation of the meninges and part of the spinal cord from a defect in the spinal column

MG. Myasthenia gravis

Micturition. The controlled act of urination

Miosis. Excessively constricted pupil

MMM. Masticatory muscle myositis

MUAP. Motor unit action potential

MUE. Meningoencephalitis of unknown etiology

Mucopolysaccharidosis. A disease resulting from an enzyme deficiency; the storage substrates are mucopolysaccharides.

Mydriasis. Excessive dilation of the pupil

Myelitis. Inflammation of the spinal cord

Myelocele. Herniation of part of the spinal cord through a defect in the spinal column

Myelodysplasia. Defective development of the spinal cord

Myelogram. A radiograph of the spinal column after a contrast agent has been injected into the subarachnoid space

Myelomalacia. Pathological softening of the spinal cord

Myoclonus. Shock-like rhythmic involuntary contractions of a muscle or group of muscles

Myositis. Inflammation of the muscle

Myotonia. Increased muscular irritability and contractility with decreased power of relaxation

Myringotomy. Surgical incision of the tympanic membrane

Narcolepsy. Excessive sleepiness and/or sudden attacks of sleep

NCV. Nerve conduction velocity

Neuroaxonal Dystrophy. A degenerative disease where the axons of the CNS accumulate swellings (spheroids)

Neuroma. A tumor growing from a nerve

Neuron. A conducting cell of the nervous system

Neuronopathy. Disease on the neuron where the primary changes are seen in the nerve cell body

Neurotmesis. Complete severance of the nerve

NLE. Necrotizing leukoencephalitis

NME. Necrotizing meningoencephalitis

Nucleus Pulposus. The central, gelatinous, portion of the intervertebral disk

Nystagmus. Movement of the eyes that may be horizontal, rotatory, vertical, or pendulous, seen with movement of the head or involuntarily without head movement

Opisthotonus. A dorsiflexion of the head with a concurrent lordosis and extension of the limbs

Palmar. The ventral surface of the thoracic limb paw

Palsy. Paralysis

Papilledema. Swelling or edema of the optic disk

Paraplegia. Paralysis of the pelvic limbs

Paresis. Incomplete paralysis or weakness

Paresthesia. Abnormal sensations, tingling, pinpricks in the skin

PEG. Polyethylene glycol

PLR. Pupillary light reflex

Polio. Having to do with the gray matter of the CNS

Polyradiculoneuritis. Inflammation of multiple nerve roots

Proprioception. Information sent to the brain from receptors in muscle, tendons, joints, and skin detailing the body's position in space

Ptosis. Dropping of the upper eyelid

Pyrexia. Abnormal elevation of body temperature

Radiculopathy. Disease of the nerve roots

Risus Sardonicus. The sardonic grin; a spasm of the facial muscles causing them to be pulled dorsally and caudally

Rostral. In the direction of the nose

Sacrococcygeal Dysgenesis. Defective development of the sacrococcygeal spinal cord and vertebra

Seizure. A sudden attack or recurrence of disease, epilepsy

SNCV. Sensory nerve conduction velocity

Spastic. Increased muscular tone

Spina Bifida. A developmental abnormality with incomplete closure of the bones around the spinal cord

Stenosis. A narrowing or stricture of a duct or canal

Storage Disease. Inherited defects, usually of an important enzyme, that results in the cell's incapability to metabolize essential compounds resulting in the accumulation of these compounds (storage) in the cell

Strabismus. Deviation of the eyeball

Stupor. Partial unconsciousness

Subluxation. Incomplete or partial dislocation

Syncope. A sudden loss of consciousness generally as a result of circulatory compromise

Syndrome. A group of clinical signs indicative of one disease

Syringomyelia. The presence on an elongated fluid-filled cavity within the spinal cord

Syrinx. A flute-shaped or linear cavity

Tetraparesis. Weakness in all four limbs

Tetraplegia. Paralysis of all four limbs

Thrombus. An obstruction/clot in the vascular system attached to the wall of the vessel

Torticollis. A twisted neck usually due to asymmetrical muscle contraction

Trismus. Difficulty in opening the mouth

UMN. Upper motor neuron; motor neurons whose cell bodies and axons lie totally within the brain or brain stem and control the activity of the lower motor neuron

Xanthochromia. Yellowish coloration

Suggested readings

Textbooks

Anatomy and physiology

DeLahunta A, Glass E. *Veterinary Neuroanatomy and Clinical Neurology*, 3rd edition, St Louis, MO: Elsevier; 2009.

Evans HE, DeLahunta A. *Miller's Anatomy of the Dog*, 3rd edition, Philadelphia, PA: W.B. Saunders; 1993.

Internal medicine

Ettinger SJ, Feldman EC. *Textbook of Veterinary Internal Medicine*, 7th edition. Philadelphia, PA: W.B. Saunders; 2010.

Greene CE. *Infectious Diseases of the Dog and Cat.* 4th edition, St Louis, MO: Elsevier; 2012.

Bonagura JD, Twedt DC. *Current Veterinary Therapy XIV.* 14th edition, St Louis, MO: W.B. Saunders; 2009.

Neurosurgery

Fossum TW. *Small Animal Surgery*, 3rd edition. St Louis, MO: Mosby; 2007.

Sharp NJH, Wheeler SJ. *Small Animal Spinal Disorders: Diagnosis and Surgery.* 2nd edition St Louis, MO: Mosby; 2005.

Slatter DH. *Textbook of Small Animal Surgery*, 3rd edition. St Louis, MO: Mosby; 2002.

Neurology

Bagley RS. *Fundamentals of Veterinary Clinical Neurology.* Ames, IA: Blackwell; 2005.

Dewey CW. *A Practical Guide to Canine and Feline Neurology.* 2nd edition Ames, IA: Blackwell; 2008.

Lorenz MD, Coates J. *Handbook of Veterinary Neurology.* 5th edition St Louis, MO: Elsevier; 2011.

Platt SR, Olby NJ. *BSAVA Manual of Canine and Feline Neurology*, 3rd edition. Wiley, 2004.

Vite CH, Braund KG. *Braund's Clinical Neurology in Small Animals: Localization, Diagnosis and Treatment.* 2006. http://www.ivis.org/advances/Vite/toc.asp.

Imaging

Assheuer J, Sager M. *MRI and CT Atlas of the Dog.* Ames, IA: Iowa State University Press; 1997.

Thrall DE. *Textbook of Veterinary Diagnostic Radiology.* 5th edition St Louis, MO: W.B. Saunders; 2007.

Journals

The Compendium of Continuing Education for the Practicing Veterinarian
Journal of Feline Medicine and Surgery
Journal of Small Animal Practice
Journal of the American Animal Hospital Association
Journal of the American Veterinary Medical Association
Journal of Veterinary Emergency and Critical Care
Journal of Veterinary Internal Medicine
Journal of Veterinary Pharmacology and Therapeutics
Veterinary Radiology & Ultrasound

Veterinary Record
Veterinary Surgery
The Veterinary Clinics of North America. Small Animal Practice
Common Neurologic Problems 1988;18(3).
Disease of the Spine 1992;22(4).

Diagnostic Imaging 1993;23(2).
Intracranial Disease 1996;26(4).
Common Neurologic Problems 2000;30(1).
Neuromuscular Diseases 2002;32(1).
Neuromuscular Diseases II 2004;34(6).

Chapter 5 Thrombotic Disorders in Small Animal Medicine

Authors: Justin D. Thomason and Clay A. Calvert

Physiology

The hemostatic system is traditionally divided into three categories: primary hemostasis, secondary hemostasis, and fibrinolysis. This division is an oversimplification but is divided based on not only the types of disorders encountered in clinical medicine but also on *in vitro* laboratory testing. The role of the hemostatic system in the normal animal is to provide effective control of endothelial damage through the generation of a "platelet plug" and fibrin clots (coagulation) to minimize blood loss. In addition, the hemostatic system is also responsible for the slow dissolution of clots through fibrinolysis in order to maintain organ perfusion. This hemostatic balance (coagulation and fibrinolysis) is maintained by physiological inhibitors in the plasma. These physiological inhibitors are responsible for localizing coagulation activity and for preventing systemic coagulation from occurring. It should be appreciated that any disorder of the hemostatic system can lead to hypocoagulation (hemorrhage), hypercoagulation (thrombosis), or both (disseminated intravascular coagulation [DIC]).

Primary hemostasis

Primary hemostasis relies on endothelium and platelets. Platelet adherence and activation represents the first step in hemostasis. Platelets adhere to damaged endothelium or collagen mediated by the von Willebrand factor and membrane glycoproteins (GPs). Once adhered, the platelets become activated to aggregate, secrete, and contract. Serotonin and thromboxane A$_2$, secreted by activated platelets, initiate smooth muscle contrac-

tion of the vessel wall. This smooth muscle contraction, in addition to platelet contraction via cytoplasmic microtubules, forms the platelet plug and initial hemostasis. However, for continued hemostasis to occur, it is necessary that secondary hemostasis (activation of coagulation factors) follows.

Secondary hemostasis

Secondary hemostasis (activation of coagulation factors) begins by the exposure of blood to negatively charged surfaces of damaged endothelium (intrinsic coagulation system) or to extravascular tissues (extrinsic coagulation system). The common end point of both the intrinsic and extrinsic coagulation systems is the conversion of prothrombin to thrombin, which is the critical step in the formation of the fibrin clot.

Intrinsic coagulation

Upon exposure to damaged endothelium, factor XII becomes activated by the enzyme kallikrein. The enzyme kallikrein is produced from a complex formed by prekallikrein, high molecular weight kininogen (HMWK), and activated factor XII. Once activated, factor XII activates factor XI. Activated factor XI activates factor IX, and the process continues involving a total of 10 serum proteins, calcium, and phospholipids (Figure 5.1).

Extrinsic coagulation

Blood exposure to extravascular tissue induces coagulation by contact of factor VII to a cell membrane factor (factor III, tissue thromboplastin, or tissue factor) and calcium. Tissue factor is abundantly present on extravascular tissues and on certain

Small Animal Internal Medicine for Veterinary Technicians and Nurses, First Edition. Edited by Linda Merrill.
© 2012 John Wiley & Sons, Inc. Published 2012 by John Wiley & Sons, Inc.

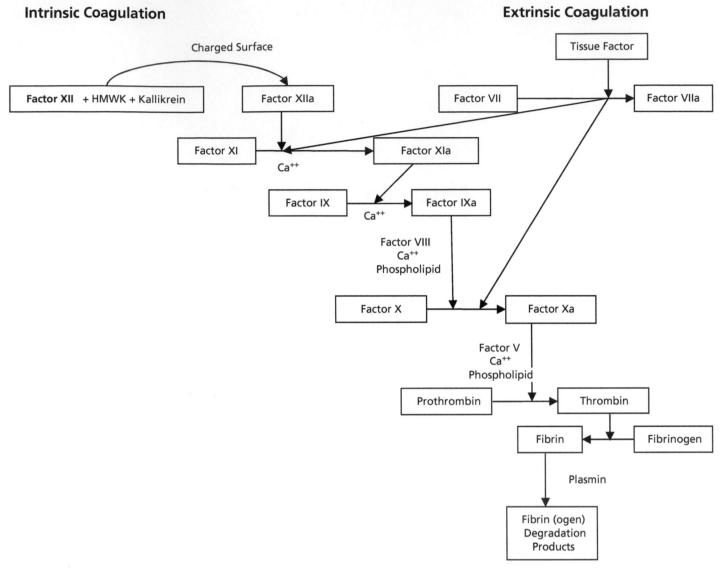

Figure 5.1 Simplification of normal hemostasis.

neoplastic cells. Endothelial cells, monocytes, and macrophages can express tissue factor in response to cytokines, especially interleukin 1, tumor necrosis factor-alpha (TNF-α), and to endotoxin. Activation of factor X leads to the common pathway and, ultimately, the formation of the fibrin clot.

Fibrinolysis

Fibrinolysis is initiated simultaneously with the activation of the coagulation cascade. Damaged endothelium and damaged extravascular tissue facilitate the conversion of plasminogen to plasmin through the release of tissue plasminogen activator (tPA) from the endothelium and urokinase plasminogen activator from the kidneys. Plasmin's role in coagulation is to degrade fibrin and fibrinogen into fibrin and fibrinogen degradation products (FDPs) and for the degradation of activated factors V, VIII, IX, and XI (see Figure 5.1). The FDPs formed are removed from circulation by the liver.

Physiological inhibitors of coagulation

There are numerous physiological inhibitors in plasma that localize the coagulation activity to the site of injury and maintain balance between coagulation and fibrinolysis in order to minimize bleeding and to ensure continuous organ perfusion. The most important inhibitor is antithrombin (AT). AT is a physiological inhibitor of blood coagulation in the normal animal. When combined with heparin, there is an acceleration of AT complex formation with thrombin. These AT–thrombin complexes are removed via the liver, therefore decreasing the concentration of circulating thrombin.

Also, circulating thrombin binds to an endothelial receptor, thrombomodulin. Through binding with thrombomodulin, thrombin's coagulation activity is lost. The thrombin–thrombomodulin complexes activate protein C to activated protein C (APC). Then, APC, with the assistance of cofactor protein S, inactivates factors V and VIII.

The fibrinolytic system is primarily opposed by alpha$_2$-antiplasmin and by plasminogen activator inhibitor. Alpha$_2$-antiplasmin binds and inactivates plasmin. Plasminogen activator inhibitor inactivates tPA and urokinase plasminogen activator, therefore regulating the conversion of plasminogen to plasmin.

Thrombotic disorders

The two most common thrombotic disorders encountered in small animal medicine are systemic and pulmonary arterial thromboembolism.

Systemic arterial thromboembolism

Feline arterial thromboembolism (FATE) is commonly associated with cardiomyopathy. FATE is a devastating complication that usually manifests as a large thrombus at the aortic trifurcation (saddle thrombus). However, thromboemboli can also occur in the tail, kidneys, in any limb (especially the right thoracic limb), or the central nervous system (CNS).

Canine arterial thromboembolism (CATE) is, in our experience, usually associated with protein-losing nephropathy (PLN). Other potential causes include protein-losing enteropathy (PLE), peracute DIC, and hyperadrenocorticism. Cardiac disease is a rare etiology of CATE. Similar to FATE, CATE usually manifests as a saddle thrombus, but thromboembolism can occur in other organs (Table 5.1).

Pathophysiology of thrombus formation with FATE

Virchow defined the pathological prerequisites for abnormal blood coagulation:

1. Endothelial injury
2. Stagnant blood flow
3. Hypercoagulation

Endothelial injury has been described in cats with left atrial dilation caused by cardiomyopathy. Such injury is most commonly associated with dilated cardiomyopathy (DCM). This is now an uncommon disorder as its etiology was identified as a taurine deficiency, and cat food manufacturers have made appropriate diet formula adjustments. Small areas of endothelial desquamation are sometimes found at necropsy in cats with hypertrophic cardiomyopathy (HCM) and restrictive cardiomyopathy (RCM). Endothelial desquamation leads to platelet aggregation and activation when subendothelial tissue is exposed. Factor III release can activate the extrinsic clotting cascade.

Stagnation of blood flow in the left atrium is a consistent finding in cats with severe left atrial dilation. During echocardiography, when low intensity signals are not rejected, a hazy or smoky pinwheel rotation within the left atrium may be seen. This spontaneous echo–contrast represents blood flow that is swirling within the left atrium and not proceeding promptly into the left ventricle. This stagnant blood flow predisposes to thrombus formation because not only are clotting factors allowed to accumulate rather than being diluted away with normal blood flow but also the "sticky" platelets of cats can accumulate and adhere to atrial endothelium.

Whether a hypercoagulable state can occur in cats with left atrial dilation is uncertain. Hypercoagulable states exist when the delicate balance between coagulation and fibrinolysis is disturbed so that the rate of coagulation exceeds the rate of fibrinolysis. Although DIC has been reported in cats with saddle thrombi, it may be a result of thromboembolism rather than a cause. The vascular occlusion and skeletal muscle ischemia resulting from the thrombus is the likely cause of the DIC.

Clinical signs of FATE

The most common historical finding in cats with arterial thromboembolism (ATE) is acute posterior paresis or paralysis. With

Table 5.1   Common sites of thrombosis

Organ involved or location	Clinical signs and clinicopathologic findings
Kidney: acute necrosis; glomerulopathy	Hematuria, oliguria–anuria, azotemia, proteinuria, granular casts, lumbar hyperesthesia
Lungs: acute respiratory distress, pulmonary thromboembolism, cor pulmonale	Dyspnea, pyrexia, cyanosis, hemoptysis, P_aO_2 <60 mmHg, respiratory acidosis
Heart: acute myocardial infarction, myocarditis, cardiomyopathy	Arrhythmias (ventricular), collapse, shock, elevated troponin I concentration
CNS (brain/spinal cord): necrosis	Coma, convulsions, blindness, tetra-/paraparesis, paralysis
Gastrointestinal tract	Melena, hematochezia, hematemesis hemoconcentration, shock, circulatory collapse
Peripheral arteritis	Hyperesthesia, lameness, swelling
Thrombophlebitis	Hyperesthesia, edema, heat

chronicity, pigmenturia (red urine) secondary to myoglobinuria may be reported. Given that FATE is most commonly seen secondary to cardiomyopathy in cats, additional signs related to cardiac disease may be present: dyspnea, anorexia, paresis, rarely coughing, and depressed mentation.

Physical examination findings in cats with ATE are paresis, hyperesthesia, poor to nonexistent pulses, cyanotic nail beds, cool extremities, and tachypnea secondary to hyperesthesia and/or pulmonary edema. With chronicity, turgid gastrocnemius muscles may be noted on palpation. Less commonly, a thrombus may affect only one leg, including a front leg (right thoracic limb most commonly). Examination findings related to myocardial disease may be present and include murmur, gallop sound, tachycardia, arrhythmia, muffled heart/lung sounds with pleural effusion, crackles and/or increased bronchovesicular sounds associated with pulmonary edema, and hypothermia.

Pulmonary arterial thromboembolism

Peripheral pulmonary artery thrombosis is common in dogs and rare in cats. Pulmonary thromboembolism (PTE) is the obstruction of pulmonary vessels with blood clots and can be acute or chronic. Rule-outs for acute dyspnea are pulmonary edema (cardiac or noncardiac), aspiration pneumonia, airway obstruction, pneumothorax, or PTE. Chronic, progressive dyspnea can be secondary to lower airway diseases or pleural effusion. Establishing the diagnosis of PTE, especially when associated with chronic dyspnea, is difficult. PTE should also be considered in patients with a diagnosis of pulmonary hypertension (PH) in which a definitive etiology is not readily apparent.

Clinical signs of PTE

Dogs with PTE variably exhibit dyspnea, exercise intolerance, depressed mentation, syncope, and ± coughing/hemoptysis. Auscultation may reveal pulmonary crackles and/or a heart murmur secondary to tricuspid regurgitation (TR). Pulmonary crackles secondary to PTE, although related to pulmonary edema, are not due to left-sided congestive heart failure (LS-CHF). Frequently, patients presenting with respiratory signs, exercise intolerance, syncope, and/or crackles are believed to have LS-CHF and are mistakenly treated with an angiotensin-converting enzyme inhibitor (ACEI) and furosemide. Splitting of the second heart sound due to delayed closure of the pulmonic valve is consistent with PH but is usually absent.

Pulmonary hypertension

PTE is a common cause of PH. PH results in a progressive increase in pulmonary vascular resistance and, in severe cases, in right-sided congestive heart failure (RS-CHF).

The causes of PH are numerous and, in some patients, the etiology is uncertain (Table 5.2).

The most common causes of PH are chronic left-sided cardiac insufficiency (i.e., elevated preload) and chronic bronchointerstitial lung disease. Primary PH is not well documented in dogs and is an exclusion diagnosis when no other etiology can be identified. In patients with a comorbid chronic disease process

Table 5.2 Causes of pulmonary hypertension

Primary (idiopathic)

Chronic alveolar hypoxia

    Bronchointerstitial lung disease

    Upper airway obstruction

    Hypoventilation: Pickwickian syndrome

Chronic left-sided cardiac insufficiency—PH seldom severe

Pulmonary thromboembolism

    Hypercoagulable states

      Antithrombin deficiency

        Protein-losing enteropathy

        Protein-losing nephropathy

      Hyperadrenocorticism

        Exogenous or endogenous

      Peracute DIC

        Bacteremia

        Pancreatitis

        Neoplasia

        Trauma

        Immune-mediated hemolytic anemia

    Endothelial damage

      Heartworm disease

    Toxins

known to predispose to thromboembolism, such as hyperadrenocorticism or PLN, PH should be suspected to be the result of chronic, progressive small pulmonary arterial thrombosis. Regardless of etiology, when PH is severe, there is always widespread small pulmonary arterial thrombosis secondary to endothelial dysfunction.

Diagnosis

Thromboembolism must be considered in patients that present with clinical signs consistent with thrombosis of one or more organ systems, with PH of an unknown etiology, or with a clinical disease known to predispose to thromboembolism.

Diagnosis of FATE

The diagnosis of saddle thrombus is most often a diagnosis made during physical examination (see above clinical signs). However, the diagnosis can be challenging in cases of partial obstruction. In these, the diagnosis can be supported by differential glucose and lactate concentrations (i.e., lower glucose and higher lactate concentrations in affected vs. nonaffected limbs).

Diagnosis of PTE

When the index of suspicion of PTE or other organ thrombosis not involving the aortic trifurcation is high, the definitive diagnosis usually relies upon other available diagnostic tests. Clinicians rely heavily on their index of suspicion and the proper interpretation of available diagnostic tests to establish a diagnosis of PTE.

Laboratory evaluation

Complete blood count, serum chemistries, and urinalysis abnormalities are frequently associated with an underlying disease process (e.g., hyperadrenocorticism, PLN, PLE, and pancreatitis). The complete blood count is frequently associated with a consumptive thrombocytopenia (thrombocytopenia with an elevated mean platelet volume). If heartworm disease is present, an inflammatory leukogram characterized by eosinophilia/basophilia and anemia (due to chronic disease or lysis secondary to microangiopathy) is possible. An inflammatory (neutrophilia with bandemia) or stress leukogram may be present with other cases of PTE. In cases of chronic PTE, polycythemia secondary to hypoxemia may be present.

When evaluating a patient with clinical suspicion of PTE, it is important to remember that thrombin activity predominates in the reaction. Although the activated partial thromboplastin time (APTT) and prothrombin times (PTs) would be expected to be decreased with increased thrombin activity, most often the times are normal. A more sensitive indicator of acute thromboembolism is D-dimer concentration. D-dimers are cross-linked fibrin-derived degradation products and are only present when fibrinolysis is activated by ongoing coagulation. D-dimers are more specific than FDPs because the presence of FDPs does not distinguish between fibrinogen- or fibrin (clot)-derived products. Given that fibrinogen concentration increases with inflammation, the presence of FDPs may only represent the breakdown of fibrinogen and not fibrin. In contrast, D-dimers indicate the breakdown of fibrin (clot) only. A positive result for D-dimers is not diagnostic for PTE but is supportive of the diagnosis. D-dimer concentrations are not reliable in cats. Samples for D-dimer concentration are collected in sodium citrate tubes. For short-time storage/transport (i.e., 24h), samples should be refrigerated. For longer-time storage/transport, freezing is recommended.

Although D-dimer concentrations have been reported to be a sensitive indicator of thromboembolism, we have identified patients with confirmed PTE in which D-dimer concentrations were normal at presentation. Whether normal D-dimer concentrations in patients with thromboembolism are truly false negatives, related to chronic/peracute thromboembolism, or a result of delayed/impaired fibrinolysis is unknown. Therefore, if the D-dimers are normal in a patient with suspected PTE, consider *serial* D-dimer assays, echocardiography, selective pulmonary arteriography, or radioisotope lung scanning. Selective pulmonary arteriography and radioisotope lung scans are limited to large referral centers.

Thromboelastography

Thromboelastography (TEG) can provide evidence of hypercoagulation in dogs and in cats by evaluating the entire coagulation system from the beginning of coagulation through fibrinolysis. Although hypercoagulation may be documented, abnormal TEG does not prove thromboembolism.

A TEG tracing is performed on citrated whole blood and has three zones that provide information about the quality and dynamics of clot formation:

1. *Procoagulation Zone.* Start of the test to the formation of the first fibrin strands.

2. *Coagulation Zone.* End of procoagulation zone to the maximum divergence of tracing lines.

3. *Fibrinolysis Zone.* End of coagulation zone to the point where tracing lines converge into a single trace (due to delayed fibrinolysis in dogs/cats, the fibrinlysis zone is rarely evaluated due to the automatic timed shutdown of the TEG machine).

The interpretation of TEG tracing relies upon the evaluation of four values:

1. *Reaction Time (R-Time).* The time from the start of tracing to 1-mm divergence of tracing lines.

2. *Clot Formation Time (K-Time).* The time from the end of R-time to 20-mm divergence of tracing lines. The K-time reflects the rapidity of clot development from the beginning of the visible phase of coagulation to a defined level of clot strength.

3. *Maximum Convergence (MA).* The maximal distance in millimeter between the diverging tracing lines. The MA reflects the final clot strength.

4. *Alpha Angle.* The angle between the midline and the tangent to the curve drawn from the 1-mm wide point. Similar to K-time, the alpha angle is also an indicator of rate of clot formation.

The values obtained from a given patient are compared to standardized normals. As an example, a short R-time, a short K-time, and an increased MA obtained on TEG are consistent with hypercoagulation (Figure 5.2).

Thoracic radiographs

Although thoracic radiographs are useful in the evaluation of lower airway and cardiovascular causes of dyspnea, they are often difficult to interpret, especially in patients that are fractious, obese, or have comorbid diseases. Minimal radiographic abnormalities, despite moderate to severe dyspnea, increase the likelihood of PTE. Two distinct radiographic changes have been associated with PTE: hypovascular lung regions and regions affected by interstitial to alveolar infiltrates commonly of the right and caudal lung lobes. PTE may also be associated with mild pleural effusion.

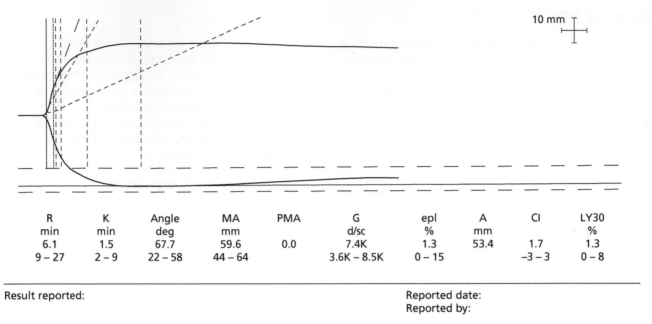

10 mm

R min	K min	Angle deg	MA mm	PMA	G d/sc	epl %	A mm	CI	LY30 %
6.1	1.5	67.7	59.6	0.0	7.4K	1.3	53.4	1.7	1.3
9 – 27	2 – 9	22 – 58	44 – 64		3.6K – 8.5K	0 – 15		–3 – 3	0 – 8

Result reported: Reported date:
                                                                     Reported by:

Figure 5.2   TEG tracing demonstrating hypercoagulation.

Electrocardiogram

The electrocardiogram (ECG) is of value only in a minority of patients. When PTE results in chronic and severe PH, high voltage S waves may be present in leads II, III, and aVF and the left thoracic leads. High voltage P waves (P-pulmonale) are occasionally present due to right atrial dilation. Right heart enlargement secondary to PH is referred to as cor pulmonale. ST segment depression/elevation may be present secondary to myocardial hypoxia. However, many patients with symptomatic PTE have normal ECGs.

Arterial blood gas analysis and pulse oximetry

Blood gas analysis and pulse oximetry may be useful in the evaluation of patients with PH and suspected chronic PTE. If normal in symptomatic patients, PTE can be ruled out. However, these tests lack specificity in that low arterial blood oxygen saturation and low hemoglobin oxygen saturation can occur with many causes of PH and pulmonary diseases.

Echocardiography

Echocardiography, in our experience, is the best, practical diagnostic test for initial evaluation of patients with suspected PTE. With acute PTE, high velocity tricuspid regurgitation (TR) and pulmonic regurgitation (PR) will be present. With chronicity, there are a number of abnormalities supportive of the diagnosis:

1. Underloaded left atrium, left ventricle, and pulmonary veins
2. High velocity TR and PR
3. Right ventricular dilation with hypertrophy
4. Right atrial dilation
5. Flattening of the interventricular septum

6. Paradoxical septal motion
7. Upward diastolic billowing of the pulmonic valve leaflets
8. Prolonged duration from initial to maximum right ventricular outflow tract (RVOT) systolic flow velocity

Underloading of the left heart, right ventricular hypertrophy, and high velocity TR and PR regurgitant jets are most common. The severity of the right ventricular hypertrophy, right ventricular dilation, and maximum regurgitant velocities correlate with the severity of PH. Severe PH is associated with TR velocities above 4 m/s and PR velocities above 2 m/s. In the absence of PH, clinical significant PTE is unlikely.

Therapy

Although the focus of therapy and prevention described here pertains to FATE, the treatment/prevention medications used in CATE and PTE are similar.

Treatment of ATE

Treatment for ATE, most often manifesting as a saddle thrombus in cats, requires attention to cardiovascular status, collateral circulation, analgesia, nutritional support, correction of hypothermia, prevention of self-mutilation, rehabilitation therapy, and to limit rethrombotic episodes. Hyperkalemia, myoglobin nephropathy, and decompensation of cardiomyopathy are potential complications of thrombolysis (especially when tPA is used). Close monitoring of renal status, electrolytes, and for congestive heart failure (CHF) is imperative.

Surgical embolectomy is occasionally performed, although pulmonary edema, pleural effusion, and atrial fibrillation must be absent. If left atrial dilation is severe, then pulmonary edema may develop soon after surgery.

Medical management

Collateral circulation refers to the establishment of blood flow through small adjacent vessels in response to the thrombosis of a main blood vessel. While some studies have indicated the importance of inhibiting platelet-derived vasoconstrictors (which may prevent and inhibit collateral circulation in cases of FATE), there are no controlled studies demonstrating improvement of collateral flow with arteriolar dilator therapy. Nevertheless, amlodipine (Norvasc®) can be used in an attempt to improve collateral circulation. However, when FATE is caused by HCM, arteriolar dilation is contraindicated in the face of severe left ventricular outflow tract obstruction (loud heart murmur). Therefore, amlodipine is not recommended if there is a loud heart murmur or if there is echocardiographic evidence of severe outflow tract obstruction. Warm compresses can also be applied with the goal of improving collateral circulation by promoting vasodilation. They may also provide some additive analgesic effects.

Analgesia must be addressed in thromboembolism cases. Butorphanol, an analgesic and a sedative, provides pain relief and may also provide a calming influence, but the necessity of frequent administration can be a disadvantage. We recommend the use of fentanyl as a constant rate infusion (CRI) to initially manage pain. A fentanyl patch can also be used, but analgesia must be addressed prior to its onset of action.

Anorexia is common in patients with thromboembolism and is associated with hyperesthesia, stress/anxiety of hospitalization, medication side effects, and/or CHF. In our experience, most cats with ATE do not drink appropriately to maintain hydration. Dehydration, coupled with myoglobinuria from ischemic myopathy, increases the risk of kidney failure. In patients with mild to no cardiomegaly, intravenous fluids (IVs) can be provided to maintain hydration. However, given that most cats have at least moderate cardiomegaly with risk of fluid overload, we recommend the placement of a nasoesophageal (NE) tube at presentation. Not only do NE tubes provide a route of fluid administration with low risk of fluid overload, but they also provide a means of nutritional support.

Hypothermia is often associated with shock (cardiogenic, distributive, and/or metabolic). Body temperature can be increased with warming blankets, warming cages, and/or heat packs. Heating devices are best applied to the glabrous skin (abdomen and groin regions). Remember when applying a heat source to cover the heat source to prevent burns. Hypothermia has been associated with a poorer prognosis in FATE.

During recovery from FATE, some cats may develop excessive licking and/or chewing of the distal limb. Application of a barrier (stockinette or bandage), coupled with effective analgesics, will usually prevent self-mutilation.

Physical therapy, via massage therapy and passive range of motion exercises, may retard or slow muscle atrophy and may also assist in the promotion of collateral circulation.

Some patients will recover from the thromboembolic effects within 3 weeks. Revascularization can occur if further thrombo-

Table 5.3 Recommended dosages—FATE

FATE therapy	Dosage
Amlodipine	0.625 mg/cat every 24 h
Fentanyl CRI	1–3 mcg/kg/hour
Sodium heparin	300 U/kg IV once followed by SQ every 8 h
tPA	0.25–0.5 mg/kg IV hourly to a total dosage of 1–10 mg/kg
FATE prevention	
Aspirin	81 mg/cat every 3–4 days
Clopidogrel (Plavix®)	18.75 mg/cat every 24 h
Warfarin	0.5 mg/cat every 24 h (starting dosage and adjusted based on PT time)
Sodium heparin	100–300 U/kg SQ every 8 h
LMWH heparin (dalteparin)	100 U/kg SQ every 6–8 h

Source: Compiled from Hogan et al. (2004), Smith et al. (2004), and Thompson et al. (2001).

sis is prevented with anticoagulants, gangrene-toxicity does not occur, and CHF can be prevented or controlled.

Pharmacology

Heparin therapy in combination with aspirin and/or clopidogrel (Plavix®) is useful to prevent additional thrombus formation (see "Prevention of ATE" for more information).

tPA is the only definitive therapy for thrombolysis. Unfortunately, the treatment is expensive and of questionable efficacy. At the university, we break down commercial vials into small aliquots that are deep frozen until used. A jugular catheter should be placed to facilitate monitoring of electrolytes and acid–base balance. A complication of thrombolysis is reperfusion syndrome; this can be lethal (due to hyperkalemia). The longer the thrombosis has been present, the greater the risk of reperfusion syndrome (Table 5.3).

Prevention of ATE

The simplest prescribed ATE prophylactic treatment is aspirin. Aspirin irreversibly acetylates cyclooxygenase and inhibits conversion of arachidonic acid to thromboxane A_2. Thromboxane A_2 is a potent platelet aggregator and vasoconstrictor. Aspirin inhibits platelet aggregation for the life span of the platelet (3–4 days).

Another class of drug that exerts an additive antiplatelet action is the thienopyridines, which can be used in conjunction with or in place of aspirin. Thienopyridines impair platelet function by irreversibly antagonizing the receptor for adenosine diphosphate (ADP). ADP is a proaggregating substance that induces changes in platelet shape and induces expression of GP IIb/IIIa receptors. Binding of protein ligands to the GP IIb/IIIa receptors is the final step in platelet aggregation. By blocking the ADP receptor, thienopyridines render the platelets unable to aggregate in response to ADP. Hepatic metabolites of the thienopyridines are the active compounds in platelet inhibition, and similar to aspirin, this inhibition is for the life of the platelet. In human trials, the combination of aspirin and a thienopyridine is superior to aspirin alone in the prevention of thrombosis. One of the thienopyridines, clopidogrel, has been studied in cats and produces dramatic antiplatelet action with a maximum activity reached in 3 days. Vomiting is the most common adverse effect reported in dogs. In humans, hepatoxicity and blood dyscrasias are uncommon adverse effects.

An alternative prophylaxis is Coumadin® (warfarin). Although warfarin may be a more effective prophylaxis than aspirin, clinical trials have not been performed. Hemorrhage complications, usually not severe, are a common complication when warfarin is used. Warfarin acts as an anticoagulant by inhibiting the synthesis of vitamin K-dependent clotting factors II, VII, IX, and X. Vitamin K is an essential cofactor for the postribosomal synthesis of these clotting factors. Warfarin also inhibits the synthesis of the anticoagulant proteins C and S. This latter effect produces a hypercoagulable state for a few days until the clotting factor levels decrease. For this reason, it is recommended to coadminister heparin for a few days to eliminate this hypercoagulable phase of warfarin therapy.

Warfarin therapy is more labor intensive and is likely to result in some hemorrhage complications. The warfarin regimen must be highly individualized for each patient and the therapeutic index is narrow. The PT should be measured frequently during the first few weeks of therapy and then monthly thereafter. Unfortunately, the drug is not evenly distributed throughout the pill; therefore, the pill should not be split but recompounded. Maintaining a PT of 1.5–2.0 times above baseline level is recommended. Daily administration, monitoring of the one-stage PT, and the risk of hemorrhage all weigh against the use of warfarin for prophylaxis. Although usually not life threatening, most treated patients will experience at least one episode of hematuria or hematoma.

Low dose unfractionated heparin administration is an alternative to warfarin, and perhaps aspirin in cats, because it rarely causes hemorrhage, requires minimal monitoring, and is not administered orally. However, it must be administered every 8h to be effective. While heparin may be a more effective ATE prophylaxis, the three times daily administration requirement makes it an impractical choice.

Low molecular weight heparin (LMWH) is an alternative to warfarin, unfractionated heparin, and aspirin, or it can be combined with aspirin in very high risk patients. The major advantages of LMWH are that it is administered only once daily (SQ) and monitoring of the coagulogram is neither required nor useful. However, recent studies suggest three to four times daily administration may be required for effective inhibition of factor Xa. LMWH enhances the inhibition of factor Xa and thrombin via antithrombin. LMWH potentiates preferentially the inhibition of coagulation factor Xa. Unlike unfractionated heparin, only 15–25% of LMWH molecules have the necessary sequence

Table 5.4   General guidelines for FATE prophylaxis

Risk	Left atrial diameter (2-D echocardiography)	Therapy
Low	<16 mm	None or aspirin or clopidogrel monotherapy
Moderate	16–20 mm	Asprin or clopidogrel monotherapy or aspirin and clopidogrel combined therapy
High	>20 mm or left atrial "smoke" or history of FATE	Aspirin and clopidogrel or aspirin or clopidogrel and heparin combined therapy or aspirin, clopidogrel, and heparin combined therapy

of 18-pentasaccharide units required for the LMWH-AT complex to bridge and bind to thrombin. This minimizes the risk of hemorrhage and largely invalidates the utility of the PT, thrombin time (TT), and APTT for monitoring efficacy. An affordable LMWH preparation is dalteparin in 9.5-mL vials. Each vial contains 10,000 U/mL of LMWH. We prescribe dalteparin via a compounding pharmacy that provides the clients with diluted (1:9 in D5W or normal saline) aliquots of sufficient volume for 1–2 months (Table 5.3).

Our general guidelines for FATE prophylaxis are outlined in Table 5.4.

Client education

Clients should be informed of the guarded short-term prognosis for patients with thromboembolism. In some patients, resolution can take many days to weeks. Should successful resolution occur, the patient is often at risk of relapse due to persistence of the predisposing etiology (i.e., cardiomyopathy). Despite the use of preventive anticoagulants, relapses are frequent.

Suggested readings

Carr AP, Johnson GS. A review of hemostatic abnormalities in dogs and cats. *Journal of the American Animal Hospital Association* 1994; 30:475.

Topper MJ and Welles EG. Hemostasis. In Duncan and Prasse's (eds): *Clinical Pathology*, 4th edition, Ames, Iowa, Iowa State University Press, 2003;4:99.

Hackner SG. Approach to the diagnosing of bleeding disorders. *Compendium on Continuing Education for the Practicing Veterinarian* 1995;17(3):331.

Triplett DA. Coagulation and bleeding disorders: review and update. *Clinical Chemistry* 2000;46(8):1260.

Mammen EF. Disseminated intravascular coagulation. *Clinical Laboratory Science* 2000;13(4):239.

Asakura H, Suga Y, Asoshima K, et al. Marked difference in pathophysiology between tissue factor and lipopolysaccharide induced disseminated intravascular coagulation models in rats. *Critical Care Medicine* 2002;30(1):161.

Herald H. Host response mechanisms in infectious diseases. *Contributions to Microbiology* 2003;10:18.

Levi M. Pathogenesis and treatment of disseminated intravascular coagulation in the septic patient. *Journal of Critical Care* 2001;16(4):167.

Cate H. Pathophysiology of disseminated intravascular coagulation in sepsis. *Critical Care Medicine* 2000;28(9):9.

Bateman SW, Matthews KA, Abrams AC. Disseminated intravascular coagulation in dogs: review of the literature. *Journal of Veterinary Emergency and Critical Care* 1998;8(1):29.

Rozanski EA, Hughes D, Scotti M, et al. The effect of heparin and fresh frozen plasma on plasma antithrombin III activity, prothrombin time and activated partial thromboplastin time in critically ill dogs. *Journal of Veterinary Emergency and Critical Care* 2001;11(1):15.

Aoki Y, Ota M, Katsuura Y, et al. Effect of activated human protein C on disseminated intravascular coagulation induced by lipopolysaccharide in rats. *Arzneimittel-Forschung/Drug Research* 2000;50(II):809.

Izutani W, Fujita M, Nishizawa K, et al. Urinary protein C inhibitor as a therapeutic agent to disseminated intravascular coagulation (DIC): a comparison with low molecular weight heparin in rats with lipopolysaccharide induced DIC. *Biological & Pharmaceutical Bulletin* 2000;23(9):1046.

Hogan DE, Andrews DA, Green HW, et al. Antiplatelet effects and pharmacodynamics of clopidogrel in cats. *Journal of the American Veterinary Medical Association* 2004;225:1406.

Smith CE, Rozanski EA, Freeman LM, et al. Use of low molecular weight heparin in cats: 57 cases (1999–2003). *Journal of the American Veterinary Medical Association* 2004;225:1237.

Smith SA, Tobias AH, Jacob KA, et al. Arterial thromboembolism in cats: acute crisis in 127 cases and long term management with low-dose aspirin in 24 cases. *Journal of Veterinary Internal Medicine/American College of Veterinary Internal Medicine* 2003;17:73.

Donahue SM, Otto CM. Thromboelastography: a tool for measuring hypercoagulability, hypocoagulability, and fibrinolysis. *Journal of Veterinary Emergency and Critical Care* 2005;15:9.

Stokol T. Plasma D-dimer for the diagnosis of thromboembolic disorders in dogs. *Veterinary Clinics of North America. Small Animal Practice* 2003;33:1419.

Thompson MF, Scott-Montcrief JC, Hogan DF. Thrombolytic therapy in dogs and cats. *Journal of Veterinary Emergency and Critical Care* 2001;11:111.

Caldin M, Furlanello T, Lubas G. Validation of an immunoturbidimetric D-dimer assay in canine citrated plasma. *Veterinary Clinical Pathology/American Society for Veterinary Clinical Pathology* 2000;29(2):51–54.

Matsuo T, Kobayashi H, Kario K, et al. Fibrin D-dimer in thrombogenic disorders. *Seminars in Thrombosis and Hemostasis* 2000;26(1):101–107.

Moresco RN, Vargas LC, Voegell CF, et al. D-dimer and its relationship to fibrinogen/fibrin degradation products (FDPs) in disorders associated with activation of coagulation or fibrinolytic systems. *Journal of Clinical Laboratory Analysis* 2003;17:77–79.

Chapter 6 Respiratory

Editor: Jennifer Garcia

SECTION 1 UPPER AIRWAY DISEASE

Anatomy and physiology

The upper airway includes the respiratory structures rostral to the trachea including the nasal passages, pharynx, and the larynx.

The larynx has two main functions: protection of the lower airway and production of the voice. The lower airway is protected against inhalation of both food and water by multiple mechanisms that include the epiglottis covering the laryngeal entrance on swallowing and closure of the glottis by adduction of the vocal folds.

Diseases of the upper airway

The most common airway diseases in dogs and cats are brachycephalic airway syndrome, laryngeal paralysis, nasopharyngeal polyps, and laryngitis.

Brachycephalic airway syndrome

Brachycephalic airway syndrome occurs in brachycephalic breeds such as English bulldogs, pugs, Boston terriers, shih tzus, and Persian cats. Brachycephalic airway syndrome results from multiple abnormalitites of the upper airway, including congenital and acquired components. The abnormalities cause upper airway obstruction and varying degrees of dyspnea. The congenital abnormalities are stenotic nares, elongation and thickening of the soft palate, and redundant pharyngeal tissue. The acquired abnormalities arise secondary to the chronically increased inspiratory effort necessary to overcome the upper airway obstruction caused by the congenital abnormalities. The acquired components of brachycephalic airway syndrome are everted laryngeal saccules, further enlargement of pharyngeal mucosal and soft palate tissues because of edema and inflammation, laryngeal edema, and potentially, laryngeal collapse as an end-stage manifestation of this syndrome. Tracheal hypoplasia is a congenital abnormality that may be seen concurrently in animals with brachycephalic airway syndrome, especially English bulldogs.

Clinical signs

The most common clinical sign of brachycephalic airway syndrome is an abnormally increased inspiratory effort, which ranges in severity from stertor to dyspnea. The increased inspiratory effort is often exacerbated by exercise and worsens over time as the acquired abnormalities develop and progress in severity. Coughing, gagging, and inspiratory stridor may also be noted.

Diagnostic testing

The diagnosis of brachycephalic airway syndrome is based on direct examination of the upper airway structures. The nares can be evaluated in the awake patient but examination of the soft palate, pharynx, and larynx requires heavy sedation or light anesthesia. The caudal edge of a normal soft palate touches the proximal portion of the epiglottis. Normal laryngeal cartilages should be firm and symmetrical and should abduct on inspiration. In dogs with brachycephalic airway syndrome, the nares are often stenotic and do not allow sufficient airflow. If the soft palate is elongated, the caudal edge often overlaps with a large portion of the epiglottis (Figure 6.1.1). Everted laryngeal saccules can be visualized on the ventrolateral aspect of either side of the larynx and look like small bubbles protruding from the surface of the mucosa. If laryngeal collapse has occurred, the laryngeal cartilages are neither firm nor symmetrical and can often be seen sagging ventrally.

Lateral radiographs of the head and neck may show elongation of the soft palate, but radiography is not generally contributory in diagnosing brachycephalic airway syndrome. Radiographs of the trachea are indicated to evaluate for concurrent tracheal hypoplasia, another congenial abnormality to which brachycephalic dog breeds, especially English bulldogs, are predisposed. Tracheal size is assessed as the ratio of tracheal diameter at the level of the thoracic inlet to thoracic inlet size on lateral thoracic radiographs. In a normal dog, the ratio is 0.16. Brachycephalic breeds have smaller tracheal sizes, and a ratio of 0.14 is considered normal in all brachycephalic breeds except in English bulldogs, where 0.12 is considered normal.

Brachycephalic airway syndrome is not usually associated with significant laboratory abnormalities. Chronic hypoxemia can occur, which may lead to a secondary polycythemia. Arterial blood gas (ABG) abnormalities such as a low PaO_2 or elevated $PaCO_2$ can occur.

Treatment

Dogs with brachycephalic airway syndrome may present in acute respiratory distress. The presence of inspiratory dyspnea in a brachycephalic breed should prompt the consideration of diagnosis of brachycephalic airway syndrome. In an emergency situation, mild sedation or an anxiolytic, and oxygen therapy are indicated. In patients with extreme dyspnea, IV catheter placement, anesthetic induction, and endotracheal intubation can be needed. These patients are also prone to development of very high body temperatures due to upper airway obstruction impairing heat dissipation. Body temperature should always be monitored and cooling measures instituted as needed. Additionally, dyspneic animals may swallow a lot of air in their effort to breathe, resulting in gastric distention that may impede movement of the diaphragm and further reduce ventilation. Patients should be monitored for gastric distention and decompression via gastric intubation or percutaneous decompression performed if needed.

Treatment of brachycephalic airway syndrome is typically surgical. Stenotic nares, everted laryngeal saccules, and an elongated soft palate can be surgically corrected (see Figure 6.1.2). Stenotic nares can be corrected with a wedge resection (see Figures 6.1.3 and 6.1.4), everted saccules can be removed, and an elongated soft palate can be shortened with a palatectomy. If

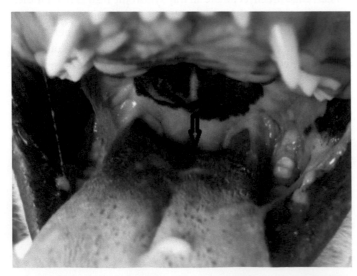

Figure 6.1.1   View of elongated soft palate (black arrow) overlapping the epiglottis (not visualized) in a bulldog.

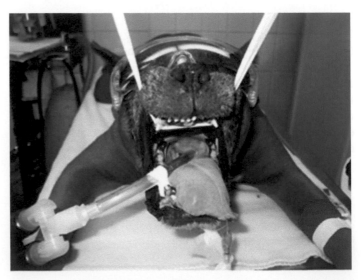

Figure 6.1.2   Typical setup for soft palate resection or everted saccule resection. Note glasses on patient to protect eyes from laser. Courtesy of Michelle Jaeger.

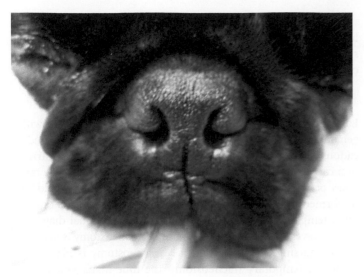

Figure 6.1.3 Before rhinoplasty to correct stenotic nares in a 1-year-old female pug.

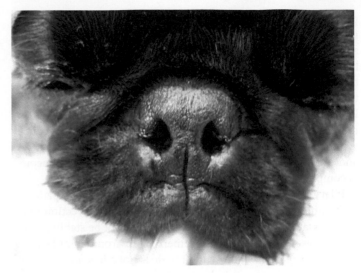

Figure 6.1.4 After rhinoplasty.

the brachycephalic airway disease progresses to laryngeal collapse, a permanent tracheostomy is needed to bypass the obstructive larynx.

Laryngeal paralysis

Laryngeal paralysis can be congenital or acquired and may manifest as either unilateral or bilateral paralysis of the muscles moving the arytenoid cartilages. Laryngeal paralysis is usually an acquired condition affecting middle-aged, medium to large dog breeds and is especially common in older retrievers. Acquired paralysis is usually idiopathic but can be secondary to polymyopathy, laryngeal trauma, injury, or disease affecting the recurrent laryngeal nerve. Congenital laryngeal paralysis has been reported in certain dog breeds including the Bouvier des Flandres, Siberian husky, and Alaskan malamute, but is rare.

Clinical signs

The most common clinical signs associated with laryngeal paralysis include inspiratory noise and exercise intolerance. The inspiratory noise is often referred to as stridor. The inability of the arytenoid cartilages to abduct results in upper airway obstruction. Dogs that have acquired laryngeal paralysis often develop clinical signs during late spring or early summer, when it begins to become warm and they are panting more frequently to dissipate heat. Dogs with laryngeal paralysis often have inspiratory stridor, gagging, and coughing. Owners may note that these dogs have a voice change or a new harsh respiratory noise.

Diagnostic testing

The diagnosis of laryngeal paralysis is made by direct laryngeal examination under heavy sedation or light anesthesia. The sedation needs to be adequate for the animal to allow access for examination but light enough to avoid depression of spontaneous respiratory effort. Normally, the arytenoid cartilages show

prompt, symmetrical abduction in inspiration. It is helpful to have an assistant watch the patient's thorax and tell the examiner when the dog inhales to correlate cartilage movement (or lack thereof) with respirations. It is important to ensure that the patient is making significant respiratory effort during the examination as depression of respiratory drive by sedatives and anesthetic agents may result in incorrect diagnosis of laryngeal paralysis because of reduced arytenoid excursion with shallow breathing. Stimulation of maximal respiratory effort by toe pinch or, ideally, by the administration of a respiratory stimulant (doxapram 2 mg/kg IV) improves the accuracy of assessment of laryngeal function by overcoming artificial depression of arytenoid motion.

Dogs with laryngeal paralysis should always have thoracic radiographs taken to evaluate for aspiration pneumonia secondary to laryngeal dysfunction, noncardiogenic pulmonary edema secondary to upper airway obstruction, and for concurrent abnormalities which may suggest an underlying cause or disease process (e.g., megaesophagus with polyneuropathies or polymyositis; inflammatory masses that may affect the recurrent laryngeal nerves).

There are no specific laboratory abnormalities associated with laryngeal paralysis; however, patients with laryngeal paralysis may be unable to protect their airway and are therefore predisposed to aspiration pneumonia, which may result in a leukocytosis.

Treatment

Dogs with laryngeal paralysis may present in acute respiratory distress. The signalment (middle-aged medium to large dog breed), time of year (hot humid weather), and the presence of inspiratory dyspnea can be suggestive of laryngeal paralysis. Emergency management includes mild sedation with an anxiolytic or sedative (e.g., acepromazine, butorphanol) to reduce the exaggerated inspiratory effort, which tends to worsen the laryngeal collapse. Intravenous access should be obtained as soon as possible. In extreme dyspnea, IV catheter placement, anesthetic induction, and endotracheal intubation are needed. Patients are also prone to the development of very high body temperatures because upper airway obstruction impairs heat dissipation. Body temperatures should be monitored and cooling measures instituted as needed. Additionally, dyspneic animals may swallow a lot of air in their effort to breathe, and resulting gastric distention may impede movement of the diaphragm and further reduce ventilation. Patients should be monitored for gastric distention and decompression via gastric intubation or percutaneous decompression if needed.

If laryngeal paralysis is bilateral, as is the case in most patients with clinical signs of laryngeal disease, surgical correction may be necessary. In particular, if the patient cannot be stabilized on initial presentation or if management of environmental factors, exercise level, and weight reduction does not adequately control clinical signs, surgery is indicated. Many surgical techniques are available, but unilateral arytenoid lateralization is the most common procedure. It should be noted that patients with laryngeal paralysis remain predisposed to aspiration pneumonia after surgical correction and should be monitored in the immediate postoperative period for the development of pneumonia. Withholding oral intake of food or water until the dog is fully recovered from anesthesia and feeding of small meatballs of food may help minimize the chance of aspiration pneumonia.

Laryngitis

Laryngitis is an inflammation, swelling, or irritation of the larynx. Laryngitis can occur in both cats and dogs, and the cause of laryngitis often differs between these two species. In dogs, laryngitis can be associated with viruses, bacteria, mycoplasma, excessive barking, intubation, insect bites, trauma, foreign bodies, or masses. In cats, laryngitis is often associated with viral infections such as feline herpesvirus or calicivirus.

Clinical signs

Clinical signs of laryngitis vary depending on the species affected and the severity of laryngitis. Dogs with laryngitis often have a mild, self-limiting cough. Cats with laryngitis often have an indication of systemic illness, and the signs include anorexia, ptyalism, fever, and dyspnea. Swelling and edema of the larynx occurs more commonly in cats than in dogs.

Diagnostic testing

A tentative diagnosis of laryngitis can be made based on history and a thorough physical examination. A laryngeal examination can be performed under sedation to evaluate both laryngeal function and the mucosa of the larynx. Biopsy and histopathology can be performed on any abnormal laryngeal mucosa and may help to discriminate inflammation from neoplasia.

Animals with laryngitis can have concurrent pneumonia, and thus thoracic radiographs should be evaluated in patients with suspected laryngitis.

There are no specific laboratory abnormalities associated with laryngitis; however, cats with laryngitis often have associated systemic illness, and thus a leukocytosis could be seen on a complete blood count (CBC).

Treatment

Laryngitis is often self-limiting, and patients are managed with general nutritional and hydration support, and antitussive medications as needed. If laryngitis is severe, upper airway obstruction can occur due to the inflammation or edema. In these rare cases of upper airway obstruction, a tracheostomy should be performed to bypass the obstructed larynx. The tracheostomy is often temporary to allow stabilization and additional diagnostics; however, occasionally, a permanent tracheostomy is needed. Special nursing care is needed if a tracheostomy is placed. In cases of a temporary tracheostomy, the tube management and cleaning technique will depend largely on the type of temporary tracheostomy tube used. If the tube is a single lumen, the tube should be gently wiped off and suctioned throughout the day. A double lumen tracheostomy tube has a removable inner tube that can be taken out of the tracheostomy tube to allow a more thorough cleaning. Initially, the tube is cleaned every 2 h, and then the cleanings can be spaced out (every 4–6 h). The time frame for cleaning often changes, and when animals begin to recover and are more mobile, the secretions often increase, requiring more frequent cleaning.

If a permanent tracheostomy is performed, nursing care is vital to a successful recovery. The permanent tracheostomy site should be cleaned by gently wiping the secretions off of the incision with moist gauze. If signs of an upper airway obstruction occur, the tracheostomy site should be suctioned to remove mucous plugs or heavy secretions.

It should be noted that reports suggest that cats develop thick airway secretions and have a higher mortality rate than dogs with this surgical procedure.

Nutritional considerations

The main nutritional consideration with upper airway disease is ensuring that the patient maintains a lean body condition. Brachycephalic breeds are predisposed to obesity, which alone can worsen respiratory function and can increase the demand for oxygen. After surgery to correct brachycephalic airway disease or laryngeal paralysis, special feeding considerations should be used until the patient has healed from the surgery. Soft food given in meatballs should be the initial food of choice. Additional information can be found in Section 7 of this chapter.

Anesthetic and analgesic considerations

Dogs with both brachycephalic airway syndrome and laryngeal paralysis can present in respiratory distress. If this occurs, a sedative and anxiolytic such as butorphanol and acepromazine may be indicated. Analgesic considerations are necessary postoperatively. It is important to control the pain associated with a surgical procedure in these animals, but heavy sedation postoperatively can lead to an unprotected airway, which could further predispose dogs with laryngeal paralysis to develop aspiration pneumonia. Additional information can be found in Section 6 of this chapter.

SECTION 2 MEDIASTINAL DISEASE

Anatomy and physiology

The mediastinum is the central compartment of the thoracic cavity, made up of a nondelineated group of structures in the thorax, surrounded by loose connective tissue. It contains the heart, the great vessels of the heart, esophagus, trachea, phrenic nerve, cardiac nerve, thoracic duct, thymus, and lymph nodes of the central chest. This section will discuss specific mediastinal diseases; however, there is much overlap with pulmonary disease. All related diseases will be covered in Section 4 of this chapter.

Mediastinitis

Mediastinitis is inflammation of the mediastinum, the area between the lungs. The most common clinical presentation in dogs and cats with mediastinitis include gagging, ptyalism (hypersalivating), dysphagia, vomiting, lethargy, respiratory distress, swelling of the head, neck, and/or front legs, weight loss, or fever.

A common scenario in which mediastinitis occurs in small animals results from the ingestion of an inedible item such as a stick or needle that causes a full or partial blockage in the esophagus or trachea. This blockage allows fluids to pass but not food. If the blockage has occurred for a period of time, the animal may lose weight and/or become lethargic. The foreign object may puncture the structure that it is lodged in, resulting in an abscess. Other routine presentations of mediastinitis may be caused by trauma such as a blow or wound to the neck or chest.

The range of diagnostic evaluators for mediastinitis are varied and typically are more of a rule-out of symptoms; among them are abdominal ultrasound, echocardiogram, CBC, chemistry panel, blood gas, chest and/or abdominal radiographs, videofluoroscopic swallow study, and ± endoscopy.

Treatment options for mediastinitis are dependent on the severity, type, and cause of infection; if severe, hospitalization for intravenous fluids, antibiotics, and chest tube placement are typical. If the cause is an abscess, then surgery is the recommended treatment along with the aforementioned treatments. If there is a foreign object causing the mediastinitis, treatment may include removal via endoscopy with surgery as a backup if noninvasive attempts at removal are unsuccessful. The medical management of mediastinitis can range from 2 weeks to 6 months, dependent on the type of infection, fungal versus bacterial.

Pneumomediastinum

Pneumomediastinum is the accumulation of air in the mediastinum. When this condition exists, the outer wall of the trachea and other cranial mediastinal structures appear in contrast radiographically. Although most cases of pneumomediastinum are self-limiting and mild, there are instances in which it can lead to pneumothorax, pneumoperitoneum, and pneumopericardium. Depending on the underlying etiology, pneumomediastinum may be either self-limiting or progressive, more often than not overlapping with some form of pulmonary disease or process. The effect of a small amount of free gas in the mediastinum alone is usually minimal. The most common underlying cause is trauma to the esophagus, trachea, pharynx, or a pulmonary injury.

Clinical presentation of pneumomediastinum can consist of respiratory distress (restrictive respiratory pattern), dyspnea, subcutaneous emphysema, tissue trauma, and/or muffled heart sounds. Disease differentials can be quite varied but oftentimes are the result of trauma. Less common causes include underlying disease processes such as pneumonia, pulmonary abscess, neoplasia, chronic granulomatous infection, or pulmonary parasitic infection. Diagnostic testing includes (but is not limited to) thoracic radiographs, ultrasound, computed tomography (CT) scan, and thoracocentesis. Treatment options include chest tube placement (pressure relief), medical management (monitoring, cage rest), and/or surgical management (repair of large, unhealing tears). Many times, cage rest is adequate for resolution or natural sealing of these tears.

Pneumomediastinum can and often does occur as a result of bite wounds about the neck or from abrupt changes in intrathoracic pressure. Common causes of intrathoracic pressure change include coughing, blunt force, excessive respiratory efforts against an obstructive airway (e.g., close pop-off valve), or tracheal tears. Iatrogenic causes include tracheal washing, tracheostomy, endotracheal tube placement, and/or overinflation of endotracheal tube cuffs.

Mediastinal masses

Masses in the mediastinum are the most common and prolific mediastinal disease seen in small animals. These masses typically cause inspiratory distress due to the displaced lung tissue and decreased lung volume; at times, secondary pleural effusion may develop.

Clinical signs include coughing, regurgitation, pleural effusion, palpable tissue mass, respiratory distress, and/or facial edema. Neoplasia is the primary differential diagnosis, although there are other non-neoplastic causes to be considered. Lymphoma, particularly (but not exclusively) in cats, is very common. Other neoplasms that are reported include thymoma, thyroid carcinoma, parathyroid carcinoma, and chemodectoma. Nonneoplastic causes include abscesses, granulomas, hematomas, or cysts.

Diagnostic evaluation typically includes thoracic radiographs, thoracocentesis and cytology (in patients with effusion), ultrasound, fine needle aspirate, CT scan, videofluoroscopic swallow study, endoscopy, and/or biopsy.

Treatment options are solely dependent on the type of mass (neoplastic vs. non-neoplastic) and are quite varied due to the large variety of diseases and can be species specific. Both medical and surgical treatments are commonly utilized when treating mediastinal masses. Medical treatment may consist of both chemotherapy and radiation therapy in addition to surgery when dealing with neoplastic masses. Non-neoplastic masses are most commonly resolved with surgical intervention.

SECTION 3 LOWER AIRWAY DISEASE

Anatomy and physiology

The lower airway includes all airway structures distal to the glottis, including the trachea, carina, bronchi, and bronchioles. The trachea bifurcates into the left and right principal bronchi at the carina. Each principal bronchus divides into lobar bronchi, which each supplies a specific lung lobe, branching into progressively smaller segmental then subsegmental bronchi and bronchioles that terminate at the alveolar sac. The airway functions principally as a conduit for air passage in and out of the lung; gas exchange (uptake of oxygen and inhalant anesthetic agents, release of carbon dioxide and other waste gases) occurs at the level of the alveoli.

The airway structure serves to keep the passageways open for unobstructed airflow to and from the alveoli. The trachea is composed of semicircular cartilage rings connected by fibroelastic annular ligaments, allowing flexibility of the neck while maintaining airway patency. In the bronchi, curved cartilage plates provide wall rigidity but are less extensive. Tracheal and bronchial walls are also composed of smooth muscle. Progressing distally in the airways there is less cartilage and more smooth muscle until the walls of the bronchioles, which are almost entirely composed of smooth muscle.

A thin layer of mucus secreted by goblet cells in the airway mucosa coats the airway lumen to moisten inspired air and to trap inhaled particles (foreign material, infectious agents). Airways are lined by ciliated epithelial cells. These cilia beat continually, which, combined with airflow, moves the mucus layer slowly toward the pharynx where the mucus is then swallowed or coughed out of the airways. Submucosal mucous glands, immune cells, and cough receptors are also present in the airways. The cough reflex is an important defense mechanism protecting the airways from injurious agents and from the accumulation of secretions. Mechanical or chemical stimulation of cough receptors results in reflex forceful expulsion of air, which also serves to expel harmful substances.

Although varied disease processes affect the lower airways, there are a limited number of ways that airways respond to injury. Airway goblet cells and submucosal mucous glands may hypertrophy and secrete excess mucus. Bronchial mucosa and submucosa may become edematous and infiltrated with inflammatory cells. Excess mucus and injurious agents may overwhelm the mucociliary clearance mechanism and stimulate cough receptors. Bronchial smooth muscle may spasm or become hypertrophied, which results in narrowing of the airways.

Clinical signs

Clinical signs of lower airway disease relate to interruption of air flow (wheezing, dyspnea), stimulation of cough receptors, or triggering of mucus secretion (crackles on auscultation, productive cough).

The most common clinical sign of primary lower airway disease is cough, which can also arise secondary to other diseases which cause compression of airways (enlarged tracheobronchial lymph nodes, cardiac enlargement, pulmonary mass) or involve terminal airways by the extension of inflammation or the accumulation of fluid or secretions (pneumonia, pulmonary edema).

Causes of primary lower airway disease in small animal patients include tracheal collapse, chronic bronchitis, feline bronchitis/asthma, airway infection (*Mycoplasma*, *Bordetella*, parasites), tracheal trauma, inhaled foreign body/foreign material, and, less commonly, tracheal hypoplasia and ciliary dyskinesia.

Diagnostic testing

History and physical examination

Most patients with lower airway disease have a history of cough, which should be characterized as to the length of time present, character (productive, dry), occurrence (nocturnal, when excited), and triggers (exercise, pulling on collar). Information on breed, age, and body size can aid in prioritizing differentials. Potential for exposure to infectious diseases (dog park, kennel), vaccination status, heartworm status and the use of heartworm prophylaxis, and potential trauma or inhaled irritant exposure should be determined.

In cats, it is important to help owners distinguish cough from other processes; owners will commonly describe cats as "bringing up a hairball" when in fact the cat is coughing.

Physical examination may reveal inspiratory (cervical trachea) or expiratory (thoracic trachea, bronchi) dyspnea or increased expiratory effort due to partial obstruction (bronchoconstriction, increased secretions, or both). Palpation of the trachea may elicit paroxysmal coughing in patients with tracheal sensitivity due to tracheal inflammation or collapse. Subcutaneous emphysema may be present secondary to penetrating injury/tear of the cervical trachea. Harsh lung sounds, crackles, or wheezes may be evident on lung auscultation.

Laboratory findings

CBC and serum chemistry results are usually normal unless systemic disease or infection is present. Leukocytosis may be present if there is parenchymal inflammation, and eosinophilia may occur with allergic or parasitic disease. Arterial blood gas analysis allows identification of the presence and severity of respiratory function impairment resulting from airway disease.

Imaging

Thoracic radiography allows for evaluation of extra-airway causes of coughing (cardiac disease, tracheobronchial lymphadenomegaly) as well as signs of lower airway disease. Bronchial inflammation may produce a bronchial radiographic pattern characterized by thickened cross-sectional end-on bronchi (doughnuts) and longitudinal sections (tram lines). In cats, bronchial disease may also be manifested by unstructured interstitial and alveolar patterns, lung hyperinflation, and lobar atelectasis.[1] Some animals with significant lower airway disease have normal thoracic radiographs. Thoracic radiographs should include the cervical as well as thoracic trachea in patients with potential tracheal disease. If tracheal collapse is suspected, both inspiratory and expiratory radiographs should be taken due to the dynamic nature of the disease.

Fluoroscopy is useful for the detection of dynamic disease processes such as tracheal or bronchial collapse. Eliciting a cough during fluoroscopic imaging of the trachea and bronchi may improve the detection of airway narrowing or collapse.

Biopsy techniques and other diagnostic tests

Transtracheal wash (TTW) allows secretion sampling from the trachea and principal bronchi for cytology and culture. TTW can be performed through a sterile endotracheal tube or by percutaneous insertion of a catheter into the tracheal lumen. An advantage of percutaneous TTW is that it can be performed awake or with sedation rather than general anesthesia. Eliciting a cough before aspirating the wash sample can improve diagnostic return. The potential for contamination of the sample by oral and pharyngeal material is a drawback to this procedure. Also, TTW does not allow evaluation of smaller airways. Complications are rare but can include exacerbation of cough and inflammation, tracheal laceration, pneumomediastinum, or subcutaneous emphysema.

Bronchoscopy allows direct visualization of airways for detection of structural abnormalities, identification and retrieval of foreign material, and collection of samples by bronchoalveolar lavage (BAL). This procedure is performed with the patient under general anesthesia. Flexible endoscopy is preferred and the endoscope may be introduced into the trachea directly (which allows examination of more distal airway structures) or through specialized adapters attached to the endotracheal tube in intubated patients. Collection of diagnostic samples is aided by direct visualization of specific lesions or regions of the lung. Endoscopic biopsy forceps and brushes facilitate sampling of luminal lesions. BAL is generally performed through the endoscope and allows sampling of more distal airways than TTW.

Evaluation for parasite infection should be a component of evaluation of respiratory disease. Several parasites can infect the lower airways of small animal patients, although they are relatively rare and typically affect young patients and those exposed to outdoor or unsanitary environments. Dogs may be affected by *Capillaria aerophila*, *Paragonimus kellicotti*, *Oslerus osleri*, and *Crenosoma vulpis*. Cats can be infected by *C. aerophila*, *P. kellicotti*, and *Aelurostrongylus abstrusus*. Diagnosis of lung parasites is based on demonstration of ova or larvae in TTW or BAL fluid, in feces, or by direct visualization during bronchoscopy.

Feces can be analyzed by direct smear, fecal flotation, or the Baermann funnel technique, which improves diagnostic yield by allowing analysis of a greater volume of feces and improves the ability to detect larvae. The Baermann technique is performed by placing gauze at the base of a funnel, suspending fecal material in water, and allowing the water to pass through the funnel overnight. The water is then centrifuged and the sediment is examined microscopically. Ideally, for fecal evaluation techniques, three fecal samples taken several days apart are analyzed to improve the chances of identifying parasites which may intermittently release ova or larvae.

Specific airway diseases and treatment

Tracheobronchial malacia: collapsing trachea

Tracheal collapse is a syndrome characterized by flattening (usually dorsoventral) of the tracheal rings and laxity of the dorsal tracheal membrane.[3] Progressive degeneration of tracheal rings with hypocellularity and softening of the cartilage leads to airway collapse during respiration. A genetic component of the disease contributing to abnormalities of the tracheal ring cartilage is presumed due to breed predispositions in toy and small dog breeds. Loss of airway support and subsequent loss of airway lumen patency lead to obstruction of airflow, mucosal inflammation, and triggering of cough by mechanical (collapse) or chemical (inflammation) stimulation. Dogs typically present as adults with a history of chronic, loud, or "honking" cough. The disease can affect the cervical trachea, intrathoracic trachea, mainstem bronchi, and bronchioles or can simultaneously involve multiple regions of the airways.

A collapsing trachea is often diagnosed by a combination of clinical and imaging (radiography, fluoroscopy) findings. Palpation of the trachea in affected dogs will often elicit a cough and may reveal a palpably abnormal flattened trachea. Endoscopy is useful in the diagnosis of tracheal collapse, grading its severity, and evaluation for collapse in lower airways (not well demonstrated by other diagnostics) by providing direct visualization of abnormal airways.

Medical management of tracheal collapse includes weight loss and use of a harness instead of a collar to eliminate pressure on the trachea.

If secondary infection is identified through cytology and/or culture, specific antimicrobial therapy should be implemented. *Pasteurella* spp., *Staphylococcus* spp., *Streptococcus* spp., *Escherichia coli*, and other gram-negative bacteria are common airway isolates. Antibiotic choice should be based on sensitivity results when possible. For empirical therapy, doxycycline (3–5 mg/kg PO q 12 h) is often selected because of its broad-spectrum activity, ability to penetrate the airway, and minimal side effects.

Antitussives are used as needed to control signs and to disrupt the cycle of self-perpetuating cough. Over-the-counter dextromethorphan-containing compounds such as Robutussin-DM® (Wyeth) or Delsym® (Reckitt Benckiser) or central acting narcotics such as butorphanol or hydrocodone may be used.

Bronchodilators (theophylline, terbutaline, albuterol) are sometimes used, but their use in tracheal collapse is controversial. These medications are usually given orally and work by relaxing the smooth muscle, especially the bronchial smooth muscle. Albuterol can also be administered by inhalation by the use of a face mask system, such as the AeroKat™, made by Trudell Medical International.

Directions on how to use this system can be found on the manufacturer's Web site at http://www.trudellmed.com/animal-health. Common side effects of bronchodilators include tachycardia, gastrointestinal (GI) upset, and hyperexcitability.

Short courses of anti-inflammatory agents such as glucocorticoids are used intermittently to control acute worsening of clinical signs attributed to flare-ups of secondary airway inflammation. Long-term steroid use is contraindicated as it can predispose to secondary bacterial infection, further degeneration of cartilage, and weight gain. An anti-inflammatory dose of prednisone or prednisolone (0.5 mg/kg PO BID) for 7–10 days should be used then tapered. Inhalant steroids may be used in dogs with concurrent chronic bronchitis requiring long-term anti-inflammatory medication. The most commonly used inhaled corticosteroid is fluticasone propionate (Flovent 110 mcg/puff by GlaxoSmithKline®), a synthetic corticosteroid. The recommended dose for dogs is one puff q 6–12 h for controlling bronchiolar inflammation.[4]

For patients failing medical management, other treatment options include surgical placement of external prosthetic supports (extraluminal polypropylene rings) for cervical tracheal collapse or placement of an intraluminal stent, which can be placed nonsurgically with endoscopic or fluoroscopic guidance.

Canine infectious tracheobronchitis

Canine infectious tracheobronchitis, also referred to as "canine respiratory disease complex" and "kennel cough," is a highly contagious infectious airway disease of dogs. Several infectious organisms are implicated as causative agents in this disease complex, including canine adenovirus-2 (CAV-2), parainfluenza virus (PIV), and the bacteria *Bordetella bronchiseptica* as primary pathogens and multiple secondary bacterial agents. Concurrent infection with more than one agent is common in this disease.

A history of exposure to groups of other dogs (animal shelter environment, dog park, dog show, recent boarding at a kennel) or exposure to a sick dog or puppy is common. Clinical signs include sudden onset of persistent, often severe cough that is exacerbated by exercise, excitement, or pressure on the cervical trachea. The cough can be productive or nonproductive and owners may describe terminal retching or gagging. Diagnosis is usually presumptive based on history and acute onset of cough. A CBC, serum chemistry, and thoracic radiographs are often unremarkable. In severe cases, disruption of the mucociliary clearance mechanism by inflammation and infection can facilitate establishment of secondary pneumonia, which may be manifested by signs of systemic illness in the patient and changes on a CBC and thoracic radiographs reflecting more severe disease and pneumonia. Infectious tracheobronchitis is usually a self-limiting disease treated with symptomatic and supportive care. To avoid exacerbation of the cough, rest for 7–10 days with restricted exercise and avoiding excitement is recommended. In uncomplicated tracheobronchitis, antitussives are used to control coughing and break the cough-inflammation cycle. If the cough is productive or the condition is complicated by pneumonia, antitussive use should be limited or avoided.

Antibiotics are not usually recommended because the disease is self-limiting and antibiotics have not been shown to alter the severity or duration of disease. If a significant bacterial component is suspected or pneumonia is present, antibiotic therapy should be based on culture and sensitivity results. Empirically, doxycycline (5–10 mg/kg PO BID for 10–14 days) is a rational choice because of its effectiveness against *Bordetella* spp. and ability to reach the bronchial epithelium.[5]

Glucocorticoids are *not* recommended for treating associated inflammation due to the infectious nature of the disease and a failure in clinical trials to demonstrate efficacy in patients with infectious tracheobronchitis.[6]

Canine chronic bronchitis

Chronic bronchitis is defined by the presence of a daily cough for at least 2 months of the year that lacks an identifiable specific cause.[4] It is a diagnosis of exclusion achieved by

1) ruling out other causes of cough and

2) identifying bronchial inflammation (radiography, bronchoscopy, BAL cytology).

The pathogenesis of the disease involves chronic inflammation that results in a continuous cycle of injury and repair, ultimately resulting in permanent damage of the airways. Chronic bronchitis is often accompanied by secondary airway collapse.

Because the clinical signs and airway injury result from airway inflammation, anti-inflammatory agents are the mainstay of treatment for chronic bronchitis. Glucocorticoids are often used and dosage is catered to patients on an individual basis: Long-term administration is often necessary. To minimize the systemic side effects of corticosteroids, local delivery to the airways may be achieved by the use of a metered-dose inhaler. Fluticasone proprionate (Flovent® by GlaxoSmithKline) is the most commonly used inhalable glucocorticoid, and dosage for dogs is one activation (puff) of the 110 mcg/puff every 6–12 h.[4] Spacing chambers for use with aerosol inhalers are available through many respiratory supply companies and can be used to facilitate administration of inhalants to dogs.

The use of bronchodilators to treat chronic bronchitis is controversial because the role of bronchoconstriction in the disease process is uncertain and bronchodilators have not been shown to effect significant improvement. There is anecdotal evidence that bronchodilators combined with glucocorticoids may be beneficial in some patients, so they are often used as adjunctive therapy.[4] The two common classes of bronchodilators used in chronic bronchitis are the methylxanthine derivatives (theophylline) and the beta-2 agonists (terbutaline, albuterol), which act by causing relaxation of the bronchial smooth muscle. Chronic bronchitis is usually *not* associated with secondary bacterial infection. If infection is identified by culture, antibiotic treatment should be implemented based on sensitivity results.

Antitussive agents may be considered in patients with chronic nonproductive cough if the cough persists despite appropriate treatment of airway inflammation. Cough suppression is contraindicated in patients with a productive cough that need to clear mucus from the lower airways. Ancillary measures such as maintenance of a lean body weight and environmental control are vital to optimal management of patients with respiratory disease in general and chronic airway disease in particular. Owners should be instructed to minimize exposure of the patient to airway irritants (dust, smoke, aerosol sprays) that can trigger coughing and initiate/exacerbate airway inflammation. Owners can be referred to Web sites for human patients with asthma for specific measures of controlling airway irritant exposure in the household environment. Owners should also be advised that dogs with airway disease are at risk of respiratory distress and overheating in hot or humid environmental conditions or with exertion.

Feline bronchial disease: "feline asthma"

Feline bronchial disease, sometimes referred to as feline asthma, is a syndrome of bronchoconstriction and airway inflammation characterized by recurrent episodes of wheezing, coughing, and respiratory distress. An allergic (type I hypersensitivity) component and genetic predisposition to developing the disease are suspected. Asthma is defined as a disorder of the lower airways that causes airflow limitation by a combination of airway inflammation, accumulated airway mucus, and smooth muscle contraction, which impede airflow[7] and trigger chronic cough. Cats are usually presented because of respiratory distress or coughing.

Feline bronchial disease is usually diagnosed by finding radiographic and bronchoscopic evidence of airway injury, inflammation (usually eosinophilic) on airway cytology, and exclusion of other causes of cough, airway inflammation, and injury (upper airway disease, lungworm infection, heartworm disease, cardiac disease, neoplasia, pneumonia). Thoracic radiographs may show bronchial (common), unstructured interstitial or alveolar lung patterns, lung hyperinflation, and lobar atelectasis but may be normal in some affected cats. Bronchoscopy may show airway inflammation and narrowing, mucus plugs, and airway collapse. Cats presenting in acute respiratory distress are managed by minimizing stress, relieving bronchoconstriction with injectable

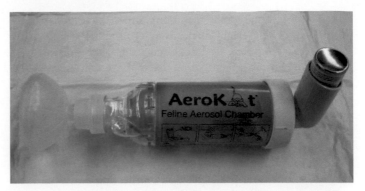

Figure 6.3.1 AeroKat (Trudell Medical International) spacer with attached metered-dose inhaler (MDI). Also available in larger size for dogs is the AeroDawg (not pictured).

bronchodilators, and supplementing oxygen to stabilize the patient for diagnostic testing. In addition, sedation with butorphanol can aid in decreasing stress and in allowing safe handling, but lower dosages should be used to avoid respiratory depression. Intravenous fast-acting anti-inflammatories such as dexamethasone (0.2–0.5 mg/kg) can be given to decrease airway inflammation, but, because glucocorticoids can impact the results of diagnostics, their use should be reserved for patients that do not respond to bronchodilators and oxygen therapy.

Maintenance therapy includes anti-inflammatories (oral or inhalant corticosteroids) and bronchodilators (oral theophylline or terbutaline, inhaled albuterol). Inhalant drugs are preferred due to reduced systemic side effects. Patient response to therapy must be monitored to guide dose adjustment to the lowest effective dose of steroids. Fluticasone propionate, a synthetic corticosteroid, is commonly used and administered at a dose of one actuation or puff (110 mcg/puff) every 12 h.[7]

Inhalant administration is best achieved by the use of a spacer such as AeroKat (Trudell Medical International) (see Figure 6.3.1). Antibiotic treatment is indicated for cats with positive culture or *Mycoplasma* PCR results on TTW or BAL. Doxycycline shows activity against *Mycoplasma* and has good distribution into airway mucosa.

Cyproheptadine (2 mg per cat PO q 12 h) has recently been used to control disease in patients with inadequate response to traditional therapies, but there is little evidence supporting its use, which should be considered as still in the experimental stage.[7] Environmental control and use of low dust cat litters are important aspects of patient management.

Ciliary dyskinesia

Ciliary dyskinesia is a condition in which the function (movement) of cilia is impaired. In the respiratory system, this results in failure of the mucociliary clearance mechanism. It may be hereditary (primary) or acquired. Primary ciliary dyskinesia (PCD) is an uncommon inherited disorder that affects microtubule formation in ciliated cells (respiratory, urogenital, and auditory epithelium). PCD may be associated with situs inversus (left–right reversal of internal organ position) and dextrocardia (heart positioned on the right instead of on the left), known as *Kartagener's syndrome*. The acquired form of the disease can result from chronic inflammation that damages cilia and ciliated cells.

The consequences of defects in ciliary function in the respiratory tract include chronic bacterial bronchopneumonia, sinusitis, and bronchitis. Due to chronic inflammation, infection, and reduced clearance of secretions, there is progressive damage to airways leading to bronchiectasis (irreversible dilation of distal airways) and further predisposition to infection.

Clinical signs are those of chronic or recurring respiratory infections including cough, often productive, and chronic nasal discharge. Patients with PCD may also show abnormalities of other systems related to ciliary dysfunction (deafness, infertility). Thoracic radiographs may show bronchiectasis, situs inversus, or dextrocardia. Definitive diagnosis of PCD requires electron microscopic examination of ciliated cells (respiratory epithelium, sperm) to demonstrate the structural defect in the cilia.

Treatment of ciliary dyskinesia centers on control of secondary infection and accumulation of secretions (antibiotics, nebulization, coupage). Because mucociliary clearance is already compromised, avoidance of smoke, aerosol sprays, and other irritant particles is important and antitussives are contraindicated.

Dietary management for weight loss and maintenance of a lean body condition is a vital component of treatment for patients with respiratory disease. Additional information can be found in the nutrition section of this chapter.

Anesthetic and analgesic considerations

Lower airway disease is not generally painful. Animals with airway disease require special consideration for general anesthesia as drug-associated decreases in respiratory rate and effort may further worsen respiratory function. Endotracheal intubation may exacerbate airway inflammation by mechanical injury to an already abnormal mucosa. Anxiety and increased respiratory rate and effort during recovery may worsen airway collapse and obstruction: Close patient monitoring is imperative and postanesthetic administration of anxiolytics may be necessary. Additional information can be found in the anesthesia and analgesia section of this chapter.

SECTION 4 PULMONARY PARENCHYMAL DISEASE

Anatomy and physiology

Conducting airways of the lung terminate in respiratory bronchioles which branch into alveolar ducts. Alveolar ducts open into alveoli, the functional gas exchange units of the lung. Each alveolus is surrounded by a network of pulmonary capillaries. Gas exchange occurs across the wall of the alveolus and the wall of the adjacent capillaries with gases diffusing in response to concentration gradients. Oxygen (O_2) diffuses out of the alveolar lumen, where oxygen concentration is highest, into capillaries, where most becomes bound to hemoglobin in red blood cells. This oxygenated blood returns via the pulmonary venous circulation to the left heart and is then pumped out into the systemic arterial circulation for distribution to tissues throughout the body. At the tissue level, O_2 diffuses from the higher concentration capillary lumen into tissues. Carbon dioxide (CO_2), produced as a waste gas of tissue metabolism, diffuses from tissues into the capillary lumen, where its concentration is initially lower. The capillaries collect into veins, which carry blood, which is now depleted of O_2 and high in CO_2, back to the right heart, where it is pumped via the pulmonary artery to the lungs and distributed into pulmonary capillaries around alveoli. CO_2 diffuses from the capillary lumen into the alveoli, where the concentration of CO_2 is lower than in venous blood, to be exhaled and removed from the body. At the level of the alveolus, the barrier to gas diffusion is normally a very thin membrane made up of a single layer of alveolar epithelial cells, the capillary endothelium and their fused basement membranes, with intermittent connective tissue fibers widening the barrier in some places. In pulmonary diseases, changes in this alveolocapillary membrane (e.g., deposition of more connective tissue, edema fluid) can interfere with diffusion/gas exchange. Because CO_2 diffuses more readily than O_2, CO_2 levels often remain normal (or low) even when diffusion barrier changes result in marked reductions of O_2 diffusion and hypoxemia. CO_2 levels become high if there is a problem with ventilation (reduced respiratory drive in anesthetized or comatose patients, upper airway obstruction, thoracic wall injury, or respiratory muscle exhaustion).

Clinical signs

Clinical signs of pulmonary parenchymal disease result from reduced oxygen diffusion from the alveoli to the bloodstream and the resultant hypoxemia. Signs of pulmonary disease may be absent or vague until the disease is advanced or the lungs are diffusely involved, and may include exercise intolerance, tachypnea, dyspnea, orthopnea, and cyanosis. Localized disease may be subclinical or may result in nonrespiratory manifestations such as fever and inappetence. Cough may be present if the disease process extends into airways, results in increased airway secretions, or causes extraluminal airway compression. Fever, anorexia, weight loss, or generalized lymphadenomegaly may be present depending on the underlying cause of pulmonary disease. Cardiac arrhythmias secondary to hypoxia may be evident. Pulmonary crackles may be auscultated in patients with pulmonary fibrosis, pulmonary edema, or if excess airway secretions or inflammation is present. Reduced heart and lung sounds on auscultation and dullness on thoracic wall percussion may be noted over regions of lung consolidation.

Diagnostic testing

Diagnostic testing should be delayed in dyspneic patients until they can be stabilized with supplemental oxygen, anxiolytics, and, when indicated, bronchodilators, diuretics, or thoracocentesis.

Laboratory findings

There are no clinicopathological changes that are specific for pulmonary parenchymal disease, but laboratory results may reflect the underlying disease process. A CBC may show leukocytosis in infectious processes or thrombocytopenia in patients with certain infectious diseases (ehrlichiosis, leptospirosis) or vasculitis. Determination of hematocrit or packed cell volume is important to help distinguish patients with elevated respiratory rate and effort associated with anemia from patients with respiratory disease. Biochemical parameters are unaffected by pulmonary disease unless the disease process is multisystemic or other tissues are negatively impacted by hypoxia secondary to respiratory dysfunction. For example, secondary hepatopathy and mild elevations of alanine aminotransferase (ALT) may be seen in hypoxemic patients. Azotemia and hyperphosphatemia are expected in patients with uremic pneumonitis secondary to severe renal disease. ABG analysis provides a sensitive assessment of respiratory function and measures the partial pressure of oxygen and carbon dioxide gases dissolved in plasma. In pulmonary disease, hypoxemia develops because of impaired gas diffusion, ventilation–perfusion mismatch, or shunting. Hypocapnia reflecting increased ventilation and enhanced discharge of waste gases is common in tachypneic patients. Hypercapnia in patients with pulmonary disease is an ominous sign resulting from respiratory muscle fatigue and subsequent ventilatory failure in patients that have a sustained increased respiratory rate and effort. Cytological evaluation of samples collected from lung tissue, airways, or tracheobronchial lymph nodes may reveal the general type of disease process (e.g., eosinophilic vs. pyogranulomatous inflammation) or the specific etiology (e.g., *Blastomyces* organisms, neoplastic lymphocytes).

Imaging

Thoracic radiographs are standard for identifying pulmonary disease and for monitoring progression or therapeutic response. They may also elucidate an underlying cause (neoplasia, cardiac disease) or may demonstrate a particular pulmonary pattern that helps narrow the list of differentials. Structured (nodules) and unstructured interstitial and alveolar patterns or a combination of these may be seen in pulmonary disease, and the distribution may be focal, regional, multifocal, or diffuse. Pneumonia often produces an unstructured interstitial pattern initially, which progresses to an alveolar pattern. Aspiration pneumonia often shows a cranioventral distribution. Fungal pneumonia typically produces a nodular or miliary pattern. In dogs, pulmonary edema due to congestive heart failure is manifested as increased pulmonary density (alveolar pattern) with a perihilar distribu-

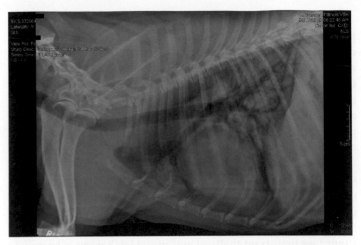

Figure 6.4.1 Noncardiogenic pulmonary edema in a dog with acute respiratory distress syndrome (ARDS)—lateral thoracic radiograph demonstrating alveolar lung pattern with a primarily caudodorsal distribution.

tion; cardiogenic pulmonary edema in cats has a less predictable radiographic appearance and may appear as patchy alveolar disease. Noncardiogenic pulmonary edema manifests as an alveolar pattern with a caudodorsal distribution (Figure 6.4.1). Smoke inhalation and near drowning are also associated with alveolar patterns. Pulmonary contusions show an alveolar pattern that is often patchy with a variable distribution depending on the angle of trauma. Neoplastic lesions may appear as distinct solitary (primary pulmonary neoplasia), multiple to diffuse (metastatic disease) pulmonary nodules or miliary changes, or as unstructured interstitial disease (lymphosarcoma). Radiographic appearance of pulmonary thromboembolism (PTE) is variable, including interstitial and alveolar changes, pleural fluid, blunting of pulmonary vessels, or a combination of patterns, but radiographs may also be normal. Acute respiratory distress syndrome (ARDS) generally produces an alveolar pattern that may be patchy or diffuse.

Thoracic ultrasonography may be useful for evaluating areas of lung consolidation or peripheral lung masses; however, the usefulness of ultrasonography may be limited because of interference by the air interface in aerated lung.

CT of the thorax may aid in the diagnosis of pulmonary disease when other techniques do not elucidate a cause. Ultrasonography of peripheral and consolidated lesions and CT of anesthetized patients can be used to guide fine needle aspiration for the collection of samples for cytology.

Other diagnostic tests and biopsy techniques

Pulse oximetry is a rapid and noninvasive technique for evaluating oxygen saturation of red blood cell hemoglobin for the detection of hypoxemia. ABG is a more accurate method of measuring changes in circulating oxygen levels and provides a more thorough evaluation of respiratory function by measuring carbon dioxide levels, an assessment of ventilation.

Lung aspiration, or fine needle aspiration of lung lesions, provides samples for cytological evaluation and is useful for evaluating diffuse disease or accessible peripheral lesions. Ultrasonographic or CT guidance can improve the diagnostic yield of this technique by allowing a more accurate placement of the needle into abnormal tissue. Pneumothorax and hemorrhage as a result of airway or blood vessel laceration are potential complications of lung aspiration, but the procedure can usually be completed safely.

TTW or bronchoscopy with BAL to collect samples for cytology and culture can be diagnostically useful for pulmonary diseases, which characteristically have an airway component (eosinophilic bronchopneumopathy, pneumonia), or diseases that involve the airway by extension. Bacterial culture and sensitivity are important to direct antimicrobial therapy in bacterial pneumonia.

Thoracoscopy provides direct visualization of thoracic structures including the lungs and can be useful for assessment and potentially for treatment of patients with pulmonary disease.

Ventilation–perfusion scintigraphy can be used to assess patients for PTE, but its availability is extremely limited. Angiography is another technique for identifying vascular occlusion in PTE patients.

Other diagnostic tests may be indicated to evaluate patients with pulmonary disease secondary to disease in another organ or for consequences of respiratory dysfunction. An electrocardiogram (ECG) serves to detect and help characterize arrhythmias resulting from hypoxia, and echocardiography is useful in defining primary cardiac disease in patients with cardiogenic pulmonary edema. Abdominal ultrasonography may demonstrate a primary neoplasm in patients with pulmonary metastases or may show lesions in other organs in patients with systemic infectious diseases with pulmonary involvement. Additionally, lesions present in abdominal organs may be more accessible and more readily aspirated for possible cytological diagnosis.

Treatment

General treatment measures for animals with pulmonary parenchymal disease may include oxygen therapy, fluid therapy, sedation, nebulization, and coupage.

Oxygen supplementation is indicated for dyspneic patients and can improve oxygenation of the blood in conditions causing hypoventilation, gas diffusion barrier problems, or ventilation perfusion mismatch. Oxygen can be provided via flow-by oxygen face mask, personal oxygen devices, or placing the animal in an oxygen cage. Humidification of the oxygen gas before it is inhaled is important to prevent drying and further injury to airway surfaces. Because oxygen can be toxic to the airways and lungs, try to avoid using levels of supplementation above 60% and limit the duration of oxygen therapy to what is necessary. This helps avoid oxygen toxicity, which may cause worsening of the respiratory function due to inflammation, edema, and decreased clearance of airway secretions. Response to oxygen therapy can be monitored by pulse oximetry or ABG.

Fluid therapy may be needed for patients unable to meet their own requirements for maintenance plus additional evaporative losses resulting from tachypnea. Intravenous fluids should be administered with caution and close monitoring is indicated due to increased vascular hydrostatic pressure or increased vascular permeability in inflamed or damaged areas of the lung. This increase may promote fluid extravasation into lung interstitium thereby worsening gas exchange resulting in respiratory distress. Anxiety can contribute to tachypnea and can exacerbate airway collapse through increased respiratory effort, further compromising gas exchange. Sedation may be beneficial in reducing these effects and improving patient comfort. Morphine is often recommended because it has beneficial effects on pulmonary vasculature as well as anxiolytic effects.

In patients with excess airway secretions, nebulization and coupage can be used to moisten (nebulization) and loosen (coupage) secretions to make them easier to remove from airways through coughing and mucociliary clearance.

Diseases

Pneumonia

Pneumonia is defined as an inflammatory disease of the terminal airways and pulmonary interstitium. It is important to recognize that pneumonia has many etiologies. Too often, the term "pneumonia" is used inappropriately as a synonym for bacterial pneumonia, and clinical findings indicative of pneumonia are erroneously ascribed to bacterial infection. Infectious agents that may cause pneumonia include bacteria (including rickettsial agents), viruses (canine distemper virus, canine influenza virus, CAV-2, canine PIV, feline herpesvirus, feline calicivirus), protozoa (*Toxoplasma, Neospora*), respiratory parasites (*Paragonimus, Aelurostrongylus, Filaroides*), and fungi (*Blastomyces, Histoplasma, Coccidioides, Aspergillus, Cryptococcus*, and *Pneumocystis*). Some viral agents predispose to secondary bacterial pneumonia (canine distemper virus, canine PIV, FeLV, and FIV). Noninfectious forms of pneumonia include aspiration pneumonia, pneumonia secondary to smoke inhalation, and lipid pneumonia (exogenous lipid pneumonia from aspiration of fatty substances or endogenous lipid pneumonia related to lipid release from breakdown of pulmonary tissues). Appropriate treatment of pneumonia requires identification of the specific etiology, including identification of specific organisms and their antimicrobial sensitivities in bacterial disease.

Bacterial pneumonia is considered a secondary condition that is established following some other pathological insult that impairs the natural defense mechanisms of the lung. Infection is usually associated with resident respiratory flora, although hematogenous spread is another potential source of bacteria (*Enterococcus*), and most cases of pneumonia involve more than one bacterial agent (polymicrobial). Common agents include *Streptococcus, Staphylococcus, E. coli, Pasteurella, Klebsiella,*

Pseudomonas, *Bordetella*, and *Mycoplasma*. Samples for bacterial culture and sensitivity can be collected by TTW, BAL, or lung aspirate. Empiric antibacterial therapy using broad-spectrum drugs with good respiratory distribution should be initiated pending culture results. A combination of (1) an aminopenicillin *or* a first-generation cephalosporin *and* (2) a fluoroquinolone *or* an aminoglycoside provides a rational empiric choice. Parenteral administration of drugs is advised for patients with severe hypoxemia that may secondarily impair gut function and absorption of orally administered drugs. Aerosol administration of antibiotics is not recommended. Response to treatment is monitored by sequential thoracic radiographs ± ABG determination and antibacterial drugs are continued until 1–2 weeks past resolution of clinical and radiographic evidence of disease.

Other forms of infectious pneumonia are also treated as indicated for the specific causative agent (i.e., long-term [months] administration of oral antifungal drugs with or without a course of injectable antifungal drug for fungal pneumonia; clindamycin or trimethoprim–sulfa with or without pyrimethamine for protozoal pneumonia). Patients with infectious or noninfectious pneumonia will often require general treatment measures such as oxygen supplementation, fluid therapy, nebulization, and coupage. Use of bronchodilators and mucolytics in the treatment of pneumonia is controversial.

Pulmonary edema

Pulmonary edema is the accumulation of fluid in the pulmonary interstitium and alveoli. It usually results from increased hydrostatic pressure in pulmonary capillaries, most commonly seen in association with congestive heart failure (cardiogenic pulmonary edema) but also as a result of fluid overload. Noncardiogenic pulmonary edema refers to edema that occurs by mechanisms other than increased vascular hydrostatic pressure in heart failure. These other mechanisms include low vascular oncotic pressure (hypoalbuminemia), increased vascular permeability (vasculitis secondary to systemic infectious or inflammatory disease, sepsis, ARDS, neurogenic edema, uremia) and decreased lymphatic drainage of the pulmonary interstitium.

The severity of clinical signs depends on the degree to which the interstitium and alveoli are flooded by fluid, impairing gas exchange. Treatment includes administration of diuretics, which can be very effective in treating cardiogenic edema but is generally less effective in managing edema secondary to increased vascular permeability. Oxygen supplementation is often necessary initially until response to diuretic therapy and specific treatment of the underlying cause is evident.

Pulmonary contusions

Pulmonary contusions are regions of hemorrhage into the pulmonary interstitium and alveoli caused by blunt trauma to the thorax and are commonly seen in animals that are hit by cars. Significant pulmonary contusion may be present even if there is no external evidence of injury. The severity of clinical signs depends on the volume of lung affected and the subsequent impairment of gas exchange and can vary from subclinical to life threatening. Radiographic changes may not be evident initially but generally appear by 24 h post-trauma. Traumatic myocarditis is often present concurrently, and ECG monitoring for cardiac arrhythmias is recommended.

Hypoventilation may occur as a result of pain or disruption of the thoracic wall or diaphragm. Treatment to stabilize or repair such injuries may be required in the form of aggressive pain management, oxygen supplementation, or ventilatory support. Antibiotics are not indicated unless there is penetrating thoracic wall injury. Improvement of respiratory abnormalities is expected within 1–2 days of onset.

Eosinophilic bronchopneumopathy and eosinophilic granulomatosis

EB, formerly known as "pulmonary infiltrates with eosinophils" (PIE), is an idiopathic inflammatory disorder of the lung characterized by eosinophilic infiltration of alveoli and bronchioles with no identifiable cause. The condition occurs in dogs, usually young to middle-aged large dog breeds, and Siberian huskies appear to be predisposed, although any age or breed can be affected. A history of chronic (months to years) respiratory signs and progressive exercise intolerance is common. Cough, which is often productive of thick green-yellow mucus, is the usual clinical presentation. Nasal discharge may also be present, and some dogs are systemically ill. Thoracic radiographics show varying lung patterns and a combination of unstructured interstitial, bronchial, and alveolar changes may be present. A CBC may show a peripheral eosinophilia, which can be marked, in some patients, and hypoxemia is often identified by ABG. EB is a diagnosis of exclusion. Important differentials include heartworm disease, lungworm infection and pulmonary migration of other parasites, respiratory fungal infections, or neoplasia that can also be associated with eosinophilic infiltration.

EB is treated with immunosuppressive doses of corticosteroids (prednisone, prednisolone) tapered over 3–6 months depending on response to therapy. Most dogs respond favorably and may eventually be taken off corticosteroids or maintained on low doses. Environmental control to reduce exposure to respiratory irritants and potential allergens should be instituted and prophylactic treatment for occult parasitism is also recommended.

Eosinophilic granulomatosis is a similar idiopathic eosinophilic inflammatory condition, but, in this condition, the inflammatory infiltrates in the lungs form nodular lesions, which must be distinguished from neoplastic or other granulomatous conditions.

Lung lobe torsion

Lung lobe torsion occurs when a lung lobe rotates around the axis of the lobar bronchus, closing off the bronchus and blocking venous drainage. Continuing inflow of arterial blood, which is less susceptible to obstruction, causes progressive congestion and enlargement of the lung lobe and exudation of bloody fluid into the pleural space. The mechanisms resulting in lung lobe torsion are unknown, but some cases arise secondary to pleural effusion, trauma, or consolidation or atelectasis of a lung lobe. The condition is usually seen in dogs, more commonly those with a deep-chested conformation, and Afghans and pugs appear to be predisposed. Radiographic findings include pleural effusion and lung lobe consolidation and, sometimes, a more specific finding of an abnormally positioned bronchus. Pleural fluid may show chyle, modified transudate, exudate, or hemorrhage. Bronchoscopy may demonstrate a twisted bronchus. Treatment includes stabilization with oxygen therapy and thoracocentesis in preparation for definitive surgical treatment (lung lobectomy).

Idiopathic pulmonary fibrosis

Idiopathic pulmonary fibrosis (IPF) is a progressive interstitial lung disease of dogs and, rarely, cats. IPF is a diagnosis of exclusion, made after ruling out alternative causes of pulmonary fibrosis. IPF may occur as an end result of pulmonary inflammation or secondary to inhaled toxins, administration of certain drugs, or neoplasia. The condition is more common in terriers, especially West Highland white terriers, and most patients are presented when they are middle-aged or older. Clinical signs include progressive exercise intolerance and dyspnea and sometimes a nonproductive cough. Patients typically show tachypnea, which may be marked, and diffuse inspiratory crackles are often found on auscultation. Patients with pulmonary hypertension, a common consequence of IPF, may have a tricuspid systolic murmur or a split-second heart sound. Thoracic radiographs usually show a diffuse interstitial pattern; right heart enlargement may be evident in patients with secondary pulmonary hypertension. Diagnosis requires lung biopsy and demonstration of interstitial fibrosis. Inflammation may or may not be present. The prognosis is poor. Treatment usually includes use of corticosteroids ± azathioprine to try to reduce inflammation and further fibrosis, pulmonary vasodilators to control secondary pulmonary hypertension, bronchodilators to control concurrent bronchitis, and general measures of weight management and environmental control.

Pulmonary thromboembolism

PTE is a condition that results from obstruction of a pulmonary vessel or vessels by a thrombus (clot) that forms locally in the vessel or by an embolus (clot, parasite, fat, neoplastic cells) that forms elsewhere and travels to the lung to lodge in the vessel lumen (embolization). PTE is a secondary condition. Predisposing factors include stasis of blood flow, injury to vascular endothelium, and hypercoagulability. PTE is generally seen in patients with diseases that impact one or more of these factors. The most common cause of PTE in dogs is heartworm infection, which causes mechanical obstruction of blood flow and injury to the vessel lining (presence of the parasite in the vessel lumen). Other associated diseases include immune-mediated hemolytic anemia (hypercoagulability, endothelial injury), protein-losing enteropathy or protein-losing nephropathy (loss of antithrombin results in hypercoagulability), hyperadrenocorticism (hypercoagulability), cardiac disease (stasis of blood flow), sepsis, and trauma (vascular stasis, endothelial injury). PTE causes hypoxemia because of ventilation/perfusion mismatch and right-to-left shunting of unoxygenated blood. Secondary edema, reduced lung compliance, and bronchoconstriction may occur and worsen the hypoxemia. The typical clinical presentation is acute onset of tachypnea and respiratory distress.

Thoracic radiographs are often abnormal, but radiographic changes are variable (patchy alveolar pattern, hyperinflation, pleural effusion, blunted pulmonary vessels, or may be normal) and not specific for PTE. Premortem diagnosis of PTE is difficult, but PTE should be suspected in patients with an associated disease condition that show acute onset of tachypnea or respiratory distress. Plasma D-dimer measurement may provide supporting evidence for PTE, but levels are elevated in a number of other disease conditions. A normal D-dimer result suggests that PTE is less likely. Scintigraphy (perfusion ± ventilation scan), angiography, CT, and MRI can be used to support a diagnosis of PTE but are rarely used in veterinary patients because of limited availability or need for general anesthesia of a high risk patient.

PTE is treated with oxygen therapy, although hypoxemia in PTE patients may be refractory to oxygen administration, and administration of anticoagulants (heparin or warfarin) to prevent further clot formation. Thrombolytic treatment with tissue plasminogen activator (tPA) or streptokinase to break down existing clots is usually NOT done in veterinary patients because of cost and potential complications but may be considered for severely affected animals with low output cardiac failure associated with PTE. Treatment of the underlying disease process that predisposed to PTE is a vital component of PTE management, and recurrence of PTE is likely if the predisposing cause cannot be resolved. See Chapter 5 for additional information.

Acute respiratory distress syndrome

ARDS is a condition of rapidly progressive acute respiratory failure due to acute lung injury. Increased pulmonary capillary permeability secondary to injury to alveolar epithelium or capillary endothelium leads to proteinaceous noncardiogenic pulmonary edema, inflammation, refractory hypoxemia, decreased lung compliance, and, later, hyaline membrane formation and fibrosis. ARDS is a secondary condition that may develop in patients with a number of other critical illnesses including sepsis (most common cause), aspiration or bacterial pneumonia, drug or transfusion reaction, severe inflammatory disease (pancreatitis), or trauma.

Patients typically present with acute severe respiratory distress. Crackles and wheezes may be detected on thoracic auscultation, and other signs related to the underlying cause (e.g., abdominal pain in patients with pancreatitis) may be evident. Thoracic radiographs show bilateral alveolar or mixed pulmonary changes, often with a caudodorsal distribution (Figure 6.4.1) and normal cardiac silhouette, which helps differentiate the changes from those of cardiogenic pulmonary edema.

Echocardiography may also be beneficial in ruling out cardiac disease and may show evidence of pulmonary hypertension, which can develop acutely in ARDS patients.

ARDS is treated aggressively with oxygen therapy and treating the underlying disease that initiated the lung injury. Mechanical ventilation with positive end-expiratory pressure (PEEP) may be necessary for improving oxygenation. Diuretics may be helpful in the early stages of lung injury, but pulmonary edema that is proteinaceous, as it is in ARDS, is characteristically nonresponsive to diuretic administration. Lung function can be monitored by serial ABG and thoracic radiography. Mortality is high in patients that do not show improvement in the first 24–36 h.

Smoke inhalation

Injury to the airways and lungs with smoke inhalation is multifactorial and results from heat, toxic gases released from burning materials, and particulates inhaled in the smoke. Initially, smoke inhalation results in tissue injury, edema, and tissue hypoxia. Ventilation may be impaired by laryngeal edema or neurological dysfunction due to carbon monoxide intoxication. Subsequently, there is an increase in mucus and other respiratory secretions and infiltration with inflammatory cells. Inflammation can contribute to chemical injury of the airways and lungs, which constitutes the main mechanism of injury in smoke inhalation. Reflex bronchoconstriction in response to chemical or particulate irritants worsens respiratory function. Carbon monoxide and other gases released in the smoke further worsen tissue oxygenation by blocking oxygen uptake by red blood cells (carboxyhemoglobin formed by carbon monoxide) and by altering cell metabolism (hydrogen cyanide). Secondary bacterial infection is common due to damage to the respiratory epithelium and disruption of mucociliary clearance.

Treatment is supportive with oxygen administration being key in the efforts to improve tissue oxygenation and to facilitate clearance of carboxyhemoglobin. Judicious use of intravenous fluids is important to prevent drying/thickening of airway secretions without promoting pulmonary edema due to increased permeability of pulmonary vessels. Nebulization and coupage are beneficial in patients with excessive accumulations of airway secretions. Bronchodilator therapy (methylxanthines, beta-2 agonists) may be beneficial by relieving reflex bronchoconstriction. The use of corticosteroids to reduce inflammation is not recommended because it has not been shown to result in improvement and may interfere with healing of injured tissues. Antibiotic use should be based on specific diagnosis of the presence of bacterial infection by culture and determination of antimicrobial sensitivity. Prophylactic antibiotic use is contraindicated by the tendency of smoke inhalation victims to develop resistant infection. The overall survival rate of dogs and cats hospitalized and treated for smoke inhalation is high.

Pulmonary neoplasia

Neoplastic pulmonary disease may be primary (adenocarcinoma, bronchialveolar carcinoma, squamous cell carcinoma,

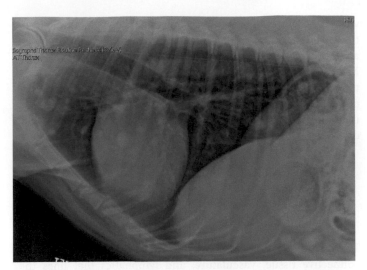

Figure 6.4.2 Pulmonary nodules in a dog with metastatic neoplasia. Nodular lesions in lung parenchyma may also be seen in other disease conditions (fungal pneumonia, eosinophilic granulomatosis), and additional diagnostic procedures are necessary to distinguish among neoplastic and infectious/inflammatory causes.

anaplastic carcinoma, sarcoma, histicytoma) or secondary (metastatic). Metastatic neoplasia is more common. Pulmonary neoplastic lesions may be radiographically indistinguishable from nodular lesions associated with inflammatory/infectious diseases especially granulomatous processes (fungal disease, eosinophilic granulomatosis) (Figure 6.4.2). Lung aspiration, TTW, or BAL may provide diagnostic samples for cytological diagnosis; otherwise, lung biopsy may be necessary to distinguish neoplastic from non-neoplastic lesions and to identify the cell type for neoplastic lesions. Treatment recommendations are based on tumor type. Solitary lesions may be amenable to surgical resection.

Nutritional considerations

Patients with pulmonary disease may experience weight loss because of increased energy expenditure due to fever, increased work of breathing, reduced gut function because of hypoxia, and decreased intake because sustained efforts to breathe preclude stopping to eat. Small frequent meals and food that is calorie dense and requires minimal chewing may be helpful in dyspneic animals. Patients that are significantly hypoxemic and experiencing reduced gut function may benefit from highly digestible diets.

Anesthetic and analgesic considerations

Alterations in respiratory and cardiac function in pulmonary disease patients are important anesthetic considerations. Hypoxemic patients are predisposed to the development of cardiac arrhythmias. Pulmonary hypertension is a potential complication of pulmonary disease that may alter right heart function. Anesthesia results in decreased spontaneous ventilation and worsening of ventilation–perfusion mismatch and shunt fractions. Patient positioning while under anesthesia contributes to atelectasis and small airway obstruction in the dependent lung. Mechanical ventilation may result in rupture of diseased lung tissue and the resultant pneumothorax. Preoxygenation and procedures to minimize the stress of handling during anesthesia induction are recommended for patients with pulmonary disease.

SECTION 5 PLEURAL DISEASE

Anatomy and physiology

The pleura is a thin layer of mesothelial cells and supporting connective tissue, vasculature, and lymphatics that lines the inner surface of the thoracic wall, anterior surface of the diaphragm and lateral mediastinum (parietal pleura), and the outer lung surface (visceral pleura). The pleural space is a potential space between the lungs and thoracic wall (visceral and parietal pleura), which normally contains a very small volume (few milliliters) of fluid that serves to lubricate pleural surfaces to facilitate their sliding movements during respiration. Pleural fluid is formed continuously from capillaries in the parietal pleura and is absorbed by lymphatic vessels in the parietal pleura and capillaries in the visceral pleura. Movement of the lungs, diaphragm, and thoracic wall during respiration facilitates lymphatic flow. Excess accumulation of pleural fluid may occur secondary to increased hydrostatic pressure, decreased oncotic pressure (serum protein) or increased permeability in pleural capillaries, decreased lymphatic drainage, or increased oncotic pressure of material within the pleural space. Pleural space disease is usually secondary to heart disease, lung disease (by extension or by rupture of air-filled structures), lymphatic/thoracic duct disease, thoracic wall injury, or migrating foreign body. Specific disease conditions of the pleura and pleural space include pleural effusion, pneumothorax, hemothorax, pyothorax, chylothorax, fibrosing pleuritis, and diaphragmatic hernia. The abnormal presence of air, fluid, or tissue in the pleural space reduces the area into which the lungs can expand and may directly compress the lungs, causing hypoventilation and reduced oxygen exchange.

Clinical signs

Clinical signs of pleural disease result from restriction of lung expansion and subsequent hypoventilation and hypoxemia but may be inapparent or subtle until pleural disease is advanced. Signs may include tachypnea, shallow breathing, dyspnea, orthopnea (shortness of breath when recumbent), and cyanosis. Cough is an inconsistent sign. Fever, anorexia, weight loss, cardiac murmurs or arrhythmias, jugular pulses, and ascites are sometimes present depending on the underlying cause of pleural space disease. External wounds may be present in animals with pyothorax or traumatic hemothorax or pneumothorax. Muffled heart sounds and ventrally decreased or muffled lung sounds may be identified in animals with pleural fluid accumulation or pleural masses (including diaphragmatic hernia). Heart and lung sounds may be dorsally decreased with pneumothorax. Thoracic wall percussion may show dullness ventrally in the presence of pleural fluid or increased resonance dorsally with pneumothorax. A restrictive respiratory pattern (rapid, shallow breaths) should prompt consideration of possible pleural or pleural space disease.

Diagnostic testing

Prior to diagnostic testing, dyspneic patients should be stabilized as needed with supplemental oxygen, anxiolytics, and thoracocentesis to remove enough fluid or air to restore adequate ventilation.

Laboratory findings

There are no clinicopathological changes that are specific for pleural disease, but laboratory results may reflect the underlying disease process. A CBC may show leukocytosis in infectious processes, thrombocytopenia in patients with vasculitis, and anemia in patients with traumatic hemorrhage or coagulopathies associated with hemothorax. Lymphopenia may be present in chylothorax or severe lymphatic disease. Hypoproteinemia and hypoalbuminemia are identified in patients with pleural effusion secondary to low vascular oncotic pressure, chylothorax, and some conditions of increased vascular or lymphatic permeability. ABG analysis may show hypoxemia and potentially hypercapnia reflecting reduced ventilation resulting from restricted lung expansion. Fluid analysis and cytology of pleural fluid is important in differentiating various disease processes causing pleural effusion. Fluid should be examined for character (chylous, hemorrhagic, clear) and evaluated for protein content and cellularity, which allows classification of the fluid as a transudate, a modified transudate, or exudate, and helps narrow down the list of possible causative diseases (Table 6.5.1).

Triglyceride concentration relative to serum triglyceride levels is used to characterize milky effusions as chyle. Low glucose concentration and a low pH in pleural fluid is consistent with a septic process (pyothorax).

Table 6.5.1 Characterization of pleural fluid

Fluid type	Appearance	Protein concentration (g/dL)	Cell count (per µL)
Transudate	Clear	<2.5	<1500
Modified transudate	Hazy	2.5–4.5	1000–3000
Exudate	Turbid to opaque	>3.0	>3000

Imaging

Thoracic radiographs are important to confirm the presence of pleural disease and may also help identify an underlying cause (neoplasia, cardiac disease, lung disease, diaphragmatic hernia). Patients may tolerate dorsoventral (DV) positioning better than the usual ventrodorsal (VD) positioning. If presence of pleural fluid or air is confirmed radiographically, radiographs should be repeated after maximal thoracocentesis to evaluate for abnormalities obscured by the fluid or air. Radiographic changes indicating pleural effusion include rounding of lung margins, visualization of and widening of interlobar fissure lines, separation of the lung from the thoracic wall, and obscuring of the cardiac silhouette (Figures 6.5.1 and 6.5.2).

A horizontal beam study may allow demonstration of a fluid line. A positive contrast lymphangiogram is sometimes used to evaluate the patency of the thoracic duct in patients with chylothorax. Fibrosing pleuritis, which may be a consequence of longstanding pleural effusion, is manifested radiographically by rounded lung lobes and prominent fissure lines. In pneumothorax, radiographs show dorsal displacement of the cardiac silhouette away from the sternum, separation of the lung from the thoracic wall with radiolucent areas free of identifiable vascular structures between the lung and thoracic wall, and increased density of the lungs due to lung tissue collapse (Figures 6.5.3 and 6.5.4).

Thoracic ultrasonography is actually facilitated by the presence of fluid in the pleural space and can be useful in guiding thoracocentesis and in identifying soft tissue abnormalities in the pleural space or mediastinum, which may indicate an underlying cause of the pleural disease. CT of the thorax may facilitate diagnosis of pleural disease when other techniques do not elucidate a cause.

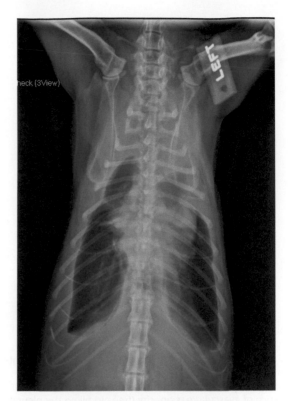

Figure 6.5.2 VD projection of same cat in Figure 6.5.1 showing retraction of the peripheral lung margins from the thoracic wall, presence of soft tissue opacity (pleural fluid) in the pleural space and delineating the interlobar fissures between lung lobes. The left cranial lung lobe is reduced in volume due to atelectasis secondary to the pleural fluid accumulation. The enlarged cardiac silhouette suggests underlying heart disease as a possible cause of the pleural effusion.

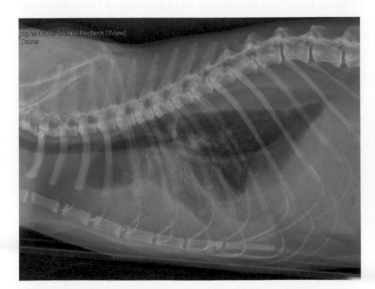

Figure 6.5.1 Pleural effusion in a cat with dilated cardiomyopathy and right-sided heart failure. This lateral radiograph shows the presence of pleural fluid obscuring the cardiac silhouette and rounding of the lung margins. The elevation of the trachea suggests cardiomegaly and possible underlying cardiac disease as an etiology for the pleural effusion.

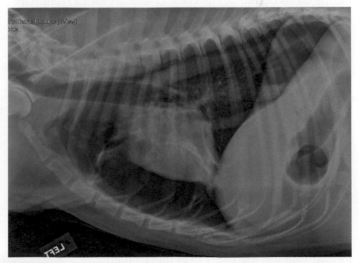

Figure 6.5.3 Lateral radiograph of a dog with pneumothorax showing elevation of the cardiac silhouette and gas opacity with no identifiable blood vessels between the sternum and the ventral margin of the heart.

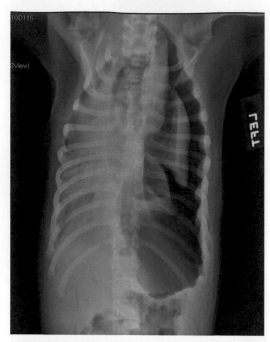

Figure 6.5.4 VD radiograph of a 6-month-old puppy with right-sided pneumothorax with secondary lung lobe collapse showing the retraction of the peripheral lung margins from the thoracic wall and the presence of avascular gas opacity (free air) filling the pleural space and compressing the lung lobes.

Other diagnostic tests and biopsy techniques

Thoracocentesis, or aspiration of the pleural space, is an important technique for both diagnosis and treatment of pleural space disease. It can be performed with a 22G needle and syringe, a butterfly catheter, or an over-the-needle intravenous catheter. Because metal needles may pose a greater risk for lacerating lung during thoracocentesis, especially in animals with a rapid respiratory rate so that the lung moves past the needle frequently during the procedure, the use of soft over-the-needle catheters is preferred for more prolonged aspiration of pleural space (therapeutic removal of air or fluid to restore respiratory function). Thoracocentesis can usually be performed in awake animals and often results in rapid improvement in respiration and anxiety level in patients with significant volumes of pleural air or fluid that are relieved by aspiration. See Chapter 14 for a detailed description of the procedure.

Thoracoscopy is another technique that may contribute to assessment, and sometimes to treatment of, patients with pleural disease. It requires general anesthesia and is generally performed similarly to laparoscopy with rigid endoscopes. Thoracoscopy provides direct visualization of structures in the thoracic cavity and allows diagnostic and therapeutic procedures to be performed with less morbidity than thoracotomy.

Treatment

Treatment of pleural disease involves two main components:

1) immediate "symptomatic" care of restoring ventilatory function and oxygenation by removing pleural fluid or air and

2) treating the underlying cause of the pleural disease, that is, definitive treatment; this varies widely depending on the specific diagnosis.

Pleural effusion

Pleural effusion, or abnormal accumulation of fluid in the pleural space, is further classified according to the character of the fluid: transudate, modified transudate, exudate, hemorrhagic (hemothorax), or chylous (chylothorax). This is a diagnostically useful classification as specific types of effusion are associated with a particular subset of differentials. Transudates are seen with diseases that cause increased capillary hydrostatic pressure (congestive heart failure, pericardial effusion/cardiac tamponade, PTE, heartworm disease) or decreased vascular oncotic pressure/hypoproteinemia (protein-losing enteropathy, protein-losing nephropathy, liver failure). Cardiac disease and hypoalbuminemic states are the most common causes of pleural transudate accumulation. Modified transudates (transudates modified by additional protein or cells) occur in conditions associated with increased vascular permeability/vasculitis (systemic infectious or inflammatory conditions), increased lymphatic permeability (inflammatory disease, lymphatic neoplasia), or increased hydrostatic pressure (lung lobe torsion, diaphragmatic hernia) and also result from the long-standing presence of transudates. Exudates (fluid with higher protein content and cell count) occur secondary to increased vascular or lymphatic permeability or reduced lymphatic drainage and are associated with systemic infectious and inflammatory conditions including FIP, neoplasia, and chronic diaphragmatic hernia.

Treatment of pleural effusion includes removal of sufficient volume of pleural fluid to relieve respiratory distress (thoracocentesis, chest tube placement) and treatment of the underlying cause. Diuretics may be beneficial in reducing hydrostatic pressure that contributes to fluid accumulation but do not reduce pleural fluid that has already formed. Hypoalbuminemic animals may require administration of colloids to increase vascular oncotic pressure. Removal of maximal volumes of pleural fluid may lead to further depletion of albumin and other fluid components. Residual pleural fluid is resorbed and pleural effusion resolves if the underlying cause can be remedied. In cases of chronic refractory pleural effusion, surgical procedures to divert the abnormal fluid from the pleural space (shunts to the peritoneum or venous vasculature, omentalization across the diaphragm) may be indicated. Pleurodesis (instillation of irritant chemicals such as tetracycline or talc into the pleural space to cause destruction of fluid-producing pleura and causing adhesions to form between the visceral and parietal pleura to obliterate the space where fluid can accumulate) is variably effective.

Hemothorax

Hemothorax, or accumulation of blood in the pleural space, may be secondary to trauma, ulcerated thoracic or lung masses, lung lobe torsion, PTE, or systemic coagulation disorders. Hemothorax is identified by finding blood via thoracocentesis.

Treatment includes removal of a sufficient volume of pleural blood to relieve respiratory distress and treatment of the underlying cause. Residual blood in the pleural space is expected to be rapidly reabsorbed and returned to the circulation by autotransfusion within a few days, which should be taken into consideration in determining the volume of blood to be removed by thoracocentesis (generally just enough to resolve respiratory restriction). Blood transfusion should be considered for anemic patients that remain tachypneic and tachycardic after therapeutic thoracocentesis.

Pneumothorax

Pneumothorax, or presence of free air in the pleural space, may be secondary to trauma to the lung or thoracic wall, lung disease (leakage of air from abnormal lung tissue or ruptured bulla), or pleural or lung infection with gas-forming bacteria. Spontaneous pneumothorax refers to pneumothorax not associated with trauma. Pneumothorax can also be iatrogenic as a result of injury to the lung following aspiration procedures or failure to properly maintain a seal against air entry into the pleural space with thoracocentesis or chest tube placement/maintenance. Some pleural air is expected following thoracic surgery. Air leakage from tracheal, bronchial, and esophageal lesions generally results in pneumomediastinum rather than pneumothorax. Management of pneumothorax varies depending on the severity and whether air leakage is ongoing. In patients with subclinical to mild pneumothorax, cage rest and monitoring is recommended as unnecessary thoracocentesis may disturb any fibrin seal over the region of air leakage. Pleural air will be absorbed from the pleural space over days to weeks. If respiratory compromise is present, thoracocentesis is performed and repeated as needed to maintain respiratory function. Chest tube placement and possibly continuous pleural drainage devices may be necessary if thoracocentesis is required frequently or beyond the first 24 h of presentation. Rarely, exploratory thoracotomy and surgical resection of the damaged lung is needed for nonresolving pneumothorax.

Chylothorax

Chylothorax, or accumulation of lipid-rich chyle in the pleural space, is often idiopathic or may be secondary to injury or obstruction of the thoracic duct, lymphangiectasia, granulomatous disease, heart disease (including hyperthyroidism and heartworm infection), lymphatic or mediastinal neoplasia, lung lobe torsion, or inflammatory abdominal disease (pancreatitis). Breed predispositions are reported for the Afghan hound, Shiba Inu, and Siamese and Himalayan cats. Chylothorax is diagnosed by identifying pleural fluid that is hazy to milky in appearance and has a higher triglyceride concentration than serum collected at the same time as the pleural fluid (Figures 6.5.5 and 6.5.6).

Diagnosis of chylothorax should trigger a diagnostic evaluation of a possible underlying cause and corresponding specific treatment; however, a definitive cause is often not found.

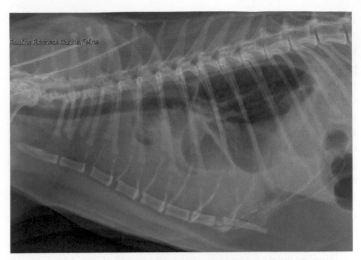

Figure 6.5.5 Pleural effusion in a cat with chylothorax. This lateral radiograph shows the presence of pleural fluid obscuring the cardiac silhouette and causing dorsal elevation of the trachea and caudodorsal displacement of the lungs with ventral scalloping of lung margins.

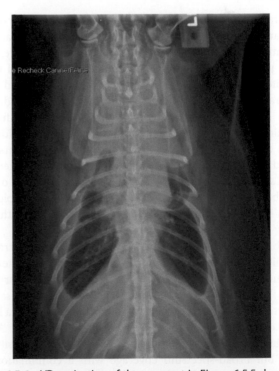

Figure 6.5.6 VD projection of the same cat in Figure 6.5.5 showing the retraction of lung lobes from the thoracic wall and the presence of soft tissue opacity (pleural fluid) in the pleural space between the thoracic wall and lung margins. The lungs are displaced caudally and the lung margins are rounded. An alveolar pattern is evident in the right cranial lung lobe, which may represent secondary atelectasis or infiltrative pulmonary disease.

Treatment includes thoracocentesis as needed to relieve respiratory distress, but removal of large volumes should be avoided because the fluid contains protein, fats, electrolytes, and lymphocytes that can become depleted through extensive and/or repeated drainage. Low fat diets are recommended to decrease the lipid content of the fluid, which may facilitate its reabsorption from the pleural space. Rutin, administered at 50–100 mg/kg PO q 8 h, may stimulate macrophage uptake of extravasated protein and thereby improve resorption of pleural fluid. Octreotide administered subcutaneously at 10 μg/kg q 8 h may decrease chyle flow through the thoracic duct, reducing the volume of chyle accumulating in the thorax, but is expensive and must be administered by injection. Chylothorax may resolve spontaneously or with treatment, but improvement takes weeks to months.

Patients not responding adequately to medical management are candidates for surgical treatment (ligation of the thoracic duct ± pericardectomy, cisterna chyli ablation, omentalization, pleuropericardial shunt placement). Fibrosing pleuritis (pleural thickening) is a potential consequence of long-standing chylothorax, which results in restriction of lung expansion and heart function, requiring removal of the abnormal pleura (decortication). Pleurodesis has sometimes been employed to treat chylothorax with limited success.

Pyothorax

Pyothorax, or accumulation of purulent pleural fluid, may occur secondary to bacterial introduction into the pleural space by penetrating thoracic wall injury, migrating foreign bodies, extension of pulmonary infections, and hematogenous spread from other sites. The most common bacterial agents associated with pyothorax are anaerobes, *Nocardia asteroides* (dogs), and *Pasteurella multocida* (cats), although other bacteria and fungal agents are reported and cytological and microbiological identification of the causative agent for each case should be pursued. Affected animals are often febrile in addition to showing general clinical signs of pleural filling. Patients with roughening of the pleura because of inflammation (pleuritis) may have a pleural friction rub evident on thoracic auscultation and pain with respiratory motion.

Pyothorax is treated by pleural drainage and administration of antibiotics. Pleural drainage is achieved by the placement of chest tubes for complete and ongoing drainage of purulent pleural fluid and lavage of the pleural space with sterile saline. In selecting a tube for placement, it is important to select a large enough diameter tube to allow drainage of thick exudates. Antimicrobial therapy should be directed by culture and sensitivity results, but broad-spectrum coverage with a combination of aminopenicillin and fluoroquinolone is appropriate pending culture results. Antibiotic therapy is usually continued for at least 4–6 weeks, longer with *Nocardia* or *Actinomyces* infections. Surgical exploration ± debridement of the thorax is indicated in patients with suspected migrating foreign bodies (based on history or the presence of *Nocardia* or *Actinomyces*) or those failing to respond adequately to medical management.

Nutritional considerations

Patients with pleural space disease may tolerate small frequent meals better than large meals because gastric filling can cause the stomach to press on and limit the excursion of the diaphragm and can further restrict thoracic and lung expansion. Patients with chylothorax should be fed a low fat diet to reduce thoracic duct flow, but, since these diets are calorie restricted and these patients have increased nutrient loss through aspirated pleural fluid, ongoing weight loss may be problematic and additional nutritional support may be necessary. Additional information can be found in the nutrition section of this chapter.

Anesthetic and analgesic considerations

Patients with pleural disease have decreased capacity for lung expansion, which impacts assisted ventilation as well as their inherent ability to ventilate. If fibrosing pleuritis is present, cardiac function may also be impaired. Additional information can be found in the anesthesia and analgesia section of this chapter.

SECTION 6 ANESTHESIC AND ANALGESIC CONSIDERATIONS IN RESPIRATORY DISEASE

Patients with respiratory disease or dysfunction can be challenging and sometimes intimidating to anesthetize. Many of the diagnostic procedures or surgical treatments involve general anesthesia. Often patients will become distressed or dyspneic with handling and require sedation for less invasive procedures—ultrasound, radiography, or even general physical exams. Specific issues pertinent to respiratory disease have been previously noted in this chapter where appropriate.

Premedication

Many anesthetic drugs have respiratory depressive effects—these side effects are usually tolerated by fairly stable patients but can be extremely significant in patients with respiratory compromise.

Phenothiazines (e.g., acepromazine) tend to have little negative effect on the respiratory system when given at low doses. Respiratory rate may slow, but patients tend to compensate with larger volume breaths. If given at higher doses, depression may occur.

Alpha-2 adrenergic agonists (e.g., dexmedetomidine) may not be the best choice for sedation. The level of respiratory depression can vary greatly and the response may be erratic. This class of drug can cause dark mucous membrane color that is unrelated to oxygenation of tissue. In patients with respiratory compromise, this can make it more difficult to visually assess potential hypoxemia.

Benzodiazepines (diazepam and midazolam) have little respiratory effect and are probably the safest choice when dealing with patients with respiratory or pulmonary compromise.

Opioids, in general, may cause respiratory depression. This is usually less so with butorphanol and buprenorphine, but those two drugs are not adequate analgesics for painful procedures. Morphine, hydromorphone, oxymorphone, and fentanyl may cause dose-dependent respiratory depression and while they should be used for patients undergoing painful procedures, they should be used with caution in especially compromised cases.

Induction

If at all possible, it is recommended to preoxygenate patients for at least 5 min before induction. This can be accomplished through a mask, nasal catheters, or an oxygen cage.

Propofol is the most common induction agent used for respiratory cases. While it does cause profound apnea when given (this is less dramatic when given slowly), the drug is eliminated very quickly and immediate intubation and assisted ventilation can negate the apnea.

Ketamine/diazepam can be used for induction, though with care. While patients usually do not become apnic after induction with this combination, they may exhibit an apneustic breathing pattern. Pharyngeal and laryngeal reflexes are still intact and laryngospasms, bronchospasms, or coughing may still occur with tracheal stimulation.

Etomidate does not typically cause much respiratory depression but can cause apnea immediately following induction. Some patients may retch or gag when given this agent.

Intubation should be performed immediately after induction. Patients with respiratory disease may have significantly compromised lung function and are less able to handle periods of apnea or hypoxia than more stable patients. Depending on the type of respiratory disorder, equipment for a tracheostomy tube may be needed. When checking the cuff or delivering an assisted breath, it is important to use caution if any kind of intrapulmonary disorder is present (e.g., pulmonary bulla, pneumothorax, flail chest) where lung expansion could be compromised. Mechanical ventilation should not exceed 20 cm of H_2O to avoid barotrauma.

Maintenance anesthesia

Isoflurane, sevoflurane, and desflurane are all acceptable choices for respiratory cases. All volatile anesthetics cause some degree of respiratory depression, often of a dose-dependent type. Nitrous oxide is not recommend for respiratory cases and in fact is contraindicated in cases such as pneumothorax. Nitrous oxide moves to internal areas of pocketing gas and will cause increasing pressure in those spaces.

Monitoring

In respiratory cases, controlling and maintaining ventilation and tissue oxygenation are going to be of utmost importance while the patient is under anesthesia. Pulse oximetry and end tidal carbon dioxide monitoring are essential tools for assessing appropriate ventilation. It is advised to check ABG levels periodically to verify adequate ventilation.

Mechanical or assisted ventilation will be necessary for most cases with pulmonary or respiratory compromise as they will be unable to achieve adequate lung expansion and maintain appropriate spontaneous ventilation.

Blood pressure monitoring via an arterial catheter is recommended for compromised cases. Not only will the invasive blood pressure monitoring give an accurate picture of the level of hypotension or normotension but it can also alert the anesthetist to the adequacy of ventilation. Excessive positive pressure ventilation can occlude venous return and may result in a state of hypotension. Alterations in the arterial waveform coinciding with the firing of the ventilator can be another clue that ventilation may be negatively affecting blood pressure.

Recovery

With few exceptions, cases with respiratory or pulmonary compromise should be recovered in a critical care unit where they can be closely monitored postoperatively.

Pulse oximetry should be monitored for as long as is feasible. If saturation falls below 95% on room air, some form of supplemental oxygen should be considered—flow by oxygen, nasal catheters, or an oxygen cage. ABGs should also be monitored in order to gain a clearer picture of ventilatory status.

Depending on the procedure, additional analgesia may be required. In order to avoid further respiratory depression, either a constant rate infusion (CRI) of fentanyl or butorphanol is recommended. If the procedure was not overly painful, the opioid agonist given can be either reversed with naloxone (which will fully reverse any analgesic provided by the opioid) or partially reversed with butorphanol (which will offer some mild analgesia but less respiratory depression). Non-steroidal anti-inflammatory drugs (NSAIDs) are an option as well for less painful procedures, as they do not adversely affect the respiratory system and offer mild pain relief.

SECTION 7 FEEDING CONSIDERATIONS FOR RESPIRATORY DISEASE

While there are no specific nutritional recommendations for animals that have either acute or chronic respiratory diseases, the value and importance of nutrition in the management of these animals should not be underestimated. Specific issues pertinent to respiratory disease have been previously noted in this chapter where appropriate.

The entire respiratory process uses many muscles and involves multiple chemical and enzymatic reactions to ensure that oxygen transfer occurs within the alveoli.

An animal with acute or chronic respiratory disease has the potential to be utilizing up to twice their normal calorie requirements. Initial caloric intake calculations are done for resting energy requirements (RER) as with other critical care hospitalized patients and adjusted based on weight changes and hydration levels.[1]

Upper GI tube placement is usually not recommended for animals with respiratory disease due to the increased incidence of vomiting and aspiration.[1] If the animal is unable to meet their caloric requirements through oral intake, then gastrostomy, jejunostomy or IV parenteral or partial–parenteral nutrition would be viable options.

Due to the difficulty with breathing, many animals are unable to consume an adequate number of calories to meet their RER or increased caloric requirements. It is difficult to eat and breathe at the same time, and most animals will chose breathing over eating. Keep in mind that many of the medications used to treat respiratory diseases may cause nausea in the animal, further decreasing their desire to consume adequate quantities of food.[2] Small meals frequently offered may help prevent vomiting associated with drug-induced nausea. An increase in appetite may also be seen when steroids are used to reduce airway inflammation—use this to your advantage by offering food frequently and monitoring the total intake of calories. It may take a couple of days to see this side effect. For animals on long-term steroid medications, there is no increased physiological need for calories, just an increased desire. A higher protein diet will not help prevent the muscle wasting commonly associated with steroid use, but this will resolve as the dose is slowly decreased over time.

To make meeting their energy requirement easier for the animal, a calorically dense, highly palatable diet is usually recommended. For most animals, this would be one of the many veterinary recovery diets. These recovery diets also have the advantage of increasing the fluid intake to help with maintaining hydration. Maintenance of airway hydration is important to facilitate mucociliary clearance.[2] Some patients will also have an increase in water loss through the respiratory process that will need to be compensated for, making a liquid recovery diet even more beneficial.

For animals with chronic respiratory diseases, weight management may need to be considered. Exercise has the benefit of helping to expand the pulmonary airways, helping in clearing out the accumulated debris in the lower airways and stimulating coughing to move the material out of the upper airways. An exercise program would need to be tailored to the individual patient's fitness level and degree of pulmonary dysfunction to keep from causing excessive respiratory effort or even death.[2] Client education in measurement of respiratory rate, assessment of mucous membrane color, and other signs of increased effort will help to improve their ability to assess their pet's status during exercise.

The key to management of patients with either acute or chronic respiratory disease is to keep them well hydrated, ensure they are receiving adequate calories in a form that they will willingly consume, and to help to move the pulmonary debris out of the airway.

Bibliography

Section 1

1. Bonagura JD, Twedt DC. *Kirk's Current Veterinary Therapy XIV*, pp. 619–621, 627–628. St. Louis, MO: Saunders Elseiver; 2009.
2. King LG. *Textbook of Respiratory Disease in Dogs and Cats*, pp. 310–338. St. Louis, MO: Saunders Elseiver; 2004.

Section 2

1. Tilley LP, Smith FWK, Jr. Mediastinitis in *The 5-Minute Veterinary Consult Canine and Feline*, 2nd edition, p. 939. Baltimore, MD: Williams & Wilkins; 2000.
2. Nelson RW, Couto CG (eds.). *Small Animal Internal Medicine*, 4th edition, St. Louis, MO: Mosby Elsevier; 2009.
3. Rogers KS, Walker MA. Disorders of the mediastinum. *Compendium on Continuing Education for the Practicing Veterinarian* 1997;19: 69–83.
4. Bauer T, Woodfield JA. Mediastinal, pleural, and extrapleural disease. In: *Veterinary Internal Medicine*, 4th edition, eds. SJ Ettinger, EC Feldman, pp. 812–842. Philadelphia, PA: W.B. Saunders; 1995.
5. Konde LJ, Spaulding K. Sonographic evaluation of the cranial mediastinum in small animals. *Journal of Veterinary Radiology and Ultrasound* 2005. DOI: 10.1111/j.1740-8261.

Section 3

1. Corcoran BM, Foster DJ, Fuentes VL. Feline asthma syndrome: a retrospective study of the clinical presentation in 29 cats. *Journal of Small Animal Practice* 1995;36:481–488.
2. Mantis P, Lamb CR, Boswood A. Assessment of the accuracy of thoracic radiography in the diagnosis of canine chronic bronchitis. *Journal of Small Animal Practice* 1998;39:518–520.
3. Herrtage M. Medical management of tracheal collapse. In: *Kirk's Current Veterinary Therapy*, 14th edition, eds. JD Bonagura, DC Twedt, pp. 630–635. Philadelphia, PA: Saunders; 2009.
4. Johnson L. Chronic bronchitis in dogs. In: *Kirk's Current Veterinary Therapy*, 14th edition, eds. JD Bonagura, DC Twedt, pp. 642–645. Philadelphia, PA: Saunders; 2009.
5. Hawkins EC. Respiratory system disorders. In: *Small Animal Internal Medicine*, 3rd edition, eds. RW Nelson, CG Couto, pp. 250–298. St. Louis, MO: Mosby; 2003.
6. Thrusfield MV, Aitken CGC, Muirhead RH. A field investigation of kennel cough: efficacy of different treatments. *Journal of Small Animal Practice* 1991;32:455.
7. Padrid P. Chronic bronchitis and asthma in cats. In: *Kirk's Current Veterinary Therapy*, 14th edition, eds. JD Bonagura, DC Twedt, pp. 650–657. Philidelphia, PA: Saunders; 2009.
8. Hawkins EC, Clay LD, Bradley JM, et al. Demographic and historical findings, including exposure to environmental tobacco smoke, in dogs with chronic cough. *Journal of Veterinary Internal Medicine* 2010;24:825–831.
9. Moise NS, Wiedenkeller D, Yeager AE, et al. Clinical, radiographic, and bronchial cytologic features of cats with bronchial disease: 65 cases (1980–1986). *Journal of the American Veterinary Medical Association* 1989;194:1467–1473.

Section 4

1. Fox PR. Approach to the coughing and dyspneic dog. Proceedings of the 32nd Annual World Small Animal Veterinary Association Congress, August 19–23, 2007, Sydney, Australia; 2007.

2. Reinero C, Cohn L. Interstitial lung diseases. *Veterinary Clinics of North America. Small Animal Practice* 2007;37(5):937–947.

3. Cohn L. Pulmonary parenchymal disease. In: *Textbook of Veterinary Internal Medicine*, 7th edition, eds. SJ Ettinger, EC Feldman, pp. 1096–1119. St. Louis, MO: Saunders Elsevier; 2010.

Section 5

1. Pawloski DR, Broaddus KD. Pneumothorax: a review. *Journal of the American Animal Hospital Association* 2010;46(6):385–397.

2. Silverstein DC. Pleural space disease. In: *Textbook of Respiratory Disease in Dogs and Cats*, ed. LG King, pp. 49–52. St. Louis, MO: Saunders Elsevier; 2004.

3. McPhail CM. Medical and surgical management of pyothorax. *Veterinary Clinics of North America. Small Animal Practice* 2007; 37(5):975–988.

4. Beatty J, Barrs V. Pleural effusion in the cat: a practical approach to determine aetiolgy. *Journal of Feline Medicine and Surgery* 2010; 12(9):693–707.

Section 6

1. Grimm K, Thurmon J, Tranquilli WJ. *Lumb and Jones Veterinary Anesthesia and Analgesia*, 4th edition, Ames, IA: Blackwell Publishing; 2007.

Section 7

1. Saker K, Remillard R. Critical care nutrition and enteral-assisted feeding. In: *Small Animal Clinical Nutrition*, 5th edition, eds. MS Hand, CD Thatcher, RL Remillard, P Roudebush, BJ Novotny, pp. 439–445. Topeka, KS: Mark Morris Institute; 2010.

2. Hawkins E. Disorders of the trachea and bronchi. In: *Small Animal Internal Medicine*, 4th edition, eds. R Nelson, CG Couto, pp. 285–290. St. Louis, MO: Mosby Elsevier; 2009.

Chapter 7 Hematology

Editors: Jennifer Garcia and Rhonda South-Bodiford

SECTION 1 ANATOMY AND PHYSIOLOGY

The circulatory system

The function of the cardiovascular system is to provide nutrient fluid (blood), oxygen, immune substances, hormones, and chemicals to distant tissues and to remove tissue waste products and carbon dioxide. Regulation of temperature and normal water and electrolyte balance is also controlled by the cardiovascular system. The heart is the central muscular organ that pumps blood through a network of joined vessels (arteries, veins, and capillaries). The lymphatic system also assists the return of fluid from the interstitial spaces back to the blood via the venous system.

The heart lies in the mediastinum and is surrounded by lungs. The rib cage protects both the heart and the lungs. The anatomy of the heart consists of the outer pericardium, the myocardium, and the inner layer, the endocardium. The pericardium has two layers, the fibrous pericardium and the serous pericardium. The fibrous pericardium is the outer layer made of fibrous connective tissue and is loosely attached to the diaphragm. The serous pericardium has two layers, the parietal layer and the visceral layer. The parietal layer lies between the fibrous pericardium and the visceral layer. The visceral layer is also called the epicardium and is closely attached to the myocardium. A thin fluid cavity exists between the parietal and visceral layers. This fluid acts as a lubricant allowing the heart to smoothly expand and contract. If this fluid space fills with excessive fluid, this pericardial effusion may interfere with the normal heart function. The increased pressure to the right heart results in the collapse of the right atrium causing pericardial tamponade. If the pericardial effusion is left untreated, right heart failure usually occurs. The myocardium is the thickest layer of the heart and consists of cardiac muscle fibers. Cardiac muscle cells are involuntary striated cells with end-to-end attachments called intercalated disks. The intercalated disks allow transmission of impulses from cell to cell, resulting in large groups of cardiac cells to contract in unison forming a syncytium. The endocardium is a thin membranous lining of the heart chambers.

Small Animal Internal Medicine for Veterinary Technicians and Nurses, First Edition. Edited by Linda Merrill.
© 2012 John Wiley & Sons, Inc. Published 2012 by John Wiley & Sons, Inc.

There are four chambers of the heart (right atrium, right ventricle, left atrium, and left ventricle). The heart is a "two-pump" organ. The low pressure right heart pumps blood through the lungs, and the left heart pumps blood to the peripheral organs. The atrium functions as a weak primer pump, while the ventricle is a much stronger pump propelling blood to the tissues.

Deoxygenated blood is received into the right atrium from the systemic and coronary veins. From the right atrium, the blood passes through the tricuspid valve into the right ventricle. The right ventricle contracts during systole, and the tricuspid valve closes to prevent backflow of the blood into the right atrium. The blood is pumped through the pulmonary valve into the pulmonary arteries. The blood continues through branching arteries to the pulmonary capillaries of the alveoli where oxygen exchange occurs. Oxygenated blood travels through merging vessels that terminate into the pulmonary veins. The pulmonary veins deliver oxygenated blood to the left atrium. Oxygenated blood then travels through the mitral valve to the left ventricle. During systole, the mitral valve closes and oxygenated blood is pumped through the aorta (the largest artery in the body). From the aorta, the blood flows from the arterial branches to the capillaries of the tissues.

There are two basic means of regulation of the heart pump. First, the intrinsic cardiac regulation occurs in response to blood volume flowing into the heart. The intrinsic ability of the heart to adapt to changing volumes of blood is called the *Frank–Starling* mechanism, which states that the greater the heart muscle is stretched during filling, the greater the force of contraction and the greater the quantity of blood pumped into the aorta. And second, the control of heart rate is determined by the autonomic nervous system. Stimulation of the sympathetic nerves can increase the heart rate and force of contraction, which increases cardiac output. Inhibition of the sympathetic nervous system can decrease heart rate and cardiac output. Parasympathetic (vagal) stimulation will slow the heart rate with minimal effect on the strength of the contraction.

The transport of nutrients to the tissues and the removal of cellular waste occur in the microcirculation. The capillaries are thin-walled vessels consisting of highly permeable endothelial cells. The blood flow is not continuous in the capillaries. The intermittent blood flow is caused by vasomotion (intermittent contractions of the metarteriole and precapillary sphincters). Each tissue has the ability to control local blood flow, and this occurs in proportion to metabolic needs. Tissues with greater metabolism (i.e., liver and kidney) have greater blood flow through the capillary bed. In the resting state, the metabolic activity of muscles is very low, resulting in low blood flow during this time.

The lymphatic system

The lymphatic system includes a network of vessels that carry lymph (a fluid similar in composition to that of interstitial fluid) to the bloodstream. The four major functions of the lymphatic system include (1) removal of excessive tissue fluid, (2) transport of waste materials to the blood, (3) filtration of lymph fluid by the lymph nodes, and (4) transport of large proteins (i.e., enzymes) to the bloodstream. The lymphatics carry proteins and large particulate matter away from tissue spaces, neither of which can be removed by direct absorption into the blood capillaries. Most tissues have lymph channels that usually align with veins. There are no lymph vessels in the brain, spinal cord, bone marrow, or skeletal muscle. The lymphatic channel is a thin-walled vessel with one-way valves. The larger lymphatic vessels are surrounded by smooth muscle and a fibrous adventitia (outer connective tissue covering). Although there are occasional intrinsic pulsations of the lymph vessels, the flow of lymph fluid depends on the movement of adjacent muscles. The lymphatic channels from the caudal body flow to the thoracic duct. The thoracic duct terminates in the vena cava.

Lymph fluid is formed when excessive interstitial fluid accumulates in the tissue. Lymphocytes are the primary cell of the lymphatic fluid when the fluid reaches the thoracic duct. Lymph from the digestive tract is known as chyle. Chyle contains microscopic particles of fat (chylomicrons).

The lymphatic structures include thymus, tonsils, gut-associated lymph tissue (GALT), lymph nodes, and spleen. The thymus is located in the caudal neck and cranial thoracic region. This organ is prominent in young animals and regresses as the animal matures. The tonsils are found in the pharyngeal region and function to prevent spread of infection to the respiratory and digestive tracts. They differ from lymph nodes in several ways. First, tonsils are found close to moist epithelial surfaces. Second, tonsils do not have a capsule. And third, tonsils are found at the beginning of a lymph drainage system but not along the lymphatic channel as are the lymph nodes. GALT is lymphoid tissue found in the lining of the intestines (mucosa and submucosa). B lymphocytes are processed through the GALT system prior to being sent to the peripheral lymphoid tissue.

The lymph nodes are small kidney bean-shaped encapsulated structures located along the lymphatic vessels. See Figure 7.1.1 for the location of common peripheral lymph nodes. The two major functions of lymph nodes include (1) the filtering of particulate material from lymph fluid and (2) the participation in immunologic processes (i.e., stimulation of B and T cells). Microscopic evaluation of the lymph node demonstrates an outer capsule and internal framework of septa and trabeculae. Internally, the lymph node contains a poorly defined cortex and medulla. Tissue macrophages are embedded in a coarse, fibrous mesh of the medulla. The cortex contains lymph nodules. T cells reside in the paracortical areas and B cells are found in the central germinal centers of the lymphoid follicles.

The spleen

The spleen is the largest lymphoid organ in the body. This tongue-shaped organ is located on the left side of the abdomen and has both lymphatic and hematologic functions. The spleen

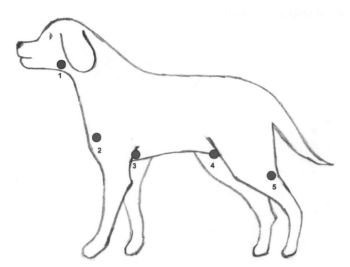

Figure 7.1.1 Location of the common lymph nodes (LNs) in the dog. 1, submandibular LN; 2, prescapular LN; 3, axillary LN; 4, inguinal LN; 5, popliteal LN.

has multiple functions including storage of blood, removal of foreign material from circulation, removal of dead, dying, and abnormal red blood cells (RBCs), and lymphocyte cloning during an immune response.

The capsule of the spleen is made of a fibrous connective tissue and smooth muscle. Trabeculae are branches of the capsule that contain blood vessels, nerves, lymph vessels, and smooth muscle cells. It is through these channels that blood is pumped in and out of the spleen. The interior of the spleen is made up of white and red pulps. The white pulp consists of lymphoid tissue that responds to immunologic challenges. The red pulp consists of blood vessels, tissue macrophages, and blood storage spaces (sinuses). In normal circumstances, the spleen can store 10–20% of the total blood volume. Certain drugs (i.e., tranquilizers and barbiturates) can relax the smooth muscle of the capsule and increase splenic pooling by up to 30% of the blood volume.

The coagulation system

Hemostasis is defined as the prevention of blood loss and is a complex series of mechanisms that maintain the integrity of a closed circulatory system. Injury to a blood vessel results in activation of the hemostatic system. Immediately after trauma, the vessel starts to contract and reduces blood flow. This vascular spasm is the first step in coagulation. The next step is the formation of the platelet plug. Exposure of the subendothelial surface by vessel trauma results in rapid platelet adhesion. The adhesion of platelets to the endothelial wall is mediated by adhesive proteins (i.e., von Willebrand factor [vWF] and fibrinogen) and allows for the formation of the platelet plug. The platelet plug is short-lived (seconds) and unstable. This primary hemostatic

plug, however, serves as the framework for clot formation. Secondary hemostasis is the development of the clot or thrombus coordinated by a tightly controlled and well-balanced interplay of hemostatic proteins. Coagulation also initiates fibrinolysis (clot removal) to restore blood flow (Table 7.1.1).

The coagulation models for the clotting cascade include the extrinsic, intrinsic, and common pathways (see Figure 7.1.2). The extrinsic pathway occurs with the release of tissue procoagulants (tissue factor [TF]). Factor X is generated via the complex of TF and factor VIIa. The intrinsic pathway consists of the contact activation of factor XII followed by the activation of factors XIa, IXa, and VIIIa. The contact pathway consists of factor XII, prekallikrein, and the cofactor high molecular weight kininogen. The role of this pathway *in vivo* is questionable as animals with factor XII deficiency have no bleeding tendencies. The common pathway consists of the formation of factors Xa and Va and the generation of thrombin. The function of thrombin is the conversion of fibrinogen to fibrin. Factor XIIIa is critical for normal clot strength and stability. The classification of the clotting cascade into these pathways is a useful model for *in vitro* laboratory evaluation; however, such divisions do not occur *in vivo*.

Fibrinolysis is defined as clot dissolution and is necessary to restore blood flow. Plasminogen, a protein synthesized by the liver, is converted to plasmin via plasminogen activators (tissue plasminogen activator [tPA] and urokinase plasminogen activator [uPA]). Excess plasmin formation can lead to spontaneous bleeding due to excessive fibrinolysis. Plasminogen activator inhibitors (plasminogen activator inhibitor 1, alpha 2-antiplasmin, and thrombin activatable fibrinolysis inhibitor) will prevent fibrinolysis leading to thrombosis. Fibrin degradation products (FDPs) result from the breakdown of fibrin. FDPs can be measured and may be useful in diagnosing disseminated intravascular coagulation (DIC).

SECTION 2 RED BLOOD CELL DISORDERS

Anemia

Anemia can be defined as a decrease in RBC concentration, a decrease in hemoglobin concentration or as a decrease in hematocrit (HCT) or packed cell volume (PCV). Anemias are usually associated with a decrease in oxygen carrying capacity. In small animals, anemia is classified as regenerative or nonregenerative. This is determined by assessing the number of polychromatophils present. Anemias are normally a secondary manifestation of a primary disease state and are not considered a primary disease.[1] A decrease in RBC concentration may be divided into a set of categories. It may present due to a lack of production (aplasia), an increase in destruction (such as an immune-mediated destruction), blood loss (trauma), or a combination of any of these. Animals may present with pale

Table 7.1.1   Summary of the hemostatic proteins in the various coagulation pathways

Pathway	Factor	Other name	Function
Extrinsic	Tissue factor	Thromboplastin	Cofactor
	Factor VII	Proconvertin	Inactive precursor
	Factor VIIa		Active enzyme
Contact	Factor XII	Hageman factor	Inactive precursor
	Factor XIIa		Active enzyme
	Prekallikrein	Fletcher factor	Inactive precursor
	Kallikrein		Active enzyme
	High molecular weight kininogen		Cofactor
Intrinsic	Factor XI		Inactive precursor
	Factor XIa		Active enzyme
	Factor IX	Christmas factor	Inactive precursor
	Factor IXa		Active enzyme
	Factor VIII		Procofactor
	Factor VIIIa		Cofactor
Common	Factor X		Inactive precursor
	Factor Xa		Active enzyme
	Factor V		Procofactor
	Factor Va		Cofactor
	Prothrombin	Factor II	Inactive precursor
	Fibrinogen	Factor I	Substrate
	Fibrin		Final product
	Factor XIII		Inactive precursor
	Factor XIIIa		Active enzyme
Fibrinolysis	Plasminogen		Inactive precursor
	Plasmin		Active enzyme

mucous membranes, exercise intolerance, rapid respiration, and/or collapse.

Regenerative anemia

A regenerative anemia is assessed by the presence of increased numbers of polychromatophils in circulation.[2] Polychromatophils are visualized on microscopy with Wright's stain. They will stain pale to moderately basophilic (Figure 7.2.1).

If a new methylene blue stain is utilized on a dog's blood, the polychromatophils will be visualized with aggregates of RNA in the cytoplasm. These cells are called reticulocytes.

Felines have two types of reticulocytes: punctate and aggregate.[3] In this text, an aggregate reticulocyte will be used synonymously with polychromatophil (Figure 7.2.2).

Polychromatophils usually have more volume than a mature RBC and thus have a larger mean corpuscular volume (MCV).

They carry less hemoglobin or have incomplete hemoglobin synthesis and therefore have a decreased mean corpuscular hemoglobin concentration (MCHC). When a complete blood count (CBC) is performed, these RBC indices accompany the HCT. A regenerative anemia is often classified as a macrocytic hypochromic anemia. However, not all regenerative anemias will fit neatly into these classifications and not all macrocytic hypochromic anemias are regenerative. Measuring reticulocyte numbers is recommended in order to properly assess the regenerative response. Most veterinary laboratories will automatically perform an automated reticulocyte count on small animals if the calculated HCT falls below a predetermined number.

In canines, reticulocyte concentration will begin to increase within 2–4 days post-RBC loss or destruction and will peak within 7–10 days.[4] With the development of anemia due to blood loss or destruction, erythropoietin (EPO) will stimulate erythroid blast-forming units and committed stem cells in the

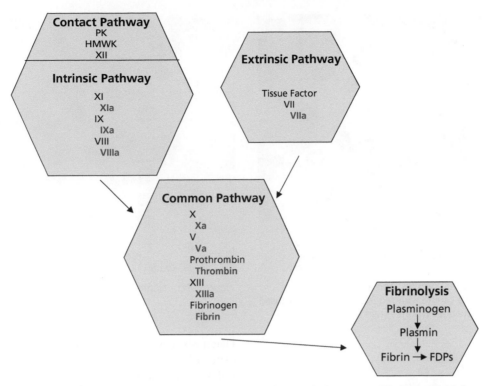

Figure 7.1.2 The coagulation pathways. PK, prekallikrein; HMWK, high molecular weight kininogen; XII, factor XII; XI, factor XI; XIa, activated factor XI; IX, factor IX; IXa, activated factor IX; VIII, factor VIII; VIIIa, activated factor VIII; VII, factor VII; VIIa, activated factor VII; X, factor X; Xa, activated factor X; V, factor V; Va, activated factor V; XIII, factor XIII; XIIIa, activated factor XIII; FDP, fibrin degradation product.

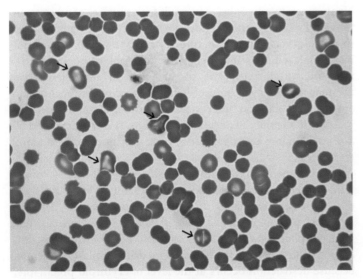

Figure 7.2.1 Polychromatophils (arrows) in a canine with regenerative anemia. Wright's stain.

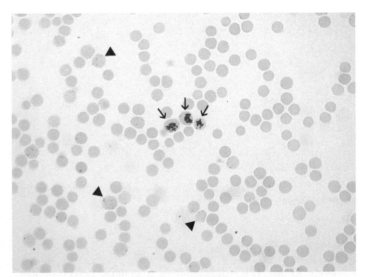

Figure 7.2.2 Aggregate reticulocytes (arrows) and punctate reticulocyte (arrowhead) in a feline with regenerative anemia. New methylene blue stain.

bone marrow, resulting in an increase in erythroid production (Figure 7.2.3).

EPO is also important in preventing apoptosis (programmed cell death) of these progenitor cells and in increasing the mass of erythroid precursors.[5] In the adult, EPO is produced by renal interstitial cells within the kidneys in response to hypoxia.[1]

With blood loss or increased destruction of the RBC, anemia will develop. With the resulting decrease in oxygen carrying ability, renal interstitial cells will produce EPO. The EPO will stimulate increased erythroid production by stimulating burst forming unit-erythroid (BFU-E) and colony forming unit-erythroid (CFU-E) cells and by decreasing apoptosis.[5] Reticulocytes will enter circulation within 2–4 days post insult and will peak within 7–10 days. The increase in aggregate reticulocytes in response to the anemia is classified as a regenerative anemia (Figure 7.2.4).

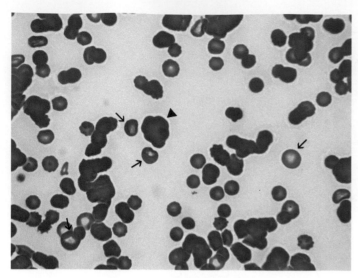

Figure 7.2.3 Polychromatophils (arrows) and agglutinating erythrocytes (arrowhead) in a canine with regenerative anemia caused by immune-mediated destruction. Wright's stain.

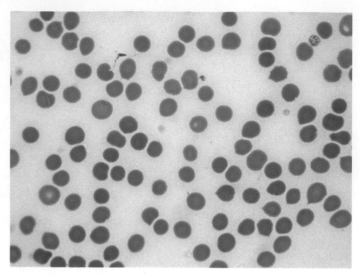

Figure 7.2.5 Nonregenerative anemia in a canine. Wright's stain.

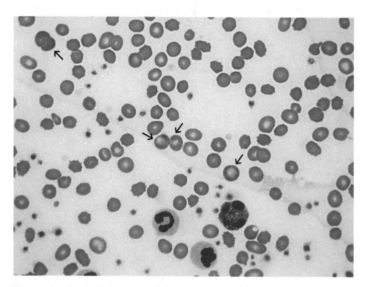

Figure 7.2.4 Polychromatophils (arrows) in a feline with regenerative anemia. Wright's stain.

Pyruvate kinase deficiency

Pyruvate kinase (PK) deficiency is a genetic defect of RBC metabolism where the lack of PK leads to shortened RBC life span, resulting in a strongly regenerative anemia. PK deficiency is seen in basenjis, West Highland white terriers, cairn terriers, pugs, Chihuahuas, miniature poodles, and many other breeds.[6] The dogs present clinically at a few months of age with exercise intolerance and weakness. Mucous membranes will be pale on exam. CBC will reveal a HCT that may range from 12% to 28% and a reticulocyte count of up to 90%.[7] In PK-deficient dogs, RBC half-life may be as little as 5–6 days. MCV is often increased due to the marked increase in reticulocytes. Affected dogs have a shortened life span, normally succumbing within 1–5 years of age. Most die from complications of anemia or hepatic failure.

Diagnosis may be made by imaging of the long bones with evidence of osteosclerosis. Bone marrow samples may be of low cellularity due to progressive myelofibrosis and osteosclerosis.[8] Affected dogs are normally treated symptomatically.

Nonregenerative anemia

Nonregenerative anemias may result for a number of reasons. In these instances, the anemia does not have a concomitant increase in reticulocytes and the mature erythrocyte population is not being replaced. This may occur due to a lack of bone marrow response or chronicity of the anemia. In nonregenerative anemias, reticulocytes are not increased in circulation. Aplastic anemia is a condition that can lead to nonregenerative anemia.[4]

Aplastic anemia can affect dogs and cats. It is characterized by a severe, nonregenerative, normocytic, normochromic anemia (Figure 7.2.5).

Aplastic anemia may result as a primary or secondary condition. Primary aplastic anemia in canines is found to be the result of an immune-mediated disorder that targets and destroys erythroid precursors in the bone marrow.[9] These animals may have peripheral erythroid agglutination, positive Coombs test, and/or spherocytes.[7] In immune-mediated aplastic anemia, because destruction occurs at the level of erythroid precursors, reticulocytes will not be present in circulation. Bone marrow exam may reveal an increase in phagocytosis of rubricytes and metarubricytes. This may result in maturation arrest at the level of rubriblast or prorubricyte stages.[7] In severe cases or in animals with chronicity, aplasia of the erythroid line may be evident in the bone marrow. As primary aplastic anemia is the result of immune-mediated destruction, animals are often treated with immunosuppressive drugs.[4]

Secondary anemia

Secondary aplastic anemias may result for various reasons, such as toxins, drugs, and estrogens. Immunosuppressive drugs and chemotherapeutic agents may lead to reversible aplastic anemias. In these situations, the stem cells within the bone marrow are damaged, but with the cessation of the drugs, the effect may be reversed.

Viruses such as feline leukemia virus (FeLV) may result in aplastic anemia.[4] FeLV may cause pure red cell aplasia or hypoplasia. It may also cause dysplastic maturation within the RBC line. Macrocytosis without regeneration may be present.

In canines, *Ehrlichia canis* can cause immune-mediated destruction of progenitor cells of the erythroid line within the bone marrow, resulting in aplastic anemia. *E. canis* may also lead to immune-mediated destruction of RBC in circulation. Diagnosis of *E. canis* should be made by serology or polymerase chain reaction (PCR). The organism is not readily seen on blood smears.[10]

Polycythemia

Polycythemia is an increase in erythrocyte concentration. This is normally indicated as an increase in PCV and/or HCT, hemoglobin concentration, or RBC count. If only RBC parameters are increased, it is more appropriate to label it as erythrocytosis. Polycythemia is more appropriately used to indicate an increase in multiple cell lines. In this text, as in common usage, the term "polycythemia" will be used to indicate an increase in RBC parameters. Polycythemia can be classified as either relative polycythemia or absolute polycythemia.[11]

Relative polycythemia

Relative polycythemia is usually due to fluid shifts or redistribution of RBCs in circulation.[12] Fluid shifting is most commonly due to dehydration. Redistribution of RBC in circulation is commonly associated with splenic contraction.

Absolute polycythemia

Absolute polycythemia is the result of an actual increase in RBC mass. This can be further classified into primary or secondary.[13]

Primary polycythemia

Primary polycythemia is also called polycythemia vera and is the result of a primary myeloproliferative disorder of the bone marrow that results in increased RBC production independent of EPO levels.[13] It is an unregulated production of the erythroid line resulting in an increase in PCV. The erythroid line will often appear without morphological abnormalities.

Secondary polycythemia

Secondary polycythemia usually occurs secondarily to other pathological conditions such as hypoxia or hypoxemia that results in a decrease in the partial pressure of oxygen (PaO_2). As a compensatory response to decreased PaO_2, the body will stimulate an increase in RBC mass. Conditions such as heart or chronic lung disease and congenital heart defects may lead to secondary polycythemia. Secondary polycythemia is also seen with animals living at high altitudes and renal masses such as renal cysts.

Diagnosis

In order to diagnose polycythemia and to differentiate it from relative, secondary, and primary polycythemia, one should assess the hydration status of the patient. If the animal is not dehydrated and an increase in PCV, HCT, or hemoglobin persists, the next step would be to measure PaO_2 and EPO levels. Within the United States at the time of this writing, commercial testing for EPO is not currently available. Testing is offered in the United Kingdom. EPO levels would be beneficial in aiding and classifying polycythemic conditions, but this is not necessary. In relative polycythemia, PaO_2 levels and EPO levels would fall within reference intervals for that species. Secondary polycythemia resulting from hypoxia or hypoxemia would have low PaO_2 levels and increased EPO levels. Primary (absolute) polycythemia (polycythemia vera) would have PaO_2 levels within reference intervals, and EPO levels may be within reference intervals or decreased.[10]

Treatment

Treatment should be aimed at the underlying pathology. If the animal is suffering from relative polycythemia due to dehydration, appropriate fluid therapy should be implemented. In animals with secondary polycythemia resulting in hypoxia or hypoxemia, diagnosing and treating the underlying disease or congenital abnormality is critical. A veterinary oncologist should be consulted if primary absolute polycythemia (polycythemia vera) is suspected or diagnosed.[10]

Transfusion medicine

The administration of blood and blood components is common among veterinary practices today, and it is most often the job of the veterinary technician to be responsible for the collection, handling, and administration of these life-saving products. This makes it important for the veterinary technician to be familiar with techniques and monitoring protocols in order to reduce the likelihood of potentially fatal transfusion reactions and/or transfusion failures. These adverse events can be minimized by careful product selection, donor screening, and careful monitoring of patients during administration.

Blood products

One of the best advances in transfusion medicine over the past few decades is the increasing availability of veterinary component products through commercial blood banking facilities. Component products are separated out from fresh whole blood (FWB) and can be used to treat very specific disorders. These products allow the veterinarian to tailor transfusion therapy to each patient's specific needs. This also allows for a higher yield of products from a single unit of whole blood and decreases the volume administered to each patient when indicated.

Whole blood

Whole blood products are either considered FWB or stored whole blood (SWB). The most common use for whole blood products is in the patient with acute blood loss, but it can be used for a variety of other disorders. The main benefits of whole blood administration are the replacement of RBCs, plasma proteins, and intravascular volume expansion. It must be noted that whole blood should not be used in patients with a normal or increased volume status due to the risk of fluid overload in these animals. See the administration guidelines later in this chapter for more information on the administration of whole blood products.

Whole blood is considered "fresh" for up to 24h after phlebotomy.[14] FWB consists of anticoagulants, RBCs, white blood cells (WBCs), platelets, plasma, and coagulation factors. FWB is usually used when stored products are not available, and/or when platelets are required. The advantages of using FWB are that platelets and coagulation factors remain intact. This may be beneficial in cases where acute blood loss is due to platelet disorders (thrombocytopenia or thrombocytopathia) or other coagulopathies. Platelet circulation time (posttransfusion) is dramatically decreased after 6–8h of refrigeration, and the hemostatic ability of platelets is completely lost after 72h of refrigeration.[15] The disadvantages of FWB are usually related to the collection process. Identification and screening of a suitable donor (if not immediately available) and the process of collection can delay the time until administration to the recipient.

SWB has been kept refrigerated (1–6°C) and differs from FWB in that platelets are destroyed within 24–72h (many are not viable after 6–8h), and some clotting factors (V and VIII within 2–4h) are lost during storage. The common use for SWB is acute blood loss due to trauma or surgery. When stored properly, the therapeutic properties of SWB remain viable for 21–35 days depending upon the anticoagulant used. Blood that has been at room temperature for 30min must be infused within 6h or returned to the refrigerator and relabeled with an expiration of 24h. Blood that has become discolored should be considered contaminated and discarded regardless of proper storage.

The dose and rate of administration of SWB and FWB are based upon the volume status of the patient. In the case of acute hemorrhage, these products can be administered at a rate to match the patient's current and ongoing losses. With the availability of packed red blood cells (pRBCs), whole blood may no longer be the preferred product to correct anemia in the normovolemic patient but might still be used in cases where pRBCs are not accessible. In these cases, caution must be used to prevent a life-threatening volume overload state. This is achieved by careful calculation of the patient's volume requirements, monitoring respiratory rate and pattern, and monitoring central venous pressure in at-risk patients. If used to correct anemia, the volume calculation for whole blood administration is as follows:

$$\text{Volume of donor blood (mL)} = \frac{\text{Recipient weight (kg)} \times [85\,(\text{dog})\,\text{or}\,60\,(\text{cat})] \times \text{desired recipient PCV} - \text{current PCV}}{\text{PCV of donor blood}}.$$

An inline blood filter (180–220 microns) should always be used during administration to eliminate any microaggregates that may have formed during storage.

Packed red blood cells

pRBCs contain RBCs, an anticoagulant, and a red cell nutrient. This product is commonly used in veterinary practices today and allows administration of the oxygen carrying capabilities of RBCs without the extra volume of plasma in whole blood products. pRBCs are often used for the treatment of symptomatic anemia in the normovolemic or hypovolemic patient. It should be noted that pRBCs do not contain viable platelets or coagulation factors; therefore, pRBCs should not be considered in patients suspected to have these deficits. pRBCs are stored in the refrigerator (1–6°C) and remain viable for up to 42 days, depending upon the type of red cell nutrient used. A single unit of pRBCs usually contains 125mL of RBCs in addition to a red cell preservative. A feline unit contains 20mL of RBCs plus a preservative.

Plasma

Plasma is the liquid portion of whole blood after the RBCs have been removed. It contains proteins, clotting factors, albumin, and immunoglobulins. The benefit of plasma products is that it allows us to administer these blood components to patients without the added volume of RBCs, which can lead to hyperviscosity, polycythemia, and the potential adverse effects of exposure to large volumes of red cell antigens. Canine single units usually contain 120mL of plasma product. Mini (60mL) and double (240mL) units are available from some commercial blood banking facilities. Feline single units usually contain about 20mL of plasma.

Fresh frozen plasma

Fresh frozen plasma (FFP) consists of all plasma proteins, albumin, and immunoglobulins contained in FWB, in addition to clotting factors (VIII, IX, X, and II). To be considered FFP, it must be separated from the FWB within 8h of collection and is given a shelf life of 1 year when stored at −18°C or colder. Common uses for FFP in dogs and cats are the replacement of labile and/or nonlabile clotting factors, and conditions that may benefit from immunoglobulin administration such as canine parvovirus enteritis.[16]

Frozen plasma

FFP is considered frozen plasma (FP) after 1 year of storage. Labile clotting factors (factors V, VII, and vWF) are lost. The plasma proteins, albumin, and immunoglobulins remain useful for an additional 4 years when stored at or below −18°C. FP can also be plasma that was separated and frozen more than 8h after collection. Common uses for FP are disorders that may benefit from immunoglobulins such as acute pancreatitis and canine parvovirus enteritis or conditions that may benefit from nonlabile clotting factors.

Cryoprecipitate

Cryoprecipitate is the precipitate of FFP after slow defrosting. It contains factor VIII, fibrinogen, fibronectin, vWF, and a small quantity of other plasma proteins. Cryoprecipitate is commonly used in the treatment of hemorrhage due to von Willebrand's syndrome and hemophilia A (factor VII deficiency). An advantage of cryoprecipitate is that the high concentration allows for low volume administration for patients at risk of volume overload. Cryoprecipitate is stable for up to 1 year when stored at −18°C.

New lyophilized (freeze-dried) cryoprecipitate has recently become available. Its uses include pretreatment of von Willebrand or hemophilia A patients prior to surgical procedures and as a topical hemostatic agent.

Cryoprecipitate poor plasma

Cryoprecipitate poor plasma (CRYOPP) or cryosupernatant is the plasma supernatant that is left after the removal of the cryoprecipitate. It contains most of the nonlabile clotting factors, albumin, immunoglobulins, and antithrombin III. Common uses of CRYOPP are the treatment of vitamin K-dependent coagulopathy and patients that will benefit from immunoglobulins as with FP and FFP. Cryosupernatants remain stable for up to 5 years when stored at −4 to 6°C, such as with FP.

Frozen platelet concentrate

Frozen platelet concentrate is collected using plateletpheresis and contains FP and DMSO as a preservative. It is used to treat disorders causing thrombocytopenia or thrombocytopathia but may not be the treatment of choice because many of these patients need the replacement of RBCs and plasma volume due to blood loss. This product can be stored for up to 6 months in the freezer (−20°C). This product should be administered slowly (over 1–2h) to prevent bradycardia due to the DMSO. A 2008 *in vitro* study showed a decrease in platelet quantity and function of this product when compared to fresh platelet-rich plasma (PRP).[17]

Platelet-rich plasma

PRP contains platelets, plasma, some leukocytes, and anticoagulant. PRP is separated from the whole blood unit within 2h of collection and has a shelf life of up to 72h under refrigeration, but the viability of the platelets can be dramatically reduced after 6–8h. Indications for the use of PRP include thrombocytopenias due to decreased production and thrombocytopathias. The use of this product for immune-mediated thrombocytopenia (IMT) is not recommended as the platelets will be readily destroyed.

Canine albumin

Lyophilized canine albumin has recently become available. This product is prepared from FFP and can be used for the temporary management of hypoproteinemia and/or hypovolemic shock until the underlying disorder can be corrected. This product is stable for up to 15 months under refrigeration (4–6°C) and for 24h after rehydration. It is important to note that lyophilized canine albumin is hyperosmolar, and careful monitoring should be provided to avoid volume overload in at-risk patients. In addition, this product should not be used in patients with dehydration or anemia without appropriate therapy to correct these conditions.

Donor selection

Careful donor selection is important for two reasons—to minimize risk of harm to the recipient as well as to the donor animal. There are many criteria to consider when selecting a donor.

Size

It is generally accepted that dogs and cats can donate up to 10% of their blood volume without any clinically significant deleterious effects. Up to 20% blood volume can be collected, but this may cause a decrease in arterial blood pressure, heart rate, and PCV. Volume replacement in the form of intravenous crystalloid administration might help to offset these effects when close to 20% blood volume is collected. Blood volume is approximately 90 mL/kg in dogs and 66 mL/kg in cats. Cats should weigh at least 4.5 kg and dogs at least 30 kg in order to donate a complete unit of blood (50 mL/cat, 500 mL/dog).

Packed cell volume

PCV should be checked on all donor animals prior to each blood collection. This is to prevent life-threatening anemia to the donor and to optimize the benefit to the recipient. Dogs should have a PCV >40% and cats >35%. Iron supplementation should be considered in all donors that are regularly used to prevent an iron deficiency anemia. Most patients can donate once every 4–6 weeks without developing anemia.

In 2005, the American College of Veterinary Internal Medicine published its consensus statement on *Canine and Feline Blood Donor Screening for Infectious Disease.*[18] The statement gives an overview of vector-borne and non-vector-borne diseases that may be transmitted through blood product transfusion and recommended testing modalities. Recommendations for donor selection, blood collection, and record keeping are also discussed, making the statement a valuable reference for facilities with a blood donor program.

Blood typing

Blood typing is the identification of antigens on the surface of an animal's RBCs. These antigens can cause an acute reaction when administered to a patient with antibodies against that particular antigen. In addition, administration of an incompatible blood type can cause the recipient to develop antibodies against that RBC antigen, which could cause delayed transfusion failures and acute transfusion reactions in the future.

In dogs, there are at least a dozen known erythrocyte antigens. Most of the antigens are labeled within the dog erythrocyte antigen (DEA) system, with the exception of the newly discovered Dal antigen. Ideally, all recipients would have a complete blood typing performed and transfused with a perfectly matched donor product. This process is time-consuming (samples must be sent out to a commercial lab) and costly. Most veterinary patients cannot afford the time it takes to perform this extensive testing. In clinical practice, the most important canine blood type is DEA 1.1, which is highly antigenic. This means that transfusion of DEA 1.1 positive blood to a DEA 1.1 negative recipient could result in antibody production against DEA 1.1, which may result in a significant acute transfusion reaction if the patient is ever exposed to this antigen again. Point-of-care tests are available to identify DEA 1.1 status in dogs and should be used prior to the administration of all RBC products. Antibodies to the other antigens (DEA 3, 4, 5, and 7) can rarely cause acute hemolytic reactions, but delayed transfusion reactions are known to occur in immunosensitized patients. Ideally, donor dogs are negative for all DEA types except DEA 4, especially if the recipient's type is unknown. Ninety-seven to ninety-eight percent of all dogs are positive for DEA 4. The Dal antigen is newly reported and of unknown significance at this time.

In cats, there are at least four known red cell antigens. These are A, B, AB, and the newly discovered Mik. Type A is by far the most common, followed by type B. Type AB is very uncommon, and the antigen Mik is of unknown prevalence. Frequency also varies among certain breeds as well as geographic locations. Naturally occurring alloantibodies against foreign red cell antigens are common in cats, and these antibodies can cause fatal hemolytic transfusion reactions. In addition, these alloantibodies are readily passed through a queen's colostrum, which can result in neonatal isoerythrolysis.

Neonatal isoerythrolysis is a potentially fatal disorder that results when a type B queen nurses type A or AB kittens. The strong anti-A antibodies are passed through the colostrum and attack the kittens' RBCs. Typing for the feline AB blood group can be performed at most reference laboratories, and point-of-care typing kits are now readily available.

Cross matching

In addition to blood typing, one of the most important procedures that can be done to reduce the likelihood of an adverse transfusion event is the recipient/donor cross match. Even with the availability of point-of-care blood typing, it is still important to perform a blood cross match on all transfused units of blood. Recipient antibodies against a donor's RBCs are a major cause of acute transfusion reaction and transfusion failure. The major cross match is used to detect the presence of these naturally occurring or induced antibodies in the recipient's plasma against the donor's RBC antigens. Since there are no known clinically significant naturally occurring alloantibodies in dogs, a major cross match will likely be negative in a dog that has never received a blood transfusion, and some may argue that a cross match is not necessary when transfusing a dog that has never been transfused before. Unfortunately, many veterinary patients have an unknown medical history and pet owners may often be unsure of the possibility of previous transfusion; therefore, cross match-

ing is recommended if time allows. The cross match should not be used as a replacement for blood typing because a recipient can develop antibodies against a foreign blood type in as few as 4 days, which will shorten the life of the transfused cells and may prime the patient for an acute transfusion reaction if ever transfused again with the same blood type in the future. These types of incompatibilities cannot be detected by cross match.

Unlike dogs, it is well documented that cats can have very strong, naturally occurring alloantibodies against foreign red cell antigens. In particular, type B cats have naturally occurring anti-A antibodies that can produce a life-threatening reaction even when administered in small amounts (just a few milliliters), making cross match imperative for all feline blood transfusions.

There are several ways to perform donor/recipient cross matching. The blood cross match procedure can be performed by most reference laboratories, but this procedure is most often performed within the hospital setting. The traditional method is to perform a major (recipient serum or plasma and donor red cells) and minor (donor serum or plasma and recipient RBCs) cross match along with a control where the red cells are washed and incubated with the respective serum or plasma and observed for macroscopic and microscopic agglutination. A new gel cross matching kit is now available, which allows the technician to perform a major cross match in much less time than the traditional method.

Administration

Careful administration of blood products is essential to reduce the incidence of adverse events. Potential complications from the administration of blood products include but are not limited to acute hemolytic transfusion reactions, thromboembolism, circulatory overload, sepsis, infectious disease, anaphylaxis, electrolyte derangements, and citrate toxicity. These events can vary in severity from very mild to life threatening, which makes it important for the nursing staff to be diligent about the proper administration and monitoring of patients receiving these products. Several steps must be taken before and during administration to reduce the likelihood of acute or delayed adverse events.

Careful storage and inspection of blood products prior to administration is a very important step that should not be overlooked. Controls should be in place to ensure that storage refrigerators and freezers maintain a consistent temperature according to the storage requirements of each product. The use of these refrigerators and freezers should be limited to product storage when possible to prevent temperature fluctuations. Each unit of blood product should be carefully inspected for signs of discoloration and current expiration date. Discolored blood products may indicate bacterial contamination and should never be administered to a patient.

Refrigerated blood products can typically be administered without warming to room temperature in most patients. Most infusion rates will allow much of the product to reach room temperature during administration. Excessive warming of RBC products can damage the cells and encourage bacterial growth, which may increase the risk of transfusion failure or sepsis. Some cases that may require warming of products to room or body temperature are hypothermic patients and when rapid infusion of large volumes is anticipated. The rapid administration of cold fluids may induce arrhythmias in some patients. When warming is required, care must be taken not to overwarm the product. Sitting at room temperature for 30–60 min is likely the safest way to warm RBCs, but placing the fluid line in a 38°C water bath can facilitate warming when delaying transfusion may threaten the patient's recovery. Microwaving is not recommended and may cause hemolysis of the RBCs. Thawing and administration instructions accompanying blood products should always be carefully followed.

Frozen products can be more rapidly warmed in a 38°C water bath. Higher temperatures should be avoided to prevent the denaturing of plasma proteins. These products can be submerged in water, but they should have an outer wrapping to avoid contamination of the injection ports. Intermittent gentle agitation can be performed to accelerate thawing by breaking up ice crystals. Microwaving of plasma has been described in some literature, but this process may increase the risk of protein denaturation due to nonuniform heating. Some products come with specific thawing instructions and these should be followed when provided.

Many blood products have the potential of containing small clots or other microaggregates that could cause harm to a patient. This hazard can be minimized by using a syringe filter or blood administration set, which should be used when administering any blood product. Filters should be changed at least every 4 h to avoid bacterial contamination and occlusion.

Transfusion reactions

Transfusion reactions are often categorized by immunologic and nonimmunologic reactions. Immune-mediated reactions can be further categorized as hemolytic or nonhemolytic. In addition, each type of reaction can be categorized as acute or delayed reaction.

Immunologic reactions

Hemolytic immunologic reactions are caused by preexisting antibodies against RBC antigens from mismatched blood products and can be acute (immediate) or delayed (2 days to 3 weeks posttransfusion) and result in the destruction of the transfused RBCs. Clinical signs of acute hemolytic immunologic reaction can include pyrexia, tachycardia, tachypnea, muscle tremors, vocalization, arrhythmia, seizures, hypotension, cardiac arrest, and a dramatic drop in PCV.

Nonhemolytic immunologic transfusion reactions are often caused by antibodies against plasma proteins, platelets, or WBCs. Signs of nonhemolytic transfusion reactions are signs of anaphylaxis, which include pyrexia, facial swelling, urticaria, pruritis, vomiting, and dyspnea.

Nonimmunologic reactions

Nonimmunologic transfusion reactions can have several causes. Hemolytic causes include overheating or mishandling of the RBC product, administration through a small bore catheter or needle, and bacterial contamination of the blood product.

Nonhemolytic, nonimmunologic transfusion reactions can be caused by citrate toxicosis in cases of large volume administration of blood products or the improper ratio of citrate containing anticoagulants during blood collection and storage. Another nonhemolytic, nonimmunologic transfusion reaction can be caused by the administration of stored blood products to patients with hepatic insufficiency due to the accumulation of ammonia during RBC storage. It has been suggested that only RBC products stored for under 2 weeks be administered to patients with liver failure.[15]

Monitoring

Early identification and treatment of an acute transfusion reaction is important in the proper nursing care of transfusion patients. A standard protocol should be developed for use by all nursing staff to ensure a standard of care for all transfusion patients. In general, the most severe and life-threatening reactions usually occur within the first 15 min of administration, and monitoring should be most diligent during this period. A baseline body temperature, pulse, respiration, mucous membrane color, and capillary refill time should be obtained prior to administration. During the first 15 min, blood products should be administered at a decreased rate (about 25% the normal rate) so that a reaction can be identified before large amounts of the products have been administered. During this time, all of the baseline parameters should be monitored every 5 min and with close, constant visual monitoring by the nursing staff. Any dramatic change from the baseline parameters should initiate discontinuation of blood product administration and veterinarian attention. After the first 15 min, the administration rate can be titrated up toward the prescribed rate and vitals can be measured every 15–30 min.

Immune-mediated hemolytic anemia

Immune-mediated hemolytic anemia (IMHA) is a relatively common disease in dogs with marked morbidity and mortality. IMHA can be primary (idiopathic) or secondary. In North America, primary IMHA is the most common form in dogs, whereas in cats, secondary IMHA (usually caused by *Mycoplasma haemofelis*) predominates. Secondary IMHA has been caused by a variety of medications (trimethoprim–sulfa, cephalosporins, etc.), neoplasia (especially lymphoma), and infections. The development of IMHA is probably influenced by genetics given that certain breeds, such as the cocker spaniel, are overrepresented in studies looking at the prevalence of IMHA. Gender may play a role as females are overrepresented (both spayed and intact).

The exact pathogenesis of IMHA is not known in each individual. What is known to occur is that the RBCs are tagged as being foreign. This results in the attachment of antibodies to the red cells, either IgG or IgM. The presence of antibodies results in the RBC being cleared partially or completely from the bloodstream by the mononuclear phagocyte system (extravascular hemolysis). In some instances, the antibodies can also fix complement resulting in the formation of membrane attack complex that leads to intravascular hemolysis. The triggers for this are uncertain. Some studies have suggested that vaccines could result in IMHA; others have determined this not to be the case.[19]

The presence of IMHA is indicative of immune system dysregulation. This means that other concurrent immune-mediated diseases could be present. By far, the most common concurrent immune-mediated disease is immune mediated thrombocytopenia (IMT). The combination of IMHA and IMT is referred to as Evans syndrome. Evans syndrome has been suggested to have a poorer prognosis than isolated IMHA.[20] Rarely have other immune-mediated diseases such as glomerulonephritis been identified as a concurrent issue in dogs with IMHA.

Both morbidity and mortality are high with IMHA, and because transfusions and careful monitoring are often needed, the costs of treatment can be quite high. This results in some patients being euthanized because of financial concerns. The other major reason for mortality in these patients is the development of widespread thrombosis, with pulmonary thromboembolism being especially common and catastrophic. The reason why thromboembolism is so common in IMHA is unclear; a variety of processes may play a role. Severe inflammation is known to favor coagulation.

Clinical signs

Clinical signs are variable with IMHA and partially are dependent on how severe the anemia is and how fast it developed. Given that anemia is usually quite marked, the clinical signs associated with this such as tachypnea, exercise intolerance, and dyspnea will often predominate over other signs. IMHA is also associated with a marked inflammatory response that may also cause significant clinical issues (Table 7.2.1).

Diagnostic testing

Diagnostic testing for patients with IMHA serves a variety of purposes. One goal is to identify if the patient truly has IMHA or some other disease process. Differential diagnosis includes zinc toxicosis, genetic diseases (phosphofructokinase deficiency, PK deficiency), or microangiopathic disease (hemangiosarcoma, hemolytic uremic syndrome [HUS]) that could be causing hemolysis. If indications are found for immune-mediated hemolysis, then diagnostic testing is also important to try to identify any causes of secondary immune-mediated disease (e.g., infections or neoplasia). Diagnostic testing also is useful in establishing a prognosis by identifying abnormalities that have been found to worsen outcome.

Laboratory

The CBC will establish that an anemia is present. With IMHA, a regenerative anemia would be expected (this can only be objectively determined by performing a reticulocyte count). In some cases, the immune reaction is to early RBC precursors so the anemia can appear nonregenerative in that either the precursors

Table 7.2.1   Clinical signs of IMHA

As noted by owners	On physical examination
Rapid respirations (cannot catch breath) or abnormal respiratory pattern (belly breaths)	Tachypnea, dyspnea (from anemia, inflammation, or pulmonary thromboembolism)
Pounding heart	Tachycardia
	Murmurs and/or gallops
White or pale gums	Pale mucous membranes
Yellow or orange gums	Jaundice
Fever	Fever
Discolored urine	Discolored urine (hemoglobinuria or bilirubinuria or both)
Lethargy, weakness, collapse, or exercise intolerance	Lethargy, weakness, collapse, or exercise intolerance
Anorexia	Weight loss
Large abdomen	Organomegaly (hepatomegaly, splenomegaly)
Lumps	Lymphadenomegaly
Skin problems	Petechia (if Evans syndrome)

to reticulocytes are targeted or alternatively the reticulocyte itself could be the target. Platelet numbers may be variable. Decreased counts could be from Evans syndrome or from consumption via DIC. WBC counts will often be elevated, either from generalized inflammation, bone marrow activation, or, if markedly elevated, because of organ necrosis. A manually reviewed blood smear is vital with the CBC to evaluate for microscopic autoagglutination and for the presence of spherocytes (small and very dense RBCs that lack central pallor, only seen in dogs). A large number of spherocytes is diagnostic for IMHA (primary or secondary).

The slide agglutination test, when positive, is definitive for IMHA. To perform this test, a drop of ethylenediaminetetracetic acid (EDTA) blood is mixed with two to three drops of saline on a microscope slide. This helps to disperse rouleaux that are similar in gross appearance to agglutination. Agglutination is caused by IgM or IgG antibodies. If gross agglutination is not seen, the slide should be examined under the microscope for microscopic agglutination.

A variety of abnormalities can be seen on the chemistry panel in patients with IMHA. A decrease in albumin may be seen, which is consistent with marked inflammation. During the acute phase response, albumin production is decreased. Hypoalbuminemia has been associated with poorer outcome.[21] Bilirubin concentration will often be elevated due to hemolysis, which results in greater hemoglobin turnover. The higher the bilirubin concentration, the poorer the prognosis. Liver enzyme activity (e.g., alkaline phosphatase [ALP] and alanine aminotransferase [ALT]) is also frequently elevated, initially probably via hypoxic injury.[21] With corticosteroid treatment, liver enzyme activity will increase in dogs, often markedly.

Many times, urinalysis with IMHA is unrewarding due to the large amount of bilirubin or hemoglobin in the urine. Hemoglobinuria and bilirubinuria can interfere with the ability to properly assess urine on the dipstick portion. The presence of marked proteinuria could be a marker of concurrent glomerular disease such as glomerulonephritis.

In those cases where IMHA is suspected but not confirmed by the presence of autoagglutination or marked spherocytosis, Coombs testing is indicated. This test is based on finding antibodies against RBCs either on the RBCs themselves (direct test) or in the serum of the patient (indirect test). This test can be negative in patients with IMHA, especially if they have received immunosuppressives prior to testing. False positives have been seen as well.

Coagulation abnormalities are not uncommon with IMHA. Assessing one-step prothrombin time (OSPT), activated partial thromboplastin time (APTT), and fibrin split products can help to determine if DIC is present. DIC is common in IMHA and can lead to thrombosis.

It is reasonable to test for tick-borne diseases in a dog with IMHA since they can be a trigger for the disease. FeLV and feline immunodeficiency virus (FIV) testing is always indicated in cats with IMHA. In cats, testing for *Mycoplasma* spp. is also indicated.

Imaging

Imaging studies are useful in patients with IMHA. Thoracic radiographs, abdominal radiographs, and abdominal ultrasound are of benefit to determine if there is disease present that could cause secondary IMHA (such as neoplasia).

Treatment and pharmacology

General supportive and nursing care is often needed as these animals can be quite ill at the time of presentation.

Treatment in dogs with IMHA focuses on several aspects. Immunosuppression is indicated to attempt to stop the hemolytic process. Blood transfusions often become necessary if the oxygen carrying capacity is severely compromised. Treatment to prevent thromboembolism is also indicated in dogs given that thromboembolism is the most common cause of death.

Treatment in cats is usually focused on the causative agent.

Supportive care

Fluid therapy is generally indicated since many patients with IMHA are debilitated. Fluid therapy maximizes perfusion, which helps to limit acid–base disturbances and reduce the chance of thromboembolism by minimizing blood sludging. Fluid therapy may also be beneficial in cases with intravascular hemolysis by minimizing the damage free hemoglobin may cause to kidney function.

Oxygen therapy is less likely to be of benefit in IMHA patients since the main issue causing hypoxemia is lack of oxygen carrying capacity. It is also of minor benefit in dogs with pulmonary thromboembolism.

Oxygen carrying support

To date, there are no specific evidence-based guidelines for when or if to administer blood products to patients with IMHA. It is generally accepted that there are no indications that transfusions worsen outcome in IMHA, though at one time there was concern about "adding fuel to the fire." Although the decision to transfuse can be based on clinical signs, it is generally advisable to transfuse patients with PCVs less than 15% even if they are not exhibiting any clinical signs. Typically, pRBCs are used since dogs with IMHA often do not need the plasma component of whole blood (unless significant coagulopathies are documented). The major cross match is not possible in dogs with autoagglutination, so ideally, blood from universal donor dogs (DEA 1.1 negative) should be used.

It is possible to use polymerized bovine hemoglobin (Oxyglobin®, Biopure Corporation) especially when blood is not available or there is a concern about incompatible transfusions. If the patient has been transfused more than 5–7 days previously, it is possible that antibodies have developed that could lead to a major transfusion reaction. If cross matching is not possible in this scenario, Oxyglobin may be a better option. The impact of Oxyglobin use on outcome in patients with IMHA is uncertain with conflicting data having been published.

Immunosuppression

In most cases, combination therapy is used, which minimizes some of the side effects that might be seen with single-agent therapy. Treatment is usually prolonged; rarely are medications used for less than 3–4 months. Glucocorticoids are almost always used (prednisone 2–4 mg/kg/day initially). If contraindicated due to nausea or vomiting, injectable dexamethasone can be used instead. Glucocorticoids have many side effects that tend to impact the pets and the owner's quality of life, such as polyuria, polydipsia, polyphagia, thin hair coat, incessant panting, and loss of muscle mass. To minimize these effects, a variety of other medications can be given concurrently. There is no strong evidence indicating if there is an advantage to any one of these drugs over the others.

Azathioprine. Used fairly commonly as it tends to be inexpensive and effective. Dosage is 2 mg/kg SID for 7 days, then reduce to every other day. There are other protocols that can be used. Rarely will adverse side effects develop, though when they do, they tend to be more serious (pancreatitis, hepatopathy, bone marrow suppression). Not usually used in cats. CBCs should be monitored initially every 1–2 weeks, then every 1–2 months.

Cyclosporine. This medication may have a faster onset of action than azathioprine. Cost may be an issue. Dosage is 5–10 mg/kg/day. It is associated with gastrointestinal (GI) side effects relatively frequently, although less so at the lower dosage ranges. Drug interactions have been noted; consult a formulary when used concurrently with other medications. Blood level monitoring is recommended, though it is uncertain if this is needed, especially when using the 5 mg/kg/day dose. Sandimmune®, Neoral®, and Gengraf® are not bioequivalent; if using generics, determine the name brand equivalent when dosing.

Intravenous Human Immunoglobulin. This product can be difficult to obtain and is exceedingly expensive. Dosage is 0.5–1.5 mg/kg, single-dose intravenous transfusion. Although effective at limiting the immune-mediated destruction, to date, there are no studies that demonstrate outcome is better when this product is used in comparison to other treatments.[22]

Cyclophosphamide. Although this has been used previously, current studies suggest that this medication may do more harm than good in IMHA patients and, as such, its use is generally not recommended in this disease.[23,24]

Others. Leflunomide, mycophenolate mofetil, and splenectomy have all been recommended for treatment of IMHA in various publications and forums. To date, there is not enough information available to routinely recommend these interventions over standard therapy.

Thrombosis prevention

Heparin. The dosages of heparin that have been recommended vary widely. The effect of a dose of heparin on a patient cannot be predicted. It has been shown that heparin therapy under close laboratory monitoring can improve outcomes.[25] Unfortunately, the monitoring needed is rarely available in practice (factor Xa activity). Although prolongation of APTT can be used as an end point for adjusting heparin dosages, this tends not to be very easy to accomplish in practice. Dosages of 100–150 units/kg SQ TID can be considered and are unlikely to cause a hypocoagulable state while still having some antithrombotic effect. Low molecular weight heparins have also been recommended for thromboprophylaxis in IMHA; however, there is no information available on optimal dosage and dosage interval with these heparin products and no data on their clinical efficacy.

Low Dose Aspirin. There has been renewed interest in using low dose aspirin in patients with IMHA. A dosage of 1–2 mg/kg/day has been suggested to improve outcomes in patients with IMHA.[26] This dosage has not been shown to worsen stomach pathology, even though glucocorticoids are being used.

Prognosis

The prognosis with IMHA in dogs tends to be guarded. Depending on the study, anywhere from one-third to two-thirds of the affected dogs will die from IMHA. Euthanasia is a major factor in mortality as well since a guarded prognosis and high cost estimates for treatment may lead some owners to not pursue treatment. Many of the dogs that succumb do so in the first few days, generally as a result of thrombotic complications, especially pulmonary thromboembolism. In one study, 80% of the dogs at necropsy had evidence of thrombosis.[21] Relapses after successful management can occur; the exact recurrence rate is unknown at this time, though it has been suggested to be as high as 15%.

A variety of factors have been found to be indicators of a poor prognosis. The presence of overt jaundice was associated with increased mortality as well as an increased risk of thrombosis in multiple studies. Jaundice is one of the most consistent factors in predicting a poor outcome. Other indicators of increased mortality include hypoalbuminemia, thrombocytopenia, and elevated ALP activity at presentation.[21]

Role of the veterinary technician

Treatment of IMHA is an intensive undertaking. These patients are often quite ill and will require considerable attention. Blood transfusions are often indicated and careful monitoring for possible adverse reactions is necessary. Aseptic techniques should be stringently followed since these patients are immunosuppressed. Intravenous catheters should be checked frequently; these patients are also at risk for thrombosis. It is important to monitor the patient's vital signs, particularly the respiratory rate and breathing pattern since thrombosis to the lungs is not uncommon and can be catastrophic for the patient. Early recognition of breathing problems may allow for medical intervention and can impact the prognosis.

SECTION 3 LEUKOCYTE DISORDERS

Evaluation of the leukogram is part of the CBC and includes quantification of the white blood cells and qualitative information via the differential count. Although a specific disease is rarely diagnosed by leukocyte evaluation, the information obtained from the CBC may be useful in narrowing the number of differential diagnoses and in predicting the severity of the disease and prognosis. Also, sequential CBCs may be useful in monitoring the response to therapy.

Methods for determining the leukogram

There are several methods of determining the leukogram portion of the CBC. Automated particle counters used in human analyzers are not validated for the veterinary patient. Newer technologies using flow cytometry provide reliable differential counts. However, when values are flagged or fall outside the normal reference range, the blood smear should be carefully evaluated by the technician or clinician. It is important to make fresh blood smears as WBC artifacts (such as hypersegmentation, pyknosis, and cytoplasmic vacuolation) may occur if the sample is allowed to sit for several hours.

All nucleated cells are counted including nucleated red blood cells (nRBCs). The following formula is used to obtain a corrected leukocyte count:

$$\text{Corrected WBC count} = \frac{\text{WBC count} \times 100}{100 + \text{nRBC}/100 \text{ WBC}}.$$

The differential WBC count may be reported in relative numbers (percentages) or absolute numbers (number per microliter). Interpretation should always be based on absolute leukocyte numbers, as the percentages may be very misleading in WBC counts that are very low or very high. Leukocytosis occurs when the WBC count exceeds the normal reference range. Leukopenia occurs when the WBC count is below the normal reference range.

Neutrophils, eosinophils, basophils, lymphocytes, and monocytes make up the major WBCs in circulation. Disorders of each cell type will be discussed.

Disorders of neutrophils

Neutrophils are the most common WBC in circulation. Neutrophil numbers are highest in the young and decrease in number with age. The primary function of neutrophils is ingestion and killing of bacteria and fungi. Many processes including margination, emigration, adhesion, chemotaxis, phagocytosis, degranulation, and bactericidal actions have important roles in these functions. Endogenous pyrogens may be secreted by neutrophils. Leukocyte-derived mediators (e.g., proteases, elastases, collagenases, leukotrienes) also play an important role in inflammation and tissue injury.

Pluripotent hematopoietic stem cells give rise to neutrophils, as well as other blood cells (RBCs, megakaryocytes, lymphocytes, eosinophils, basophils, and monocytes). Differentiation is regulated by specific protein factors (colony-stimulating factors). Granulocyte colony-stimulating factor (G-CSF) stimulates the proliferation of neutrophils from the late progenitor stages.

Neutrophils are produced primarily in the bone marrow with occasional production extramedullary in the spleen and liver. There are three theoretical neutrophil compartments in the bone marrow. The proliferation compartment is composed of myeloblasts, progranulocytes, and myelocytes. The approximate maturation time from myeloblast to metamyelocyte is 48–60 h. The maturation compartment consists of metamyelocytes and band neutrophils. The transit time through this compartment is 46–70 h. The storage compartment is made up of mature neutrophils. Transit time in this compartment is approximately 50 h. There is a 5- to 6-day supply of neutrophils in the storage compartment. Mature neutrophils leave the bone marrow by a random process that involves changes in cell deformability and adhesiveness.

In the vascular compartment, there are two neutrophil pools. The marginal neutrophil pool (MNP) consists of neutrophils that adhere to the vascular endothelium. The circulating neutrophil pool (CNP) consists of neutrophils in circulation, and the WBC count and differential count are estimations of the CNP. In dogs, the CNP is approximately equal to the MNP; however, in cats, the MNP is approximately two to three times the size of the CNP. The neutrophil has the average transit time of approximately 6–8 h in dogs and 10–12 h in cats, with all of the blood neutrophils being replaced every 2.0–2.5 days. Once the neutrophil leaves the blood vessel, it normally does not return to the circulation and may be lost in the lungs, gut, urine, skin, saliva, and other tissues.

Abnormal morphological characteristics of neutrophils may have considerable clinical significance. Neutrophils become toxic and poorly functional in response to injury. Toxic changes occur during maturation and are caused by toxic substances generated by strong inflammatory conditions (endotoxemia, sepsis, acute inflammatory disease, burns, etc.). These changes are most frequently associated with systemic rather than local inflammatory/infectious disease. Toxic neutrophils contain cytoplasmic vacuoles, basophilic granules, and Döhle bodies. Döhle bodies are blue-to-gray cytoplasmic granules that are lamellar aggregates of the retained rough endoplasmic reticulum. Resolution, with treatment, of the toxic change in the neutrophils suggests a favorable prognosis.

Intracytoplasmic organisms and inclusion bodies are uncommonly seen in neutrophils of dogs and cats. Bacterial rods and cocci may be seen during sepsis. *Histoplasma capsulatum* organisms have been seen in WBCs from dogs with systemic infections (see Figure 7.3.1). Other organisms that may be seen in neutrophils include distemper inclusion bodies, *Hepatozoon canis*, *Hepatozoon americanum*, *Leishmania donovani*, and *Anaplasma phagocytophilia*.

Nuclear hypersegmentation (i.e., five or more distinct nuclear lobes) may result from prolonged transit time. Hyperadrenocorticism, corticosteroid therapy, and chronic inflammatory disease may be associated with this change. Hypersegmentation has been seen in some poodles with macrocytosis and in feline sample when the EDTA blood sample sat for several hours prior to making the blood smear.

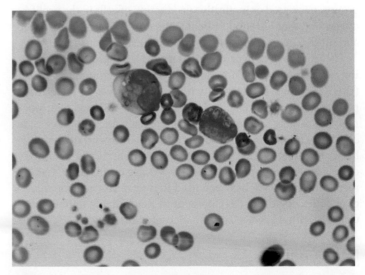

Figure 7.3.1 *Histoplasma capsulatum* in a white blood cell in a dog. Courtesy of Stan Krogman, Site Manager, Marshfield Veterinary Labs, Marshfield, Wisconsin.

Pelger–Huët anomaly

The Pelger–Huët anomaly occurs when the nucleus fails to undergo division but the nuclear chromatin and cytoplasmic maturation are complete (i.e., the nucleus has a bandlike appearance with clumped chromatin). Affected females lack Barr bodies (sex chromatin "drumstick") in circulating neutrophils. This disorder has been reported more commonly in dogs and rarely in cats. Often these animals are diagnosed with extreme left shifts; however, upon careful evaluation of these neutrophils, normal cytoplasm and hyposegmentation are identified. These changes may also be apparent in the eosinophils and basophils. This anomaly may be inherited (suspected to be autosomal dominant in Australian cattle dogs) or acquired (seen in dogs undergoing chemotherapy). Homozygous genetic expression has been rarely observed and is thought to be lethal *in utero*. In cats, the homozygous form has been associated with skeletal deformities. Latimer et al. found a 9.8% incidence of Pelger–Huët anomaly in 892 Australian shepherds over a 6-year period.[6] Other breeds reported with this anomaly include the American foxhound, basenji, border collie, Boston terrier, cocker spaniel, German shepherd dog, samoyed, and various coonhounds.

Neutrophil granulation anomaly

A neutrophil granulation anomaly was identified in Birman cats by Hirsch and Cunningham.[8] The neutrophils contained numerous fine, reddish-purple cytoplasmic granules similar to granules seen in promyelocytes. There are no clinical signs associated with this finding. *In vitro* studies demonstrated that affected cats exhibit bactericidal activity against *E. coli* similar to normal cats. Inheritance via an autosomal recessive manner was found.

Neutropenia

Neutropenia is an absolute decrease in circulating neutrophil numbers. Causes of neutropenia can be classified into three groups: decreased or ineffective production of cells in the proliferating pool, sequestration of neutrophils in the marginating pool, and sudden excessive tissue demand or consumption (Table 7.3.1).

The treatment of neutropenia is aimed at treating the underlying cause. A recombinant granulocytic colony stimulating factor (rhG-CSF) has been used with some success in veterinary patients with parvovirus and chemotherapy-induced neutropenia. The dose is 5 µg/kg/day subcutaneously for 5–20 days. Side effects include pain at the injection site and neutralizing antibody formation. The development of neutralizing antibody occurs more frequently with prolonged use of this drug. Canine recombinant G-CSF has been used to treat cyclic neutropenia in gray collie dogs. The development of neutralizing antibodies is unlikely with a species-specific recombinant drug.

Neutrophilia

Neutrophilia is an absolute increase in neutrophil numbers and is the most common cause of leukocytosis. A mature neutrophilia is an increase in neutrophils without an increase in the immature forms (i.e., band neutrophils). Neutrophilia with a left shift occurs when both mature and immature neutrophils are increased. A regenerative left shift occurs when the number of mature neutrophils exceeds the number of immature forms. A degenerative left shift occurs when the number of immature neutrophils exceeds the number of mature forms. Neutrophilia may or may not be present. A degenerative left shift usually implies a severe disease process and poor prognosis. A leukemoid response is defined as a marked neutophilia with a severe left shift that includes metamyelocytes and myelocytes. Such a response indicates severe inflammatory disease and may be difficult to distinguish from chronic granulocytic leukemia. The causes of neutrophilia can be classified into three groups: physiological or epinephrine-induced neutrophilia, stress or corticosteroid-induced neutrophilia, and inflammation or increased tissue demand. Physiological or epinephrine-induced neutrophilia is associated with a release of neutrophils from the MNP. This form of neutrophilia is transient and occurs only in normal animals (most common in cats). Other changes in the CBC include erythrocytosis and lymphocytosis (primarily in cats). Stress or corticosteroid-induced neutrophilia is associated with long transit time in circulation and increased bone marrow release of neutrophils in the storage pool. Other CBC changes include lymphopenia, eosinopenia, and monocytosis (the latter occurring only in dogs). Inflammation or increased tissue demand results in variable increases in neutrophil counts. The magnitude of the response, which is determined by the balance between the rate of bone marrow release and tissue emigration, may vary with the species, location of inflammation, virulence of the causative agent, and inciting cause of the inflammation (Table 7.3.2).

The treatment is directed at the underlying cause of the neutrophilia.

Neutrophil function defects

Neutrophil function defects result in decreased host defense against bacterial invaders. Adherence, chemotaxis, phagocytosis, and bacteriocidal activities are important functions of the neutrophil. Both congenital and acquired neutrophil dysfunctions have been reported (Table 7.3.3). Additional information on breed-related disorders may be found in Section 4.

Chédiak–Higashi syndrome

Chédiak–Higashi syndrome is characterized by enlarged neutrophilic and eosinophilic granules in the cytoplasm (see Figure 7.3.2). Other associated abnormalities include partial albinism, photophobia, increased susceptibility to infections, bleeding tendencies, and abnormal melanocytes. This lethal autosomal recessive condition has been documented in Persian cats with smoke-colored fur and yellow eyes. A mutation in the lysosomal trafficking gene (*LYST*) results in the lysosomal storage disorder. Diagnosis is based on history, physical exam, and evaluation of WBCs for large cytoplasmic eosinophilic granules, prolonged bleeding of the buccal mucosal bleeding test, and increased melanin pigment in hair shafts. Supportive medical therapy for

Table 7.3.1 Causes of neutropenia

Decreased production in the proliferating pool				
Myelophthesis	**Drug-induced marrow effects**	**Toxins**	**Infectious disease**	**Others**
Myeloproliferative disorders	Chemotherapy drugs	Inorganic solvents	Parvovirus	Idiopathic bone marrow aplasia/hypoplasia
Lymphoproliferative disease	Chloramphenicol	Benzene	Retrovirus (FeLV, FIV)	Cyclic neutropenia of gray collies
Myelofibrosis	Griseofulvin	*Fusarium sporotrichioides* toxin	Ehrlichiosis	Acquired cyclic neutropenias
Systemic mast cell disease	Trimethoprim/sulfa		Toxoplasmosis	Steroid-responsive neutropenia
Metastatic carcinoma	Estrogen		Early canine distemper virus	
Malignant histiocytosis	Phenylbutazone		Early canine hepatitis virus	
	Phenobarbital		Anaplasmosis	
	Others			

Sequestration in marginating pool
Anaphylactic shock
Endotoxic shock
Anesthesia

Excessive tissue demand or consumption
Peracute overwhelming infections
Drug induced
Immune mediated
Paraneoplastic
Hypersplenism

Table 7.3.2 Causes of neutrophilia

Physiological or epinephrine induced	Stress or corticosteroid induced	Inflammation or increased tissue demand
Fear	Pain	Infection
Excitement	Anesthesia	Tissue trauma and/or necrosis
Exercise	Trauma	Immune-mediated disorders
Seizures	Neoplasia	Neoplasia
Parturition	Hyperadrenocorticism	Metabolic disorders (uremia, diabetic ketoacidosis)
Hypertension	Metabolic disorders	Burns
	Chronic disorders	Neutrophil function disorders
		Other (acute hemorrhage, hemolysis)

Table 7.3.3   Neutrophil function defects

Congenital disease	Acquired disease
Chédiak–Higashi syndrome in blue smoked Persians	Metabolic or nutritional disease resulting in poor adherence (e.g., poorly controlled diabetes mellitus)
Neutrophil defect of Doberman pinschers	Infectious disease resulting in decreased chemotaxis (bacterial pyodermas, FeLV, feline infectious peritonitis [FIP])
Canine leukocyte adhesion deficiency in Irish setter dogs	Toxins resulting in decreased bacteriocidal function (lead, turpentine)
Lysosomal storage disease	Metabolic abnormalities resulting in decrease chemotaxis, phagocytosis, and bactericidal activity (hypophosphatemia)
Canine cyclic hematopoiesis of gray collie dogs	
Immunodeficiency of Weimaraners	

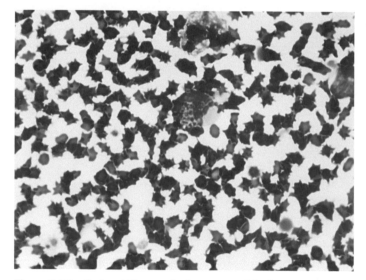

Figure 7.3.2   Eosinophilic granules in a neutrophil of a cat with Chédiak–Higashi syndrome. Courtesy of Stan Krogman, Site Manager, Marshfield Veterinary Labs, Marshfield, Wisconsin.

secondary infections and anemia secondary to bleeding may prolong survival. Shielding cats from sunlight is also advised. The prognosis is poor.

Neutrophil defect of Doberman pinschers

Breitschwerdt et al. identified a neutrophil function defect in eight closely related Doberman pinschers with chronic rhinitis and pneumonia.[11] Although the neutrophils phagocytized the bacteria normally, there was impaired bactericidal activity. One of eight dogs had decreased lymphocyte transformation indices

for three mitogens. The cause of this dysfunction is unknown, and the inheritance pattern was not reported.

Canine leukocyte adhesion deficiency

Canine leukocyte adhesion deficiency (CLAD) is a rare disease affecting Irish setters, Irish setter crosses, and Irish red and white setters. The disease is characterized by recurrent infections with a marked leukocytosis occurring shortly after birth. Recurrent pyoderma, pododermatitis, pneumonia, thrombophelbitis, and osteomyelitis with minimal pus formation are common. The defect is caused by a genetic mutation resulting in a CD18 deficiency. As an autosomal recessive trait, carrier dogs do not exhibit signs of disease. Affected dogs respond poorly to medical therapy even with aggressive antibiotic therapy. Successful treatment of four out of five affected dogs using foamy virus vectors expressing canine CD18 was achieved by Bauer et al.[13] OptiGen, LLC (Ithaca, New York) offers genetic testing using PCR amplification of the gene to identify affected and carrier dogs.

Lysosomal storage diseases

The lysosomal storage diseases are rare, inherited disorders caused by the deficiency of one or more enzymes within the lysosome. The consequence of this dysfunction is the inability to activate the protein or cofactor necessary for enzymatic activity. This disruption of the catabolic pathway results in accumulation of storage material (glycoproteins, oligosaccharides, sphingolipids, mucopolysaccharides, etc.). The inheritance pattern is autosomal recessive in most veterinary patients. Although puppies and kittens are normal at birth, progressive accumulation of lysosomal storage products can lead to skeletal abnormalities, growth retardation, visual defects, and organomegaly. Abnormal findings include neurological abnormalities (seizures, behavioral abnormalities, tremors, cerebellar signs, hypermetria), ocular changes (corneal opacification, cataract development, impaired vision), skeletal and connective tissue changes (dwarfism, coarse facial features, collapse of intervertebral disk spaces, dysostoses multiplex, long bone deformation), and hepatomegaly. An early clue to diagnosis is the presence of abnormal vacuoles or cytoplasmic granules in peripheral blood leukocytes. Cytology of aspirates of the lymph node, spleen, and liver may help identify abnormal cytoplasmic vacuoles. Radiographic changes include skeletal deformities (dysmorphism, vertebral changes, and fractures). Cerebrospinal fluid may reveal vacuolated macrophages or lymphocytes. Specific diagnosis of canine fucosidosis, globoid cell leukodystrophy, mucopolysaccharidosis (MPS) I and VII and feline MPS VI is available through DNA-based molecular testing. The long-term prognosis is poor due to the progressive nature of these diseases (Table 7.3.4).

Canine cyclic hemopoiesis of gray collies

Cyclic hemopoiesis is a rare autosomal recessive disorder of stem cells in gray collies. A genetic mutation results in a neutrophil elastase-processing defect. This disease is characterized by a regular 12- to 14-day cyclic decrease of neutrophils, monocytes, eosinophils, lymphocytes, platelets, and reticulocytes. Puppies are usually smaller than normal littermates and develop clinical

Table 7.3.4   Lysosomal storage diseases

Storage disease	Enzyme defect	Breeds affected
Fucosidosis	Alpha L fucosidase	English springer spaniel
Mannosidosis	Alpha D mannosidase	Domestic shorthair (DSH), Persian cat
Pompe's disease	Alpha-glucosidase	Lapland dog, DSH
GMI gangliosidosis	Beta D galactosidase	Siamese, DSH, Korat, English springer spaniel, beagle, Portugese water dog, Alaskan malamute, husky, mixed breed dog
GMII gangliosidosis	Beta D hexosaminidase	DSH, Korat, Siamese German shorthair pointer
	Activator protein	Japanese spaniel
Gaucher's disease	Beta D glucocerebrosidase	Sydney silky terrier
Globoid cell leukodystrophy	Beta D galactocerebrosidase	West Highland white terrier, cairn terrier, beagle, poodle, DSH
Sphingomyelinosis (Niemann–Pick disease)	Sphingomyelinase (type A)	Balinese, Siamese cats Poodle
	Cholesterol esterification deficiency (type C)	Boxer DSH
Mucopolysaccharidosis (MPS) MPS I	Alpha L iduronidase	DSH, Plott hound
MPS II	Iduraonate-2-sulfate sulfatase	Labrador retriever
MPS III	Sulfamidase	Wire-haired dachshund
MPS VI	Arylsulfatase B	Siamese cat
MPS VII	Beta D glucuronidase	Mixed breed dog
Ceroid lipofuscinosis	Unknown but several gene defects identified in some breeds	Siamese cat, many breeds (dachshund, American Staffordshire terrier, American bulldogs, border collies, English setters, Labrador retriever, Tibetan terrier)

signs by 8–12 weeks of age. Fever, diarrhea, respiratory and skin infections, and epistaxis may occur during the cytopenia phase. Without treatment, affected dogs usually die by 2–3 years of age. Improvement of the neutrophil nadir and control of the clinical signs have been seen with high dose oral lithium carbonate and recombinant human G-CSF and canine G-CSF injections. Bone marrow transplantion has resulted in resolution of the cyclic hematopoiesis and coat color change toward normal. Yanay et al. successfully treated an affected collie with a lentivirus-mediated G-CSF delivery method for 17 months.[19] Several companies (HealthGene, Toronto, Canada; VetGene, Ann Arbor, Michigan) offer DNA testing for this disorder.

Immunodeficiency of Weimaraners

Chronic recurrent infections in young Weimaraner dogs have been reported worldwide since the 1980s. The exact pathogenesis is unknown but suspected to be related to an immunodeficiency syndrome. Although the mode of inheritance is unknown, the disease is suspected to be inherited. Some studies suggest that affected dogs have an intrinsic functional defect (decreased phagocytosis and destruction of pathogens). However, a failure to produce serum immunoglobulins (IgG and IgA) has been documented in many studies. The lack of response to produce adequate vaccine titers following immunizations also suggests an abnormality in immunoglobulin production. There has been concern that this disease may be triggered by vaccinations as the timing of puppy vaccination protocols correlates with the time of disease development. The onset of clinical signs usually occurs at 12–15 weeks of age when maternal antibody wanes. Involvement of multiple body systems has been described and includes the skin (pyoderma), GI tract (diarrhea), joints (hypertrophic osteodystrophy), bone (osteomyelitis), lung (pneumonia), central nervous system (seizures, behavioral changes), and eye (conjunctivitis). Anorexia, lethargy, diarrhea, lameness, and coughing are commonly noted by owners. Physical examination findings of fever, lymphadenophathy, bone pain, and hypoplasia of dental enamel are typical. Diagnosis is based on history, physical findings, radiographic evidence of hypertrophic osteodystrophy and pneumonia, CBC findings of mild anemia, mild thrombocytopenia, neutrophilia with a left shift, monocytosis, and decreased gammaglobulins. Measurement of serum immunoglobulins, especially IgG and IgA, is usually decreased. The treatment for this disease is supportive care. Anti-inflammatory doses of glucocorticoids have been reported to be beneficial in dogs with hypertrophic osteodystrophy. Vaccination protocols are usually modified using killed products and separating vaccine components.

Disorders of eosinophils

The eosinophil is produced in the bone marrow and, like neutrophils, they function to phagocytize and kill pathogens (bacteria, mycoplasmas, yeasts, etc.). Additional functions of the eosinophil included parasitical activity, modulation of type I hypersensitivity reactions, and activation of plasminogen resulting in thrombosis. Eosinophil production occurs in response to GM-CSF, IL-3, and IL-5. Normally, there are only a small number of eosinophils in the peripheral circulation. Eosinophils migrate to tissues (gut, skin, and lung) that have a close interaction with foreign material. Like neutrophils, eosinophils do not recirculate. The transit time within the blood is approximately 24–35 h. The tissue eosinophil pool is significantly larger than the circulating pool, and eosinophils are predominant in the mucous membranes.

Eosinphilia is defined as an absolute increase in eosinophils (>1300/µL in dogs and >1500/µL in cats). Parasitism (endoparasites and ectoparasites) is the most common cause of eosinophilia in dogs. Other causes include inflammatory and hypersensitivity reactions of the GI, respiratory and genitourinary systems, and in the skin eosinophilic infiltrative disease. Neoplasia-associated eosinophilia has been associated with mast cell tumors and lymphoma. Uncommonly, eosinophilia has been associated with hypereosinophilic syndrome, tetracycline and recombinant interleukin-2 administration, and canine estrus. In 1990, Center et al. retrospectively surveyed 312 cats with eosinophilia over an 11-year period.[23] The eosinophil count ranged from 1500 to 46,200/µL (median 2400/µL). Skin-related disease accounted for 27.6% of cats with eosinophilia. Respiratory disorders (20.8%) and neoplasia (6.4%) were the second and third most common causes of feline eosinophilia. Other conditions included cardiac disease, feline urological syndrome, toxoplasmosis, feline panleukopenia, renal disease, feline infectious peritonitis, myeloproliferative disease, IMHA, and hyperimmune serum reaction.

Hypereosinophilic syndrome

Hypereosinophilic syndrome has been reported in cats and rarely in dogs. The cause is unknown, but possible mechanisms suggested include abnormal regulation of eosinophil production, abnormal immunoregulatory ability, and/or inappropriate response to an antigen. This disease is characterized by marked eosinophilia (>50,000/µL). Purebred felines are unlikely to develop this disease. Ages affected have ranged from 10 months to 12 years. Females are overrepresented in a study by Helmond et al.[25] The most frequently affected organs or tissues include bone marrow, spleen, lymph nodes, and the gut. Anorexia, vomiting, diarrhea, and weight loss are commonly reported. Physical exam findings include emaciation, hepatosplenomegaly, thickened intestinal tract, mesenteric lymphadenopathy, fever, and rarely, eosinophilic granulomatous lesions of lymph nodes and organs. Hematologic abnormalities include marked eosinophilia, basophilia, and occasional anemia. Biochemical abnormalities may be seen with organ dysfunction. Imaging often reveals thickened intestines, mesenteric lymphadenopathy, and hepatosplenomegaly. Bone marrow aspirate findings are consistent with a hyperplastic marrow with eosinophilic hyperplasia and an increased myeloid/erythroid ratio. Histopathology of affected tissues demonstrates pronounced eosinophilic infiltration. Therapy includes corticosteroids and chemotherapeutic agents; however, the prognosis is poor with mean survival from diagnosis to death being 7.5 weeks reported from several studies.

Eosinopenia

Eosinopenia is difficult to document in dogs as the normal range of eosinophils is 0–1300/µL. Endogenous glucocorticoids from stress and inflammation and exogenous glucocorticoids are often the cause of suspected eosinopenia in dogs. In cats, the eosinophil range is 0–1500/µL and as in dogs, the cause of eosinpenia is associated with endogenous and exogenous glucocorticoids.

Disorders of basophils

Basophils are the least numerous circulating blood cell. The function of basophils appears to be similar to mast cells as both contain histamine and other vasoactive substances. Basophils play an important role in type 1 hypersensitivity reactions, cell-mediated delayed-type hypersensitivity response, and development of IgE-mediated chronic allergic reactions. Basophils are produced in the bone marrow with maturation completed in 2.5 days. Peripheral circulation in the blood lasts approximately 6 h; however, some may live for as long as 2 weeks. Interleukin-3 is the major basophil growth factor and cytokine effector of basophil function.

Basophilia is defined as an absolute increase in peripheral basophils (>140/µL in dogs and >200/µL in cats). Usually, basophilia accompanies eosinophilia. The most common cause of basophilia in dogs is heartworm disease. Other causes of basophilia in dogs and cats include allergic respiratory disease, parasitic disease, disseminated mast cell disease, other neoplasias (basophilic leukemia, myeloid leukemia, thymoma), and pulmonary granulomatous disease.

Disorders of monocytes

Monocytes with free and fixed macrophages and their progenitor cells in the bone marrow make up the mononuclear phagocyte system. Monocytes emigrate from the blood into peripheral tissues and, depending on the tissue and inflammatory response, differentiation into free, fixed tissue and inflammatory macrophages may occur. Functions of the macrophage include phagocytosis of pathogens, senescent cells, and cellular debris; presenting antigen to lymphocytes; cytotoxic effects against some tumor cells; and secretion of cytokines, interleukins, chemokines, endogenous pyrogens, lysosomal hydrolases, prostaglandins, and complement procoagulation factors. The half-life of circulating monocytes in cats and dogs is unknown; however, it is 20–23 h in cattle and 70 h in humans. Monocytes leave circulation in a random manner or in response to inflammation. Free macrophages may migrate to other tissues or may reenter the circulation. The exact life span of macrophages is unknown, but tissue macrophages appear to be long-lived.

Monocytosis is defined as >1400/μL in dogs and >850/μL in cats and is associated with necrosis, suppuration, pyogranulomatous lesions, internal hemorrhage, trauma, immune-mediated disease, and malignant neoplasia (monocytic and myelomonocytic leukemia). Excessive glucocorticoids (endogenous and exogenous) are a common cause of monocytosis in dogs but not in cats.

Monocytopenia is clinically unimportant as the low end of the reference range is zero.

Disorders of lymphocytes

The lymphocyte is the second most common WBC in circulation. There are two morphologically indistinguishable types of lymphocytes (T and B cells) in circulation. T lymphocytes (derived from the thymus) participate in cell-mediated immunity, and B lymphocytes (derived from the bursa) are associated with humoral immunity. Only 10% of the total lymphocyte pool circulates in the peripheral blood. Unlike other WBCs, lymphocytes are long-lived and are capable of transformation to more functional active forms. Lymphoid precursors are present in the central compartment (thymus, bone marrow, and bursa equivalent). These lymphocytes may differentiate or may provide precursors to the peripheral compartment (lymph nodes, spleen, and Peyer's patches). The lymphocytes of the peripheral compartment respond to antigenic stimulation and develop into B or T lymphocytes. Lymphocytes can recirculate into the bloodstream via efferent lymphatics and the thoracic duct. The number of circulating lymphocytes declines with age.

Several morphological alterations of lymphocytes can occur. Reactive lymphocytes (also termed immunocytes) are produced in response to antigenic stimulation. Morphologically, these cells have an intense basophilic cytoplasm and perinuclear Golgi zone. Azurophilic granules and vacuoles may also be present. Large granular lymphocytes (natural killer cells, null lymphoid cells) have azurophilic granules and, occasionally, vacuoles. Granular lymphocytes have been reported in association with lymphoma and canine ehrlichiosis. Plasma cells are large lymphocytes with intensely basophilic cytoplasm and a prominent, pale staining perinuclear Golgi zone; these lymphocytes are rare in the peripheral circulation. Severe antigenic stimulation or neoplasia (plasmacytoma, multiple myeloma) has been associated with circulating plasma cells. Lymphoblasts are large lymphocytes with a large nucleus that has a vesicular chromatin pattern of the nucleus and prominent nucleoli. Circulating lymphoblasts are associated with lymphoblastic leukemia and disseminated lymphoma.

Lymphocytosis is defined as circulating lymphocytes >2900/μL in dogs and >7000/μL in cats. Causes of lymphocytosis include chronic antigenic stimulation, hypoadrenocorticism, lymphoid neoplasia, feline hyperthyroidism, and physiological leukocytosis (more common in cats).

Lymphopenia occurs when circulating lymphocyte numbers are decreased (<400/μL in dogs and <1500/μL in cats). Causes of lymphopenia include acute systemic bacterial infections, glucocorticoids (endogenous and exogenous), disruption of the lymph node architecture, immunosuppressive drugs, loss of lymphocyte-rich fluids, malignant neoplasia, GI disease, radiation, and viral infections.

Immunodeficiency disorders occur when one or more components of the immune system are defective and result in an increased susceptibility to infection. Decreased immunoglobulins have been recognized in several canine breeds.

Selective IgA deficiency

Selective IgA deficiencies have been identified in Chinese sharpei, beagle, German shepherd, English cocker spaniel, and Irish wolfhound dogs. There are several consequences of decreased concentrations of IgA. A failure to mount a local immune response to pathogens (bacteria and virus) results in recurrent infections. These animals also have an increased risk of allergic and autoimmune disease due to increased absorption of antigens. The mode of inheritance is unknown. The most common clinical signs are respiratory infections, staphylococcal dermatitis, and atopic dermatitis. Although these signs occur at an early age, life-threatening infections are uncommon. The diagnosis is based on quantitation of serum IgA. Normally, serum IgA concentrations are low in all dogs until 12–18 months of age; therefore, comparison of serum results with age-matched controls is necessary in dogs less than 18 months of age. Approximately 20% of dogs diagnosed with IgA deficiency before 1 year of age will revert to normal IgA concentrations between 12 and 18 months. However, approximately 10% of dogs diagnosed with IgA deficiency after 1 year of age will revert to normal. Treatment of this disease is limited to supportive care.

X-linked severe combined immunodeficiency (XSCID)

Severe combined immunodeficiency (SCID) has been reported in Cardigan Welsh corgis and basset hounds. Infections begin to occur when maternal antibody levels decline (usually between 4 and 8 weeks of age). These puppies fail to thrive and are usually stunted. Physical examination reveals small or absent lymph nodes and tonsils. Lymphopenia may be seen in the CBC. Measurement of serum IgM is usually normal; however, serum IgG and IgA are very low to absent once maternal antibodies are gone. Postmortem findings include a small thymus and a lack of tonsils, lymph nodes, and Peyer's patches. Mutations in the common gamma chain gene result in a deficiency of several interleukins (IL-2, IL-4, IL-7, IL-9, IL-15) and in a lack of normal development and function of B and T cells. The mode of inheritance is an X-linked recessive pattern. Successful treatment has been achieved with bone marrow transplantation and *in vivo* retroviral gene therapy.

Combined immunodeficiency of Jack Russell terriers

Bell et al. described SCID in a family of Jack Russell terriers.[31] Twelve puppies died between 8 and 14 weeks of age. Six other puppies died within 50 h of vaccination with modified live vaccines. Decreased immunoglobulins (IgA, IgM, and IgG) and lymphopenia were found in affected dogs. Necropsy revealed hypoplasia of all lymphoid tissue. The pedigree analysis suggested that the pattern of inheritance was autosomal recessive. Prognosis is very poor.

C3 deficiency of Brittany spaniels

Deficiency of the third component of complement (C3) was identified in a closed colony of Brittany spaniels by Blum et al.[32] Twenty dogs with C3 deficiency were monitored for 6 years. Five of these dogs developed severe bacterial infections (pneumonia, sepsis, and pyometra), and two of these developed renal disease (amyloidosis and membranoproliferative glomerulonephritis). This disorder is inherited as an autosomal recessive trait.

Immunodeficiency associated with respiratory disease

Several breeds have been described with chronic respiratory disease and immunodeficiency. Reported breeds include young Irish wolfhounds with chronic rhinitis and/or bronchopneumonia and decreased serum IgA levels, several related miniature dachshunds with *Pneumocystis carinii* (an opportunistic organism usually associated with immunodeficiency), and several Cavalier King Charles spaniels (CKCS) with respiratory signs and generalized demodicosis. Decreased immunoglobulin concentrations have been reported in these dogs.

SECTION 4 PLATELET, COAGULATION, AND INHERITED DISORDERS

Diseases of coagulation

Inherited

Hemophilia

Hemophilia A is the most common inherited coagulopathy and represents a deficiency of factor VIII. Factor VIII is part of the intrinsic pathway and is linked to the normal function of vWF.

The deficiency is more common in large dog breeds and German shepherds are overrepresented.

Hemophilia B (factor IX deficiency) is the second most common inherited coagulopathy and Labrador retrievers may be overrepresented. Factor IX is also part of the intrinsic pathway. Inheritance for both conditions is X-linked recessive and males are more commonly affected than females. Identification of female carriers may be difficult. Clinical disease is only seen in those animals that are homozygous recessive. Initial episodes of abnormal hemorrhage may be seen with minor surgical procedures or loss of deciduous teeth. Both forms of hemophilia have been diagnosed in cats. As these conditions are genetic, breeding of affected animals is not recommended.

Pharmacology, treatment, and contraindications

Basic nursing care should be employed for animals with active hemorrhage, consisting of compression bandages, cold compresses, and strict cage rest. Hospitalized animals should be clearly identified as having a coagulopathy. Jugular venipuncture should be avoided and venous access should be obtained with the smallest possible needle. Intramuscular injections should be avoided in animals with coagulopathies to avoid the formation of painful intramuscular hematomas. For animals with more extensive hemorrhage, transfusion therapy is indicated. Factor VIII is found in fresh whole blood and fresh frozen plasma. If available, cryoprecipitate has higher levels of factor VIII, along with vWF, but does not contain factor IX. Factor IX may be successfully transfused via whole blood, plasma, and fresh serum. If hemorrhage has been significant, additional RBC transfusions may be required. However, in animals that require repeated transfusions, factor VIII inhibitor antibodies have been shown to develop and can complicate therapy.

Diagnostic testing: laboratory, imaging, biopsy

Prolonged partial thromboplastin time (PTT) with normal prothrombin time (PT) should increase suspicion for hemophilia A or B. Specific assays for factor VIII and factor IX analysis are available. Clinically significant bleeding is noted when factor concentration is <5% when compared to normal control. Spontaneous bleeding, with no identified traumatic episode, may be seen with levels <2%.

Feline factor XII deficiency

Factor XII (Hageman factor) deficiency is the most common inherited coagulopathy identified in domestic cats. The reported incidence is three to four times that of hemophilia A and B. Factor XII is also part of the intrinsic pathway, but in contrast to hemophilia, factor XII deficiency is an autosomal recessive inheritance, and thus there is no sex predilection. Siamese cats may be predisposed. Also, the deficiency is clinically silent and cats do not have hemorrhagic tendencies.

No therapy is required and no blood products or transfusion support is necessary.

Diagnostic testing: laboratory, imaging, biopsy

A prolonged PTT with normal PT in a cat with no clinical signs of bleeding should increase the suspicion for factor XII deficiency. As with other individual coagulation factors, factor XII levels can be measured specifically.

Acquired

Toxicity

The major toxicities associated with coagulation deficits are rodenticide (vitamin K antagonists) and non-steroidal anti-inflammatory drug (NSAID) ingestion. Vitamin K antagonism affects secondary hemostasis (hemostasis associated with coagulation factors), while NSAID intoxication results in abnormalities with primary hemostasis (hemostasis due to platelets). As with any coagulopathy, gentle handling and nursing care of hospitalized animals and clear communication with hospital staff is imperative.

Pharmacology, treatment, and contraindications

For rodenticide intoxication, bleeding is primarily associated with deep body cavities (hemothorax, hemoabdomen, hemomediastinum), though hemorrhage may be seen in numerous locations (joints, spinal cord, etc.). Clinical signs of hemorrhage may be delayed for days to weeks after ingestion, depending upon the substance ingested. Thus, obtaining an accurate and complete history is imperative. When possible, the identity of the specific rodenticide should be ascertained. Immediate therapy is administered via subcutaneous injection of vitamin K_1. Intravenous injection of vitamin K_1 has been associated with anaphylaxis and is not recommended. Intramuscular injections are contraindicated so as to prevent intramuscular hematomas. In severe cases, animals may require transfusion support with coagulation factors or RBCs. Hemorrhage in and around the pulmonary system is common, so animals may present with dyspnea and may require supplemental oxygen therapy. Once the animal is stable, therapy is continued with oral vitamin K_1, and the length of treatment is based on the specific toxin ingested. After discontinuation of vitamin K_1 therapy, coagulation times should be rechecked to ensure additional therapy is not necessary.

With NSAID intoxication, evidence of platelet dysfunction may be seen as petechiation, ecchymosis, or other mucosal hemorrhage (epistaxis, hematochezia, etc.). All NSAIDs should be immediately discontinued in animals with signs of toxicity. As a general recommendation, NSAIDs should be used with caution in animals with underlying renal or GI disease as they may exacerbate the potential for renal and GI toxicity. Excessive hemorrhage may be seen during surgical procedures on animals that have had recent NSAID therapy. Due to the GI effects of NSAIDs, GI upset, erosions, and ulcers may also be seen. Therefore, gastroprotectant (sucralfate) and antacid therapy (famotidine, omeprazole, etc.) may be required. Misoprostol is a prostaglandin analogue that is especially effective at preventing the GI side effects seen with NSAID administration. Animals with NSAID intoxication and GI distress may have nausea and vomiting and may require antiemetic or antinausea medication. Sudden onset or significant abdominal pain should increase the suspicion for GI perforation; pain relief is indicated. In severe cases, GI perforation and septic peritonitis may result. As with rodenticide intoxication, transfusion therapy may be indicated in animals with severe disease.

Diagnostic testing: laboratory, imaging, biopsy

Vitamin K antagonism affects those coagulation factors that are vitamin K dependent (factors II, VII, IX, and X). As factor VII has the shortest half-life, the extrinsic pathway is the first pathway affected, evidenced by prolonged PT. With time and consumption of other factors, PTT also becomes prolonged. The diagnosis is made via abnormal coagulation testing with prolonged PT, PTT, or activated clotting time (ACT) in an animal with consistent clinical signs and known or suspected rodenticide exposure. Other tests of coagulation include proteins induced by vitamin K antagonism (PIVKA) and thromboelastography (TEG). Normal ranges for coagulation testing are specific to each laboratory, so it is recommended to become familiar with the normal ranges and testing recommendations for your laboratory.

With NSAID toxicity, the hemorrhagic tendency is due to platelet dysfunction. Therefore, tests of platelet function are recommended (buccal mucosal bleeding time, platelet aggregation, TEG).

Nutritional considerations

Vitamin K is a fat-soluble vitamin, so appropriate dietary fat is necessary for adequate absorption.

Uremia

Uremia (the clinical syndrome associated with renal failure) has hemorrhagic consequences. The main sources of bleeding include inhibition of normal platelet function due to uremic toxins and blood loss from GI erosions and ulcerations. This condition causes alterations in both primary and secondary hemostasis. Anemia, due to blood loss, decreased RBC production, and decreased RBC life span, can be a significant contributing factor to disease progression with renal failure.

Pharmacology, treatment, and contraindications

Treatment is supportive, centered on reducing uremic toxins and on providing circulatory support as indicated by patient status. Options for therapy include crystalloid fluid administration, gastroprotectants, EPO therapy, RBC transfusions, and supplemental iron administration.

Anesthesia and analgesia

Topical (oral) anesthetics may be utilized if oral ulceration is severe enough to impact normal prehension and mastication. The placement of indwelling feeding tubes (esophagostomy, gastrostomy) allows administration of water, nutrition, and medication for animals with uremia. Tube placement should be performed cautiously in animals with underlying hemorrhagic tendencies.

Diagnostic testing: laboratory, imaging, biopsy

Anemia is readily diagnosed on routine blood work. Azotemia is identified as elevations in blood urea nitrogen, creatinine, and phosphorus. Urine specific gravity may be concentrated in cases of prerenal azotemia or may be isosthenuric. Platelet dysfunction and prolonged bleeding times are diagnosed as described above.

Hepatic

Animals with severe acute or chronic hepatic disease may have clinical hemorrhage. In most cases, this will be due to decreased production of coagulation factors, which results in a syndrome similar to that of rodenticide toxicity.

Pharmacology, treatment, and contraindications

In addition to coagulation support, therapy may need to be directed toward the primary hepatic disease itself. It should be noted that stored canine RBC products have higher ammonia concentrations. It is uncertain if administration of stored RBCs to animals with hepatic disease may result in hyperammonemia and neurological signs. Low protein diets may be required for severe hepatic disease or for those animals with hepatic encephalopathy. However, it is important to ensure that diets are nutritionally complete and protein malnutrition does not result.

Diagnostic testing: laboratory, imaging, biopsy

In addition to prolonged bleeding times as described above, potential laboratory indications for hepatic disease include hypoglycemia, hypoalbuminemia, elevated liver enzymes, hyperbilirubinemia, and hypocholesterolemia. If hepatic biopsy is pursued, coagulation status needs to be determined prior to invasive techniques and coagulation support may be necessary. Most, if not all, systemic anesthetics and analgesics require some degree of hepatic metabolism. Dosage adjustments may be necessary and close monitoring for side effects and drug interactions is recommended.

Disorders of platelets

Platelets are the first line of defense against bleeding at the sites of vascular injury and play a critical role in the initiation, regulation, and localization of hemostasis. These small, anucleated cells originate in the bone marrow from megakaryocytes and are the second most numerous cells in circulation. Thrombopoietin is the major cytokine that regulates all stages of megakaryocyte and platelet production. Platelet production is regulated by total platelet mass rather than platelet numbers. Approximately 30% of the platelet circulating mass can be transiently compartmentalized in the spleen. Platelets circulate in the bloodstream for approximately 5–9 days. Macrophages in the spleen and liver remove aging platelets. In the healthy body, there is a steady state between platelet production and platelet destruction.

Thrombocytopenia

Thrombocytopenia is defined as a decrease in circulating platelet numbers and results from one or more of four basic mechanisms. See Table 7.4.1 for causes of thrombocytopenia.

Decreased production disorders are uncommon and result from disorders or radiation therapy that directly affects the megakaryocyte or bone marrow microenvironment (e.g., tumor infiltration, fibrosis, and necrosis). Infiltrative neoplasia or leukemia may decrease platelet numbers due to the destruction of the bone marrow architecture. Acquired megakaryocytic hypoplasia occurs as a consequence of immune-mediated destruction or secondary to infections or drug reactions. See Table 7.4.2 for drugs that may affect platelet function or numbers.

Increased platelet loss or consumption results in a mild to moderate decrease in platelet number. Thrombocytopenia with external hemorrhage is usually self-limiting and resolves once the hemorrhage is stopped. Massive trauma may result in utilization of platelets in areas of vascular damage. The thrombocytopenia associated with massive trauma is usually mild to moderate and transient. DIC occurs secondarily to a wide variety of systemic diseases (septicemia, neoplasia, and severe metabolic disease). DIC is characterized by overwhelming activation of coagulation and subsequent disruption of normal regulatory mechanisms. The degree of thrombocytopenia with DIC is variable. Hemolytic uremic syndrome is rare in veterinary patients but has been reported in dogs. Acute renal failure and microangiopathic hemolytic anemia and thrombocytopenia are preceded by hemorrhagic diarrhea in these cases.

Increased platelet destruction results as a consequence of platelet lysis, phagocytosis, or aggregation. IMT is the most common cause of increased platelet destruction. Primary IMT occurs independent of predisposing factors (drugs, infectious agents, and neoplasia). Secondary IMT results when there is a clear association of thrombocytopenia with an underlying condition.

Thrombocytopenia associated with platelet sequestration is rare. Hypersplenism occurs when 90% of the circulating platelets become sequestered in the spleen and is characterized by splenomegaly, the presence of one or more cytopenias, and bone marrow hyperplasia. Mild thrombocytopenia may develop with severe hypothermia. This condition adversely affects platelet morphology, leading to platelet pooling in the spleen.

It is important to note that several breeds have nonclinical thrombocytopenia. The greyhound platelet count normally ranges between 80,000 and 120,000/μL. An inherited thrombocytopenia has been reported in the CKCS. An autosomal recessive trait has been identified and as many as 50% of CKCS may be affected. Macroplatelets are often present and may result in unreliable platelet counts when using automated machines; therefore, hand platelet evaluation is more reliable in assessing platelet numbers in this breed (see Figure 7.4.1). Although the circulating platelet number is decreased, the total platelet mass remains normal and the thrombocytopenia in this breed is considered benign and clinically insignificant.

Table 7.4.1 Causes of thrombocytopenia

Decreased production (primary bone marrow disease)	Increased platelet loss or consumption	Increased platelet destruction	Platelet sequestration
Megakaryocytic hypoplasia	Hemorrhage	Immune-mediated thrombocytopenia	Hypersplenism
Immune mediated			
Cytoxic drug effect			
Infections			
Infection	Massive trauma	Infections	Severe hypothermia
Viral (e.g. parvo, FIV, FeLV)		Bacterial	
Rickettsial (e.g. ehrlichia)		Rickettsial	
		Viral	
Myelopthisis	Disseminated intravascular coagulation (DIC)	Neoplasia	
Neoplasia		Hemangiosarcoma	
Myelofibrosis		Lymphoproliferative tumors	
		Myeloproliferative tumors	
		Hemophagocytic	
		Histiosarcoma	
Myelonecrosis	Hemolytic uremic syndrome (HUS)	Drugs	
		Various antibiotics	
		Chemotherapy drugs	
		Phenobarbital	
		NSAIDs	
		Estrogen	
Radiation therapy			

Clinical signs

The approach to the thrombocytopenic patient should include a detailed history, thorough physical examination, and an initial minimum database (CBC, biochemical panel, coagulation panel, urinalysis, chest and abdominal radiographs). The severity of the thrombocytopenia may also help narrow the list of rule-outs. Treatment of thrombocytopenia is aimed at eliminating or managing the underlying disease.

Primary IMT is the most common cause of severe thrombocytopenia in the author's clinic. It is important to obtain a detailed history to rule out drug reactions (including vaccination schedule) and exposure to infectious agents (tick infestation, geographic location). Clinical signs reported by the owner include lethargy, anorexia, weakness, collapse, hematuria, hemorrhage (skin, eyes, gums, nose), and GI bleeding. Some animals may be asymptomatic and the thrombocytopenia is detected in a CBC. Physical findings may include petechial and ecchymotic hemorrhages, epistaxis, melena, oral hemorrhage, and hematuria (see Figures 7.4.2 and 7.4.3). Pale mucous membranes, tachycardia, and a heart murmur may occur with severe hemorrhage.

The diagnosis of primary IMT is one of exclusion. Blood work, body imaging, infectious disease panels, and bone marrow evaluation are necessary to rule out other causes of thrombocytopenia. Flow cytometry has been utilized to detect platelet surface-associated immunoglobulin (PSAIg) in dogs and cats. PSAIg are found in patients with IMT and other secondary disorders (secondary IMT) and are not pathognomonic for primary IMT. A major disadvantage of this test is false-positive results due to a number of factors such as low storage temperature, improper blood drawing, tube agitation, and storage time.

Treatment

Immunosuppressive doses of glucocorticoids are the mainstay of treatment for IMT. Other immunosuppressive agents such as azathioprine, cyclosporine, cyclophosphamide, danazol, mycophenolate, vincristine, and human gammaglobulin have been used. Platelet transfusion (PRP) may be used in life-threatening situations. The life span of transfused platelets is relatively short due to the increased consumption and destruction by circulating antiplatelet antibodies. Splenectomy may be a consideration

Table 7.4.2 Drugs that have been associated with platelet disorders

Drug	Effect on platelet
Antibiotics	
Cephalosporins	Altered platelet function
Chloramphenicol	Decreased platelet number
Penicillin	Decreased platelet number
Sulfonamides	Decreased platelet number
Anti-inflammatory drugs	
Aspirin	Altered platelet function
Ibuprofen	Altered platelet function
Naproxen	Altered platelet function
Phenylbutazone	Altered platelet function, decreased platelet number
Cardiac and respiratory drugs	
Aminophylline	Altered platelet function
Diltiazem	Altered platelet function
Procainamide	Decreased platelet number
Propranolol	Altered platelet function
Verapamil	Altered platelet function
Cytotoxic drugs	
Azathioprine	Decreased platelet number
Chlorambucil	Decreased platelet number
Cyclophosphamide	Decreased platelet number
Doxorubicin	Decreased platelet number
Miscellaneous	
Dextran	Altered platelet function
Estrogen	Decreased platelet number
Methimazole	Decreased platelet number

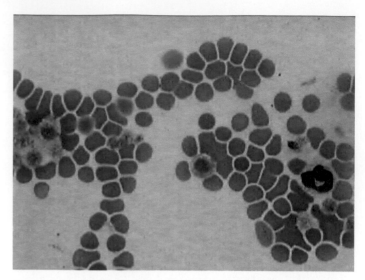

Figure 7.4.1 Macroplatelets in a Cavalier King Charles spaniel. Courtesy of Stan Krogman, Site Manager, Marshfield Veterinary Labs, Marshfield, Wisconsin.

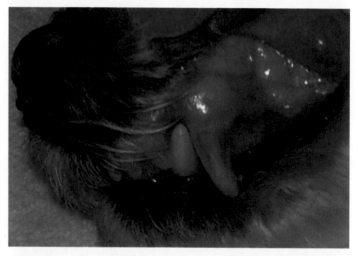

Figure 7.4.2 Petechial hemorrhage in the oral mucosa of a dog with IMT.

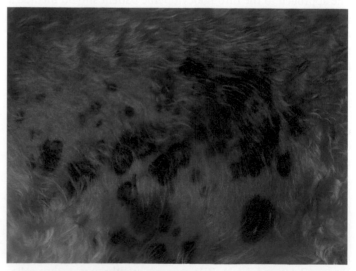

Figure 7.4.3 Ecchymotic hemorrhages of the lateral body wall of a miniature poodle with IMT.

when there is poor response to medical therapy. Supportive care utilizing intravenous fluids, antiemetics, gastroproctectant agents, and RBC transfusions may also be necessary. Antibiotics must be used with caution due to potential side effects. Patients should be handled with care due to the increased risk of bruising. Injections, venipunctures, and needle aspirations (e.g., for cysto-centesis) should be avoided. A peripheral vein should be used for blood samples, and a pressure bandage should be applied to the site used. Liquid and soft diets are used to prevent damage to the gingival surfaces.

Prognosis

The prognosis with IMT is guarded. Survival rates reported have ranged from 10% to 43%; however, relapses of the thrombocytopenia may occur, requiring chronic therapy.

Thrombocytosis

Thrombocytosis is defined as an increased platelet count above the reference range. Causes of thrombocytosis are listed in Table 7.4.3.

Psuedothrombocytosis occurs when cell fragments are counted as platelets. Evaluation of the blood smear is helpful to verify the platelet count and to identify any morphological changes.

Reactive thrombocytosis is the most common cause of increased platelet numbers in dogs and cats. Cytokine stimulation of thrombopoietin is suspected to induce the thrombocytosis. Physiological thrombocytosis may develop secondary to splenic contraction, which can be secondary to excitement, exercise, and trauma. In humans, a transient or persistent thrombocytosis occurs after splenectomy. This phenomenon is not a consistent finding in dogs. Several drugs (vinca alkaloids, epinephrine, and glucocorticoids) have been associated with thrombocytosis. Inflammation, infections, and trauma are another cause of thrombocytosis. Several retrospective studies reported that GI disorders (pancreatitis, inflammatory bowel disease, chronic hepatitis) were only second to neoplasia (lymphoma, carcinoma) as a cause of thrombocytosis. Other causes of reactive thrombocytosis include iron deficiency, endocrine disorders (hyperadrenocorticism, diabetes mellitus, hypothyroidism), and a rebound phenomenon associated with recovery from thrombocytopenia disorders. Treatment of reactive thrombocytosis is directed at the cause of the underlying disease.

Essential thrombocytosis is a clonal disorder of hematopoiesis that affects megakaryocytes. The disease is characterized by a marked thrombocytosis in peripheral blood and megakaryocytic hyperplasia of the bone marrow. This disease is rare in dogs and cats and must be differentiated from reactive thrombocytosis.

Other bone marrow disorders associated with thrombocytosis include polycythemia vera and basophilic leukemia, which are rarely reported in dogs and cats.

Table 7.4.3 Causes of thrombocytosis

Psuedothrombocytosis
Reactive thrombocytosis
Physiological—redistribution
Epinephrine
Postsplenectomy
Drug induced
Vinca alkaloids
Epinephrine
Glucocorticoids
Inflammation, infection, trauma
Rebound effect from thrombocytopenia
Iron deficiency
Paraneoplastic (lymphoma, lung carcinoma)
Endocrine disorders (hyperadrenocorticism, diabetes mellitus, hypothyroidism)
Neoplasia involving megakaryocytes
Primary (essential) thrombocytosis
Acute megakaryocyte leukemia (M7)
Myeloproliferative disease
Polycythemia vera
Basophilic leukemia

Platelet function disorders

Thrombocytopathia is defined as platelet dysfunction. The clinical significance of platelet function abnormalities is variable. The pathogenesis is complex and multifactorial. Many disease processes (anemia, liver failure, uremia, DIC, and paraproteinemia) may result in platelet dysfunction. Many drugs are associated with thrombocytopenia and/or platelet dysfunction (see Table 7.4.2).

Congenital defects of platelet dysfunction are rare. Intrinsic platelet disorders are characterized by defects of membrane glycoproteins, storage granules, signal transduction proteins, or structural proteins. Extrinsic platelet disorders are characterized by abnormalities in plasma or subendothelial proteins that are necessary for platelet adhesion or aggregation. von Willebrand disease (vWD) and hypo- or dysfibrinogenemia are examples of extrinsic platelet disorders.

Glanzmann's thrombobastenia (GT) occurs when platelet glycoprotein complex IIb–IIIa is absent or markedly reduced. This disorder has been reported as an autosomal recessive trait in otterhounds and Great Pyrenees dogs. Basset hounds and Eskimo spitz dogs have been reported to have an inherited signal transduction platelet disorder. The lack of procoagulant expression on the surface of platelets has been recognized in a family of German shepherd dogs. Although the clinical signs are typical of a coagulopathy (e.g., epistaxis, hyphema, and intramuscular hemorrhage), this is a platelet defect.

von Willebrand disease

vWD is the most common hereditary hemostatic defect in dogs; it is an autosomal trait. There are both incomplete dominance and recessive patterns seen. Multiple breeds have been reported with this disease and include the Doberman pinscher, Airedale terrier, Akita, dachshund, Bernese mountain dog, Coton de Tuléar, German shepherd, golden retriever, greyhound, Irish wolfhound, Kerry blue terrier, papillon, Pembroke Welsh corgi, schnauzer, Shetland sheepdog, Chesapeake Bay retriever, and Scottish terrier.

The bleeding tendency of vWD is caused by functional deficiencies of von Willebrand factor. vWF is a large plasma glycoprotein necessary for platelet adhesion at the site of vascular damage. The major site of vWF synthesis is the endothelial cell. vWF subunits combine to form dimers then multimers. These multimers act as a carrier for the coagulation factor VIII. When vascular injury occurs, vWF binds to the subendothelial collagen and supports platelet adherence and platelet plug formation. There are three subtypes classified in dogs, based on the vWF multimers, plasma vWF antigen concentration (vWF : Ag), and the severity of clinical signs. Type 1 is characterized by normal multimer distribution, low plasma vWF : Ag, and mild to moderate bleeding. Type 2 occurs when there is a disproportionate loss of high molecular weight multimers, a variable decrease in plasma vWF : Ag, and moderate to severe bleeding. Type 3 occurs due to a total lack of vWF and results in severe bleeding.

Clinical signs

Clinical signs are characterized by mucosal bleeding (e.g., epistaxis, hematuria, GI bleeding, gingival bleeding, and prolonged estral bleeding in intact females), cutaneous bruising, and prolonged hemorrhage after injury or surgery. Petechial hemorrhage is uncommon in this disease.

Diagnostics

The diagnosis of vWD is made in patients with low plasma vWF : Ag, a normal platelet count, normal coagulation tests, and a prolonged buccal mucosal bleeding time. vWF antigen (vWF : Ag), the most common test used, is an enzyme-linked immunosorbent assay (ELISA). The blood sample should be drawn directly into the citrated blood tube via a Vacutainer® blood collection needle (BD Diagnostics, Franklin Lakes, NJ). Once blood is drawn directly into a syringe, the clotting cascade begins and may cause inaccurate test results. Within 30 min, the blood sample should be spun and the plasma separated and placed into another tube to be sent to the lab. Results are reported as a percentage of normal. Each laboratory determines the reference range; however, in general, normal animals have greater than 50% vWF : Ag.

Treatment

Treatment of vWD includes control of the active sites of hemorrhage and the use of blood products (FWB 20 mL/kg), FFP (10 mL/kg), and/or cryoprecipitate (1 U/10 kg). Desmopressin acetate (deamino-8-d-arginine vasopressin [DDAVP]) can be used in dogs with type 1 VWD. This drug may act by stimulating endothelial V2 vasopressin receptors, resulting in the release of vWF. Desmopressin has been recommended as a presurgical treatment in dogs with type 1 VWD. The dose is 1 mcg/kg subcutaneously 1 h prior to surgery. Close surgical monitoring is advised as additional blood products (FFP or whole blood) may be necessary.

Breed-related disorders

Defective neutrophil function in Dobermans

Defective neutrophil function in Dobermans is also called bactericidal neutrophil defect. Inheritance (carriers, disease expression, and litter issues) has not been determined for this disease. Neutrophils appear to phagocytize bacteria normally, but bacterial killing is impaired. Some affected animals may live for years with therapy; thus, it is suspected that the defect may be partial, as compared to complete, in those animals. The most common clinical syndrome is chronic rhinitis and pneumonia, evidenced by sneezing, coughing, and nasal discharge. The earliest reported age of presentation is 9 months.

Pharmacology, treatment, and contraindications

Affected animals may respond well, though temporarily, to antimicrobial therapy. As repeated treatments are necessary, antibiotic choices should be based on culture and sensitivity results when possible. Samples should be obtained under sterile conditions. Sulfa-based antibiotics should be used with caution in Doberman pinschers. This breed appears to be overrepresented with sulfa drug side effects such as blood dyscrasias, polyarthritis, and decreased tear production.

Diagnostic testing

The CBC is variable. RBC indices are primarily within normal limits. Neutrophilia with a left shift may be seen, and eosinophilia is reported, though concurrent parasitism may affect eosinophil counts. Serum biochemistry panels and urinalysis are also primarily within normal limits. Thoracic radiographs of affected dogs may have radiographic signs of cardiomyopathy and may show evidence of bronchopneumonia. If histopathology is performed on the affected lung tissue, results are consistent with chronic pneumonia. Ciliary lesions (as may be seen with ciliary dyskinesia) have not been identified.

Anesthetic and analgesia

As for any animal with significant pulmonary disease, anesthesia should be carefully planned. Ensuring a patent airway and providing adequate oxygen supplementation are essential. If concurrent cardiomyopathy is present, judicious fluid administration during anesthesia is warranted.

Combined immunodeficiency in Jack Russell terriers

Inheritance is most consistent with an autosomal recessive disease. There is no evidence for sex-linked inheritance, and carrier animals are clinically normal. Some affected puppies may become ill and may die after vaccination with modified live vaccines as early as 8 weeks of age. Puppies that are not vaccinated begin to show clinical signs of illness at 14–15 weeks of age, including pneumonia, diarrhea, and neurological disease.

Treatment

There is no known treatment for this disease and the genetic defect is uniformly fatal.

Diagnostic testing

Affected puppies have little to no detectable B lymphocytes and, as a result, are severely lymphopenic on CBC. In animals with lymphopenia, serum immunoglobulins are also significantly reduced when compared to normal litter mates. If biopsy or necropsy is pursued, lymphoid tissue (spleen, thymus, lymph node) is markedly reduced in affected puppies.

Birman cat neutrophil granulation anomaly

This is an autosomal recessive trait identified in purebred Birman cats. Affected cats have azurophilic granules seen in the cytoplasm of neutrophils, and these granules must be differentiated from other cytoplasmic inclusion bodies. Neutrophil function is normal and immunity is not impaired. Affected animals have no clinical signs.

Immunodeficiency of shar-peis

Inheritance is unknown and dogs present with signs of illness at an average of 3 years of age. Affected dogs present with a variety of recurrent illnesses, including cutaneous (pyoderma, demodecosis, otitis), intestinal (inflammatory bowel disease, ulcerative colitis, adenocarcinoma), and respiratory diseases and fever.

Pharmacology and treatment

Treatment should be directed based on results of diagnostic evaluation, including histopathology. As there is no cure, therapy is primarily supportive and aimed at disease control. Animals may be lethargic and febrile, so appropriate nursing care with analgesic support is recommended.

Diagnostic testing

Affected dogs have deficiencies in one or multiple immunoglobulins (IgA, IgM, and IgG). Lymphocytes show abnormal responses and proliferation indices, though specific laboratory testing is required to demonstrate these abnormalities. The immunodeficiency affects both cell-mediated and humoral immune responses.

Immunodeficiency of Weimaraners

The mode of inheritance is unknown, though a genetic basis for the disease is suspected on the basis of young age of presentation (median age at presentation is 4 months) and familial predisposition. There is no apparent gender predilection, so a sex-linked trait is less likely. The most common clinical signs include pyrexia, vomiting and diarrhea, joint pain and swelling, long bone pain, subcutaneous swelling at injection sites, lymphadenopathy, urinary tract infection, and pyoderma. Bronchopneumonia and meningitis have also been reported.

Pharmacology and treatment

Clinical presentation is variable, though some cases present soon after vaccination and are treated with steroids for presumptive vaccine reactions. When possible, therapeutic decisions should be based on culture and sensitivity, cytology, and/or histopathology results. Osteopathic manifestations of the disease may be painful, and therapy with NSAIDs and steroids has been reported. The concurrent use of steroids and NSAIDs should be avoided due to increased risk of GI side effects. As most affected animals are young, nutritional calculations should take musculoskeletal growth into account. Nutrient-dense diets may be recommended to minimize the volume of diet that would need to be fed to an animal with clinical illness.

Diagnostic testing

Leukocytosis with a neutrophilia is commonly seen on CBC. There is evidence that a neutrophil phagocytic defect may also be present; however, this has not been thoroughly elucidated. There are no consistent changes noted on serum biochemistry analysis. However, when specific immunoglobulins are measured, significant decreases in IgG are noted in affected dogs. Other immunoglobulins (IgA, IgM) may also be decreased below the standard reference range. Additional testing, including histopathology, should be pursued depending upon the clinical presentation of the animal.

Bibliography

Section 1

1. Colville T, Bassert JM. *Clinical Anatomy and Physiology for Veterinary Technicians*, 2nd edition, pp. 205–246. St. Louis, MO: Mosby Elsevier; 2008.
2. Guyton AC, Hall JE. *Textbook of Medical Physiology*, 10th edition, pp. 96–106, 162–174, 419–429. Philadelphia, PA: W.B. Saunders; 2000.
3. Nelson RW, Couto CG. *Small Animal Internal Medicine*, 4th edition, pp. 1242–1244, 1260–1264. St. Louis, MO: Mosby Elsevier; 2009.
4. Evans HE, Christensen GC. *Miller's Anatomy of the Dog*, 2nd edition, pp. 802–841. Philadelphia, PA: W.B. Saunders; 1980.
5. Weiss DJ, Wardrop KJ. *Schalm's Veterinary Hematology*, 6th edition, pp. 635–653. Ames, IA: Blackwell Publishing; 2010.

Section 2

1. Stockham SL, Scott MA. *Fundamentals of Veterinary Clinical Pathology*. Ames, IA: Blackwell Publishing; 2008.
2. Kociba GJ. Erythrocytes. *Veterinary Clinics of North America. Small Animal Practice* 1989;19:627–635.
3. Alsaker RD, Laber J, Stevens J, Perman V. A comparison of polychromasia and reticulocyte counts in assessing erythrocytic regenerative response in the cat. *Journal of the American Veterinary Medical Association* 1977;170:39–41.
4. Weiss DJ. New insights into the physiology and treatment of acquired myelodysplastic syndromes and aplastic pancytopenia. *Veterinary Clinics of North America. Small Animal Practice* 2003;33:1317–1334.

5. Lappin T. The cellular biology of erythropoietin receptors. *The Oncologist* 2003;8 Suppl 1:15–18.

6. Giger U, Mason GD, Wang P. Inherited erythrocyte pyruvate kinase deficiency in a beagle dog. *Veterinary Clinical Pathology* 1991;20:83–86.

7. Feldman BV, Zinkl JG, Jain NC, Schalm OW. *Schalm's Veterinary Hematology*. Philadelphia, PA: Lippincott Williams & Wilkins; 2000.

8. Harvey JW. Pathogenesis, laboratory diagnosis, and clinical implications of erythrocyte enzyme deficiencies in dogs, cats, and horses. *Veterinary Clinical Pathology* 2006;35:144–156.

9. Weiss DJ. Bone marrow pathology in dogs and cats with non-regenerative immune-mediated haemolytic anaemia and pure red cell aplasia. *Journal of Comparative Pathology* 2008;138:46–53.

10. Thrall MA. *Veterinary Hematology and Clinical Chemistry*. Philadelphia, PA: Lippincott Williams & Wilkins; 2004.

11. Kessler M. Secondary polycythaemia associated with high plasma erythropoietin concentrations in a dog with a necrotising pyelonephritis. *Journal of Small Animal Practice* 2008;49:363–366.

12. Hsia CC, Johnson RL, JR, Dane DM, Wu EY, Estrera AS, Wagner HE, Wagner PD. The canine spleen in oxygen transport: gas exchange and hemodynamic responses to splenectomy. *Journal of Applied Physiology* 2007;103:1496–1505.

13. Gray HE, Weigand CM, Cottrill NB, Willis AM, Morgan RV. Polycythemia vera in a dog presenting with uveitis. *Journal of the American Animal Hospital Association* 2003;39:355–360.

14. Feldman BF, Sink CA. *Practical Transfusion Medicine for the Small Animal Practitioner*. Jackson, WY: Teton NewMedia; 2006.

15. Abrams-Ogg A. Practical blood transfusion. In: *Manual of Canine and Feline Haematology and Transfusion Medicine*, eds. M Day, A Mackin, J Littlewood, pp. 263–303. Gloucester: British Small Animal Veterinary Association; 2008.

16. Mischke R. Plasma transfusion and automated plasmapheresis—possibilities and limitations for veterinary medicine. *Veterinary Journal* 2005;169(1):102–107.

17. Guillaumin J, Jandrey KE, Norris JW, et al. Assessment of a dimethyl sulfoxide–stabilized frozen canine platelet concentrate. *American Journal of Veterinary Research* 2008;Dec;69(12):1580–1586.

18. Wardrop JK, Reine N, Birkenheuer A, et al. Canine and feline blood donor screening for infectious disease. *Journal of Veterinary Internal Medicine* 2005;Jan-Feb;19(1):135–142.

19. Duval D, Giger U. Vaccine-associated immune-mediated hemolytic anemia in the dog. *Journal of Veterinary Internal Medicine* 1996;10:290–295.

20. Goggs R, Boag AK, Chan DL. Concurrent immune-mediated haemolytic anaemia and severe thrombocytopenia in 21 dogs. *Veterinary Record* 2008;163(11):323–327.

21. Carr AP, Panciera DL, Kidd L. Prognostic factors for mortality and thromboembolism in canine immune-mediated hemolytic anemia: a retrospective study of 72 dogs. *Journal of Veterinary Internal Medicine* 2002;16:504–509.

22. Scott-Moncrieff JCR, Reagan WJ, Snyder PW, Glickman LT. Intravenous administration of human immune globulin in dogs with immune-mediated hemolytic anemia. *Journal of the American Veterinary Medical Association* 1997;210:1623–1627.

23. Burgess K, Moore A, Rand W, Cotter SM. Treatment of immune-mediated hemolytic anemia in dogs with cyclophosphamide. *Journal of Veterinary Internal Medicine* 2000;14:456–462.

24. Grundy SA, Barton C. Influence of drug treatment on survival of dogs with immune-mediated hemolytic anemia: 88 cases (1989–1999). *Journal of the American Veterinary Medical Association* 2001;218:543–546.

25. Helmond SE, Polzin DJ, Armstrong PJ, Finke M, Smith SA. Treatment of immune-mediated hemolytic anemia with individually adjusted heparin dosing in dogs. *Journal of Veterinary Internal Medicine* [0891-6640] SE 2010;24(3):597–605.

26. Weinkle TK, Center SA, Randolph JF, Warner KL, Barr SC, Erb HN. Evaluation of prognostic factors, survival rates, and treatment protocols for immune-mediated hemolytic anemia in dogs: 151 cases (1993–2002). *Journal of the American Veterinary Medical Association* 2005;226(11):1869–1880.

Section 3

1. Fenner WR. *Quick Reference to Veterinary Medicine*, 3rd edition, pp. 149–158. Philadelphia, PA: Lippincott, Williams and Wilkins; 2000.

2. Nelson RW, Couto CG. *Small Animal Internal Medicine*, 4th edition, pp. 1228–1235. St. Louis, MO: Mosby Elsevier; 2009.

3. Weiss DJ, Wardrop KJ. *Schalm's Veterinary Hematology*, 6th edition, pp. 263–365. Ames, IA: Blackwell Publishing; 2010.

4. Ettinger SJ, Feldman EC. *Textbook of Veterinary Internal Medicine*, 7th edition, Chapters 801–809. St. Louis, MO: Saunders Elsevier; 2010.

5. Latimer KS, Campagnoli RP, Danilenko DM. Pelger–Huët anomaly in Australian shepherds: 87 cases (1991–1997). *Comparative Haematology International* 2000;10:9–13.

6. Latimer KS, Duncan JR, Kircher IM. Nuclear segmentation, ultrastructure, and cytochemistry of blood cells from dogs with Pelger–Huët anomaly. *Journal of Comparative Pathology* 1987;97:61–72.

7. Latimer KS, Rakich PM, Thompson DF. Pelger–Huët anomaly in cats. *Veterinary Pathology* 1985;22:370–374.

8. Hirsch VM, Cunningham TA. Hereditary anomaly of neutrophil granulation in Birman cats. *American Journal of Veterinary Research* 1984;45(10):2170–2174.

9. Prieur DJ, Collier LL. Neutropenia in cats with the Chédiak–Higashi syndrome. *Canadian Journal of Veterinary Research* 1987;51:407–408.

10. Prieur DJ, Collier LL. Inheritance of the Chédiak–Higashi syndrome in cats. *Journal of Heredity* 1981;72(3):175–177.

11. Breitschwerdt EB, Brown TT, De Buysscher EV, Andersen BR, Thrall DE, Hager E, Ananaba G, Degen MA, Ward MD. Rhinitis, pneumonia, and defective neutrophil function in the Doberman pinscher. *American Journal of Veterinary Research* 1987;48(7):1054–1062.

12. Foureman P, Whiteley M, Giger U. Canine leukocyte adhesion deficiency: presence of the Cys36Ser beta-2 integrin mutation in an affected US Irish setter cross-breed dog and in US Irish red and white setters. *Journal of Veterinary Internal Medicine* 2002;16(5):518–523.

13. Bauer TR, Allen JM, Hai M, Tuschong LM, Khan IF, Olson EM, Adler RL, Burkholder TH, Gu Y, Russell DW, Hickstein DD. Successful treatment of canine leukocyte adhesion deficiency by foamy virus vectors. *Nature Medicine* 2008;14:93–97.

14. Skelly BJ, Franklin RJM. Recognition and diagnosis of lysosomal storage diseases in the cat and dog. *Journal of Veterinary Internal Medicine* 2002;16:133–141.

15. Pacheco JM, Traulsen M, Antal T, Dingli D. Cyclic neutropenia in animals. *American Journal of Hematology* 2008;83:920–921.

16. Abkowitz JL, Holly RD, Hammond WP. Cyclic hematopoeisis in dogs: studies of erythroid burst-forming cells confirm an early stem cell defect. *Experimental Hematology* 1988;16:941–945.

17. Lothrop CD, Warren DJ, Souza LM, Jones JB, Moore MAS. Correction of canine cyclic hematopoiesis with recombinant human granulocyte colony-stimulating factor. *Blood* 1988;72:1324–1328.

18. Hammond WP, Boone TC, Donahue RE, Souza LM, Dale DC. A comparison of treatment of canine cyclic hematopoiesis with recombinant human granulocyte-macrophage-colony stimulating factor (GM-CSF), G-CSF, interleukin-3, and canine G-CSF. *Blood* 1990;76:523–532.

19. Yanay O, Barry SC, Katen LJ, Brzezinski M, Flint LY, Christensen J, Liggitt D, Dale DC, Osborne WR. Treatment of canine cyclic neutropenia by lentivirus-mediated G-CSF delivery. *Blood* 2003;102:2046–2052.

20. Krakowka S, Johnson G, Ciekot P, Hill R, Lafrado L, Kociba G. In vitro immunologic features of Weimaraner dogs with neutrophil abnormalities and recurrent infections. *Veterinary Immunology and Immunopathology* 1989;23:103–112.

21. Hansen P, Clercx C, Henroteaux M, Rutten PM, Bernakina WE. Neutrophil phagocyte dysfunction in a Weimaraner with recurrent infections. *Journal of Small Animal Practice* 1995;36:128–131.

22. Harrus S, Waner T, Aizenberg I, Safra N, Mosenco A, Radoshitsky M, Bark H. Development of hypertrophic osteodystrophy and antibody response in a litter of vaccinated Weimaraner puppies. *Journal of Small Animal Practice* 2002;43:27–31.

23. Center SA, Randolph JF, Erb HN, Reiter S. Eosinophilia in the cat: a retrospective study of 312 cases (1975–1986). *Journal of the American Animal Hospital Association* 1990;26:349–358.

24. Wilson SC, Thomson-Kerr K, Houston DM. Hypereosinophilic syndrome in a cat. *The Canadian Veterinary Journal* 1996;37:679–680.

25. Neer M. Hypereosinophilic syndrome in cats. *Compendium of Continuing Education Small Animal Practice* 1991;13:549–555.

26. Uivas AL, Tintle L, Argentieri D, Kimball ES, Goodman MG, Anderson DQ, Capetola RJ, Quimby FW. A primary immunodeficiency syndrome in shar-pei dogs. *Clinical Immunology and Immunopathology* 1995;74:243–251.

27. Felsburg PJ, Glickman LT, Jezyk PF. Selective IgA deficiency in the dog. *Clinical Immunology and Immunopathology* 1985;36:297 305.

28. Jezyk PF, Felsburg PJ, Haskins ME, Patterson DF. X-linked severe combined immunodeficiency in the dog. *Clinical Immunology and Immunopathology* 1989;52:173–189.

29. Pullen RP, Somberg RL, Felsburg PJ, Henthorn PS. X-linked severe combined immunodeficiency in a family of Cardigan Welsh corgis. *Journal of the American Animal Hospital Association* 1997;33:494–499.

30. De Ravin SST, Kennedy DR, Naumann N, Kennedy JS, Choi U, Hartnett J, Linton GF, Whiting-Theobald NL, Moore PF, Vernau W, Malech HL, Felsburg PJ. Correction of canine X-linked severe combined immunodeficiency by in vivo retroviral gene therapy. *Blood* 2006;107:3091–3097.

31. Bell TG, Butler KL, Sill HB, Stickle JE, Ramos-Vara JA, Dark MJ. Autosomal recessive severe combined immunodeficiency of Jack Russell terriers. *Journal of Veterinary Diagnostic Investigation* 2002;14:194–204.

32. Blum JR, Cork LC, Morris JM, Olson JL, Winkelstein JA. The clinical manifestations of a genetically determined deficiency of the third component of complement in the dog. *Clinical Immunology and Immunopathology* 1985;34:304–315.

33. Ameratunga R, Winkelstein JA, Brody L, Binns M, Cork LC, Colomabani P, Valle D. Molecular analysis of the third component of canine complement (C3) and identification of the mutation responsible for hereditary canine C3 deficiency. *Journal of Immunology* 1998;160:2824–2830.

34. Clercx C, Reichler I, Peeters D, McEntee K, German A, Dubois J, Schynts F, Scaff-Lafontaine N, Willems T, Jorissen M, Day MJ. Rhinitis/bronchopneumonia syndrome in Irish wolfhounds. *Journal of Veterinary Internal Medicine* 2003;17:843–849.

35. Watson PJ, Wotton P, Eastwood J, Swift S, Jones B, Day MJ. Immunoglobulin deficiency in Cavalier King Charles spaniels with pneumocystosis pneumonia. *Journal of Veterinary Internal Medicine* 2006;20:523–527.

36. Lobetti RG, Leizewitz JA. *Pneumocystis carinii* in the miniature dachshund: case report and literature review. *Journal of Small Animal Practice* 1996;37(6):280–285.

Section 4

1. O'Kelley BM, Whelan MF, Brooks MB. Factor VIII inhibitors complicating treatment of postoperative bleeding in a dog with hemophilia A. *Journal of Veterinary Emergency and Critical Care* 2009;19(4):381–385.

2. Brooks M, DeWilde L. Feline factor XII deficiency. *Compendium* 2006;28(2, February):148–156.

3. Feldman BF, Zinkl JG, Jain NC. *Schalm's Veterinary Hematology*, 5th edition, Philadelphia, PA: Lippincott, Williams and Wilkins; 2000.

4. Smith JW, Day TK, Mackin A. Diagnosing bleeding disorders. *Compendium* 2005;27(11, November):828–843.

5. Berry CR, Gallaway A, Thrall DE, Carlisle C. Thoracic radiographic features of anticoagulant toxicity in fourteen dogs. *Veterinary Radiology & Ultrasound* 1993;34(6):391–396.

6. Sheafor SE, Couto CG. Anticoagulant rodenticide toxicity in 21 dogs. *Journal of the American Animal Hospital Association* 1999;35:38–46.

7. Waddell LS, Holt DE, Hughes D, Giger U. The effect of storage on ammonia concentration in canine packed red blood cells. *Journal of Veterinary Emergency and Critical Care* 2001;11(1):23–26.

8. Nelson RW, Couto CG. *Small Animal Internal Medicine*, 4th edition, pp. 1248–1250. St. Louis, MO: Mosby Elsevier; 2009.

9. Weiss DJ, Wardrop KJ. *Schalm's Veterinary Hematology*, 6th edition, pp. 561–631. Ames, IA: Blackwell Publishing; 2010.

10. Ettinger SJ, Feldman EC. *Textbook of Veterinary Internal Medicine*, 7th edition, pp. 777–783. St. Louis, MO: Saunders Elsevier; 2010.

11. Pedersen HD, Haggstrom J, Olsen LH, Christensen K, Selin A, Burmeister ML, Larsen H. Idiopathic asymptomatic thrombocytopenia in Cavalier King Charles spaniels is an autosomal recessive trait. *Journal of Veterinary Internal Medicine* 2002;16:169–173.

12. Davis B, Toivio-Kinnucan M, Schuller S, Boudreaux MK. Mutation in beta 1- tubulin correlates with macrothrombocytopenia in Cavalier King Charles spaniels. *Journal of Veterinary Internal Medicine* 2008;22:540–545.

13. Putsche JC, Kohn B. Primary immune-mediated thrombocytopenia in 30 dogs (1997–2003). *Journal of the American Animal Hospital Association* 2008;44:250–257.

14. Botsch V, Kuchenhoff H, Hartmann K, Hirshberger J. Retrospective study of 871 dogs with thrombocytopenia. *Veterinary Record* 2009;164:647–651.

15. Dircks BH, Schuberth HJ, Mischke R. Underlying diseases and clinicopathologic variables of thrombocytopenic dogs with and without platelet-bound antibodies detected by use of a flow cytometric assay: 83 cases (2004–2006). *Journal of the American Veterinary Medical Association* 2009;235:960–966.

16. Hammer AS. Thrombocytosis in dogs and cats: a retrospective study. *Comparative Haematology International* 1991;1:181–186.

17. Rizzo F, Tappin SW, Tasker S. Thrombocytosis in cats: a retrospective study of 51 cases (200 = 2005). *Journal of Feline Medicine and Surgery* 2007;9:319–325.

18. Bass MC, Schultze AE. Essential thrombocythemia in a dog: case report and literature review. *Journal of the American Animal Hospital Association* 1998;34:197–203.

19. Dunn JK, Heath MF, Jefferies AR, Blackwood L, McKay JS, Nicholls PK. Diagnostic and hematologic features of probable essential thrombocythemia in two dogs. *Veterinary Clinical Pathology* 1999;28:131–138.

20. Hogan DF, Dhaliwal RS, Sisson DD, Kitchell BE. Paraneoplastic thrombocytocysis-induced systemic thromboembolism in a cat. *Journal of the American Animal Hospital Association* 1999;35:483–486.

21. Boudreaux MK, Crager C, Dillon AR, et al. Identification of an intrinsic platelet function defect in Spitz dogs. *Journal of Veterinary Internal Medicine* 1994;8:93–98.

22. Boudreaux MK, Kvam K, Dillon AR, et al. Type I Glanzmann's thrombobasthenia in a Great Pyrenees dog. *Veterinary Pathology* 1996;33:503–511.

23. Boudreaux MK, Catalfamo JL. The molecular basis fro Glanzmann's thrombobasthenia in otterhounds. *American Journal of Veterinary Research* 2001;62:1797–1804.

24. Brooks MB, Catalfamo JL, Brown HA, et al. A hereditary bleeding disorder of dogs caused by a lack of platelet procoagulant activity. *Blood* 2002;99:2434–2441.

25. Breitschwerdt EB, Brown TT, DeBuysscher EV, Andersen BR, Thrall DE, Hager E, Ananaba G, Degen MA, Ward MDW. Rhinitis, pneumonia, and defective neutrophil function in the Doberman pinscher. *American Journal of Veterinary Research* 1987;48(7):1054–1062.

26. DeBey MC. Primary immunodeficiencies of dogs and cats. *Veterinary Clinics of North America. Small Animal Practice* 2010;40:425–438.

27. Bell TG, Butler KL, Sill HB, Stickle JE, Ramos-Vara JA, Dark MJ. Autosomal recessive severe combined immunodeficiency of Jack Russell terriers. *Journal of Veterinary Diagnostic Investigation* 2002;14:194–204.

28. Hirsch VM, Cunningham TA. Hereditary anomaly of neutrophil granulation in Birman cats. *American Journal of Veterinary Research* 1984;45(10):2170–2174.

29. Feldman BF, Zinkl JG, Jain NC. *Schalm's Veterinary Hematology*, 5th edition, pp. 467–594, 953–1054. Philadelphia, PA: Lippincott, Williams and Wilkins; 2000.

30. Rivas AL, Argentieri D, Kimball ES, Goodman MG, Anderson DW, Capetola RJ, Quimby FW. A primary immunodeficiency syndrome in shar-pei dogs. *Clinical Immunology and Immunopathology* 1995;74(3):243–251.

31. Foale RD, Herrtage ME, Day MJ. Retrospective study of 25 young Weimaraners with low serum immunoglobulin concentrations and inflammatory disease. *Veterinary Record* 2003;153:553–558.

32. Hansen P, Clercx C, Henroteaux M, Rutten VP, Bernadina WE. Neutrophil phagocyte dysfunction in a Weimaraner with recurrent infections. *Journal of Small Animal Practice* 1995;36(3):128–131.

Chapter 8 Gastrointestinal

Editors: Peter J. Bondy, Jr. and Ann Wortinger

SECTION 1 CLINICAL SIGNS AND EXAMINATION OF THE GI PATIENT

Gastrointestinal (GI) problems are one of the most common reasons pet owners bring their pet to a veterinary hospital. The main challenge to the veterinary health-care team presented with such a case is to determine whether this is an emergency or a potentially serious problem versus a chronic or intermittent problem.

While many cases of acute vomiting and/or diarrhea resolve uneventfully, some without any supportive care may become life-threatening disorders that, if not identified and treated, can lead to poor patient management and/or death of the pet.[1] It is imperative that the health-care team approach all patients presenting with GI concerns in a consistent, thorough manner. One of the most important steps in the process is a thorough physical examination, and that begins with an accurate history.

Patient history

The first step in patient evaluation is to obtain a complete history, starting with the signalment (i.e., species, breed, age, gender,

Small Animal Internal Medicine for Veterinary Technicians and Nurses, First Edition. Edited by Linda Merrill.
© 2012 John Wiley & Sons, Inc. Published 2012 by John Wiley & Sons, Inc.

reproductive status, activity level, and environment).[2] Next, questions to help assess GI signs should include the following:

- Duration and description of clinical signs
- Content of the vomitus
- Time in relation to eating
- Nature and frequency of vomiting (e.g., distinguish vomiting from retching, drooling, or regurgitation)
- Nature and frequency of diarrhea (mucus or blood in stool, frequency, tenesmus?)
- Dietary and environmental history

A nutritional history should also be performed to ascertain the quality and adequacy of the food, the feeding protocol (e.g., whether the pet is fed at designated meals or has free choice, the amount of food given), and the type or types of food given to the pet. When evaluating a pet presenting with GI signs, the technician should ask the owner the following questions:

- What brand and type of food do you feed your pet?
- What brand and type of snacks or treats do you give your pet?
- Do you give your pet any supplements? If so, what kind?
- Is your pet on any chewable medications? If so, what are they?
- What type of chew toys does your pet play with?
- What human foods does your pet consume?
- Does your pet have access to other sources of food?

It is also important to remember to discuss the potential that the pet could have eaten something from the trash or something out of the ordinary (e.g., rodenticides, pesticides, human medications).

Physical examination

A complete physical examination should be performed and the patient's overall attitude, posture, and energy level should be assessed. Patients with nausea will swallow frequently and may salivate. Patients with serious conditions such as foreign body obstruction, pancreatitis, or gastric neoplasia are often subdued upon examination. The mucous membranes should be observed as findings may suggest loss of blood or dehydration. An oral exam is necessary to rule out the potential of an oral or pharyngeal mass or foreign body that may be contributing to the GI disease. Cardiac auscultation should be performed to assess rate and rhythm abnormalities that may occur with metabolic disturbances such as hypoadrenocorticism, infectious enteritis with septic shock, or gastric dilatation–volvulus (GDV). Careful assessment and palpation of the abdomen should be performed and notice taken of generalized or localized pain. Remember to evaluate and note other abdominal factors such as organ size, presence of a mass, gastric distention, and altered bowel sounds. Rectal examinations should always be performed to examine

stool characteristics (e.g., fresh blood, mucus, or melena), to obtain a fresh stool sample for parasite and cytological examination and to evaluate the mucosa for sensitivity and/or abnormal texture.

The pet's body condition scoring (BCS) and weight should be documented at every visit as part of the physical examination. BCS is a subjective assessment that is important when determining whether a dog or a cat is at a healthy weight and when substantiating a weight loss or gain in a pet suffering with GI symptoms. It allows assessment of a patient's fat stores and muscle mass and helps in evaluating weight changes. The two most common BCS systems are the five- and nine-point scales. Both rating scales use nine points, but the five-point scale is scored to the nearest half-point, whereas the nine-point scale is scored to the whole point. It is important for all members of the health-care team to use the same scoring system from the outset so as not to confuse or miscalculate the patient's body condition.

Clinical signs of gastrointestinal disorders

When performing a history and physical examination on a potential GI patient, there are a number of clinical signs of which to be aware and to document (Table 8.1.1).

Oral manifestations of GI disease

Dysphagia (difficult or painful swallowing) may be present in an animal due to a foreign body, pain, motility disturbance, mass, trauma, or a combination of these. Dysphagia is most commonly indicative of a disorder in the oral cavity or in the pharynx, but esophageal disorders can cause dysphagia as well. The importance of taking a history is paramount as it is the history that most often differentiates oropharyngeal dysphagia from esophageal dysphagia. Oropharyngeal disorders typically include acute gagging, increased frequency of swallowing, and exaggerated swallowing movements. It is also common for food to be dropped from the mouth as the pet tries to pick up food to eat. Patients with esophageal dysphagia do not drop food from the mouth and do not exhibit the exaggerated swallowing motions seen with oropharyngeal dysphagia.[1]

Halitosis is associated with a proliferation of bacteria secondary to tissue necrosis, tartar, periodontitis, or retention (orally or esophageally) of food or noxious substances (eating of feces). Ptyalism (drooling) arises when animals are unable or are in too much pain to swallow. It is also attributed to nausea and can be seen in patients suffering from hepatic encephalopathy, hyperthermia, chemical or toxic stimulation of salivation, and seizures.[3]

Nature of vomiting

When dealing with patients presenting with potential GI disorders, it is imperative to distinguish regurgitation from vomiting.

Table 8.1.1 Clinical signs of gastrointestinal disease

Gastrointestinal sign	Definition of GI sign
Anorexia	Loss of appetite/not interested in eating
Borborygmus	Rumbling sound in the gut, caused by moving gas–fluid interface, from stomach through intestines
Constipation	Dry, hard feces; difficulty and straining to defecate
Diarrhea	Passage of feces containing excessive amount of water, increasing daily fecal weight
Dyschezia	Difficulty or painful passing of feces
Dysphagia	Difficult or painful swallowing
Flatulence	Presence of large amounts of intestinal air/gas, leading to distention of organs
Hematemesis	Vomiting of digested and/or fresh blood
Hematochezia	Bright red blood in feces
Melena	Black, tarry stools as a result of digested blood
Obstipation	Intractable constipation, typically with progressive enlargement and hardening of the feces
Polyphagia	Excessive eating or ingestion of food
Ptyalism	Excessive salivation
Regurgitation	Passive, upward movement of ingested material from the esophagus
Tenesmus	Ineffective and painful straining to pass stool

Regurgitation refers to the passive, retrograde movement of ingested material to a level above the upper esophageal sphincter. Typically, regurgitation happens before the ingested material reaches the stomach and is not an active process. Vomiting is the forceful discharge of ingested material from the stomach and sometimes proximal small intestines. Vomiting involves three stages: nausea, retching, and, subsequently, vomiting. Vomiting is a clinical sign—not a diagnosis.

Expectoration refers to the expulsion of material from the respiratory tract and is generally associated with coughing. However, careful history taking is important as some dogs that cough and gag excessively may stimulate themselves to vomit.

Hematemesis refers to vomiting with the presence of blood in the vomitus and may involve the expulsion of digested blood (commonly referred to as "coffee grounds") or fresh blood. Digested blood is indicative of erosions or ulcerations along the GI tract. Fresh blood can be altered in the stomach to the brown or black coffee ground appearance in a matter of minutes. Blood in the vomitus that is bright red in appearance is indicative of very recent or active hemorrhage.

Defecation

In addition to vomiting, diarrhea is one of the most common reasons owners bring their pets to the veterinary hospital.[1] Diarrhea is the passage of feces containing an excessive amount of water, thus resulting in an abnormal increase in stool liquidity and weight. Diarrhea best correlates with an increase in stool weight; stool weights above normal for the species per day generally indicates diarrhea. This is mainly due to excess water, which normally makes up 60–85% of fecal matter. In this way, true diarrhea is distinguished from diseases that cause only an increase in the number of bowel movements (hyperdefecation) or incontinence (involuntary loss of bowel contents). Some patients may have an increase in the frequency of defecation or may exhibit an increased urgency to defecate. A pet owner may describe this as very loose stools that appear to suddenly affect the pet or "come on" quickly. It is important to gain a thorough understanding of the owner's definition of diarrhea as it may not be the same as the health-care team's definition. Specific history-taking questions when investigating diarrhea can be found in Table 8.1.2.

Diarrhea is the trademark sign of intestinal dysfunction. It is important for health-care team members to determine acute from chronic problems when assessing animals with diarrhea.

Acute diarrhea is typically the result of diet, parasites, or infectious disease (e.g., parvovirus, coronavirus). Diarrhea is considered chronic when it has not responded to conventional therapy within a 2- to 3-week time frame. All patients with chronic diarrhea should be checked for parasites with multiple fecal flotation tests looking for nematodes, *Giardia*, and *Tritrichomonas*.

Determination of the origination of the diarrhea, small intestine (SI) or large intestine (LI), should be made. Increased frequency of defecation resulting in larger than normal amounts of soft to watery stool is often seen in small bowel diarrhea. Weight loss usually indicates small bowel disease, although severe large bowel diseases such as malignancy, histoplasmosis, and pythiosis may result in weight loss. Failure to lose weight or body condition is typically indicative of large bowel disease. Animals with weight loss from severe large bowel disease usually have signs associated with colonic involvement such as fecal mucus, marked tenesmus, and hematochezia.

Fresh blood (bright red in color) in the stool or evidence that the pet is straining to defecate is indicative of a large bowel disorder. Hematochezia (bright-red blood) typically originates in the anus, rectum, or descending colon. Melena is described as coal tar black stools that result from digested blood. Melena may originate from the pharynx, lungs (coughed up and swallowed), esophagus, stomach, or upper SI. Tarry stools are the result of the bacterial breakdown of hemoglobin.

Dyschezia is difficult and/or painful defecation, while tenesmus refers to persistent and/or prolonged straining, typically with no effect. Dyschezia and tenesmus are most often associated with large bowel disorders. Owners may mistake tenesmus with

Table 8.1.2 History-taking questions for patients presenting with diarrhea

1. Was the onset recent?
2. Was the onset acute?
3. Any other animals at home? If yes, are others showing signs of diarrhea?
4. Has the patient been to areas where there are large numbers of other animals? Obedience, dog parks, pet stores, pet shows, and so on?
5. Has there been access to drinking from a pond or streams?
6. What is the environment like where the pet spends its time?
7. What is the breed? Typical temperament of the pet?
8. Did the patient get into/ingest any of the following: trash, toxins, other pet foods, foods that have spoiled, and so on?
9. Have any drugs been prescribed or administered recently that could result in diarrhea, for example, antibiotics?
10. Have there been any changes in the pet's environment that may be stressful to the pet? New pet, change in family dynamics, alteration in home environment, boarding, day care, and so on.
11. Has there been any change in diet?

    Dry to can?

    Raw food?

    Treats?

    People foods? Added? Part of diet?
12. Describe the diarrhea.
13. What is the size and volume of the feces?
14. Consistency of the stool? Watery? Soft, formed?
15. Are there any normal stools passed during the day?
16. Frequency of stools?
17. Blood or mucus seen?
18. Timing? Increased defecation? Unable to make it outside? Increased during nighttime? Urgency?
19. If feline—does the cat use litter box? Does it defecate near the box or away from the litter box?
20. Other symptoms present? Lethargy, fever, vomiting?

constipation, so it is important to question the owner further to determine which clinical sign truly is manifesting in their pet. Constipation is the infrequent and difficult evacuation of feces. Obstipation is intractable constipation.

The cause of fecal incontinence or the inability to control defecation is typically a neuromuscular disease such as cauda equina syndrome or lumbosacral stenosis. A partial rectal obstruction may also result in fecal incontinence.[3]

Bowel auscultation

Borborygmus is described as a rumbling sound in the gut. The cause is a moving gas–fluid interface in the gut, and the sounds originate in the stomach. Borborygmi commonly are heard in the dog and are very rarely heard in cats. Flatulence refers to the excessive buildup of gas in the GI tract and oftentimes is associated with eructation, borborygmus, or flatus. Eructation is known as the expulsion of gas from the stomach, whereas flatus is the anal passage of intestinal gas.[4]

Food consumption and caloric intake

The consumption of food exceeding normal caloric intake is known as polyphagia. Regions of the central nervous system

(CNS) control an individual's hunger, satiety, and eating behavior.[5] However, there are many factors that control the function of the CNS regions. Polyphagia can be primary or secondary. Primary polyphagia would be indicative of a CNS abnormality. Secondary polyphagia is characterized by a systemic problem affecting the CNS. Secondary polyphagia is more common and typically is concurrent with clinical signs of the underlying disease.

Weight loss may or may not be a sign of GI disease. Weight loss can be attributed to one or a combination of many different etiologies (see Table 8.1.3). If non-GI factors are present in a patient with weight loss, the detection of the underlying disease process and treatment as appropriate to the findings should be provided. By using a muscle condition scoring system, the health-care team will also be able to evaluate whether any weight loss has caused a secondary muscle wasting.

If no other disease process is discovered, then an approach to determining the weight loss should begin with the determination of when the weight loss began and the patient's weight prior to the start of the weight loss. Almost any disease can result in weight loss. If the patient exhibits a good appetite while concurrently losing weight, then the rule-outs include maldigestion, malabsorption, excessive utilization of calories (e.g., hyperthyroidism, lactation), or excessive loss of calories (e.g., diabetes mellitus). The accurate history and complete

Table 8.1.3   Etiology of weight loss

Food
- Quantity
  - Not enough—multiple animals
- Quality
  - Poor
  - Low caloric density
- Inedible

Anorexia
- Inflammatory disease
- Alimentary tract disease
- Metabolic disease
- Central nervous system disease
- Cachexia
- Psychological/behavioral disorders

Dysphagia
- Oral pain
- Oral mass
- Oral trauma
- Neuromuscular disease

Regurgitation/vomiting

Maldigestive disease
- Exocrine pancreatic insufficiency
- Malabsorptive disease
  - Small intestinal disease

Organ failure
- Cardiac failure
- Hepatic failure
- Renal failure
- Adrenal failure

Cachexia
- Cancer
- Cardiac

Excessive utilization of calories
- Lactation
- Pregnancy
- Working
- Cold environment
- Fever/inflammation
  - Increased catabolism
- Hyperthyroidism

Increased loss of nutrients
- Diabetes mellitus
- Protein-losing neuropathy
- Protein-losing enteropathy

Neuromuscular disease
- Lower motor neuron disease

Source: Compiled from Willard MD. Clinical Manifestations of gastrointestinal disease. In: *Small Animal Internal Medicine*, 4th edition, pp. 351–373. St. Louis, MO: Mosby; 2009; Medinger TL. Clinical evaluation of patients with chronic weight loss. In: *Small Animal Gastroenterology*, ed. JM Steiner, pp. 133–136. Germany: Schlutersche; 2008.

physical examination can be crucial when determining the cause of weight loss.

Anorexia, which is the lack or loss of appetite for food, is another clinical sign that causes pet owners to frequently visit the veterinary hospital. Hyporexia may actually be a more accurate term to use as this is a reduction of appetite versus a complete loss of appetite; furthermore, the differentiation of not wanting to eat as opposed to not being able to eat needs to be made. There are a number of diseases that may result in the patient losing the ability to eat, such as severe dental disease, a foreign body in the mouth or pharyngeal area, and masticatory muscle myositis.[6]

Cachexia differs from anorexia in that cachexia is described as weight loss, loss of muscle mass, and anorexia in a patient. It is important to note that cachexia is not caused simply by inadequate nutrient intake and that it differs from starvation in several physiological processes. There are two important biochemical features that differentiate cachexia-induced malnutrition from starvation-induced malnutrition. First, inflammation is a feature of cachexia. Cachexia causes marked activation of the inflammatory cascade, characterized by an acute phase inflammatory response and an excessive production of proinflammatory cytokines. Second, malnutrition from cachexia is associated with a rise in resting energy expenditure, which is increased secondary to altered protein, fat, and carbohydrate metabolism. A marked loss of body muscle and adipose tissue occurs and an insulin-resistant state may develop in cachectic patients. Although the clinical appearance of the patient may be similar to starvation, activation of the inflammatory cascade and increased energy expenditure are not commonly equated with starvation.[7] Cachexia should be considered for any pet that exhibits marked weight loss, severe muscle loss, and decreased appetite with a chronic inflammatory process or cancer.

Conclusion

It has been established that GI problems are one of the most common reasons pet owners visit the veterinary hospital. Performing a complete and accurate history and physical examination are crucial to the proper diagnosis and subsequent treatment of the GI patient, as is the comprehension of the numerous signs that pets experience when faced with a GI issue.

SECTION 2 SELECTED DIAGNOSTICS IN GASTROINTESTINAL DISEASE

It has already been established that a complete history and physical examination should be performed on each patient presenting with clinical signs of GI disease. Beyond the history and physical examination, a number of diagnostic evaluations may be indicated.

Laboratory evaluation

Clinical pathology testing

In order to differentiate primary GI disease from non-GI disease, clinicopathological testing is utilized on patients presenting to the hospital with any type of GI sign. Clinicopathological testing will also help to determine the metabolic consequences of GI disease.

Prior to beginning any therapy, baseline blood and urine samples should be obtained from the patient.[1] In sick patients, the swift evaluation of packed cell volume (PCV), total solids (TS), blood glucose, blood urea nitrogen (BUN), urine specific gravity, glucose, ketones and protein, and plasma concentrations of sodium and potassium help to detect life-threatening disease, such as renal failure and hypoadrenocorticism. The results of this initial evaluation should serve as a guide to initial management pending more definitive testing.

Complete blood count

Abnormalities in the complete blood count (CBC) are uncommon when dealing with primary gastric disease. Hemoconcentration as a consequence of dehydration or shock typically is seen in conditions such as GDV, gastric ulceration, or gastric obstruction. In dogs with hemorrhagic gastroenteritis, a hematocrit level greater than 55% is seen in conjunction with normal or decreased protein concentrations. Anemia, erythrocyte microcytosis, and thrombocytosis may be present in dogs with chronic gastric bleeding. Basophilic stippling of red cells is suggestive of lead toxicity.

Chemistries

Biochemical abnormalities in primary GI disease are mainly restricted to alterations in electrolytes and acid–base balance, prerenal increases in creatinine and BUN, and occasionally hypoproteinemia. Vomiting of gastric and intestinal contents typically results in the loss of chloride, potassium, sodium, and bicarbonate-containing fluid. Dehydration is often accompanied by hypochloremia, hypokalemia, and hyponatremia.[1,2]

Through the determination of acid–base status by measurement of total CO_2 or venous blood gas analysis, the ability to detect the presence of metabolic acidosis or alkalosis is enabled. Metabolic acidosis is generally more common than metabolic alkalosis in dogs with GI disease.[2] When the gastric outflow tract or proximal duodenum is obstructed, the loss of chloride may exceed that of bicarbonate, thus resulting in hypochloremia, hypokalemia, and metabolic alkalosis. Metabolic alkalosis is enhanced by elevated HCO_3^- conservation due to volume and potassium and chloride depletion. The end result is a preferential conservation of volume at the expense of the extracellular pH. The renal reabsorption of almost all filtered bicarbonate and the exchange of sodium for hydrogen in the distal tubule promote an acid urine pH despite an extracellular alkalemia ("paradoxical aciduria").

Metabolic alkalosis in patients with GI signs is not invariably associated with outflow obstruction and has been encountered in dogs with parvovirus enteritis and acute pancreatitis.[1] Diseases characterized by acid hypersecretion, such as gastrinoma, may also be associated with metabolic alkalosis and aciduria. Venous blood gases and plasma osmolality are often determined in animals suspected of ethylene glycol ingestion, with the findings of metabolic acidosis and a high osmolal gap (calculated by subtracting calculated from measured osmolality) supportive of ingestion.

Elevated BUN without the elevation of creatinine may indicate gastric bleeding. Low albumin levels may be found in any dog with protein-losing gastroenteropathy or pythiosis, and dogs or cats with gastric neoplasia. Also of note, elevated globulin concentrations have been observed in basenji gastroenteropathy, *Pythium* infection, and gastric plasmacytoma. Elevations in creatinine, urea, calcium, potassium, glucose, liver enzymes, bilirubin, cholesterol, triglycerides, and globulin and decreases in sodium, calcium, urea, or albumin often predict non-GI causes of vomiting.

Coagulation testing is indicated in patients with melena or hematemesis to detect underlying coagulopathies and in those with acute abdomen to detect disseminated intravascular coagulation (DIC).

Infectious diseases associated with vomiting and diarrhea may require fecal enzyme-linked immunosorbent assay (ELISA) testing for diagnosis to detect *Giardia*, parvovirus, or serologic testing for feline leukemia virus (FeLV) and feline immunodeficiency virus (FIV).

Urinalysis

Urine should be evaluated for specific gravity, pH, glucose, casts, crystals, and bacteria. A complete urinalysis is important. For example, discovering white cell casts in the microscopic evaluation of the urine may aid in the diagnosis of pyelonephritis which can be responsible for GI clinical signs such as vomiting.

Additional clinical pathology tests are required to detect hypoadrenocorticism (adrenocorticotropic hormone [ACTH] stimulation), liver dysfunction (preprandial and postprandial bile acids), hyperthyroidism in cats (T_4), pancreatitis (amylase and lipase, pancreas-specific, if possible), and intestinal disease (serum cobalamin and folate).

Microscopic fecal evaluation

Fecal examination is an important part of the investigation of GI disease.[3] Feces may be preserved in a mixture of 10% neutral buffered formalin mixed with an equal quantity of feces. Commercial kits are also available and these kits use polyvinyl alcohol as the preservative, which allows for the feces to be preserved for weeks to months.

Direct fecal smear

Unstained wet mounts may be helpful to identify motility and protozoal trophozoite forms (e.g., strongyloides, giardia). The addition of Lugol's iodine will kill the parasites and stain some of the internal structures, which may aid in identification.

Fecal cytology

The staining of fecal smears for undigested starch granules (Lugol's iodine), fat globules (Sudan stain), and muscle fibers (Wright's or Diff-Quik stain) may be indicative of malabsorption but overall is nonspecific. Campylobacteriosis should be considered when short, curved, gram-negative rods are seen. Enterotoxin production by *Clostridium perfringens* is a potential cause of diarrhea and fungal elements (e.g., histoplasmosis) and sporulating clostridia may be seen in fecal cytology smears, but the significance is uncertain. The presence of a large number of clostridial endospores (more than five per oil field) on Diff-Quik-stained smears may be more significant (a positive fecal enterotoxin ELISA assay or reverse passive latex agglutination is likely to be more significant).

Rectal cytology

When the rectal examination is completed, the gloved finger manually abrades the rectal mucosa; the material on the glove is rolled onto a microscope slide and the smear stained. Although neutrophils are seldom seen, if found, they are indicative of large intestinal disease, and an increased number of neutrophils may be suggestive of a bacterial problem, indicating the possible need for fecal culture. Fungal elements may also be identified (e.g., histoplasmosis). The test is fast and simple, but in all cases, confirmatory tests are indicated.

Fecal flotation concentration

A fecal flotation concentration test is indicated in every pet presenting with GI signs. If parasitism is not the main cause of the presenting sign, it is highly likely to cause additional problems in pets with GI signs. Concentrated salt or sugar solutions are the typical solutions used in fecal flotation tests. Correctly formulated concentrated salt solutions are believed to be superior to sugar solutions. The centrifugation concentration method is superior to the simple flotation method to detect low levels of ova in a sample. When attempting to detect nematode ova and *Giardia* cysts, a zinc sulfate solution should be used, resulting in a more sensitive fecal exam. Examination of three samples by zinc sulfate flotation enhances detection of *Giardia* oocysts.

If negative, follow-up fecal evaluations should be performed in suspect cases as some parasites intermittently shed small numbers of ova or cysts.

Fecal sedimentation

Fecal sedimentation detects fluke ova missed by other techniques, especially the ova of *Eurytrema* spp., *Platynosomum* spp., *Amphimerus* spp., and *Heterobilharzia*. For a sedimentation test, the feces is suspended in water, centrifuged, and the sediment is examined.

Bacteriologic examination

Routine culture

It is not considered worthwhile to attempt to grow all the bacteria from a fecal sample; however, the targeted identification of potential pathogens may be helpful. In animals with hemorrhagic diarrhea, pyrexia, an inflammatory leukogram, or neutrophils on rectal cytology, culturing the patient feces may be considered. The importance of a positive result should always be interpreted in light of the clinical history because potential pathogens may be present in clinically healthy animals. Additionally, the fecal flora does not necessarily reflect the GI flora and cannot be used to diagnose small intestinal bacterial overgrowth (SIBO). Feces can be cultured for fungi, such as *Histoplasma capsulatum*, but fungal cultures are considered to be of questionable value.

When compared to routine fecal flotations, the ELISA test for detecting cryptosporidial antigens (ProSpecT® Cryptosporidium Microplate Assay, Meridian Diagnostics, Inc., and ProSpecT® Cryptosporidium Microplate Assay, Remel Inc.) in feces appears to be more sensitive.

When investigating *Tritrichomonas foetus* in feline feces, there are culture techniques (InPouch® TF, BioMed Diagnostics) and polymerase chain reaction (PCR) tests. The culture technique is easily done in the veterinary hospital and is reportedly sensitive and specific.

Molecular fingerprinting

It is important to note that many intestinal bacteria are unculturable and can only be identified by comparative gene sequencing of the bacterial 16S rRNA.[3] This method can identify a single species or it can look at the pattern of the flora in both duodenal fluid and feces.

Virologic examination

Diarrhea of a viral nature is usually acute and self-limiting and does not require a positive diagnosis. Electron microscopy can be used to identify the characteristic viral particles of rotavirus, coronavirus, and parvovirus. Fecal ELISA tests for parvovirus are also available and will be discussed further in this section. A commercially available ELISA can be used to detect *Giardia* antigen in feces, although PCR is likely to be more sensitive.[1,4]

Occult blood

This test is used to search for intestinal bleeding before melena is seen. Unfortunately, it tests nonspecifically for any hemoglobin and is very sensitive, reacting with any dietary meat as well as with patient blood. Therefore, the patient must be fed a meat-free diet for at least 72 h for a positive result to have any significance. The sensitivity of different techniques used in this analysis varies, thus making it very difficult to compare results with any accuracy. Blood is not distributed homogenously throughout the feces and a negative result could occur from a sampling error, especially in pets suffering from a lower intestinal tract problem. Tests using guaiac reagents have been found to be more specific and thus are preferred over other reagents.[5]

Alpha₁-protease inhibitor

This test assays the presence in feces of alpha₁-protease inhibitor (α_1-PI), a naturally occurring endogenous serum protein that is resistant to bacterial degradation if lost into the intestine.[6] In order to improve diagnostic accuracy, three fresh fecal samples are examined. The assay is only valid if there is no GI bleeding. Samples must be collected by voluntary evacuation since abrasion of the colonic wall during digital evacuation is enough to liberate α_1-PI. The test is of value for the diagnosis of protein-losing enteropathy (PLE), correlating with testing by fecal radioactive chromium-labeled albumin excretion. It is likely a more sensitive marker of early disease than measuring serum albumin.[6–10]

Imaging

Historically, imaging of the intestinal tract has been limited to plain and contrast radiographs. This has been dramatically altered by the use of ultrasound and endoscopy. Scintigraphy, computed tomography (CT), and magnetic resonance imaging (MRI) scanning are rapidly being adopted, and "virtual endoscopy" by helical CT is becoming available.

Plain radiography

During physical examination, there may be some structures that are not easily accessible to palpation and some abnormalities may not be palpable; therefore, imaging may be indicated as a diagnostic tool. Survey or plain radiographs are most useful in the investigation of diarrhea associated with vomiting, abdominal pain, and palpable abnormalities. Diagnostic results are improved if both lateral views are taken, although a single lateral view may be adequate if combined with ultrasonography. The value of plain radiographs in malabsorption is reportedly minimal, particularly if ascites is present, as the majority of detail is obscured by fluid. Generally, the aim is the detection of (acute) surgical disease (e.g., foreign bodies, free gas, displacement, masses, obstructions), decreased serosal detail, and ileus. Ileus is an abnormal dilatation of an immotile segment of intestine, and the differential diagnosis depends on whether it is localized or generalized and whether an accumulation of gas or fluid is present. Interpretation should be cautious if the patient has been treated with drugs that affect the GI tract.[3,5,11]

Follow-through examinations

GI studies using microfine barium suspensions can recognize ulcers and irregular mucosal detail. They may confirm the presence of radiolucent foreign bodies but are of limited use in identifying mural masses and partial obstructions and rarely provide more information than good quality survey films.

Enteroclysis (fluoroscopic contrast) provides additional information, but this type of examination is technically demanding and has not truly been adopted in the veterinary community. Although contrast studies allow assessment of the intestinal transit rate, this does not correlate closely to movement of ingesta assessed by scintigraphy. Additionally, dysmotility may occur secondary to other causes, and studies provide limited etiologic information. Administration of barium may delay endoscopy for at least 24 h. If perforation is suspected, an iodine-based contrast should be used.[3]

Barium-impregnated polyethylene spheres

Barium-impregnated polyethylene spheres (BIPS) are solid-phase radiopaque markers that are dispensed in capsule form to provide information on gastric emptying, intestinal transit, and obstructive disorders. Given that the transit time of BIPS is highly variable, their use for transit studies is limited. They may be most helpful in the detection of partial obstructions.[3,12]

Ultrasonography

Ultrasonography may be performed in conjunction with initial survey radiographs, although certain diagnosticians may opt to only use ultrasonography.

The use of ultrasound may be indicated in animals with the following clinical signs: vomiting, diarrhea, abdominal effusion, acute abdominal pain, anorexia of unknown origin, weight loss, and when an abdominal mass is palpated or suspected. Ultrasonography is especially advantageous in the identification of pancreatitis, infiltrative disease, mesenteric lymphadenopathy, motility disorders, and intussusceptions that are difficult to appreciate with radiography. In addition, effusions enhance the ultrasonographic contrast, as opposed to radiographs where effusions mask the details of the viscera. Another advantage of ultrasound is that needle aspirations and/or biopsies can be performed in real time with guidance from the ultrasound, thus potentially avoiding laparoscopic or surgical exploration.[5,11,12]

Transabdominal ultrasound examination of the GI tract is now a routine part of the investigation of GI disease, especially in suspected cases of pancreatitis. A conventional abdominal examination of the GI tract can image peristalsis, ileus, lumenal contents, layering of the bowel wall, and it can measure SI wall thickness. It has excellent sensitivity for the detection of masses, radiolucent foreign bodies, lesions such as intussusceptions, and intestinal wall thickening and lymphadenopathy in chronic inflammatory, lymphatic, and neoplastic enteropathies. Endoscopic ultrasound will allow the mucosal wall and adjacent viscera, such as the pancreas, to be examined in more detail.

Intussusceptions are usually recognized in the transverse plane as multiple concentric rings and longitudinally as a thick, multilayered segment. Values for normal SI wall thickness have been reported for dogs and cats; thickness decreases from proximal (5–6 mm) to distal (4–5 mm) but depends on body size, with the thickest being observed in the largest dogs. Disturbance of the normal five-layered sonographic appearance (mucosal surface, mucosa, submucosa, muscularis, serosa) is typical of neoplasia, while wall thickening can also result from other infiltrative disorders and edema. Ultrasound-guided fine needle aspiration for cytological examination is possible.

Endoscopy

Endoscopy is very commonly performed and is a relatively simple and a minimally invasive means of examination. Endoscopy allows for the collection of multiple tissue samples without the need for invasive surgery.[3,5,13,14] Videocapsule endoscopy is an emerging technology, but currently, flexible endoscopy is the standard method. Optimal, well-maintained equipment and operator experience are more important than pharmacological manipulation in achieving successful small intestinal intubation. Foreign bodies below a certain size can be visualized and removed endoscopically. The proximal SI is viewed during gastroduodenoscopy, and the distal SI can be sampled by passing the endoscope retrograde through the ileocolic valve. Truly, only the mid-jejunum cannot be examined adequately by routine endoscopy. This limitation may not be significant given that most cases of malabsorption involve diffuse disease. Enteroscopy uses a much longer, thinner endoscope with or without an oversleeve and/or advancement balloons and can allow examination of most of the jejunum, as does a videoendoscopic capsule that passes from mouth to anus and transmits images by telemetry. The SMART capsule allows collection of physiological data (pH, pressure) by telemetry but does not provide images.[15] Abnormal findings on gross endoscopic examination include mucosal granularity and friability, erosions and ulcers, retained food, mass lesions, and hyperemia/erythema. However, none of these characteristics is pathognomonic for a particular disease condition, and findings frequently do not correlate with histopathologic results. A milky white exudate or dilated lymphatics are suggestive of lymphangiectasia, and the presence of intraluminal parasites may be diagnostic in some cases.

Special tests

In cases of malabsorption, intestinal biopsy is usually necessary to obtain a definitive diagnosis. However, exocrine pancreatic insufficiency (EPI) should be ruled out before biopsy because signs of malabsorption are nonspecific and do not permit differentiation of cause. Thus, serum trypsin-like immunoreactivity (TLI) measurement must be performed in all cases. It is well documented that biopsies from up to 50% of patients are considered normal by light microscopy. Therefore, usually before biopsy, a number of indirect tests are performed to assess GI damage, permeability, and dysfunction.[3]

Tests of intestinal absorption

Attempts to assess intestinal function by measuring the mediated absorption of numerous substrates (e.g., lactose, glucose, starch, triglyceride, and vitamin A) are no longer performed because of a lack of sensitivity and specificity. The D-xylose test has also been abandoned due to its being nondiscriminatory in cats and its insensitivy in dogs. The differential absorption of two sugars (xylose/3-O-methyl-D-glucose) eliminates nonmucosal effects that blight other tests.

Conclusion

The diagnostic tests for the GI tract section have provided a basic overview of how to proceed with a patient that presents with the GI signs outlined earlier. The next section will take a look at actual disease conditions, clinical signs, treatment, and nursing care and, where applicable, will outline further diagnostic tests.

SECTION 3 GASTROINTESTINAL DISEASE

Oral disease

Feline eosinophilic granuloma complex

Feline eosinophilic granuloma complex (FEGC) is a common syndrome in cats that includes occurrence of a linear eosinophilic granuloma, an eosinophilic plaque, or an eosinophilic ulcer (indolent ulcer, rodent ulcer).[1] FEGC is the common terminology for this syndrome, although a definitive relationship between the three lesions has not been determined. Typically, oral lesions consist of a linear granuloma or an eosinophilic ulcer and intraoral lesions present as one or more defined, firm, raised nodules. It is estimated that 80% of eosinophilic granulomas occur on the maxillary lips.[1]

The etiology of this complex remains unknown, although associations have been determined with bacterial and viral infections and hypersensitivity and immune-mediated disorders.

Clinical signs

Cats typically present with increased salivation and changes in eating behaviors. Oral examination may reveal lesions on the lips, chin, or intraoral structures, typically distinct and notably different from inflammatory lesions associated with gingivitis, periodontal inflammation, or stomatitis.

Diagnostics

Diagnosis is usually based on history and clinical findings. A CBC usually shows an eosinophilia and, although characteristic of this disease, should be differentiated from other causes of eosinophilia. Biopsy with histopathology may be indicated to identify the lesions and to rule out oral neoplasm.

Treatment and patient care

Any underlying allergies should be identified and controlled. Lesions typically resolve in cats with underlying allergies that are successfully managed. Corticosteroid therapy, either intralesional, oral, or systemic, administered until the lesions resolve, is the standard mode of treatment. Significant improvement should be noted in 2–4 weeks; however, it may take several more weeks for the lesions to completely resolve.[2] In severe cases involving coalescing lesions on the tongue or palates, aggressive medical intervention may be necessary. Systemic antibiotic treatment may be indicated to control secondary bacterial infections in ulcerated lesions, and surgical resection may be indicated for unresponsive lesions. Clients should be counseled that lesions take several weeks to resolve, may recur, and ongoing control of any hypersensitivities (flea bite, food sensitivity, etc.) is important.

Analgesia considerations

Cats with intraoral lesions may be painful and have difficulty eating or swallowing. Supportive care and feeding moist foods are helpful in recovery; administration of a topical chlorhexidine gel may provide some relief. Untreated, unresolved, or recurring eosinophilic ulcers may become disfiguring but are typically not pruritic or painful.

Prognosis

Prognosis is variable. Lesions associated with hypersensitivity as an underlying cause are usually well managed with successful allergy management. When no associated cause is determined, the lesions are more apt to recur; long-term therapy may be required, and these lesions have a less favorable prognosis.

Feline gingivitis–stomatitis–pharyngitis complex

This painful oral disease is often seen in cats with clinical signs of inflammation of the oral tissues, which may be generalized or localized to specific areas such as the glossopalatine mucosa and fauces. Inflammation is often accompanied by ulceration and proliferation of the oral mucosa, and histopathologically dense infiltrations of lymphocytes and plasma cells are present. The cause of this disease remains unknown; however, based on the cellular infiltrate and tissue involvement, this disease is referred to by a variety of names including feline gingivitis–stomatitis–pharyngitis complex (GSPC), lymphoplasmacytic gingivitis–stomatitis (LPGS), gingivostomatitis (GS), chronic ulcerative paradental stomatitis (CUPS), and similar variations.

The degree of inflammation is variable and may involve the gingiva, buccal mucosa, fauces, and pharyngeal areas. A specific etiology remains unknown and is most likely multifactorial with an immune-mediated component resulting in an excessive inflammatory response. Research studies evaluating associations with feline viruses, bartonella, periodontal disease, and tooth resorptive lesions have found positive associations but no direct correlations.

Clinical signs

Clinical signs vary and are typically progressive with the severity of the inflammatory changes. Clients may notice that their cat seems interested in food but is reluctant to eat or may only eat moistened or softer foods. As the lesions become more severe, cats typically present with excessive salivation, halitosis, extreme changes in eating behavior, anorexia, and weight loss. Behavior changes including decreased activity and reluctance to groom are commonly noted.

Clinical examination should begin with an examination of the regional lymph nodes and external head and facial tissues. Oral examination can be difficult as affected cats may demonstrate extreme aversion to any type of mouth manipulation and severe pain on opening the mouth. Initially, gentle retraction of the lips while keeping the cat's mouth closed should be performed. If possible, the mouth is then carefully opened to examine the gingival tissues and the oral mucosa. In severe cases, the oral tissues may be prolific, ulcerated, and bleed easily, and a complete oral examination may require sedation or general anesthesia.

Diagnostics

The history and clinical signs accompanied by the specific oral pathology support a diagnosis of GSPC. Additional laboratory testing that should be performed to evaluate and identify contributing or underlying conditions includes a CBC, biochemical profile, urinalysis, and serologic testing for FeLV and FIV. A complete dental examination including dental radiographs should be performed to identify any potential causes/contributors such as periodontal disease, retained roots and tooth resorption. Biopsies of oral lesions should be obtained and submitted for histopathology.

Treatment and patient care

Therapeutic options are targeted at meticulous plaque control and management of the inflammatory and immunologic responses. The degree of treatment will depend on the severity of the disease, the ability of the client to apply oral homecare medications, and the tolerance of the patient to oral manipulations. Primary treatment protocols typically involve a combination or progression of processes including periodontal management, meticulous plaque control, antibiotic, anti-inflammatory and analgesic administration, and tooth extraction. There is a lack of consensus on primary treatment for this disease and a more conservative approach is often the first step. Extraction of all premolars and molars is emerging as the preferred treatment to provide the best long-term results. Careful extraction, including complete root removal (which eliminates the plaque-retentive surfaces), decreases the inflammatory response.

If the client is unwilling to proceed with extractions, periodontal therapy should be provided, including removal of supra- and subgingival plaque and calculus deposits, treatment/extraction of compromised teeth, topical and systemic antimicrobial administration, and prescription of effective home plaque control to control oral inflammation. Antibiotics are administered for 4–6 weeks, often in conjunction with corticosteroids and analgesics to reduce and manage the inflammation and pain. Response to more conservative medical management has been poor and is reported to lose effectiveness over time. In addition, client compliance is often poor as it is difficult for clients to provide meticulous plaque control to their cats.

Treatment recommendation should be made based on the current pathology, laboratory results, patient presentation, and client commitment. This disease can be difficult to manage and a progression of therapeutic options may be necessary. Therapy can be frustrating for the health-care team, the client, and the patient, and successful treatment may be control of the clinical signs that allows the cat to have an acceptable quality of life. Client support includes training on the application of oral and topical medications as well as plaque control techniques.

Immediate inflammation and pain support should be provided in severe cases where the patient is not eating. In these cases, most cats will require immunosuppressive doses of glucocorticoids to decrease the inflammation and to provide sufficient pain reduction. Offering soft food or syringe feeding may be necessary, and in severe cases, enteral nutrition may be required to maintain adequate energy intake and balanced nutrition.

Prognosis

GSPC is a difficult disease to manage with a guarded prognosis. Clients should be advised of the treatment options, associated response rates, and the potential need for more aggressive, long-term therapy.

Neoplasms of the oral cavity

Oral neoplasia accounts for approximately 6% of all canine tumors and about 3% of all feline tumors. These tumors may arise from any region of the mouth and include nonodontogenic and odontogenic tumor types. The most common nonodontogenic tumor types include malignant melanoma, squamous cell carcinoma, and fibrosarcoma. Odontogenic tumors are typically rare and include epulides (acanthomatous ameloblastomas), fibromas, and odontomas.

Malignant melanoma is the most common type of oral tumor in dogs and occurs more commonly in old, male, small breed dogs. These tumors grow rapidly, are invasive, and have a high rate of metastasis. Malignant melanomas are rare in cats and carry a poor prognosis in both species.

Squamous cell carcinoma is the most common oral tumor in cats and the second most common oral tumor in dogs. Squamous cell carcinoma often originates on the gingiva and typically presents as a red, ulcerative, cauliflower-like growth. These tumors grow rapidly, are invasive, and infiltrate deeply. Regional lymph node metastasis is common in cats, less common in dogs, and in both species, distant metastasis is infrequent.

Fibrosarcoma is the second most common oral tumor in cats and is less common in dogs. These tumors generally occur in the gingiva of cats and in the gingival and hard palates of dogs, with bony involvement very common. There is a low incidence of regional lymph node involvement with occasional metastasis to pulmonary tissues.

Clinical signs

Often, oral tumors are unnoticed by the pet owner until an advanced stage of development is reached. Clinical signs in dogs and cats with oral tumors range from no obvious symptoms to halitosis, changes in eating behavior, salivation or bleeding, or a noticeable growth observed by the pet owner. General physical examination may reveal nasal congestion, asymmetrical facial swelling, necrotic odor, regional lymph node enlargement, weight loss or muscle atrophy, and an unthrifty appearance.

Diagnostics

A CBC, biochemical profile, and urinalysis should be performed to evaluate the patient's overall health status, and in feline patients, retrovirus tests are recommended to accurately assess the prognosis. A definitive oral examination under anesthesia is recommended to determine the exact location, physical appearance, tooth mobility, tongue or bony structure involvement, and presence of any other abnormal oral conditions.

Diagnostic imaging, biopsy with histopathology, and clinical staging of oral tumors are important in selecting the appropriate treatment protocol and in determining the prognosis. The tumor–node–metastasis (TNM) system is a systematic approach recommended for an accurate assessment. The TNM involves careful evaluation of the mass, regional lymph nodes, and distant metastasis. The primary tool for determining the type and nature of an oral tumor is incisional biopsy with histopathology and is indicated for all oral masses and any suspicious oral lesions. Incisional biopsies provide the greatest diagnostic accuracy. Fine needle aspirates of oral masses are often contaminated with inflammatory cells and cellular debris and are therefore inconclusive. Fine needle biopsy with cytology should be performed on regional lymph nodes regardless of size. Excisional biopsy of small oral masses and regional lymph nodes may also be indicated.

Diagnostic imaging includes intraoral dental radiographs and extraoral skull radiographs. These radiographs help identify the extent of the tumor and the involvement of tooth and bony structures. Thoracic and abdominal radiographs should be taken to determine if metastasis has occurred. Additional imaging including ultrasound, CT, or MRI may be necessary to determine the extent of involvement of soft tissues, lymph nodes, and intranasal and periorbital structures.

Treatment and patient care

Treatment is determined by the stage and nature of the tumor. Surgical resection of malignant oral tumors and benign, locally invasive masses is the preferred treatment. Adequate excision with tumor-free margins and the absence of metastasis typically result in a curative outcome. Postsurgical care including pain management, wound care, and nutritional support is critically important to minimize complications and to support successful recovery and healing. In cases where surgical resection is not an option, palliative surgery or surgical debulking may be performed to improve the patient's quality of life or to reduce the size of the mass prior to the application of other therapeutic modalities.

If resection is not an option, either due to the invasiveness or nature of the tumor or if not elected by the client, radiation therapy may be indicated. Chemotherapy has generally been ineffective in the treatment of oral malignant tumors; however, new protocols may be under investigation.

Prognosis

The success rate and prognosis are generally determined by the tumor type and the aggressiveness of the surgical resection with the presence of tumor-free margins. Odontogenic tumors are often cured with surgical resection. In dogs, the prognosis for nonodontogenic tumors is good for squamous cell carcinoma, fair for fibrosarcoma, and poor for malignant melanoma. Cats do not seem to tolerate aggressive surgical resections as well as dogs, and prognosis for nonodontogenic tumors is generally poor. Treatment options, prognosis, postsurgical physical appearance, functional outcomes, quality of life, and expected survival time should be thoroughly discussed with the client.

Esophageal disorders

The esophagus is a muscular tube (both striated and smooth) with an upper esophageal sphincter and a lower esophageal sphincter (also called the cardiac sphincter). They work in concert to transport food boluses by peristaltic waves, from the mouth to the stomach. The esophagus is responsive to both hormonal influences (e.g., gastrin, secretin) and innervation (e.g., vagus nerve, branches of laryngeal, pharyngeal, and glossopharyngeal).

Megaesophagus

Megaesophagus is a syndrome manifested by the generalized loss of motor function to the esophagus. This results in esophageal dilatation and loss of normal peristaltic motility. The loss of motility can be severe, resulting in food and fluid accumulation in the esophagus. Megaesophagus may be congenital, idiopathic, or acquired (secondary to other disease processes).[1–3]

Congenital megaesophagus

Congenital megaesophagus is an uncommon type of megaesophagus in dogs and in cats.[4] The syndrome typically manifests in puppies and kittens at the time of weaning. The site and pathogenesis of the lesion in congenital megaesophagus is unknown. The congenital form, also known as esophageal weakness, may be due to a delay in maturation of the esophageal neuromuscular system, which explains why young animals have shown improvement when feeding is carefully managed. There does not appear to be evidence of demyelination or neuronal degeneration. It is suggested that the underlying defect may lie in the vagal afferent innervation to the esophagus.[5] Congenital megaesophagus has been shown to be inherited in the wire-haired fox terrier and the miniature schnauzer. A breed predisposition also exists for the German shepherd, Great Dane, Irish setter, retriever breeds, and Siamese cats, although it is rarely seen in cats.[6]

Typically, patients present to the hospital after weaning for what owners perceive to be vomiting, when in fact the patient is regurgitating. Others signs noted are coughing or fever secondary to aspiration pneumonia and possible weight loss.[1]

Idiopathic megaesophagus

Idiopathic megaesophagus, also known as adult-onset primary megaesophagus, is a common form of megaesophagus, mainly seen in dogs. A defect in the afferent neural pathway responsive to esophageal distention is suspected.[7,8] The age of onset is frequently 8 years or older; however, it has been reported in younger patients.

Presentation is similar to congenital idiopathic megaesophagus in that patients typically present for regurgitation, which often occurs immediately after or several hours after eating. Dysphagia is not generally present. Anorexia, drooling, and pain on swallowing may be seen secondary to esophagitis, which can develop due to the accumulation of food in the esophagus. Animals with megaesophagus are predisposed to aspiration pneumonia. However, there is one major difference seen with idiopathic megaesophagus, and that is the loss of body condition.[1] Weight loss and emaciation take place secondarily to insufficient food intake and/or insufficient food digestion. Inappetance may be the result of discomfort caused by regurgitation.

Acquired secondary megaesophagus

Acquired secondary megaesophagus may result from a number of systemic diseases, especially those that lead to diffuse neuromuscular dysfunction (e.g., myasthenia gravis, polymyositis, polymyopathies, polyneuropathies, dysautonomia, and distemper).[4] Lead and organophosphate toxicity, thymoma, systemic lupus erythematosus, hiatal hernia, hypoadrenocorticism, and esophagitis can also result in megaesophagus.

Many obstructive esophageal diseases (e.g., neoplasia, granuloma, vascular ring anomaly, stricture, periesophageal masses and foreign bodies) can also lead to megaesophagus if they are of sufficiently chronic duration.[1–3,6]

Diagnostic testing

Megaesophagus generally is diagnosed based on the history, physical examination, clinical signs, and thoracic radiography of the patient. Once a diagnosis of generalized megaesophagus is established, further diagnostic testing should be performed to identify an underlying etiology.

Laboratory tests

Diagnostic tests that may be considered to evaluate animals with generalized megaesophagus include a CBC, biochemical panel, and urinalysis. Additional laboratory tests to rule out secondary causes of megaesophagus include blood lead level and cholinesterase activity (toxicity), creatine kinase concentration (polymyositis/polymyopathy), acetylcholine receptor antibody test and Tensilon® test (myasthenia gravis), antinuclear antibody

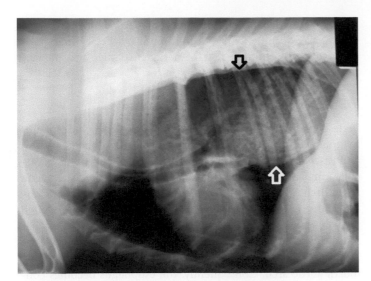

Figure 8.3.1 Ten-year-old mixed breed dog with severe megaesophagus (between arrows) (containing food) and resolving aspiration pneumonia.

test (systemic lupus erythematosus), and evaluation of adrenal and thyroid gland function.

Imaging

Survey neck and thoracic radiographs are indicated in suspected cases of megaesophagus. The cervical esophagus may be dilated with air and the thoracic esophagus will contain large amounts of food or fluid; however, it is considered normal for dogs that are excited or animals that are anesthetized to have some air in the esophagus (Figure 8.3.1).

Positive contrast studies (i.e., barium esophagram) may be required to differentiate esophageal obstructive pathology, stricture, hernia, diverticula, fistula, or vascular ring anomaly from megaesophagus.[4,5] Barium sulfate or barium mixed with food can be utilized for the esophagram. If esophageal perforation is suspected, a water-based contrast agent should be utilized (e.g., iohcxol).

Videofluoroscopy is necessary for the diagnosis of functional esophageal disorders (esophageal dysmotility) or cricopharyngeal dysphagia. An esophageal stricture is suspected when there is an enlargement of the proximal esophagus with normal function of the distal esophagus. Videofluoroscopy has some prognostic value in megaesophagus not associated with esophageal dilation via assessment of the severity of peristaltic dysfunction.[9] Esophagoscopy is less reliable than radiography and fluoroscopy, although it can be used to rule out underlying causes of megaesophagus, such as esophagitis, stricture, neoplasia, and radiolucent foreign bodies.

Additional diagnostics

If neurological or muscular pathology is suspected, additional diagnostics to consider include electromyogram (EMG), nerve conduction velocities, and muscle biopsies.

Patient care

The treatment of megaesophagus is dependent on the underlying cause and any secondary disease conditions. Treatment may include surgery (e.g., foreign body retrieval, surgical resection of neoplasia, balloon dilatation), drug therapy (e.g., immunosuppression, anti-inflammatory, pyridostigmine), and antibiotic therapy for aspiration pneumonia.

The key objectives of medical management of megaesophagus/regurgitation are to remove the initiating cause as early as possible, to minimize aspiration, and to maximize nutrient intake to the GI tract. Medical management of generalized megaesophagus involves modification of feeding practices. Foods of differing consistency should be used to determine the best texture for individual patients. A liquid or gruel consistency is usually best for patients with cricopharyngeal dysphagia, esophageal obstructive lesions, and/or esophagitis and may be effective in patients with megaesophagus. Dry food or moist food formed into large boluses may act as a stimulus (secondary peristalsis) to any remaining normal esophageal tissue, and some improvement in esophageal performance may be noted when the swallowing reflex is maximally stimulated. Gruels or liquids may not stimulate secondary peristalsis, thereby increasing the risk of aspiration pneumonia.

Esophageal obstruction

Obstructions of the esophagus may be intraluminal, intramural, or periesophageal and may be congenital or acquired.

Intraluminal obstruction

Most intraluminal obstructions are the result of foreign bodies, typically bones and fish hooks. Objects tend to lodge in the thoracic inlet, at the base of the heart, and at the diaphragmatic hiatus, which are the areas of least distensibility.[2–4] Foreign bodies stimulate peristalsis and may result in severe ulcerative esophagitis, esophageal perforation (causing pleuritis or mediastinitis), or stricture formation.

Possible clinical signs of an esophageal foreign body are anorexia, adipsia, lethargy, and ptyalism (hypersalivation). Occasionally, regurgitation is observed.

Diagnostic testing

To definitively diagnose an obstruction in the esophagus, radiography should be performed. Survey radiographs are typically diagnostic, as most foreign objects are radiopaque. However, radiolucent objects may require radiographic contrast for full visualization. Barium should be avoided if esophageal perforation is suspected as this can cause granulomas should the barium leak into the mediastinum. In this case, an iodinated compound should be administered. The option of using endoscopy to visualize the foreign body, if available, is preferable to barium contrast studies even if perforation is not suspected as diagnosis and removal can often be accomplished in one procedure.

Patient care

Treatment involves removal of the foreign body by either endoscopy or surgery.[10,11] Endoscopy is the technique of choice unless the object is deeply embedded or has perforated the esophageal wall. Esophageal foreign bodies can lead to complications such as mediastinitis secondary to perforation, aspiration pneumonia, stricture formation, or segmental hypomotility.

Intramural obstructions

Intramural esophageal obstruction is usually a result of stricture formation. A circumferential stricture (e.g., a ring of scar tissue) may develop when esophageal erosions extend into the muscle layer of the esophagus, thus stimulating the production of fibrous tissue. Typical causes of benign stricture formation are esophageal foreign body trauma and severe esophagitis from gastroesophageal reflux (which may occur during anesthesia). The location, length, and number of strictures can vary, although most commonly, single strictures are noted. Strictures may also be the result of malignant disease.

The primary clinical sign is progressive regurgitation, especially after a meal. Ptyalism, repeated or exaggerated swallowing attempts, and extension of the head and neck may also be noted.

Diagnostic testing

Positive contrast radiography and endoscopic visualization are recommended for diagnosis. Esophageal dilatation may occur cranial to the stricture, and abnormal esophageal motility may also occur.[1-3]

Patient care

Treating esophageal stricture(s) is multimodal. Surgical management involves dilatation of the stricture using balloon catheter dilators (passed through an endoscope under direct vision or under fluoroscopic guidance). Esophageal strictures may require repeated dilation every 3–4 days and may potentially require up to six procedures to prevent restricturing. Surgical resection is the option of choice for benign strictures but may be reserved for those cases in which no response is seen to medical treatment or when the lesion is very near to the gastroesophageal junction.[1-3] The risks from dilation surgery are excessive hemorrhage and esophageal rupture (rare).

Medical management to prevent further reflux and to treat esophagitis if indicated, are started following dilatation or resection. Antibiotics may also be used if indicated. To increase the intragastric pH and to minimize esophageal mucosa damage from refluxed gastric secretions an H_2-receptor antagonist (e.g., famotidine) and a proton pump inhibitor (PPI) (e.g., omeprazole) are commonly administered. Sucralfate (Carafate') is used to treat and prevent ulcers in patients with strictures associated with esophagitis. It is also recommended that corticosteroids at anti-inflammatory doses be administered after dilation to inhibit the formation of new fibrous connective tissue. Decreasing esophagitis by feeding the animal through a gastrostomy tube may also be indicated.

Total resolution of strictures may not be possible; however, clinical signs can be kept to a minimum by dietary manipulations such as feeding a soft or a liquefied diet and medical management.

Periesophageal obstructions

Periesophageal causes of esophageal obstruction include inflammation, neoplasia, severe cardiomegaly, hilar lymphadenopathy, and vascular ring anomalies, which will be discussed here. Vascular ring anomalies are congenital defects and persistent right aortic arch (PRAA) is the most common vascular ring anomaly (95%) that is seen in dogs and cats.[1-3] PRAA is seen more often in Irish setters, German shepherds, and Boston terriers and has also been reported, albeit rarely, in cats. In cases of PRAA, the aortic arch develops from the right rather than from the left fourth aortic arch. Consequently, the esophagus becomes constricted by a ring formed by the aorta on the right, the pulmonary artery on the left, the ligamentum arteriosum dorsally, and the trachea ventrally. Food is unable to pass through the vascular ring and accumulates in the cranial esophagus, resulting in dilatation and loss of esophageal motility.

Clinical signs of regurgitation and poor weight gain are typically first observed in puppies during the weaning phase. The animal usually appears healthy otherwise and has a good appetite.

Diagnostic testing

Thoracic radiographs frequently reveal esophageal dilation cranial to the base of the heart, a normal esophagus caudal to the heart, and a leftward deviation of the trachea near the cranial edge of the heart. A positive contrast esophagram, fluoroscopy, or endoscopy may be needed to fully characterize the anomaly.

Patient care

Therapy involves surgical resection of the ligamentum arteriosum. Esophageal hypomotility and regurgitation may persist, but significant clinical improvement is seen in most patients (>90%) following corrective surgery.[4] If esophageal hypomotility or regurgitation is seen following corrective surgery, it is recommended that owners manage their pets with elevated feedings. Early diagnosis, normal or near normal BCS, no complicating diseases (e.g., aspiration pneumonia), and prompt surgical correction favor the outcome.

Key nutritional factors in patients with esophageal disease

Patients with swallowing disorders are often debilitated and the growth of very young patients may be underdeveloped. The health-care team needs to be mindful of the fact that in addition to the key nutritional factors discussed here, other nutritional factors may be important depending on the life stage and the body condition of the patient.

Energy density

In patients with motility and obstructive disorders, a relatively high energy density is helpful in meeting the patient's caloric requirement in a small volume of food comparative to lower fat foods. Foods with at least 25% dry matter (DM) fat and energy densities of at least 4.5 kcal/g (18.8 kJ/g) DM are recommended. However, a lower fat content (≥15% DM for dogs and ≥20% DM for cats) is a better option for cases of esophagitis due to gastric reflux. It is important to note that high dietary fat delays gastric emptying and reduces lower esophageal sphincter pressure, which can lead to reflux of food and gastric secretions into the esophagus. However, these patients also need relatively energy dense foods (at least 4 kcal/g DM [16.7 kJ/g]). For patients with esophagitis/gastroesophageal reflux, an energy dense, moderate fat food is recommended. Foods with these characteristics tend to be highly digestible.

Protein

Protein is required in amounts adequate for tissue repair and to support growth in young patients. In addition, dietary protein may play an essential role in reducing occurences of gastro-esophageal reflux secondary to protein stimulating an increase in gastroesophageal sphincter pressure.[6] This effect is linked to dietary protein's stimulatory effect on gastrin and gastric acid secretion. By increasing the pressure in the lower esophageal sphincter, episodes of gastroesophageal reflux are decreased and the potential for further esophageal injury or aspiration pneumonia is lessened. For these reasons, dietary protein content should be at least 25% DM for foods for adult dogs and at least 35% DM for foods for adult cats.

Feeding protocols

In patients with swallowing or esophageal disorders, the current feeding protocol of one to three meals per day, fed in a bowl on the floor is rarely appropriate, and special feeding methods are often required. The key tools of nutritional management are a change in the feeding method and a change to the appropriate food (including form). Veterinary technicians play a key role in developing the feeding protocol and in communicating the importance of the changes to the owner. Small-volume, frequent meals are recommended and gruel-type foods are often necessary.

Feeding a high calorie food to a patient in an upright position, and maintaining this position for 20–30 min after feeding, provides ample time for gravitational flow of the food through the esophagus to the stomach. Upright feeding can be accomplished by several methods. The most common technique is to elevate the food bowl so that the dog or cat has to sit down or stand on its hind legs to eat. Pets can also be trained to eat on the stairs or from a counter or stool. Another option is to cradle small dogs and cats in an upright position in the arms while eating. Dogs can be trained to sit after eating or to lie in sternal recumbency on an inclined board for the required period of time. The use of a Bailey chair (see http://www.caninemegaesophagus.org/index.htm) is another option.

Feeding tubes

These suggestions will not work in all cases as upright feeding may be inadequate to control regurgitation or impractical because of the pet's temperament or the owner's schedule. In those cases, placement of a gastrostomy or enterostomy tube is recommended to bypass the esophagus entirely. This will involve extensive counseling with the owner. Nasoesophageal (NE), nasogastric, and esophagostomy tubes are not appropriate in this situation because they deliver food into the esophagus where it can be regurgitated. Patients with ongoing signs of malnutrition at presentation should receive a large-bore gastrostomy feeding tube, if possible, and immediate alimentation via the tube until adequate oral intake can be achieved. Gastrostomy tubes have been used successfully for long periods of time to maintain the nutritional status of dogs with megaesophagus. In those cases where owners are willing to feed their pet long term via a gastrostomy tube, a permanent button-type gastrostomy tube should be considered. Even with the use of gastrostomy tubes, regurgitation of saliva and food refluxed from the stomach may still occur, which can result in aspiration pneumonia. For this reason, some clinicians prefer feeding via enterostomy tube. Owners should be counseled that regurgitation might not entirely cease even if all food and water is administered through the gastrostomy tube. Many patients will continue to regurgitate fluid (most likely salivary secretions), but the likelihood of aspiration pneumonia is reduced greatly.

As discussed, the feeding plan is often used in conjunction with other therapeutic modalities including surgery (e.g., cricopharyngeal myotomy, esophageal stricture, vascular ring anomaly, esophageal foreign bodies), esophageal ballooning (e.g., esophageal stricture), endoscopy (e.g., foreign body removal), and drugs (e.g., antibiotics, prokinetic agents, corticosteroids, PPIs, H_2-receptor antagonists, mucosal protective agents).

Gastric disease

The stomach is a hollow, muscular (smooth) organ that stores, mixes, and begins the digestive process. It is composed of four regions: the *cardia*, where the esophagus connects to the *body* of the stomach; the *fundus* is the upper curvature of the stomach (often gas filled); and the *antrum*, which connects to the duodenum at the pylorus. The layers of the stomach are the serosal (outer layer), muscularis (muscle layer), and the mucosa (inner layer). The functions of the stomach are under the complex influence of many hormonal and neural pathways that regulate gastric acid production, gastric motility, and the initial digestion of proteins, fats, and micronutrients.

Acute gastritis

One of the most common causes of vomiting in dogs and cats is acute gastritis. The prevalence of gastritis in the pet population is unknown but is believed to be high, as many different insults can result in gastric mucosal inflammation.[1] Dogs are affected with acute gastritis more often than cats. Factors to consider that

Table 8.3.1 Acute gastritis etiology

Dietary
- Indiscretion
- Spoiled food
- Intolerance/sensitivity

Foreign bodies
- Bones
- Toys
- Hair balls

Drugs and toxins
- Non-steroidal anti-inflammatory drugs (NSAIDS)
- Corticosteroids
- Heavy metals
- Antibiotics
- Plants
- Cleaners
- Ethylene glycol
- Bleach
- Herbicides
- Fertilizers
- Petroleum distillates
- Organophosphates

Systemic disease
- Uremia
- Liver disease
- Hypoadrenocorticism

Parasites
- *Ollulanus*
- *Physaloptera* spp.

Bacteria
- Bacterial toxins
- *Helicobacter*

Viral
- Parvovirus
- Distemper
- Infectious hepatitis
- Coronavirus

may result in gastritis are dietary indiscretion; food intolerance or allergy; ingestion of foreign material, chemicals, plant irritants; viral or parasitic infections; and drugs (Table 8.3.1).

The clinical sign most commonly associated with acute gastritis is vomiting; typically, the vomitus contains food and bile. Animals with gastritis are usually not interested in food, and they may or may not feel nauseous. Abdominal pain and fever seldom accompany gastritis—especially acute gastritis.

Diagnostic testing and patient care

Acute gastritis is a diagnosis of exclusion, so it is imperative to obtain a thorough history; many patients respond to symptomatic treatment and a definitive diagnosis is never ascertained.

Unless the pet was observed eating an irritating substance, the diagnosis is a presumptive one based upon the history and physical examination findings. Dependent on these findings, abdominal imaging may be recommended. If the clinical signs are mild and the patient's examination is unremarkable, supportive therapy may be instituted. Symptomatic care consists of parenteral fluid therapy if the patient is dehydrated, antinausea medication, and the withholding of food and water for approximately 24 h. At home, the owner observes the patient closely and continues any prescribed medication. If the patient's condition continues to improve after 24 h, the reintroduction of small amounts of water is indicated. Water is the key nutrient in patients with gastritis due to the risk of dehydration. If the hydration status of the patient is not closely monitored, the life-threatening state of dehydration may result. If after ~12 h the patient is able to keep the water down, it is recommended to begin reintroducing small amounts of a bland diet. If the clinical signs worsen or do not improve after a few days, a reexamination and further diagnostics are indicated. At this time, a minimum database (CBC, serum biochemistry profile, and a complete urinalysis) is warranted.[2-5]

Chronic gastritis

Chronic gastritis is defined as intermittent vomiting that occurs for more than 1–2 weeks' duration. Vomiting of food or bile is also the primary clinical sign of chronic gastritis. Decreased appetite, weight loss, hematemesis, or melena may suggest the presence of chronic gastritis. Chronic gastritis is seen more often in cats than in dogs.

Diagnostic testing

Diagnosis is based on laboratory findings (to rule out metabolic causes of vomiting), radiography and/or ultrasonography, and endoscopic or surgical biopsy. Abnormal laboratory values that may be seen include anemia, leukocytosis, eosinophilia, and hypoproteinemia. Survey radiographs seldom identify gastric lesions but will help to rule out foreign bodies. Contrast radiographs may aid in the diagnosis by identifying a thickened gastric wall, mucosal ulceration, mass lesions, and/or evidence of a delay in gastric emptying.[3]

A definitive diagnosis of chronic gastritis is based on histopathologic examination of gastric biopsy specimens. The histopathology (e.g., cellular infiltrate, architectural abnormalities, and severity) and etiology, if identified, determine the type of chronic gastritis affecting the patient. Chronic gastritis may be lymphocytic-plasmacytic, eosinophilic, granulomatous, or atrophic. Lymphocytic-plasmacytic gastritis may be an immune and/or inflammatory reaction to a variety of antigens. *Helicobacter* organisms might be responsible for such a reaction in some animals (especially cats). *Physaloptera rara* has been associated with a similar reaction in some dogs. Eosinophilic gastritis may represent an allergic reaction, most likely to food antigens. Atrophic gastritis may be the result of chronic gastric inflammatory disease and/or immune mechanisms. *Ollulanus tricuspis* may cause granulomatous gastritis in cats.

Even so, the cause of chronic gastritis in dogs and cats is not fully understood. In some cases, an underlying etiology, such as parasitism or a metabolic disorder (e.g., uremia, liver disease), can be identified. In the majority of cases though, an immune-mediated response is hypothesized to be responsible for inflammatory infiltrates within the gastric mucosa.

Chronic idiopathic gastritis is probably a subset of the inflammatory bowel disease (IBD) syndrome or may arise as an adverse reaction to food antigens. Chronic idiopathic gastritis may be localized or may occur with more diffuse IBD of the small or large bowel. Once present, inflammation interferes with gastric motility and reservoir function leading to vomiting. Nutrients, including proteins, can be lost through the inflamed mucosal surface.

Patient care

The following treatment options should be considered when treating a pet with chronic gastritis. Lymphocytic-plasmacytic gastritis sometimes responds to dietary therapy (e.g., low fat, low fiber, elimination diets) alone. If dietary therapy alone is not efficacious, corticosteroids (e.g., prednisolone, 2.2 mg/kg/day) can be used as a concurrent treatment option. Although corticosteroids are required, dietary therapy may ultimately allow a substantially decreased dose, thus avoiding glucocorticoid adverse effects. If corticosteroid therapy is necessary, the dose should be gradually decreased to find the lowest effective dose. The dose should not be tapered too quickly after obtaining a clinical response or the clinical signs may return and be more difficult to control than they were initially. In rare cases, azathioprine and cyclophosphamide have been used sporadically in dogs. These drugs should not be used for treating chronic idiopathic gastritis in cats. Concurrent use of H_2-receptor antagonists is sometimes beneficial.

Canine eosinophilic gastritis usually responds well to a *strict* elimination diet. If dietary therapy alone fails, corticosteroid therapy (e.g., prednisolone, 1.1–2.2 mg/kg/day) in conjunction with diet is usually effective.

Atrophic and granulomatous gastritis has been reported to be more difficult to treat than lymphocytic-plasmacytic or canine eosinophilic gastritis. Diets low in fat and fiber may help control signs. Atrophic gastritis may respond to anti-inflammatory, antacid, and/or prokinetic therapy, with the latter being intended to keep the stomach empty, especially at night.[2,4]

Gastrointestinal ulceration and erosions

Acute gastritis is characterized by sudden-onset vomiting, resulting from gastric mucosal injury or inflammation. If hematemesis is present, it is safe to presume that gastroduodenal erosions or ulcerations are also present. Gastroduodenal ulceration takes place following disruption of the gastric mucosal barrier, which is a group of physical and chemical defense mechanisms. It is these defense mechanisms that protect the gastric mucosa from injury. If not protected, erosions or ulcers may develop. Disruption of the gastric mucosal barrier may involve direct injury, decreased mucosal blood flow, alterations in protective prostag-

landins (prostaglandin E2 [PGE2]) or oversecretion of gastric acid (e.g., secondary to a gastrinoma).

Acute gastritis and gastroduodenal ulceration may be associated with a number of metabolic disorders. Uremia potentially can result in diffuse GI tract hemorrhage from uremic toxins or increased gastrin concentrations. Typically, the kidneys excrete up to 40% of circulating gastrin, and clearance of gastrin is decreased with chronic kidney disease resulting in increased acid production. In dogs with chronic kidney disease, GI signs and histopathologic changes have been noted.

Liver disease is another cause of GI ulceration, which may manifest as hematemesis. Liver disease was one of the two most common risk factors (the other being treatment with nonsteroidal anti-inflammatory drugs [NSAIDs]) in a retrospective study of 43 dogs with gastroduodenal ulceration.[6] The pathogenesis of mucosal ulceration associated with hepatopathies is multifactorial, and associated coagulopathies may worsen clinical signs. Potential mechanisms include altered gastric blood flow due to portal hypertension, delayed epithelial turnover, gastric hyperacidity, and hypergastrinemia.[6]

It is a well-known fact that dogs that have been prescribed NSAIDs may have a variety of adverse drug reactions. These drug reactions include GI bleeding, ulceration, hepatotoxicity, and nephrotoxicity. The adverse GI effects occur because several NSAIDs have a topical irritant effect on the gastric mucosa and can inhibit protective prostaglandins. Experimentally induced and spontaneous gastritis and gastroduodenal ulcerations have been reported to occur in dogs prescribed these uncommon NSAIDs, including aspirin, indomethacin, naproxen, ibuprofen, phenylbutazone, flunixin meglumine, piroxicam, sulindac, and meclofenamic acid. The ulcerogenicity of NSAIDs is attributed to inhibition of the enzyme cyclooxygenase (COX) in the prostaglandin synthesis pathway, resulting in the loss of the gastric protective effects of prostacyclin and prostaglandin E.

COX-1 is a constitutive form that is found in many tissues (e.g., gastric mucosa), where it is involved in the production of protective prostaglandins. COX-2 is primarily an inducible enzyme that is involved in the production of inflammatory mediators, including proinflammatory prostaglandins. Newer NSAIDs have been developed to minimize the effects on COX-1 and consequently to decrease the adverse effects on gastric mucosa. The newer NSAIDs are selective inhibitors of COX-2 and generally are considered to be "gastric sparing." However, despite the selective inhibition of COX-2, these newer NSAIDs still carry the risk of GI ulceration and perforation. Newer veterinary-approved selective COX inhibitors include flunixin, meloxicam, carprofen, etodolac, ketoprofen, tepoxalin, previcox, and deracoxib. Prescribing NSAIDs in patients with underlying renal or hepatic insufficiency may increase the risk of GI ulcerative disease. Concurrent NSAID and corticosteroid use should also be avoided due to the risk of gastric injury.

GI ulcers are recognized complications of critical illnesses (e.g., hypotension, coagulopathy, sepsis) in people. They are believed to develop as a response to the stress of the critical illness and are thus termed "stress ulcers,"[6] but this is a poorly defined process in veterinary patients. However, gastroduodenal ulcerations have been noted in cats and dogs in conjunction with severe burns, heat stroke, multiple trauma, head injuries, and spinal cord disorders.[1,6] In addition, hypovolemic shock and sepsis may be complicated by the development of GI ulcers. Experimentally, endotoxin in septic dogs decreases gastric blood flow resulting in mucosal ischemia. Histamine release stimulated by catecholamines worsened the mucosal damage.[6] Gastrin-producing pancreatic tumors, histamine-producing tumors (e.g., mast cell tumors, basophilic leukemia), and a polypeptide-producing pancreatic tumor have been associated with gastric or duodenal ulceration in dogs and cats.

Gastric motility disorders

After ingestion of a normal meal, on average, the stomach should be empty in 6–8 h for dogs and 4–6 h for cats.[7] Gastric emptying rates are influenced by the nutrient content of the food, formulation of the food, size of the meal, and the pet's body size. Gastric motility disorders result from conditions that directly or indirectly disrupt one or more of the three functions of the stomach:

1. Storage of ingesta
2. Mixing and dispersion of food particles
3. Timely expulsion of gastric contents into the duodenum

Various processes can affect gastric emptying; however, not all disruptions lead to clinical signs.[7]

In general, delayed gastric motility can be divided into outflow obstructions (e.g., stenosis, foreign bodies, hypertrophy of pyloric mucosa, granulomas, and neoplasia including both intragastric and extragastric masses) or defective propulsion (e.g., gastritis, ulcers, gastroenteritis, pancreatitis, and metabolic). Delayed gastric emptying may also be involved in the etiopathogenesis of GDV.

Certain breeds are associated with gastric motility disorders. Congenital pyloric stenosis most often is encountered in brachycephalic dogs and Siamese cats. Chronic hypertrophic pyloric gastropathy usually affects small, purebred, middle-aged dogs, such as the Lhasa Apsos, Maltese, shih tzus, and Pekingese. Young animals typically are at greater risk for gastric foreign bodies, while older pets are more likely to have neoplastic lesions that may lead to obstruction of gastric outflow. Young, large breed dogs living in states that border the Gulf of Mexico may be infected with *Pythium insidiosum* (a fungus-like parasite), resulting in gastric pythiosis and possible gastric outflow obstruction.

Clinical signs

Delayed gastric emptying typically results in vomiting, regardless of the cause. When taking a history from owners, vomiting of undigested or partially digested food more than 12 h after the pet eats may be reported. The onset of clinical signs may be gradual, as in patients with acquired chronic hypertrophic pyloric gastropathy, or acute, as in the case of foreign body ingestion. In dogs and cats with congenital pyloric stenosis, clinical signs may have been present since the pet was weaned. Pets suffering from a chronic condition often have poor body condition and weight loss. Sporadic gastric bloating, nausea, partial or complete inappetence, and belching may also be seen. If patients present with unrelenting or projectile vomiting, complete gastric outflow obstruction should be suspected.

Diagnostic testing

Physical examination findings are typically unremarkable beyond evidence of possible weight loss. However, body condition should be assessed and used as a reassessment tool. Gastric distention and tympany may be evident in some cases. Patients with unrelenting vomiting may be dehydrated, depressed, and lethargic. Electrolyte abnormalities, resulting from continual vomiting, may manifest as weakness.

Laboratory evaluation

In patients with gastroparesis or gastric obstruction, hematologic and serologic findings are typically nonspecific and may be more reflective of the underlying disorder. Chronic, persistent vomiting may precipitate dehydration, electrolyte disturbances (hypokalemia, hypochloremia), and acid–base abnormalities. It is not uncommon to see prerenal azotemia secondary to dehydration. Hypochloremic metabolic alkalosis with paradoxical aciduria may be present in dogs and cats with complete pyloric outflow obstruction.

Imaging

Survey abdominal radiographs are often helpful for evaluating dogs and cats with gastric motility disorders. Findings include a stomach distended by fluid, air, or food; gastric wall thickening may also be recognized. The presence of food in the stomach 12–18 h after the last meal is indicative of an emptying disorder.

GI contrast studies can confirm delayed gastric emptying if liquid contrast media (i.e., barium sulfate) remains in the stomach. Gastroparesis or mechanical obstruction should be suspected if contrast remains in the stomach longer than 4 h in dogs or 30 min in cats.[8] Liquid contrast media is not representative of a typical meal; for that reason, it is recommended to feed barium mixed with food or to administer radiopaque particles (e.g., BIPS) to more completely assess gastric function. Studies have demonstrated that radiopaque markers exit the stomach at a rate proportional to the disappearance of food (DM basis) in dogs. GI contrast studies also may identify thickened gastric walls and intraluminal foreign bodies.

Endoscopy frequently is preferred over radiographic studies in evaluating delayed gastric emptying and gastric outflow obstruction by allowing direct visualization of the outflow tract and surrounding the mucosa. However, endoscopy should be performed before the administration of barium contrast media as barium can make endoscopy much more difficult by obscuring vision. In cases such as antropyloric or proximal duodenal foreign bodies, endoscopy can be both a diagnostic and a curative procedure (with endoscopic removal of the foreign body).

Ultrasonography is a noninvasive method for evaluating both outflow obstructions and propulsion disorders, but the presence of excessive gas in the stomach lumen can make imaging challenging and may negatively affect the resulting image quality. In dogs, gastric contractions can be visualized using ultrasonography, allowing for the evaluation of liquid- and solid-phase gastric emptying in dogs.

Patient care

Care of patients with delayed gastric emptying or outflow obstruction is based on the cause of the disorder. Surgical and medical care may both be required. The administration of prokinetics (e.g., metoclopramide, cisapride) may be indicated. Close monitoring of hydration status and electrolytes is warranted, especially in cases of protracted vomiting. Total parenteral nutrition (TPN) or partial parenteral nutrition (PPN) may be necessary in patients that are NPO due to prolonged nausea and vomiting.

Infiltrative gastric disease

Neoplastic infiltrations such as adenocarcinoma, lymphoma, leiomyomas, and leiomyosarcomas in dogs and lymphoma in cats may produce gastric ulceration/erosion through direct mucosal disruption. Usually, gastric lymphoma is a diffuse lesion, but it can produce distinct masses. The cause and significance of benign gastric polyps are unknown at this time and seem to occur mostly in the antrum.[2]

Dogs and cats with gastric tumors are generally asymptomatic until the disease is advanced. The most common sign is anorexia, vomiting is the next sign noted. Vomiting secondary to gastric neoplasia usually signifies advanced disease or gastric outflow obstruction. Adenocarcinomas are typically infiltrative and decrease emptying by impairing motility and/or obstructing the outflow tract. Weight loss may be due to nutrient loss or to cancer cachexia syndrome. Hematemesis intermittently is seen, but leiomyomas seem to be the tumor most likely to cause severe acute upper GI bleeding. Other bleeding gastric tumors are more likely to cause iron deficiency anemia and melena even if GI blood loss is not obvious. Polyps infrequently cause clinical signs unless the pylorus is obstructed.[3] Iron deficiency anemia in a dog or cat without noticeable blood loss is suggestive of GI bleeding; this is typically caused by a tumor.

Diagnostic testing

Imaging

Plain and/or contrast imaging may reveal gastric wall thickening, decreased motility, and/or mucosal irregularities. Ultrasonography can be utilized to detect gastric masses and mesenteric lymphadenopathy. Endoscopically, these areas may appear as multiple mucosal folds extending into the lumen without ulceration or erosion.

Biopsy

Ultrasound-guided aspiration of thickened areas in the gastric wall or enlarged mesenteric lymph nodes may be diagnostic for adenocarcinoma or lymphoma. When biopsy of such lesions is performed endoscopically, the sample must be deep enough to ensure that submucosal tissue is included. Mucosal lymphomas and nonscirrhous adenocarcinomas often produce GI ulceration/erosions; therefore, endoscopically obtained tissue samples are usually diagnostic, but full-thickness biopsies may be needed in some cases. Polyps are usually obvious endoscopically, but a biopsy specimen should always be obtained and evaluated to ensure that adenocarcinoma is not present.[9]

Patient care

Unfortunately, the majority of adenocarcinomas are advanced before clinical signs manifest, thus resulting in difficult (or impossible) surgical excision. Leiomyomas and leiomyosarcomas are more likely to be resectable than adenocarcinomas. Gastroduodenostomy may palliate gastric outflow obstruction caused by an nonresectable tumor. Except for dogs and cats with lymphoma, chemotherapy is rarely helpful.

Unless diagnosed very early, the prognosis for adenocarcinomas and lymphomas is poor. If diagnosed early, leiomyomas and leiomyosarcomas can be alleviated surgically. It does not appear to be necessary to resect gastric polyps unless they are causing outflow obstruction.

Pythiosis

Pythiosis is a fungal infection caused by *P. insidiosum*. This species is predominantly found along the Gulf Coast area of the southeastern United States. Any area of the alimentary tract or skin may be affected. The fungus typically causes intense submucosal infiltration of fibrous connective tissue and a purulent, eosinophilic, granulomatous inflammation causing gastric ulcerations/erosions. This infiltration prevents peristalsis, resulting in stasis.

Seen typically in dogs, the clinical signs of pythiosis are vomiting, anorexia, diarrhea, and/or weight loss. Gastric outflow obstruction frequently occurs commonly resulting in vomition. If the colon is involved, tenesmus and hematochezia are seen.

Diagnostic testing

Laboratory

To aid in the diagnosis, serological, cytological, or histological tests may be performed. ELISA and PCR tests are available to look for antibodies or antigen, respectively. Gastric, intestinal, or colonic biopsy samples need to include the submucosa because the organism is more likely to be in the submucosa than in the mucosa. Such diagnostic biopsy specimens can be procured by way of rigid endoscopy, but full-thickness samples may be indicated. Cytological analysis of a tissue sample obtained by scraping an excised piece of submucosa with a scalpel blade may be diagnostic. The organisms can be sparse and difficult to find histologically even in large tissue samples.

Patient care

Complete surgical excision provides the best chance for a cure. Itraconazole (5 mg/kg administered orally q 12 h) or liposomal amphotericin B (2.2 mg/kg per treatment) may benefit some animals.[2] Immunotherapy has recently become available, but critical evaluation of the efficacy of this therapy is not currently available.

Pythiosis often spreads to or involves structures that cannot be surgically removed (e.g., root of the mesentery, pancreas surrounding the bile duct), resulting in a grim prognosis.

Key nutritional factors in patients with gastric disease or gastric motility disorders

Water

Water is the most important nutrient for patients with acute or chronic vomiting due to the potential for life-threatening dehydration. Dehydration results from excessive fluid loss combined with the patient's inability to replace those losses. Patients with persistent nausea and vomiting should be supported with subcutaneous or intravenous fluids as oral fluids will not suffice to replace loss in most cases. The hydration status of patients with persistent vomiting should be closely monitored and dehydration should be corrected with appropriate parenteral fluid therapy. Once vomiting has resolved, water should be offered in small amounts initially at room and body temperatures (as colder water delays gastric emptying). If well tolerated, water can be made available free choice.

Electrolytes

Gastric and intestinal secretions differ from extracellular fluids in electrolyte composition, so the loss of these fluids may result in systemic electrolyte abnormalities. Dogs and cats with vomiting and diarrhea may have abnormal serum potassium, chloride, and sodium concentrations. Whether or not this occurs depends on several factors, such as the severity of the disease, the nutritional status of the patient, and the site of the disease process as well as the absence or presence of an acid–base disturbance. Serum electrolyte concentrations are helpful in tailoring appropriate fluid therapy and nutritional management of these patients. Mild hypokalemia, hypochloremia, and either hypernatremia or hyponatremia are the electrolyte abnormalities most commonly associated with acute vomiting and diarrhea, while severe or chronic GI disease typically results in a depletion of potassium as the concentration of this electrolyte in gastric and intestinal secretions is high.

Electrolyte disorders should be corrected initially with appropriate parenteral fluid and electrolyte therapy. Foods for patients with acute gastroenteritis should contain levels of potassium, chloride, and sodium above the minimum allowances for normal dogs and cats. Recommended levels of these nutrients are 0.8–1.1% DM potassium, 0.5–1.3% DM chloride, and 0.3–0.5% DM sodium.[1] Once the patient has recovered, the food should contain levels appropriate for the patient's life stage.

Protein

It is suggested that foods for patients with acute gastritis and/or gastroduodenal ulcers should not contain excess protein (no more than 30% for dogs and 40% for cats).[1] Products of protein digestion (peptides, amino acids, and amines) increase gastrin and gastric acid secretion.

Recommendations of "hypoallergenic" or elimination foods for patients with chronic idiopathic gastritis are made because dietary antigens are assumed to play a role in the cause of the gastritis. Potentially, elimination foods may be used successfully without pharmacological intervention because mild to moderate chronic gastritis may respond to dietary management alone. Ideally, elimination foods should avoid protein excess (16–26% for dogs; 30–40% for cats). Also, elimination foods should have high protein digestibility (≥87%) and should contain a restricted number of novel protein sources to which the patient has never been exposed.[1]

Fat

Animals with chronic vomiting are often underweight due to inadequate caloric intake. As stated previously, the energy density of foods is related to dietary fat content. Increasing dietary fat normally results in increased caloric intake when consuming the same amount of food. However, both solid and liquid foods with increased fat levels usually have slower gastric emptying times than similar foods with lower fat content. Fat in the duodenum stimulates the release of cholecystokinin, a hormone that stimulates the release of bile from the gallbladder, which can delay gastric emptying. Accordingly, foods for cats and dogs with gastric emptying, motility disorders, gastritis, or gastroduodenal ulcers should not provide excess fat.[1] It is recommended that foods with 15% or less (dogs) or 25% or less (cats) DM fat are appropriate for patients with gastric emptying or motility disorders.

Fiber

Gelling agents such as gums or hydrocolloids found in some moist food are added to enhance the aesthetic characteristics of the food for the owners. Pet foods containing gel-forming soluble fibers should be avoided in patients with gastric emptying and motility disorders because they increase the viscosity of ingesta and subsequently slow gastric emptying. Such fibers include pectins and gums (e.g., gum arabic, guar gum, carrageenan, psyllium gum, xanthan gum, carob gum, gum ghatti, and gum tragacanth). It has been shown that increased levels (>8% DM crude fiber) of insoluble fiber (powdered cellulose) in dry foods fed to cats had no effect on gastric emptying.[10] Other reports show that the ratio of slowly to rapidly fermentable fibers is important. As a result of the variability of fiber types on gastric emptying, the crude fiber content of foods for patients with gastritis and gastroduodenal ulcers should not exceed more than 5% DM.[1]

Energy density

It has been established that patients with chronic vomiting are often underweight due to inadequate caloric intake. To ensure the intake of sufficient energy with small amounts of food, the energy density of the food should be moderately increased

(4.0–4.5 kcal/g [DM]). High energy density foods may help patients maintain or regain body weight and condition but will also require higher dietary fat levels, which can adversely affects gastric emptying and should be avoided.

Food forms

In cats and dogs, larger meals are emptied more slowly from the stomach as compared to smaller meals. Liquids are emptied from the stomach more quickly than solids due to lower digesta osmolality with water being emptied the fastest. High osmolality fluids are emptied more slowly than dilute fluids, with solids being the slowest to be emptied. Cold meals slow gastric emptying; therefore, food should be offered between room and body temperature (70–100°F [21–38°C]).

The ideal food form for patients with gastric emptying disorders would be small, frequent meals of liquid or semiliquid consistency. Moist foods are recommended in patients with gastritis and/or ulcerations because they reduce gastric retention time.

Acid load

Alkalemia (i.e., a plasma pH > 7.45) should be expected if vomiting patients lose hydrogen and chloride ions in excess of sodium and bicarbonate. Hypochloremia continues the alkalosis by increasing renal bicarbonate reabsorption. Mild alkalemia is common, but severe alkalemia is not when dealing with gastritis patients. Profound alkalemia is more likely to occur with pyloric or upper duodenal obstruction.

Acidemia (i.e., a plasma pH < 7.35) may occur in vomiting patients if the vomited gastric fluid is relatively low in hydrogen and chloride ion content (e.g., during fasting) or if concurrent loss of intestinal sodium and bicarbonate occurs. It is recommended to correct severe acid–base disorders with parenteral fluid and electrolyte therapy. Foods for patients with acute vomiting and diarrhea should avoid excess dietary acid load. Foods that normally produce alkaline urine are less likely to be associated with acidosis.

Alimentary tract parasites

Whipworm

Whipworm (*Trichuris vulpis*) infection can cause acute, chronic, or intermittent signs of large bowel diarrhea. Whipworms are a parasite of the cecum and large bowel and have a direct life cycle. Female adults pass ova in the feces (diagnostic stage), which mature in the environment into the embryonated, infective stage. Animals acquire the infection by ingesting ova, and once ingested, the life cycle repeats. The adults burrow into the colonic and cecal mucosa where the distinctive "whip" head firmly embeds into the mucosa and feeds on blood and tissue fluids. This parasite infection can cause inflammation, bleeding, and intestinal protein loss.[1–4] Whipworms are known to infect dogs of all ages. Ova may survive and remain infectious in the environment for up to 5 years; therefore, whipworm infections are typically the result of exposure to contaminated ground.

Dogs, and rarely cats, acquire whipworms which produce a wide spectrum of mild to severe colonic disease that can include hematochezia and PLE. Severe trichuriasis may cause severe hyponatremia and hyperkalemia, mimicking hypoadrenocorticism. Marked hyponatremia might even be responsible for CNS signs (e.g., seizures).[2] The feline whipworms, *Trichuris campanula* and *Trichuris serrata*, are very rare and typically do not produce clinical signs.

In dogs presenting with bloody stools or other colonic diseases, *T. vulpis* infection should be considered. Diagnosis is made through observation of the ova in a fecal flotation test. Ova are relatively dense and float only in properly prepared flotation solutions; furthermore, ova are shed intermittently and sometimes can be found only if multiple fecal examinations are performed. Up to 50% of dogs presenting with whipworm infestation and diarrhea are ova-negative.[3] It is also possible to visualize adult *T. vulpis* through colonoscopic evaluation.

Due to the potential difficulty in diagnosing *T. vulpis*, it is practical to empirically treat dogs with chronic large bowel disease with fenbendazole (50 mg/kg PO qd × 3 days) before proceeding to endoscopy. If a dog is treated for whipworms, it should be treated again in 3 weeks and then again in 3 months to kill worms that were not in the intestinal lumen at the time of the first treatment. Febantel/pyrantel is an alternative treatment for whipworm infections. Regular administration of milbemycin for heartworm prevention also has been shown to control whipworm infections in dogs.[3] When properly treated, the prognosis for recovery is good.

Roundworms

Roundworms are common in both dogs (*Toxocara canis* and *Toxascaris leonina*) and cats (*Toxocara cati* and *T. leonina*). Dogs and cats can obtain roundworms from ingesting the ova (either directly or via paratenic hosts). *T. canis* is often obtained transplacentally from the mother; *T. cati* may use transmammary passage, and *T. leonina* can use intermediate hosts. The parasite can burrow through the wall of the GI tract, entering the blood vessels, and migrate to the lungs or other organs, and, as mentioned, can be transmitted through the colostrum. Migration through the host's tissue by immature larval forms can cause hepatic fibrosis and significant pulmonary lesions. Adult roundworms live in the small intestinal lumen and migrate against the flow of ingesta. They can cause inflammatory infiltrates (e.g., eosinophils) in the wall of the intestine.[2,5] Female adults pass ova in the feces (diagnostic stage), which mature in the environment into the embryonated, infective stage.

Roundworms can cause or contribute to diarrhea, stunted growth, poor hair coat, and poor weight gain, especially in young animals. A runt with a "potbelly" appearance is suggestive of severe roundworm infection. At times, roundworms may gain access to the stomach, in which case they may be produced in vomitus. If roundworms are numerous, they may cause obstruction of the intestines or the bile duct.

Diagnosis is relatively easy because ova are produced in large numbers and readily float in fecal flotation tests. On occasion, neonates develop clinical signs of roundworm infestation, but ova cannot be found in the feces. In these cases, transplacental migration of immature larva results in large worm burdens, causing clinical signs in these animals before the parasites mature and are able to produce ova.[6,7]

Various anthelmintics are effective, but pyrantel (10 mg/kg) is typically prescribed as a first line of defense because it is safe for young dogs and cats, particularly those with diarrhea. Affected animals should be retreated at 2- to 3-week intervals to kill roundworms that were initially in the host's tissues but migrated into the intestinal lumen since the previous treatment.

High dose fenbendazole therapy (i.e., 50 mg/kg/day from day 40 of gestation until 2 weeks postpartum) has been suggested to reduce the somatic roundworm burden in bitches and to lessen transplacental transmission to puppies. Newborn puppies can be treated with fenbendazole (100 mg/kg for 3 days), which kills more than 90% of prenatal larvae. This treatment can be repeated 2–3 weeks later. Preweaning puppies should be treated at 2, 4, 6, and 8 weeks of age to lessen contamination of the environment. *T. canis* and *T. cati* pose a zoonotic risk (i.e., visceral and ocular larval migrans); preventing environmental contamination can help decrease this potential.[2] Preweaning kittens should be treated at 6, 8, and 10 weeks of age. The prognosis for recovery is good unless the animal is already severely stunted when treated, in which case it may never attain its anticipated body size.

Hookworms

Ancylostoma spp. and *Uncinaria* spp. are more common in dogs than in cats. Infestation is usually from one of two routes, via ingestion of the ova or through transcolostral transmission. Also, although not as common, freshly hatched larvae may also penetrate the skin. The adults live in the small intestinal lumen, where they attach to the mucosa. Plugs of intestinal mucosa and/or blood are ingested, depending on the worm species. In severe infestations, hookworms may be found in the colon. The mature female lays ova that are expelled in the feces (diagnostic phase); then in the environment the larva hatch (rhabditiform larva) and grow into third-stage larva (filariform, infective stage).

Dogs are more severely affected than cats. Young animals may have life-threatening blood loss or iron deficiency anemia, melena, frank fecal blood, diarrhea, and/or failure to thrive. Senior dogs hardly ever have primary disease caused by hookworms unless they harbor a massive infestation. However, these worms may still contribute to disease caused by other intestinal problems.

Finding ova in the feces using fecal flotation is diagnostic and relatively easy because hookworms are prolific egg producers. However, 5- to 10-day-old puppies may be exsanguinated by feeding hookworms obtained transcolostrally before ova appear in their feces. Such prepatent infections rarely occur in older animals that have received a sudden, massive exposure. Diagnosis is suggested by signalment and clinical signs in these animals. Iron deficiency anemia in a puppy or kitten free of fleas is highly

suggestive of hookworm infestation. Eosinophilia is an ancillary but common finding on the CBC of patients with hookworm parasites.

Various anthelmintics are effective with the following commonly prescribed doses: fenbendazole 50 mg/kg PO qd × 3 days; febantel 10–20 mg/kg PO qd × 3 days; pyrantel pamoate 5–10 mg/kg PO once.[5,7] Treatment should be repeated in approximately 3 weeks to kill parasites entering the intestinal lumen from the tissues. The use of heartworm preventives containing pyrantel or milbemycin helps to minimize hookworm infestations. In anemic puppies and kittens, blood transfusions may be necessary. Application of moxidectin to pregnant bitches on day 55 of pregnancy reduces transcolostral transmission to puppies.

Hookworms are a potential human health hazard (i.e., cutaneous larval migrans) and it is imperative that owners are educated of this zoonotic risk. The prognosis in mature dogs and cats is good but can be guarded in severely anemic puppies and kittens. Owners of puppies or kittens that are severely stunted in their growth from hookworm infections should be advised that they may never attain their anticipated body size.

Tapeworms

There are several tapeworms known to infect dogs and cats, with the most common being *Dipylidium caninum*. Tapeworms usually have an indirect life cycle; the dog or cat is infected when it eats an infected intermediate host. Fleas and lice are intermediate hosts for *D. caninum*, whereas wild animals (e.g., rabbits) are intermediate hosts for some *Taenia* spp.

Aesthetically offensive, tapeworms are rarely pathogenic in small animals, although it should be mentioned that *Mesocestoides* spp. can reproduce in the host and cause disease such as abdominal effusion. The most common sign in infested dogs and cats is anal irritation associated with shed segments "crawling" on the area. A segment may enter an anal sac and cause inflammation, but this is very uncommon. Very rarely, large numbers of tapeworms cause intestinal obstruction or vomiting.

Taenia spp. and especially *D. caninum* eggs are typically confined in segments not detected by routine fecal flotations. This is a very important part of client education on parasites as owners may become confused why a fecal flotation test does not diagnose all worms in their pets. *Echinococcus* spp. and some *Taenia* spp. ova may be found in the feces. Tapeworms are usually diagnosed when tapeworm segments (e.g., "rice grains") are observed on the feces or in the perineal area.

Praziquantel and episprantel are effective against all species of tapeworms. Prevention of tapeworms involves controlling the intermediate hosts (i.e., fleas and lice for *D. caninum*). *Echinococcus* spp. are also considered to be a human health hazard, so treatment, prevention (through flea, lice, and rodent control), and education are indicated.

Strongyloidiasis

Strongyloides stercoralis and *Strongyloides planiceps* infect dogs, principally puppies, occurring most commonly in crowded conditions. *Strongyloides felis* and *Strongyloides tumefaciens* infect cats. These parasites produce motile larvae that can penetrate unbroken skin or mucosa (infective stage). Subsequently, the animal may be infested from its own feces even before the larvae are evacuated from the colon. Because of this, animals can quickly acquire large parasitic burdens. Most animals are infested after being exposed to fresh feces containing the motile larvae (diagnostic phase). Likely sources for infestation are humane shelters and pet stores.[2,3,5] The clinical signs of strongyloidiasis are mucoid or hemorrhagic diarrhea and lethargy. Respiratory signs (i.e., verminous pneumonia) may be present if parasites have penetrated the lungs.

S. stercoralis can be diagnosed by finding the larvae in fresh feces, either by direct fecal examination or by Baermann sedimentation. *Strongyloides* larvae must be differentiated from *Oslerus* spp. larvae. It is important to use fresh feces because old feces may contain hatched hookworm larvae, which resemble those of *Strongyloides* spp.

Effective anthelmintics such as fenbendazole, thiabendazole, and ivermectin should be used to treat strongyloides. The owner must be educated that this parasite is a human health hazard because larvae penetrate unbroken skin. Immunosuppressed people are at risk for severe disease if they become infected. The prognosis is guarded in young animals with severe diarrhea and/or pneumonia.

Coccidiosis

Isospora spp. are obligate intracellular parasites that infect the intestine, predominantly seen in young cats and dogs, and more often in dogs than in cats. The pet is usually infested by ingesting infective oocysts from the environment, and the coccidia invade and destroy villous epithelial cells.

Coccidia may be clinically insignificant as with an asymptomatic, older animal, or they may be responsible for mild to severe diarrhea, sometimes with blood. Rarely, a kitten or puppy loses enough blood to require a blood transfusion. Conversely, small numbers of oocysts do not ensure that the infestation is insignificant.

Coccidiosis is diagnosed by finding oocysts on fecal flotation examination. These oocysts should not be confused with giardial cysts. In coprophagic dogs, special attention should be paid to the potential presence of coccidian oocysts from other animals.[5] Occasionally, *Eimeria* oocysts will be seen in the feces of dogs that eat deer or rabbit excrement.

If coccidia are believed to be a problem, sulfadimethoxine or trimethoprim–sulfa should be administered for 10–20 days. The sulfa drug does not eradicate the coccidia but rather inhibits it in order for body defense mechanisms to reestablish control. Amprolium (25 mg/kg administered orally q 24 h for 3–5 days) can be used in puppies but is not approved for use in dogs. It is not to be used in cats as it is potentially toxic. Toltrazuril (15 mg/kg q 24 h for 3 days) has been found to decrease oocyst shedding, at least temporarily.[2] The prognosis for recovery is usually good unless there are underlying problems that allowed the coccidia to become pathogenic in the first place.

Cryptosporidia

The *Cryptosporidium* spp. are obligate intracellular protozoan parasites that infect enterocytes. *Cryptosporidium parvum* may infect animals that ingest the sporulated oocysts originating from infested animals. The oocysts may also be carried in water. Thin-walled oocysts are produced, which can rupture in the intestine and produce autoinfection. The organism infests the brush border of small intestinal epithelial cells, leading to diarrhea in the animal.

Diarrhea is the most common clinical sign in dogs and cats; however, many cats infested with *Cryptosporidium* spp. are asymptomatic.[7] Dogs presenting with diarrhea are frequently under 6 months of age, but a similar age predilection has not been recognized for cats.[2,5]

Diagnosis requires finding the oocysts in the feces or a positive ELISA test. *C. parvum* is the smallest of the coccidians and is therefore easy to miss on fecal examination. Examination should be performed at ×1000 magnification. The use of acid-fast stains on fecal smears and fluorescent antibody techniques has been reported to improve sensitivity. It is recommended to submit the feces to a laboratory experienced in diagnosing cryptosporidiosis. When submitting the fecal sample, the laboratory must be notified that the feces may contain *C. parvum* as this is potentially infective for people. The ELISA is more sensitive than fecal examination. A PCR-based test developed for the detection of *Cryptosporidium* spp. in cat feces has proven to be more sensitive than the available immunoassays.[8]

In dogs and cats, there are no known reliable treatments. Immunocompetent people and cattle often spontaneously eliminate the infestation, but whether cats and dogs also eliminate the infestation is unknown. Most young dogs with diarrhea associated with cryptosporidiosis die or are euthanized. Many cats have asymptomatic infestations, and those with diarrhea have an unknown prognosis.

Trichomoniasis

Trichomoniasis in cats appears to be caused by *T. foetus/Tritrichomonas suis*, an intestinal pathogen. Animals most likely become infected by the fecal–oral route.

Trichomoniasis typically is associated with large bowel diarrhea, which rarely contains blood or mucus. While cats of any age, breed, or gender can become infected, this intestinal pathogen is seen more frequently in young cats that are housed in community or densely populated situations (e.g., catteries, shelters). Exotic cat breeds (e.g., Somalis, ocicats, Bengals) seem to have a higher percentage of clinical signs.

T. foetus colonizes the surface of the mucosa in the colon, which leads to chronic large bowel diarrhea. Affected cats are typically otherwise normal, but there may be anal irritation, defecation in inappropriate places, or fecal incontinence. Although it may persist for months, the diarrhea typically resolves spontaneously. Even in cats whose diarrhea resolves, infected cats most likely will represent with bouts of diarrhea after being exposed to stress.[2,9]

Diagnosis requires identifying the motile trophozoite in the feces. Care must be taken as *Tritrichomonas* trophozoites can be mistaken for *Giardia* trophozoites. Diagnosis can be made by the identification of trophozites on a direct fecal smear, fecal culture, PCR analysis of fecal material, or by colonic mucosal biopsy.[9] Timely examination of fresh feces diluted with warm saline solution is the easiest technique, but it is insensitive. Fecal culture using the pouch technique developed for bovine venereal trichomoniasis is more sensitive.[2]

Ronidazole (30–50 mg/kg q 12 h for 14 days) is the only drug currently known to safely and effectively eliminate *Tritrichomonas* and to resolve the diarrhea associated with the infestation. However, neurological signs have been reported with its use; discontinuing the drug has been reported to stop the adverse effects. If trichomoniasis is diagnosed, it is important to rule out other causes of diarrhea (e.g., *C. perfringens*, diet, *Cryptosporidium* spp.) because treatment for one of these other causes may cause resolution of the diarrhea. Treatment can reduce the number of organisms and improve clinical signs; however, it seldom eliminates the infection.[3] As previously stated, most affected cats will eventually resolve the clinical signs of trichomoniasis, although diarrhea may recur if the patient undergoes stressful events.

Diseases of the small intestine

The SI is the part of the digestive tract from the pylorus of the stomach to the ileocolic valve where it joins to the LI. It is roughly divided into three segments (proximal to distal): the duodenum, the jejunum, and the ileum. There are four layers to the SI: The serosal layer is the outer most, followed by the muscularis, the submucosa, and the inner most layer, the mucosa. The SI, working with the microflora of the gut, functions to digest (e.g., breaks down carbohydrates and continue the digestion of proteins and fat) and to absorb nutrients, and serves as a physical and immune barrier to prevent exposure to any harmful elements. Peristaltic waves provide for mixing of the ingesta and for propelling the ingesta onward through the GI tract. The SI both secretes and is under the influence of hormones.

Protein-losing enteropathy

PLE is a general term applied to GI disease whereby serum proteins (albumin and globulins) are lost due to leakage into the intestinal lumen. Blood chemistry typically reveals a panhypoproteinemia. In contrast, decreased protein due to renal disease (due to loss of albumin through a damaged glomerulus) or liver disease (due to lack of production of albumin by the liver) usually results in only hypoalbuminemia.

There are many underlying causes for PLE, which include (but are not limited to) IBD (lymphoplasmacytic, eosinophilic, or granulomatous enteritis), lymphangiectasia, parvovirus, histoplasmosis, phycomycosis, giardiasis, intussusception, GI erosion/ulceration, and lymphoma.[1,2] Panhypoproteinemia due to GI disease is uncommon in the cat.[1] Biopsy of the GI tract is required for definitive diagnosis of the underlying cause for most cases of PLE.[1]

Certain breeds appear to be predisposed: basenji, soft-coated wheaten terrier, shar-pei, rottweilers, Yorkshire terriers, and Lundehund.[1,2]

Clinical signs

Chronic, intermittent small bowel diarrhea, anorexia, vomiting, and weight loss are all common clinical signs of PLE. Occasionally, affected dogs will not have diarrhea, weight loss, or vomiting. When serum albumin is below 2.0 g/dL, ascites and edema can develop.[1] The owner may notice a distended abdomen due to ascites. Fluid accumulation can also occur in the pleural space, causing dyspnea, tachypnea, and decreased lung sounds. Enteric loss of antithrombin may lead to a hypercoagulable state, which can cause thromboembolic disease. Dyspnea can be seen when pulmonary thromboemboli occur. Rarely, thromboemboli can occur in the CNS, causing seizures or twitching.[1]

Diagnostics

A database on these patients should include CBC, serum biochemistry profile, urinalysis, +/− urine protein : creatinine ratio, serum bile acid assay, abdominal and thoracic radiographs, abdominal ultrasound, fecal flotation, abdominal effusion analysis (if present), and serum cobalamin and folate measurements. Additional diagnostics may be performed depending on signalment (parvoviral testing in puppies) or diseases endemic to an area (rectal scrape or urine antigen testing for histoplasmosis). Diagnosis of PLE is made on the basis of clinical signs and a finding of low albumin and globulins. Occasionally, increased globulins and a low albumin can occur with PLE. This can be seen with histoplasmosis and immunoproliferative enteropathy in the basenji.[1,2] Low albumin caused by renal protein loss should be ruled out with a urinalysis and urine protein : creatinine ratio. Low albumin due to liver disease is ruled out in many cases with normal pre- and postprandial serum bile acids. Once these other etiologies of low albumin are ruled out, a diagnosis of PLE may be made by exclusion. Other common abnormalities on serum biochemistry include low cholesterol, low calcium (total and ionized should be measured), and low magnesium. Lymphopenia can be seen on CBC.[1,2] Cobalamin (vitamin B_{12}) is frequently decreased due to poor absorption in the ileum from diffuse disease. Fecal α_1-PI may be measured to confirm protein loss in the feces, especially in cases where there is concurrent renal protein loss or hepatic insufficiency.[1] Survey abdominal radiographs may be normal or may indicate peritoneal effusion. Chest radiographs are usually normal but can show pleural effusion or evidence of histoplasmosis or metastatic neoplasia. Abdominal ultrasound may show enlarged mesenteric lymph nodes, intestinal wall thickening, and abdominal effusion. Analysis of abdominal effusion, if present, reveals a pure transudate.

To definitively diagnose the underlying cause of PLE, intestinal biopsy is required. Biopsy may be obtained via endoscopy, laparoscopy, or laparotomy. Due to the diffuse nature of most underlying causes associated with PLE and the risks associated with poor healing due to low albumin, endoscopic biopsy is often preferred as a means to obtain intestinal biopsies for definitive diagnosis,[1,2] unless abdominal ultrasound reveals a lesion that cannot be reached with the scope (distal small intestinal thickening or mass lesion), a surgical lesion is found (intussusception), or a liver biopsy is needed to determine if hepatic disease as a cause of low albumin is present.[1] Additionally, endoscopy allows the clinician to visualize the mucosa.[1]

Treatment

Treatment includes identification and removal or management of the underlying cause when possible (e.g., immunosuppressive drugs for IBD, surgery for intussusception, antifungals for histoplasmosis, and chemotherapy for GI lymphoma).[1,2] Hypocobaliminemia requires parenteral cobalamin supplementation. Additional supportive care may be necessary (fluid therapy, transfusion), especially prior to diagnostic procedures such as gastroduodenoscopy.

Prognosis

Prognosis is dependent on the underlying cause but is considered guarded to poor in most cases.

Anesthetic complications

Hypotension is the main complication when anesthetizing animals with PLE. Colloidal support with hetastarch or other colloids prior to and during the anesthetic procedure is recommended. Careful blood pressure monitoring during the procedure is necessary. Drugs that are highly protein bound should not be used or should be used with extreme caution and require dose reduction.

Short bowel syndrome

Extensive surgical resection of the SI with associated clinical signs results in short bowel syndrome (SBS). The amount of intestine that must be removed before SBS develops has not been clearly defined in veterinary medicine. In humans, it is thought that removal of ≥50% of the SI leads to SBS.[3] SBS in animals frequently results when 75% or more of the SI is resected.[2] The decreased absorptive surface area of the SI that results from extensive resection often causes inadequate digestion and malabsorption.[2–4] Common causes for extensive bowel resection in veterinary medicine include intestinal foreign bodies, volvulus, intussusception, trauma, infarction, and fungal infection.[2–4]

Clinical signs

Clinical signs after extensive bowel resection include very loose, watery diarrhea, malabsorption, and weight loss.[2–4] During the first 24–48 h post-op, diarrhea may be severe and may lead to dehydration and abrupt weight loss due to significant water loss. Severe diarrhea may also lead to electrolyte imbalances such as hyponatremia and hypokalemia.[4] As post-op shock subsides, animals with SBS become more alert and may develop polyphagia.[4] Chronically, the patient may experience persistent diarrhea,[2–4] weight loss, or lack of weight gain to preoperative levels, malnutrition, hypergastrinemia, and steatorrhea (excess fat in the stool).[2,4] Over the following several months, as intestinal hyperplasia and adaption may occur, clinical improvement can be seen.[2–4] This is manifested by decreased defecation frequency, with more formed stool, leading to less water loss. The patient may regain weight but may still not reach optimal weight.[2,4]

Diagnostics

Diagnosis is based on clinical signs and length of intestine resected. Particularly in the immediate postoperative period, the patient may experience hyponatremia, hypokalemia, azotemia, and metabolic acidosis.[4] GI contrast studies can show dilated intestinal segments and decreased intestinal transit time.[4] Blood work at this time may continue to show anemia and hypoalbuminemia.[4] Clinical signs of SBS may persist when the remaining intestines are unable to undergo adequate compensatory changes. Diarrhea and steatorrhea persist in these patients and can be severe, especially if the ileocolic valve has not been preserved.[2] The response of a particular patient to extensive bowel loss is unpredictable and is not always related to the amount of bowel that has been resected.[2–4]

Treatment

Treatment is directed at maintaining adequate nutritional support, minimizing electrolyte abnormalities, and controlling diarrhea.[2,4] During the initial post-op period, ideal nutritional support may be provided via TPN. PPN can also be utilized. Intravenous fluid therapy and electrolyte support are important during the initial period after resection to maintain hydration and to minimize electrolyte abnormalities.[4] Sodium and potassium levels should be evaluated at least every 24 h.[4] Limited oral intake should be started as early as possible after surgery to help stimulate intestinal adaptation.[2,4] In the initial phase, elemental or polymeric diets can be fed. Polymeric diets can be fed via an NE or gastrostomy tube. Some animals with SBS will have an increased appetite soon after surgery. Care should be taken to not feed these animals large amounts as this can contribute to diarrhea.[2,4]

Low fat, highly digestible diets should be fed long term. Supplementation with parenteral vitamin B_{12} (cobalamin) is recommended long term. Other fat-soluble vitamins should be supplemented indefinitely. Calcium, zinc, and magnesium may also need to be supplemented long term.[2,4]

Additionally, gastric acid hypersecretion can occur, which can be an important contributor to diarrhea. This is managed with the use of H_2-receptor antagonists such as famotidine. Intestinal bacterial overgrowth is common and should be managed with antibiotics (metronidazole and amoxicillin or enrofloxacin initially; choices for long-term management include metronidazole and tylosin). Occasionally, pancreatic enzyme replacement is useful (Pancrezyme*) if extensive resection of the duodenum has disrupted the pancreatic duct. Persistent, loose, watery diarrhea can be treated with an antidiarrheal such as loperamide. Other treatments that have been found to be beneficial include urso-deoxycholate (UDCA).[5] In one experimental study, dogs receiving UDCA (300 mg every other day) experienced significant improvements in fecal characteristics, body weight, and overall nutritional state versus the control group.[5] Hydrophilic laxatives may decrease fluidity of existing bowel content and may increase fecal bulk. Compounds that may be tried for this purpose include methylcellulose (Citrucel'), psyllium (Metamucil'), and calcium polycarbophil (Fiberall').[2,4] The animal's nutritional status and food tolerance should be closely monitored long term to avoid starvation.[4]

Prognosis

Factors involved in determining the clinical course are status of the ileocolic valve (if resected, symptoms are consistently worse), extent and site of bowel resection, functional capacity of remaining bowel and other digestive organs, degree of adaptation that occurs in the remaining intestine,[2] and client determination to pursue management with significant cost. A decision to euthanize should not be made too hastily as time is needed for remaining intestines to adapt.[2] The prognosis seems to be better in patients with early aggressive management.[2] Persistent malabsorption and steatorrhea are associated with a poor prognosis if enough time has passed for adaptation of the intestinal tract to occur. This is especially common in patients whose ileocolic valves have not been preserved.[2]

In one retrospective study, most animals had diarrhea or loose stools for a few weeks to months postoperatively and then developed normal fecal consistency or had only mild clinical signs that were deemed acceptable to the owner.[3]

It is important to keep in mind that each patient should be treated on an individual basis and that care should be taken to not make a hasty decision regarding euthanasia.

Intestinal obstruction

Simple intestinal obstruction

Simple intestinal obstruction (i.e., the intestinal lumen is obstructed without peritoneal leakage, severe venous occlusion, or bowel devitalization) is usually caused by foreign objects in dogs and linear foreign bodies in cats. Infiltrative disease, intussusception, and torsion are also possible etiologies.[6,7]

Clinical signs

Vomiting with or without anorexia, depression, or diarrhea are common clinical signs. Abdominal pain is not typically noted upon physical examination. The clinical findings of intestinal obstruction are related to the site, severity, and cause of the obstruction. A complete upper intestinal obstruction can result in severe acute vomiting, which may lead to dehydration and fluid loss. If the intestines become devitalized and septic peritonitis results, the obstruction becomes complicated and the animal may be presented in a moribund state or in septic shock (systemic inflammatory response syndrome [SIRS]). Partial obstructions are more of a challenge to diagnose as the pet presents with an insidious onset of vomiting and intermittent diarrhea.

Diagnostic testing

A complete history is crucial when a foreign body is suspected as the cause of an obstruction. Abdominal palpation, plain abdominal radiographs, or ultrasonographic imaging can be diagnostic if they reveal a foreign object, mass, dilated intestinal loops, or obvious obstructive ileus. Abdominal ultrasonography is preferred as the more sensitive technique and can reveal dilated or thickened intestinal loops that are not obvious on palpation or radiographs due to poor serosal contrast caused by abdominal fluid or lack of abdominal fat. The sensitivity of the ultrasound will be lessened by gas-filled loops of bowel. In cases where it is difficult to distinguish obstruction from physiological ileus, abdominal contrast radiographs may be considered. Many intestinal foreign bodies cause hypochloremic, hypokalemic metabolic alkalosis, a metabolic change that is suggestive of gastric outflow obstruction.[6,7]

If a foreign object is found and an intestinal obstruction is diagnosed, surgical intervention is warranted. If an abdominal mass or an obvious obstructive ileus is found, a presumptive diagnosis of obstruction is made, and further diagnostics may be needed to completely characterize the obstructive process. Fine needle biopsy and cytological evaluation of an intestinal mass prior to surgery may be warranted to rule out certain diseases (e.g., lymphoma).

Once intestinal obstruction is diagnosed, routine preanesthetic laboratory tests should be performed as serum electrolyte and acid–base abnormalities are common in vomiting animals. The animal should be stabilized and then promptly prepared for surgery. Vomiting of gastric origin classically produces a hypokalemic, hypochloremic metabolic alkalosis and paradoxical aciduria, whereas vomiting caused by intestinal obstruction may produce metabolic acidosis and varying degrees of hypokalemia. However, these changes cannot be predicted even when the cause of the vomiting is known, making serum electrolyte and acid–base determinations important in therapy planning. If septic peritonitis is absent and massive intestinal resection is not necessary, the prognosis is usually good.

Neoplasms of the small intestine

Overall, tumors of the SI are not common but are usually malignant when found. In cats, lymphomas (most common), adenocarcinomas, and mast cell tumors are the most common, whereas in dogs, adenocarcinomas, smooth muscle tumors, and other stromal cell tumors are more common. Other neoplasia of the SI are rare but have been noted (e.g., intestinal fibrosarcomas [dogs], hemangiosarcomas [cats], schwannomas, neuroendocrine tumors, carcinoids, and plasma cell tumors).[8] Small intestinal neoplasia appears more frequently in older dogs and cats with the mean age being approximately 9 years of age. However, it should be noted that some tumors, such as leiomyosarcomas, have been seen in very young animals; therefore, age should not exclude a diagnosis of SI cancer.[2,6,9]

Alimentary lymphoma

Alimentary lymphoma (lymphosarcoma, malignant lymphoma) is a neoplastic proliferation of lymphocytes in the intestinal tract; it can be either focal or diffuse disease. In cats, it may be caused by FeLV, but the etiology in dogs is unknown. Lymphocytic-plasmacytic enteritis (LPE) has been suggested to be prelymphomatous in some animals, but the frequency of malignant transformation of LPE to lymphoma is unknown.[8] Alimentary lymphoma appears to be more common in cats, and the incidence of intestinal lymphoma is increasing. The extraintestinal forms of lymphoma (e.g., arising from the lymph nodes, liver, spleen) are more common in dogs. Intestines affected by alimentary lymphoma may appear grossly normal or may exhibit nodules, masses, diffuse intestinal thickening (resulting from infiltrative disease), dilated sections, and/or focal constrictions. Mesenteric lymphadenopathy is often noted, but it is not constant, and it is important to note that IBD can cause mild to moderate mesenteric lymphadenopathy. A PLE may also occur.

Chronic, progressive weight loss, anorexia, small intestinal diarrhea, and vomiting are typically the presenting signs. Inappetance may be present in advanced stages of disease. Clinical signs are typically slow to progress, and owners may attribute this to the aging process.

Diagnostic testing

The diagnosis of alimentary lymphoma is through the identification of neoplastic lymphocytes, which may be obtained by fine needle aspiration cytology or histopathology via biopsy. Histopathologic evaluation of intestinal biopsy specimens is the most reliable diagnostic method. Biopsy samples may be collected via endoscopy (partial thickness) or surgery (full thickness). When collecting endoscopic biopsy samples, it is of utmost importance to obtain multiple, deep samples. A sample that is not sufficiently deep may lead to the erroneous diagnosis of LPE instead of lymphoma. On histopathology, lymphocytes found in the submucosa are not specific for lymphoma; lymphocytes can be also found in the submucosa of cats with IBD. However, cats with IBD generally do not have the dramatic numbers that can be found in some cases with lymphoma. Occasionally, neoplastic lymphocytes are found only in the serosal layer, thus necessitating full-thickness surgical biopsy specimens. If collecting full-thickness biopsy samples, it is important to biopsy the ileum because many patients (especially cats) do not have lymphoma in the duodenum.[8]

Animals with extremely well-differentiated lymphocytic lymphoma may be impossible to distinguish from those with LPE using routine histopathology, even with multiple full-thickness biopsy samples. This seems to be more of a problem in cats. In these cases, diagnosis often depends on finding evidence of lymphoma in other organs (e.g., liver) or in running immunohistochemical studies to determine if the lymphoid population is monoclonal. Paraneoplastic hypercalcemia occasionally occurs but is neither sensitive nor specific for lymphoma.

Patient care

Cats with well-differentiated small cell lymphomas, treated with prednisolone and chlorambucil, may do as well as cats with IBD that receive the same therapy. There is a much better prognosis in cats with low grade small cell lymphoma as compared with the intermediate or high grade lymphoma. A more aggressive form of intestinal lymphoma, lymphoblastic large cell, also is more resistant to treatment. The long-term prognosis is very poor, but some cats with well-differentiated intestinal lymphoma will live years with therapy.[2,6,9]

Chemotherapy (cyclophosphamide, hydroxydoxorubicin, Oncovin, prednisone [CHOP] protocol 21-day cycle)[10] may be of value in dogs, but this value has been questioned as some patients have become quite ill if given aggressive chemotherapy.[6]

Intestinal adenocarcinoma

Adenocarcinoma is a malignant neoplasia of the epithelium arising from glandular tissue that can be further characterized by the tissue of origin. Both the gastric form and the intestinal form of adenocarcinoma are seen. Intestinal adenocarcinoma may affect either the SI or LI. Both adenoma and adenocarcinoma are more common in the canine LI than in the SI, with the converse being true in cats.[8] In dogs SI carcinoma has a predilection for the duodenum, whereas the jejunum and ileum are more commonly affected in cats. Adenocarcinoma is most common in older dogs (mean age 9 years) and cats (mean age 11 years).[8]

Diagnostic testing

Clinical signs at presentation are weight loss and vomiting caused by partial or complete intestinal obstruction. Dogs with intestinal adenocarcinoma occasionally present with acute signs of obstruction. Physical examination findings aid in the diagnosis as a palpable mass is found in approximately half of all cases.[11,12] If significant ulceration has occurred (local infiltration), melena and anemia may be present. If the intestinal wall is perforated, clinical signs associated with peritonitis or intracoelomic carcinomatosis may be noted. Diagnosis requires demonstrating neoplastic epithelial cells. Endoscopy, surgery, and ultrasound-guided fine needle aspiration may be diagnostic. Adenocarcinomas are locally infiltrative and may extend to the serosa and mesentery and may metastasize to local lymph nodes and/or the peritoneal cavity. Carcinomatosis as well as metastasis to the liver, testes, skin, and other organs have been reported.[8] Diagnostic imaging, particularly ultrasound, may delineate a mass lesion. Ultrasound-guided fine needle aspirations may be diagnostic, although adenocarcinomas may not exfoliate well and a definitive diagnosis via percutaneous or surgical biopsy may be needed.

Patient care

Surgical resection, if feasible, is the treatment of choice, but the prognosis is usually grave due to local metastasis at the time of diagnosis.[8] Remission times from surgery of up to 2 years have been reported, but survival time is usually less than 6 months.[8] COX-2 expression has been documented in canine but not in feline intestinal epithelial tumors and may play a role in future therapy; standard adjunctive chemotherapy has not been demonstrated to be effective.[6,8,12–14]

Intestinal leiomyomas and leiomyosarcomas

Intestinal leiomyomas and leiomyosarcomas are connective tissue tumors that usually form a distinct mass and are primarily found in the SI and stomach of older dogs. Leiomyomas and leiomyosarcomas originate from the smooth muscle and are reportedly the most frequent mesenchymal tumors affecting the canine GI tract.[6,9]

Primary clinical signs are intestinal hemorrhage, iron deficiency anemia, melena, and obstruction. These tumors can also cause hypoglycemia as a paraneoplastic effect.[8]

Diagnosis requires identification of neoplastic cells, often at the time of surgical resection. Evaluation of ultrasound-guided fine needle aspiration may be diagnostic, but these tumors do not exfoliate as readily as many carcinomas or lymphomas. For this reason, surgical biopsy is often necessary. Surgical excision may be curative if there are no metastases. Metastases make the prognosis poor, although some animals are palliated by chemotherapy.

Inflammatory bowel disease

IBD describes a chronic, immune-mediated group of disorders of the SI and/or the LI that is distinguished by persistent, recurrent GI signs and histological evidence of intestinal inflammation. The term *IBD* can be overused and the disease may be overdiagnosed. A number of diseases are associated with chronic intestinal inflammation, and the failure to eliminate other causes of mucosal inflammation coupled with the difficulties in the interpretation of histopathologic specimens exacerbates the problem. The etiology of IBD is unknown, hence the term idiopathic, but environmental, genetic, and immune factors may play a role in the disease process. Histological variation in the appearance of the inflammation suggests that idiopathic IBD is not a single disease but a group of disorders. The terminology used reflects the predominant cell type of inflammation present and the affected location in the GI tract. The most common form of IBD is LPE, followed by eosinophilic gastroenteritis (EGE) and the rarer forms, granulomatous enteritis and neutrophilic infiltration.[2,6,8,15]

Manifestations of inflammatory bowel disease

LPE is the most common manifestation of intestinal inflammation.[8] Mucosal infiltration of lymphocytes and plasma cells coupled with architectural changes characterizes the inflammation on histopathology. German shepherds, shar-peis, and purebred cats may be predisposed to LPE, and the basenji and Ludenhund have a severe, hereditary form of LPE (basenji enteropathy and diarrheal syndrome in Ludenhund). LPE is most often seen in older animals but has rarely been reported in younger animals.

The second most common form of idiopathic IBD is eosinophilic enteritis (EE). Architectural changes coupled with mucosal infiltration of eosinophils on histopathology characterize the inflammation. There is no age predilection for EE but Dobermans, rottweilers and German shepherds may be overrepresented.

Granulomatous enteritis is uncommon and is characterized by mucosal infiltration of macrophages resulting in the formation of granulomas. It has been suggested that intracellular bacterial infection similar to the attaching and invading *Escherichia coli* seen in the histiocytic ulcerative colitis of boxers may underlie these conditions.[8]

Proliferative enteritis is a rare inflammatory enteritis characterized by segmental mucosal hypertrophy of the intestine. An underlying infectious etiology has been suggested (e.g., *Lawsonia intracellularis*, *Campylobacter* spp., and *Chlamydophila*).[8]

Clinical signs

Idiopathic IBD typically presents as persistent or reoccurring vomiting and diarrhea in dogs and in cats, but an individual case may present with other GI signs (e.g., appetite changes, lethargy, weight loss, abdominal pain) (see Table 8.3.2). Clinical signs may be constant or they may wax and wane, with or without a precipitating reason. In general, the clinical signs are associated with the affected region of the GI tract. Patients with inflammation in the gastric region or upper SI commonly present with vomiting as the predominate sign. This is especially true in cats. Diarrhea may be the result of large intestinal inflammation or chronic SI inflammation. Anorexia is typically thought of as the predominant change in appetite (possibly due to inflammation), although polyphagia may be present in the patient with weight loss. Changes in appetite may not even be reported in milder cases of IBD. Postprandial pain may be present in some patients and may need to be managed, even without any other clinical signs.[8,16,17] Hematemesis, hematochezia, or melena may be associated with more severe inflammation and/or EGE. Severe, chronic disease may also be associated with weight loss and PLE.

Taking a thorough history is the crucial first step in the diagnostic process as sometimes, an obvious precipitating event (e.g., stress, dietary change) is uncovered. Educating owners on the use of a pet diary may be helpful in discovering these events and will also prove useful in monitoring a response to therapy.

Etiology

The etiology of small animal IBD remains unknown, even with the extensive research in the human analogues of Crohn's disease and ulcerative colitis. Suggested factors include environmental (e.g., drugs, diet, altered flora in the gut), genetic (i.e., shown to be an issue in human disease), and immune response. The altered immune response may include such factors as the response to antigens formed by the microflora of the gut during the digestive process and a disruption in the mucosal barrier.

Diagnostics

The diagnosis of idiopathic IBD is made by ruling out all other etiologies (e.g., parasitic, infectious, diet-responsive, and

Table 8.3.2 Inflammatory bowel disease signs

Vomiting
- Bile
- Food
- Cats—with or without hair
- Dogs—with or without grass
- Hematemesis

Small intestinal-type diarrhea
- Large volume
- Watery
- Melena

Large intestinal-type diarrhea
- Hematochezia
- Mucoid
- Frequency
- Tenesmus

Thickened bowel loops

Abdominal discomfort/abdominal pain

Excessive borborygmus and flatulence

Weight loss

Alterations in appetite
- Polyphagia
- Decreased appetite/anorexia
- Eating grass
- Pica

Hypoproteinemia
- Ascites
- Subcutaneous edema
- Hydrothorax

Source: Hall EJ, German AJ. Diseases of the small intestine. In: *Textbook of Veterinary Internal Medicine*, 7th edition, eds. SJ Ettinger, EC Feldman, pp. 1526–1572. St. Louis, MO: Elsevier; Hall EJ, German AJ. Inflammatory bowel disease. In: *Small Animal Gastroenterology*, ed. JM Steiner, pp. 312–329. Germany: Schlutersche; 2008.

antibacterial-responsive conditions), ruling out intestinal and extraintestinal disease (e.g., tumor, pancreatitis), demonstrating intestinal inflammation on histopathology, and pairing these findings with the clinical signs. Infection that is not diagnosed remains a possibility, particularly after the identification of adhering and invading *E. coli* in histiocytic ulcerative colitis of boxers and human Crohn's disease.[8]

Clinical indices, used in human medicine, are a clinical scoring system that measures quantifiable and repeatable measures of disease. Canine and feline IBD activity indices, (CIBDAI and FIBDAI), respectively, have been developed. Six GI signs (attitude, appetite, vomiting, stool consistency, stool frequency, and weight loss) are scored on a scale of 0–3 (0 = none, 3 = severe). The composite score is used to stage the disease from clinical insignificant disease (0–3), to mild (4–5), moderate (6–8), or severe IBD (>9). The CIBDAI has been shown to correlate with

histological severity and serum concentrations of C-reactive proteins.[8] CIBDAI and FIBDAI may also be utilized to monitor response to treatment.[18–23]

Laboratory assessment of the minimum database

The diagnosis of IBD starts with the exclusion of other causes of inflammation. The minimum database should include the CBC, serum chemistries, urinalysis, and serial fecal flotation tests.

The CBC is typically within normal limits, although occasionally, neutrophilia, eosinophilia, anemia, or thrombocytopenia may be noted. No changes are typically seen on serum chemistries either, but hypocholesterolemia, hypocalcemia, and hypomagnesemia may be found, and in dogs, a mild elevation in liver enzymes may be noted. In cases of PLE, hypoalbuminemia and hypoglobulinemia are noted.[8,15,16]

Fecal examination is important to rule out parasitic causes of inflammation (e.g., hookworms, whipworms, and *Giardia*). However, even if fecal tests are negative, empirical treatment for occult *Giardia* infection is recommended in all cases.[16]

Additional laboratory diagnostics

Additional fecal tests may be indicated depending on the clinical presentation (e.g., fecal culture, acid fast stain, rectal scraping). Additional serum chemistries may also be indicated to help rule in/rule out other causes of inflammation. Both folate and cobalamin are affected by intestinal absorption and serum concentrations will reflect these alterations. Folate is absorbed in the proximal intestine and cobalamin is absorbed in the distal SI. Low blood levels of either can help to localize the inflammatory response or, if both are depressed, can indicate diffuse inflammation. However, it is important to remember that inflammation does not necessarily indicate IBD.

Other diagnostic tests that may be utilized in cases where the diagnosis is in question (e.g., poor response to therapy, discerning IBD from lymphoma), and newly emerging diagnostic tests include detection of perinuclear antineutrophilic cytoplasmic antibodies (pANCAs) or increased serum acute phase proteins (to detect inflammation), altered GI hormone concentrations, increased intestinal permeability, fecal excretion of calprotectin, immunohistochemistry or flow cytometry (to analyze immune cell subsets), reverse transcriptase polymerase chain reaction (RT-PCR) (to measure cytokine mRNA expression), and clonality testing (to distinguish lymphoma from severe IBD).

Imaging

Plain radiographs may be useful for detecting diffuse disease and to discern gross anatomical disease, but ultrasonographic examination is the superior modality for detecting focal disease, particularly in cats. Intestinal wall thickness, changes to the layers of the SI, mesenteric lymphadenopathy, and pancreatitis can all be imaged and evaluated with ultrasound. In addition, real-time guided aspirations, if indicated, are possible and may be useful in diagnosing certain conditions (e.g., lymphoma). Increased intestinal wall thickness is noted in some but not all cases of idiopathic IBD; this is particularly true in the dog.[16]

Biopsy and histopathology

Intestinal biopsy is necessary to document intestinal inflammation and to characterize the inflammatory cell type; however, the diagnosis of IBD is not made on histopathology alone. Biopsy can be accomplished with either endoscopic or surgical biopsy (laparoscopic or laparotomy). Endoscopy is the least invasive biopsy technique but has limitations both in the depth of the sample (not full thickness) and in the sampling locations (gastric, proximal duodenum or colon). Scope diameter is another limitation, being more of an issue in cats and in small dogs. Full-thickness surgical biopsy may be indicated, especially in cases with multiorgan involvement, but may be contraindicated in patients with PLE.

The gold standard for the diagnosis of intestinal inflammation is the histopathologic assessment of biopsy material. The current limitations of histopathologic interpretation of intestinal biopsies may limit the histopathologic diagnosis. One limitation is the variability in specimen quality; this may be especially true for endoscopic samples due to small sample size, instrumentation, and the skill of the operator. The experience level of the pathologist can also affect interpretation as the current set of standards (inflammation, architectural changes, increased cellularity, evidence of cellular damage) have not been universally adopted and the differentiation between normal specimens, IBD, and lymphoma can be difficult.[8,15,16]

Treatment and patient care

The treatment of IBD, regardless of cell type or location, involves therapy with a combination of dietary modification and medical management that is tailored to the severity of clinical signs and client compliance. Empirical treatment with antiparasiticides is recommended for all patients. Medical management typically begins with antibacterials and, if indicated, an immunosuppressive medication is utilized. Mild cases of IBD often respond to diet therapy and metronidazole alone, especially in cats.[8] Severe cases (where clinical signs or mucosal inflammation are severe) may require early intervention with immunosuppressives.

Patients with IBD need a highly digestible diet (decreases the intestinal antigenic load and thus may reduce mucosal inflammation) and one that meets their dietary requirements. In order to eliminate adverse food reactions, the diet should also be antigen limited and based on a single-source protein preparation.

The treatment of patients with antimicrobials is usually indicated, at least short term, except in very mild cases that may be controlled with dietary therapy alone. Metronidazole is the first choice not only for its broad spectrum anaerobic antibacterial and antiprotozoal effects but also for its inhibition on cell-mediated immunity. Other antibacterials (e.g., oxytetracycline, tylosin, trimethoprim–sulfa) may also have immunomodulatory effects and some efficacy.[8]

Immunosuppression and the control of inflammation is used in chronic and acute episodes of IBD, although due to adverse effects with long-term use, it is utilized only as a last resort. Oral glucocorticoids (e.g., prednisone and prednisolone) are the most frequently utilized. An initial dosage of 1–2 mg/kg is given orally every 12 h for 2–4 weeks and then tapered slowly over the subsequent weeks to months. If possible, patients should be weaned off of glucocorticoids and their use reserved for relapse or at least reduced to a low dose given every 48 h. Monitoring for the adverse effects of glucocorticoids is indicated, keeping in mind that feline patients tolerate long-term therapy with less adverse effects than dogs.

Other medications used in the treatment of IBD are budesonide, sulfasalazine, azathioprine, 5-aminosalicylate (mesalamine), cyclophosphamide, and cyclosporine. In addition, probiotics and prebiotics may reduce intestinal inflammation, although no canine or feline trials have been run.

Prognosis

The prognosis for idiopathic IBD has many variables and is dependent on species, degree of severity, cell type, area affected, focal or diffuse disease, and responsiveness to therapy. In addition, since the diagnosis of idiopathic IBD is a diagnosis by exclusion, it is theorized that some positive and poor outcomes are actually attributable to misdiagnosis rather than failure to respond to therapy. In general, the more severe the disease, and if concurrent pancreatic disease, hypocobaliminemia, or hypoalbuminemia are present, the poorer the response.

The health-care team must remember that clinical improvement, histological improvement, and response to therapy may not correlate.

Key nutritional factors for IBD

Water

Dehydration is a frequent problem in patients with IBD. Reduced water consumption is often aggravated by fluid losses from vomiting and/or diarrhea. Whenever possible, fluid balance should be maintained via oral consumption of fluids. However, dehydrated patients and those with persistent vomiting often need parenteral fluid administration.[24]

Electrolytes

Serum electrolyte concentrations should be assessed regularly to allow early detection of abnormalities as vomiting and diarrhea persist. A common finding in IBD patients is hypokalemia. Thus, foods containing 0.8–1.1% DM potassium are preferred for dogs and cats with IBD. Initially, potassium levels should be restored with intravenous potassium supplementation. IBD patients often lose large amounts of sodium through fluid feces; however, sodium deficits may be masked by dehydration.

Energy density and fat

When managing patients with chronic enteropathies, energy dense foods are favored. Energy dense foods allow for smaller volumes of food, which minimize GI distention and secretions. Unfortunately, energy dense foods are also high in fats. High fat foods may contribute to osmotic diarrhea and GI protein losses, further complicating IBD. Dogs and cats should begin therapy with a food with moderate energy density (4.0–4.5 kcal/g

[16.7–18.8 kJ/g] DM). The fat levels should be as follows: 12–15% DM for dogs and 15–25% DM for cats. Only if the patient can tolerate them should foods with higher fat levels be offered.[24]

Fiber-enhanced foods are typically lower in fat and thus have lower energy density levels than highly digestible foods. The DM energy density of fiber-enhanced foods for IBD should be at least 3.2 kcal/g for dog foods and at least 3.4 kcal/g for cat foods. In fiber-enhanced foods, the fat content for dogs and cats with IBD should be 8–12% and 9–18% DM, respectively. Dogs and cats with GI disease tolerate dietary fat differently. Cats in general can tolerate much higher concentrations of dietary fat than dogs.[24,25]

Protein

Fecal losses may contribute to protein malnutrition in dogs and cats with IBD. Protein sources that have a high biological value and are highly digestible (≥87%) should be used. If patients are not experiencing high protein loss, protein should be provided at levels sufficient for the appropriate life stage (at least 25% for adult dogs and 35% for adult cats [DM]).

Dietary antigens are assumed to play a role in the pathogenesis of IBD; therefore, hypoallergenic novel protein elimination foods or foods containing a protein hydrolysate are often utilized.[24,26–28] In some cases, elimination foods have been used successfully without adding pharmacological intervention.[29] If patients are managed with "hypoallergenic foods," protein levels can be lower. Ideal elimination foods should (1) avoid protein excess (16–26% for dogs and 30–45% for cats), (2) have high protein digestibility (≥87%), and (3) contain a limited number of novel protein sources to which the patient has never been exposed or contain a protein hydrolysate.[24]

Fiber

Beet pulp, soy fiber, inulin, and fructooligosaccharides (FOSs) have been confirmed by *in vitro* fermentation to generate volatile fatty acids. These fatty acids are considered beneficial in patients with IBD of the distal SI and colon.[30–32] Fermentable fibers may also serve as prebiotics, which promote the growth of beneficial bacterial organisms such as *Bifidobacterium* and *Lactobacillus*, at the expense of more pathogenic microbes such as *Desulfovibrio* and *Clostridium* spp. In commercial products, these fibers are incorporated at rates of 1–5% DM.[24]

There are several physiological characteristics in fiber that are beneficial in the management of small bowel diarrhea as increased fiber content normalizes intestinal motility, water balance, and microflora. Transit time through the small bowel can be normalized with the addition of fiber, thus slowing a hypermotile state and/or improving a hypomotile state to reestablish normal peristaltic action. Fiber also provides intraluminal stimuli, which help to reestablish the coordinated actions of hormones, neurons, smooth muscle, enzyme delivery, digestion, and absorption.[24] Finally, dietary fiber adds nondigestible bulk, which buffers toxins and holds excess water. Moderate levels (7–15% DM) of insoluble fiber (e.g., cellulose) are suggested; however, this level of fiber reduces the energy density and digestibility of a food.

Digestibility

The feeding of highly digestible (fat and digestible [soluble] carbohydrate ≥90% and protein ≥87%) foods provides a number of advantages when managing dogs and cats with IBD. Highly digestible foods are associated with reduced osmotic diarrhea (secondary to fat and carbohydrate malabsorption) and reduced intestinal gas (due to carbohydrate malabsorption), and smaller amounts of protein are absorbed intact (leading to decreased antigen loads). Furthermore, the proximal gut is able to absorb nutrients more completely from low residue foods. Foods for IBD patients should be free of lactose so as to avoid the complication of lactose intolerance. Digestibility percentages of protein, fat, and carbohydrate in fiber-enhanced foods should be at least 80, 80, and 90%, respectively.[24]

Vitamins

In patients with IBD, the intake of water-soluble and fat-soluble vitamins is critical. Typically, water-soluble vitamins have been significantly reduced or depleted by diarrheic losses and the large fluid flux through the patient.[24] Dogs and cats with chronic enteropathies may have cobalamin (vitamin B_{12}) deficiency, which can result in severe metabolic abnormalities including increased serum methylmalonic acid and disturbances in serum amino acid levels.[33] Hypocobaliminemia usually results when specific cobalamin receptors in the ileum become damaged secondary to inflammatory disease. Ongoing GI losses and a reduction in cobalamin consumption further exacerbate the deficiency. It is important to assess serum cobalamin in patients with chronic small intestinal disease, and patients found to be deficient (cobalamin level <300 ng/L) should receive weekly subcutaneous cobalamin therapy (250 µg in cats and 500 µg in dogs) for 4–6 weeks or until serum levels return to the normal range.[34] For long-term maintenance, once or twice monthly therapy may be required. Absorption of dietary folate (Vitamin B_9), which is present in foods in the polyglutamate form, may be inhibited secondary to disease of the proximal SI, including chronic inflammatory disease of the small bowel. Low values are a result of jejunal mucosal damage, reduced folate absorption, and depletion of folate stores.[24]

In patients with steatorrhea (increased fat in the stool), loss of fat-soluble vitamins may be significant (e.g., vitamin K-deficient coagulopathies may occur in patients with IBD) and parenteral administration of fat-soluble vitamins may be necessary. If a vitamin K-responsive coagulopathy is suspected, vitamin K_1 at a dosage of 0.5–1.0 mg/kg subcutaneously is recommended. The dietary intake of vitamins is often sufficient when the disease responds to treatment and fat absorption is reestablished.[24]

Zinc

In humans, zinc deficiency is a well-recognized complication of IBD as the SI is the primary site of zinc homeostasis.[35] Zinc may provide benefits by enhancing brush border enzyme activity, water and electrolyte absorption, and regeneration of the gut epithelial surface.[24] The veterinary health-care team should consider supplementing dietary zinc intake if dogs and cats with IBD are exhibiting dermatitis or poor hair coat quality.

Acute and chronic diarrhea

Diarrhea is defined as a change in the frequency, consistency, or volume of bowel movements or stools.[1] There are four major mechanisms for diarrhea; they are osmotic, altered mucosal permeability, abnormal motility, and secretory diarrhea. Under normal circumstances, absorption exceeds secretion; when this does not occur, the patient produces large volumes of fluid diarrhea, which can cause rapid dehydration.[1]

Diarrhea can present as either a small bowel disorder involving the duodenum, jejunum, and ileum or as a large bowel disorder involving the colon. Presenting signs are the easiest way to distinguish the two causes. Small bowel diarrhea typically presents as diarrhea with weight loss, poor body condition, vomiting, borborygmus, and flatulence. Large bowel diarrhea typically presents as diarrhea with mucous and blood, tenesmus, severe cramping, discomfort, and dyschezia (straining to defecate) (Table 8.3.3).[1]

Causes of diarrhea

Diarrhea can be caused by anything that disrupts the normal function of the intestinal tract, usually affecting one of the four mechanisms of action.

Osmotic diarrhea

Osmotic diarrhea is associated with retention of water within the intestine due to failure in absorption or digestion and when additional water is pulled into the intestinal tract.[1,2] This type of diarrhea can be seen with EPI, small intestinal diseases such as SIBO and viral diseases that cause villus atrophy, such as parvovirus and coronavirus. Diseases that cause severe inflammation can change the permeability of the intestinal tract, increasing hydrostatic pressure. This change in pressure can lead not only to an increase in fluid loss but can also create a PLE.[2]

Altered mucosal permeability

The intestinal tract is composed of epithelial cells, lymphatic and blood vessels, and the local immune system. When any of these fail to perform properly, the water and other nutrients typically found in the intestines are not able to pass through the intestinal wall as they normally would and diarrhea can result. Failure can result from diseases that cause erosions, ulcerations, inflammation, or infiltration of the mucosa. Causes can be NSAID or other drug uses, infectious agents (e.g., bacteria and viruses), IBD, and cancers (e.g., especially with diffuse cancer such as lymphoma).[1]

Abnormal GI motility

Abnormal motility can be seen either as an ileus, causing a "pipe effect" with little resistance to ingesta passing through the intestinal tract, or as increased peristaltic contractions pushing the ingesta through the intestinal tract prior to complete absorption of water.[1] The pipe effect can be seen secondary to infiltrative

Table 8.3.3 Acute and chronic diarrhea tables

Acute causes	Chronic causes
Dietary	Dietary
• Dietary indiscretion	• Adverse reaction to food
• Foreign bodies	• Carbohydrate intolerance in cats
• Garbage/compost toxicity	
• Contaminated raw food diets	
Infectious agents	Infectious agents
• Bacteria	• Bacteria and small intestinal bacterial overgrowth
• Parasites	• Fungi
• Rickettsia	• Parasites
• Virus	
Miscellaneous	Miscellaneous
• Hemorrhagic gastroenteritis	• Juvenile diarrhea of cats
	• Pancreatic exocrine insufficiency
Toxin or drug induced	IBD
• Chemotherapeutic agents	• Lymphoplasmacytic eosinophilic, lymphocytic, suppurative gastroenteritis/enteritis
• Laxatives	
• NSAIDs in dogs	
	Neoplasia
	• Lymphosarcoma
	• Mast cell tumor

Source: Davenport DJ, Remillard RL, Carroll M. Large bowel diarrhea: colitis. In: *Small Animal Clinical Nutrition*, 5th edition, eds. MS Hand, CD Thatcher, RL Remilliard, P Roudebush, BJ Novotny, pp. 1101–1107. Marceline, MO: Walsworth Publishing; 2010.

disease (e.g., IBD), severe abdominal pain, parvoviral enteritis, or postoperative due to ileus from anesthesia or analgesia. Increased peristaltic contractions can be seen with IBD. A change in intestinal motility can also predispose the patient to developing SIBO.[1]

Secretory diarrhea

Secretory diarrhea is relatively uncommon in dogs and cats compared to people and food animals. Crypt epithelial cells lining the intestinal tract produce intestinal fluid, while enterocytes lining the villous tips are responsible for absorption of nutrients and water. Factors that can affect the production of intestinal fluid are hormones within the body, bacterial enterotoxins, certain medications, deconjugated bile acids (i.e., those that have not be "conjugated" with albumin in the liver), and hydroxy fatty acids (such as butyric acid and acetic acid).[1] In people, this type of diarrhea is typically seen with bacterial and viral infections such as cholera, dysentery, and salmonella infections.[1]

Acute versus chronic diarrhea

Acute diarrhea is usually caused by diet, parasites, or infectious diseases (e.g., *Salmonella* or *E. coli*). Chronic diarrhea is more commonly caused by maldigestion of nutrients (e.g., EPI), non-protein-losing malabsorption and protein-losing malabsorption.

Differentiation between non-protein-losing and protein-losing enteropathies is determined by evaluating the plasma albumin levels. In non-protein-losing disease, plasma albumin levels will be within normal limits. In patients with protein-losing diseases with normal hepatic and renal function, plasma albumin levels are ≤2.0–2.2 g/dL.[1]

Acute cases of diarrhea may be a component of a chronic disease, meaning the signs started and presented as an acute disease, but the causative disease has been present for a long period of time, as seen with parasitic infections.

There are no definitive time limits assigned to acute or chronic diarrhea, though generally, acute diarrhea is seen as a disease that has a length of symptoms usually less than 7–14 days, while chronic diarrhea is often measured in weeks to months.[3]

Diagnostics

Obviously, not all causes of diarrhea will be responsive to dietary manipulation, but nutrition is still important for all animals presenting with diarrhea. The most important step in the diagnosis and treatment of both acute and chronic diarrhea is a complete physical exam and history, playing close attention to the number, characteristics, and frequency of defecations seen by the owner. BCS and weight also need to be evaluated. Large-volume, fluid stools are more typical of small bowel diarrhea. Bloody or tarry stools could indicate a potentially life-threatening condition such as intestinal bleeding or an ulcer.[4]

Careful attention should be paid to the dietary history as diet-induced diarrhea is one of the most common etiologies seen in dogs and cats. This can include recent diet changes to a moist, high fat or meat-based diet, as well as feeding table scraps, and access to garbage, dead animals, or abrasive materials. Cats that hunt can also be exposed to salmonella from the birds they eat.[4]

Husbandry issues also need to be evaluated. Vaccination and anthelmintic administration records should be reviewed to see if they are current. The health of other pets and people in the house should be questioned. A positive answer to any of these questions would increase the likelihood of the involvement of an infectious organism as opposed to dietary indiscretion.[4]

Determining the laboratory tests that would be most helpful in diagnosing the cause of the diarrhea is dependent on the presenting signs. It is important to determine if the condition is self-limiting, as with dietary indiscretion, or life threatening, as with parvoviral infection. Signs consistent with a life-threatening problem would include abdominal pain, dehydration, depression, fever, and red and white blood cells in the stool.[1] Initial diagnostics often include assessment of dehydration through a PCV and TS and fecal examination for parasites and bacteria not commonly seen in the stool.[4] Centrifugation of fecal flotation samples is the preferred method for the detection of parasitic ova. A dried and stained fecal smear is required for the assessment of bacterial populations. If the veterinarian suspects a pancreatic enzyme deficiency, a 12-h fasted serum sample should be collected to evaluate the TLI (trypsin-like immunoassay). B_{12} (cobalamin) and B_6 (folate) levels are commonly run with TLI to evaluate GI bacterial populations and whether they are in adequate numbers to produce these vitamins normally. These tests, while not giving an assessment of the EPI, do indicate overall GI health. Serum chemistry can be used to evaluate other organ dysfunctions that may be present.

Radiographs of the intestinal tract are usually unrewarding, unless there is a suspicion for intestinal foreign body. Mucosal changes do not produce significant radiographic changes, and the presence of ileus and air within the intestines is nonspecific. Ultrasound can be more helpful as the individual layers of the intestinal walls may be evaluated to determine if they are within normal limits. This can help to rule in or rule out inflammatory conditions where wall thickness changes can occur. Unfortunately, ultrasound is not able to identify what is causing these changes but may be helpful in pinpointing what area is affected. Endoscopic (partial thickness) or surgical biopsies (full thickness) may be required to thoroughly evaluate the changes that are occurring in the intestines (Figure 8.3.2).

Patient care

In general, the more of the clinical signs that are present, the more aggressive the therapy that will be required. If a history of dietary indiscretion is uncovered and the patient is still eating and is not clinically dehydrated, usually time will take care of the irritation causing the diarrhea. Switching the animal to a highly digestible, low residue food for 5–7 days may help the inflamed intestinal tract absorb the nutrients in the food while the healing process is ongoing.

Typically, the digestibility of an intestinal diet should be >87% overall, with >87% digestibility for protein content and >90% digestibility for the fat and carbohydrate content. If using a fiber-enhanced diet, overall digestibility will be affected. Digestibility

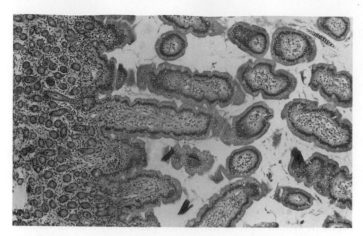

Figure 8.3.2 Histopathologic image of normal intestinal villi via endoscopy. Image courtesy of Dr. Barb Powers, Colorado State University.

should be no lower than 80% for protein and fat, while the digestibility of carbohydrates remains the same (at least 90%).[4]

Sometimes, a secondary bacterial or fungal infection (e.g., compost gut) will develop because of the dietary indiscretion. A fecal culture is required to identify either bacterial or fungal infections. Since the intestinal tract is already populated with bacteria and fungi, identifying causative pathogens is difficult and often unrewarding. Cases of suspected bacteria or fungal infection should be empirically treated with the appropriate antibiotics or antifungals if cultures are not pursued. This type of diarrhea may not clear up on just dietary manipulation and medical therapy will be needed for full recovery.

Food poisoning, secondary to bacterial infection, can be life threatening. Food poisoning is not always the result of dietary indiscretion. The feeding of raw food diets can introduce bacteria into the intestinal tract. There have been documented cases of both animals and humans dying because of food poisoning.[5] The bacterial infection, as well as potential endotoxins, needs to be treated. The introduction of a highly digestible bland diet is also indicated. The addition of probiotics may also be beneficial in reestablishing the proper bacterial population in the SIs.

Obviously, foreign body obstruction will not be responsive to dietary manipulation. Radiographs and abdominal ultrasound offer some help in locating foreign bodies, but unfortunately, not all foreign bodies show up on abdominal radiographs. Sometimes, endoscopic or surgical identification and removal may be the only option. The reintroduction of a highly digestible diet following surgery is essential for tissue healing and to restore positive nitrogen balance.[4] While we cannot always predict what objects an animal will eat, limiting their access to foreign bodies is always a good suggestion, especially with the more oral breeds (e.g., retrievers) and with animals who are "repeat offenders." The judicious use of a basket muzzle may be needed.

Dietary sensitivity can be caused either by a true food allergy (rarely) or by food sensitivity. There is no breed, age, or sex predisposition to either condition. The problem can occur at any time and without a change in food. Dermatologic signs are com-

monly seen, but GI signs can appear on their own or in conjunction with skin changes.[2] Intestinal changes are reversible with appropriate treatment and removal of the inciting food item. Normal intestinal function can return in approximately 6–8 weeks. Dietary changes include switching to a novel protein diet or to a modified protein diet, such as the hydrolyzed protein diets. When using novel or modified protein diets, it is important to offer a diet that the animal has not been exposed to before, and this would include foods given as treats and table foods.

While not actually a dietary sensitivity, some cats are carbohydrate intolerant and will develop a diarrhea from high carbohydrate diets; a low carbohydrate diet often will resolve the problem. The lower the level of carbohydrates, the better, and there are some foods with as low as 15% carbohydrates available. To find a low carbohydrate diet, look for ones that are high in protein and moderate to high in fats.

While intestinal cancers are not responsive to dietary manipulation (with the exception of high levels of fish oils in some forms of lymphoma), the inclusion of a high quality diet will aid the patient in healing, responding to the chemotherapeutic agents, and will ensure adequate nutrients in a form the body can utilize.[1]

Medications

Anti-inflammatory and immunosuppressive drugs (e.g., corticosteroids, cyclophosphamide, azathioprine, chlorambucil) are commonly used in the treatment of intestinal diseases that cause diarrhea. In patients with SIBO, antibiotics (metronidazole, tetracycline, tylosin, or sulfasalazine) are used concurrently with anti-inflammatory and diet therapy to improve the overall treatment effectiveness.[6]

Corticosteroids (prednisone, prednisolone, and budesonide)

The efficacy of corticosteroids in the management of intestinal disease relates primarily to their anti-inflammatory and immunosuppressive properties; appetite stimulation is a secondary benefit. In cases of chronic administration, the dose should be slowly decreased over 4–6 months. Relapses can occur if the dose reduction occurs too quickly and sometimes are so severe that corticosteroids alone can no longer control the signs associated with a relapse of the disease. In these situations, stronger immunosuppressive agents, such as azathioprine, cyclophosphamide, or cyclosporine may need to be added.[6]

It is ideal that steroids not be given without a definitive pathological diagnosis. Changes in the intestines that can obscure diagnosis can occur even with a short course of use and will render endoscopic biopsies possibly nondiagnostic.

Antibiotics: metronidazole, tetracycline, tylosin

Metronidazole, tetracycline, and tylosin are antibiotics that can be used alone, in combination, or in conjunction with the anti-inflammatory/immunosuppressive agents. Metronidazole can cause nausea, anorexia, and, occasionally, vomiting and diarrhea. Hepatic and encephalopathic problems can occur in sensitive animals or when doses are too high. Metronidazole is also very bitter tasting. If the animal does not swallow the pill the first time, considerable drooling can occur. This can cause the pill to dissolve too quickly, preventing redosing with the same pill. Except for the hepatic problems, the side effects of tetracycline and tylosin are similar to those of metronidazole.[6]

Acid Neutralizers

Gastric reflux, esophagitis, and gastritis can commonly occur secondary to chronic gastric or intestinal inflammation. This increased acidity can also exacerbate inflammation in the duodenum.[1] Famotidine and cimetidine are useful in cases of severe GI inflammation, gastric reflux, and esophagitis. Both are readily available over-the-counter. Cimetidine must be administered more frequently in dogs and in cats than in humans. Ranitidine also provides gastric motility actions in cats; this has not been evaluated in dogs.[6]

Role of the veterinary technician and client education

Most, if not all, of the care for a patient with diarrhea can and should be provided by the veterinary technician. Ensuring that our patients remain clean, dry, and comfortable and that they are in a positive nutritional status is equally important for their long-term recovery.

Technicians are also important in client education. Many times, this is not "simple diarrhea." Ensuring that the clients understand the pathophysiology of the disease as well as the goal of treatment recommendations will help increase client compliance and, ultimately, patient outcome.

Key nutritional factors in patients with small bowel diarrhea

Protein manipulation

Protein quality determines the availability of the various amino acids for utilization by the body. The highest quality protein is egg with a biological value of 100; all other proteins are compared to this. Protein quality is determined by the amino acid that is found in the lowest quantity and this is termed the limiting amino acid (see Table 8.3.4).

Every species has a different essential amino acid profile. Cats, as obligate carnivores, have a larger amino acid profile and have a higher protein requirement than do dogs.[4,7] Due to cats' amino acid and fatty acid requirements, they must have a meat-based source of protein in their diets.[4,7]

Protein energy malnutrition can occur when feeding a diet that is inappropriate for the age or disease state of the animal. This can be seen when a cat is fed a canine diet, when a pregnant or nursing animal is fed a maintenance diet, or when a restricted protein diet is fed during a disease state requiring increased protein intake.

Fatty acid manipulation

Fats are classified by their physical state of matter while at room temperature and by the location of the first set of double bonds that occur within the molecule. Lipids are a solid at room temperature, and fats are a liquid at room temperature. The double

Table 8.3.4 Protein energy source comparison

Protein type	Biological value	Percentage of protein (%)	Protein quality
Egg	94	45–49	Excellent
Casein	80	80	Good
Beef, lamb, pork, chicken	74	29	Good
Soybean meal	73	48	Good
Rice (white)	64	7	Adequate
Collagen	0	88	Poor

Source: Gross KL, Jewell DE, Yamka RM, et al. Macronutrients. In: *Small Animal Clinical Nutrition*, 5th edition, eds. MS Hand, CD Thatcher, RL Remilliard, P Roudebush, BJ Novotny, pp. 49–104. Marceline, MO: Walsworth Publishing; 2010.

bonds are located at the terminal or omega end of the molecule and are given an "n" designation within the molecule. The main fatty acid families include the n-3, n-6, and n-9 fatty acids. In common usage, the "n" is replaced with the term "omega," hence the common classification of omega-3, omega-6, and omega-9 fatty acids. The n-3 and n-6 fatty acids are essential fatty acids (EFAs) because they cannot be synthesized from other fats in the animal. The n-9 fatty acids can be synthesized in the body from the n-3 and n-6 fatty acids. Fats elongate during digestion rather than breaking down during digestion, so the longer fatty acids are easier for the body to produce than the shorter ones. Fatty acids also cannot be converted from one family to another.[8,9]

Increasing the amount of n-3 fatty acids found in the diet, specifically eicosapentaenoic acid (EPA) and docosahexaenoic acid (DHA), has been found to help decrease the inflammatory responses of the animal. The n-6 EFAs are seen as proinflammatory, and by increasing the amount of n-3 in a diet, the n-6's have less space available to exert their negative effects.[8,9]

Altered n-3:n-6 fatty acid ratios can be found in many of the commercially available intestinal and critical care diets. By adjusting the fatty acid ratios in the foods rather than adding supplements, the animal receives the correct EFAs and has better absorption of these nutrients.[8]

Fiber manipulation

Dietary fibers predominately affect the large bowel, though they can also affect gastric, small intestinal, and pancreatic structure and function. Fibers in diets are responsible for modifying gastric emptying time, ensuring normal intestinal motility and intestinal transport time, buffering toxins, binding and holding excess water within the intestinal tract, supporting the growth of normal intestinal bacterial flora, buffering gastric acidity after transport into the intestinal tract, altering the viscosity of the intestinal contents, and adding nondigestible bulk to the diet.[10,11]

Carbohydrates and fibers can be divided into three classes depending on their digestibility in dogs and in cats. There are highly fermentable fibers, such as guar gum and pectin, which can aggravate diarrhea by increasing the osmolality within the intestinal tract. This can cause additional fluid to be pulled into the intestinal lumen. These carbohydrates can be found in some of the canned and saucy foods.[10,11]

Moderately fermentable fibers, though not actually digested well by the animal, can be broken down by the intestinal bacterial flora into short-chain fatty acids (SCFAs), such as butyric acid and acetic acid. Butyric acid is a significant energy source for the enterocytes lining the intestinal tract. One class of moderately fermentable fibers that has received much attention is the fructooligosaccharides (FOSs). These fibers not only provide energy for the enterocytes but they can also exert a "prebiotic" effect on the bacterial flora. This prebiotic effect selects for the presence of certain bacteria over others, helping to maintain an optimal bacterial population within the gut. Pea fiber, beet pulp, and oat fiber are examples of moderately fermentable fibers.[10,11]

Nonfermentable or slowly fermentable fibers are typically added to foods to dilute calories and to provide bulk. Cellulose, peanut hulls, and soybean hulls are examples of nonfermentable fibers. Though these fibers are not very water soluble, they do have significant water-holding capacity and can be useful in some fiber-responsive diarrheas.[10,11]

Many diets contain a combination of these fiber sources to provide the best of each, without the problems associated with the use of a single fiber source. Other diets may contain minimal fiber sources to increase digestibility and to decrease stool volume.

Digestibility

The term "highly digestible" does not have a regulatory definition, but the term is generally used to describe a diet that has protein digestibility of ≥87%, and fat and carbohydrate digestibility of ≥90%. Veterinary therapeutic diets formulated for patients with intestinal disease usually contain meat and carbohydrate sources that have been highly refined to increase digestibility.[4,11] The digestibility of diets fed to patients with intestinal disease should be higher than normal because digestion and the absorption of nutrients are often compromised. Additionally, since tissue damage and immune function may be side effects of the disease process, the use of high quality nutrients is even more important.[4,11]

Digestibility can be found in the product reference guide for most therapeutic diets. If this information is not available, call the client service representative for additional help. If a feeding trial has not been done on the food, digestibility information will not be available.

Probiotics

Probiotics are a class of supplements that can be used in animals with diarrhea. Probiotics are typically live bacteria or yeast that are beneficial to the animal. Probiotics may be recommended after a course of antibiotics to allow the gut microflora to reestablish healthy numbers of beneficial bacteria (rather than allowing the "bad" bacteria to flourish). Problems that stress the immune system may also affect the bacterial numbers in the intestines and may benefit from a course of probiotics. One of the primary problems with probiotics is getting live organisms past the gastric acids. Most, but definitely not all, bacteria are killed by the high acidity found in the stomach.

When using probiotics on a patient, ensure that the product has been evaluated in animals; ascertain if significant numbers of the bacteria have been documented to survive the stomach's high acidity and if they will grow in the host animal. There are a number of veterinary products available that meet these criteria. While there are usually no problems associated with administering probiotics, they are an expensive source of protein if the bacteria do not survive.

Lymphoma versus severe IBD in cats

Occasionally, the clinician is unable to distinguish between well-differentiated lymphosarcoma and severe IBD despite excellent biopsies and competent histological evaluation. For these patients, aggressive medical treatment protocols should be tried, including prednisolone, metronidazole, chlorambucil, and dietary manipulation. Chlorambucil should probably be initiated at the same time as the prednisolone so as to avoid acquired chemotherapy resistance in lymphosarcoma, which occurs with prednisolone therapy alone.[12]

Conclusion

The therapy of choice for treating a patient with diarrhea is dependent on a number of conditions. By performing a complete physical exam, gathering a good diet history and conducting all appropriate laboratory tests, the veterinary health-care team can better define the right treatment plan for each patient.

Infectious diarrhea

Canine parvoviral enteritis

Canine parvovirus (CPV) is a small, nonenveloped DNA virus that is highly resistant in the environment. There are two types of parvoviruses that infect dogs. Canine parvovirus-1 (CPV-1) is a somewhat nonpathogenic virus that may be associated with gastroenteritis, pneumonitis, and/or myocarditis in puppies 1–3 weeks of age. Canine parvovirus-2 (CPV-2) is responsible for classic parvoviral enteritis. CPV-2 usually causes clinical signs 5–12 days after the dog is infected via the fecal–oral route. CPV-2 preferentially invades and destroys rapidly dividing cells (e.g., bone marrow progenitors, intestinal crypt epithelium).[13,14]

The virus has mutated since it was first recognized, and the most recently recognized mutation, CPV-2b, may be more pathogenic in some dogs. CPV-2b and the even more recently identified CPV-2c can also infect cats. The clinical signs are dependent upon the virulence of the virus, the size of the inoculum, the patient's defenses, the age of the patient, and the presence of other enteric pathogens (e.g., parasites). Doberman pinschers, rottweilers, pit bulls, Labrador retrievers, and German shepherds may be more susceptible to parvoviral infection than other breeds. Viral destruction of intestinal crypts may produce villus collapse, diarrhea, vomiting, and intestinal bleeding, leading to bacterial invasion; however, some animals may have mild or even subclinical disease. Many dogs are initially presented because of depression, anorexia, and/or vomiting (which can resemble foreign object ingestion) without diarrhea. Diarrhea is often absent for the first 24–48 h of illness and when diarrhea does occur, it may or may not be bloody. Secondary to inflammation, intestinal protein loss may be present, causing hypoalbuminemia. Vomiting is prominent and the severity may cause esophagitis and dehydration. Transient or prolonged neutropenia may be present due to damage to bone marrow progenitors, thus making the animal susceptible to serious bacterial infection. This is especially true if the damaged intestinal tract allows bacteria access to the body (via bacterial translocation through the GI wall). Fever and septic shock (i.e., SIRS) are common in severely ill dogs but are often absent in less severely affected animals. It is important to note that puppies infected *in utero* or before 8 weeks of age may develop myocarditis.

Diagnostic testing

Diagnosis is often tentatively made on the basis of a complete history and physical examination. Neutropenia is suggestive but is neither sensitive nor specific for CPV enteritis since salmonellosis or any overwhelming infection can cause similar changes in the CBC. Regardless of whether diarrhea occurs, infected dogs shed large numbers of viral particles in the feces (i.e., >10^9 particles/g). Therefore, ELISA for CPV-2 in the feces is the best diagnostic test although vaccination with a modified live parvoviral vaccine may cause a weak positive result for 5–15 days after vaccination. It is important to remember that the ELISA result may be negative if the assay is performed early in the clinical course of the disease; this test should be repeated in dogs that seem likely to have parvoviral enteritis but that initially have negative findings. Shedding decreases rapidly and may be undetectable 10–14 days after infection. The real benefit to testing is that either a presumptive diagnosis of parvoviral enteritis is confirmed or other diseases that can mimic parvovirus but require different therapy (e.g., salmonellosis, intussusception) must be considered.[14–16]

Electron microscopic evaluation of feces detects the presence of the virus, but CPV-1 (which is usually nonpathogenic except perhaps in neonates) is morphologically indistinguishable from CPV-2. Definitive diagnosis requires demonstration of CPV-2 virus or viral antigens either in feces or in tissues (e.g., intestine, tongue) postmortem.[15] Also on necropsy, intestinal biopsy will demonstrate typical histological lesions (i.e., crypt necrosis).

Patient care

Fundamentally, the treatment of canine parvoviral enteritis is similar to any severe, acute, infectious enteritis. Fluid and electrolyte therapy is crucial and is typically combined with antibiotics. With appropriate care of sufficient duration, the outcome is usually positive. However, very young puppies, dogs in severe septic shock and certain breeds may have a more guarded prognosis. Common treatment problems include inadequate fluid therapy (common), overzealous fluid administration (especially in dogs with severe hypoproteinemia), failure to administer glucose to hypoglycemic patients, failure to supplement adequate potassium, unrecognized sepsis, and unsuspected concurrent GI disease (e.g., parasites, intussusception). Close attention and monitoring of the patient to avoid these pitfalls can favorably affect the prognosis and outcome.

It is beneficial to administer plasma if the serum albumin concentration is less than 2.0 g/dL. Colloids such as hetastarch may be substituted for plasma; however, they usually do not contain antibodies that might be beneficial. Antibiotic therapy is warranted if there is evidence of infection (e.g., fever, septic shock) or if the patient is at risk of infection (i.e., severe neutropenia). It is reasonable to administer a first-generation cephalosporin if the animal is neutropenic but afebrile. If the animal is in septic shock (i.e., SIRS), then an antibiotic combination with a broad spectrum aerobic and anaerobic spectrum is recommended (e.g., ticaricillin or ampicillin plus amikacin or enrofloxacin). Aminoglycosides should be avoided until the patient is rehydrated and renal perfusion is reestablished. Remember to use caution when administering enrofloxacin to young, large breed dogs as cartilage damage may occur. Severe vomiting complicates therapy and may require administration of antiemetics such as dolasetron, ondansetron, or maropitant. If esophagitis occurs, H_2-receptor antagonists may be useful.

Feeding small amounts of liquid diet via an NE tube appears to help the intestines to heal more rapidly. Care must be exercised if placing an NE tube in a puppy that is still vomiting as the tube can be vomited up from the esophagus and can end up in the trachea. A bland diet may be fed once vomiting has ceased for 18–24 h. Parenteral nutrition can be lifesaving for patients that are not able to keep food down via the oral route or for patients unable to accept any enteral nutrition. PPN is an easier option for many situations as the nutrition can be administered through a peripheral catheter and acts as fluid resuscitation as well.

In order to minimize the spread of parvoviral enteritis, both veterinary personnel and the pet owner need to understand the modes of transmission of the disease: (1) Parvovirus persists for long periods of time (i.e., months) in the environment, making it difficult to prevent exposure; (2) asymptomatic dogs may shed virulent CPV-2; (3) maternal immunity sufficient to inactivate vaccine virus may be present in some puppies; and (4) dilute bleach (1 : 32) is one of the few readily available disinfectants that kills the virus, but it can take 10 min to achieve effectiveness. Client education on the severity and contagiousness of parvovirus should be provided. The home environment should be cleaned and disinfected prior to discharge of the animal from the hospital, and the owners should be encouraged to be conscientious about the disposal of feces. At home, the animal should be isolated from other susceptible animals for 2–4 weeks following discharge.

Vaccination of puppies should begin at 6–8 weeks of age. The antigen density and immunogenicity of the vaccine as well as the amount of antibody transferred from the bitch determine when the pup can be successfully immunized. Inactivated vaccines generally are not as successful as attenuated vaccines, and giving a series of these vaccinations is typically best for the patient. In general, attenuated vaccines appear more successful in producing a long-lasting immunity. When the immune status of the pup is unknown, it is recommended to administer three doses of an attenuated vaccine, 3–4 weeks apart between 6 and 16 weeks of age. If a vaccination needs to be administered prior to 5–6 weeks of age, an inactivated vaccine is safer. All puppies should be revaccinated 1 year later, then at intervals of 3 years.[13–15] Regardless of the vaccine used, there appears to be a 2- to 3-week window during which the puppy is susceptible to parvovirus infection and yet cannot be successfully immunized. Adults that were previously not vaccinated usually receive two doses 3–4 weeks apart.

There is no strong evidence that parvoviral vaccination should be given separately from modified live canine distemper vaccinations. However, modified live vaccinations should not be administered to patients younger than 5 weeks of age or those suspected of incubating or being affected with distemper. If parvoviral enteritis develops in one dog in a multiple-dog household, it is practical to administer booster vaccinations to the other dogs. However, in this instance, the vaccination of preference is an inactivated vaccine in case the other dogs are incubating the infection at the time of immunization. The client must be educated to keep a new puppy elsewhere if bringing this puppy into a house with a dog that has recently had parvoviral enteritis. See canine vaccination recommendations in Chapter 12 for more information.

CPV is a serious disease, but dogs that are treated in a timely fashion with proper therapy typically survive, especially if they survive the first 4 days of clinical signs. Dogs that have recovered from CPV-2 enteritis develop long-lived immunity of at least 20 months and potentially lifelong. Whether immunization against CPV-1 will be needed is unknown.

Feline parvoviral enteritis

Feline parvoviral enteritis, more commonly known as feline distemper or feline panleukopenia, is caused by feline panleukopenia virus (FPV), which is distinct from CVP-2b. FPV is a very stable virus without an envelope that has the ability to survive in the environment for up to a year. However, CPV-2a, CPV-2b, and CPV-2c can infect cats and cause disease.[13,14]

Many infected cats never demonstrate any clinical signs of the disease. The virus is shed in the feces for up to 6 weeks postinfection. The virus typically spreads from the tonsils to other lymphoid tissues, then to the bone marrow, and to intestinal crypt cells. Clinical signs in affected cats are usually similar to those described for dogs with parvoviral enteritis. Kittens affected *in utero* may develop cerebellar hypoplasia.[15]

Diagnostic testing

Diagnosis of feline parvovirus enteritis is similar to that as described for CPV. The ELISA test for fecal canine CPV is also a good test for feline parvovirus. However, it is important to note that the test may be positive for only 1–2 days after infection, and by the time the cat is clinically ill, this test may not be able to detect viral shedding in the feces. A presumptive diagnosis can be made based on clinical signs and a severe leukopenia (50–3000 leukocytes/mL).

Patient care

Cats with parvoviral infection are treated in much the same way as described for dogs with the disease. Supportive therapy with parenteral fluid therapy is a must when treating FPV. A major difference between dogs and cats centers on immunization: Parvoviral vaccine seems to engender a better protective response in cats than in dogs. However, kittens younger than 4 weeks of age should not be vaccinated with modified live virus vaccines or risk the occurrence of cerebellar hypoplasia. The vaccine cannot be administered orally, but intranasal administration has been found to be effective. See feline vaccination recommendations in Chapter 12 for more information.

As with dogs, many affected cats live with aggressive supportive care and if overwhelming sepsis is prevented.

Canine coronaviral enteritis

Canine coronaviral enteritis occurs when coronavirus invades and destroys mature cells on the intestinal villi, causing diarrhea and, occasionally, vomiting. Because the intestinal crypts remain intact, villi are able to regenerate more quickly in dogs with coronaviral enteritis than in dogs with parvoviral enteritis. A distinguishing feature of canine coronaviral enteritis is that bone marrow cells are not affected.

Usually, coronaviral enteritis is not as severe as classic parvoviral enteritis; it rarely causes hemorrhagic diarrhea, septicemia, or death. Dogs of any age may be infected. Typically, clinical signs are seen for less than 1 to 1½ weeks. It is important to remember that any small or very young dog may die as a result of dehydration or electrolyte abnormalities caused by diarrhea; therefore, evaluation and treatment, if indicated, is important. Dual infections with parvovirus and coronavirus may produce a high incidence of morbidity and mortality.

Diagnostic testing

Canine coronaviral enteritis is usually much less severe than many other enteritises. Thus, it is seldom definitively diagnosed. Most dogs are treated symptomatically for acute enteritis until they improve. Electron microscopic examination of feces obtained early in the course of the disease can be diagnostic. However, this virus is fragile and easily disrupted by inappropriate handling of the feces. A history of contagion and the elimination of other causes are reasons to suspect canine coronaviral enteritis.

Patient care

Fluid therapy, motility modifiers, and time should resolve most cases of coronaviral enteritis. Symptomatic therapy is usually successful except, perhaps, for very young animals. A vaccination is available, but the value of this vaccination is uncertain, except perhaps in animals at high risk of infection (e.g., those in infected kennels or dog shows).

The prognosis for recovery in an animal suffering from canine coronaviral enteritis is usually good.

Feline coronaviral enteritis

Infections in adults are often asymptomatic, whereas kittens may have mild, transient diarrhea and fever. Deaths are rare, and the prognosis for recovery is excellent. This disease is important because affected animals seroconvert and may become positive on feline infectious peritonitis serologic analysis. It is theorized that mutation by the feline coronavirus may be the cause of feline infectious peritonitis. Testing is done through PCR evaluating titers. However, a positive titer only indicates exposure to coronavirus and may not necessarily indicate actual disease.

Feline leukemia virus: associated panleukopenia

FeLV-associated panleukopenia (myeloblastopenia) may be caused by coinfection with FeLV and FPV.[13] Histological comparison of the intestinal lesions of myeloblastopenia resembles the lesions produced by feline parvovirus. However, the bone marrow and lymph nodes are not consistently affected as they are in cats with parvoviral enteritis.

Owners will present their cats with signs of chronic weight loss, vomiting, and diarrhea (often characteristic of large bowel disease). Anemia is also commonly noted in affected cats.

Diagnostic testing

Finding FeLV infection in a cat with chronic diarrhea is suggestive of the disease. Neutropenia and anemia is typically noted on the CBC of these cats. Histological lesions of FPV in a cat with FeLV are definitive for diagnosis.

Patient care

Symptomatic therapy involves fluid/electrolyte therapy, antibiotics, antiemetics, and highly digestible bland diets. Elimination of other problems that compromise the intestines (e.g., parasites, poor diet) may be beneficial.

Unfortunately, this disease has a poor prognosis due to other FeLV-related complications.

Feline immunodeficiency virus: associated diarrhea

FIV may be associated with severe, purulent colitis. The pathogenesis is unclear and may involve multiple mechanisms.

Severe large bowel disease is common and can occasionally result in colonic rupture. These cats will present with the appearance of being very ill, whereas most cats with chronic large bowel disease caused by IBD or dietary intolerance seemingly feel fine. The severe purulent colitis in conjunction with the detection of antibodies to FIV allows for a presumptive diagnosis.

Therapy is supportive and includes fluids/electrolytes, antiemetics, antibiotics, and/or highly digestible bland diets. The long-term prognosis is very poor, although some cats can be maintained for months.

Bacterial diseases

The following bacterial diseases all have certain aspects in common. It is important to remember that the bacteria discussed below may be found in the feces of clinically normal dogs and cats. Demonstrating the bacteria, or the toxin produced by the bacteria, in the patient's feces is insufficient to definitively diagnose a particular organism as the causative agent of intestinal disease.

The diagnosis of bacterial enteritis can be made if the finding of clinical disease is consistent with a particular organism, there is evidence of the organism or its toxin, thereby eliminating other causes of the clinical signs, and appropriate therapy produces the expected response. If a fecal culture is to be performed, the veterinary laboratory should be consulted ahead of time as to the appropriate media and protocol for the submission of the sample. In many cases, the best chance of making a definitive diagnosis involves following the guidelines described and using molecular techniques on isolates to demonstrate toxin production.

Campylobacteriosis

There are several species of *Campylobacter*. Typically, *Campylobacter jejuni* is the species associated with GI disease. However, in certain cases, *Campylobacter upsaliensis* has been implicated. These organisms prefer high temperatures (i.e., 39–41°C); consequently, poultry is probably a reservoir. *Campylobacter* infections appear less frequently in cats than in dogs. These organisms may be found in the intestinal tract and feces of healthy dogs and cats.[17]

Symptomatic campylobacteriosis is primarily diagnosed in animals younger than 6 months old, living in crowded conditions (e.g., kennels, humane shelters) or as a nosocomial infection. Although clinical signs are variable, mucoid diarrhea (with or without blood), anorexia, and/or fever are the primary signs. Campylobacteriosis tends to be self-limiting in dogs, cats, and in humans; however, it occasionally causes chronic diarrhea.

Occasionally, classic *Campylobacter* forms such as "commas" or "seagull wings" may be found during cytological examination of a fecal sample. This cytology is thought to be specific but of uncertain sensitivity. PCR analysis of the feces is also available.

If campylobacteriosis is suspected, erythromycin (11–15 mg/kg administered orally q 8 h) or neomycin (20 mg/kg administered orally q 12 h) is usually effective. β-Lactam antibiotics (i.e., penicillins, first-generation cephalosporins) are reportedly ineffective.[13] The length of treatment needed for a cure has not been definitively established. The animal should be treated for at least 1–3 days beyond resolution of clinical signs. It is important to remember that antibiotic therapy may not eradicate the bacteria, and reinfection is probable in kennel conditions. Chronic infections may require prolonged therapy.

This bacterium is potentially transmissible to people, and there are cases in which there is convincing evidence of transmission from pets to people. Infected dogs and cats should be isolated and individuals working with the animal, its environment, or its waste products should wear protective clothing. Thorough hand washing after handling the animal or any objects in close proximity is indicated.

With appropriate antibiotic therapy and removal from the contaminated environment, the prognosis for these patients is good.

Salmonellosis

There are a number of *Salmonella* serotypes that may cause disease. These serovars occur across the globe and have the potential to infect not only mammals but also birds and reptiles.[14] *Salmonella typhimurium* is one of the serovars that is more commonly associated with disease. The bacteria may originate from infected dogs or cats shedding the organism or from contaminated food sources (especially poultry, swine meat, and eggs).

Salmonella spp. may generate acute or chronic diarrhea, septicemia, and/or sudden death, especially in pediatric or geriatric animals. Salmonellosis in young animals can produce a syndrome that closely mimics parvoviral enteritis (including severe neutropenia), which is one reason that ELISA testing for parvovirus is useful in ruling in/out this disease.

Culture of *Salmonella* spp. from normally sterile areas (e.g., blood), identification by PCR, or fecal isolation of *Salmonella* serotypes in a patient with clinical signs can be used for diagnosis.[13,15]

Treatment of salmonellosis is dependent upon the severity of the clinical signs. In animals with diarrhea as the sole presenting sign, only supportive fluid therapy may be needed. Antibiotic treatment may promote bacterial resistance and a carrier state; thus, it is not recommended when *Salmonella* bacteria are isolated from healthy infected animals or stable animals with diarrhea. In animals with severe hemorrhagic diarrhea, marked depression, shock, persistent pyrexia, or sepsis, parenteral antibiotics need to be given. The choice of antibiotic should be governed by sensitivity testing when possible, but fluoroquinolones appear to be effective against many *Salmonella* spp. Therapy initially should be given for 10 days, but prolonged therapy may be required. The feces should be recultured on several occasions to ensure that the infection has been eliminated.[18] Aggressive plasma therapy should be considered as it is often beneficial in septicemic patients.[13]

Infected animals are a risk to public health (especially for infants and older adults) and should be isolated until they are asymptomatic. When signs disappear, it is prudent to reculture the feces to ensure that shedding has stopped. It is necessary to properly educate all individuals in contact with the animal, its environment, and its waste products. Such persons should wear protective clothing and should wash all contaminated surfaces with disinfectants such as phenolic compounds or bleach (1:32 dilution).

The prognosis in *Salmonella*-affected patients is usually good if diarrhea is the only clinical sign but is guarded in septicemic dogs and cats.

Clostridial diseases

C. perfringens and *Clostridium difficile* can be found in clinically normal dogs but appears to cause diarrhea in others. In order for *C. perfringens* to produce disease, environmental conditions must be such that the bacteria have the ability to produce toxin and that the toxin is produced. Clostridial disease is mostly recognized in dogs.

C. perfringens may result in an acute, bloody, self-limiting nosocomial diarrhea; an acute, potentially fatal hemorrhagic diarrhea; or a chronic large bowel or small bowel (or even both) diarrhea—with or without blood or mucus. Disease associated with *C. difficile* is not well characterized in small animals but may include large bowel diarrhea, especially after antibiotic therapy.

Finding spore-forming bacteria on fecal smears is not diagnostic. Commercially available toxin assays for *C. difficile* toxin have not been validated for the dog or cat, and results do not always correlate with the patient's clinical condition. The basis for presumptive diagnosis lies in determining that the patient has large bowel diarrhea without weight loss or hypoalbuminemia, elimination of other causes, and resolution of signs when treated appropriately.

If *C. perfringens* disease is suspected, the animal may begin treatment with tylosin or amoxicillin. A positive response is expected soon after initiating treatment. In some patients, clinical signs resolve after a 1- to 3-week course of therapy. It is important to remember that antibiotic treatment does not necessarily eliminate the bacteria, and some animals may need therapy to continue indefinitely. Tylosin (20–80 mg/kg/day, divided, q 12 h) or amoxicillin (22 mg/kg q 12 h) seem to be effective and so far have been shown to have minimal adverse effects. Eventually, some animals can be maintained with once-daily or every-other-day antibiotic therapy. Metronidazole is not as consistently effective as tylosin or amoxicillin. Some dogs with chronic diarrhea, seemingly caused by *C. perfringens*, respond well to fiber-supplemented diets. The prognosis in these cases is good, and there appears to be no obvious public health risk, but anecdotal evidence of transmission between people and dogs does exist.

If disease caused by *C. difficile* is suspected, supportive fluid and electrolyte therapy may be necessary dependent upon the severity of signs in the animal. Metronidazole typically is effective in killing this bacterium, but a sufficiently high dose to achieve adequate metronidazole concentrations in the feces is needed for effective therapy. Vancomycin is often used to treat humans with this disease but has not generally been needed in the treatment of dogs or cats.

Dogs suffering from diarrhea caused by *C. perfringens* have an excellent prognosis, but if diagnosed with *C. difficile*, the prognosis is uncertain.

Miscellaneous bacteria

Yersinia enterocolitica, *Aeromonas hydrophila*, and *Plesiomonas shigelloides* have been shown to cause acute or chronic enterocolitis in dogs and/or in cats as well as in people. However, these bacteria are uncommonly diagnosed in the United States.

Y. enterocolitica is primarily found in swine (which may serve as a reservoir) and in cold environments. Due to its ability to grow in cold temperatures, it is also a cause of food poisoning. Enterohemorrhagic *E. coli* (EHEC) may seemingly be associated with canine and feline diarrhea, although it does not appear to be especially common.

Small bowel diarrhea may be caused by any of these bacteria. Yersiniosis frequently affects the colon and results in chronic large bowel diarrhea. Abdominal pain may also be present as this symptom is reported to occur in humans.

It would be reasonable to culture for *Y. enterocolitica* if animals present with persistent colitis, especially if they have been in contact with pigs.

Supportive therapy should be initiated and the affected animal should be isolated from other animals. Persons in contact with the affected animal and/or its environment and waste products should be advised to wear protective clothing and to follow strict hand washing protocols. Antibiotics would seem indicated; however, in cases of EHEC, their use has not shortened clinical disease. Even so, appropriate antibiotics as determined by culture and sensitivity are often utilized (e.g., *Y. enterocolitica* is often sensitive to tetracyclines). The preferred length of antibiotic therapy has not been established, but it is suggested that treatment should be continued for 1–3 days beyond clinical remission.

The prognosis is uncertain but appears to be good if the bacteria can be identified by culture and the infection treated appropriately.

Histoplasmosis

Histoplasmosis is a mycotic infection caused by *H. capsulatum*. This infection can affect the GI, respiratory, and/or reticuloendothelial systems, as well as the bones and eyes. It occurs in a number of areas but is mainly found in animals from the Mississippi and Ohio River valleys. It is typically seen in young dogs and cats, and it is acquired through the inhalation or ingestion of microconidia. Please refer to Chapter 11, Section 2 for more information.[13,14]

Alimentary tract involvement is primarily found in dogs; diarrhea (with or without blood or mucus) and weight loss are the commonly seen and reported signs. It is important to note that the lungs, liver, spleen, lymph nodes, bone marrow, skeletal system, and/or eyes may also be affected. Symptomatic alimentary involvement is much less common in cats; respiratory dysfunction (e.g., dyspnea, cough), fever, and/or weight loss are seen more often in cats. In GI histoplasmosis, the colon is usually the most severely affected segment. Diffuse, severe, granulomatous, ulcerative mucosal disease can produce bloody stool, intestinal protein loss, intermittent fever, and/or weight loss. Small intestinal involvement may be seen, but this is infrequent. The disease may linger for long periods of time, causing mild to moderate, nonprogressive signs. On occasion, histoplasmosis may result in focal colonic granulomas or may be present in grossly normal-appearing colonic mucosa.

Histoplasmosis is most consistently diagnosed by identifying the organism on cytological smears from lymph node aspiration, rectal scrapings, or histological samples. Dogs from endemic areas with chronic large bowel diarrhea are especially suspect. PLE is common in dogs with severe histoplasmosis, and hypoalbuminemia in dogs with large bowel disease is suggestive of the disease, regardless of the location.

A rectal examination may reveal thickened rectal folds; these can easily be scraped with a dull curette or syringe case cap to obtain material for cytological preparations. Evaluation of colonic biopsy specimens is usually diagnostic, but special stains may be necessary. Fundic examination of the eye occasionally reveals active chorioretinitis. Abdominal radiographs may show hepatosplenomegaly, and thoracic radiographs sometimes reveal pulmonary involvement (e.g., miliary interstitial involvement and/or hilar lymphadenopathy). Cytological evaluation of hepatic or splenic aspirates may be diagnostic. Rarely, a CBC may demonstrate yeast in circulating WBCs. Thrombocytopenia may occur. Cytological examination of bone marrow or of buffy coat smears may reveal the organism. It is important to note that serologic tests and fecal culture for the yeast are unreliable.

It is crucial to look for histoplasmosis before beginning empiric corticosteroid therapy for suspected canine colonic IBD. Corticosteroid therapy diminishes the animals' defenses and may allow a previously treatable case to rapidly progress and kill the animal. Treatment with itraconazole by itself or preceded by amphotericin B is often effective. Treatment should be continued long enough (i.e., at least 4–6 months) to lessen chances for relapse.

Many animals can be cured if treatment begins relatively early. Multiple organ system involvement and CNS involvement worsens the prognosis.

Giardiasis

Giardia sp. is a protozoan that causes giardiasis. Animals become infected when they ingest cysts shed from infected animals, typically through water. Organisms are principally found in the SI, where they interfere with digestion through uncertain mechanisms.

Animals present with signs that vary from mild to severe diarrhea, which may be persistent, intermittent, or self-limiting. Typically, the diarrhea is of "cow patty" consistency, without blood or mucus. There can be substantial variation in the presentation of clinical signs. Some animals experience weight loss; others do not. Diarrhea caused by *Giardia* can mimic large bowel diarrhea in some patients, making diagnosis difficult. In cats, there may be an association between shedding giardial oocysts and shedding either cryptosporidial or coccidian oocysts.

Diagnostic testing

Giardiasis can be diagnosed by finding motile trophozoites in saline smears of fresh feces or duodenal washes, by finding cysts with fecal flotation techniques, or by finding giardial proteins in feces using an ELISA test. Zinc sulfate solutions appear to be the best fecal flotation medium for identifying cysts, especially when centrifugal flotation is performed (as other solutions may cause distortion). It is recommended to perform at least three fecal examinations over the course of 7–10 days before discounting giardiasis. Some fecal ELISA techniques (e.g., SNAP Giardia Test®, Idexx Laboratories) appear to have excellent sensitivity and are easier than centrifugal fecal flotation examinations. Performing washes of the duodenal lumen (endoscopically or surgically by instilling and then retrieving 5–10 mL of physiological saline solution from the duodenal lumen) or cytological evaluation of the duodenal mucosa occasionally reveals *Giardia* organisms when other techniques do not. Trophozoites and cysts may also be found on stained fecal smears.

Patient care

It is often difficult to identify *Giardia* organisms (especially in animals that have had various symptomatic antidiarrheal medications), and the response to treatment is often the retrospective basis of diagnosis. This approach certainly has limitations. Quinacrine is effective but is no longer available. Metronidazole has few adverse effects and seems reasonably effective (approximately 85% cured after 7 days of therapy); however, clinical response to metronidazole therapy may occur in animals without giardiasis.[13] Furazolidone (5 days of therapy) is probably as effective as metronidazole and is available as a suspension, thus making it easier to treat infected kittens. Albendazole (3 days of therapy in dogs, 5 days of therapy in cats) and fenbendazole (5 days of therapy in dogs or cats) are also effective, and recent data suggest that ronidazole may also be effective. None of these drugs are 100% effective, meaning that failure to respond to drug therapy does not rule out giardiasis.

It can be difficult to eliminate *Giardia* spp. for a variety of reasons. *Giardia* organisms may apparently become resistant to some drugs; patient immunodeficiency or concurrent disease may make it difficult to eliminate the organism; and reinfection is easy because giardial cysts are rather resistant to environmental influences, and only a few are needed to reinfect a dog or person. Client education on prevention includes bathing the patient (to remove cysts from the fur and perineal area) and cleaning the environment (quaternary ammonium compounds and pine tars are effective disinfectants for the premises). These techniques may be very important to the successful treatment in many patients. Finally, sometimes other protozoal agents (e.g., *Tritrichomonas*) are mistaken for *Giardia*. Vaccination is not recommended (see vaccine recommendations).

The prognosis for recovery is usually good, although in some cases, the organism is difficult to eradicate. More information is available in Chapter 11.

Key nutritional factors in patients with large bowel diarrhea

Water

Water is the most important nutrient for patients with acute large bowel due to the potential for life-threatening dehydration. Dehydration results with from excessive fluid loss combined with the patient's inability to replace those losses. Patients with chronic diarrhea and mild acute diarrhea should be monitored for signs of dehydration, but usually, the oral route is sufficient for their needs. Parenteral fluid therapy may be indicated when the patient presents with moderate to severe diarrhea.

Electrolytes

Potassium depletion is a predictable consequence of severe and chronic enteric diseases because the potassium concentration of intestinal secretions is high. Hypokalemia in association with large bowel diarrhea or colitis will be particularly profound if losses are not replaced through sufficient dietary intake of potassium. Electrolyte disorders should be corrected initially with appropriate parenteral fluid and electrolyte therapy. Foods for patients with colitis should contain levels of sodium, chloride, and potassium above the minimum allowances for normal dogs and cats. Recommended levels of these nutrients are 0.3–0.5% DM sodium, 0.5–1.3% DM chloride, and 0.8–1.1% DM potassium.[10]

Protein

Protein should be provided at levels sufficient for the appropriate life stage of the patients unless PLE is present. Thus, DM protein levels in foods for adult dogs and cats should be between 15% and 30% and between 30% and 45%, respectively.[10] Protein levels for growing puppies and kittens should be in the ranges of 22–32% and 35–50% DM, respectively.[10] High biological value, highly digestible (≥87%) protein sources are ideal. The use of elimination foods are recommended because of the suspected role of dietary antigens in the pathogenesis of chronic colitis.[19,20] In some cases, elimination foods may be used successfully without pharmacological intervention.

Fat

Compared with the processes involved with other macronutrients, fat digestion and absorption are relatively complex and may be disrupted in patients with GI disease. The action of bacterial flora on unabsorbed fats in the colon resulting in hydroxy fatty acid production is an important cause of large bowel diarrhea. Thus, foods indicated for patients with colitis and many other GI diseases often contain low to moderate amounts of fat (i.e., 8–15% DM for dogs and 9–25% DM for cats). However, dogs and cats digest fat very efficiently and the process is rarely disrupted except in malassimilative disorders. Therefore, colitis patients can be fed foods containing higher concentrations of fat when greater caloric density is required.[10]

Fiber

Dietary fiber predominantly affects the large bowel of dogs and cats. Beneficial effects of dietary fiber include (1) normalizing colonic motility and transit time, (2) buffering toxins (e.g., bile acids and bacterial enterotoxins) in the GI lumen, (3) binding or holding excess water, (4) supporting growth of normal GI microflora, (5) providing fuel for colonocytes, and (6) altering the viscosity of GI luminal contents.

Fibers are often categorized as soluble, insoluble, or mixed. Mixed fibers include beet pulp, brans (rice, wheat, or oat), pea and soy fibers, soy hulls, and mixtures of soluble and insoluble fibers. Insoluble fibers include purified cellulose and peanut hulls. Soluble fiber sources include fruit pectins, guar gums, and psyllium.

Various types and levels of dietary fiber have been advocated for use in patients with large bowel diarrhea or colitis. Some veterinarians recommend low fiber foods (5% DM crude fiber) to enhance DM digestibility and to reduce quantities of ingesta presented to the colon. Results have also been seen when using moderate levels (10–15% DM crude fiber) to high levels (>15%

DM crude fiber) of insoluble fiber.[10] If a food with an increased fiber level is being considered, a crude fiber content of at least 7% DM is advisable. These strategies have been used successfully in managing patients with colitis and each strategy is patient dependent.

Small amounts (1–5% DM fiber) of a mixed-fiber (i.e., soluble/insoluble) type can also be added to a highly digestible food. Many clinicians select foods enhanced with insoluble fiber as their first food option in the management of acute and chronic colitis and large bowel diarrhea.

Digestibility

Feeding highly digestible (fat and digestible carbohydrate ≥90% and protein ≥87%) foods offer several advantages for managing dogs and cats with long-standing inflammatory colitis. Nutrients from highly digestible, low residue foods are more completely absorbed from the proximal gut. Low residue foods are associated with (1) reduced osmotic diarrhea due to fat and carbohydrate malabsorption, (2) reduced production of intestinal gas due to carbohydrate malabsorption, and (3) decreased antigen loads because smaller amounts of protein are absorbed intact. Fiber-enhanced foods inherently have somewhat lower digestibility values. These foods should have protein and fat digestibilities of at least 80% and carbohydrate digestibility of at least 90%.[10]

Acid load

Acidemia (i.e., normal anion gap hyperchloremic acidosis) is common in patients with acute large bowel diarrhea because fluid secreted in the caudal SI and LI contains bicarbonate concentrations higher than those in plasma and sodium in excess of chloride ions. Hypovolemia (i.e., severe dehydration) compounds the acidosis in some patients. Severe acid–base disorders are best corrected with appropriate parenteral fluid therapy. Foods for patients with acute colitis should, as a rule, produce an alkaline urinary pH. These foods preferably contain buffering salts such as potassium gluconate and calcium carbonate.

Omega-3 fatty acids

Omega-3 (n-3) fatty acids derived from fish oil or other sources may have a beneficial effect in controlling mucosal inflammation in patients with chronic inflammatory colitis.[19] There is clinical evidence that dietary omega-3 fatty acid supplementation may modulate the generation and biological activity of inflammatory mediators.

Vitamins

Folic acid supplementation is recommended for patients receiving long-term sulfasalazine therapy.[10]

Diseases of the large intestine

The LI begins at the ileocolic junction and terminates at the anus; it is composed of the cecum, ascending, transverse, and descending colon, and the rectum. The main functions of the LI are to extract fluid and electrolytes, fermentation, and to store feces. The four layers of the LI are the serosal, muscularis, submucosa, and the mucosa. The LI is innervated by the vagus and pelvic nerves, and the blood supply is through the cranial and caudal mesenteric arteries.

Inflammation of the large intestine

Acute colitis/proctitis

Acute colitis can be attributed to many causes (e.g., bacteria, diet, parasites) or it may be idiopathic in origin. The underlying cause is seldom diagnosed as this problem tends to be self-limiting.[1] Acute proctitis (inflammation of the lining of the rectum) most likely has similar causes but, in addition, can be the resultant of passage of a rough foreign object that traumatizes the rectal mucosa.[2]

Animals with acute colitis often present feeling well despite large bowel diarrhea (i.e., hematochezia, fecal mucus, tenesmus). These animals tend to have an increase in the frequency of defecation and often a reduced volume of feces despite the increased "need" to defecate. Although reported in both cats and dogs, colitis is seen more frequently in dogs. Vomiting may occur but is not a frequently reported sign. The major clinical signs of acute proctitis are constipation, tenesmus, hematochezia, dyschezia, and/or depression.

A rectal examination is a very important part of the physical examination as animals with acute colitis may have rectal discomfort and/or hematochezia. The elimination of obvious causes such as diet and parasites and subsequent resolution of the problem with symptomatic therapy leads to a presumptive diagnosis. Colonoscopy and biopsy are required to make a definitive diagnosis; however, colonoscopy and biopsy are not often indicated unless the patient's initial presentation is severe. Rectal examination of animals with acute proctitis may reveal roughened, thick, and/or obviously ulcerated mucosa. Proctoscopy and rectal mucosal biopsy are definitive for diagnosis but, again, are seldom indicated.[1,2]

Because acute proctitis and colitis are usually idiopathic in nature, symptomatic therapy is typically warranted. Withholding food for 24–36 h lessens the severity of clinical signs. The animal should then be fed small amounts of a bland diet or a low residue formulation. After resolution of the clinical signs, the animal may be gradually returned to its original diet. Any areas of anal excoriation should be cleansed, and an antibiotic–corticosteroid ointment should be applied. Most animals recover within 1–3 days. For proctitis, stool softeners such as lactulose or dioctyl sodium sulfosuccinate (DSS) may be necessary.

Treatment for proctitis also includes antibiotic therapy (e.g., metronidazole) and anti-inflammatory medications. Anti-inflammatory medications such as prednisolone and the aminosalicylates are recommended. Sulfasalazine and olsalazine can also be used; however, both of these (particularly sulfasalazine) are associated with side effects such as keratoconjunctivitis sicca. Topical therapies such as Proctofoam-HC, which contains a local anesthetic and hydrocortisone, have also been recommended for proctitis but may be difficult for owners to apply.

Chronic colitis

Chronic colitis is typically attributable to *Clostridium* spp., parasites, dietary intolerance, and fiber-responsive diarrhea. As discussed earlier, *C. perfringens* and *C. difficile* may be found in clinically normal dogs. However, in some patients, *C. perfringens* and *C. difficile* may result in diarrhea. For *C. perfringens* to produce disease, the bacteria must possess the ability to produce toxin, and environmental conditions must be such that toxin is produced.

Chronic colitis may be the reason that most cases have been diagnosed previously as having "intractable" large bowel "IBD." One common type of chronic colitis is lymphocytic-plasmacytic colitis (LPC). Dogs with LPC usually present with large bowel diarrhea (i.e., soft stools with or without blood or mucus). In cats with LPC, hematochezia is the most common clinical sign, and diarrhea is the second most common sign. Feline LPC may occur by itself or concurrently with LPE.

The diagnosis of chronic colitis is through exclusion of other causes and through documenting mucosal histological changes. When diagnosing chronic colitis in cats, it is important to remember that *Tritrichomonas* can cause substantial mononuclear infiltrates into feline colonic mucosa.[2]

Dietary modification plays a large role in therapy. Hypoallergenic and fiber-enriched diets have been found to be very helpful in both dogs and cats. Reportedly, the most intractable feline LPC cases are ultimately determined to be related to diet.[2] The majority of cats with LPC also respond well to prednisolone and/or metronidazole. Sulfasalazine is rarely needed. Steroids, metronidazole, sulfasalazine (Azulfidine), mesalamine, or olsalazine may be used in dogs with moderate to severe LPC. The prognosis for patients with chronic colitis or LPC tends to be better than for patients suffering from small bowel IBD.

Large intestinal cancers

In dogs, tumors of the LI are more common than tumors of the stomach or SI. Large intestinal cancer, when found, is more commonly diagnosed in middle age or older dogs. Most colonic tumors of dogs are malignant and include adenocarcinomas, lymphosarcomas, and GI stromal tumors (leiomyosarcoma, neurofibrosarcoma, fibrosarcoma, and ganglioneuroma). Most colonic neoplasias develop in the descending colon and rectum, although leiomyosarcomas more frequently develop in the cecum. Local tumor invasion apparently occurs at a slower rate with canine colonic neoplasia as compared to intestinal neoplasia, and metastasis to distant sites is relatively uncommon. Benign colonic neoplasia such as adenomas, adenomatous polyps, and leiomyomas are much less common than malignant tumors. Malignant transformation of adenomatous polyps to carcinoma *in situ* and invasive adenocarcinoma has been demonstrated in dogs. In cats, adenocarcinoma is the most common tumor of the LI (46%), followed by lymphosarcoma (41%), and mast cell tumors (9%). The mean age of cats affected with colonic neoplasia is 12.5 years. The most common sites of colonic neo-

plasia in cats are the descending colon (39%) and the ileocolic sphincter (28%). Unlike dogs, cats with colonic tumors have a high rate (63%) of local metastasis, which is associated with decreased survival time.[4]

Adenocarcinoma

These tumors can extend into the lumen or can be infiltrative and produce a circumferential narrowing. In cats, the most common large intestinal tumor is adenocarcinoma; the age of the cat is typically older, with an average age of 12 years.[2,4,5]

Presenting signs may include hematochezia, dyschezia, and/or intermittent rectal bleeding not associated with defecation. Infiltrative tumors are likely to cause tenesmus and/or constipation secondary to obstruction. Cats typically present with weight loss, anorexia, vomiting, and diarrhea.[2,5,6]

Rectal examination, as part of the complete physical examination, is useful in identifying colorectal masses because most colonic neoplasms arise in or near the rectum. Digital examination is the best screening test.

Histopathologic evaluation is often preferable to cytological analysis. This is due to epithelial dysplasia (possibly being present in benign lesions), which may cause a false-positive cytological diagnosis of carcinoma. Moderately deep biopsies obtained with rigid biopsy forceps are usually required to diagnose submucosal carcinomas and to differentiate benign polyps from carcinomas (invasion of the submucosa is an important feature of rectal adenocarcinomas). Imaging may be used to detect sublumbar lymph node enlargement or pulmonary involvement (i.e., metastases) but is not typically helpful in the visualization of the colon due to gas and bone interference.

Complete surgical excision is the treatment of choice and may provide excellent long-term outcomes for patients with a single mass. Nevertheless, most malignancies cannot be surgically cured because of their location in the pelvic canal, extent of local invasion, and/or tendency to metastasize to regional lymph nodes. The prognosis for unresectable adenocarcinoma is poor. Preoperative and intraoperative radiotherapy may be palliative for some dogs with nonresectable colorectal adenocarcinomas.[2,5,6]

Rectal polyps

Rectal polyps are benign adenomatous growths. Polyps are rare but are more commonly reported in dogs. Clinical signs include hematochezia (and this may be considerable) and tenesmus. Obstruction secondary to polyps in the rectum is very uncommon.

Rectal polyps are usually detected during rectal palpation. It is important to discern polyps from adenocarcinomas as some adenomatous polyps resemble sessile adenocarcinomas (because they are so large that the narrow, stalk-like attachment cannot be readily discerned). Rarely, multiple small polyps may be palpated throughout one segment of the colon, usually within a few centimeters of the rectum. Histopathology must be performed for diagnosis to distinguish polyps from malignancies.

Complete excision via surgery or endoscopy is recommended and has been reported to be curative. A thorough endoscopic or imaging evaluation of the colon should be done prior to surgery to rule out the presence of any additional polyps. If polyps are incompletely excised, they will return and will need to be re-excised at some point in the future. Multiple polyps within a defined area may necessitate segmental colonic mucosal resection.[2,5,6]

Megacolon

Megacolon is hypertrophy and dilation of the colon and is associated with chronic constipation and obstipation. The cause is not completely understood, but most cases are either idiopathic, orthopedic, or neurological in origin. A review of cases in the literature found that 96% of cases of obstipation are accounted for by idiopathic megacolon (62%), pelvic canal stenosis (23%), nerve injury (6%), or Manx sacral spinal cord deformity (5%).[7] Other theories involve behavior (i.e., refusal to defecate) or altered colonic neurotransmitters.[2,8]

Idiopathic megacolon is predominantly a feline disease, although on occasion, dogs are affected. Affected animals may be depressed and anorectic and are often presented because of infrequent defecation. Upon physical examination, colonic impaction is often found. Other signs are dependent upon the severity and pathogenesis of the constipation. In cats with severe megacolon, signs such as dehydration, weight loss, abdominal pain, and mild to moderate mesenteric lymphadenopathy may be seen.

Although most cats with obstipation and megacolon are not likely to have significant changes in laboratory data (e.g., CBC, serum chemistry, urinalysis), these tests should nonetheless be performed in all cats with constipation. Metabolic causes of constipation, such as dehydration, hypokalemia, and hypercalcemia, may be detected in some instances. Basal serum T_4 concentration and other thyroid function tests should also be considered in cats with recurrent constipation and other signs consistent with hypothyroidism.[4]

Abdominal radiography should be performed in all constipated cats to characterize the severity of colonic impaction and to identify predisposing factors, such as intraluminal radiopaque foreign material (e.g., bone chips), intraluminal or extraluminal mass lesions, pelvic fractures, and spinal cord abnormalities. Ancillary studies may be indicated in some cases. Extraluminal mass lesions may be further evaluated by abdominal ultrasonography and guided biopsy, whereas intraluminal mass lesions are best evaluated by endoscopy. Finally, colonic biopsy is necessary to diagnose suspected cases of aganglionic megacolon (Hirschsprung disease), a congenital condition described once in a young cat.[9]

Idiopathic megacolon is diagnosed by elimination of dietary, behavioral, metabolic, and anatomic causes. A complete neurological evaluation should be performed, with special emphasis on caudal spinal cord function, to identify any neurological causes of constipation.

Impacted feces must be removed, and this can be accomplished through the use of rectal suppositories, enemas, or through manual extraction. Due to the severity of the constipation, multiple warm water retention and cleansing enemas with manual extraction of fecal matter has the best chance of relieving the obstruction and this may be a multiday process.

To aid in the prevention of future fecal impaction, the addition of fiber to a moist diet (e.g., Metamucil, pumpkin pie filling) and medicating with osmotic laxatives (e.g., lactulose) and/or prokinetic drugs is recommended. A large body of anecdotal experience suggests that cisapride is useful in stimulating colonic propulsive motility in cats affected with mild to moderate idiopathic constipation. However, cats with long-standing obstipation and megacolon are not likely to show much improvement with cisapride therapy. Cisapride was withdrawn from the American, Canadian, and certain Western European countries in July 2000 after reports of cardiac side effects in people. Two new prokinetic agents, tegaserod and prucalopride, are in differing stages of drug development and may prove useful in the therapy of GI motility disorders of several animal species.[4,10]

Tegaserod is a potent partial nonbenzamide agonist at 5-HT$_4$ receptors and a weak agonist at 5-HT$_{1D}$ receptors. Tegaserod has definite prokinetic effects in the canine colon, but it has not yet been studied in the feline colon. Prucalopride is a potent 5-HT$_4$ receptor agonist that stimulates giant migrating contractions (GMCs) and defecation in the dog and cat.[11] There are no data available on its usefulness in cats with megacolon.

Lubricant enemas are not recommended because they are not helpful, as they do not change fecal consistency. At home, owners should make sure that litter boxes are plentiful, clean, and in low traffic areas in order to prevent litter box aversions. If this conservative therapy fails or if the client is unable to comply, colectomy may be indicated. Postoperatively, cats typically have soft stools for a few weeks, but some may have soft stools for the rest of their lives. Following the recommendations above and if treated early, many cats respond well to conservative therapy and have a fair to good outcome.[11]

Key nutritional factors for patients with chronic constipation and obstipation

Key nutritional factors for chronic constipation differ from key nutritional factors for obstipation and the differences will be outlined below.

Water

Maintaining normal hydration status is important for managing patients with chronic constipation or obstipation. Water is a key nutrient and its intake is often overlooked. A variety of methods should be used to encourage water intake. These include providing multiple bowls of potable water in prominent locations in the pet's environment, feeding moist (>75% water) rather than dry forms of foods, adding small amounts of flavoring substances such as bouillon or broth to water sources, and offering ice cubes as treats or snacks. Adding canned pumpkin and/or sweet potato to the current food has been successfully implemented in some cases of constipation. These canned vegetables consist primarily of water (90%), which adds a significant quantity of water to the digesta. Beneficial effects resulting from canned pumpkin or sweet potato are likely the result of an increase in total daily water consumption, although fiber intake is also increased.

Fiber

Many patients with constipation improve clinically when the fiber content of their food is increased. Dietary fibers are poorly digestible polysaccharides, derived from a variety of sources. Fiber sources typically used in commercial pet foods include sugar beet pulp, cereal grains, cellulose, soy hulls, peanut hulls, and pea fiber. Increasing fiber intake typically increases fecal water content, colonic motility, and intestinal transit rate, all of which may benefit patients with constipation. Both fermentable and nonfermentable fiber sources have been advocated for the management of constipation.[13] Fiber acts as a bulk-forming laxative. Insoluble fibers (e.g., purified cellulose, peanut hulls) normalize colonic motility by distending the colonic lumen, increasing colonic water content, diluting luminal toxins (e.g., bile acids, ammonia, and ingested toxins) and increasing the rate of passage of digesta. This change in colonic transit time reduces colonocyte exposure to toxins while softening the stool and increasing the frequency of defecation. Several gel-forming fibers have been recommended as an aid in managing constipation in people and in animals. Soluble (fermentable) fibers (fruit pectins, guar gum, psyllium) are readily fermented by bacteria, producing SCFAs, which promote colonic health. These fibers, whether added to or incorporated into food, are reported to swell to form emollient gels and facilitate passage of fecal matter.[14] However, fermentable fibers may not be as laxative as insoluble or mixed fibers because they have little ability to increase fecal bulk or dilute luminal toxins. Flatulence, diarrhea, and abdominal cramping are potential adverse effects to be aware of when using fermentable, gel-forming fibers. These adverse effects can be reduced by a gradual transition to fiber supplementation, slowly increasing the level of added fermentable fiber until efficacy is achieved with minimal side effects. Such fibers should be added at no more than 5% of the total food because soluble fibers can significantly reduce the availability of minerals, including zinc, calcium, iron, and phosphorus. Ingredients such as beet pulp, brans (rice, wheat, or oat), pea fiber, soy fibers, soy hulls, or mixtures of soluble and insoluble fiber sources are intermediate in their fermentability and have moderate attributes of both fermentable and poorly fermentable fibers. They are referred to as mixed fibers.

For patients with chronic constipation that still have some level of colonic motility, the crude fiber content of a food should be at least 7% DM initially, and the fiber source should be insoluble or mixed. Fiber sources can be added to a patient's current food, but it is generally better to switch to a fiber-enhanced food. Feeding additional dietary fiber is preferable to the use of laxative medications alone. Dietary fiber is more physiological, better tolerated, and often more effective than nonfiber laxatives.

The motility patterns of patients with obstipation are completely abolished (e.g., severe end-stage megacolon in cats). In these patients, fiber-enhanced foods and fiber supplements are no longer effective stimulants of colonic motility and, worse, may contribute to obstipation. Foods for patients with megacolon should have no more than 5% DM crude fiber.

Digestibility and caloric density

For patients suffering from obstipation (including feline megacolon), wherein colonic motility patterns are completely abolished, feeding a highly digestible food (fat and digestible [soluble] carbohydrate $\geq 90\%$ and protein $\geq 87\%$) with an increased energy density ($\geq 4.0\,\text{kcal/g}$ [$\geq 16.7\,\text{kJ/g}$] DM) will provide adequate nutrition and distinctly reduce the fecal mass.[14] A food's energy density and digestibility are inversely related to its fiber content. Reducing fiber results in increased caloric density, which in turn helps to meet the patient's requirements in a small volume of food. Calorically dense foods can markedly reduce the burden of home management (i.e., administering stool softeners and enemas) for pet owners. Fecal production is reduced to such an extent that owners can generally remove feces by cleansing enemas once or twice weekly. The energy density and digestibility of a food are not as important in constipated patients.

SECTION 4 PHARMACOLOGY

Antacids

Antacids reduce gastric acid production, thereby increasing gastric pH. These drugs are used in the treatment of gastric ulcers and erosions due to drugs such as non-steroidal anti-inflammatories and steroids, uremic gastritis, esophagitis, esophageal reflux disease, gastrinomas, and mast cell tumors.[1,2] Increased acid production can occur secondarily to chronic gastric or intestinal inflammation and may also exacerbate inflammation in the duodenum.[3] The two classes of antacids generally utilized in veterinary medicine are H_2-receptor antagonists and proton pump inhibitors.

H_2-receptor antagonists

H_2-receptor antagonists competitively inhibit histamine at the level of the H_2 receptor of the gastric parietal cell, thereby reducing gastric acid output.[1,2] Examples of antacids in this class include cimetidine, ranitidine, and famotidine.

Cimetidine (Tagamet®)

Adverse effects with this drug are uncommon. However, cimetidine inhibits the hepatic microsomal enzyme system, causing reduced metabolism, longer serum half-lives, and increased serum levels of several drugs if given concurrently.[1,2] The following drugs may be affected: beta blockers, lidocaine, diazepam, metronidazole, and theophylline, among others.[2]

Ranitidine (Zantac®)

Ranitidine inhibits gastric acid secretion to a greater extent than cimetidine.[1] In addition, ranitidine has prokinetic activity and increases lower esophageal pressure.[1,2]

Famotidine (Pepcid®)

Famotidine is similar in potency to ranitidine, but it has no prokinetic effects.[1,2] It can cause bradycardia with rapid intravenous infusion.[2] There have been reports of intravascular hemolysis when given to cats.[2] Famotidine for injection should be stored in the refrigerator.[2]

Proton pump inhibitors

PPIs inhibit the H^+/K^+ ATPase enzyme at the parietal cell surface, thereby inhibiting transport of hydrogen ions into the stomach.[1,2] They are more potent at inhibiting gastric acid secretion than the H_2-receptor antagonists.[1,2] The drug used most commonly in veterinary medicine in this class is omeprazole (Prilosec®).

Omeprazole (Prilosec)

Omeprazole can inhibit the cytochrome P450 enzyme system, causing reduced hepatic clearance of specific drugs such as diazepam, which may enhance its effects or may cause toxicity.[2] There is a delay in inhibition of gastric acid secretion of 3–4 days after starting treatment with omeprazole, so it is recommended to use an H_2 antagonist concurrently with omeprazole during the first few days if rapid inhibition of gastric acid is needed.[1] PPIs are recommended as the first line of treatment for patients with excessive gastric acid secretion due to mast cell tumors and gastrinomas.[1]

Antiemetics

Antiemetics are widely used in veterinary medicine to symptomatically treat vomiting due to a variety of causes. Underlying causes for which antiemetics are prescribed include primary GI disease (e.g., IBD and motility disorders), pancreatitis, uremia, drug-induced vomiting, and motion sickness. The antiemetic chosen depends on the underlying disease process and how vomiting is stimulated, species differences, and adverse effects of the drug. The classes of antiemetics used in veterinary medicine include α-adrenergic antagonists, D_2-dopaminergic antagonists, H_1-histaminergic antagonists, 5-HT_3 serotonergic receptor antagonists, 5-HT_4 receptor agonists, and NK-1 receptor antagonists.

α-Adrenergic antagonists

The commonly used drug in this group is chlorpromazine (Thorazine®). Chlorpramizine acts on several receptors (including serotonergic and histaminic), mainly in the chemoreceptor trigger zone (CRTZ).[4] Drugs in this class can cause hypotension, cardiac rate abnormalities, and hyper- or hypothermia.[5] Contraindications for use include hypotension or shock.

D_2-dopaminergic receptor antagonists

Metoclopramide (Reglan®) is the most commonly used drug in this group. Metoclopramide stimulates upper GI motility without stimulating gastric, biliary, or pancreatic secretions. Metoclopramide given 30 min prior to a meal will increase the tone and amplitude of the gastric contractions, relax the pyloric canal, and increase the contraction in the proximal SI. This drug has prokinetic activity[4,5] and therefore should not be used in animals with GI obstruction from foreign bodies, perforation, or GI hemorrhage.[5] It is often used as a constant rate infusion (CRI). Potential adverse effects include hyperreactivity and occasional drowsiness and sedation.[5]

This is often the drug of choice for motility disorders in dogs. Cats appear to be less sensitive to the effects of metoclopramide due to decreased receptors sites in the CRTZ in the brain.[3] Ranitidine may be a better motility agent in cats.[6]

H_1-histaminergic receptor antagonists

Dimenhydrinate and diphenhydramine (Dramamine® and Benadryl®, respectively) are examples of drugs in this class. Dimenhydrinate has been used for motion sickness in dogs. In addition, nausea and vomiting associated with vestibular disease can be managed with dimenhydrinate.[5] These drugs should be used with caution in patients with hypertension, hyperthyroidism, cardiovascular disease, and angle closure glaucoma.[5] Potential adverse effects of drugs in this class include sedation, urinary retention, and occasional GI effects.[5]

5-HT_3 serotonergic receptor antagonists

The two drugs commonly used from this group are dolasetron and ondansetron (Anzemet® and Zofran®, respectively). Drugs in this class are potent antiemetics and are used when other antiemetics do not control vomiting. Ondansetron works best against acute vomiting from peripheral causes, such as with cisplatin administration.[4,5] Collie-type breeds may be more sensitive to the effects of ondansetron.[5] The expense of Zofran limits its use in veterinary medicine.[4,5]

5-HT_4 receptor agonists

The main example in this group is cisapride, a potent promotility drug. Cisapride is different from metoclopramide in that it does not cross the blood–brain barrier. It has no known central antiemetic effects; rather, it acts to enhance gastric emptying and to stimulate smooth muscle contraction throughout the GI tract. It can be used for GI stasis and reflux esophagitis. The drug is no longer available and must be obtained from a compounding pharmacy. Cisapride is contraindicated in patients with GI obstruction, hemorrhage, and perforation.[5]

NK-1 receptor antagonists

Maropitant (Cerenia®) is approved for use in dogs, in both injectable (SQ) and oral formulations. It is used for a wide variety of causes of vomiting, including motion sickness, which requires a higher dose.[4,7] It works well for both peripheral and central causes of vomiting.[4] Cerenia injections SQ have been associated with pain, and recent evidence suggests that refrigeration of the drug prior to injection may help.[5]

Anti-inflammatory and immunosuppressive drugs

Anti-inflammatory and immunosuppressive drugs are used in the treatment of intestinal diseases. In some instances, these medications are used concurrently with antibiotics and diet therapy to improve the overall treatment effectiveness.[6]

Corticosteroids (prednisone, prednisolone, and budesonide)

The efficacy of corticosteroids in the management of intestinal disease relates primarily to their anti-inflammatory and immunosuppressive properties; appetite stimulation is a secondary benefit. In cases of chronic administration, the dose should be slowly decreased over 4–6 months. Relapses can occur if the dose reduction occurs too quickly and sometimes are so severe that corticosteroids alone can no longer control the signs associated with a relapse of the disease. In these situations, stronger immunosuppressive agents, such as azathioprine, cyclophosphamide, or cyclosporine, may need to be added.[6]

It is ideal that steroids not be given without a definitive pathological diagnosis. Changes in the intestines that can obscure diagnosis can occur even with a short course of use and will render endoscopic biopsies useless.

Prednisone and prednisolone

Prednisone is the primary anti-inflammatory agent used to treat intestinal inflammation. It is preferred because of its low cost, easy availability, and its efficacy. The side effects are dose related and include increased thirst and appetite, increased urination, weight gain, muscle weakness (seen as exercise intolerance, a potbelly appearance, and muscle wasting), and possible agitation or mood changes. These signs are more prominent in dogs than in cats and resolve as the dose of medication is slowly decreased over time. A certain percentage of cats (~15–20%) lack the glutathione pathways in their livers to convert prednisone to the active form of the medication (prednisolone); because of this, it is good medical practice to use prednisolone instead of prednisone when treating any cat (since there is no reliable way of knowing which cats can convert this and which ones cannot).

Budesonide

Budesonide is a poorly absorbed topical steroid that has been developed for use in humans with GI inflammation. When given orally, the site of action remains in the GI tract with fewer systemic effects than seen with other oral steroid medications. This can be very helpful in diabetic animals and those with severe systemic side effects.[8]

Cyclophosphamide (Cytoxan®)

Cyclophosphamide is an immunosuppressive medication that may be used in patients that are nonresponsive to corticosteroids or in cases in which corticosteroids cannot be used (i.e., diabetes mellitus, hyperadrenocorticism). Side effects include bone marrow suppression and hemorrhagic cystitis. It is very important that a CBC and platelet count be performed regularly (every 30–90 days) for any animal receiving this medication. Since cyclophosphamide can be absorbed through the skin and is excreted unchanged in the urine, owners should be instructed to wear gloves when administering this drug and when cleaning up urine.[9]

Cyclosporine (Atopica®, Neoral®, Sandimmune®, Cyclosporine-A®)

Cyclosporine has been used to treat immune-mediated diseases in small animals. Cyclosporine primarily inhibits cellular immunity. Cyclosporine is primarily metabolized by the liver and excreted into the bile. It is contraindicated for use in dogs with malignancies, in dogs and cats with renal or liver disease, and in pregnant or nursing patients as it can cause adverse fetal effects and can be found in the milk. The adverse effects of cyclosporine are primarily GI and may include vomiting, anorexia, and diarrhea (which typically occurs within the first week of therapy). With extremely high blood levels (>3000 ng/mL), nephrotoxicity and hepatoxicity is possible. Cyclosporine administration has been associated with the development of neoplasia in humans and in dogs.[10]

The dosing of cyclosporine is varied depending on the form chosen. The Neoral/Atopica or modified forms have a higher bioavailability in small animals and are recommended for use over Sandimmune. Cyclosporine should be administered on an empty stomach; liquid forms have limited palatability, so they may need to be mixed with juices/broths for administration.

Oral absorption of cyclosporine can vary among patients. Therapeutic drug monitoring ensures the dose administered is achieving therapeutic levels (usually 300–500 ng/mL)[11] while not reaching toxic levels. A trough level can be measured 72 h after starting treatment and is performed on blood obtained immediately before the next dose is due. Routine monitoring of drug levels (e.g., every 2–4 weeks) is likely not necessary once the effective dose is achieved but is recommended if treatment efficacy is poor or if adverse effects are suspected. Serial CBC and serum biochemical panels should also be performed at least every 3 months or in accordance to guidelines for the disease being treated.

Azathioprine

Azathioprine is typically used for dogs that are either not responsive to or are having problems with the side effects of corticosteroids. Azathioprine takes 2–3 weeks to become fully effective, and thus corticosteroids should not be tapered off for at least 1 week after starting azathioprine treatment. Azathioprine can also cause bone marrow suppression, so CBC and platelet counts need to be monitored on a regular basis, preferably monthly. GI distress, pancreatitis, and hepatotoxicity can also be seen; consider monitoring for these adverse effects with periodic blood chemistries or if clinical signs are noted. This drug is toxic for bone marrow in cats and should be used with extreme caution.[6]

Chlorambucil

Like azathioprine, chlorambucil takes 2–3 weeks to become fully effective and should be reserved only for those cases where severe disease is present or lack of response is seen with steroid use. It has a much less toxic effect in cats, and if serial CBC and platelet counts are monitored for myelosuppression, it is much safer for use than cyclophosphamide.[6]

Sulfasalazine

The anti-inflammatory sulfasalazine is a salicylate, not a corticosteroid. It is most useful in the treatment of colonic IBD as colonic bacterial cleavage is necessary to release the active form of the drug. Animals taking sulfasalazine can develop keratoconjunctivitis sicca (dry eye), anorexia, nausea, vomiting, diarrhea, and abdominal pain. Since many of the GI signs are present already, proper monitoring and a thorough patient history can control these problems.[6]

Antibiotics

Many antibiotics may be prescribed for patients with GI disease and this chapter will not specifically cover them all (e.g., amoxicillin, enrofloxacin). Of these antibiotics, metronidazole, tetracycline and tylosin are antibiotics that can be used alone in combination with or in conjunction with the anti-inflammatory/immunosuppressive agents.

Erythromycin

Erythromycin is a macrolide antibiotic that is also used as a prokinetic agent (medication that promotes gastric motility). It enhances gastric emptying by inducing antral contractions and may be used in patients with gastric reflux esophagitis.[2] It is available in both oral and injectable forms. Adverse effects include pain on IM injection, thrombophlebitis on IV injection, and possible intestinal distress (increased gastric emptying of larger food particles).

Metronidazole

Metronidazole is both an antibacterial (anaerobes) and an antiprotozoal medication available in both injectable and oral forms. Adverse effects include lethargy, nausea, anorexia, and, occasionally, vomiting and diarrhea. Hepatic and encephalopathic problems can occur in sensitive animals or when doses are too high. Metronidazole is very bitter tasting. If the animal does not swallow the pill the first time, considerable drooling can occur. This can cause the pill to dissolve too quickly, preventing redosing with the same pill.

Tetracycline

This antibiotic may be utilized in cases of SIBO, primarily in dogs as cats do not tolerate it very well. Tetracycline should not be used in young animals as it can cause discoloration of the teeth. The adverse effects are similar to metronidazole.

Tylosin

This macrolide antibiotic is used primarily for chronic colitis. It is also used in cases of SIBO, antibiotic enteropathy, and diarrhea caused by *C. perfringens*, and as an adjunctive treatment for IBD. The adverse effects are mild and include anorexia and diarrhea.

Gastromucosal protectants

Sucralfate is a locally acting treatment for ulcers and may also be a gastromucosal protectant. This medication works best if administered on an empty stomach and in an acidic environment. For this reason, it is best to administer sucralfate at least 0.5 h prior to H_2 antagonist or antacids. Sucralfate may reduce the bioavailability of other medications, and separating concurrent medication administration by up to 2 h is advised. The use of sucralfate slurry, made by dissolving the tablet (or partial tablet) in 3–5 mL of water, may be advantageous. The exact mode of action for sucralfate is unknown, but it is believed to react with stomach acid to form a paste-like complex that binds selectively to proteins at the ulcer site by way of electrostatic interactions. It may also have cytoprotective effects. Adverse effects are uncommon; rarely, constipation may occur.

Digestive enzymes

Pancreatic enzymes in the form of pancrelipase pancretin (more commonly known by the brand names Pancreazyme® and Viokase®) may be prescribed to test for or to treat exocrine pancreatic enzyme deficiency. The enzymes help to digest and absorb fats, proteins, and carbohydrates. Usually in powder form (although tablets and capsules are available), this medication is mixed with the food; some manufacturers advise to allow the food to stand for 15–20 min prior to feeding. Adverse effects are usually only seen with high dosages and are primarily GI distress. If given in tablet form, food and/or water should be given afterward to prevent oral or esophageal ulceration. Humans handling this medication should avoid inhalation of the powder and may develop skin irritation; hand washing is advised after handling.

Laxatives

Hydrophilic laxatives

These over-the-counter laxatives may decrease fluidity of existing bowel content and increase fecal bulk. Compounds that may be tried for this purpose include methylcellulose (Citrucel), psyllium (Metamucil), and calcium polycarbophil (Fiberall).

Emollient laxatives

These laxatives, also called surfactant stool softeners, are usually dioctyl sodium, calcium, or potassium sulfosuccinate. They are anionic detergents that reduce surface tension, which enhances fat absorption and impairs water absorption.[12] This allows the water to penetrate the ingesta, thereby softening the stool. They are available over-the-counter in oral, suppository, and enema forms. These laxatives should be used with caution in animals with preexisting dehydration or electrolyte imbalances as these conditions may be exacerbated. Common names are D-S-S® and Colace® and these laxatives are often in disposable enemas such as Enema-DSS®.

Lubricant laxatives

Mineral oil and white petrolatum are the most commonly utilized lubricants; they are also found in hair ball remedy products such as Laxatone® and Kat-A-Lax®. If the liquid form is administered orally, the use of a stomach tube is advised to avoid the possibility of aspiration lipid pneumonitis.[2,12] The majority of the oil will pass through the GI tract into the colon. Lubricant laxatives act by easing the passage of stool and inhibiting water absorption by the colon. Mineral oil or petrolatum may also be administered as an enema, either as is or diluted with warm water; the dosage varies based on the size of the patient, the degree of constipation, the response to previous enemas, and clinician preferences.

Osmotic laxatives

The osmotic laxatives work by stimulating colonic fluid secretion, thereby increasing bulk and water content of the ingesta. Lactulose is the most common osmotic laxative used; colonic bacteria metabolize the lactulose forming acids which exert osmotic pressure, drawing fluid into the colon.[2] Lactulose is also utilized in patients with hepatic encephalopathy due to its acidification effects, which draws ammonium from the blood into the colon where it is trapped as ammonium ions and expelled in the feces.[2] Lactulose should be used with caution in patients with diabetes mellitus as there is free lactose in the syrup. The solution is slightly sweet, which may make administration difficult in cats. The dose is adjusted based on efficacy (e.g., consistency of the stool).

SECTION 5 FEEDING TUBES

Addressing the nutritional needs of our hospitalized and critical care patients can dramatically improve their outcomes, and it may also allow them to return home sooner. Oral enteral nutrition is the ideal route, but if the patient is unable or unwilling to consume at least 85% of their calculated resting energy requirements (RERs), then another feeding route needs to be utilized.

Feeding tubes

When oral nutrition is not an option, what other options are available? There are a number of feeding tube options available; the choice of tube will be dependent on the condition of the patient, the disease being addressed, the expense of administration, the availability of intensive care facilities, the preferred food, and the anticipated length of feeding assistance (Table 8.5.1).

The best feeding tubes for prolonged use are made of polyurethane or silicone. For short-term feeding, usually less than 10 days, polyvinylchloride (PVC) tubes can be used. These are not appropriate for long-term feeding because they tend to become stiff with prolonged use, causing additional discomfort for the patient. Silicone is softer and more flexible than other tube materials and has a greater tendency to stretch and collapse. Poly-

Table 8.5.1 Tube feeding comparisons

Type of tube	Condition	Disease	ICU costs	Food type used	Length of time
Nasoesophageal or nasogastric	Not recommended for patients that are vomiting or those with respiratory disease	Short-term anorexia, supplement oral intake	$	Liquid ± thinning required, CRI, or bolus	Short term, in-hospital use only (3–7 days)
Esophagostomy	Not recommended for patients that are vomiting or those with respiratory disease	Hepatic lipidosis, anorexia, oral surgery or trauma, cancer	$$	Liquid, recovery diet, or gruel commercial diet based on tube size, CRI, or bolus	Long term, in-hospital and at-home use, (1–20 weeks, depending on tube type used)
Gastrostomy	Can be used on patients that are vomiting or that have respiratory diseases	Pancreatitis, hepatic lipidosis, anorexia, esophageal strictures, oral surgery or trauma, cancer	$$$	Liquid, recovery diet, or gruel commercial diet based on tube size; CRI or bolus	Long-term use, can be permanent, depending on tube type used
Jejunostomy	Can be used on patients that are vomiting or that have respiratory disease	Pancreatitis, intestinal anastomosis, coma	$$$$	Liquid diet, CRI or bolus	Short term, in-hospital use only (3–10 days)

urethane is stronger than silicone, allowing for thinner tube walls and a greater internal diameter despite the same French size. Both the silicone and polyurethane tubes do not disintegrate or become brittle *in situ*, providing a longer tube life. The French unit measures the outer lumen diameter of a tube and is equal to 0.33 mm.[1]

While assisted feeding (force feeding) can be used to provide the necessary nutrition, this is usually too stressful to the patient, not to mention also stressful to the owner. Seldom is this method able to deliver the volume of nutrients necessary to meet the patients' needs on a regular basis.

Nasoesophageal and nasogastric tube placement

NE tubes are useful for providing short-term nutritional support, usually less than 10 days. They can be used in patients with a functional esophagus, stomach, and intestines. NE tubes are contraindicated in patients that are vomiting, comatose, or lack a gag reflex.[1,2]

Supplies needed include lidocaine drops (ophthalmic drops can be used); 5- to 8-Fr tube with length sufficient to reach the distal esophagus, sterile lubricant, suture or glue, Luer slip catheter plug, and Elizabethan collar.

The length of tube to be inserted is determined by measuring from the nasal planum along the side of the patient to the caudal margin of the last rib. This indicates the ideal tube placement; mark this area with either a piece of tape or a permanent marker. After instilling a few drops of the lidocaine into the nose, wait 10–15 min for full analgesic effect. A sterile catheter of sufficient length (8 Fr × 42 in. in dogs >15 kg, 5 Fr × 36 in. in dogs <15 kg) is advanced into the nose. The tube should be passed with the tip directed in a caudoventral, medial direction into the ventrolateral aspect of the external nares. The head should be held in a normal static position. As soon as the tip of the catheter reaches the medial septum at the floor of the nasal cavity in dogs, the external nares are pushed dorsally; this opens the ventral meatus, ensuring passage of the tube into the oropharynx. In cats, the tube can be inserted initially in a ventromedial direction and continued directly into the oropharynx. The tube is inserted until the tape tab or marked area is reached. To evaluate proper tube placement, 3–15 mL or sterile water or saline can be injected through the tube and the animal evaluated for coughing. Coughing would indicate the tube is placed in the lungs, not the esophagus. Lateral radiographs may also be taken to confirm tube location. After confirmation of position, the tube is secured with either glue or sutures at the external nares and along the dorsal midline along the bridge of the nose. Continue to direct the tube over the head and secure with a bandage around the neck. Place the catheter plug into the catheter. An Elizabethan collar is used in most animals to prevent inadvertent removal of the tube (Figure 8.5.1).[1–3]

Complications include epistaxis, lack of tolerance of the procedure, and inadvertent/intentional removal by the patient. These tubes should not be used in vomiting patients or in those with respiratory disease.[1–4]

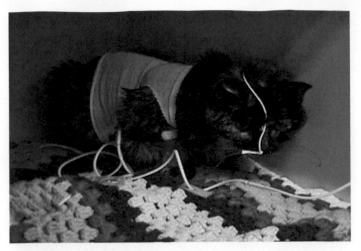

Figure 8.5.1   Nasoesophageal tube in a cat receiving CRI infusion of diet.

To place a nasogastric tube, follow the same procedure but measure the length to 3–4 in. past the last rib. Nasogastric tubes increase the risk of gastroesophageal reflux, increasing the incidence of esophageal strictures. This is due to passage through the cardiac sphincter of the stomach, allowing reflux of gastric acids into the esophagus.

Due to the small internal diameter of these tubes, only liquid enteral diets can be used. They can either be fed through a syringe pump as a continuous rate infusion or bolus fed. If feeding through a syringe pump, completely change the delivery equipment every 24 h to help prevent bacterial growth within the system. Tube clogging is a common problem; a syringe pump may help to decrease the incidence as will flushing well before and after bolus feeding. If the tube becomes clogged, replacement may be necessary. Diluting the liquid with water may also help, though this further decreases the caloric concentration of the diet, increasing the volume necessary to meet the caloric needs.

When removing, the tube may be simply pulled out after the glue or sutures are removed. Ensure that the tube is kinked prior to removal to decrease the chance of inadvertently aspirating fluid into the lungs during removal.

Esophagostomy tube placement

Esophagostomy tube placement does require anesthesia to be performed, but it does not need to be to a surgical depth of anesthesia. The animal should be deep enough to allow placement of a mouth gag to protect the placer's hand and equipment. The patient should be heavily sedated or anesthetized, intubated, and placed in lateral recumbency (usually, right lateral is easier for placement if you are right-handed). The entire lateral cervical region from ventral midline to near dorsal midline is clipped and surgically prepped.

Supplies needed include large Kelly or Carmalt forceps, scalpel blade, appropriately sized tube, tape or suture to secure, and Luer slip catheter plug.

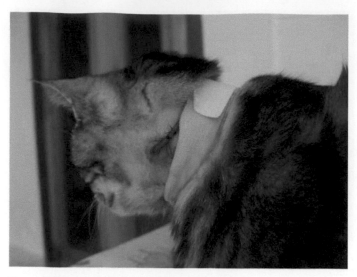

Figure 8.5.2 Esophagostomy tube placement.

One technique uses a large curved Kelly or Carmalt forceps inserted into the proximal cervical esophagus. The tip of the forceps is turned laterally and pressure is applied in an outward direction, causing a bulge in the cervical tissue so the instrument tip can be seen and palpated externally. A small skin incision, just large enough to accommodate the feeding tube, is made over the tip of the forceps. In small dogs and cats, the tip of the forceps is forced bluntly through the esophagus; in larger dogs, a deeper incision is made to allow passage of the tip of the forceps through the esophagus. The tube is premeasured as with an NE tube, except the exit is in the mid- to caudal esophagus. A convenient landmark would be the wings of the atlas; the exit hole should be in line with this reference point. The distal tip of the tube is grasped with the forceps, pulled in to the esophagus and out through the mouth, then turned around and redirected into the esophagus. The tube is secured with tape and sutures. A light bandage is applied around the neck; whether to apply triple antibiotic ointment to the site is an individual choice. Place the catheter plug into the catheter (Figure 8.5.2).[1-4]

There are also tube placement systems commercially available for esophagostomy tube placement.

Complications include tube displacement due to vomiting or removal by the patient, skin infection around the exit site, and biting off of the tube end by the patient after vomiting.

Depending on the technique used and the size of the patient, an 8- to 20-Fr catheter may be used; the large bore of these catheters allow for feeding of a gruel recovery diet, sometimes without dilution with water. These catheters are also easy for clients to use and to maintain as long as vomiting is not a problem.

When removing, the tube may be simply pulled out after the sutures are removed. The exit hole is allowed to heal by second intension. A light bandage may be applied for the first 12 h.

Gastrostomy tube placement

Gastrostomy tubes can be placed either endoscopically, blindly, or surgically. All three techniques require general anesthesia; this does not need to be a surgical depth of anesthesia. Endoscopic placement allows for visualization of the esophagus and stomach as well as biopsy collection from the stomach and proximal duodenum and foreign body removal. Blind placement allows a gastrostomy tube to be inserted without the investment in an endoscopic unit. Surgical placement is useful during surgical exploratory laparotomy or when the scope cannot be passed through the esophagus due to trauma or esophageal strictures.

Supplies needed include an endoscope, endoscopic grabbers, Pezzer catheter, 14-ga. needle or catheter, 1–2 lengths of #2 suture material ~3 ft long, catheter guide, sterile lubricant, and Luer slip catheter plug.

For percutaneous endoscopic gastrostomy (PEG) tube placement, the patient is anesthetized, placed in right lateral recumbency. The left flank is clipped and surgically prepped from 1–2 in. above the last caudal rib to 2–3 in. beyond the last caudal rib. The area should be 4–6 in. in diameter. A 20- to 24-Fr Pezzer catheter is used for placement; these are available singly and as kits. The endoscope is advanced into the stomach and is used to insufflate air. This helps to ensure that the spleen or omentum does not become entrapped between the stomach and the body wall. An assistant digitally palpates the external body wall ~1–2 cm behind the ninth rib; the palpation can be seen internally and can be used to confirm correct placement of the feeding tube. When the site is confirmed, a 14-ga. needle or catheter is introduced into the stomach through the body wall; a length of #2 suture is threaded through the needle into the stomach and grasped with endoscopic grabbers; and the string and scope are removed from the stomach. Ensure that assistants maintain a hold on their end of the suture and that it does not get pulled thorough as the scope is removed. The catheter guide is slid onto the suture and used to secure the Pezzer catheter (it helps to bevel the end of the Pezzer catheter to help it fit into the catheter guide). Using the 14-ga. needle, push it through the Pezzer catheter then thread the suture through the needle; remove the needle and secure the suture. Pull everything tautly; apply the sterile lubricant to the feeding tube liberally, and using firm and steady pressure, pull the catheter guide with the Pezzer catheter attached through the body wall; it may be necessary to use a scalpel blade to enlarge the hole in the body wall to allow passage of the tube assembly. It is important to maintain firm and steady pressure throughout the entire passage of the feeding tube from the mouth through the body wall. Once the tube is through the body wall, pull the mushroom tip firmly against the stomach wall; in most animals, this can be felt from the outside. An external tube assembly should be made to prevent the tube from migrating back into the stomach; be sure to leave a little extra room (~1 in.) to allow for tube movement and for weight gain. Place the Luer plug into the catheter (Figure 8.5.3).[1-4]

A minimum of 12 h is needed for a temporary stoma to form before feeding can begin; the feeding tube should be left in place for a minimum of 7–10 days to allow a permanent stoma to form before removal. The tubes can be left in a long term (1–6 months) without replacement; when replaced with another PEG tube, a low profile silicone tube, or a foley-type feeding tube, the stoma can be used for the rest of the patient's life (Figure 8.5.4).

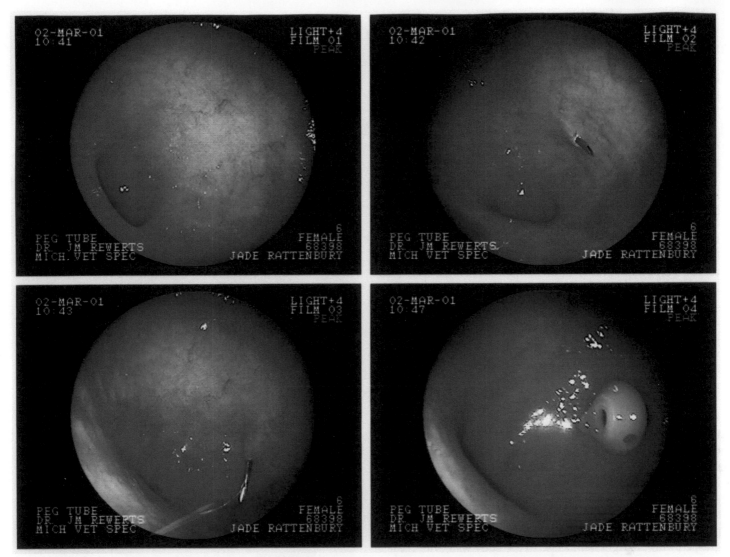

Figure 8.5.3 View via gastroscopy of PEG tube placement. Image courtesy of Dr. Jennifer Rewerts from Michigan Veterinary Specialists.

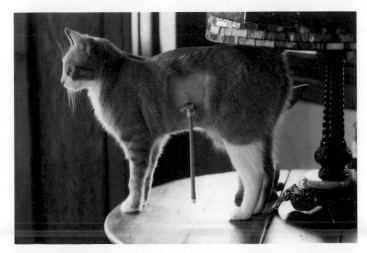

Figure 8.5.4 Author's cat (Benny) at home with PEG tube in place.

Complications associated with PEG tubes include those seen from tube placement such as splenic laceration, gastric hemorrhage, and pneumoperitoneum. Delayed complications can also be seen, such as vomiting, aspiration pneumonia, tube removal, tube migration, and peritonitis and stoma infection.[1]

Blind percutaneous gastrostomy tube placement involves basically the same technique as endoscopic placement, but a large plastic or steel tube is used instead of the endoscope and a firm wire is used instead of the suture. The catheter is the same as in the endoscopic insertion technique. Reported complications are the same as for PEG tubes, though the risk of splenic, stomach, or omental laceration is greater. Contraindications to using the blind technique include severe obesity, which would make palpation of the end of the tube difficult, and esophageal disease.

Surgical placement has been largely superseded by endoscopic placement because of the ease and speed of placement, lower cost, and decreased morbidity. A surgical approach may be indicated in obese animals, in those with esophageal disease, or when laparotomy is already scheduled. To place a surgical gastrostomy, a larger incision is needed into the stomach, and the exit location is sometimes hard to locate because of the position on the surgical table. Surgical placement involves placing purse string sutures around the catheter to secure it as well as attaching the stomach to the body wall.

Gastrostomy tube placement is the technique of choice for long-term enteral support. These tubes are well tolerated by the patient, produce minimal discomfort, allow feeding of either gruel recovery diets of blenderized commercial foods, and can be easily managed by owners at home.[2] Patients are able to eat normally with gastrostomy tubes in place and can easily be used as a nutritional supplement until the patient is totally self-feeding. For patients that are difficult to medicate and require long-term medications, many medicines can also be given through the feeding tube. Gastrostomy tubes can also be used for rehydration therapy as with renal failure. It is typically less stressful for clients to administer fluids through a feeding tube as opposed to under the skin or intravenously. An additional benefit to this use is that regular tap water can be used, further reducing the cost to the clients. The major disadvantage of gastrostomy tubes is the need for general anesthesia and the risk of peritonitis (Figure 8.5.5).[2]

For animals requiring long-term management, the initial Pezzer catheter can be replaced with either low profile silicone tubes or with foley-type gastrostomy tubes. Both of these types can be placed through the external stoma site without the endoscope. Sedation or anesthesia may be necessary based on the individual patient (Figures 8.5.6–8.5.8).

For removal, if the tube has been in place 16 weeks or less, the tube may be simply removed. This is best accomplished by placing the patient in right lateral recumbency. The tube is grasped with the right hand close to the body wall, with the left hand holding the animal. Pull firmly and consistently to the right in an upward motion. Some force may be required for this. It is also helpful to ensure that the patient has been fasted, and to place a towel over the tube site to catch any gastric contents that may be removed along with the feeding tube. If the tube has been in longer than 16 weeks, the incidence of tube breakage is much higher. Depending on where the breakage occurs determines the need to be endoscopically retrieved. Larger patients can easily pass retained parts; smaller patients may need to have them retrieved.

Alternately, tubes may also be endoscopically removed, but this would require anesthesia. The feeding tube is cut off at the

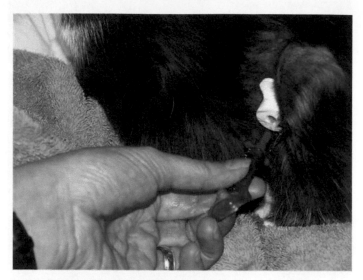

Figure 8.5.6   Low profile feeding tube in place.

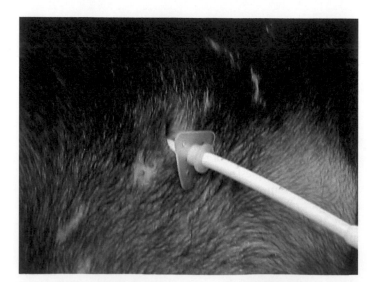

Figure 8.5.5   Great Dane with feeding tube in place for over 3 years. Note mature stoma site.

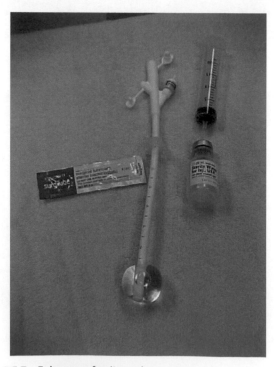

Figure 8.5.7   Foley-type feeding tube.

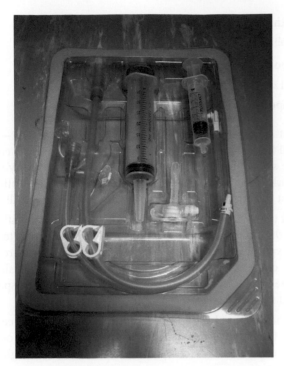

Figure 8.5.8   Low profile (button-type) feeding tube.

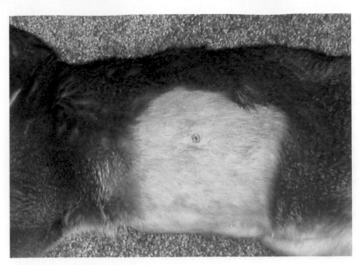

Figure 8.5.9   PEG tube site 24 h after removal.

level of the skin and pushed into the stomach from the outside. Using the endoscopic grabbers, the remaining parts are grabbed and removed through the esophagus (Figure 8.5.9).

The exit site is cleaned well with soap and water and then dried. Antibiotic ointment may be applied to the site, with the primary purpose to stop the flow of gastric contents out of the hole rather than protect from an infection. The exit hole is allowed to heal by second intension. A light bandage may be applied for the first 12 h or however long the animal will allow.

Jejunostomy tube placement

Jejunostomy feeding is indicated when the upper GI tract must be rested or when pancreatic stimulation must be decreased. Jejunal tubes can be placed either surgically or threaded through a gastrostomy tube for transpyloric placement. Standard gastro-jejunal tubes designed for humans are unreliable in dogs due to frequent reflux of the jejunal portion of the tube back into the stomach. Investigation is ongoing involving endoscopic place-ment of transpyloric jejunal tubes through PEG tubes. This tech-nique requires skill and patience to be successful in animals.

Supplies needed for placement include 5- to 8-Fr PVC tubing, suture, and Luer slip catheter plug.

Due to the small diameter of these tubes and the location, liquid enteral diets are recommended. Because the jejunum has minimal storage capacity compared to the stomach, continuous rate infusion using a syringe pump is the preferred method of delivery.

Common complications include osmotic diarrhea and vomit-ing. It is recommended that the jejunal tube be left in place for

7–10 days to allow adhesions to form around the tube site and to prevent leakage back into the abdomen.[2,4] Completely chang-ing the delivery equipment every 24 h will help prevent bacterial growth within the system. Clogging is a common problem; a syringe pump may help to decrease the incidence as will flushing well every 4 h.

When removing, the tube may be simply pulled out after the sutures are removed. The exit hole is allowed to heal by second intension. A light bandage may be applied for the first 12 h.

Conclusion

The enteral route is the preferred method of nutritional support in patients with functional GI tracts. Many tube and food choices are available and can be tailored to fit the individual patient and condition. Do not let ignorance or fear prevent you from provid-ing your patients with nutritional support; appropriate nutrition should not be treated as an afterthought.

Feeding tube management and complications

A complete feeding plan should be done for each animal in which a feeding tube has been placed with written feeding direc-tions given to the owner.[5,6] Since many owners are unfamiliar with the use of syringes and the feeding procedure itself, plan on an extended discharge for each animal. This appointment should include instructions on care of the feeding tube, how to feed, amount and frequency of the feedings, and potential complica-tions; this typically takes 30–45 min.

There are multiple veterinary recovery diets that are available in a gruel form, which easily pass through most of the larger-bore feeding tubes (12 Fr and higher). Sometimes, adding as little as 1–2 tablespoons of water (15–30 mL) to the can of food will greatly increase ease of passage. However, it should be noted that adding excessive amounts of water will dilute the diet and result in lower calories (kilocalories) per milliliter. If needed, home-made gruel diets can be prepared from commercial diets. The disadvantage of using these diets is not knowing the caloric amount found in each milliliter of the final mixture or the final volume achieved after mixing. Additional math is required to calculate the caloric content of the final product. The total volume achieved after mixing with water is measured, and this amount is divided by the kilocalories per can or cup used to make the final product. This will give you the final kilocalories per millimeter (kcal/mL) amount. These diets also tend to fall out of suspension after they have been mixed with water if not well blended and increases the possibility of tube blockage due to larger food particles in the mixture.

Mechanical complications

Mechanical complications include both tube obstruction and premature removal or dislodgement of the tube from the site of placement. The most common problem, tube obstruction, can be prevented in most cases by proper tube maintenance and blending of food.[6,7] Food should never be allowed to sit in the tube and the tube should be flushed with warm water after *every* feeding, administration of medications, or whenever GI contents are aspirated through the tube, as when checking residuals. When using the feeding tube to administer medications, only one medication at a time should be given through the tube, and some advise that it should be given separately from the food.[6,8] This will help to prevent drug-to-drug interactions as well as drug-to-food interactions, as not all medications and enteral foods are compatible with one another. Certain medications can form solid obstructions in feeding tubes after mixture and prior to getting to the stomach Therefore, even though it is common practice to administer certain medications with food, it may not be advisable. If administered in this fashion, instruct clients to crush all pills in a mortar and pestle prior to adding to the food.

There may be increased difficulty in passing the food through the feeding tube if the holes in the feeding tube become clogged, due to either insufficient flushing after feeding or the accumulation of hair swallowed while grooming. If after massaging the length of the tube to break up any obstructions it is still obstructed, the first attempt to open the tube is to try to flush the clog out using warm water and the feeding syringe. Hold the tube firmly and push the water with moderate force. If the clog is not bad, this technique may work. If it is still clogged, try switching to a carbonated beverage (anecdotally, colas work the best). Instill the cola into the feeding tube and allow it to sit for a period of time (approximately 5 min). As an alternative, some practitioners have suggested the use of pancreatic enzymes mixed with water and various other mixtures instilled into the tube to break up the clog.[6,9]

This following technique is used by the author for stubborn clogs and has proven to be very effective in the removal of the clogs. This technique is used after the above techniques have failed to relieve the clog in a feeding tube. This tube unplugging technique can be used with 20 Fr or larger Pezzer gastrostomy tubes and 20 Fr or larger esophagostomy tubes:

Use with *extreme* caution . . .

Supplies:

10-Fr polypropylene catheter

10- to 12-mL Luer slip syringe

1-in. tape

1. Cut a bevel on the end of the polypropylene catheter—this will be sharp! Measure the length of the catheter to either the site of the obstruction or the outside of the body wall. Mark with a piece of 1-in. tape. Do not pass the cut catheter past the body wall—it will perforate the stomach wall!

2. Fill the syringe with warm water then pass the cut catheter to the level of the obstruction. Attach the syringe to the polypropylene catheter and use your fingers to pinch around the end of the feeding tube to prevent backflow. Flush the water into the catheter with force. You may need to aspirate and flush repeatedly.

3. If the plug has been in the tube for >12 h, you may need to carefully "ream" out the plug with the beveled end of the catheter; continue to try to flush the water through the catheter.

4. This technique has always worked for me, and I have never had to replace a tube because it was plugged. The sooner the clients bring the animal in, the better (Figures 8.5.10 and 8.5.11).

Premature tube removal or dislodgement is best prevented by choosing the most appropriate tube for the animal, properly securing the tube, and by judicious use of collars and wraps when appropriate. Other factors that may influence premature tube removal or dislodgement are durability of the particular tube, pruritus from site infection, activity level of the patient, owner compliance, damage to the tube from animal bites, and balloon breakage. Whenever the location of the tube is in doubt, it should be checked radiographically. While most tubes are

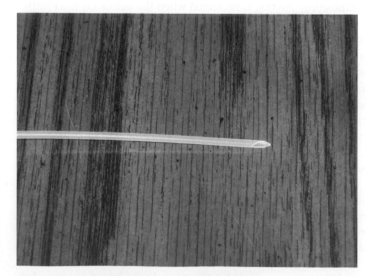

Figure 8.5.10   Bevel cut to polypropylene catheter.

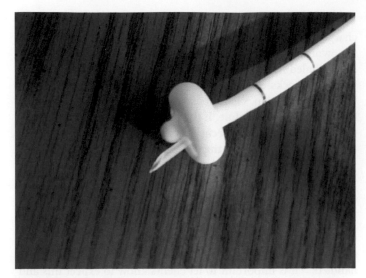

Figure 8.5.11 Example of what not to do. The catheter has passed through the end of the feeding tube. This could result in puncture of the stomach wall.

radiopaque, a sterile contract media (e.g., Omnipaque') can be infused through the tube to check for leaks into the peritoneal or thoracic cavity.[9,10] Barium should not be used to check tube placement due to the irritating effect of barium when outside of the GI tract.

Gastrointestinal complications

Some of the GI complications seen with tube feeding are related to the feeding itself. Food that is administered too quickly, in too large of a quantity or at the wrong temperature, can all cause nausea, vomiting, or abdominal discomfort. These signs can also be related to the patient's underlying disease process or to a complication of medications the patient is receiving.[8,10]

Liquid enteral diets are typically very low residue and are likely to cause a soft stool, if not actual diarrhea, in a normal animal, let alone in one who is already ill. Likewise, most recovery diets, in both liquid and gruel forms, are high in fat; a patient with impaired fat digestion and absorption may develop steatorrhea when fed these diets.[6]

Another cause of diarrhea not typically thought of is the medications that we are giving to the animals, whether they are orally administered or administered through the feeding tubes. Many liquid oral forms of medications are hypertonic or contain sorbital (a nonabsorbable sugar) and may cause, at least in part, diarrhea.[6] Canned pumpkin, 5–15 mL per feeding, will usually resolve the diarrhea. Aliquots of pumpkin can be prepared ahead of time in ice cube trays and stored in a freezer bag until needed. The total amount of each feeding will need to be adjusted accordingly.

We also need to remember that a number of commonly used antibiotics, analgesic agents, and other drugs can cause nausea, vomiting, and GI ileus. This can contribute to the discomfort our patients are feeling.

Constipation is not an unusual complication seen in patients with feeding tubes. As these patients can be fairly weak from muscle loss and metabolic derangement, the development of constipation is not unexpected. Adding lactulose to the diet will often solve this problem, 1–2 mL per meal; adjust as needed to maintain stool consistency.[8,9]

Metabolic complications

There are two types of metabolic complications that patients with feeding tubes can develop. The first is the result of the patient's inability to assimilate certain nutrients. This can best be anticipated by doing a proper nutritional assessment of the patient before developing the nutritional plan. The other type of metabolic complication is called refeeding syndrome. For more information on the refeeding syndrome, please refer to Chapter 14.

Metabolic complications of any type are less likely to occur if estimated caloric needs are conservative. Current recommendations are to initiate feeding at caloric amounts equal to the patient's calculated RERs without the addition of any "illness requirements."[6,9]

Infectious complications

The types of infectious complications that can occur in tube-fed patients include contamination of the enterally fed formulas, peristomal cellulitis, septic peritonitis, and aspiration pneumonia.

Microbial contamination of the food is easily avoided by following basic hygiene in the preparation and storage of the food. Blenderized foods should be prepared daily, and opened commercial liquid diets should be kept refrigerated and discarded after 48 h. When food is being delivered via a syringe pump, no more than 6-h worth of food should be set up at a time. One of the biggest sources of contamination is inadequate cleaning of the equipment used for the preparation and delivery of foods.[6,8,9] Syringes, containers, and tubing used for preparing, storing, and delivering food should be discarded after use. Items that are reused, such as blenders and storage containers, should be cleaned thoroughly and preferably sterilized each time they are used. The equipment used to deliver the food should also be replaced every 24 h. This includes the syringes and delivery tubes and, if the food is hung, the administration bag.

Peristomal cellulitis can be seen with esophagostomy, gastrostomy, and jejunostomy tubes. This can usually be avoided by ensuring that the tube is not secured too tightly to the body wall and by keeping the site clean and protected. Septic peritonitis can develop in patients where the gastrostomy or jejunostomy tube has become dislodged or removed before a permanent stoma had formed (Figure 8.5.12).[9,10] Less commonly, but more of a concern, is the development of septic peritonitis associated with dislodgement of the stomach from the gastric portion of the feeding tube without any external evidence of problems. In these situations, the patient is fed through the feeding tube; however, instead of the food being delivered into the stomach,

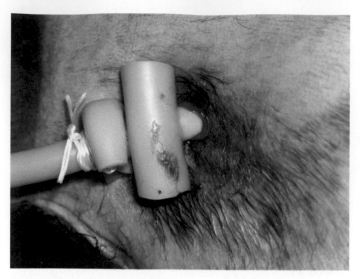

Figure 8.5.12 Peristomal cellulitis.

it is deposited in the abdominal cavity. These patients often display marked and rapid abdominal pain. Proper tube selection can help prevent these problems. Proper button or balloon size is determined as one that is large enough to secure the tube in the stomach lumen but not so small so as to easily become displaced out of the stomach and into the abdomen. Some clinicians add a second "inner flange" to avoid premature removal, dislodgement, or displacement. Body wraps, shirts, or Elizabethan collars may be necessary to prevent the patient from accidentally or intentionally prematurely removing the tube. Ensuring that a mature stoma has formed prior to tube removal can help to prevent peritonitis. Patients that are malnourished or are receiving medications that impair wound healing may take longer to develop a mature stoma than would healthy patients.

Aspiration pneumonia can be seen in patients that have previously developed aspiration pneumonia, laryngeal paralysis, or prior surgery for laryngeal paralysis, patients with impaired mental status, patients with neurological injuries, patients with reduced or absent cough or gag reflexes, and those on mechanical ventilation.[5,7,9] Feeding patients in any of these categories prepylorically puts them at risk of aspiration of food. Viable alternatives would include jejunostomy tubes (although even these patients are at risk for retrograde reflux into the stomach) and parenteral nutrition. Lastly, caution should be used when feeding patients with NE or esophagostomy tubes using CRI.[6] These types of tubes can be regurgitated and the tip of the tube could relocate in the pharynx and place the patient at risk for pulmonary aspiration.

Hospital management

Patients should be allowed out to exercise for 20–30 min approximately 1 h before feeding, two to three times daily. This can be started even while the CRI feedings are being done; just disconnect the syringe pump, flush the line with water, and cap. Exercise has been found to greatly enhance both gastric motility and patient attitude.[9]

Very few patients do poorly with their feeding tube after discharge, particularly if good communication is established with the owners and regular rechecks are scheduled. Rechecks should be scheduled with the technician managing the case. This author prefers rechecks every 2 weeks until the tube is removed, but individual clinician, client, or patient preference may dictate a different recheck schedule. If the tube will be in place long term (months to years), these rechecks can become less frequent once the animal stabilizes and the owners become more comfortable with tube maintenance and management.

Potential postdischarge complications

Granulation tissue normally forms around the tube site on the outside and may be quite pink and can even bleed when handled.[8,9] It is important to let clients know to expect this and that it is normal. This is the tissue that allows the hole to close after the tube is removed. Cats with dark hair coats (including tabbies) will often have hair growth in a dark ring around the tube site, and it may be thicker than the surrounding hair. Many clients will think that this is necrosis and become very concerned; a quick warning to expect this will greatly ease their minds.

What do you do about the patient that insists on chewing on its tube? A simple solution is to place a baby's T-shirt or onesie on a cat; usually, an infant's size 6–9 months works well. For large patients, larger shirts can be used. Use a T-shirt that has a fitted neck, not the lap shoulders type. Once the T-shirt is on, place a piece of 1-in. porous tape near the end of the feeding tube, tuck the tube up under the T-shirt, and use a safety pin to pin the tape to the T-shirt. This makes removal easier for feeding and decreases the risk of pinning through the tube and damaging it.

Once the patient goes home, tube feedings are continued even after the patient begins oral self-feeding. Owners are given instructions to always have fresh food and water available for the convalescing patient. When the desired weight is reached, tube feedings are decreased by 25–50% depending on the oral intake. The tube can be removed after the patient has reached its desired weight, has recovered from the trauma, or has finished chemotherapy treatment and has been totally self-feeding for 2 weeks without showing any signs of weight loss. Many feeding tubes can be maintained long term, and the same stoma hole can be used for repeated tube placements.

Conclusion

Typically, animals feel much better and the owners are very happy with the results they see when using a feeding tube. Feeding tubes do require routine daily care such as cleaning around the tube site and flushing of the feeding tube with water, but the tubes need not be used every day to feed the patient. The use of feeding tubes can give many clients the benefit of enjoying their pet for a longer period of time and of having a better quality of life for both of them.

SECTION 6 FOOD INTOLERANCE AND FOOD ALLERGY

An adverse reaction to food is an abnormal response to an ingested food or food additive.[1] These reactions can be divided up into immunological and nonimmunological in origin. An immunological reaction is caused by an antibody immune complex or a cell-mediated immune reaction. An adverse reaction that is nonimmune based can be caused by enzyme deficiencies, food toxicities, or pharmacological reactions to food ingredients.[2]

Adverse food reactions are a common cause of chronic GI disease.[3] In cats, this is the second most common dermatologic disorder, after flea allergy hypersensitivity, and is seen more commonly in cats than in dogs.[4]

Nonimmunological reactions to foods can be seen with nutrient excesses (vitamin A or D toxicosis), food contamination with bacteria, metabolites or endotoxins, specific foods (e.g., onions, chocolate), and toxic food preservatives (benzoic acid, propylene glycol in cats).[1]

Clinical signs

Clinical signs may affect more than one body system, with the most common sites being dermatologic (pruritus) and GI (primarily vomiting and diarrhea).[3] GI signs with concurrent cutaneous signs may also be seen. GI signs are seen in 10–15% of dogs and cats presenting with cutaneous signs. A peripheral eosinophilia is also seen in 20–50% of feline cases.[1]

Clinical response to treatment can be slow, and risk of reoccurrence with dietary indiscretion is an ongoing concern.[3] Strict owner compliance is essential to successful treatment. Eosinophilic granulomas and respiratory and other GI signs can be seen in addition to the above-mentioned vomiting, diarrhea, and dermatologic signs. Concurrent hypersensitivities (e.g., flea bite hypersensitivity) may present a complicating factor in diagnosis and management and is seen in up to 30% of cats with food allergies.[1,4]

Allergies may develop after prolonged exposure to one brand, one type, or one form of food. Adverse reactions may develop after a single exposure as immune amplification is not necessary (Table 8.6.1).[1]

Causes

Risk factors associated with development of food allergies are difficult to document but include certain foods or food ingredients, poorly digestible protein sources, diseases that increase intestinal mucosal permeability (e.g., viral enteritis), selective immunoglobulin A deficiency, certain breeds (Irish setters), age (less than 1 year old), and concurrent allergic diseases.[1] According to Drs. Case and Daristotle, German shepherd dogs, Chinese shar-peis, and Irish setters with adverse food reactions have an increased incidence of developing GI signs that may accompany the dermatologic signs typically seen.[2]

Table 8.6.1 Primary dermatologic responses

Severe generalized pruritus without lesions
Military dermatitis
Pruritus with self-trauma centered around head, neck, ears
Traumatic alopecia
Moist dermatitis
Scaling dermatitis

Source: Roudebush P, Guilford WG, Shanley KJ. Adverse reactions to food. In: *Small Animal Clinical Nutrition*, 4th edition, eds. MS Hand, CD Thatcher, RL Remillard, P Roudebush, pp. 431–453. Topeka, KS: Mark Morris Institute; 2000.

Physical defenses against hypersensitivity to food antigens include effective mucosal barrier and oral tolerance generated by the cellular immune system gut-associated lymphoid tissue (GALT). An effective mucosal barrier includes effective digestive enzymes, adequate mucus layer, as well as intact and functioning epithelial cells and immunoglobulin A.[1] This interaction between luminal factors of dietary and bacterial origin and the gut wall itself is important in preventing food allergies.[3]

Exogenous food antigens (including peptides, glycoproteins, lectins, and microorganisms) have the ability to interact with the gut wall and to induce reactions as well as regulatory and counter-regulatory processes. Interactions of luminal factors with the gut wall influence digestion (secretion, absorption, motility), immune functions (exclusion of antigens, regulation of the GI immune system, antigen processing, sensitivity, allergy), and neuroendocrine processes.[3]

Diagnostics

The clinical feature most sensitive for diagnosis of food allergies is concurrent GI signs and cutaneous signs.[4]

Elimination trials remain the gold standard for diagnosis. A positive response to an exclusion diet with subsequent relapse with challenge of the food product is diagnostic.[3] Intradermal skin testing tends to be unreliable and no evidence is available to justify the use of this test for the diagnosis of food allergies.[4] Radioallergosorbent testing (RAST) and ELISA are likewise unreliable for diagnosis of food hypersensitivity, especially with concurrent dermatologic disease.[1,4]

Treatment

For an adverse food reaction, removal of the inciting cause will usually resolve the problem (if you can identify the source). The inciting cause can be poor quality ingredients (rancid fat), bacterial enterotoxins or fungal mycotoxins, or an inability to digest the ingested product (foreign bodies).[5]

Many clients complain of a transitory diarrhea associated with a sudden diet change. Initially, with sudden diet changes, the animal may be unable to digest or absorb certain nutrients until the brush border enzymes adapt to the new diet as these enzymes are produced in response to the presence of specific substrates in the diet. In some cases, they may be unable to produce the necessary enzymes, as seen with lactose intolerance in some adult animals.[5]

Elimination diets

The ingredients found to most commonly cause hypersensitivity reactions in cats is fish, beef, and dairy products in ~89% of the cases. For dogs, the list includes beef, dairy products, and wheat in ~65% of the cases, and chicken, egg, lamb, and soy in ~25% of the cases.[1,2] There may be single or multiple sensitivities found.[2]

The primary requirements for an elimination diet are that it is complete and balanced, has high digestibility in the SIs, and has limited ingredients.[3] This can either be a homemade diet, a commercial limited ingredient diet, or a hydrolyzed protein diet.

A detailed diet history should help to guide to which diet ingredient the animal has not previously been exposed. Be sure to ask about treats as well as any table foods the animal may be fed. The elimination diet should ideally include only food items to which the animal has not previously been exposed. Ask about other animals in the environment, specifically for past exposure to the novel food source (pet rabbits, ducks, etc.). Selection of an appropriate elimination diet can be challenging in some animals, and a hydrolyzed protein diet may be a consideration.

There are a number of sources for balanced homemade diets. Unbalanced diets should not be fed for longer than a few weeks, especially to young animals.[3] No raw meats should be fed in any homemade diet as potential for contamination is high.[4]

In multiple pet households, if they are all the same species, all may be fed the elimination diet. If other dietary restrictions exist, then a strict food quarantine must be established. Outdoor cats will need to be transitioned to strictly indoors to eliminate hunting and seeking of alternate food source behaviors.[3]

The new diet should be fed as the sole source of nutrition for at least 3–4 weeks with GI signs, and potentially for as long as 3 months for dermatologic conditions.[3] A typical trial lasts at least 6–8 weeks; after this time, the owners may start reintroducing food ingredients. Only one ingredient should be added every 7 days, if a reaction is seen that food is considered a causative ingredient.[3] Many clients are unwilling to try the reintroduction food trials once the clinical signs have resolved, which is not a problem as long as the animal and the clients are satisfied with the diet.

Lastly, a new diet may have positive effects on intestinal digestion by decreasing potentially harmful bacteria and thereby decreasing the concentration of bacterial metabolites found in the gut. Increased digestibility may also be helpful in the management of other GI diseases.[3]

Proteins

Single-source protein choices are ideal, with usually only one ingredient selected for the diet. Depending on the diet history, this may include chicken, turkey, venison, duck, rabbit, lamb, or fish; soy (a vegetable protein) can be used if properly processed.[3] Poorly digestible protein sources retain their inherent antigenicity during the heat processing of the food and should be avoided.[2] Selecting a highly digestible protein as evidenced by feeding trials is ideal.

Gluten is a protein found commonly in grains, primarily wheat, rye, and barley. It is a cause of food intolerance in humans and has been found to have a genetic component in some Irish setters.[1,3] If these grains have not been previously fed to the animal, then there is no reason to exclude them from an elimination diet as gluten allergies are rare in dogs and cats.

Though not commonly thought of as a protein, the gelatin used in some medications as well as in the encapsulation of vitamins is usually derived from beef and pork protein.[3] The fact that it is minimally digestible does not affect its antigenic potential.

Protein hydrolysates

Protein hydrolysates are produced by enzymatic proteolysis of dietary proteins. This produces peptides that, in theory, are less likely to interact with the immune system because they are small enough not to be recognized by nor trigger a reaction by the immune system. By decreasing the molecular weight of the proteins, digestibility is also increased. Because of the predigestion of the proteins, the actual base source of the protein no longer matters.[1,6] More work needs to be done to confirm that these proteins are truly hypoallergenic in dogs and cats.

Diets with protein hydrolysates are usually reserved for animals with adverse food reactions, allergies, or maldigestion problems. Unlike elimination diets, the commercial diets using protein hydrolysates are complete and balanced, decreasing the concern for dietary imbalance.[1,6]

Carbohydrates

As with proteins, a single-source diet is ideal. The carbohydrates most commonly selected include corn, potato, rice, and tapioca.[3] As noted above, grains are an important source of protein as well as carbohydrates. Their inclusion in a diet should be based on exposure.

Carbohydrate intolerance can be seen and most commonly involves lactose. The lack of the enzyme lactase can cause diarrhea, bloating, and abdominal discomfort.[1] It is usually related to volume consumed rather than to just exposure.

Fats

Fats are an important source of calories, especially in an elimination diet. Usually, fats are not seen as allergenic, but they may contain small amounts of either plant or animal proteins dependent on their source.[3] For most animals, this is not a concern, but for extremely sensitive animals, this should be a consideration.

Minerals and trace elements

These are essential to make a diet complete and balanced, but some sources of mineral salts may contain small amounts of protein. It is important to look at the extender and carrier for these ingredients as protein and carbohydrates can often be found in them.[3]

Conclusion

As with most things, once the source of the problem has been identified, avoidance is the most effective treatment. Animals can be maintained on commercial limited ingredient diets long term. It is important to know that the food has undergone feeding trials and, if possible, that those trials were conducted on animals with either dermatologic or GI disease.[1] Feeding trials done on healthy animals may not adequately represent the digestibility and absorption of a diseased GI tract.

Prebiotics and probiotics

According to the currently adopted definition by the Food and Agriculture Organization (FAO) and the World Health Organization (WHO), probiotics are "live microorganisms which when administered in adequate amounts confer a health benefit on the host,"[7] whereas prebiotics are "non-digestible food ingredients that selectively stimulate the growth and activities of specific bacteria in the gastrointestinal tract and exert beneficial effects on the host."[8] The Food and Drug Administration (FDA) defines nutraceuticals as "nondrug substances produced in a purified or extracted form and administered orally to provide agents required for normal body structure and function with the intent of improving health and well-being."[9]

Prebiotics and probiotics are either bacteria or substances that benefit bacteria in the intestinal tract. There are millions of bacteria that typically reside in the SIs and LIs of normal, healthy animals that help with digestion of food, maintain intestinal mucosal integrity, participate in metabolism, as well as local and systemic immune stimulation.[10] When disease, parasites, stress, or dietary changes affect these beneficial bacteria, imbalances can occur, causing changes in the digestion of food, mucosal integrity, metabolism, and immunity (both local and systemic). One other common cause of changes within the GI microflora is the use of broad-spectrum antibiotics to treat infections. When the GI microflora is disturbed, potentially harmful and pathogenic bacteria can become more prolific and can cause antibiotic-induced diarrhea.[10]

The intestines

The intestines are seen as the largest component of the immune system in the body, comprising ~70% of the total immune system. The mucosal barrier found in the intestines helps to block the entrance of most pathogenic bacteria into the body while allowing the entrance of permeable nutrients.[10] As most pathogens enter the body through the mouth, these intestinal defenses must be working optimally to cope with the onslaught of foreign substances and pathogens to which they are constantly exposed.[10]

This defense involves the coordination of three different systems within the intestines. The first is the resident intestinal microflora, which provides an environment that favors the growth and functioning of beneficial bacteria. The second is the intestinal mucosa, which provides a protective barrier against pathogenic bacteria. Last is the GALT, which provides the cellular protection for containment of bacteria within the intestinal tract.[10]

Prebiotics

Typically, prebiotics are a type of carbohydrate called oligosaccharides, though by definition, noncarbohydrates can also be classified as prebiotics. The ones used most frequently are classified as soluble fibers. These were first identified as a functional food in 1995 by Marcel Roberfroid. In 2007, Dr. Roberfroid clarified that only two classes of FOSs fully meet the definition of a prebiotic. These are oligofructose and inulin.[11]

Oligofructose is a short-chain prebiotic (two to eight fructose links per saccharide molecule) that undergoes fermentation fairly quickly in the colon, providing nourishment to the bacteria of that area. Examples of food sources for FOSs are soybeans, oats, beets, and tomatoes.

Inulin is a longer-chain prebiotic (9–64 fructose links per saccharide molecule) that tends to be fermented more slowly, benefiting bacteria farther down the colon. Inulin is composed of the same fructose base as is FOS but is a much larger molecule. The length of the molecule will affect the digestibility and therefore its availability for use by the intestinal bacteria. It can also be broken down into the FOSs by the intestinal bacteria to provide both FOS and inulin. Inulin can be found in Jerusalem artichoke, jicama, and chicory root.

These two fibers are seen as minimally digestible because of their beta-bond base connecting the fructose molecules. Dogs and cats lack the enzyme in their intestines to break down the beta bond; instead, they break down alpha saccharide bonds. The resident bacteria of dogs and cats do have the ability to break this beta bond, which produces SCFAs. The SCFAs seen most commonly include acetate, proprionate, and butyrate.

Plants have more than one type of carbohydrate in them, so both FOS and inulin can be found in varying amounts in the same plant. Conversely, neither type may be found in other carbohydrates. The addition of fiber to the diet may or may not provide prebiotic effects, depending on the types of fibers found in the product. All fibers are carbohydrates, but not all carbohydrates are fibers. Different fibers provide different benefits. Cellulose is minimally digestible and will usually only provide bulking, whereas chicory or beet pulp does not provide much fiber but does make for happy bacteria in the guts.

The SCFAs produced by the breaking of the beta bond (through bacterial fermentation) serve as an energy source to the colonocytes, act to lower the colonic pH, and stimulate

Table 8.6.2 Intestinal bacteria

Beneficial	Pathogenic
Lactobacilli	Pseudomonas aeruginosa
Eubacteria	Proteus species
Bifidobacteria	Staphylococci
Enterococci	Clostridia
	Veillonella

Source: Kelly M. *The Role of Probiotics in GI Tract Health.* St. Louis, MO: Nestle Purina Pet Care;2006.

sodium and water absorption.[8] One SCFA in particular, butyrate, serves as the primary energy source for colonocytes but may also directly enhance cell proliferation of normal cells while suppressing proliferation of transformed cells. Since FOS and inulin are both fibers, there can be negative side effects to their addition to the diet. Both FOS and inulin have been shown to cause a decrease in the intestine's ability to break down and digest proteins when fibers are at higher levels in the diet.[8]

Studies have shown that there are generally positive effects when FOSs and fructose-based inulins are added to the diet.[12] These effects can be seen in the gut microflora, host health (as evaluated through gut integrity and bacterial colonization), animal performance (as evaluated through digestion), body weight gain, and feed efficiency when FOSs and fructose-based inulins are added to the diet (Table 8.6.2).[12]

Probiotics

Probiotics, rather than encouraging the growth of beneficial bacteria and suppressing the growth of pathogenic bacteria, actually introduce these beneficial bacteria into the environment. To be able to function as a probiotic, certain criteria must be met by the bacteria being used. They must be able to

– survive the acid and bile found in the GI tract;

– adhere to the intestinal cells and transiently colonize various areas within the GI tract;

– exclude or reduce pathogenic bacterial adherence;

– produce acids, hydrogen peroxide, and/or bacteriocins that antagonize the growth of pathogens;

– coaggregate to help achieve normal balanced microflora population; and

– be safe, noninvasive, noncarcinogenic, and nonpathogenic to the animal.[10]

Initially, the GI tract of a newborn is sterile but is colonized within hours of birth. These bacteria find their individual niches within the intestinal tract and reach a state of equilibrium. Once this neonate "grace period" is over, introduction of bacteria is significantly more difficult due to the gastric acidity and the introduction of bile acids to the chyme leaving the stomach.

Though yogurt and a number of other bacterial fermented products contain beneficial bacteria, these bacteria seldom survive the stomach and therefore do not provide any benefit to the intestinal bacteria.[7] The beneficial effects of probiotics depend on the number of live bacteria that make it to the intestines and are able to transiently colonize there.[10]

The primary bacterial populations that are seen to benefit cats and dogs are the lactic acid bacteria, especially *lactobacilli*, *bifidobacteria*, and *enterococci*. These bacteria use fermentation to transform some sugars into organic acids, particularly lactic and acetic acids. These acids serve to lower the pH in the intestinal tract and inhibit the growth of pathogenic bacteria.[10]

Probiotics can benefit the intestinal microflora in a number of ways. They can increase fecal bacteria counts of good bacteria while decreasing the numbers of pathogenic bacteria. Some probiotics have been shown to minimize adherence of pathogenic bacteria to the intestinal epithelial cells, thereby minimizing the establishment of pathogenic bacteria populations.

Probiotics can also help to control diarrhea caused by bacterial overgrowth or parasitic infection. This uses the principles of competitive exclusion, competition for nutrients and binding sites, and an increase in specific and nonspecific immune response.[10] One of the biggest challenges for manufacturers of probiotic products is survivability of the bacteria. Most commercially available products suffer tremendous loss of activity during storage. After 5–6 months of storage, virtually no live organisms are present. Those bacteria that are present still have to survive the gastric pH and the duodenal bile acids before they can colonize the SIs. To address these concerns, some manufacturers have developed microencapsulation processes to protect the bacteria, while others provide a variety of bacteria to cover more bases.

Conclusion

Prebiotics are used as both a source of nutrition for the colonocytes and as a fiber source for the animal; inclusion in the diet is relatively easy. This is because adding a fiber to the diet during manufacturing is much easier than adding actual bacteria to the diet. The fiber source used should be listed on the ingredient panel but may not state whether it is a source of FOS or inulin. Increasing your familiarity with the different fiber sources used and their relative FOS and inulin contents can help when evaluating a diet. When in doubt, contact the manufacturer for further information.

Unlike the prebiotics, the use of probiotics is more of a transient process based on need rather than a long-term process. Ideally, through ingestion, the bacterial population most beneficial to the animal and the one that supports the best intestinal health will take up residence. But when this does not occur, or when challenges are expected that could affect intestinal health, probiotics can be easily added into the diet to help support the bacterial populations there. There have been no detrimental effects seen with long-term prebiotic or probiotic use, as opposed to the detrimental effects seen with the long-term use of antibiotics.

SECTION 7 ANESTHESIA AND ANALGESIA CONSIDERATIONS IN GASTROINTESTINAL DISEASE

Patients with GI disorders often require general anesthesia in order to facilitate complete examination, obtain necessary diagnostic testing or imaging, or in cases where surgical intervention is required. Specific considerations regarding the type of GI dysfunction should be made for each step in the anesthetic process from premedication and induction to maintenance and monitoring, and to the recovery and postoperative phases.

Premedication

When creating an anesthetic plan, the premedication combination typically consists of a sedative and an analgesic. The sedative or analgesic chosen will depend greatly on the type and severity of the GI issue and the personality of the patient.

Standard choices for sedatives include benzodiazepines, phenothiazines, and alpha-2 adrenergic agonists. Benzodiazepines (diazepam and midazolam) provide adequate sedation but no analgesia for most patients with relatively calm personalities and have the benefit of little negative effect on cardiovascular, respiratory, or GI systems. Benzodiazepines are able to be reversed using flumazenil.

Phenothiazines, acepromazine being the most commonly used, provide good sedation (but again, no analgesia) for most patients, particularly those that are aggressive or extremely anxious. They are potent antiemetics, which may be beneficial when considering the gastrointestinally compromised patient. They may also decrease sensitivity to some ventricular arrhythmias. Phenothiazines have little effect on respiratory function but can result in dramatic reduction in cardiovascular output. It may cause some decrease in the time of gastric emptying.

Alpha-2 adrenergic agonists, most commonly dexmedetomidine, provide excellent sedation for most patients and provide very minor analgesia (not enough for any surgical purpose). Other potential effects include profound bradycardia, vasoconstriction, and cardiac sensitization to arrhythmias. GI effects include decreased gastric motility and emesis in some dogs and in most cats. Alpha-2 adrenergic agonists are reversible.

The second part of the premedication mixture is an appropriate opioid analgesic. There are many choices available for a variety of different situations. Butorphanol is an agonist-antagonist and buprenorphine is a partial agonist. Both drugs provide some sedation and are less likely to cause vomiting. They can cause decreased GI motility but less markedly than other opioids. Both drugs can be reversed but with difficulty as they bind with very high affinity to receptor sites. The analgesia provided is mild and, in the case of butorphanol, very short-acting (30–60 min), so these drugs are only appropriate for short, relatively painless procedures like endoscopy, diagnostic imaging, or minor biopsies.

Opioid agonists such as morphine, hydromorphone, oxymorphone, and fentanyl are better choices for painful, long, or invasive procedures such as abdominal exploratory or esophageal foreign body removal. Morphine and hydromorphone, when given intramuscularly, often cause emesis and excessive salivation. When given intravenously, the incidence of vomiting is dramatically decreased (if giving morphine IV, it should be done very slowly to prevent sudden histamine release) but is still a possibility. Fentanyl given IV is the best choice for any case where risk of vomiting would be detrimental.

All opioid agonists can cause depression of the cardiovascular and respiratory centers and are known to slow GI transit time. This category of drug does provide sedation and excellent analgesia for varying periods of time. All can be given intraoperatively as CRIs (though it may be cost prohibitive to do so with oxymorphone) and are reversible.

Induction

The most common choices for anesthetic induction are propofol, ketamine/diazepam, and etomidate. Propofol is a sedative-hypnotic that is relatively safe for use in most patients. It does cause transient apnea and a dose-dependent cardiovascular depression. In cats, it is known to cause Heinz body formation following repeated administration.

Ketamine/diazepam is readily available and relatively inexpensive. It is safe for use in most patients (there have been reports of ketamine-related seizures in some patients, so this particular combination should be avoided if there is any epileptic history or known seizure activities). Ketamine does cause an increase in cardiac contractility, which can lead to an increase in heart rate and blood pressure.

Etomidate is an imidazole derivative that has a minimal cardiovascular or respiratory effect. It is more expensive and tends to be used for traumatized or extremely critical patients. Etomidate can cause suppression of adrenal functioning and acute hemolysis. Most importantly, when considering this agent for gastrointestinally dysfunctional cases, it often causes nausea, retching, and vomiting at induction particularly if the patient is not appropriately sedated or if underdosing of the drug occurs.

Intubation of patients should be done quickly and the cuff of the endotracheal tube checked and inflated as soon as possible. To check the seal of an endotracheal tube cuff, intubate the patient and secure the tube. Close the pop-off valve and squeeze the reservoir bag. Watch the manometer gauge—the needle should hold at 20–25 cm H_2O. If the needle falls or air can be heard escaping around the endotracheal tube, the cuff should be inflated slightly and the process repeated until an adequate seal is achieved. Lubricating the endotracheal tube cuff prior to intubation can facilitate a less traumatic intubation and may prevent the passage of liquid into the trachea. This group of patients is at high risk of regurgitation under anesthesia, and it is important to avoid aspiration of any fluid or material. It is advisable to check the cuff again after full anesthetic depth has been reached as further muscle relaxation may occur, allowing additional air/gas to escape around the endotracheal tube.

Considerations should be made if the patient has any comorbidity that could make intubation difficult, such as an oropharyngeal mass or esophageal foreign body displacing the trachea; in challenging cases, supplies for a tracheostomy should be ready.

Maintenance anesthesia

Isoflurane, sevoflurane, or desflurane are all acceptable choices for anesthetic maintenance in these patients. In volvulus cases, nitrous oxide is not an acceptable option because the gases will try to reach equilibrium and will increase volume and pressure within the stomach and GI tract.

Monitoring

Abdominal distention can impair cardiac function and impede appropriate ventilation requiring mechanical ventilation for adequate gas exchange. Once decompression has occurred, it should be significantly easier to ventilate the patient.

Many patients that suffer dehydration from excessive vomiting/diarrhea or those with a GDV may have electrolyte imbalances and/or acid–base disturbances. These abnormalities should be corrected before anesthesia if at all possible. If stabilization is not possible prior to anesthesia, aggressive fluid therapy with appropriately balanced solutions should begin immediately. Electrolyte panels and, if possible, arterial blood gas parameters should be checked regularly during the intraoperative period.

As ventilation and tissue perfusion can be impaired in bloated or metabolically disturbed patients, end tidal carbon dioxide and oxygen saturation should be closely monitored.

Respiratory disturbances causing acidosis or alkalosis occur when a patient is hyperventilating (in response to pain, fever, or overcompensation with manual/mechanical ventilation) or hypoventilating (as a result of drug administration, CNS trauma, or restricted thoracic movement). Metabolic disturbances causing acidosis or alkalosis occur in response to electrolyte imbalances. Acidosis is common in conjunction with shock, sepsis, pancreatitis, hypoxemia, and some toxins. Alkalosis commonly occurs in conjunction with vomiting, hypokalemia, steroid therapy, or bicarbonate therapy.

Cardiac arrhythmias are extremely common in volvulus cases and may be seen in patients with severe electrolyte imbalances, so electrocardiogram (ECG) monitoring is strongly recommended. Cardiac output can be affected by distention and dehydration, so for critical cases, arterial blood pressure monitoring is advised.

Recovery

Serious cases should be recovered and maintained in a critical care unit for continued fluid support and postoperative monitoring. Cardiac dysrhythmias are common postoperatively in many surgical cases and ECG monitoring may be necessary. It is also essential to monitor for both electrolytes and acid–base disturbances in the postoperative period. Shock, hypo/hyperkalemia, acidosis/alkalosis, respiratory impairment, and hypovolemia can all be consequences associated with GI dysfunctions. Depending on the severity of the case, additional analgesia may be needed. CRIs of fentanyl or morphine–lidocaine–ketamine are often used, as are fentanyl patches and IV or IM doses of opioid analgesics.

Noncritical cases may not need any additional analgesia or may be sent home with butorphanol (which is only appropriate for cases where the duration of discomfort is not expected to be very long) or NSAIDs. EXTREME caution should be used when administering NSAIDs to patients with GI abnormalities. NSAIDs mediate inflammatory processes by blocking the activity of COX enzymes in the body. However, COX enzymes also function as GI protectors and are necessary for maintaining the health of the GI tract. NSAIDs are strictly contraindicated in any patient that is dehydrated, hypovolemic, has evidence of coagulation disorders, or any suggestion of gastric lesions, ulcerations, or intestinal compromise.

Bibliography

Section 1

1. Tams TR. *Handbook of Small Animal Gastroenterology*, 2nd edition, St. Louis, MO: Saunders; 2003.
2. Burns KM. Managing overweight or obese pets. *Veterinary Technician* 2006;27(6):385–389.
3. Willard MD. Clinical manifestations of gastrointestinal disorders. In: *Small Animal Internal Medicine*, 4th edition, eds. RW Nelson, CG Couto, pp. 351–373. St. Louis, MO: Mosby; 2009.
4. Matz ME. Flatulence. In: *Textbook of Veterinary Internal Medicine*, 7th edition, eds. SJ Ettinger, EC Feldman, pp. 210–212. St. Louis, MO: Saunders Elsevier; 2010.
5. Behrend EN. Polyphagia. In: *Textbook of Veterinary Internal Medicine*, 7th edition, eds. SJ Ettinger, EC Feldman, pp. 175–179. St. Louis, MO: Saunders Elsevier; 2010.
6. Forman MA. Anorexia. In: *Textbook of Veterinary Internal Medicine*, 7th edition, eds. SJ Ettinger, EC Feldman, pp. 172–175. St. Louis, MO: Saunders Elsevier; 2010.
7. Schermerhorn T. Cachexia. In: *Textbook of Veterinary Medicine*, 7th edition, eds. SJ Ettinger, EC Feldman, pp. 124–126. St. Louis, MO: Saunders Elsevier; 2010.

Section 2

1. Simpson KW. Diseases of the stomach. In: *Textbook of Veterinary Internal Medicine*, 7th edition, eds. SJ Ettinger, EC Feldman, pp. 1504–1526. St. Louis, MO: Elsevier; 2010.
2. Cornelius LM, Rawling CA. Arterial blood gas and acid–base values in dogs with various diseases and signs of disease. *Journal of the American Veterinary Medical Association* 1981;178:992.
3. Hall EJ, German AJ. Diseases of the small intestine. In: *Textbook of Veterinary Internal Medicine*, 7th edition, eds. SJ Ettinger, EC Feldman, pp. 1526–1572. St. Louis, MO: Elsevier; 2010.
4. Desario C, Decaro N, Campolo M, et al. Canine parvovirus infection: which diagnostic test for virus? *Journal of Virological Methods* 2005;126:179.
5. Willard MD. Diagnostic tests for the alimentary tract. In: *Small Animal Internal Medicine*, 4th edition, eds. RW Nelson, CG Couto, pp. 374–394. St. Louis, MO: Mosby; 2009.

6. Williams DA. Evaluation of fecal alpha1 protease inhibitor concentration as a test for canine protein-losing enteropathy. *Journal of Veterinary Internal Medicine* 1991;5:133.

7. Fetz K, Steiner JM, Ruaux CG, et al. Development and validation of an enzyme-linked immunosorbent assay (ELISA) for the measurement of feline alpha1-proteinase inhibitor in serum and feces. *Journal of Veterinary Internal Medicine* 2004;18:424.

8. Fetz K, Steiner JM, Ruaux CG, et al. Increased fecal alpha1-proteinase inhibitor concentrations in cats with gastrointestinal disease. *Journal of Veterinary Internal Medicine* 2005;19:474.

9. Melgarejo T, Williams DA, Asem EK. Enzyme-linked immunosorbent assay for canine alpha1-protease inhibitor. *American Journal of Veterinary Research* 1998;59:127.

10. Murphy KF, German AJ, Ruaux CG, et al. Fecal alpha1-proteinase inhibitor concentration in dogs with chronic gastrointestinal disease. *Veterinary Clinical Pathology* 2003;32:67.

11. Konde LJ, Green PA, Pugh CR. Radiology and ultrasonography of the digestive system. In: *Handbook of Small Animal Gastroenterology*, 2nd edition, ed. TR Tams, pp. 51–96. St. Louis, MO: Saunders; 2003.

12. Tams TR. Gastrointestinal symptoms. In: *Handbook of Small Animal Gastroenterology*, 2nd edition, ed. TR Tams, pp. 1–50. St. Louis, MO: Saunders; 2003.

13. Tams TR, Webb CB. Endoscopic examination or the small intestine. In: *Small Animal Endoscopy*, 3rd edition, eds. TR Tams, CA Rawlings, pp. 27–40. St. Louis, MO: Elsevier/Mosby; 2011.

14. DeNovo RC. Diseases of the stomach. In: *Handbook of Small Animal Gastroenterology*, 2nd edition, ed. TR Tams, pp. 159–194. St. Louis, MO: Saunders; 2003.

15. Andrews F, Denovo R, Reese R, et al. The evaluation of the wireless capsule (SmartPill) for measuring gastric emptying and GI transit in normal dogs. *Journal of Veterinary Internal Medicine* 2008; 22:751.

Section 3.1

1. Smith MM. Oral and salivary gland disorders. In: *Textbook of veterinary internal medicine*, 6th edition, eds. SJ Ettinger, EC Feldman, pp. 1294–1295. St. Louis, MO: Elsevier Saunders; 2005.

2. DeBowes LJ. Feline caudal stomatitis. In: *Kirks' Current Veterinary Therapy*, 14th edition, ed. JD Bonagura, pp. 476–478. St. Louis, MO: Saunders; 2009.

3. Robson M, Crystal MA. Gingivitis-stomatitis-pharyngitis. In: *The Feline Patient*, 4th edition, ed. GD Norsworthy, pp. 199–201. Ames, IA: Blackwell Publishing; 2011.

4. Lyon KF. Gingivostomatitis. In SE Holmstrom, ed., *Veterinary Clinics of North America. Small Animal Practice* 2005;35: 891–911.

5. Schmidt BR, Crystal MA. Oral neoplasia. In: *The Feline Patient*, 4th edition, ed. GD Norsworthy, pp. 361–363. Ames, IA: Blackwell Publishing; 2011.

6. Verstraete FJM. Mandibulectomy and maxillectomy. In SE Holmstrom, ed., *Veterinary Clinics of North America. Small Animal Practice* 2005;35:1009–1039.

7. Cherry B. Malignant oral cancer: open wide for early detection. *The NAVTA Journal* 2010;Summer:48–54.

8. McEntee M. Summary of results of cancer treatment with radiation therapy. In: *Cancer in Dogs and Cats Medical and Surgical Management*, ed. WB Morrison, pp. 389–424. Jackson, WY: Teton NewMedia; 2002.

9. Salisbury SK. Principles of oncologic surgery. In: *Cancer in Dogs and Cats Medical and Surgical Management*, ed. WB Morrison, pp. 209–225. Jackson, WY: Teton NewMedia Jackson; 2002.

Section 3.2

1. Tams TR. Diseases of the esophagus. In: *Small Animal Endoscopy*, 3rd edition, eds. TR Tams, CA Rawlings, pp. 118–158. St. Louis, MO: Elsevier/Mosby; 2011.

2. Willard MD. Disorders of the oral cavity, pharynx, and esophagus. In: *Small Animal Internal Medicine*, 4th edition, eds. RW Nelson, CG Couto, pp. 414–426. St. Louis, MO: Mosby; 2009.

3. Marks SL. Diagnosis and management of esophagel disorders. 2011. Proceedings of the North American Veterinary Conference, January 15–19, 2011, Orlando, FL.

4. Jergens AE. Diseases of the esophagus. In: *Textbook of Veterinary Internal Medicine*, 7th edition, eds. SJ Ettinger, EC Feldman, pp. 1487–1499.. St. Louis, MO: Elsevier; 2010.

5. Holland CT, Satchell PM, Farrow BR. Selective vagal afferent dysfunction in dogs with congenital megaesophagus. *Autonomic Neuroscience* 2002;99(1):18–23.

6. Davenport DJ, Leib MS, Remillard RL. Pharyngeal and esophageal disorders. In: *Small Animal Clinical Nutrition*, 5th edition, eds. MS Hand, CD Thatcher, RL Remillard, R Roudebush, BJ Novotny, pp. 1013–1022. Topeka, KS: MMI; 2010.

7. Moore LE. Esophagus. In: *Small Animal Gastroenterology*, ed. JM Steiner, pp. 139–150. Hannover, Germany: Schlutersche; 2008.

8. Gaynor AR, Shofer FS, Washabau RJ. Risk factors for acquired megaesophagus in dogs. *Journal of the American Veterinary Medical Association* 1997;211:1406–1412.

9. Bexfield NH, Watson PJ, Herrtage ME. Esophageal dysmotility in young dogs. *Journal of Veterinary Internal Medicine* 2006;20: 1314–1318.

10. Sherding RG, Johnson SE. Esophagoscopy. In: *Small Animal Endoscopy*, 3rd edition, eds. TR Tams, CA Rawlings, pp. 41–198. St. Louis, MO: Elsevier/Mosby; 2011.

11. Tams TR, Spector DJ. Endoscopic removal of gastrointestinal foreign bodies. In: *Small Animal Endoscopy*, 3rd edition, eds. TR Tams, CA Rawlings, pp. 245–292. St. Louis, MO: Elsevier/Mosby; 2011.

Section 3.3

1. Davenport DJ, Remillard RL, Jenkins C. Gastritis. In: *Small Animal Clinical Nutrition*, 5th edition, eds. MS Hand, CD Thatcher, RJ Remillard, P Roudebush, BJ Novotony, pp. 1025–1032. Topeka, KS: MMI; 2010.

2. Willard MD. Disorders of the stomach. In: *Small Animal Internal Medicine*, 4th edition, eds. RW Nelson, CG Couto, pp. 427–439. St. Louis, MO: Mosby; 2009.

3. DeNovo RC. *Handbook of Small Animal Gastroenterology*, 2nd edition, pp. 159–194. St. Louis, MO: Saunders; 2003.

4. Neiger R. Disease of the stomach. In: *Small Animall Gastroenterology*, ed. JM Steiner, pp. 159–175. Hannover, Germany: Schlutersche; 2008.

5. Simpson KW. Diseases of the stomach. In: *Textbook of Veterinary Internal Medicine*, 7th edition, eds. SJ Ettinger, EC Feldman, pp. 1504–1526. St. Louis, MO: Elsevier; 2010.

6. Henderson AK, Webster CRL. Disruption of the mucosal barrier in dogs. *Compendium* 2006(May);28(5):340–356.

7. Twedt DC. Gastric or gastrointestinal motility disorders. In: *The 5 Minute Veterinary Consult*, 3rd edition, eds. LP Tilley, FWK

Smith, pp. 494–495. Baltimore, MD: Lippincott Williams & Wilkins; 2004.

8. Davenport DJ, Remillard RL, Jenkins C. Gastric motility and emptying disorders. In: *Small Animal Clinical Nutrition*, 5th edition, eds. MS Hand, CD Thatcher, RJ Remillard, P Roudebush, BJ Novotony, pp. 1041–1046. Topeka, KS: MMI; 2010.

9. Tams TR. *Handbook of Small Animal Gastroenterology*, 2nd edition, pp. 97–117. St. Louis, MO: Saunders; 2003.

10. Armbrust LJ, Hoskinson JJ, Lora-Michiels M, et al. Gastric emptying in cats using foods varying in fiber content and kibble shapes. *Veterinary Radiology & Ultrasound* 2003;44:339–343.

Section 3.4

1. Allenspach K. Diseases of the large intestine. In: *Textbook of Veterinary Internal Medicine*, 7th edition, eds. SJ Ettinger, EC Feldman, pp. 1573–1594. St. Louis, MO: Elsevier; 2010.

2. Willard MD. Disorders of the intestinal tract. In: *Small Animal Internal Medicine*, 4th edition, eds. RW Nelson, CG Couto, pp. 441–476. St. Louis, MO: Mosby; 2009.

3. Sherding RA. Diseases of the large intestine. In: *Handbook of Small Animal Gastroenterology*, 2nd edition, ed. TR Tams, pp. 251–285. St. Louis, MO: Saunders; 2003.

4. Leib MS. Large intestine. In: *Small Animal Gastroenterology*, ed. JM Steiner, pp. 217–240. Hannover, Germany: Schlutersche; 2008.

5. Allenspach K, Gaschein FP. Small intestinal disease. In: *Small Animal Gastroenterology*, ed. JM Steiner, pp. 187–202. Hannover, Germany: Schlutersche; 2008.

6. Triolo A, Lappin MR. Acute medical diseases of the small intestine. In: *Handbook of Small Animal Gastroenterology*, 2nd edition, ed. TR Tams, pp. 195–250. St. Louis, MO: Saunders; 2003.

7. Hall EJ, German AJ. Diseases of the small intestine. In: *Textbook of Veterinary Internal Medicine*, 7th edition, eds. SJ Ettinger, EC Feldman, pp. 1526–1572. St. Louis, MO: Elsevier; 2010.

8. Scorza AV, Brewer MM, Lappin MR. Polymerase chain reaction for the detection of *Cryptosporidium* spp. in cat feces. *The Journal of Parasitology* 2003;89:423–426.

9. Sucholdoski JS. *Tritrichomonas foetus* infection. In: *Small Animal Gastroenterology*, ed. JM Steiner, pp. 225–226. Hannover, Germany: Schlutersche; 2008.

Section 3.5

1. Peterson PB, Willard MD. Protein-losing enteropathies. *Veterinary Clinics of North America. Small Animal Practice* 2003;33(5): 1061–1082.

2. Tams T. Chronic diseases of the small intestine. In: *Handbook of Small Animal Gastroenterology*, 2nd edition, ed. T Tams, pp. 211–250. St. Louis, MO: W.B. Saunders; 2003.

3. Gorman SC, Freeman LM, Mitchell SL, Chan DL. Extensive small bowel resection in dogs and cats: 20 cases (1998–2004). *Journal of the American Veterinary Medical Association* 2006;228(3):403–407.

4. Kouti VI, Papazoglou LG, Rallis T. Short-bowel syndrome in dogs and cats. *Compendium : Continuing Education for Veterinarians* 2006;28(3):182–195.

5. Imamura M, Yamauchi H. Effects of massive bowel resection on metabolism of bile acids and vitamin D_3 and gastrin release in dogs. *The Tohoku Journal of Experimental Medicine* 1992;168: 515–528.

6. Willard MD. Disorders of the intestinal tract. In: *Small Animal Internal Medicine*, 4th edition, ed. RW Nelson, CG Couto, pp. 441–483. St. Louis, MO: Mosby; 2009.

7. Triolo A, Lappin MR. Acute medical diseases of the small intestine. In: *Handbook of Small Animal Gastroenterology*, 2nd edition, ed. TR Tams, pp. 195–210. St. Louis, MO: Saunders; 2003.

8. Hall EJ, German AJ. Diseases of the small intestine. In: *Textbook of Veterinary Internal Medicine*, 7th edition, eds. SJ Ettinger, EC Feldman, pp. 1526–1572. St. Louis, MO: Elsevier; 2010.

9. Henry CJ. Neoplastic diseases of the small intestine. In: *Small Animal Gastroenterology*, ed. JM Steiner, pp. 211–215. Hannover, Germany: Schlutersche; 2008.

10. Couto CG. Disorders of the intestinal tract. In: *Small Animal Internal Medicine*, 4th edition, eds. RW Nelson, CG Couto, pp. 1174–1185. St. Louis, MO: Mosby; 2009.

11. Birchard SJ, Couto CG, Johnson S. Nonlymphoid intestinal neoplasia in 32 dogs and 14 cats. *Journal of the American Animal Hospital Association* 1986;22:533–537.

12. Crawshaw J, Berg J, Sardinas JC, et al. Prognosis for dogs with nonlymphomatous, small intestinal tumors treated by surgical excision. *Journal of the American Animal Hospital Association* 1998;34:451–456.

13. Beam SL, Rassnick KM, Moore AS, et al. An immunohistochemical study of cyclooxygenase-2 expression in various feline neoplasms. *Veterinary Pathology* 2003;40:496.

14. Esplin DG, Wilson SR. Gastrointestinal adenocarcinomas metastatic to the testes and associated structures in three dogs. *Journal of the American Animal Hospital Association* 1998;34:287.

15. Hall EJ, German AJ. Inflammatory bowel disease. In: *Small Animal Gastroenterology*, ed. JM Steiner, pp. 312–329. Hannover, Germany: Schlutersche; 2008.

16. Allenspach K, Wieland B, Grone A, et al. Chronic enteropathies in dogs: evaluation of risk factors for negative outcome. *Journal of Veterinary Internal Medicine* 2007;21:700.

17. Jergens AE, Moore FM, Haynes JS, et al. Idiopathic inflammatory bowel disease in dogs and cats: 84 cases. *Journal of the American Veterinary Medical Association* 1992;201:1987–1990.

18. Gaschen L, Kircher P, Stussi A, et al. Comparison of ultrasonographic findings with clinical activity index (CIBDAI) and diagnosis in dogs with chronic enteropathies. *Veterinary Radiology & Ultrasound* 2008;49:56.

19. Crandell JM, Jergens AE, Morrison JA, et al. Development of a clinical scoring index for disease activity in feline inflammatory bowel disease. *Journal of Veterinary Internal Medicine* 2006;20:788.

20. Jergens AE. Clinical assessment of disease activity for canine inflammatory bowel disease. *Journal of the American Animal Hospital Association* 2004;40:437.

21. Jergens AE, Schreiner CA, Frank DE, et al. A scoring index for disease activity in canine inflammatory bowel disease. *Journal of Veterinary Internal Medicine* 2003;17:291.

22. McCann TM, Ridyard AE, Else RW, et al. Evaluation of disease activity markers in dogs with idiopathic inflammatory bowel disease. *Journal of Small Animal Practice* 2007;48:619.

23. MüNSTER M, Horauf A, Bilzer T. Assessment of disease severity and outcome of dietary, antibiotic, and immunosuppressive interventions by use of the canine IBD activity index in 21 dogs with inflammatory bowel disease. *Berliner und Munchener tierarztliche Wochenschrift* 2006;119:493.

24. Davenport DJ, Jergens AE, Remillard RJ. Inflammatory bowel disease. In: *Small Animal Clinical Nutrition*, 5th edition, eds. MS Hand, CD Thatcher, RJ Remillard, P Roudebush, BJ Novotony, pp. 1065–1076. Topeka, KS: MMI; 2010.

25. Lewis LD, Boulay JP, Chow FHC. Fat excretion and assimilation by the cat. *Feline Practice* 1979;9:46–49.

26. Nelson RW, Dimperio ME, Long GG. Lymphocytic-plasmacytic colitis in the cat. *Journal of the American Veterinary Medical Association* 1984;184:1133–1135.

27. Nelson RW, Stookey LJ. Nutritional management of idiopathic chronic colitis in the dog. *Journal of Veterinary Internal Medicine* 1988;2:133–137.

28. Guilford WG, Jones BR, Markwell PJ, et al. Food sensitivity in cats with chronic idiopathic intestinal problems. *Journal of Veterinary Internal Medicine* 2001;15:7–13.

29. Allenspach K, Rüfenacht S, Sauter S, et al. Pharmacokinetics and clinical efficacy of cyclosporine treatment of dogs with steroid-refractory inflammatory bowel disease. *Journal of Veterinary Internal Medicine* 2006;20:239–244.

30. Sunvold GD, Fahey GC, Jr., Merchen NR, et al. Dietary fiber for cats: in vitro fermentation of selected fiber sources by cat fecal inoculum and in vivo utilization of diets containing selected fiber sources and their blends. *Journal of Animal Science* 1995;73: 2329–2339.

31. Sunvold GD, Fahey GC, Jr., Merchen NR, et al. Dietary fiber for dogs: IV. In vitro fermentation of selected fiber sources by dog fecal inoculum and in vivo digestion and metabolism of fiber-supplemented diets. *Journal of Animal Science* 1995a;73: 1099–1109.

32. Sunvold GD, Fahey GC, Jr., Merchen NR, et al. In vitro fermentation of selected fibrous substrates by dog and cat fecal inoculum: influence of diet composition on substrate organic matter disappearance and short-chain fatty acid production. *Journal of Animal Science* 1995b;73:1110–1122.

33. Ruaux CG, Steiner JM, Williams DA. Metabolism of amino acids in cats with severe cobalamin deficiency. *American Journal of Veterinary Research* 2001;61:1852–1858.

34. Ruaux CG, Steiner JM, Williams DA. Early biochemical and clinical response to cobalamin supplementation in cats with signs of gastrointestinal disease and severe hypocobalaminemia. *Journal of Veterinary Internal Medicine* 2005;19:155–160.

35. Hendricks KM, Walker A. Zinc deficiency in inflammatory bowel disease. *Nutrition Reviews* 1988;46:401–408.

36. Allenspach K, Gaschen FP. Small intestinal disease. In: *Small Animal Gastroenterology*, ed. JM Steiner, pp. 187–202. Hannover, Germany: Schlutersche; 2008.

37. Martin L, Matteson V, Wingfield W. Abnormalities of serum magnesium in critically ill dogs: incidence and implications. *Journal of Veterinary Emergency and Critical Care* 1994;4:15–20.

38. Toll J, Erb H, Birnbaum N, et al. Prevalence and incidence of serum magnesium abnormalities in hospitalized cats. *Journal of Veterinary Internal Medicine* 2002;16:217–221.

Section 3.6

1. Davenport DJ, Remilliard RL. Introduction to small intestinal disease. In: *Small Animal Clinical Nutrition*, 5th edition, eds. MS Hand, CD Thatcher, RL Remilliard, P Roudebush, BJ Novotny, pp. 1047–1049. Marceline, MO: Walsworth Publishing; 2010.

2. Simpson JW, Anderson RS, Markwell PJ. Dietary management of clinical diseases. In: *Clinical Nutrition of the Dog and Cat*, eds. JW Simpson, RS Anderson, PJ Markwell, pp. 59–62. Cambridge, MA: Blackwell Publishing; 1993.

3. Nelson RW, Couto CG. Clinical manifestations of gastrointestinal disorders. In: *Small Animal Internal Medicine*, 4th edition, eds. RW Nelson, CG Couto, GR Grauer, EC Hawkins, pp. 360–361. St. Louis, MO: Mosby; 2009. 2009.

4. Davenport DJ, Remillard RL. Acute gastroenteritis and enteritis. In: *Small Animal Clinical Nutrition*, 5th edition, eds. MS Hand, CD Thatcher, RL Remilliard, P Roudebush, BJ Novotny, pp. 1053–1061. Marceline, MO: Walsworth Publishing; 2010. 2010.

5. LeJeune JT, Hancock DD. Public health concerns associated with feeding raw meat diets to dogs. *Journal of the American Veterinary Medical Association* 2001(November 1);219(9):1222–1225.

6. Nelson RW, Couto CG. General therapeutic principles. In: *Small Animal Internal Medicine*, 4th edition, eds. RW Nelson, CG Couto, GR Grauer, EC Hawkins, pp. 395–412. St. Louis, MO: Mosby; 2009. 2009.

7. Case LP, Carey DP, Hirakawa DA, Daristotle L. Protein and amino acids. In: *Canine and Feline Nutrition*, 2nd edition, pp. 23–28. St. Louis, MO: Mosby; 2000b. 2000.

8. Gross KL, Jewell DE, Yamka RM, et al. Macronutrients. In: *Small Animal Clinical Nutrition*, 5th edition, eds. MS Hand, CD Thatcher, RL Remilliard, P Roudebush, BJ Novotny, pp. 49–104. Marceline, MO: Walsworth Publishing; 2010. 2010.

9. Case LP, Carey DP, Hirakawa DA, Daristotle L. Fats. In: *Canine and Feline Nutrition*, 2nd edition, pp. 19–22. St. Louis, MO: Mosby; 2000c. 2000.

10. Davenport DJ, Remillard RL, Carroll M. Large bowel diarrhea: colitis. In: *Small Animal Clinical Nutrition*, 5th edition, eds. MS Hand, CD Thatcher, RL Remilliard, P Roudebush, BJ Novotny, pp. 1101–1109. Marceline, MO: Walsworth Publishing; 2010c. 2010.

11. Case LP, Carey DP, Hirakawa DA, Daristotle L. Carbohydrates. In: *Canine and Feline Nutrition*, 2nd edition, pp. 16–18. St. Louis, MO: Mosby; 2000a. 2000.

12. Jergens AE. (2005) *Canine and feline inflammatory bowel disease—what's new*. AAHA Proceedings CD.

13. Willard MD. Disorders of the intestinal tract. In: *Small Animal Internal Medicine*, 4th edition, eds. RW Nelson, CG Cuoto, pp. 441–476. St. Louis, MO: Mosby; 2009.

14. Allenspach K, Gaschein FP. Small intestinal disease. In: *Small Animal Gastroenterology*, ed. JM Steiner, pp. 187–202. Hannover, Germany: Schlutersche; 2008.

15. Hall EJ, German AJ. Diseases of the small intestine. In: *Textbook of Veterinary Internal Medicine*, 7th edition, eds. SJ Ettinger, EC Feldman, pp. 1526–1572. St. Louis, MO: Elsevier; 2010.

16. Triolo A, Lappin MR. Acute medical diseases of the small intestine. In: *Handbook of Small Animal Gastroenterology*, 2nd edition, ed. TR Tams, pp. 195–250. St. Louis, MO: Saunders; 2003.

17. Sandberg M, Bergsjo B, Hofshagen M, et al. Risk factors for *Campylobacter* infection in Norwegian cats and dogs. *Preventive Veterinary Medicine* 2002;55:241–253.

18. Van Immerseel F, Pasmans F, De Buck J, et al. Cats as a risk for transmission of antimicrobial drug-resistant *Salmonella*. *Emerging Infectious Diseases* 2004;10:2169.

19. German AJ. *Diagnostic Tree: large bowel diarrhea*. North American Veterinary Conference Clinician's Brief. 2006: pp. 54–55.

20. Guilford WG. Effect of diet on inflammatory bowel diseases. *Veterinary Clinical Nutrition* 1997;4:58–61.

21. Graham-Mize CA, Rosser EJ. Bioavailability and activity of prednisone and prednisolone in the feline patient. *Veterinary Dermatology* (2004) Issue 15(s1):10. 2004.

Section 3.7

1. Leib M. In: *Small Animal Gastroenterology*, ed. JM Steiner, pp. 230–236. Hannover, Germany: Schlutersche; 2008.

2. Willard MD. Disorders of the intestinal tract. In: *Small Animal Internal Medicine*, 4th edition, eds. RW Nelson, CG Couto, pp. 441–476. St. Louis, MO: Mosby; 2009.

3. Craven M. Rectoanal disease. In: *Textbook of Veterinary Internal Medicine*, 7th edition, eds. SJ Ettinger, EC Feldman, pp. 1595–1608. St. Louis, MO: Elsevier; 2010.

4. Allenspach K. Diseases of the large intestine. In: *Textbook of Veterinary Internal Medicine*, 7th edition, eds. SJ Ettinger, EC Feldman, pp. 1573–1594. St. Louis, MO: Elsevier; 2010.

5. Henry CJ. Neoplastic diseases of the large intestine. In: *Small Animal Gastroenterology*, ed. JM Steiner, pp. 236–240. Hannover, Germany: Schlutersche; 2008.

6. Sherding RA. Diseases of the large intestine. In: *Handbook of Small Animal Gastroenterology*, 2nd edition, ed. TR Tams, pp. 251–285. St. Louis, MO: Saunders; 2003.

7. Washabau RJ, Hasler A. Constipation, obstipation, and megacolon. In: *Consultations in Feline Medicine*, 3rd edition, ed. JR Agust, pp. 104–112. Philadelphia, PA: Saunders; 1997.

8. Washabau RJ. Feline megacolon. In: *Small Animal Gastroenterology*, ed. JM Steiner, pp. 230–236. Hannover, Germany: Schlutersche; 2008.

9. Haricharan RN, Georgeson KE. Hirschsprung disease. *Seminars in Pediatric Surgery* 2008;17(4):266–275.

10. Hall JA, Washabau RJ. Diagnosis and treatment of gastric motility disorders. *Veterinary Clinics of North America. Small Animal Practice* 1999;29(2):377–395.

11. Prins NH, Briejer MR, Schuurkes JA. Characterization of the contraction to 5-HT in the canine colon longitudinal muscle. *British Journal of Pharmacology* 1997;120(4):714–720.

12. Davenport DJ, Remillard RL, Jenkins C. Gastritis. In: *Small Animal Clinical Nutrition*, 5th edition, eds. MS Hand, CD Thatcher, RJ Remillard, P Roudebush, BJ Novotony, pp. 1025–1032. Topeka, KS: MMI; 2010.

13. Davenport DJ, Remilliard RL, Carroll M. Constipation/obstipation/megacolon. In: *Small Animal Clinical Nutrition*, 5th edition, eds. MS Hand, CD Thatcher, RL Remilliard, P Roudebush, BJ Novotny, pp. 1116–1126. Topeka, KS: MMI; 2010.

14. Lembo A, Camilleri M. Chronic constipation. *The New England Journal of Medicine* 2003;349:1360–1368.

Section 4

1. DeNovo RC. Diseases of the stomach. In: *Handbook of Small Animal Gastroenterology*, 2nd edition, ed. T Todd, pp. 159–194. St. Louis: W.B. Saunders; 2003.

2. Plumb DC. *Plumb's Veterinary Drug Handbook*, 5th edition, Ames, IA: Blackwell Publishing; 2005.

3. Nelson RW, Couto CG. General therapeutics principles Sm. Anim IM, 4th edition, pp. 405–406.

4. Elwood C, Devauchelle P, Elliott J, Freiche V, German AJ, Gualtieri M, Hall E, den Hertog E, Neiger R, Peeters D, Roura X, Savary-Bataille K. Emesis in dogs: a review. *Journal of Small Animal Practice* 2010;51(1):4–22.

5. Narishetty ST, Galvan B, Coscarelli E, Aleo M, Fleck T, Humphrey W, McCall RB. Effect of refrigeration of the antiemetic Cerenia (maropitant) on pain on injection. *Veterinary Therapeutics* 2009;10(3):93–102.

6. Nelson RW, Couto CG. General therapeutic principles. In: *Small Animal Internal Medicine*, 4th edition, eds. RW Nelson, CG Couto, GR Grauer, EC Hawkins, pp. 395–412. St. Louis, MO: Mosby; 2009.

7. Ramsey DS, Kincaid K, Watkins JA, Boucher JF, Condor GA, Eagleson JS, Clemence RG. Safety and efficacy of injectable and oral maropitant, a selective neurokinin 1 receptor antagonist, in a randomized clinical trial for treatment of vomiting in dogs. *Journal of Veterinary Pharmacology and Therapeutics* 2008;31(6):538–543.

8. Jergens AE. 2005. Canine and feline inflammatory bowel disease—what's new. *AAHA proceedings CD*.

9. Davenport DJ, Remillard RL. Acute gastroenteritis and enteritis. In: *Small Animal Clinical Nutrition*, 5th edition, eds. MS Hand, CD Thatcher, RL Remilliard, P Roudebush, BJ Novotny, pp. 1053–1061. Marceline, MO: Walsworth Publishing; 2010.

10. Blackwood L, German AJ, Stell AJ, O'Neill T. Multicentric lymphoma in a dog after cyclosporine therapy. *Journal of Small Animal Practice* 2004;45(5):259–262.

11. Al-Ghazlat S.. Immunosuppressive therapy for canine immune mediated hemolytic anemia. *Compendium* 2009;31(1).

12. Allenspach K. Diseases of the large intestine. In: *Textbook of Veterinary Internal Medicine*, 7th edition, eds. SJ Ettinger, EC Feldman, p. 1594. St. Louis, MO: Saunders; 2010.

Section 5

1. Marks SL. Enteral and parenteral nutritional support. In: *Textbook of Veterinary Internal Medicine*, Vol. 1., 5th edition, eds. SJ Ettinger, EC Feldman, pp. 275–282. Philadelphia, PA: W.B. Saunders; 2000.

2. Guilford WG, Center SA, Strombeck DR et al. Nutritional management of gastrointestinal disease. In: *Strombeck's Small Animal Gastroenterology*, 3rd edition, pp. 904–908. Philadelphia, PA: W.B. Saunders; 1996.

3. Saker KE, Remillard R. Critical care nutrition and enteral-assisted feeding. In: *Small Animal Clinical Nutrition*, 5th edition, eds. MS Hand, CD Thatcher, RL Remillard, P Roudebush, BBJ Novotny, pp. 439–471. Marceline, MO: Walsworth Publishing; 2010.

4. Willard M. The GI system. In: *Essentials of Small Animal Internal Medicine*, eds. RW Nelson, CG Couto, pp. 305–309. St. Louis, MO: Mosby; 1992.

5. Donoghue S. Nutritional support of hospitalized patients. *Veterinary Clinics of North America. Small Animal Practice* 1989;19(3):475–493.

6. Michel KE. 2006. Monitoring the enterally fed patient to maximize benefits and minimize complication. In: *IVECCS Proceedings*, pp. 495–498.

7. Dimski DS, Taboada, J. Feline idiopathic hepatic lipidosis. In: *The Veterinary Clinics of North America Small Animal Practice: Liver Disease*, ed. DS Dimski, pp. 357–373. Philadelphia, PA: W.B. Saunders; 1995.

8. Hill RH. Critical care nutrition. In: *Waltham Book Clinical Nutrition of the Dog & Cat*, eds. JM Wills, KW Simpson, pp. 39–57. Cambridge, MA: Blackwell; 1994.

9. Remillard RL, Armstrong PJ, Davenport DJ. Assisted feeding in hospitalized patients; enteral and parental nutrition. In: *Small Animal Clinical Nutrition*, 4th edition, eds. MS Hand, CD Thatcher, RL Remilliard, P Roudebush, pp. 351–399. Marceline, MO: Walsworth Publishing; 2000.

10. Guilford G, Center S. Nutritional management of gastrointestinal disease. In: *Strombecks's Small Animal Gastroenterology*, 3rd edition, pp. 889–910. Philadelphia, PA: W.B. Saunders; 1996.

Section 6

1. Roudebush P, Guilford WG, Shanley KJ. Adverse reactions to food. In: *Small Animal Clinical Nutrition*, 4th edition, eds. MS Hand, CD Thatcher, RL Remillard, P Roudebush, pp. 431–453. Topeka, KS: Mark Morris Institute; 2000.

2. Case LC, Carey DP, Hirakawa DA, Daristotle L. Nutritionally responsive dermatoses. In: *Canine and Feline Nutrition*, 2nd edition, pp. 443–450. St. Louis, MO: Mosby; 2000.

3. German A, Zentek J. The most common digestive diseases: the role of nutrition. In: *Encyclopedia of Canine Clinical Nutrition*, eds. P Pibot, V Biourge, D Elliott, pp. 115–118. Aimargues, France: Aniwa SAS; 2006.

4. Mueller RS, Dethioux F. Nutritional dermatoses and the contribution of dietetics in dermatology. In: *Encyclopedia of Feline Clinical Nutrition*, eds. P Pibot, V Biourge, D Elliott, p. 58. Aimargues, France: Aniwa SAS; 2008.

5. Nelson RW, Couto CG. Disorders of the intestinal tract. In: *Small Animal Internal Medicine*, 4th edition, eds. RW Nelson, CG Couto, p. 442. St. Louis, MO: Mosby Elsevier; 2009.

6. Simpson KW. The role of nutrition in the pathogenesis and the management of exocrine pancreatic disorders. In: *Encyclopedia of Canine Clinical Nutrition*, eds. P Pibot, V Biourge, D Elliot, p. 171. Aimargues, France: Aniwa SAS/Royal Canin; 2006.

7. Weese JS, Arroyo L. Bacteriological evaluation of dog and cat diets that claim to contain probiotics. *The Canadian Veterinary Journal* 2003;44(March):212–216.

8. Pan X, Chen F, Wu T, Tang H, Zhao Z. Prebiotic oligosaccharides change the concentrations of short-chain fatty acids and the microbial population of mouse bowel. *Journal of Zhejiang University. Science. B* 2009;10(4):258–263.

9. Lerman A, Lockwood B. Nutraceuticals in veterinary medicine. *Pharmacy Journal* 2007;278:51.

10. Kelly M. *The role of probiotics in GI tract health*. St. Louis, MO: Nestle Purina Pet Care; 2006.

11. Roberfroid M. Prebiotics: the concept revisited. *The Journal of Nutrition* 2007;137:830s.

12. Verdonk JMAJ, Shim SB, van Leeuwen P, Verstegan MWA. Application of inulin-type fructans in animal feed and pet food. *The British Journal of Nutrition* 2005;93 Suppl 1:s125–s138.

Section 7

1. Grimm K, Thurmon J, Tranquilli WJ. *Lumb and Jones Veterinary Anesthesia and Analgesia*, 4th edition, Ames, IA: Blackwell Publishing Inc; 2007.

Chapter 9 Liver

Editors: Jocelyn Mott and Ann Wortinger

SECTION 1 HEPATIC DISEASE

Acute hepatitis

Acute hepatitis is defined as acute hepatic inflammation. This may be due to viral, bacterial, protozoal, or fungal agents, or to immune-mediated diseases.

Anatomy and physiology

The liver is a metabolically active organ with numerous functions critical for survival. Due to its unique anatomic position and blood supply, it acts as the main filter for portal blood from the gastrointestinal (GI) tract. Thus, it is the main site for drug metabolism and immunologic surveillance. As such, the liver is also susceptible to various toxic entities and infectious agents.

Clinical Signs

The clinical signs of acute hepatitis may have a very rapid onset; therefore, affected animals may present on an emergency basis. Clinical signs may include vomiting, diarrhea, anorexia, lethargy, and depression. Jaundice and dehydration may be detected on physical examination. Animals may also be painful on abdominal palpation and hepatomegaly can be present in some cases.

With severe disease, affected animals may present with evidence of derangements in coagulation (prolonged bleeding from venipuncture sites, epistaxis, melena) and/or with central neurological signs (dull mentation, blindness, obtunded, comatose, seizure activity) consistent with hepatic encephalopathy (HE). Animals with acute hepatitis due to infectious agents such as bacteria, parasites, or viruses may also be febrile at presentation.

Small Animal Internal Medicine for Veterinary Technicians and Nurses, First Edition. Edited by Linda Merrill.
© 2012 John Wiley & Sons, Inc. Published 2012 by John Wiley & Sons, Inc.

Diagnostic testing

Laboratory

The most consistent laboratory finding with acute hepatitis is a markedly elevated alanine aminotransferase (ALT). This is consistent with recent and ongoing hepatocyte damage. Significant elevations in alkaline phosphatase (ALP) and total bilirubin may also be seen and may be severe. With significant hepatic impairment, decreased blood urea nitrogen (BUN), albumin, and cholesterol may be present. This is most likely due to decreased hepatic ability in functions such as protein synthesis, protein breakdown, and bile acid production. Hypoglycemia can be the result of an overwhelming infection or decreased hepatic function.

If jaundice is present, a fasting blood ammonia level should be performed to confirm hepatic dysfunction or to help determine if an animal is encephalopathic. In the absence of jaundice, fasting and postprandial bile acids may be performed and may be elevated. Bile acids would not be recommended if visible icterus is seen. Isosthenuria and bilirubinuria may be seen on urinalysis. Various compositions of urine crystals may also be noted.

Hematocrit or packed cell volume (PCV) may be normal, increased if dehydration is severe, or decreased if blood loss has occurred due to hemorrhage secondary to diminished coagulation factors. White blood cells may be normal, increased due to inflammation or response to infection, or decreased if infection is becoming overwhelming.

The number and morphological characteristics of mature and band neutrophils should be determined. With significant inflammatory disease, toxic changes may be seen in mature neutrophils in the form of increased vacuoles and Döhle bodies. Similarly, platelets may be normal, increased as a response to hemorrhage, or decreased due to consumption or possible disseminated intravascular coagulation (DIC). Prothrombin time (PT) and partial thromboplastin time (PTT) may be prolonged as a result of consumption in DIC or a lack of hepatic production of coagulation factors. D-dimers may be elevated and could provide additional evidence for DIC. When appropriate, serum should be submitted for leptospirosis serology.

Imaging

Abdominal radiographs may be relatively normal, but hepatomegaly may be demonstrated by extension of the liver past the caudal rib margin and with caudal deviation of the gastric axis. GI contents should be evaluated radiographically for foreign or potentially toxic material that may exhibit different densities from normal stomach contents. On ultrasound, the liver may appear normal or may be diffusely altered in echotexture. If the animal is jaundiced, the gallbladder and biliary tree should be assessed for evidence of obstruction.

Biopsy

Coagulation status should always be assessed prior to biopsy to limit bleeding complications. Tissue and, where appropriate, bile samples should routinely be collected for histopathology, aerobic and anaerobic (in cats) bacterial culture and sensitivity, and fungal culture (where appropriate). Options for obtaining the necessary diagnostic samples include surgical laparotomy, minimally invasive laparoscopy, and percutaneous ultrasound-guided techniques. Ascites and prolonged coagulation profiles may be contraindications to ultrasound-guided liver biopsy, necessitating surgical biopsies instead.

Pharmacology

The management of acute hepatitis may vary significantly, depending on the underlying etiology of the disease. Supportive care and, in some cases, aggressive measures, are likely to be required in the majority of cases. General supportive measures consist of crystalloid (for correction of dehydration and replacing ongoing fluid losses) and colloid fluid support (for animals unable to maintain oncotic pressure due to hypoalbuminemia), normalization and maintenance of plasma electrolyte levels, antioxidant therapy, and antacid and antiemetic medications.

Additional therapies may include intravenous dextrose if hypoglycemia is present, vitamin K administration, and plasma transfusions for coagulation support, oral or rectal therapy with lactulose for HE, antibiotics in cases of bacterial hepatitis, and even specific antidote or chelation therapy in cases of toxic hepatitis. Immunosuppressive therapy may be indicated when an immune-mediated hepatitis is diagnosed. Animals may be prescribed multiple medications, and the potential for drug interactions and toxicities may be higher with severe liver disease due to decreased metabolism and excretion of metabolites. Close monitoring for medication side effects and client education is imperative.

Anesthetic and analgesic considerations specific to acute hepatitis

Animals with acute hepatitis may experience abdominal pain, which may be exacerbated by vomiting. Analgesic therapy should be considered when abdominal pain is documented or suspected, using agents that require minimal hepatic metabolism. During anesthetic events, particular attention should be paid to monitoring blood glucose levels, blood pressure, and body temperature. Dextrose infusions, pressor support, and external warming may be required.

Nutritional considerations

Animals with acute hepatitis may have life-threatening diseases, but this does not decrease the need for adequate nutritional support. There may also be an increased risk for feline patients to develop secondary hepatic lipidosis due to decreased appetite or total anorexia. Whenever possible, the enteral route should be used for nutritional support. Feeding tubes should be utilized if animals will not ingest at least 85% of the recommended calories as calculated by resting energy requirement (RER). The type of tube (nasoesophageal, nasogastric, esophagostomy, percutaneous endoscopic gastrostomy tube [PEG] tube, or jejunostomy tube) to be placed depends on patient size, ability to tolerate sedation or anesthesia, and cardiovascular status. Total or partial parenteral nutrition may be pursued if the animal does not tolerate enteral feedings or is not consuming at least 85% of RER.

Chronic hepatitis

The key components of the disease appear to include a subclinical phase of variable length, advanced disease at the time of diagnosis, and an overall poor response to therapy. The response to therapy may be prolonged with early identification and intervention, while in the subclinical phase. The etiology of the disease is unknown. Several canine breeds (Dobermans, cocker spaniels, Labrador retrievers, etc.) have been shown to have an increased susceptibility to chronic hepatitis, and there may be a genetic component to the disease.

Clinical signs

The clinical signs of chronic hepatitis relate to a loss of normal liver function, so clinical signs are variable. Signs are typically vague and nonspecific (polyuria and polydipsia [PU/PD], weight loss, vomiting, and anorexia), though the presence of jaundice may be a more specific indicator of potential liver dysfunction. With progressive disease, the liver will become small and irregular, and abdominal effusion may be present. Ascites may be a result of portal hypertension or a result of loss of oncotic pressure due to low serum albumin. HE, characterized by central neurological signs, and coagulopathies may also be seen with severe disease.

Diagnostic testing

Laboratory

The most consistent laboratory finding with chronic hepatitis is an elevated ALT, especially in the subclinical stage of the disease. Elevations in ALP and total bilirubin are seen more consistently in the clinical stage of the disease. Additional laboratory findings include decreases in BUN, albumin, cholesterol, and glucose. Changes in serum electrolytes (hyperkalemia, hyponatremia) may represent third spacing of fluids if ascites is present. Specific liver function testing (fasting and postprandial bile acids or fasting ammonia level) may be significantly abnormal, though these changes are not specific for chronic hepatitis. Isosthenuria is a common finding on urinalysis, and bilirubinuria and ammonium urate or biurate crystals may also be seen.

The complete blood count (CBC) may be normal or may show a nonregenerative anemia, consistent with chronic disease. A mild thrombocytosis can be seen with chronic hemorrhage. PT and PTT may be prolonged due to lack of hepatic production of coagulation factors. A coagulation panel should always be performed prior to invasive procedures.

Imaging

Abdominal radiographs may demonstrate microhepatica with cranial displacement of the gastric axis and other abdominal organs (spleen, intestines). If ascites is present, the abdominal viscera may be effaced with a soft tissue/fluid effect and abdominal detail may be very poor.

In chronic hepatitis, the liver should appear diffusely affected and abnormal on abdominal ultrasound. Normal tissue architecture is lost and the liver parenchyma may appear irregular and nodular. The liver capsule loses its expected smooth appearance and becomes undulant or "lumpy-bumpy." The gallbladder and biliary tree should be assessed for evidence of obstruction if the animal is jaundiced. If ascites is present, in most cases, the fluid will appear hypocellular to acellular; however, hemorrhage may be present, causing the fluid to be more cellular than otherwise expected. Fluid may be sampled via abdominocentesis for cytological analysis, protein content, and cell count. Due to the concerns for possible hemorrhage, a smaller-gauge butterfly catheter should be used for abdominocentesis and fluid should be collected under sterile conditions.

Biopsy

Hepatic biopsy is required for the diagnosis of chronic hepatitis and the coagulation status should always be assessed prior to biopsy. Samples should routinely be collected for histopathology, bacterial culture and sensitivity (liver and bile samples), and copper quantification. This requires larger amounts of tissue, and thus requires surgical exploratory or laparoscopic procedures. Ultrasound-guided techniques are generally not indicated for this disease. This is due to the limited amount of tissue that can be obtained via ultrasound-guided biopsy. Ascites and prolonged coagulation profiles are also contraindications to ultrasound-guided liver biopsy.

Treatment and pharmacology

Chronic hepatitis is a medically managed disease and while therapy is primarily supportive, animals may be on multidrug therapies. It is generally not possible to avoid medications that have some degree of hepatic metabolism. In addition, dosing strategies may be affected by loss of lean body mass, presence of ascites, and changes in drug binding due to hypoalbuminemia. It is prudent to monitor animals closely for signs of drug toxicities or untoward drug interactions. Client education regarding pharmacological side effects is vital.

Multidrug protocols are commonly employed. Antioxidant medications increase hepatocyte concentrations of glutathione and are generally well tolerated. Oral absorption is variable, depending on the formulation used. Ursodiol (ursodeoxycholic acid) is a hydrophilic bile acid that increases bile flow in cases with cholestasis. It is contraindicated with biliary obstruction and can cause GI side effects (inappetence, diarrhea). Chelating agents (e.g., penicillamine) may be useful in cases with significant metal (copper) accumulation based on results from tissue quantification as discussed above. Colchicine is an antifibrotic agent that may be helpful in cases with hepatic fibrosis and cirrhosis identified on histopathology. The efficacy of this medication is relatively unknown in the veterinary field, but myelosuppression has been identified in human patients. If affected animals have bleeding tendencies, oral or injectable vitamin K therapy may be beneficial. Additionally, animals may benefit from antinausea and antiemetic therapy as discussed elsewhere. For animals with HE, lactulose therapy (orally or via enema) is recommended. Dosing should be adjusted to avoid diarrhea.

Anesthetic and analgesic considerations

Anesthesia will generally only be pursued for obtaining liver samples for analysis. If a coagulopathy is present, transfusions of plasma and therapy with vitamin K may be indicated. There is a risk for hemorrhage with hepatic biopsy, so whole blood or packed red blood cell transfusions may also be necessary. Postprocedural PCVs should be routinely monitored.

Nutritional considerations

For animals with a primary or secondary copper disorder, the most significant component of nutritional therapy is limiting dietary copper. Protein restriction is especially recommended for animals with HE, though protein malnutrition may result from aggressive protein restriction. Changes in lean body mass and serum albumin should be monitored. Additional supplementation with antioxidants, zinc, and vitamin K may be beneficial.

Copper-associated chronic hepatitis

Copper-associated chronic hepatitis (CACH) is a disease in which an abnormal accumulation of copper in hepatocytes causes toxic injury and incites inflammation and hepatocellular necrosis, which progresses to chronic hepatitis and cirrhosis. In CACH, copper accumulation is the *primary* abnormality and results in secondary hepatic injury and hepatitis, as distinguished from other forms of hepatic disease, in which copper accumulation is *secondary* and occurs as a *consequence* of hepatitis, hepatocellular dysfunction, and cholestasis. CACH is principally a disease of dogs, although one affected cat has been reported,[1] and there are distinct breed predispositions, supporting a genetic basis for abnormal copper handling in affected dogs. Hereditary copper toxicosis has been best described in the Bedlington terrier, where the genetic defect has been identified as a mutation in the *COMMD1* (previously called *MURR1*) gene. Breed-related hepatic copper accumulation with secondary hepatitis is also reported in West Highland white terriers, Skye terriers, Labrador retrievers, and Dalmatians. Other breeds (Doberman pinschers, cocker spaniels) are reported to have chronic hepatitis associated with high hepatic copper concentrations, but it is unclear in these breeds if the copper accumulation is primary or secondary.

Anatomy and physiology

Copper is an essential nutrient that is a component of many proteins and serves as a cofactor for critical enzymes involved in hematopoiesis, pigmentation, neurotransmission, maintenance of connective tissues (cardiovascular system, lung, bone), oxidative metabolism, and free radical scavenging. Dietary copper is absorbed in the intestine, especially in the small intestine. Absorbed copper is complexed to albumin and transported to the liver, which is the central organ for copper metabolism. Copper is taken up from the bloodstream into hepatocytes, which may handle the now intracellular copper by a number of routes, including (1) formation of ceruloplasmin (copper–protein complex) and export from the liver to the circulation to serve as a carrier of copper to other tissues, (2) utilization within the hepatocyte including mitochondrial enzyme systems, (3) excretion of excess copper into the bile for elimination from the body in the feces, or (4) metallothionein-bound storage in hepatocytes. Because copper is a reactive substance (oxidant), it is maintained in the body complexed to other compounds to control its reactivity, and its absorption is somewhat regulated by intestinal metallothionein (a metal-binding protein). Abnormal accumulation of copper within hepatocytes can result from increased intestinal and hepatocellular uptake of copper, abnormal intracellular copper metabolism, or defects in elimination of copper via biliary excretion. In patients with CACH, the underlying abnormality is most likely a genetic defect causing abnormal copper transport or storage. The specific defect has been defined only in the Bedlington terrier breed, where a mutation in the *COMMD1* gene results in defective biliary excretion of copper. Excess intracellular copper causes oxidative injury to hepatocytes and triggers inflammation (hepatitis), which causes further liver damage and promotes collagen deposition (fibrosis, cirrhosis), potentially progressing to liver failure. Additionally, during periods of active hepatocellular necrosis, excess copper can be released from hepatocytes into the circulation in high enough levels to cause hemolytic anemia. This is sometimes clinically seen in the Bedlington terrier.

Clinical signs

Affected dogs may remain clinically normal in the initial stages (years) as copper is progressively accumulating in the liver. Generally, the clinical signs are those of liver dysfunction. Initially, the signs may be subtle and nonspecific, such as inappetence and lethargy, which may wax and wane. Owners often do not recognize these vague early changes and may later present the patient as having an "acute" disease when the chronic liver injury and loss of function has progressed to a point where more severe clinical signs develop. In more advanced disease, intermittent to persistent anorexia, depression, weight loss, vomiting, diarrhea, PU/PD, icterus, and ascites may be manifested. Less commonly, some dogs (Bedlington terriers) present with acute fulminant disease resulting from acute hepatic necrosis, precipitated by periods of extreme physiological stress (whelping, intercurrent disease). Bedlington terriers may present with hemolytic anemia associated with these episodes of acute hepatic necrosis. Patients with advanced liver disease may also show neurological abnormalities (mental dullness, circling, head pressing) consistent with HE.

Diagnostic testing

Laboratory

Clinicopathologic abnormalities are similar to those associated with liver disease in general. Elevated serum ALT is the most consistent finding and is often evident in the earlier stages of disease before clinical signs appear. Milder elevations of ALP are sometimes present. Other less consistent findings include low BUN, hypoalbuminemia, hyperbilirubinemia, elevated serum bile acids, and abnormal coagulation. These parameters reflect the degree of liver dysfunction. The CBC commonly shows leukocytosis, thrombocytopenia, and mild anemia. Urinalysis may demonstrate bilirubinuria and, in patients with severe liver dysfunction, ammonium biurate crystals. Blood copper levels are not helpful in identifying or monitoring affected animals. Bedlington terriers can be tested for the *COMMD1* mutation, which accounts for most (but not all) of the copper-associated disease in this breed by genetic testing of a mouth swab sample (VetGen Veterinary Genetic Services, http://www.vetgen.com). Absence of this mutation does not rule out copper-associated disease.

Imaging

There are no imaging findings that are specific for CACH. Ultrasonographic findings may include hypoechogenicity of the liver associated with inflammation and/or reduced liver size as a result of hepatocyte loss and cirrhosis. Patients with advanced disease may have portal hypertension and ascites, which can manifest as decreased serosal detail on abdominal radiographs.

Biopsy techniques

Definitive diagnosis requires liver biopsy for histopathology and quantification of liver copper. Care should be taken to obtain tissue samples of sufficiently large size for inclusion of six to eight portal triads on histopathology and for quantitative copper analysis (1 g). Special stains (rhodanine or rubeanic acid) are used to demonstrate copper in liver histopathology specimens. In animals with primary copper accumulation and secondary hepatitis, copper accumulation occurs first in centrilobular regions (zone 3) with associated mononuclear to mixed inflammatory infiltrates and copper-laden macrophages[2] as opposed to periportal copper accumulations that occur secondary to primary hepatitis and cholestasis. Fibrosis or cirrhosis may also be identified. Copper concentrations should be evaluated using breed-specific reference ranges whenever possible as normal liver copper concentrations vary between breeds.[3]

Pharmacology and treatment

Specific treatment of CACH is directed at reducing levels of the toxic principle, copper. This entails treatment to remove copper that has already accumulated in the liver coupled with treatment to reduce absorption of additional copper from the intestine. Therapy to reduce copper concentrations in the liver consists of administration of chelating agents that bind copper and facilitate its urinary excretion. Penicillamine or trientene may be used. Chelator therapy results in a decrease in accumulated copper, which may take months to years to show a significant effect, and lifelong treatment may be needed. Serial hepatic copper level determinations should be done to demonstrate a response and to prevent copper depletion. Treatments to reduce absorption of additional copper include dietary zinc administration, low copper diets, and selected water sources. Dietary zinc supplementation induces intestinal metallothionein, which binds dietary copper to prevent its absorption. Copper then remains bound to the metallothionein until the intestinal cell is sloughed and eliminated in the feces, carrying the bound copper from the body. Zinc and penicillamine should not be used concurrently. Zinc therapy is typically reserved for maintenance treatment of patients completing chelator therapy or for treating asymptomatic patients. Animals receiving zinc supplementation should have zinc levels monitored to prevent zinc toxicity and resulting hemolytic anemia. Animals with CACH should be fed a low copper diet. Because copper induces oxidative injury, addition of antioxidant agents (N-acetylcysteine [NAC], S-adenosylmethionine [SAMe], silymarin, vitamin E) to the treatment protocol may be considered. Additional treatment for hepatitis and hepatic dysfunction may be needed depending on the degree to which liver damage has advanced.

Because reducing hepatic copper levels is a difficult and slow process and because associated liver injury may not be reversible in advanced cases, screening dogs at risk is indicated. Bedlington terriers can be genetically screened as puppies for the *COMMD1* mutation linked to copper toxicosis. A positive result indicates that the individual is at risk, but a negative result does not mean that the patient will be unaffected. Other breeds at risk can have their liver copper levels measured via biopsy as early as 12 months of age. Dogs with abnormal results in initial screening can be placed on a high zinc, low copper diet to minimize hepatic copper accumulation if copper levels have not yet reached toxic levels requiring chelation therapy.

Anesthetic and analgesic considerations

Animals with impaired liver function may decompensate when anesthetized and are prone to development of cerebral edema.

Nutritional considerations

Diets for animals with CACH should exclude copper-rich foods such as organ meat, eggs, shellfish, and legumes. Commercial prescription diets formulated for patients with liver disease (Royal Canin Hepatic Support, Hill's l/d) are appropriately copper restricted, but, in young growing dogs, protein levels may need to be supplemented with low copper proteins (dairy based, egg whites, white meat from poultry). Avoid water from copper pipes. Bottled water may be used to assure low copper content.

Hepatic lipidosis

Hepatic lipidosis is a well-recognized disease syndrome in cats. The disease may be idiopathic or it may develop secondary to some other underlying medical problem. Many affected cats were formerly obese and significant weight loss of up to 25% of body weight may occur by the time they are presented for complaints of anorexia and weight loss. Hepatic lipidosis is the most common hepatobiliary disorder affecting cats in the United States.[4–6] The disease typically affects middle-aged cats but ranges from 0.5 to 15.0 years. There is no breed predisposition for this disease.[4,6]

Anatomy and physiology

The liver is responsible for a variety of important functions within the body, including metabolism of carbohydrates and fats, synthesis of proteins and vitamins, storage of vitamins and iron, production of coagulation factors, and removal and excretion of toxins.[7] The liver is involved in many crucial biological functions; as such, a cat with liver disease may show a wide variety of signs including lethargy, anorexia, weight loss, weakness, jaundice, vomiting, diarrhea, and behavioral changes.

Etiology

Factors that may be associated with the onset of hepatic lipidosis include stress, obesity, anorexia, cancer, changes in the diet, nutritional deficiencies, or any other disease that affects the cat's willingness to eat. Hepatic lipidosis is seldom a primary cause of disease but is most often seen secondary to other diseases such as diabetes mellitus, pancreatitis, renal disease, inflammatory bowel disease, and cancer. Hepatic lipidosis is caused by severe energy (calorie) and/or protein restriction, or rapid weight loss in obese cats.[5,6] To help prevent the occurrence of hepatic lipidosis in dieting cats, weight loss should not exceed 1 lb/month, or 10% of their body weight per month (depending on their starting weight).

Anorexia can cause mobilization of free fatty acids from the adipose tissue. Free fatty acids are taken up by the liver and converted to ketone bodies, or if glycerol is available, reassembled into triglycerides. Triglycerides are further converted into lipoproteins if enough protein is available for use. Ketone bodies and lipoproteins are used by the brain and muscle for 5% of their energy requirements during absolute starvation.[6,8]

Healthy obese cats have excessive hepatic lipid accumulation because the normal liver has the ability to extract fatty acids and to convert them into triglycerides at a rate greater than that required for their use in energy or lipoprotein dispersal.[6,8] Since obese cats have the underlying tendency favoring hepatic lipid accumulation, starvation will exacerbate hepatic triglyceride accumulation due to the release of large amounts of fatty acids from the adipose stores during periods of rapid weight loss.

Reduced availability of lipotropic proteins, amino acids, and other nutrients during periods of marginal food intake or anorexia can further limit lipoprotein synthesis and promote hepatic lipid accumulation. This excessive accumulation of triglycerides in the liver eventually interferes with hepatic function and liver failure results.[4,6]

In situations of less than absolute starvation (marginal food intake), adaptation to fatty acid metabolism is also lost and excessive hepatic triglyceride accumulation results.[8] This is important because ingestion or force feeding of some diets with insufficient calories or intravenous administration of dextrose will worsen hepatic triglyceride storage. Feeding a balanced diet with sufficient caloric and protein content is essential to facilitate recovery from hepatic lipidosis syndrome.

The disease is characterized by extensive vacuolation of hepatocytes. In healthy cats, ~5% of the liver tissue contains lipids; however, in cats with hepatic lipidosis, greater than 50% of the liver tissue contains lipids. This lipid is stored as vacuoles in the liver tissue. Lipid vacuolation of more than 50% is consistent with feline hepatic lipidosis syndrome (Figures 9.1.1 and 9.1.2).[4]

Clinical signs

The history usually discloses a cat that has been either totally or partially anorexic over a period of days to weeks and as a result has undergone a sudden weight loss. The cats may be jaundiced upon presentation, but the absence of jaundice does not rule out hepatic lipidosis. There may be intermittent vomiting, diarrhea or constipation, and dehydration. Palpable liver margins may be found on physical exam. The clinical signs vary based on any secondary disease processes and on the duration of the illness. Cats may be unkempt, lethargic, weak, and may have weight loss. With severe disease, HE may be seen with head pressing, depression, and ptyalism.[9]

Diagnostic testing

Laboratory

Laboratory evaluation demonstrates biochemical changes that are consistent with hepatic lipidosis. The serum alkaline phosphatase (SAP), ALT, and AST will be elevated with the gamma-glutamyl transferase (GGT) normal to low. The serum bilirubin levels will usually be increased; if it is greater than 2 mg/dL, visible jaundice may be seen. If this increase is significant enough, there may be spillover of direct bilirubin in the urine causing the presence of bilirubin crystals in the urinalysis. Unlike dogs, any bilirubin in the urine of cats is significant.[9]

Imaging

On ultrasound examination, a normal liver will be isoechoic to the kidney (the same echogenicity) and hypoechoic to the surrounding fat. In patients with hepatic lipidosis, the liver will be hyperechoic, with respect to the falciform fat and the kidney[4,6] (see Figure 9.1.3). A tentative diagnosis may be made based on the ultrasound findings of a diffuse hyperechoic hepatopathy.

Biopsy

Definitive diagnosis of hepatic lipidosis requires examination of either aspirations or biopsies of the liver.

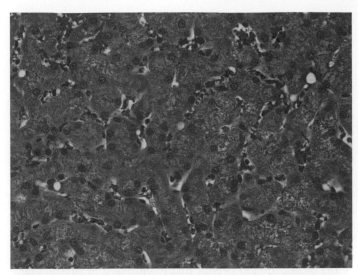

Figure 9.1.1 Normal fat vacuoles in the liver. Image courtesy of Dr. Barb Powers, Colorado State University Histopathology Laboratory.

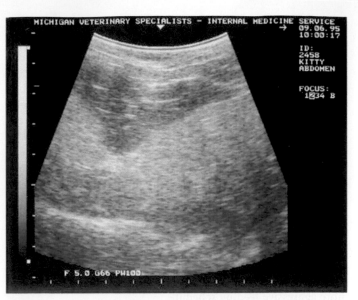

Figure 9.1.3 Ultrasound image showing echogenicity comparison of falciform fat and a fatty liver. Image courtesy of Dr. Ned F. Kuehn, Michigan Veterinary Specialists.

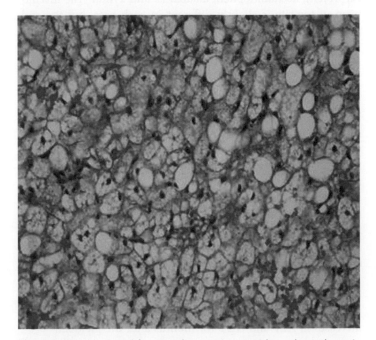

Figure 9.1.2 Increased fat vacuoles consistent with moderate hepatic lipidosis. Image courtesy of Dr. Barb Powers, Colorado State University Histopathology Laboratory.

Fine needle aspiration (FNA) of the liver is performed for cytological evaluation. This can be done without anesthesia if the cat will remain still during the procedure. Ultrasound-guided biopsy is performed under sedation or anesthesia if the cat is fractious or too mobile. Also, the larger-sized biopsy samples are preferred if there are any questions as to whether hepatic lipidosis is the primary problem. Ultrasound-guided biopsy does require profound sedation or general anesthesia. Because the liver is responsible for the production of coagulation factors, a clotting profile should be performed prior to any biopsy to ensure the patient has the ability to form a blood clot after the biopsy has been completed.[9]

The cytology or biopsy results for hepatic lipidosis show a highly vacuolated cytoplasm consistent with lipid accumulation, resulting in a vacuolar hepatopathy. The pathologist should grade the lipidosis as mild, moderate, marked, or severe. This will be one of the best prognostic indicators for the recovery of the cat. The more severe the changes, the poorer the prognosis.[4,6,7]

Treatment and pharmacology

Regardless of the etiology, the basic treatment for hepatic lipidosis remains the same. Many cats will be dehydrated and completely anorexic when brought into the hospital. Intravenous fluids, type dependent on electrolyte status, are used to correct the dehydration.[5,7,10] Normal nutrition must be restored to reverse the disease. If the disease is caught early enough, appetite stimulants may be used to reestablish adequate nutrition. Cyproheptadine and mirtazapine are used most commonly. Any underlying or concurrent disease should also be addressed to ensure this is not negatively affecting appetite. As liver failure progresses, it exerts a strong appetite-suppressant effect, placing the veterinary health-care team in a difficult position. The cat needs to eat to reverse the disease, but the disease itself is suppressing the appetite, making self-feeding more unlikely.[9] Since most cats refuse to eat, it is often necessary to place a feeding tube in order to provide adequate nutritional support.

Feeding tubes should be placed as soon as possible after diagnosis. If placing a PEG tube, feeding should not begin for at least 12 h to allow formation of a temporary stoma around the tube. This is not necessary when placing an esophagostomy tube as peritonitis is not a concern.[7,8] More information on feeding tubes can be found in Chapter 8.

At this time, the cat will shift from catabolic metabolism to anabolic metabolism; in doing this, it will shift from using protein as the preferred energy source to using carbohydrates and fats.[4,6]

By providing adequate nutrition, the liver will be allowed to regain its normal function. A veterinary recovery diet is typically fed through the feeding tube for the entire time it takes the cat to recover from hepatic lipidosis, typically 8–16 weeks. Daily energy requirements (DERs) should be calculated as you would for any other critical care patient, with your initial calculation done at the patient's current weight, progressing up to the amount for the desired weight.

Generally, these cats require 7–10 days of hospitalization to allow the food to be slowly increased until they are receiving their calculated daily kilocalorie requirements per day. A quicker increase in feeding can be done if finances necessitate, but the incidence of complications increases significantly with a shorter, more aggressive feeding schedule.

The slow increase in food is necessary due to villus atrophy and ileus in the GI tract. Nausea is often seen secondary to the reintroduction of food. The faster the food is given, the worse the nausea can be. This can be due to the GI changes or may be secondary to the liver disease. GI motility agents such as metoclopramide and ranitidine can be used to help with the ileus.

When the cat is receiving 100% DER of food divided into three equal feedings, it can be discharged from the hospital to the care of their owners. As the liver function recovers, the appetite will gradually improve and the cat will begin to eat a regular diet on its own. The degree of recovery is related to and measured by the increase in appetite. When the cat is consistently eating normal amounts of food, without supplemental tube feeding and without weight loss, the tube can be removed. In this author's experience, waiting to remove the tube for 2 weeks after the cat is totally self-feeding is prudent. The clinician may also want to recheck blood work to ensure that the values have returned to normal levels.

Role of the veterinary technician

After the initial diagnosis, the patient's recovery from hepatic lipidosis is primarily nursing related. As technicians, we need to be able to assess response to feeding, anticipate common complications, and direct owners in at-home care. After discharge from the hospital, the primary care is transferred to the owners but should still be overseen by the technician. This supervision needs to include regular recheck examinations and frequent phone calls to monitor progress and to help prevent setbacks in recovery. This process should be like a well-choreographed dance between the hospital staff, the owners, and the patient in order to ensure a successful outcome in the management of this disease.

Toxic hepatopathy

The liver's central role in drug and toxin metabolism and elimination makes it a particularly vulnerable organ to the negative effects of these substances. The liver receives a major portion of the venous drainage from the abdominal cavity and therefore receives direct delivery of toxins and chemicals that have been absorbed via the GI tract. Drug-induced liver injury can affect any part of the liver and can mimic any form of spontaneous liver disease. The most common pathophysiological response is necrosis. In addition to hepatocellular necrosis, cholestasis, lipidosis, and steatosis can all be seen.

Toxic substances

There are hundreds of known hepatic toxins and the specific pathophysiology is not necessarily known in all cases. This section will focus on a few of the most common toxins affecting dogs and cats with a treatment section that will be helpful for any cause of hepatic failure.

The most common hepatic toxins witnessed in clinical practice include the anticonvulsants phenobarbital and diazepam, non-steroidal anti-inflammatory drugs (NSAIDs) (particularly carprofen), acetaminophen, aflatoxins, and xylitol. The mechanism of toxicity is slightly different in each case, but the end points, acute hepatic damage, are similar.

Drug-related hepatopathies
Anticonvulsants

Phenobarbital toxicity seems to be an idiosyncratic reaction in dogs that can occur anytime in relation to starting the drug, even years later. Most dogs that will develop toxicity do so within the first year of starting the drug. Initial clinical signs are generally related to impaired drug metabolism and manifest as sedation and ataxia. In some cases, stopping the drug leads to complete resolution of symptoms. Necropsy changes reported include cirrhosis or nodular vacuolar hepatopathy.

Diazepam toxicity has been reported in cats (but not in dogs) and appears to be more common with the oral form of the drug. It can cause a panlobular hepatocellular necrosis that spares the biliary epithelium. Clinical signs are generally reported within 1 week of administration. Some cats that have survived have had increases in ALP and GGT for months after the incident.

Non-steroidal anti-inflammatory drugs and analgesics

NSAIDs, particularly carprofen, can cause an idiosyncratic cytotoxic hepatopathy in dogs. The severity varies considerably, and most dogs have been on the drug for over 2 weeks when clinical signs appear.

Acetaminophen is oxidized by cytochrome P450 to its toxic metabolite, N-acetyl-p-benzoquinoneimine (NADPQI). This toxin causes a centrilobular necrosis if it is not eliminated by glutathione. Glutathione is an essential antioxidant required by the liver for detoxification purposes and is composed of three amino acids: glutamine, glycine, and cysteine. Cysteine is the rate-limiting amino acid as the other two are thought to be ubiquitous. N-acetylcysteine (NAC) provides the cysteine available for the body to be able to produce glutathione in most mammals.

Contaminants

Aflatoxin, a fungal toxin, was a contaminant in many commercial dog foods in 2005. It caused inconsistent increases in liver enzymes and hepatocellular lipid vacuolar injury along with diffuse hepatic lipidosis in the dogs that were necropsied.

Human food additives

Xylitol is a sugar substitute found in many candies, gum, and baked goods made for human consumption. It does not appear to cause insulin release in people but does cause a profound insulin release in dogs. The toxicity is thought to be related to increased reactive oxygen species (i.e., free radicals) causing cellular damage and, eventually, necrosis. The toxicity seems to be biphasic with the first clinical signs (within 1 h of ingestion) being related to acute hypoglycemia, which is often accompanied by seizures. Anywhere from 9 to 72 h later, many dogs develop acute, severe hepatic failure.

Inappropriate consumption

There are numerous substances that can cause hepatoxicity if ingested. The cycad (sago) palm is an indoor/outdoor plant that contains cycasin, a liver toxin, in high concentration in the seeds. Ingestion of as little as one to two seeds has been reported to cause death in dogs. GI signs (vomiting and diarrhea) often precede the classic signs of hepatic failure (abdominal pain, icterus, dull mentation, seizures, and coma). Laboratory tests may not become abnormal for 24–48 h after ingestion. Thrombocytopenia and alterations in white blood cell counts may be seen along with elevated liver enzymes and total bilirubin, decreases in total protein and blood glucose, and prolongations in the PT.

Several types of mushrooms can cause hepatotoxicity if ingested in sufficient numbers. Owner often reports observation of the animal eating "wild" mushrooms. Clinical signs usually begin with GI disturbances (vomiting, diarrhea, abdominal pain) and then proceed to include hepatic failure.

Clinical signs

In the early stages, clinical signs are generally nonspecific. Hepatotoxins can cause vague GI symptoms within hours after ingestion. Anorexia, lethargy, and vomiting appear to be common and may be associated with circulating hepatotoxins. In many cases of mild toxin ingestion, the clinical signs are self-limiting and do not progress. In later stages of moderate to severe toxin ingestion, clinical signs that are liver specific are apparent. Jaundice will frequently develop along with coagulopathy, hypoglycemia, and encephalopathy. In many cases, abdominal distention will occur from ascites. Severe generalized or partial focal seizures can occur due to hypoglycemia and/or toxin accumulation. The one exception is xylitol, which causes rapid, severe hypoglycemia that frequently leads to seizures and a subsequent onset of liver failure.

Diagnostic testing

Laboratory testing

Diagnostic testing is aimed at evaluating if and to what extent liver injury has occurred, not necessarily identifying a specific toxin. A CBC, biochemistry panel, and coagulation panel are essential first steps in attempting to diagnose liver injury. On a chemistry panel, albumin, BUN, bilirubin, glucose, and cholesterol are five markers that indicate the functionality of the liver, and evaluation of these markers can be very helpful in diagnosing failure. Sequential evaluation of liver enzymes along with bilirubin is very helpful to follow the progression of liver disease and resolution of injury; however, ALP and GGT can often remain elevated for weeks after clinical improvement. Serum bile acids may be helpful in diagnosing and monitoring hepatic injury if the bilirubin is normal.

Imaging

Abdominal radiographs and ultrasound are frequently required imaging modalities to evaluate the liver and abdominal cavity more thoroughly. Abdominal radiographs may show hepatomegaly and free abdominal fluid. Abdominal ultrasound may reveal changes in echogenicity and is very helpful to evaluate the biliary tract.

Biopsy

Liver biopsy may be helpful to characterize the hepatic lesion histologically and may be especially helpful in cases of chronic carprofen or phenobarbital toxicity when unsure if the cause is hepatotoxicity, chronic active hepatitis, or a combination of the two.

Treatment and pharmacology

If the toxin was ingested within 1–2 h and the patient is conscious, emesis is recommended. If the toxin was ingested over 2 h ago and the patient is conscious, administration of activated charcoal is recommended. Caution is recommended when inducing emesis followed by administration of activated charcoal as the animal will frequently vomit the charcoal and may aspirate it. If encephalopathy is a concern, a lactulose retention enema is recommended.

Eliminating the offending toxin or drug is paramount to treating the toxicity. A thorough history to determine any and all medications the patient has received, including over-the-counter supplements, is indicated. All drugs should be checked for their potential effects on the liver before continuing to administer them in an animal showing signs of liver toxicity.

A constant rate infusion (CRI) of a balanced crystalloid solution (e.g., Normosol-R') will assist in maintaining hydration and in biliary and renal excretion of toxins. Supplementation of the fluids with B complex vitamins (2 mL/L) and other additives (e.g., potassium chloride, dextrose) as needed is helpful.

Glutathione is the most important antioxidant used by the liver. It acts to prevent free radical damage and is an essential component in responding to any type of liver damage. Glutathione levels can be increased via the administration of NAC or SAMe. The products listed here have not been associated with any adverse events when given in the appropriate dose. NAC can be administered intravenously through a nonpyrogenic 0.2-mm filter, at 140 mg/kg, diluted 1:2 in 0.9% NaCl, and given over 1 h. Subsequent doses should be decreased to 70 mg/kg and given every 6 h for a minimum of 48 h. SAMe can be given orally at 20 mg/kg on an empty stomach, q 24 h. Silymarin and its main active ingredient, silibinin, are derived from milk thistle. Silibinin helps to prevent toxic liver damage and aids in faster liver regeneration.

The liver produces most of the coagulation factors needed to form a stable fibrin clot and has a central role in glucose metabolism. Complete hepatic failure may be accompanied by hypoglycemia and bleeding. Depending on the presence of these clinical signs, the animal may need to have a dextrose infusion (i.e., generally 2.5–5.0% dextrose in isotonic crystalloids) and administration of fresh frozen plasma (FFP) to replace coagulation factors. Administration of vitamin K_1 (2.5 mg/kg SC q 12 h) is also helpful. If the animal is actively bleeding and administration of FFP has not helped the bleeding, it may be alleviated by the administration of cryoprecipitate, which has a higher concentration of fibrinogen.

Anesthetic and analgesic considerations

There are significant risks associated with the administration of anesthesia to animals in hepatic failure. Ideally, coagulation tests, blood glucose, and albumin, will be normalized prior to induction.

Nutritional considerations

Nutritional support is essential for animals recovering from acute hepatic toxicity and protein restriction should be limited to animals that are showing clinical or laboratory (e.g., increased ammonia) evidence of HE. Enteral nutrition is superior if the animal can handle it.

Monitoring in hospital

The most important monitoring parameter will be the serial physical exam. Mentation, appetite, abdominal pain, and energy level are all essential tools to assist in prognosis. Animals will often improve clinically before their blood work improves. In addition to monitoring the heart rate, respiratory rate, and body temperature, evaluation of blood pressure, perfusion (pulse quality, extremity temperature, urine output), oxygenation parameters (pulse oximetry), and body weight are also essential and should be monitored at least every 12 h.

Role of the veterinary technician

The veterinary technician is often the "frontline" person who has the most "face" time with the patient. The veterinary technician, therefore, is often the first person to detect subtle changes in behavior or a change in clinical signs that may, if caught early, be reversed or minimized before permanent damage is done. Veterinary technicians should always trust their intuition as they will often suspect changes that are occurring before overt and obvious clinical changes. This comes from a combination of experience and spending many hours over many days with an individual patient. Alerting the primary clinician to suspected changes may help avert a downward spiral.

Client education

Clients are often unaware that seemingly harmless, over-the-counter substances (e.g., Tylenol) or foods (e.g., baked goods or candy with xylitol) are extremely toxic. Ideally, an information sheet, with a thorough list of these substances, will either be created or downloaded to give to the client. At the time of discharge, an information sheet on the clinical signs associated with liver failure should be sent home with the clients so they can monitor their pet appropriately. All client educational materials need to be documented in the medical record.

Hepatocutaneous syndrome

Hepatocutaneous syndrome (HCS), also known as superficial necrolytic dermatitis, in most animals is associated with significant hepatic disease of unknown etiology, though a minimum of cases have been seen in conjunction with glucagon-secreting tumors. Clinical signs refer to the cutaneous manifestations of the disease or signs of the underlying hepatic dysfunction, including amino acid dysregulation and hypoalbuminemia.

Clinical signs

Animals with HCS may present with dermatologic lesions or with signs of hepatic disease. The dermatologic lesions are usually localized to mucocutaneous junctions, on and around footpads, and over anatomical pressure points. The footpad lesions may make affected animals reluctant to walk and animals may be painful on palpation of the affected skin. Lesions are characterized by open, draining, and crusting wounds (Figure 9.1.4). Signs of hepatic disease are variable and include polyuria, polydipsia, vomiting, diarrhea, lethargy, depression, anorexia, and weight loss .

Diagnostic testing

Laboratory

HCS is seen with chronic, severe liver disease and there is also an association with glucagon-secreting tumors and diabetes mellitus in advanced stages. The laboratory abnormalities are similar to those that are seen with chronic liver disease such as liver enzyme elevations and/or hyperbilirubinemia and/or hypoalbuminemia. Additional findings with HCS may include leukocytosis due to the pyoderma associated with skin lesions. Hypoalbuminemia may also be exacerbated with excessive cutaneous losses of protein.

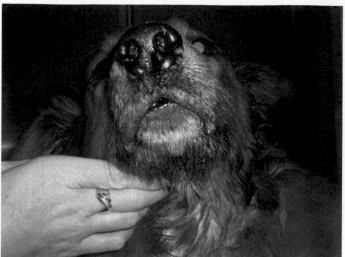

Figure 9.1.4 Dog with HCS showing alopecia and erythematous lesions at the mucocutaneous junctions of the oral cavity.

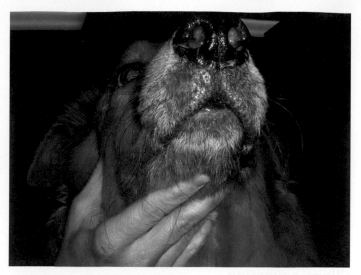

Figure 9.1.5 Same dog as in Figure 9.1.4 showing resolution of previous mucocutaneous lesions.

Imaging

As with chronic liver disease, abdominal radiographs may show peritoneal effusion and microhepatica. Abdominal ultrasound reveals a characteristic "Swiss cheese" appearance to the liver. This is considered by some to be a pathognomonic finding for HCS.

Biopsy

Coagulation status should always be assessed prior to biopsy to limit bleeding complications. Options for obtaining the necessary diagnostic samples include surgical laparotomy and minimally invasive laparoscopy. Percutaneous ultrasound-guided techniques do not provide adequate tissue amounts for the required analysis for HCS. Ascites and prolonged coagulation profiles may also be contraindications to ultrasound-guided liver biopsy. Approaches and limitations for hepatic biopsy are similar to those for chronic hepatitis. In addition to hepatic biopsy, skin biopsies are also required for a diagnosis of HCS. Skin biopsies should be obtained in affected areas, avoiding obviously necrotic tissue, and at interfaces of affected and nonaffected skin. Skin from affected animals has a characteristic "red, white, and blue" appearance on histopathology. Samples should also be obtained for tissue culture. Superficial swabs of skin are not appropriate samples. Rather, a portion of deep tissue should be submitted for bacterial culture and sensitivity. Tissue samples may be submitted in sterile red top tubes, Petri dishes, or culturettes. Technicians should inquire of their microbiology laboratory regarding the preferred transport of tissue samples for analysis.

Pharmacology and treatment

In addition to supportive measures for chronic liver disease, animals with HCS may benefit from intravenous infusions of amino acids. Many of the cutaneous lesions are a result of amino acid loss and dysregulation. While the prognosis for HCS is considered poor to grave, there have been reports of animals having prolonged survival times with aggressive, multimodal therapy (Figure 9.1.5). However, providing an intravenous protein load, via amino acid infusions, has the potential to precipitate a neurological crisis in the form of HE. Additional components of therapy include zinc (for hepatic and cutaneous components) and, potentially, antibiotic therapy for pyoderma where appropriate.

Anesthetic and analgesic considerations

The cutaneous lesions in animals with HCS may be painful and analgesic therapy should be considered. As with other forms of severe liver disease, agents with minimal hepatic metabolism should be utilized when available and appropriate. Local or topical anesthesia may be a consideration for cutaneous lesions. If animals show reluctance to walk, footpads or booties may be beneficial.

Nutritional considerations

If animals with HCS are encephalopathic (central neurological signs, elevated fasting blood ammonia level), then dietary protein should be restricted. However, animals with HCS have clinical illness due to amino acid loss and dysregulation. Therefore, additional protein restriction may be problematic. Intravenous amino acids provide a therapeutic benefit and will also provide a nutritional benefit to affected animals. Nutritional requirements, starting with basal energy and protein requirements, should be calculated. Supplemental zinc may be provided by the diet or may be an additional oral medication. Dietary antioxidants and omega-3 fatty acids are indicated as omega-3 fatty acids may particularly benefit the cutaneous lesions. Diarrhea is an uncommon component of the disease, but in cases where it is present, dietary fiber may be manipulated to assist in the control of GI signs.

Nursing considerations

Animals with HCS have severe, life-threatening disease and require extensive nursing care. Debilitation may be significant, animals may be in pain, and some will show profound neurological signs. Special attention should be paid to meeting nutritional goals and providing pain relief. While animals are undergoing amino acid therapy for HCS, they should receive especially close monitoring with serial neurological examinations, focusing on mentation status. If mentation status worsens during amino acid infusion, therapy for HE should be administered immediately as this is a life-threatening condition. Therapy should include immediate discontinuation of amino acid infusions and, potentially, administration of lactulose via oral route or enema.

Client education

Clients need to be aware of the long-term prognosis for HCS. Even if therapy is successful in the short term, prolonged survival is not a realistic goal. Therapy and hospitalization may be extensive and complications with therapy can arise and can be life threatening. Intensive nursing care may be required in the hospital and at home. Repeated and realistic client education is imperative. Quality of life issues may arise and honest communication is essential.

Congenital vascular anomaly

Congenital vascular anomalies, more commonly known as portosystemic shunts (PSSs), are abnormal vascular channels that divert blood from the portal vein to other vessels (e.g., caudal vena cava, azygos vein). This aberrant communication allows blood to reach the systemic circulation without traveling through the liver. Thus, certain substances (ammonia, bile acids, etc.) are present in higher concentrations than would be normally found in the circulation.

Congenital shunts are found much more commonly in dogs than in cats. As a general rule, congenital shunts tend to be single vessels. Large breed dogs are more likely to have intrahepatic shunts, and smaller breed dogs more commonly exhibit extrahepatic shunts. Yorkshire terriers are the most commonly affected breed.

Anatomy and physiology

Anatomically, the portal vein drains blood from the abdominal viscera (spleen, intestines) and courses to the liver. The portal blood then flows through the liver for metabolism and detoxification, before distribution to the systemic circulation.

PSSs are named for the vessels they join. For example, a PSS between the portal vein and the caudal vena cava would be named a portocaval shunt.

Clinical signs

Clinical signs are variable, but the most commonly reported include small body stature, failure to thrive, and poor body condition. Neurological signs such as lethargy, depression, seizures, blindness, and head pressing represent HE and may be reported more commonly after eating. Polyuria, polydipsia, and lower urinary tract signs (hematuria, pollakiuria) are also seen. Ptyalism (excessive salivation) may be more commonly noted in cats.

Diagnostic testing

Laboratory

The most common finding on the CBC is a microcytic anemia. This is due to mechanisms not completely understood but may include abnormalities of iron metabolism. A normal serum biochemistry panel does not rule out a PSS, but common abnormalities include decreases in BUN, glucose, cholesterol, creatinine, and albumin. ALT and ALP may be mildly elevated or may be normal. Total bilirubin is more commonly found in the normal range. Isosthenuria and ammonium urate or biurate crystals may be findings on a urinalysis.

The fasting and postprandial bile acid profile is considered the best indicator of hepatic function. The expected result, for an animal with a PSS, is an elevation in both fasting and postprandial samples. The postprandial sample is typically more elevated than the fasting sample, but both may be >100 µmol/L in an animal with a PSS.

Imaging

The most consistent finding on abdominal radiographs is microhepatica. Other radiographic findings may include renomegaly and potentially cystic calculi, although the majority of urate uroliths are radiolucent. Abdominal ultrasound done by a skilled ultrasonographer will be successful in identifying a congenital PSS in >85% of cases. Computed tomography (CT) scan, portal scintigraphy, and contrast portography are other imaging options where available.

Treatment and pharmacology

The recommended therapy for congenital PSS is surgical ligation. Multiple samples of liver should be taken for analysis at the time of surgery. Prior to invasive procedures, the coagulation status of the patient should be ascertained via PT and PTT. Additionally, a presurgical protein C level may provide diagnostic and prognostic information. Protein C is a vitamin K-dependent glycoprotein affecting blood clotting factors, such as prothrombin, factor VII, factor IX, and factor X. With concurrent diagnostic testing, protein C helps differentiate PSS from other hepatobiliary diseases (such as microvascular dysplasia) and can be used to monitor the success of treatment.

Medical stabilization prior to surgery is recommended to reduce anesthetic and surgical complications. Lactulose is used to lower blood ammonia levels and is the initial treatment for HE. This medication is typically given orally, but if the animal is unable to swallow (or is comatose), then lactulose may be administered rectally as an enema. Lactulose acidifies colonic contents causing ammonia to migrate from the blood into the colon where it is trapped and excreted in the feces. Antimicrobial therapy is prescribed to reduce ammonia-producing bacteria in the GI tract. If clinical signs include seizures, then anticonvulsant therapy with potassium bromide is recommended, as this medication has no hepatic metabolism. Coagulation support may be indicated and may consist of oral or injectable vitamin K therapy.

Anesthetic and analgesic considerations

Internal and external warmings should be utilized to maintain patient temperature. Caution should be exercised with external warming as patients may be of poor body condition and may be prone to burns over pressure points.

Nutritional considerations

Those animals with congenital PSSs, and particularly those with signs of HE, benefit from dietary protein restriction. The amount of protein restriction should be balanced with the protein needs of a growing animal. Long-term, significant protein restriction may not be indicated or necessary if medical and surgical treatments are successful. A diet should be mildly copper restricted, and supplementation with antioxidants and vitamin K is generally recommended. Commercial diets are available as are recipes for nutritionally complete homemade diets.

Liver neoplasia

Primary hepatic and biliary tract tumors in dogs and cats

Primary hepatobiliary tumors are uncommon in companion animals and account for only about 2% of canine and feline tumors.[11,12] Metastatic or secondary cancerous processes involving the liver occur more frequently than primary liver tumors in dogs, and the majority of primary hepatobiliary tumors in dogs are malignant.[13,14] In contrast, primary hepatobiliary tumors are more common than metastatic disease in cats, and up to 65% of primary hepatobiliary tumors in cats are benign.[12,15,16]

Primary liver tumors can arise from the hepatocyte (hepatocellular adenoma or carcinoma), biliary epithelium (biliary adenoma or carcinoma), neuroendocrine cells (carcinoid), or stromal cells (sarcoma). Hepatocellular carcinoma accounts for more than 50% of all primary liver tumors in dogs and is the second most common liver tumor in cats.[13,17] Biliary adenomas, also called biliary cystadenomas due to their cystic appearance, are most common in cats, accounting for more than 50% of feline liver tumors (Figure 9.1.6).[12]

In general, there are three morphological subtypes of primary liver tumors: massive, nodular, and diffuse. Massive liver tumors are defined as a large tumor affecting a single liver lobe, whereas nodular and diffuse tumors involve multiple liver lobes.[17,18]

Clinical signs and physical exam findings

Nearly one-third of dogs and one-half of cats with hepatobiliary tumors are asymptomatic, and cats with malignant tumors are more likely to show clinical signs than those with benign tumors.[16,19] Many of the clinical signs are nonspecific and include inappetence, weight loss, lethargy, vomiting, polyuria–polydipsia, ascites, and seizures. Seizures are generally associated with hypoglycemia or HE. Physical exam may be unrewarding but may reveal icterus, an abdominal fluid wave, or a cranial abdominal mass, which is palpable in up to three-fourths of dogs and cats with liver tumors.[12,14,15,17–21]

Diagnostic testing

Laboratory

It is important to perform a thorough clinical evaluation, including a CBC, serum chemistry profile, and urinalysis in all dogs and cats suspected of having neoplastic hepatobiliary disease. Mild to moderate anemia may be present, but hematologic abnormalities are nonspecific.[19] Liver enzymes are commonly elevated in dogs with hepatobiliary tumors; however, this finding is not specific for hepatic neoplasia.[22] Elevations in ALP and ALT as well as hypoglycemia and hypoproteinemia occur more commonly in dogs with primary liver tumors, whereas hyperbilirubinemia occurs more consistently in dogs with metastatic liver tumors.[20,23] Azotemia is often present in cats with hepatobiliary tumors, and ALT, aspartate aminotransferase (AST) and total bilirubin tend to be higher in cats with malignant versus benign tumors.[16,21]

Imaging

Abdominal radiographs can be useful to evaluate hepatomegaly. A common radiographic pattern observed with hepatobiliary

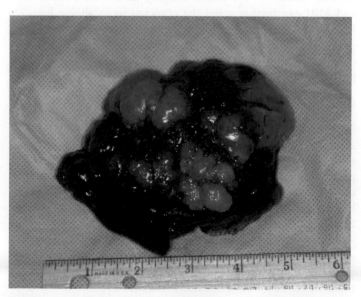

Figure 9.1.6 Hepatic neoplasia. Appearance of a biliary adenoma from a cat following liver lobectomy surgery. Surgical resection was curative in this cat. Image courtesy of Dr. Laura Garrett.

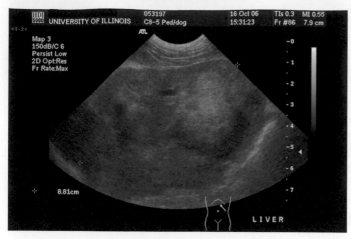

Figure 9.1.7 Hepatic neoplasia. Ultrasound image of a heterogeneous and cavitated massive liver tumor in an 11-year-old mixed breed dog that was presented for evaluation of elevated liver enzymes. The tumor was confined to the papillary process of the caudate lobe of the liver. Following liver lobectomy, the histological diagnosis of the hepatic mass was hepatocellular carcinoma.

tumors is a cranial abdominal mass with caudal and lateral displacement of the stomach.[24] Abdominal ultrasound is more useful than radiographs to evaluate the liver parenchyma itself and to guide aspiration of abnormal regions (see Figure 9.1.7).[25] However, benign lesions, such as nodular hyperplasia, and some malignant lesions may have a similar appearance ultrasonographically in dogs.[10,26]

Contrast-enhanced ultrasonography using Sonovue® or Sonazoid®, second-generation contrast agents administered intravenously, can aid in differentiation between malignant liver tumors and benign nodules with very high accuracy based on evaluation of echogenicity of the nodules following contrast administration.[27–29] Advanced imaging modalities such as CT and MRI can further assist the clinician in localizing hepatic lesions and in determining potential for resectability (relationship to the caudal vena cava and gallbladder). MRI has also been used to differentiate between benign and malignant hepatic lesions in dogs.[30]

Cytology and histology

FNA of hepatic masses is relatively easy to perform and is usually associated with minimal complications. Most FNAs are obtained under ultrasound guidance using a 1.5-in. disposable 20- to 22-ga. injection needle attached to a 6- or 12-mL syringe.[31] Overall, the sensitivity of cytology for diagnosing hepatic tumors is low; however, a correct diagnosis can be obtained in up to 60% of liver aspirations.[32–34]

Biopsy samples of the liver may be necessary for definitive diagnosis. A coagulation profile and platelet count should be performed prior to hepatic biopsy as hemorrhage can occur. The incidence of major complications is reduced in patients that have greater than 80,000/µL platelets and normal coagulation parameters prior to biopsy.[35] Several different needles and biopsy techniques can be used to obtain liver tissue for histopathology. A

Tru-Cut-type needle is most commonly used under ultrasound guidance; however, laparoscopic and surgical biopsies may also be obtained.[31,36] Histopathology provides a definitive diagnosis in up to 83–90% of liver biopsy samples.[37]

Prognosis and treatment

If anatomically feasible, liver lobectomy surgery remains the recommended treatment for cats and dogs with a liver tumor that has a massive appearance.[38] Up to 75% of a normal liver can be resected without impairing hepatic function, and complete regeneration of the parenchyma can occur within 8 weeks following surgical resection.[39] Surgical excision of massive liver tumors may provide prolonged disease-free intervals in dogs and cats. In dogs, even incomplete excision of massive hepatocellular carcinoma is associated with prolonged survival.[19]

Prognosis is poor for cats with malignant liver tumors and for dogs with nodular and diffuse malignant liver tumors.[14,16,21] Systemic chemotherapy is considered relatively ineffective for treating hepatobiliary tumors.[12]

SECTION 2 POSTHEPATIC DISEASE

Feline cholangitis complex

Anatomy and physiology

Feline inflammatory liver disease is termed feline cholangitis complex and is the second most common hepatic disorder in cats. Recently, the disease has been renamed from feline cholangiohepatitis complex to feline cholangitis complex. The disease in cats is a primary cholangitis with inflammation centered on the intrahepatic biliary system. In some cases, inflammation does extend into the hepatic parenchyma, but it is an extension of the cholangitis.

Feline cholangitis complex has been classified into several groups based on liver pathology. A neutrophilic cholangitis with acute and chronic forms occurs and is thought to result from ascending infections from the intestine. Neutrophilic cholangitis is often associated with pancreatitis and/or inflammatory bowel disease. Another group is the lymphocytic cholangitis. The etiology of lymphocytic cholangitis is unknown; however, an immune-mediated mechanism is suspected. The final group is chronic cholangitis associated with infestation by liver flukes.[1]

Clinical signs

Clinical signs associated with feline cholangitis complex can be quite variable with an acute or a chronic onset. Cats with acute neutrophilic cholangitis are often febrile, lethargic, vomiting, and anorexic. Jaundice and abdominal pain may or may not be present. These cats tend to be middle-aged or older.

In contrast, cats with lymphocytic cholangitis tend to be young, with 50% of them being less than 4 years of age.[1] Jaundice is the most common clinical sign. Ascites may also be present and is often indicative of end-stage liver disease or cirrhosis.

Some cats may have no clinical signs of disease other than weight loss.

Hepatomegaly may be evident in some cats with cholangitis complex. Evidence of bruising or bleeding may also be present in cats with concurrent coagulopathies.

Diagnostic testing

Laboratory

There can be several different changes in the complete blood cell count (CBC), chemistry panel, urinalysis, and bile acids, which can be supportive of the feline cholangitis complex. The CBC may be normal or may show an inflammatory neutrophilia. A left-shifted neutrophilia with or without toxic changes is often an indication of concurrent inflammatory or infectious disease. Nonregenerative anemia consistent with anemia of chronic disease may also be documented.

Elevations in liver enzymes are common in feline cholangitis complex. Serum alanine transaminase (ALT) often has a moderate to marked increase compared to a mild to moderate increase in serum ALP and GGT. If biliary obstruction is present, as is possible with concurrent pancreatitis or cholelithiasis, then GGT and ALP may be markedly increased. Hyperbilirubinemia is a common biochemical abnormality. Hyperglobulinemia with or without hypoalbuminemia may occur in lymphocytic cholangitis.

Bile acids (pre- and post-) are a liver function test that is usually abnormal with feline cholangitis complex. Urinalysis may show bilirubinuria. Some cats develop bilirubinuria before the onset of hyperbilirubinemia. Coagulation panels often reveal at least one abnormality in the PT or PTT. These prolongations in coagulation may be due to vitamin K malabsorption or to decreased hepatic production of coagulation factors.

Imaging

Diagnostic imaging such as abdominal radiographs and abdominal ultrasound are critical to further assess feline cholangitis and to help identify any other concurrent diseases. Abdominal radiographs often divulge hepatomegaly and, less commonly, cholelithiasis, ascites, and/or pancreatitis. Abdominal ultrasonography allows detailed evaluation of hepatic parenchyma and the biliary system. Cats with cholangitis may have none to variable echogenicity changes in the hepatic parenchyma. Ultrasound can differentiate between focal hepatic disease and more diffuse hepatic disease. Abdominal ultrasound can also detect other concurrent diseases such as extrahepatic bile duct obstruction, pancreatitis, cholelithiasis, and cholecystitis.

Biopsy

The definitive diagnosis of feline cholangitis complex is obtained through liver biopsy and cholecystocentesis. Biopsy rather than FNA of the liver is recommended as the pathologist needs to examine the liver architecture to determine the diagnosis. Any underlying coagulopathies should be identified and addressed prior to biopsying the liver. Liver biopsies can be obtained by ultrasound-guided, laparoscopic, or surgical techniques.

Generally larger tissue samples are more likely to be diagnostic than smaller ones. Both laparoscopy and surgery allow the clinician to obtain good-sized and diagnostic liver biopsies. Ultrasound-guided liver biopsies may be diagnostic in feline cholangitis, but small sample size can be an issue.[2] Hepatic tissue should be collected for histopathology and aerobic and anaerobic culture and sensitivity.

Cholecystocentesis should also be performed and bile submitted for cytology and aerobic and anaerobic culture and sensitivity in cats suspected to have neutrophilic cholangitis.

Pharmacology and treatment

Antibiotics are the mainstay of treatment for neutrophilic cholangitis. A broad-spectrum antibiotic should be instituted until culture and sensitivity results return. Beta lactams, fluoroquinolones or cephalosporins, and metronidazole are commonly used.[3] Antibiotic treatment should be continued for 2 months or longer.

Glucocorticoids are indicated when cats with neutrophilic cholangitis do not respond to antibiotics after 2–3 weeks or when cats have been diagnosed with lymphocytic cholangitis. Immunosuppressive doses are initiated with lymphocytic cholangitis and then tapered depending on response. In some cases, additional immunosuppressive drugs may be necessary. Anti-inflammatory doses of prednisone are used in cases of non-antibiotic-responsive cases of neutrophilic cholangitis.

Ursodeoxycholic acid has immunomodulating, antifibrotic, anti-inflammatory, and choleretic effects (increases fluidity of bile secretions).[3] This drug is often beneficial for cats with cholangitis. Ursodeoxycholic acid should not be given in cases with complete bile duct obstruction.

Very ill cats often require hospitalization with intravenous fluids and supportive care. Cats with ascites may require diuretics such as furosemide and spironolactone and periodic abdominocentesis for control.

Any underlying or concurrent diseases should be addressed as well. Surgery may be recommended for bile duct obstruction or removal of inspissated bile.

Anesthetic and analgesic considerations

Sedation and/or anesthesia are required for liver biopsy depending on the method used to procure the sample. Anesthetic agents with minimal hepatic metabolism are recommended.

Some cats with neutrophilic cholangitis will have abdominal pain, and the use of analgesics such as buprenorphine is recommended.

Nutritional considerations

A complete, balanced, palatable, highly digestible diet with moderate to high protein levels is recommended for cats with cholangitis unless there is concurrent renal impairment or HE. Cats with HE or renal impairment will require a protein-restricted diet. Enteral nutrition is preferred unless the cat is anorexic. Feeding tubes may need to be placed in order to nutritionally support some anorexic cats.

Biliary cysts

A biliary cyst is a benign cystic dilation of a bile duct structure. It is an uncommon lesion that can occur in the liver of dogs and cats. Biliary cysts arise from bile ducts that lack normal wall strength or lack normal connections to the biliary tree. These dilations or blind ducts accumulate fluid to form cystic structures. Biliary cysts may be congenital or acquired and may occur as solitary or multiple lesions. Acquired cysts (secondary to trauma, inflammation, or obstruction) are usually solitary. Congenital cysts are often multiple.

Multiple cysts (polycystic form) may occur in association with polycystic disease of other organs, especially the kidneys: This may be seen as a heritable congenital/developmental disorder in Persian cats (autosomal dominant polycystic kidney disease with liver cysts seen in up to 70% of affected animals) and in cairn and West Highland white terrier dogs (autosomal recessive polycystic disease): Affected animals often have significant hepatic fibrosis and may develop portal hypertension, acquired PSSs, and ascites.[4-7]

Anatomy and physiology

The biliary tree serves to carry bile from its site of production (hepatocytes) to the duodenum, where bile constituents are important for aiding digestion/absorption of nutrients, especially fats. In the normal biliary tree, microscopic bile canaliculi, which carry bile from cords of hepatocytes within hepatic lobules, unite to form interlobular bile ducts, which then join to form intrahepatic lobar ducts.

Lobar ducts transport bile to the left and right hepatic ducts, which join with the cystic duct serving the gallbladder and with the common bile duct, which enters the duodenum. Biliary cysts are abnormal dilatations of intrahepatic and/or extrahepatic bile duct structures. Cyst formation may result from abnormal proliferation of biliary epithelium or abnormal remodeling of embryonic duct tissue (congenital cysts) or may result from bile duct obstruction, distension, or injury secondary to refluxed pancreatic secretions (congenital or acquired cysts).

Clinical signs

Biliary cysts are usually asymptomatic. When present, clinical signs are usually referable to compression of adjacent tissues or secondary infection of the cysts and include intermittent abdominal pain, jaundice, and sometimes fever. Large cysts may be palpable as an abdominal mass and must be distinguished from neoplastic lesions.

Abdominal distension is sometimes noted and may be due to hepatomegaly, ascites, or the presence of a large cyst. Cysts that occur within the common bile duct or hepatic duct may cause intraluminal bile duct obstruction. Bile duct obstruction may also occur as a result of extraluminal compression of the biliary tract by large cysts. In these patients, clinical signs are those of bile duct obstruction (jaundice, hepatomegaly, abdominal pain, vomiting). Cysts that impede portal blood flow by compression of portal vessels may cause portal hypertension and ascites.

In congenital polycystic disease, hepatic fibrosis is a common finding and may result in portal hypertension, ascites, and acquired PSS formation. Ascites may also occur due to cyst rupture, releasing cystic fluid into the abdominal cavity. Cysts may become secondarily infected, resulting in systemic signs of lethargy, fever, and vomiting. Animals with congenital polycystic disease may present at an early age (months) with signs of renal insufficiency.

Diagnostic testing

Biliary cysts are usually an incidental finding in patients evaluated for another disease process and must be distinguished from hepatic cysts associated with parasitic or neoplastic lesions, congenital polycystic conditions affecting multiple organs, and hepatic abscesses.

Laboratory

Fluid aspirated from cystic lesions in the liver should be evaluated for evidence of infection or neoplasia. Biliary cyst content is usually clear serous fluid, but blood or bile may be present (if present, it is usually associated with acquired cysts). A CBC, serum chemistry, and urinalysis may be normal or may show evidence of renal insufficiency in patients with congenital polycystic disease. Elevated ALT may be seen as a result of pressure necrosis of hepatocytes adjacent to cysts, and elevations of bilirubin, ALP, and GGT are expected in patients with bile duct obstruction.

Imaging

Ultrasonography is sensitive and specific for diagnosing larger cysts, which appear as focal circular thin-walled anechoic structures, and for evaluating the extent of involvement (focal or diffuse, concurrent renal lesions) and the presence or absence of biliary obstruction. Cysts associated with congenital polycystic disease may be microscopic and may not be evident with ultrasonography. Imaging diagnoses should be confirmed with other techniques to rule out neoplasia or parasitic disease.

Biopsy

Ultrasound-guided percutaneous aspiration of cyst and/or adjacent hepatic parenchyma for cytological evaluation is adequate for the diagnosis of biliary cyst.

Pharmacology and treatment

Asymptomatic cysts do not require treatment. Cysts that are problematic because of impingement on adjacent tissues (diaphragm, hepatic vascular or biliary structures) or causing abdominal pain may be treated initially by aspiration of cyst contents to reduce the volume of the cyst, but recurrence rates are high and introduction of infection is a possible complication.

If the cyst contents rapidly reaccumulate, the patient may be treated by repeated aspiration of the cyst, by surgical or laparoscopic deroofing (fenestration) of the cyst (lesion may still recur and procedure is contraindicated if cyst contains bile), or by surgical excision of the cyst or affected liver lobe. Intracystic administration of sclerosing agents is employed successfully in treating humans. Polycystic conditions are often diffuse and are not amenable to surgical management, although fenestration techniques may be used to limit compression injury to tissue adjacent to larger cysts.

Anesthetic and analgesia considerations

Cysts that impinge on the diaphragm or that are associated with ascites formation may impair the patient's ability to ventilate properly with spontaneous respiration; preoperative abdominocentesis or cyst aspiration should be considered if respiratory function is compromised. Patients with biliary obstruction may have bleeding tendencies as a result of fat-soluble vitamin (vitamin K) malabsorption, which should be corrected before surgery.

Extrahepatic biliary obstruction

Extrahepatic biliary obstruction (EHBO) is a condition that arises when bile flow through the extrahepatic elements of the biliary tree is blocked, leading to retention of bile constituents, liver distension, and secondary injury to liver cells.

Anatomy and physiology

The biliary tract serves as a conduit through which bile (produced by the hepatocytes and secreted into the bile canaliculi) flows into the interlobular ducts, the lobar ducts, the left and right hepatic ducts, and eventually, the cystic duct. From the cystic duct, the bile can either continue on to the duodenum via the common bile duct or be stored in the gallbladder. The gallbladder is located between the right medial and the quadrate lobes of the liver. It is a thin-walled structure made up of four layers. The gallbladder contracts when stimulated by cholecystokinin (CCK) (a peptide hormone of the duodenum) and in response to vagal parasympathetic stimulation. This causes the bile to pass through the common bile duct and the sphincter of Oddi into the duodenum. Other hormones involved in emptying the gallbladder are gastrin and motilin. Somatostatin inhibits the contraction of and facilitates the filling of the gallbladder. In the duodenum, bile (bile acid) is an important component for the proper digestion and absorption of fats and fat-soluble vitamins. Bile also carries waste products including bilirubin, excess cholesterol, and copper. These are removed from the body by secretion into the bile and are eliminated in the feces.

The extrahepatic components of the biliary tree include the left and right hepatic ducts, the cystic duct serving the gallbladder, and the common bile duct. The distal common bile duct runs adjacent to the pancreas. In cats, the common bile duct and the pancreatic duct fuse before entering the duodenum; in dogs, the common bile duct and the pancreatic duct enter the duodenum separately but in close proximity to each other. When bile flow is blocked, the retained bile fluid causes distension of the biliary tree and liver swelling, accumulation of wastes normally eliminated via bile, and secondary injury to liver cells by retained bile constituents (bile acids, copper). Bilirubin accumulates because of the inability to eliminate it into the intestine, leading to a yellow discoloration of the serum (icterus) and tissues (jaundice). Additionally, failure to deliver bile to the intestine results in impaired digestion and absorption of fats, leading to diarrhea, and poor absorption of fat-soluble vitamins. This can result in vitamin K deficiency and subsequent defects in clotting because vitamin K-dependent clotting factors (factors II, VII, IX, X) cannot be activated.

Clinical signs

The most common clinical signs of EHBO are jaundice, inappetence, lethargy, and vomiting. Some patients may be febrile. With complete biliary obstruction, fecal color may be abnormally light (acholic) because of the absence of bile pigments, which gives feces its normal brown color. Hepatomegaly may be noted on physical examination and abdominal pain may be present due to distention of bile ducts and liver swelling or may be referable to the underlying disease process causing the bile duct obstruction (e.g., pancreatitis).

Diagnostics

The most common cause of EHBO is pancreatitis (swelling of the pancreas causes extraluminal compression of the common bile duct) followed by neoplasia (pancreatic or hepatobiliary mass causing extraluminal compression or intraluminal obstructive mass). Other causes include gallbladder mucocoele (GBM), cholelithiasis (gallstone), biliary cyst, intestinal mass or foreign body obstructing the duodenal papilla, common bile duct entrapment in a diaphragmatic hernia, parasite infestation of the common bile duct (liver fluke), or stricture of the common bile duct secondary to trauma or inflammation

Laboratory

Hyperbilirubinemia is the most consistent clinicopathologic abnormality, and serum bilirubin elevations may be quite severe in patients with complete obstruction (20- to 50-fold increase). Marked increases in cholestatic liver enzymes (ALP and GGT) and hypercholesterolemia are also common findings. Increased ALT may be present, reflecting secondary injury to hepatocytes by retained bile salts and other toxic bile constituents. ALT elevations are usually milder than the changes in cholestatic enzyme levels but may be marked in some patients. On a CBC, a significant number of patients show a leukocytosis with a mature neutrophilia; anemia is less common but may occur secondary to coagulopathy and bleeding (regenerative) or as anemia of chronic disease (normocytic normochromic nonregenerative). Patients with EHBO should be tested for coagulation disorders associated with vitamin K malabsorption by evaluation of PT and activated partial thromboplastin (aPTT) (PT is the first to be prolonged) or by proteins induced by vitamin K antagonism/absence (PIVKA) test.

Imaging

Ultrasonography may provide evidence of the presence of EHBO and may help elucidate the underlying cause of the obstruction (e.g., pancreatitis, mass compressing the common bile duct, cholelith). Ultrasonographic findings that support a diagnosis of EHBO include distension of the common bile duct (85–97% of cases), gallbladder distension (45–60% of cases), tortuous bile ducts, and distension of hepatic ducts.[9–11] The absence of ultrasonographic abnormalities does not rule out EHBO. In patients with chronic disease resulting in fibrosis, the common bile duct may not distend in EHBO. In patients with long-standing bile duct dilation from EHBO, biliary distension may persist even after the obstruction has been relieved and therefore is not in itself indicative of current obstruction. Ultrasonographic findings should always be interpreted in light of concurrent clinical status and clinicopathologic findings.

Treatment and pharmacology

Patients should be stabilized with intravenous fluid therapy to correct dehydration and appropriate pain management. Coagulopathies are treated with parenteral administration of vitamin K_1. Definitive treatment of EHBO is directed at the underlying cause of the obstruction. In patients with partial biliary obstruction secondary to pancreatitis, the obstruction may resolve as pancreatic inflammation and swelling resolve with supportive medical management for pancreatitis. In most other patients, treatment is surgical. The biliary obstruction must be relieved by removing the obstruction (e.g., duodenal foreign body, mass resection) or by performing a diversionary procedure connecting the biliary tract to the intestine in a manner to divert bile flow around the site of obstruction (cholecystoduodenostomy, cholecystojejunostomy).[9,10,12]

Restoring patency of the common bile duct by placement of intraluminal stents has also been successful in managing patients with extraluminal compression secondary to pancreatitis or neoplastic masses.[13] Percutaneous ultrasound-guided aspiration of the gallbladder contents has been described as an alternative means of decompressing the biliary tree in dogs with EHBO secondary to acute pancreatitis.[14]

Anesthetic and analgesia considerations

Patients with biliary obstruction may have bleeding tendencies as a result of fat-soluble vitamin K malabsorption, which should be corrected before surgery. Additionally, patients with obstructive jaundice are at an increased risk for endotoxemia, hypotension, cardiac dysfunction, and renal ischemia and have a greater risk of anesthetic complications.

Gallbladder mucocoeles

Gallbladder mucocoeles (GBM) are a noninflammatory condition in which the gallbladder becomes distended by an abnormal accumulation of mucus and inspissated bile, which forms a gelatinous mass in the gallbladder lumen.

GBM is principally a disease of dogs, although the condition has been reported in a domestic shorthair cat[15] and in a ferret.[16] They rarely occur in humans. GBM is most commonly diagnosed in older adult small- to medium-sized dogs. There appears to be a breed predisposition to GBM in Shetland sheepdogs and cocker spaniels,[17,18] although other breeds and mixed breed dogs may be affected. Breed predisposition to GBM may be secondary to other heritable problems such as familial hyperlipidemia. Hyperlipdemia, through high biliary cholesterol levels, promotes more viscous bile and may stimulate mucin secretion, thereby increasing bile viscosity and the potential for impaired gallbladder emptying, both of which are thought to predispose to mucocoele formation.

Several studies have supported an association of hyperadrenocorticism (HAC) and GBM: One study reported the odds of GBM in dogs with HAC to be 29× that of dogs without HAC.[19] It has been shown that people with HAC have altered bile composition and abnormal gallbladder motility, but it is unknown if similar abnormalities occur in dogs with HAC. There is no evidence that hypothyroidism, diabetes mellitus, or chronic pancreatitis predispose to the development of GBM. Concurrent liver disease is present in about half of GBM patients. This association may be coincidental or may be the result of secondary cholestatic liver injury caused by GBM-related biliary obstruction.

Pathophysiology

Normally, the gallbladder serves to store bile during fasting periods. With meals, the presence of fatty acids and amino acids in the duodenal lumen trigger the duodenal release of CCK, which in turn stimulates gallbladder contraction and emptying of stored bile into the duodenum. In the duodenum, bile constituents aid in the digestion and absorption of dietary fats.

Gallbladder epithelial cells secrete mucin and concentrate stored bile by the absorption of water from the gallbladder lumen. Delayed gallbladder emptying (primary motility disorder allowing for excessive dehydration of gallbladder bile) or changes in mucin production may result in more viscous bile, both of which impair bile flow from the gallbladder and may predispose to GBM.

The underlying cause of GBM in dogs is unknown. In people, mucocoeles develop secondary to gallbladder outflow obstruction, most often associated with choleliths. In dogs, biliary obstruction, cholecystitis, and bacterial infection do not appear to be inciting factors. Dogs may, instead, develop GBM due to a primary dysfunction of mucus-secreting cells in the gallbladder mucosa, resulting in secretion of excessive amounts of mucus. Cystic mucosal hyperplasia of the gallbladder is a consistent biopsy finding in dogs with GBM. Progressive accumulation of excess mucus may cause increased intraluminal pressure, pressure necrosis of the gallbladder wall, gallbladder rupture, and bile peritonitis. Gallbladder hypomotility with subsequent biliary stasis has also been implicated as a possible factor in the development of GBM. EHBO sometimes occurs secondary to GBM as a result of extension of the accumulated mucus and inspissated bile into the cystic duct and the biliary tree.

Clinical signs

Dogs with GBM usually present with vague nonspecific signs of inappetence, vomiting, and lethargy, which have been present for a relatively short time (mean of 5–8 days but up to 3 weeks) at the time of presentation. Abdominal pain and diarrhea are reported in approximately one-fourth of cases, and, less commonly, dogs show abdominal distension as a result of organomegaly or ascites (pancreatitis, bile peritonitis). GBMs may present with signs of biliary obstruction with acute abdominal pain and icterus. A smaller proportion of dogs have a history of PU/PD, which probably relates to concurrent disease (endocrinopathy, renal disease) rather than the gallbladder disease itself.

A significant number of dogs (23–44%) with GBM are asymptomatic, especially in the earlier stages of development of the mucocoele, and the GBM is identified as an incidental finding during abdominal ultrasonography performed to evaluate another disease.

Physical examination may be normal, especially in asymptomatic dogs, but hepatomegaly, abdominal pain/discomfort (87%), and icterus (56.5%) are common in clinically ill dogs. Fever is present in about 25% of clinical cases. Abdominal distension and ascites are less common.[17,20–22] Dogs with gallbladder rupture may present with fever, acute severe abdominal pain, and septic shock.

Diagnostic testing

GBMs are being diagnosed in dogs with increasing frequency, probably due, at least in part, to the now widespread use of ultrasonography in small animal practice. Because presenting clinical signs of GBM are usually nonspecific and could relate to a myriad of other conditions, a suspicion of GBM usually arises only after initial diagnostic test results indicate biliary disease.

Laboratory findings

Most dogs have elevated liver enzyme (ALT, ALP, AST, and GGT) levels (80–95% of all dogs) and hyperbilirubinemia (60–65%); approximately 40% show hypoalbuminemia. Leukocytosis is seen in roughly 50% of cases, and about one-third are anemic. The severity of the laboratory abnormalities is not predictive of outcome. Generally, no biochemical or hematologic parameter has been shown to predict severity or outcome in GBM cases, although gallbladder rupture may be associated with greater elevations of liver enzymes and bilirubin and with more severe leukocytosis.[17,20–22]

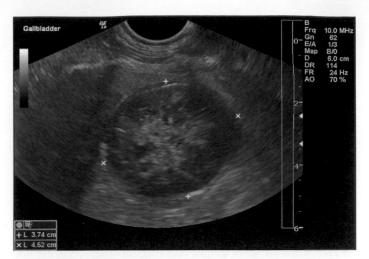

Figure 9.2.1 Ultrasonographic image of a gallbladder mucocoele in a Shetland sheepdog.

Imaging

Abdominal radiography may show hepatomegaly or abdominal fluid and occasionally a mass-like effect in the right cranioventral abdomen produced by a distended gallbladder, but this rarely contributes to establishing a diagnosis of GBM.

Abdominal ultrasonography is a sensitive and definitive test for GBM and is the diagnostic procedure of choice. A diagnosis of GBM is confirmed by the ultrasonographic finding of immobile (not moving with ballottement or patient repositioning) echogenic material in the gallbladder lumen, often with a characteristic finely striated or stellate ("kiwi fruit") appearance considered being pathognomonic for GBM (Figure 9.2.1).

If the gallbladder is ruptured, echogenic peritoneal fluid may be found around the gallbladder. Focal thinning or discontinuity of the gallbladder wall is a good predictor of gallbladder rupture, but, in many dogs with GBM, gallbladder rupture is present but not detected on ultrasound examination. Other variable ultrasonographic findings include thickened gallbladder wall and bile duct dilation (20% of dogs).

Other diagnostic tests

Abdominocentesis and abdominal fluid analysis should be performed in patients with ascites to evaluate for bile peritonitis. A canine pancreatic lipase (cPLI) assay is indicated to assess for concurrent pancreatic disease. Aerobic and anaerobic culture of bile collected via ultrasound-guided percutaneous gallbladder aspiration or at surgery should be performed to direct antibiotic treatment.

Biopsy findings

Cystic mucinous hyperplasia of the gallbladder mucosa is consistently present. Thickening of the gallbladder wall may or may not be noted. Inflammation (cholecystitis) or bacterial infection of the gallbladder is *uncommon* in dogs with GBM. Concurrent hepatitis or other hepatopathies are *common*.

Treatment

Surgical

Clinically ill dogs should be stabilized with fluid therapy to correct dehydration and electrolyte imbalances, antiemetics to control vomiting, and treatment of peritonitis when present. GBM is generally considered to be a surgical disease, with complete removal of the diseased gallbladder (cholecystectomy) considered to be the treatment of choice.

Patients with known or suspected gallbladder rupture should be treated as surgical emergencies because of the risk of septic bile peritonitis. Patients without clinical evidence of rupture may be scheduled routinely. Most (80%) of the affected gallbladders show microscopic evidence of rupture or gallbladder wall necrosis even when ultrasonography and surgical observation did not show evidence of rupture; therefore, resection of the diseased gallbladder is preferable to biliary diversion techniques, which have a higher postoperative mortality rate. GBM is associated with high perioperative mortality (20–40%), especially in the immediate postoperative period. Patients should remain hospitalized for careful monitoring and treatment of common complications such as bile leakage, bile peritonitis, postoperative pancreatitis, sepsis, and pneumonia.

Duration of hospitalization following surgery is generally 1–7 days (mean 3.5 days). Most complications occur immediately post-op but have been reported up to 3 weeks after surgery. In surviving dogs, clinical pathological abnormalities improve or resolve within 2 weeks to 3 months. GBM carries a good long-term prognosis if the patient survives the perioperative period.[21,23]

Medical

As noted earlier, delayed gallbladder emptying or changes in mucin production may result in more viscous bile. While GBM has traditionally been treated surgically, multiple reports of successful nonsurgical management of dogs with GBM have emerged.[24,25] Medical management may be considered for asymptomatic or mildly affected patients with no indication of gallbladder rupture. The key features of medical treatment are choleretics (ursodiol 10–15 mg/kg PO divided into two doses per day), fat-restricted diet if hyperlipidemic, and ultrasonographic monitoring. Although bacterial infection is rarely present in GBM, antibiotics are commonly used in the medical management of GBM because of concerns that biliary stasis could predispose to secondary bacterial infection by enteric organisms. Additionally, antibiotics are used because of grave consequences should the gallbladder rupture and establish septic peritonitis.

Ideally, culture of bile collected by FNA should direct antimicrobial choice; otherwise, empiric treatment should include broad-spectrum coverage using antibiotics with good distribution into bile. Reported regimens include ampicillin or amoxicillin alone, ampicillin or amoxicillin and enrofloxacin, ampicillin or amoxicillin and enrofloxacin and metronidazole, ampicillin or amoxicillin and metronidazole, and cefazolin alone. Hepatoprotectants such as SAMe are often administered due to the potential for hepatic injury by bile acids retained secondary to bile stasis and because many dogs with GBM have concurrent inflammatory hepatic diseases.

Patients must be closely monitored for complications such as gallbladder rupture. Owners opting for medical management must be advised of the potential for acute decompensation because of gallbladder rupture, EHBO, or sepsis.

In patients managed medically, gallbladder rupture remains a potential complication, but, in the limited published reports of medically managed dogs, it appears to be infrequent and to occur within 2 weeks of diagnosis. In dogs monitored ultrasonographically, complications were uncommon and GBM is often resolved within 2–6 months. Once resolved, GBM almost never recurs. Complete resolution of clinical signs, normalization of bilirubin levels, and improvement in liver enzyme levels are expected, but many recovered dogs have persistent elevations of liver enzymes, which may reflect concurrent hepatic disease or HAC. In dogs with bile duct dilation, the common bile duct may remain distended, but dogs remain clinically normal.

Nutritional considerations

Dogs with hyperlipidemia should be fed a fat-restricted diet (7–15%) such as

- Hill's Prescription Diet Canine r/d
- Hill's Prescription Diet Canine w/d
- Iam's Veterinary Formula Weight Loss Restricted-Calorie Canine Formula
- Purina Veterinary Diet EN Gastroenteric
- Purina Veterinary Diet OM Overweight Management
- Purina Veterinary Diet HA Hypoallergenic
- Royal Canin Veterinary Diet LF Canine Gastrointestinal Low Fat

Conclusion

In the future, additional studies are needed to address potential roles for gallbladder dysmotility and endocrine disease in the development of GBM. In addition, further elucidation of the pathogenesis of GBM and its predisposing factors is needed to inform recommendations for prevention, which will hopefully improve outcomes for affected dogs. Finally, the significance of biliary sludge as a possible preliminary stage of GBM, if biliary sludge should be treated, and if treatment for biliary sludge will help to prevent the possible progression to GBM should be addressed.

SECTION 3 NUTRITION IN LIVER DISEASE

The liver is essential for the digestion, absorption, metabolism, and storage of nutrients required by the body.[1] Because of this, liver disease can result in secondary malnutrition, which further aggravates the disease process and can negatively affect the ultimate outcome of treatment.[2]

Early and aggressive nutritional intervention can decrease morbidity and mortality.[2] Potential causes for malnutrition can include (1) anorexia, nausea, and vomiting; (2) impaired nutrient digestion, absorption, and metabolism; (3) increased energy requirements; and (4) accelerated protein catabolism and impaired protein synthesis.[3]

Liver disease can be divided into acute and chronic forms, with chronic being the most common form seen in dogs and cats.[2] The goals for nutritional management of liver disease are (1) to maintain normal metabolic processes, (2) to correct any electrolyte disturbances, (3) to avoid toxic by-product accumulation, and (4) to provide necessary substrates to support hepatocellular regeneration.[2,3]

The liver is the primary site for detoxification of endogenous and exogenous substances absorbed by the GI tract. This ability plays a role in the development of HE. Unfortunately, plasma ammonia levels correlate poorly with the degree of HE seen in the patient.[1] Delayed or altered drug metabolism can also be seen with liver disease and may necessitate a change in dose or administration frequency.[2]

The liver synthesizes the majority of the circulating plasma proteins and is the only site for the synthesis of albumin. Because of this, albumin can be used as an indirect marker for liver function. The plasma concentration can reflect the hepatic synthesis, rate of degradation, pathological excretion, and volume distribution of albumin within the body.[3] The liver is the primary organ for glycogen storage and glucogenolysis, as well as for the storage of fat-soluble vitamins and the synthesis of coagulation factors.[1,2]

When introducing food to an animal with liver disease, care must be taken to not overwhelm the remaining metabolic capacity of the liver. Alternately, negative protein/energy balance can have a harmful influence on hepatocellular regeneration and repair. This can be due to a decrease in the immune response and altered intermediary metabolism resulting in the promotion of HE and an increased incidence of mortality.[2]

The use of appetite stimulants such as anabolic steroids and benzodiazepine derivatives should be used cautiously due to the potential for hepatotoxicity.[3] Force feeding and appetite stimulants are not recommended in cats in order to avoid food aversions.[2] The best course of action is to select a highly palatable diet with high energy density. This allows the animal to eat small amounts of food and still meet their energy requirements.[3] If they are unable to meet at least 85% of their calculated RERs on a daily basis, feeding intervention needs to be considered.

Protein

Protein restrictions should only be done when signs of HE are seen. If this is the case, protein levels can be decreased to 20–25% of the calories being fed (metabolizable energy [ME]).[2] Inappropriate protein restriction in dogs and cats with liver disease causes catabolism of endogenous protein, decreased muscle mass, and increased potential for HE.[1]

A high quality protein (high biological value) is better digested and has an amino acid profile closer to what the animal requires. Whether the protein is animal or plant based is not as important as the quality of the protein. Milk- and soy-based protein tend to be better tolerated than animal-based proteins because of their increased digestibility.[1]

Cats, unlike dogs, are unable to downregulate their enzymes responsible for breaking down proteins into their base amino acids. Because of this, cats maintain a higher protein requirement at all times compared with dogs.[3]

Fats

Fats are important in liver disease because they are essential for fatty acid and triglyceride synthesis, phosopholipid and cholesterol production, lipoprotein metabolism, and bile acid synthesis.[3]

The use of nonprotein calories is important to prevent the utilization of amino acids for energy and to decrease the need for gluconeogenesis. This can best be accomplished through the use of fats as they provide almost three times the amount of calories when compared to proteins or carbohydrates. Fat intake should only be decreased when severe cholestatic disease is seen or with fat malabsorption.[2]

Severe cholestatic disease causes a decrease in the production of bile acids, which results in malabsorption of fats, fat-soluble vitamins, and some minerals.[1]

Medium-chain triglycerides (MCTs) such as coconut and palm kernel oils are not recommended, especially in cats, due to their decreased palatability. They have been implicated in the development of hepatic lipidosis in cats because of their refusal to eat the food.[2,3]

Carbohydrates

Carbohydrates should not be more than 35% of the calories found in the diet due to a limited ability to digest, absorb, and metabolize the resulting monosaccharides. With cirrhosis, this is even more important.[2] The liver plays a key role in the use of the monosaccharides glucose, fructose, and galactose. In humans, glucose intolerance is seen more commonly than hypoglycemia with severe hepatic dysfunction.[3]

Fiber

Moderate amounts of fiber can have beneficial effects in the management of liver disease. Soluble fibers (fructooligosaccharides [FOSs]) are fermented by the colonic bacteria, causing a decrease in the local pH. This results in a decrease in the production and absorption of ammonia from the colon. Soluble and insoluble fibers also bind bile acids in the small intestinal lumen, promoting excretion from the body rather than reabsorption into the bloodstream.[2]

Insoluble fibers, such as those found in lignin and cellulose, help to increase GI transit time. This can decrease the incidence of constipation and helps to absorb and remove intestinal toxins from the body.[2]

Vitamins and minerals

Vitamin deficiencies are common with liver disease, especially the B complex vitamins. As these vitamins are essential for the hepatic metabolism of nutrients, supplementation of the diet may be necessary. Additional supplementation with B$_{12}$ (cobalamin) is suggested in feline hepatic lipidosis.[2] Cobalamin is not included in most B complex vitamin mixes and must be given separately.

The fat-soluble vitamin stores in the liver are usually sufficient for several months, but with chronic disease, these, too, may become depleted.[3] Decreases can also be seen with cholestatic disease as absorption is dependent on the presence of the bile salts in the intestines.[2]

Feeding plan

Diet plans are best formulated on an individual basis. Consideration needs to be given to the type and origin of the liver disease and the extent of the dysfunction seen.[1] Additional information specific to the liver disease can be found in the appropriate chapter (Table 9.3.1).

Early, adequate, and aggressive nutritional support is essential for the long-term survivability of the patient. Typically, commercial, therapeutic diets are selected by the clinician as it is difficult to create a balanced homemade diet that will meet the animal's needs over a prolonged period of time.[2] If significant nutrient modifications are necessary, select a therapeutic diet closest to the nutrient distribution desired and supplement accordingly. There is no one diet that is ideal for all liver diseases; let the patient and the disease guide your diet selection. In cases where the animal is unable or unwilling to eat the selected diet, assisted feeding through the use of feeding tubes is recommended.

Table 9.3.1   Goal of liver diets

The basic goals for a diet in patients with liver disease
Maintain metabolic balance
Provide nutrients for healing and regeneration of damaged tissues
Correct and/or prevent malnutrition
Decrease the need for hepatic "work" through the use of highly digestible foods
Avoid production of hepatotoxic and neurotoxic compounds
Eliminate underlying cause

Source: Roudebush P, Davenport DJ, Dimski DS. Hepatobiliary disease. In *Small Animal Clinical Nutrition*, 4th edition, eds. MS Hand, CD Thatcher, RL Remillard, P Roudebush, pp. 811–835. Topeka, KS: Mark Morris Institute; 2000.

SECTION 4 ANESTHESIA AND ANALGESIA CONSIDERATIONS IN HEPATIC DISEASE

The liver is one of the most important and versatile organs in the body and is heavily involved in the processes important to each phase of general anesthesia. When hepatic function is compromised, it can be something of an obstacle course choosing an appropriate anesthetic protocol for surgical or diagnostic purposes.

Premedication

Biotransformation and breakdown of most drugs occur primarily in the liver, whereas actual clearance of the drugs from the body usually occurs through the renal system. Much of the breakdown process is dependent on blood flow to the liver, so drugs that can cause hypotension should be avoided.

Benzodiazepines are considered the safest choice for tranquilization in hepatically compromised patients. Midazolam has little effect on the cardiovascular system; thus, hepatic blood flow is not affected. However, this class of drug is broken down by the liver, and patients with moderate to severe liver dysfunction could have more exaggerated sedation and extremely prolonged recoveries from benzodiazepine administration. In these cases, much lower doses should be used.

Opioids are considered relatively safe to use in patients with hepatic disease except in patients with HE. All opioids come with the associated risk of bradycardia and decreased cardiac output, but this side effect can be nullified by the use of an anticholinergic, such as atropine or glycopyrrolate, when needed. Morphine, hydromorphone, oxymorphone, and fentanyl are all appropriate choices for painful procedures. Fentanyl as a CRI may be the best choice because it can be titrated to effect and is quickly eliminated from the system. Butorphanol and buprenorphine have the least amount of respiratory or cardiovascular depression and are good choices for minimally invasive procedures. Opioids can be fully reversed using naloxone; full mu opioids can be partially reversed using butorphanol.

Phenothiazines, such as acepromazine, should be not be used primarily because of their hypotensive effects. This category of drugs may also interfere with platelet aggregation. Alpha-2 adrenergic agonists, such as xylazine and dexmedetomidine, are also a poor choice due to initial vasoconstriction, which is followed by potentially profound vasodilation. Both states may negatively affect hepatic blood flow.

Induction

The most common induction agents are propofol, ketamine/ diazepam, and etomidate. Propofol is very rapidly eliminated from the body. Propofol is primarily metabolized by the liver, although other sites of extrahepatic metabolism, such as the lungs, contribute. Thus, propofol is considered relatively safe as an induction agent in patients with liver disease. Propofol can cause apnea and transient hypotension, but these side effects can be lessened with slow administration.

Ketamine/diazepam can be used for induction also. Both drugs are heavily metabolized by the liver and thus take much longer to be eliminated with hepatic compromised patients. As there have been reports of ketamine-related seizures in some patients, this particular combination should be avoided if there is any epileptic history or known seizure activities.

Etomidate has little effect on the respiratory or cardiac systems and is rapidly metabolized by both the liver and plasma esterases.

All the induction drugs are metabolized by the liver to some degree, therefore repeated boluses are not recommended. Anesthesia should be maintained using inhalant anesthetics (Table 9.4.1).

Maintenance anesthesia

Isoflurane, sevoflurane, and desflurane are all good choices for maintaining anesthesia in hepatic cases. Very nominal amounts

Table 9.4.1 Anesthetic and analgesic drug dosages for hepatic patients

Drug	Canine	Feline
Midazolam	0.1–0.3 mg/kg IV[a] or IM	0.05–0.3 mg/kg IV[a] or IM
Morphine	0.5–2 mg/kg IM or SQ	0.05–0.2 mg/kg IM or SQ
Hydromorphone	0.1–0.2 mg/kg	Same as canine
Oxymorphone	0.1–0.2 mg/kg IV,[a] IM, or SQ	0.05–0.1 mg/kg IV,[a] IM, or SQ
Fentanyl	5–45 mcg/kg/hr CRI IV only	2–20 mcg/kg/hr CRI IV only
Butorphanol	0.2–0.4 mg/kg IV,[a] IM, or SQ	Same as canine
Buprenorphine	50–200 mcg/kg IV,[a] IM, or SQ	50–100 mcg/kg IV,[a] IM, or SQ
Propofol	Up to 6 mg/kg IV only	Same as canine
Ketamine/ diazepam	10 mg/kg ketamine plus 0.5 mg/kg diazepam IV only	Same as canine
Ketamine/ midazolam	10 mg/kg ketamine plus 0.22 mg/kg midazolam IV only	Same as canine
Etomidate	1–2 mg/kg Rapidly IV	Same as canine

[a] When administered IV, lower dosage should always be used.
Source: Plumb D. *Veterinary Drug Handbook*, 5th edition. Ames, IA: Blackwell Publishing; 2005.

of these inhalant anesthetics are metabolized by the liver. Inhalants can cause vasodilation and hypotension, which may affect hepatic blood flow. This can be combated by using opioid analgesics to decrease inhalant requirements and by maintaining appropriate fluid support.

Nitrous oxide can also be used in patients with liver dysfunction. When used with inhalant anesthetics, it can decrease the concentration of inhalant required and can potentially offset associated hypotension.

Monitoring

Patients with hepatic dysfunction are prone to several potential anesthetic complications. Patients with ascites or fluid in the abdomen may have difficulty with proper lung expansion and ventilation. Slow, partial removal of abdominal fluid may be indicated and if performed, IV isotonic crystalloids and/or colloids (depending on the albumin concentration) should be administered. End tidal carbon dioxide and oxygen saturation should be closely monitored. If the patient is not able to spontaneously ventilate adequately (this would be indicated if the CO_2 is greater than 45 mmHg or the oxygen saturation is less than 95%), then assisted or mechanical ventilation is needed.

Hypoalbuminemia is commonly seen with liver dysfunction and can cause dramatic hypotension. If albumin is low (below 1.5 g/dL), plasma oncotic pressure is low and the force keeping fluid within the vascular system is decreased. Patients are at an increased risk of pulmonary edema. Measuring arterial blood pressure is recommended and aggressive fluid therapy delivered as needed. Colloidal support may be needed during anesthesia and caution should be used to avoid fluid overload. Monitoring central venous pressure is the best way to achieve an accurate picture of volume. However, some signs of fluid overload include hypertension, pitting edema, increased or "bounding" pulse quality, crackles heard in the lungs, and decreased oxygen saturation.

Patients with low albumin often require lower doses of anesthetic drugs. Many drugs, such as propofol, are highly protein bound, and in a hypoalbuminemic patient, this means that there is less protein available to bind to the drug and thus more active drug circulating in the system.

Hepatic impairment can have detrimental effects on clotting function and production of coagulation factors. A coagulation profile should be run before any surgery or liver biopsy occurs. Arterial blood pressure and heart rate monitoring can be early indicators of a hemorrhagic episode. While arterial blood pressure monitoring is the gold standard, it is not always available. All patients undergoing anesthesia should have some form of blood pressure monitoring and should have peripheral pulse quality routinely assessed. If an arterial line is not feasible, then oscillometric or Doppler ultrasound monitoring is needed. If the patient becomes acutely hypotensive (mean arterial pressure [MAP] below 60 mmHg) and tachycardic (heart rate above 240 in cats, 220 in neonatal canines, 180 in small dogs, and 160 in average sized dogs), it could indicate hypovolemia. It is recommended that FFP and/or whole blood be on hand if necessary.

Hypoglycemia is present in many hepatic cases and periodic glucose monitoring under anesthesia is recommended. If hypoglycemia occurs (glucose reading below 60 mg/dL), an intravenous dextrose bolus (given slowly) and the addition of 2.5–5.0% dextrose to crystalloid fluids is indicated.

Elimination of drugs given before and during anesthesia is dependent on metabolism. Hypothermia (temperatures below 96°) can cause a decrease in the rate of metabolism and can lead to prolonged recovery. In addition, hypothermia can impair coagulation, which may already be abnormal in patients with liver injury. Temperature should be closely monitored intraoperatively and combative measures taken if the patient becomes hypothermic (hot water circulation mats or blankets, convective air warming units, or warmed fluids are all useful tools).

Recovery

Many patients with hepatic disease will need to recover in a critical care unit so they have continued monitoring, fluid therapy, and postoperative analgesia.

Temperature should be closely monitored and maintained in the postoperative period to aid in the metabolism of circulating anesthetic drugs. Blood glucose levels should also be watched and dextrose added to fluids if necessary.

In patients that are hypotensive, arterial (preferred) or systolic blood pressure monitoring should be continued until the patient is normotensive. Central venous pressures can be monitored through jugular central lines to prevent overhydration.

Continuous rate infusions of fentanyl or morphine–lidocaine–ketamine are standard for painful cases as they can be given at very low doses and maintain a constant level of analgesia. Fentanyl patches are often used as are IV or IM doses of opioid analgesics. Noncritical cases may not need any additional analgesia or may be sent home with butorphanol or buprenorphine. NSAIDs should not be given to patients with hepatic dysfunction. They are specifically contraindicated in patients with liver disease, as well as in patients with hypotension or coagulation disorders.

Bibliography

Section 1

1. Meertens NM, Bokhove CAM, van den Ingh TSAM. Copper-associated chronic hepatitis and cirrhosis in a European shorthair cat. *Veterinary Pathology* 2005;42:97–100.
2. Rothuizen J, Bunch SA, Charles JA, et al. *WSAVA Standards for Clinical and Histological Diagnosis of Canine and Feline Liver Disease.* St. Louis, MO: Saunders Elsevier; 2006.
3. Hoffmann G. Copper-associated liver diseases. *Veterinary Clinics of North America. Small Animal Practice* 2009;39:489–511.
4. Dimski D, Taboada J. Feline idiopathic hepatic lipidosis. in *Veterinary Clinics of North America. Small Animal Practice* 1995; 25(2):357–373. ISSN: 0195-5616.
5. Donoghue S. Nutritional support of hospitalized patients. *Veterinary Clinics of North America. Small Animal Practice* 1989; 19(3):475–493.
6. Guilford G, Center S. Nutritional management of gastrointestinal disease. In: *Strombecks's Small Animal Gastroenterology*, 3rd edition, eds. DR Strombeck, WG Guilford, SA Center, pp. 889–910. Philadelphia, PA: W.B. Saunders; 1996.
7. Roudebush P, Davenport D, Dimski D. Hepatobiliary disease. In: *Small Animal Clinical Nutrition*, 4th edition, eds. T Hand, R Remillard, pp. 816–833. Topeka, KS: Mark Morris Institute; 2000.
8. Marks SL, Rogers QR, Strombeck DR. Nutritional support in hepatic disease part 1 & 2. *Compendium on Continuing Education for the Practicing Veterinarian* 1994;16(8, 10):971–979. 1287–1296.
9. Center SA. Chronic liver disease: current concepts of disease mechanisms. *Journal of Small Animal Practice* 1999;40:106–114.
10. Feeney DA, Johnston GR, Hardy RM. Two-dimensional, gray-scale ultrasonography for assessment of hepatic and splenic neoplasia in the dog and cat. *Journal of the American Veterinary Medical Association* 1984;184:68–81.
11. Hammer AS, Sikkema DA. Hepatic neoplasia in the dog and cat. *Veterinary Clinics of North America. Small Animal Practice* 1995; 25:419–435.
12. Liptak JM. Hepatobiliary tumors. In: *Withrow & MacEwen's Small Animal Clinical Oncology*, 4th edition, eds. SJ Withrow, DM Vail, pp. 483–491. St. Louis, MO: Saunders; 2007.
13. Cullen JM, Popp JA. Tumors of the liver and gallbladder. In: *Tumors in Domestic Animals*, 4th edition, ed. DJ Meuten, pp. 483–508. Ames, IA: Iowa State Press; 2002.
14. Balkman C. Hepatobiliary neoplasia in dogs and cats. *Veterinary Clinics of North America. Small Animal Practice* 2009;39: 617–625.
15. Patnaik AK. A morphologic and immunocytochemical study of hepatic neoplasms in cats. *Veterinary Pathology* 1992;29: 405–415.
16. Lawrence HJ, Erb HN, Harvey HJ. Nonlymphomatous hepatobiliary masses in cats: 41 cases (1972 to 1991). *Veterinary Surgery* 1994;23:365–368.
17. Patnaik AK, Hurvitz AI, Lieberman PH, et al. Canine hepatocellular carcinoma. *Veterinary Pathology* 1981;18:427–438.
18. Patnaik AK, Hurvitz AI, Lieberman PH. Canine hepatic neoplasms: a clinicopathological study. *Veterinary Pathology* 1980;17: 553–564.
19. Liptak JM, Dernell WS, Monnet E, et al. Massive hepatocellular carcinoma in dogs: 48 cases (1992–2002). *Journal of the American Veterinary Medical Association* 2004;225:1225–1230.
20. Strombeck DR. Clinicopathologic features of primary and metastatic neoplastic disease of the liver in dogs. *Journal of the American Veterinary Medical Association* 1978;173:267–269.
21. Post G, Patnaik AK. Nonhematopoietic hepatic neoplasms in cats: 21 cases (1983–1988). *Journal of the American Veterinary Medical Association* 1992;201:1080–1082.
22. Alvarez L, Whittemore J. Liver enzyme elevations in dogs: physiology and pathophysiology. *Compendium on Continuing Education for the Practicing Veterinarian* 2009;31(9):408–414.
23. McConnell MF, Lumsden JH. Biochemical evaluation of metastatic liver disease in the dog. *Journal of the American Animal Hospital Association* 1983;19:173–178.
24. Evans SM. The radiographic appearance of primary liver neoplasia in dogs. *Veterinary Radiology* 1987;28:192–196.
25. Guillot M, D'Anjou MA, Alexander K, et al. Can sonographic findings predict the results of liver aspirates in dogs with suspected liver disease? *Veterinary Radiology & Ultrasound* 2009; 50(5):513–518.

26. Stowater JL, Lamb CR, Schelling SH. Ultrasonographic features of canine hepatic nodular hyperplasia. *Veterinary Radiology* 1990;31: 268–272.

27. O'Brien RT, Iani M, Matheson J, et al. Contrast harmonic ultrasound of spontaneous liver nodules in 32 dogs. *Veterinary Radiology & Ultrasound* 2004;45(6):547–553.

28. Kanemoto H, Ohno K, Nakashima K, et al. Characterization of canine focal liver lesions with contrast-enhanced ultrasound using a novel contrast agent—Sonazoid. *Veterinary Radiology & Ultrasound* 2009;50(2):188–194.

29. Nakamura K, Takagi S, Sasaki N, et al. Contrast-enhanced ultrasonography for characterization of canine focal liver lesions. *Veterinary Radiology & Ultrasound* 2010;51(1):79–85.

30. Clifford CA, Pretprius ES, Weisse C, et al. Magnetic resonance imaging of focal splenic and hepatic lesions in the dog. *Journal of Veterinary Internal Medicine* 2004;18:330–338.

31. Rothuizen J, Twedt DC. Liver biopsy techniques. *Veterinary Clinics of North America. Small Animal Practice* 2009;39: 469–480.

32. Roth L. Comparison of liver cytology and biopsy diagnoses in dogs and cats: 56 cases. *Veterinary Clinical Pathology* 2001;30: 35–38.

33. Cohen M, Bohling MW, Wright JC, et al. Evaluation of sensitivity and specificity of cytologic examination: 269 cases (1999–2000). *Journal of the American Veterinary Medical Association* 2003;222: 964–967.

34. Wang KY, Panciera DL, Al-Rukibat RK, et al. Accuracy of ultrasound-guided fine-needle aspiration of the liver and cytologic findings in dogs and cats: 97 cases (1990–2000). *Journal of the American Veterinary Medical Association* 2004;224:75–78.

35. Bigge LA, Brown DJ, Penninck DG. Correlation between coagulation profile findings and bleeding complications after ultrasound-guided biopsies: 434 cases (1993–1996). *Journal of the American Animal Hospital Association* 2001;37:228–233.

36. Vasanjee SC, Bubenik LJ, Hosgood G et al. Evaluation of hemorrhage, sample size, and collateral damage for five hepatic biopsy methods in dogs. *Veterinary Surgery* 2006;35:86–93.

37. Barr F. Percutaneous biopsy of abdominal organs under ultrasound guidance. *Journal of Small Animal Practice* 1995;36: 105–113.

38. Trout NJ, Berg J, McMillan MC et al. Surgical treatment of hepatobiliary cystadenomas in cats: five cases (1988–1993). *Journal of the American Veterinary Medical Association* 1995;206: 505–507.

39. Kosovsky JE, Manfra-Marretta S, Matthiesen DT, et al. Results of partial hepatectomy in 18 dogs with hepatocellular carcinoma. *Journal of the American Animal Hospital Association* 1989;25: 203–206.

40. Dunayer EK, Gwaltney-Brant SM. Acute hepatic failure and coagulopathy associated with xylitol ingestion in eight dogs. *Journal of the American Veterinary Medical Association* 2006;229(7): 1113–1117.

41. Cooper J, Webster C. Acute liver failure. *Compendium* 2006;28(7): 498–515.

42. Weiss DJ, Gagne J, Armstrong PJ. Inflammatory liver diseases in cats. *Compendium* 2001;23(4):364–372.

43. Shih JL, Keating JH, Freeman LM, Webster C. Chronic hepatitis in Labrador retrievers: clinical presentation and prognostic factors. *Journal of Veterinary Internal Medicine* 2007;21:33–39.

44. Poldervaart JH, Favier RP, Penning LC, Van Den Ingh TSGAM, Rothuizen J. Primary hepatitis in dogs: a retrospective review

(2002–2006). *Journal of Veterinary Internal Medicine* 2009;23: 72–80.

45. Raffan E, McCallum A, Scase TJ, Watson PJ. Ascites is a negative prognostic indicator in chronic hepatitis in dogs. *Journal of Veterinary Internal Medicine* 2009;23:63–66.

46. Rutgers HC, Harte JG. Hepatic disease. In: *Waltham Book of Clinical Nutrition of the Dog & Cat*, eds. JM Wills, KW Simpson, pp. 265–269. Tarrytown, NY: Elsevier; 1994.

47. Grubb TL. Anesthesia for patients with special concerns. In: *Small Animal Anesthesia and Analgesia*, ed. G Carroll, pp. 193–239. Ames, IA: Blackwell; 2008.

48. Scherk MA, Center SA. Toxic, metabolic, infectious, and neoplastic liver diseases. In: *Textbook of Veterinary Internal Medicine*, 6th edition, eds. SJ Ettinger, ED Feldman, pp. 1464–1478. St. Louis, MO: Elsevier Saunders; 2005.

49. McMichael MA. *Handbook of Veterinary Emergency Protocols: Dog and Cat*. Jackson, WY: Teton NewMedia; 2008.

50. Byrne KP. Metabolic epidermal necrosis-hepatocutaneous syndrome. *Veterinary Clinics of North America. Small Animal Practice* 1999;29(6):1337–1355.

51. Jacobsen LS, Kirberger RM, Nesbit JW. Hepatic ultrasonography and pathological findings in dogs with hepatocutaneous syndrome: new concepts. *Journal of Veterinary Internal Medicine* 1995;9(6):399–404.

52. Tobias KM, Rohrbach BW. Association of breed with the diagnosis of congenital portosystemic shunts in dogs: 2400 cases (1980–2002). *Journal of the American Veterinary Medical Association* 2003;223(11):1636–1639.

53. Mehl ML, Kyles AE, Hardie EM, Kass PH, Adin CA, Flynn AK, De Cock HE, Gregory CR. Evaluation of ameroid ring constrictors for treatment for single extrahepatic portosystemic shunts in dogs: 168 cases (1995–2001). *Journal of the American Veterinary Medical Association* 2005;226(12):2020–2030.

54. Proot S, Biourge V, Teske E, Rothuizen J. Soy protein isolate versus meat-based low protein diet for dogs with congenital portosystemic shunts. *Journal of Veterinary Internal Medicine* 2009;23: 794–800.

55. Toulza O, Center SA, Brooks MB, Erb HN, Warner KL, Deal W. Evaluation of plasma protein C activity for detection of hepatobiliary disease and portosystemic shunting in dogs. *Journal of the American Veterinary Medical Association* 2006;229(11): 1761–1771.

56. Cellio LM, Dennis J. Canine superficial necrolytic dermatitis. *Compendium* 2005;27(11):820–825.

Section 2

1. Harvey AM, Gruffydd-Jones TJ. Feline inflammatory liver disease. In: *Textbook of Veterinary Internal Medicine*, Vol. 2, 7th edition, eds. SJ Ettinger, EC Feldman, pp. 1643–1648. St. Louis, MO: Saunders Elsevier; 2010.

2. Cole TL, Center SA, Flood SN, et al. Diagnostic comparison of needle and wedge biopsy specimens of the liver in dogs and cats. *Journal of the American Veterinary Medical Association* 2002; 220(10):1483–1490.

3. Sartor LL, Trepanier LA. Rational pharmacologic therapy of hepatobiliary disease in dogs and cats. *Compendium of Continuing Education* 2003;25:432–447.

4. Bosje JT, van den Ingh TS, van der Linde-Sipman JS. Polycystic kidney and liver disease in cats. *The Veterinary Quarterly* 1998;20:136–139.

5. Eaton KA, Biller DS, DiBartola SP et al. Autosomal dominant polycystic kidney disease in Persian and Persian-cross cats. *Veterinary Pathology* 1997;34:117–126.

6. McAloose D, Casal M, Patterson DF, Dambach DM. Polycystic kidney and liver disease in two related West Highland white terrier litters. *Veterinary Pathology* 1998;35:77–81.

7. McKenna SC, Carpenter JL. Polycystic disease of the kidney and liver in the cairn terrier. *Veterinary Pathology* 1980;17:436–442.

8. Rothuizen J. Diseases of the biliary system. In: *BSAVA Manual of Canine and Feline Gastroenterology*, 2nd edition, eds. EJ Hal, JW Simpson, DA Williams, p. 277. Quedgeley, Gloucester, UK: British Small Animal Veterinary Association; 2005.

9. Mayhew PD, Holt DE, McLear RC, Washabau RJ. Pathogenesis and outcome of extrahepatic biliary obstruction in cats. *Journal of Small Animal Practice* 2002;43:247–253.

10. Buote NJ, Mitchell SL, Penninck D et al. Cholecystoenterostomy for treatment of extrahepatic biliary tract obstruction in cats: 22 cases (1994–2003). *Journal of the American Veterinary Medical Association* 2006;228:1376–1382.

11. Gaillot H, Penninck D, Webster CRL, Crawford S. Ultrasonographic features of extrahepatic biliary obstruction in 30 cats. *Veterinary Radiology & Ultrasound* 2007;48:439–447.

12. Fahie MA, Martin RA. Extrahepatic biliary tract obstruction: a retrospective study of 45 cases (1983–1993). *Journal of the American Animal Hospital Association* 1995;31:478–482.

13. Mayhew PD, Weisse CW. Treatment of pancreatitis-associated extrahepatic biliary tract obstruction by choledochal stenting in seven cats. *Journal of Small Animal Practice* 2008;49:133–138.

14. Herman BA, Brawer RS, Murtaugh RJ, Hackner SG. Therapeutic percutaneous ultrasound-guided cholecystocentesis in three dogs with extrahepatic biliary obstruction and pancreatitis. *Journal of the American Veterinary Medical Association* 2005;227:1782–1786.

15. Bennett SL, Milne M, Slocombe RF, Landon BP. Gallbladder mucocoele and concurrent hepatic lipidosis in a cat. *Australian Veterinary Journal* 2007;85:397–400.

16. Reindel JF, Evans MG. Cystic mucinous hyperplasia in the gallbladder of a ferret. *Journal of Comparative Pathology* 1987;97:601–604.

17. Pike FS, Berg J, King NW, Penninck DG, Webster CRL. Gallbladder mucocele in dogs: 30 cases (2000–2002). *Journal of the American Veterinary Medical Association* 2004;224:1615–1622.

18. Aguirre AL, Center SA, Randolph JF et al. Gallbladder disease in Shetland sheepdogs: 38 cases (1995–2005). *Journal of the American Veterinary Medical Association* 2007;231:79–88.

19. Mesich MLL, Mayhew PD, Paek M, Holt DE, Brown DC. Gallbladder mucoceles and their association with endocrinopathies in dogs: a retrospective case-control study. *Journal of Small Animal Practice* 2009;50:630–635.

20. Besso JG, Wrigley RH, Gliatto JM, Webster CRL. Ultrasonographic appearance and clinical findings in 14 dogs with gallbladder mucocele. *Veterinary Radiology & Ultrasound* 2000;41:261–271.

21. Worley DR, Hottinger HA, Lawrence HJ. Surgical management of gallbladder mucoceles in dogs: 22 cases (1999–2003). *Journal of the American Veterinary Medical Association* 2004;225:1418–1422.

22. Crews LJ, Feeney DA, Jessen CR, Rose ND, Matise I. Clinical, ultrasonographic, and laboratory findings associated with gallbladder disease and rupture in dogs: 45 cases (1997–2007). *Journal of the American Veterinary Medical Association* 2009;234:359–366.

23. Amsellem PM, Seim HB, MacPhail CM et al. Long-term survival and risk factors associated with biliary surgery in dogs: 34 cases (1994–2004). *Journal of the American Veterinary Medical Association* 2006;229:1451–1457.

24. Reed WH, Ramirez S. What is your diagnosis? *Journal of the American Veterinary Medical Association* 2007;230:661–662.

25. Walter R, Dunn ME, d'Anjou M-A, Lècuyer M. Nonsurgical resolution of gallbladder mucocele in two dogs. *Journal of the American Veterinary Medical Association* 2008;232:1688–1693.

Section 3

1. Rutgers C, Biourge V. Nutrition of dogs with liver disease. In: *Encyclopedia of Canine Clinical Nutrition*, eds. P Pibot, V Biourge, D Elliott, pp. 134–152. Aimargues, France: Aniwa SAS; 2006.

2. Rutgers C, Biourge V. Nutritional management of hepatobiliary and pancreatic diseases. In: *Encyclopedia of Feline Clinical Nutrition*, eds. P Pibot, V Biourge, D Elliott, pp. 140–157. Aimargues, France: Aniwa SAS Aimargues; 2008.

3. Roudebush P, Davenport DJ, Dimski DS. Hepatobiliary disease. In: *Small Animal Clinical Nutrition*, 4th edition, eds. MS Hand, CD Thatcher, RL Remillard, P Roudebush, pp. 811–835. Topeka, KS: Mark Morris Institute; 2000.

Section 4

1. Grimm K, Thurmon J, Tranquilli WJ. *Lumb and Jones Veterinary Anesthesia and Analgesia*, 4th edition. Ames, IA: Blackwell Publishing; 2007.

2. Thurman J, Tranquilli W, Benson G. *Essentials of Small Animal Anesthesia and Analgesia*, 1st edition. Philadelphia, PA: Lippencott, Williams, and Wilkins; 1999.

Chapter **10** Urinary and Renal Diseases

Editors: Ale Aguirre and Tracy Darling

SECTION 1 URINARY ANATOMY AND PHYSIOLOGY

The kidneys are reddish brown organs that mark the start of the urinary tract. They are located dorsally in the abdomen within the retroperitoneal space. The kidneys are covered by a fibrous capsule and are held in place by connective tissue. The left kidney lies at the level of the 13th rib. The right kidney is located farther cranially under the ribs and touches the liver. The kidneys have three major components. The cortex, or the outer layer, filters blood and starts the process of urine formation. The medulla is located centrally within the kidney. It is in the medulla that urine gradually becomes concentrated. The renal pelvis, or the most central part of the kidney, is an open space where urine collects before it exits the kidneys. Urine flows from the renal pelvis into the ureters. The left and right ureters connect the kidneys to the bladder. The ureters enter the bladder at the trigone (Figure 10.1.1).[1]

The urinary bladder is a balloon-shaped organ situated in the caudal abdomen and is held in place by several ligaments. The bladder is a reservoir where urine is stored until it can be voided. The bladder has a body and neck. The urethra arises from the neck of the bladder and ushers urine outside the body. The urethral sphincter is located just beyond the bladder in the proximal urethra. It is this sphincter that maintains urine in the bladder until it is released by conscious urination. In male dogs, the prostate completely surrounds the neck of the bladder and the proximal urethra. The urethra passes through the penis and eventually leaves the body. The prepuce envelops the penis and provides support and protection. In the female, the urethra courses caudally until it enters the vestibule. The vulva marks the end of the urinary tract in the female.

Physiology

Urine is formed and concentrated by filtering blood through millions of nephrons, the functional units of the kidney. The nephron consists of a glomerulus, Bowman's capsule, a proximal tubule, the loop of Henle, a distal tubule, and the collecting ducts (Figure 10.1.2).

Small Animal Internal Medicine for Veterinary Technicians and Nurses, First Edition. Edited by Linda Merrill.
© 2012 John Wiley & Sons, Inc. Published 2012 by John Wiley & Sons, Inc.

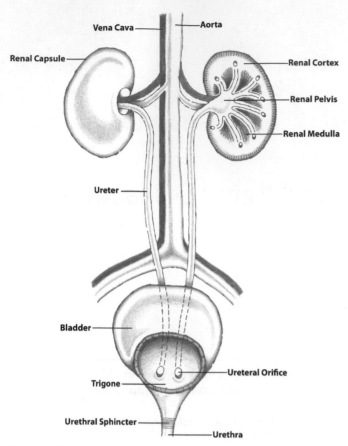

Figure 10.1.1 Diagram displaying the normal anatomical structures of the urinary system.

The glomerulus is a modified capillary bed that filters blood. The glomeruli are located in the cortex of the kidney. High blood pressure (BP) in the glomerular capillaries forces plasma through small pores in the capillary walls. The glomerular filtration rate (GFR) is a term used to describe how fast plasma is filtered through the glomerulus. The glomerular filtration system is completely permeable to water and small dissolved substances (electrolytes, amino acids, glucose, and urea). However, larger molecules like proteins are unable to pass through the filter. Albumin is approximately the same size as the pores in the filter. In a normal animal, albumin stays in the plasma. However, when disease of the glomerulus ensues, it is often the first protein to be found at high levels in the urine. Criteria that determine if a substance is going to be filtered include its size and electrical charge. The glomerular capillaries have a negative electrical charge and therefore repel proteins since they are of the same charge. Most electrolytes are positively charged or are of small enough size that they easily transverse the barrier. The fluid that completes its journey through the glomerulus enters Bowman's capsule and is known as the ultrafiltrate.[2,3]

From Bowman's capsule, the ultrafiltrate flows into the renal tubules. The tubules are responsible for maintaining fluid balance, electrolytes, acid–base status, and for the excretion of waste products and drugs. The proximal convoluted tubule is a continuation of Bowman's capsule. The proximal tubule has specialized cells that work to return many of the filtered substances back to the blood. Approximately 60–65% of the filtered substances are reabsorbed in the proximal convoluted tubule. These include amino acids, glucose, and many of the electrolytes.

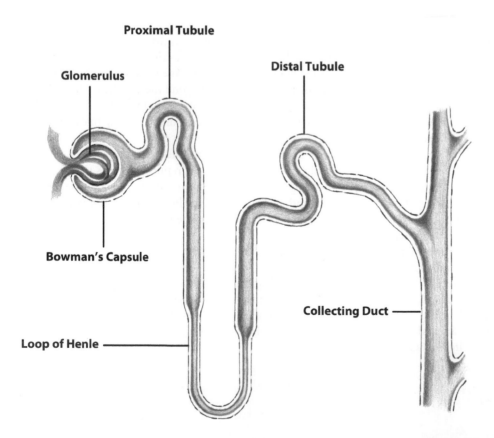

Figure 10.1.2 Diagram displaying the normal anatomical structures of the nephron.

Secretion also occurs in the proximal convoluted tubule, and it is primarily responsible for eliminating drugs and hydrogen ions, which are important for maintaining a normal blood pH.

Following modification in the proximal convoluted tubule, the ultrafiltrate enters the loop of Henle. The loop of Henle begins in the cortex and descends into the medulla. It then makes a sharp U-turn before heading back to the cortex. The loop of Henle is instrumental in the formation of concentrated urine. Water passively moves out of the descending loop of Henle due to a concentration gradient in the interstitium surrounding the nephron. Sodium and chloride are actively pumped out of the tubules in the ascending limb under the influence of aldosterone, a hormone secreted by the adrenal glands. The movement of sodium out of the ascending tubules helps to maintain the interstitial concentration gradient.

Specialized cells in the ascending loop of Henle, known as the macula densa, are responsible for the secretion of erythropoietin. Erythropoietin is a hormone essential for new red blood cell (RBC) production and for preventing premature RBC death.

Once the ultrafiltrate has been modified in the loop of Henle, it enters the distal convoluted tubule in the cortex of the kidney. Antidiuretic hormone (ADH) is secreted by the pituitary gland but exerts it effect in the distal convoluted tubule. Its primary function is to reabsorb large quantities of water, thereby regulating urine volume. A deficiency of ADH results in severe polyuria (PU) and is known as diabetes insipidus (DI). Hydrogen, potassium, and ammonia are eliminated by secretion into the distal tubule.

From the distal convoluted tubules, the ultrafiltrate then enters the collecting duct system. The collection ducts carry urine from the cortex through the medulla to the renal pelvis. The ducts become progressively larger as they descend into the renal pelvis. The collecting ducts work to further absorb electrolytes, water, and bicarbonate, thereby regulating electrolyte and acid–base balance.

SECTION 2 CLINICAL SIGNS

The complete evaluation of a patient with a primary complaint suggestive of renal or urinary disease often begins with the client interview. Specific questions to investigate the status of the urinary system should include those pertaining to water intake (frequency and volume) as well as descriptive characteristics of the patient's urination (ease of urination as well as color, quantity, and frequency of urination). Disorders of the upper and lower urinary tract can produce nonspecific clinical signs including anorexia, gastrointestinal (GI) disturbances, and weight loss. Several signs can be helpful in localizing disorders, and the following terminology is useful in describing clinical signs associated with disorders of the urinary tract.

Lower urinary tract disorders often present with a combination of clinical signs including *pollakiuria* (frequent episodes of urination), *stranguria* (straining while urinating), and *dysuria* (difficulty urinating). These clinical signs can be suggestive of many disorders that affect the bladder and the urethra, including lower urinary tract infections (UTIs), urethral obstruction, neoplasia, and feline idiopathic cystitis.

Hematuria (RBCs in the urine) can arise from upper or lower urinary tract disorders and may be macroscopic (grossly visible) or only observed microscopically. Macroscopic hematuria must be differentiated with a sediment examination from other causes of discolored urine (including hemoglobin or myoglobin in the urine; termed hemoglobinuria or myoglobinuria, respectively).

The timing of the appearance of blood in the urine stream can indicate the general location of the source. Urethral disorders can cause hematuria at the beginning of the urine stream. Hematuria in the later part of the urine stream is more suggestive of disorders in the bladder or kidneys. Additionally, hematuria concurrent with clinical signs of pollakiuria, stranguria, and/or dysuria can help localize a disorder to the lower urinary tract. Hematuria can also arise from systemic coagulation disorders and from disorders of the genital tract. Heat stroke and excessive exercise can lead to hematuria, hemoglobinuria, and/or myoglobinuria.

Normal urine output for cats and dogs is 20–40 mL/kg/day. *Polyuria* (PU) occurs when urine output is greater than normal. The true definition of PU is urine output >40–50 mL/kg/day. This is usually difficult to measure, and a clinically useful definition of PU is observation of an increase in urine volume output. For example, PU may be noted by dogs asking to go outside more frequently and producing large volumes of urine (not to be confused with pollakiuria—which also results in more frequent urination, but only small volumes of urine are produced). Owners of polyuric cats may find that the litter box needs to be cleaned more frequently.

Polydipsia (PD), an increase in water intake, usually accompanies PU as a compensatory mechanism. The true definition of PD is water intake >80–100 mL/kg/day. Clinically, water intake can be measured or PD may be noted by owners having to fill water dishes more frequently. Primary polyuric conditions (e.g., secondary to renal insufficiency or endocrine disorders) are more common than primary polydipsic conditions (e.g., psychogenic PD). However, the two conditions usually exist concurrently (e.g., primary PU with compensatory PD).

When urine output falls below the normal level, the patient can be described as having *oliguria*. *Anuria* is a term to describe the patient with no urine output. Oliguria and anuria can result from acute kidney injury. Additionally, bilateral ureteral obstruction or urethral obstruction can cause oliguria or anuria.

Urinary incontinence occurs when a patient loses voluntary control of urination, resulting in leakage of urine. Urinary incontinence results either from an anatomic abnormality bypassing the normal urethral sphincter mechanism or from pressure in the bladder becoming greater than the urethral pressure.

Urinary incontinence must be distinguished from inappropriate urination associated with PU, dysuria, or pollakiuria. Signs suggestive of true urinary incontinence can include urination while sleeping or observing that the animal does not appear to be aware of the leakage of urine (e.g., not posturing to urinate). It should be noted that disorders resulting in PD/PU can exacerbate urinary incontinence.

Common causes of urinary incontinence in younger animals include ectopic ureter(s) or other congenital abnormalities. Middle-aged to older dogs with urinary incontinence, especially spayed females, are typically affected by hormonal responsive urethral sphincter mechanism insufficiency (also known as urethral mechanism incompetence).

Some disorders of the urinary tract can lead to systemic clinical signs. Specifically, acute kidney injury may be associated with anorexia, lethargy, and depression. These signs are often a feature of chronic kidney disease (CKD), also known as renal insufficiency (CRI), with poor body condition being a feature, especially in more advanced stages. GI signs such as vomiting and diarrhea may accompany the clinical signs of acute and CKD. This can be due, in part, to the lack of gastrin clearance by the dysfunctional kidneys, resulting in hyperacidity of the stomach and secondary ulceration. Advanced azotemia can produce uremic oral ulceration. This is most commonly a feature of feline CKD and can present as halitosis as well as ulcerative lesions on the tongue and/or gingiva.

A thorough history with an accurate description of the patient's clinical signs, when presenting with renal or urinary problems, will assist the clinician in formulating the diagnostic plan. This may be especially helpful to the process when determining if the problems are behavioral or medical in nature.

SECTION 3 URINARY DISEASES

Chronic kidney disease

Chronic kidney disease (CKD) is the most commonly recognized renal disorder in dogs and cats. CKD is defined as kidney damage or decreased kidney function that has persisted for at least 3 months.[1] Kidney disease, kidney insufficiency, kidney failure, azotemia, and uremia are all terms that have been previously used to describe disorders of the kidney, but CKD is the preferred terminology. CKD generally refers to an irreversible and progressive loss of kidney function. Unlike acute renal failure (ARF), patients with CKD have already sustained permanent injury and have exceeded the maximal amount of compensatory glomerular hypertrophy. In most patients, the kidney function slowly declines over several months to years as the kidney damage continues. CKD is managed with supportive care, which often helps to slow the progression of the disease. With appropriate management, dogs and cats can often survive for long periods of time with a good quality of life.

Uremia and azotemia are important terms used when describing kidney disease. *Azotemia* classically describes blood work changes, particularly elevations in blood urea nitrogen (BUN) and creatinine. In contrast, *uremia* is a descriptive term that encompasses the clinical signs associated with declining renal function. Important clinical signs include vomiting, lethargy, anorexia, weight loss, halitosis, and neurological abnormalities.

CKD encompasses a wide variety of kidney problems. Some of the disorders are congenital, while others arise during the patient's life. Some diseases result in changes to the size and shape of the kidneys, while others may cause problems while leaving the kidney architecture intact. Some disorders are better detected in blood work, while others are best identified in urine samples. Often, the initiating cause of the CKD cannot be identified. However, a thorough investigation to find an underlying cause is beneficial. Potentially treatable disease processes include pyelonephritis, obstructing kidney or ureteral stones, lymphoma (especially in cats), and glomerular diseases. Therapy should be directed toward the inciting cause if possible. Treating the underlying disease process may not reverse the existing damage, but it may help to limit further kidney injury.

There are several consistent findings in patients with CKD. Most canine and feline patients lose the ability to concentrate their urine when more than two-thirds of the kidney function has been lost. Creatinine and BUN generally rise with approximately three-fourths loss in function. Proteinuria and hypertension play a more important role in the progression of canine CKD. Cats with chronic kidney disease often far outlive their canine counterparts.

The International Renal Interest Society (IRIS) has proposed a four-tier system for staging CKD in order to better determine a patient's prognosis and treatment (Table 10.3.1).[2]

In its simplest form, the stage is determined by the level of kidney function, particularly creatinine. However, the patient's clinical status also plays an important role in the classification scheme despite the strict cutoff points for laboratory values. Stage 1 includes dogs and cats with PU and PD, but with normal blood creatinine. Patients with stage 2 disease are polyuric and polydipsic and have mild blood work abnormalities. Some patients in stages 1 and 2 may have very high BP, which could include hyphema (blood in the eye), sudden blindness due to retinopathy and retinal detachments, lethargy, and weakness. Patients with significant protein loss in the urine may show signs of weight loss and a poor hair coat. Careful monitoring is advised in these patients to see if the disease is progressing. Patients with stage 3 disease often show signs including weight loss, vomiting, decreased appetite, PU, and PD. However, many of the signs improve or resolve with symptomatic therapy. The disease is generally progressive in these patients, so careful monitoring and adjustment of medications is necessary. Stage 4 disease results in clinical signs that are difficult to control with therapy.

Table 10.3.1 Stages of chronic kidney disease in dogs and cats

Serum creatinine values (mg/dL)		
Stage	Dogs	Cats
Stage 1	<1.4	<1.6
Stage 2	1.4–2.0	1.6–2.8
Stage 3	2.1–5.0	2.9–5.0
Stage 4	>5.0	>5.0

Source: Brown S. Evaluation of chronic renal disease: a staged approach. *Compendium on Continuing Education for Veterinarians* 1999; 21:752–763; http://www.iris-kidney.com.

CKD often progresses rapidly when patients enter stage 4. Evaluating quality of life issues in these patients is important.

There are a variety of clinical signs associated with CKD both in dogs and in cats. PU and PD are the predominant signs noted by the owner. Some patients may also be incontinent or may urinate inappropriately in the house. Many patients show GI signs as part of their disease. Vomiting, gastric ulceration, halitosis, diarrhea, and intestinal bleeding are increasingly more common in the advanced stages of CKD. Weight loss, muscle tremors, hypothermia, and muscle wasting are other important physical exam findings. Neurological consequences of CKD may include difficultly walking or stumbling, altered mentation, lethargy, and seizures. Cats with low potassium due to their kidney disease may manifest with cervical ventroflexion and a plantigrade stance. Other signs of hypokalemia include muscle tremors, cramps, weakness, and pain. Anemia occurs in patients with CKD because of decreased erythropoietin, a hormone produced by the kidneys that is vital in RBC production. Pale gums, lethargy, and lack of appetite are important warning signs. Alterations in the calcium and phosphorus balance in patients can lead to renal secondary hyperparathyroidism particularly in young dogs and cats.

Renal secondary hyperparathyroidism

The origin of renal secondary hyperparathyroidism is multifactorial but may have devastating effects in its advance stages. Phosphorus is retained in the blood as renal function declines. Phosphorus retention is the principal driving force for renal secondary hyperparathyroidism because it induces the production of parathyroid hormone (PTH). PTH enhances the release of calcium from bone, aids in the reabsorption of calcium from the renal tubules, and augments the absorption of calcium from the intestines. The combination of hyperphosphatemia and increased calcium absorption leads to the formation of calcium phosphorus crystals in soft tissues, joints, and vessels. The kidney, stomach, and liver seem to be particularly sensitive to mineralization. It is important to note that renal secondary hyperparathyroidism often starts before phosphorus levels rise outside the normal range.

Calcitriol is the most active form of vitamin D. Calcitriol is formed in the renal tubular cells. PTH promotes the formation of calcitriol, and calcitriol in return reduces PTH production through a negative feedback system. High phosphorus levels reduce the formation of calcitriol in the renal tubules. Without the negative feedback of calcitriol, PTH levels rise, leading to renal secondary hyperparathyroidism. As CKD progresses, there are fewer and fewer renal tubular cells to produce calcitriol, leading to further increases in PTH. Therefore, declining calcitriol levels play an important role in the development of renal secondary hyperparathyroidism.

Other important factors in renal secondary hyperparathyroidism include impaired intestinal absorption of the calcium due to low levels of calcitriol. Uremic toxins also accumulate as renal function declines. Uremic toxins limit the effectiveness of calcitriol to inhibit PTH secretion.

Renal secondary hyperparathyroidism can result in a variety of visible derangements throughout the body. Clinical signs may include mental dullness, lethargy, weakness, anorexia, and impaired muscle function. Renal secondary hyperparathyroidism manifests more severely in young growing patients. Changes in bone density are most frequently observed, and the bones of the skull and the mandible are often affected. Bone is reabsorbed from these areas, leading to a soft jaw (rubber jaw) and freely movable teeth. In particularly severe cases, the jaw can actually fracture. Distortion of the face may also be seen due to the deposition of fibrous tissue where bone has been reabsorbed.

Acute renal failure

Acute renal failure (ARF) is defined as a rapid loss of kidney function leading to the accumulation of nitrogenous waste, fluid imbalances, and electrolyte disturbances. Approximately 75% of the kidney function must be altered to increase creatinine. Thus, even a mild rise in creatinine may signal important disruptions in kidney function.[3] As opposed to CKD, acute renal failure is potentially reversible either by resolution of the injury or by adaptation of the kidney (hypertrophy) or by both mechanisms.

Renal azotemia can be categorized as prerenal, renal, or postrenal.[4] In some patients, the categories overlap.

Prerenal azotemia

Prerenal azotemia occurs because of insufficient blood flow to the glomeruli preventing adequate filtering and removal of uremic toxins. Dehydration, hypotension, anesthesia, hypoadrenocorticism, trauma, surgery, and shock are just a few of the disorders that can reduce perfusion to the kidney. Prerenal azotemia causes a rise in BUN and creatinine, but unlike the other categories, the urine is generally very concentrated. Prerenal azotemia is best treated by replenishing fluid volume and by restoring normal BP.

Renal azotemia

Renal azotemia results from injury to any part of the kidney (glomeruli, tubules, interstitium, or vessels). Most cases of ARF in this category are due to decreased perfusion, toxins, medications, or infection. Perfusion problems arise for the same reason as those described for prerenal azotemia but are typically more severe and occur for a long duration, resulting in renal azotemia.

Toxins can damage any part of the kidney. Potential toxins include ethylene glycol (antifreeze), lilies (in cats), grapes, and raisins. Some medications can inadvertently injure the kidneys. The renal tubule is particularly sensitive to the adverse effects of medications. ARF can arise from the use of non-steroidal anti-inflammatory drugs (NSAIDs), amikacin, gentamicin, amphotericin B, chemotherapy drugs, and diuretics, to name a few (Table 10.3.2).

Infectious causes of renal azotemia include pyelonephritis, leptospirosis, and Lyme disease. Leptospirosis is caused by the bacteria *Leptospira interrogans*, which has a predilection for inducing hepatic and renal injury. It is generally acquired from slow-moving or standing water. Wildlife such as raccoons,

Table 10.3.2   Causes of acute renal failure

Antibiotics

  Trimethoprim–sulfa

  Gentamicin

  Amikacin

  Polymyxin

  Rifampin

Medications

  Amphotericin B

  Cyclosporine

  Allopurinol

  Penicillamine

  NSAIDs

  Diuretics

Heavy metals

  Lead

  Mercury

  Chromium

  Arsenic

Toxins

  Ethylene glycol (antifreeze)

  Grapes

  Raisins

  Lillies (cats)

  Mushrooms

  Snake venom

  Spider venom

Chemotherapeutics

  Cisplatin

  Carboplatin

  Doxorubicin

  Azathioprine

  Methotrexate

opossums, and skunks carry the organism and spread the disease by shedding it in their urine. Water sources may be contaminated by infected urine, but soil, food, and bedding have also been shown to be a source of the disease.[5,6] The peak incidence occurs between July and November.[6] Leptospirosis organisms induce kidney injury by colonizing and multiplying directly in the renal tubules and interstitum as well as by a direct toxic effect on renal cells and secondary inflammation. Lyme disease is caused by the bacterial organism *Borrelia burgdorferi* and is endemic in many parts of the United States and Europe. Lyme disease is transmitted by the bite of an *Ixodes* tick. Lyme disease typically causes fever, lethargy, and polyarthritis. However, many severely affected patients develop a severe protein-losing nephropathy (PLN) and rapidly progressive ARF.[7] The mechanism by which *Borrelia* injures the kidney is likely inflammatory or immune mediated rather than by direct infection.[7,8] For more information on leptospirosis and Lyme disease, please see Chapter 11.

Postrenal azotemia

Postrenal azotemia arises most commonly from obstruction or rupture of the urinary tract. Uroliths or crystalline sludge may obstruct the ureters or urethra, leading to postrenal azotemia. Obstruction induces back pressure on the kidneys, thereby reducing glomerular filtration. If the obstruction is longstanding, then direct kidney injury or renal azotemia may occur. Neoplasia, particularly of the lower urinary tract, may also lead to obstruction. Rupture of the urinary tract allows leakage of the uremic toxin into the abdomen and surrounding tissues. Although glomerular filtration continues, uremic toxins enter the abdomen and quickly diffuse into the bloodstream. Treatment for postrenal azotemia is centered on alleviating the obstruction or correcting the rupture.

Historical findings for patients with ARF are variable and are often determined by the length of time that has transpired since the onset of the insult. In the early stages of ARF, the patient may be completely normal. As the injury and uremia progress, patients often become anorexic and begin to vomit. Lethargy, weakness, and diarrhea are common. The patient may initially be polyuric, but oliguira or anuria may develop as the severity of the insult increases. Neurological side effects may also occur particularly with toxin ingestion.

Physical examination findings are often determined by the severity of ARF. Halitosis and oral ulceration are noted with severe azotemia. Enlarged kidneys and renal pain may be noted on abdominal palpation. Bradycardia occurs particularly with severe hyperkalemia. A large painful bladder may be present in the case of obstruction. A rectal examination may reveal a prostatic or urethral mass causing obstruction. Stones can occasionally be palpated in the bladder or urethra.

Urinary tract infections

UTIs most commonly arise from organisms ascending into the urinary tract from the skin or tissues surrounding the external urinary opening. Bacteria are the most frequently documented pathogens to invade the urinary tract, but fungi and viruses may also cause infections. Individual terms have been developed to describe the location of the infection. They include pyelonephritis (infection of the kidney), ureteritis (infection of the ureter), cystitis (infection of the bladder), urethritis (infection of the urethra), prostatitis (infection of the prostate), and vaginitis (infection of the vagina). UTIs are more frequently identified in females. The urethra is shorter in females, predisposing them to

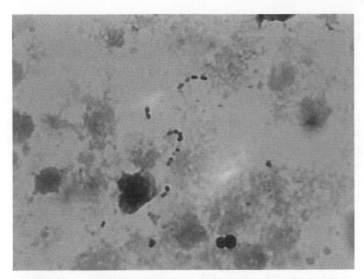

Figure 10.3.1 Urine sediment stained with Dip Quick from a patient with a lower urinary tract infection. Chains of bacteria are readily seen along with degenerative neutrophils. The patient was diagnosed with an *Enterococcus* UTI.

ascending infection. The vestibule and the vagina also have resident populations of bacteria in close proximity with the urethra. In cats, urinary infections are more likely in patients over the age of 10 years.[9]

Approximately 70% of UTIs are caused by a single organism.[10] The most common gram-negative organisms include *Escherichia coli*, *Proteus*, *Klebsiella*, *Pseudomonas*, and *Enterobacter*.[11] The most common gram-positive organisms include *Staphylococcus*, *Streptococcus*, and *Enterococcus* (Figure 10.3.1).[11]

UTIs can arise for a variety of reasons. Particularly virulent organisms have the ability to overcome normal host defense mechanisms. Adaptations that make bacteria more likely to colonize the urinary tract may include protective outer layers (capsules, cell walls), structures to increase attachment and movement in the urinary tract (fimbriae, flagella), ability to break down urea (urease producing), and genetic adaptations that make them antibiotic resistant (plasmid-mediated resistance). If the host defense mechanisms are weakened, then normal resident bacteria can invade and cause infection. Natural host defenses against infections include concentrated acidic urine, normal commensal bacterial populations inhabiting the distal urinary tract, frequent normal volume urinations, complete bladder emptying, and antibacterial secretions in the urinary tract (defensins).

UTIs may be complicated or uncomplicated. Uncomplicated UTIs occur in patients that lack structural, neurological, or functional abnormalities that may predispose them to infection.[12] Most uncomplicated UTIs can be treated successfully with a 10- to 14-day course of an appropriate antibiotic. Signs of infection quickly improve within the first few days of starting antibiotics. Complicated UTIs occur in patients with underlying disease processes that make them more susceptible to infection. Cushing's disease, diabetes mellitus, and CKD are all well-known risk factors. Intact dogs and patients with predisposing causes are all considered to have complicated UTIs. Patients with complicated UTIs generally require longer durations of treatment; 4–6 weeks of therapy and multiple antibiotics are frequently necessary.

Several other terms have been developed to describe the nature of UTIs. A relapsed infection is a UTI caused by the same organism within days to weeks of finishing antibiotics. Reinfection is another UTI following an initial infection, but with a different organism. A superinfection occurs in a patient that is already on antibiotics for a UTI when a second infection with a different organism is isolated. Patients with indwelling urinary catheters are at high risk for superinfections.

Many patients with UTIs demonstrate a number of signs. Symptoms most frequently include pollakiuria, hematuria, and stranguria. Many patients will urinate inappropriately in the house. A foul odor or cloudy urine may be associated with infection. Frequent licking of the perivulvar area may be observed by some owners.

Physical examination findings in patients with UTIs are usually lacking. Some patients may have perivulvar dermatitis or evidence of perivulvar saliva staining. Palpation of the abdomen is often unremarkable, but caudal abdominal pain may be noted. A hooded vulva may be observed in patients with recurrent infections.

Pyelonephritis

Pyelonephritis is defined as an infection of the renal pelvis (Figure 10.3.2).

Pyelonephritis often results in more severe symptoms when compared with a traditional lower UTI and its treatment is often more complicated. Pyelonephritis generally results from an ascending bacterial bladder infection, but hematogenous spread is possible particularly in patients with discospondylitis or sepsis. *E. coli* is the most commonly isolated bacteria causing pyelonephritis.[13,14] Predisposing disease processes include diabetes mellitus, hyperadrenocorticism, and chronic kidney disease.

Pyelonephritis can be acute or chronic in nature. Patients with acute pyelonephritis present with high fevers, a hunched posture suggestive of abdominal pain, lethargy, and vomiting. Foul-smelling urine and inappropriate urination may be noted by some owners. Patients tend to be polyuric and polydipsic rather than pollakiuric as in patients with lower urinary tract disease. Advanced cases may present with oliguria or anuria suggestive of severe ARF. Physical exams in patients with acute disease may reveal large painful kidneys on abdominal palpation. Symptoms in patients with chronic pyelonephritis may vary from no presenting complaints to signs of chronic renal failure (vomiting, weight loss, and poor hair coat). Physical exam findings in these patients may be unremarkable or the kidneys may palpate small and irregular.

Urolithiasis

Uroliths, also known as calculi or stones, in the urinary tract result from supersaturation of urine with particular

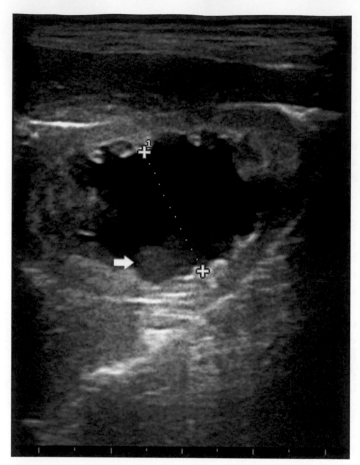

Figure 10.3.2 Ultrasonographic image of a dog with severe pyelonephritis. The renal pelvis is markedly dilated (dotted white line between plus marks). Sediment is also seen ventrally in the dilated pelvis (white arrow).

stone-forming substances or crystalline components. The bladder is a common place for uroliths to form since urine is stored there for long periods of time, thereby giving the components more time to interact. The kidney is another frequent location for stone (nephrolith) formation (Figure 10.3.3).

The higher the concentration of urolith components and the longer they are in contact with each other, the higher the risk of stone formation. Uroliths form around a nidus, which can consist of white blood cells (WBCs), bacteria, organic matrix, or crystals. It is possible for the nidus to be made of a different type of crystal than the rest of the stone. Uroliths can grow slowly layer by layer or they can increase in size when larger crystals come together and conglomerate. Other contributing factors to urolith formation include diet, frequency of urination, genetics, current medications, and the presence of a UTI.

Many dogs and cats with concentrated urine develop crystals, but only a small fraction of those patients ever develops a true urolith. It is important to remember that just because a patient has crystals in its urine does not mean that that patient will go on to develop uroliths.

Preventing or dissolving uroliths is based on the principles of increasing urine flow and minimizing the particular components that form a urolith. Interestingly, there are certain components of the urine that actually inhibit the formation of crystals and uroliths. Inhibitors of urolith formation may be either organic (proteins) or inorganic (other minerals). Although not much is known about urolith inhibitors, this may be a potential therapeutic area in the future.

Patients with bladder or urethral stones tend to manifest with signs of lower urinary tract disease. Stranguria, pollakiuria, and dysuria are common. Hematuria, malodorous urine, and inappropriate urination may also be signs that are observed by

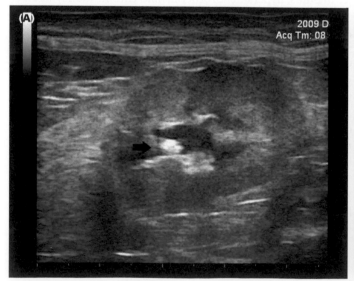

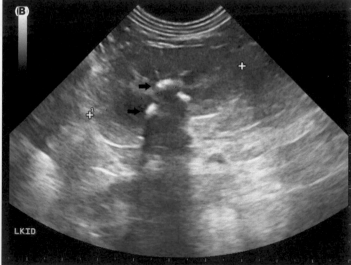

Figure 10.3.3 Ultrasonographic images of cats with nephroliths (black arrows). (A) Cat with a markedly dilated renal pelvis and central nephrolith. (B) Cat with nonobstructing diverticular nephroliths.

owners. In rare cases, patients can present for a complete urinary obstruction (anuria) or bladder rupture (lethargy, vomiting, bloated abdomen), particularly if a stone lodges in the urethra.

Physical exam findings in patients with bladder and urethral stones can vary widely. Many patients lack any significant physical findings. In very compliant patients, uroliths may be felt in the bladder on deep palpation of the caudal abdomen. If a urolith is lodged in the neck of the bladder or the urethra, then a large firm and often painful bladder may be detectable. Blood or blood-tinged urine may be present around the vulva or the penile urethra. A urethral stone can occasionally be palpable in the perineal region of male dogs or on rectal exam in females. In rare cases, an abdominal fluid wave can be observed if the bladder has ruptured.

Struvite urolithiasis

Struvite uroliths are formed primarily of magnesium ammonium phosphate and smaller amounts of calcium phosphate. In dogs, struvite uroliths form most commonly as a result of UTIs. Urease-producing bacteria have long been incriminated as a source of struvite urolithiasis because they are able to hydrolyze urea to form ammonia and bicarbonate. Ammonia goes on to precipitate with magnesium and phosphate to form a stone. Bicarbonate increases the pH of the urine making struvite stones more likely to precipitate. *Staphylococcus*, *Klebsiella*, *Pseudomonas*, and *Proteus* are among the most common urease-producing bacteria that are isolated on culture.[15] Bacteria become incorporated into the urolith as it grows. Recurrent urinary infections are common in patients with uroliths and vice versa; patients that get recurrent infections are at high risk for struvite uroliths. Sterile struvite uroliths are extremely rare in dogs but have been known to occur.[16] In contrast, feline struvite uroliths are usually not infection induced.

The etiology of struvite urolithiasis is likely multifactorial and includes gender, breed, and dietary factors. Most struvite uroliths are radiopaque and can therefore be seen on abdominal radiographs. They can be smooth, spiculated, spherical, and often conform to the shape of the urinary tract where they lodge (Figure 10.3.4).

Struvite uroliths account for approximately 41% of analyzed stones,[17] and they most frequently occur in the lower urinary

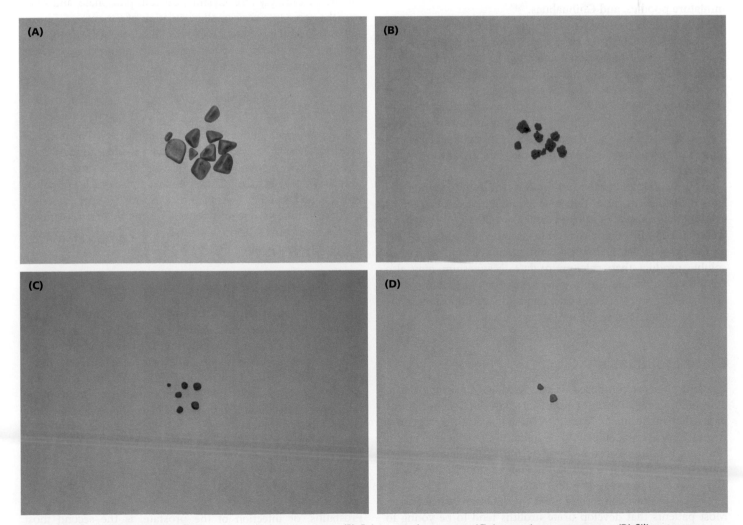

Figure 10.3.4   Different canine urinary stones. (A) Struvite stones. (B) Calcium oxalate stones. (C) Ammonium urate stones. (D) Silica stones.

tract. Approximately 71–85% of struvite uroliths occur in female dogs.[18] A longer urethra and a lower incidence of UTIs in male dogs likely explain the female predominance. Breed predilections include mixed breed dogs, miniature schnauzers, Lhasa apsos, bichon frises, shih tzus, miniature poodles, and cocker spaniels.[17]

Calcium oxalate urolithiasis

Calcium oxalate uroliths are formed primarily from calcium, oxalate, and varying amounts of calcium phosphate. Calcium oxalate uroliths can be smooth, lobulated, or spiculated.

These uroliths tend to form on the surface of cellular debris in the urine or on other crystals. Calcium oxalate uroliths form most frequently in the lower urinary tract of dogs and cats. However, most feline nephroliths and ureteroliths are composed of calcium oxalate. Neutered male dogs form more oxalate uroliths than females (approximately 70% males and 30% females).[18,19] Overweight patients are at increased risk. Certain breeds are known to form calcium oxalate uroliths more readily and include miniature schnauzers, Lhasa apsos, Yorkshire terriers, bichon frises, Pomeranians, shih tzus, cairn terrier, Maltese, miniature poodles, and Chihuahuas.[18,20]

Most calcium oxalates are radiopaque and can therefore be seen on abdominal radiographs. Calcium oxalate uroliths do not form as a result of bacterial infection of the urinary tract. However, like all uroliths, calcium oxalates may be secondarily infected. The occurrence of calcium oxalate uroliths in dogs and cats has been steadily increasing over the past 20 years. It is now estimated that approximately 41% of the stones that are removed from patients are calcium oxalate.[17] It is thought that the frequent use of struvite prevention diets may be shifting the dynamics toward the formation of oxalate uroliths.

In humans, citrate, magnesium, pyrophosphate, glycosaminoglycan, nephrocalcin, and Tamm–Horsfall mucoprotein (THM) inhibit the formation of calcium oxalate uroliths.[21] Although not well studied, it is thought that these components also likely play a role in dogs. Citrate complexes with calcium and forms a more soluble product than calcium oxalate. Magnesium may also complex with oxalate, limiting the formation of calcium oxalate crystals. As a result, citrate and magnesium are important in the dietary management of calcium oxalate uroliths.

Urate urolithiasis

Urate uroliths are composed of uric acids and its principal salt, ammonium urate. Purines comprise two of the four nucleotide bases that make up DNA and RNA, but like all nitrogenous wastes, they are still subject to degradation. Uric acid is one of the final breakdown products of purine metabolism. Ammonium urates tend to be small stones that are smooth and round. They also tend to have a greenish hue.

Urates are most commonly found in the lower urinary tract. Most patients that develop urate uroliths tend to be young to middle-aged. They occur more often in males than in females.[22]

Ammonium urates are radiolucent and are therefore not readily seen on abdominal radiographs. Urate uroliths are not frequently associated with infection, but urease-producing bacteria increase the incident of urolith formation. Approximately 6.4% of all analyzed stones are purine based.[17] A diet high in purine and acidic urine tends to increase the formation of these uroliths.

The Dalmatian and English bulldog are overrepresented. Genetic defects in urate metabolism have been identified in the Dalmatian and are highly suspected in the English bulldog.[23,24] Although all purebred Dalmatians seem to carry the defect, only approximately 25% ever develop uroliths.[25] A few other breeds seem to be at increased risk and include Yorkshire terriers, miniature schnauzers, and shih tzus.[23,26]

Severe liver disease and patients with portosystemic shunts are also at higher risk of developing urate uroliths. In these patients, the liver is unable to convert ammonia to urea and uric acid, leading to higher levels of these substances in the urine.

Other uroliths

Several other uroliths have been observed in the urinary tract but are exceedingly rare. Cystine, calcium phosphate, and silica uroliths occur in a very small population of patients.

Drugs and their metabolites have also been known to form uroliths. Ciprofloxacin, primidone, and tetracycline uroliths have been previously identified.[27]

Prostatic diseases

The prostate is a bilobed organ that completely encircles the proximal urethra and neck of the urinary bladder in male dogs. The prostate is surrounded by a thick capsule. The prostate is the only accessory sex organ that produces fluid which nourishes, protects, and prolongs sperm survival during it journey in reproduction. A testosterone derivative is responsible for the growth and development of the prostate. In a neutered male, the prostate is typically very small.

Benign prostatic hyperplasia

Benign prostatic hyperplasia (BPH) is the most common clinical abnormality of older intact male dogs.[28] In BPH, the prostate gradually enlarges over a dog's lifetime as a result of the influence of testosterone and its derivatives. The constant hormonal influence can lead to the formation of cysts and fluid within the prostate. It is estimated that 80% of intact male dogs over the age of 5 have BPH.[28] Unlike humans, BPH tends *not* to cause any significant signs unless the prostate becomes infected with bacteria. The prostate is symmetrically enlarged and is nonpainful on rectal exam.

Prostatitis

Prostatitis, or infection of the prostate, is the second most common prostatic disorder. Prostatitis can be acute or chronic in nature. Acute prostatitis is a rare disorder in dogs. In acute prostatitis, the prostate tends to be normal in size, but it is often very painful on rectal palpation. Chronic prostatitis is a frequent disorder that is often found in patients with BPH. Patients with chronic prostatitis can have normal to large prostates on rectal exam. The prostate may or may not be painful on palpation. Mild asymmetry may also be noted if one side of the prostate is more severely affected.

Prostatic infections

Infections of the prostate most frequently arise from ascending urethral infections. However, hematogenous infections may also occur. Most prostatic infections are due to *E. coli*, but *Pseudomonas*, *Proteus*, *Staphylococcus*, and *Streptococcus* may also be isolated.[28] Chronic prostatitis is often suspected when a male patient has recurrent UTIs with the same organism following the discontinuation of antibiotics. In these patients, the prostate acts as a reservoir for infection. Antibiotics that cross the blood–prostate barrier and achieve high concentration in the prostatic fluid are needed to eliminate the infection.

Lower urinary tract disease in cats

Lower urinary tract disease in cats has had a variety of names over the years. Synonyms include feline lower urinary tract disease (FLUTD), feline urological syndrome (FUS), and feline idiopathic cystitis or feline interstitial cystitis (FIC). FIC is currently the most commonly used term to identify the disorder. FIC affects approximately 4.6% of cats in the United States.[29] Approximately 45% of cats with FIC will have a recurrence of their disease within weeks to months of diagnosis.[30] Indoor cats in multicat households are at higher risk. Increased body weight and inactivity are also described risk factors. Environmental issues including the number of litter boxes, the type of litter, exposure to toys, and the hierarchy of the cats in the household have also been implicated in the pathogenesis of the disease. Recent relocation to a new house, construction, changes in furniture, and visiting houseguests are known stressors that trigger symptoms in some patients. Therefore, the pathophysiology of FIC is multifactorial and involves complex interactions between the anatomic, hormonal, and environmental factors.

The role of infectious organisms in FIC has been investigated. Viral disease does not seem to be the cause of the disorder in a large majority of cats.[31] Despite the widely held belief that many FIC cats have a UTI, an important study showed that less than 2% of cats are found to have bacteria in their urine when a urine culture was performed at the time of diagnosis.[32] Therefore, infectious organisms are unlikely to play a role in the majority of cats with FIC.

FIC occurs most commonly in young to middle-aged indoor cats. FIC can be obstructive or nonobstructive. Obstructive feline idiopathic cystitis occurs most frequently in male cats. The narrow penile urethra of male cats predisposes to obstruction with plugs, stones, or by urethral spasms. Urethral plugs are typically composed of struvite crystals and a protein matrix. The incidence of calcium oxalate stones seems to be rising and now comprises approximately 40% of analyzed stones.[17,33] Nonobstructive disease occurs in both female and male cats. Approximately 92% of cats have spontaneous resolution of their signs in 5–7 days.[34,35]

Clinical signs of lower urinary tract disease in cats may wax and wane. Signs may include inappropriate urination, stranguria, and hematuria. Many patients are pollakiuric and some may present for anuria.

Physical exam findings may be negligible in most patients with nonobstructive disease. The most common finding on examination in patients with obstructive disease is a large turgid bladder. Occasionally, stones are palpable in the bladder. In males, the penis can be rigid and purple with prolonged obstruction.

Ectopic ureters

A ureter that opens in a location other than the bladder trigone is considered ectopic. Developmental defects in the fetus result in a variety of ureteral abnormalities. The location of the ureteral opening can vary widely and may occur anywhere along the urethra, vagina, or uterus. Ectopic ureters may be unilateral or bilateral. Extramural ectopic ureters completely bypass the urinary bladder and directly insert at a more distal location. Intramural ectopic ureters enter the bladder trigone on the external surface but tunnel through the bladder wall to exit at more distal locations, particularly in the urethra (Figure 10.3.5).

An ectopic ureter may have one or more openings at its final destination. Anatomic abnormalities of the urethra, vagina, and vestibule are common in female patients with ectopic ureters. Urethral sphincter mechanism incompetence (USMI) occurs commonly in patients with intramural ectopic ureters and is often due to disruption of the sphincter by the tunneling ectopic ureter.

Ectopic ureters are most frequently diagnosed in female patients. Although ectopic ureters occur in males, the longer urethra and urethral sphincter likely result in fewer clinical signs and diagnosed cases. A genetic basis is likely because particular breeds appear predisposed. High risk breeds include Siberian huskies, Labrador retrievers, golden retriever, Newfoundlands, English bulldogs, West Highland white terriers, fox terriers, Skye terriers, and miniature and toy poodles.[36,37] Ectopic ureters have been reported in cats but are exceedingly rare.[38]

Owners of patients with ectopic ureters frequently report intermittent or continuous dribbling of urine. Many owners resort to the use of diapers to avoid constantly cleaning up urine. The incontinence associated with ectopic ureters occurs regardless of whether the patient is awake or asleep.

Physical examination findings may include a urine-soaked perineum or evidence of urine staining. A perivulvar dermatitis and saliva staining may also be noted. Erythema of the vulva may occur and is often the result of urine scalding. Some patients have normal physical exams.

Ectopic ureters have traditionally been diagnosed by excretory urography or ultrasonography. However, both methods

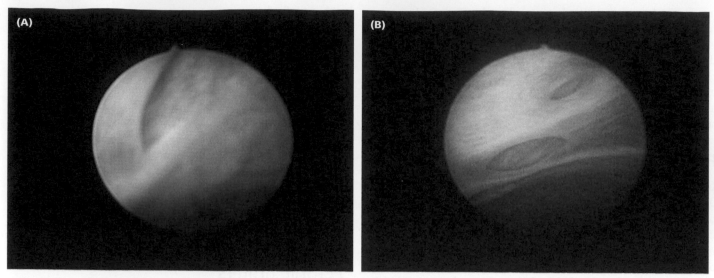

Figure 10.3.5 Ureteral orifice as seen from the bladder during cystoscopy. (A) Normal ureteral orifice. (B) An intramural ectopic ureter tunneling in the bladder wall with multiple openings in the bladder neck.

have a tendency to underdiagnose the problem. Recent studies have compared traditional imaging to that of contrast-enhanced computed tomography (CT) scans, fluoroscopy, and cystoscopy for the detection of ectopic ureters. Contrast-enhanced CT scans and cystoscopy were found to be the most successful in identifying the type and location of ectopic ureters.[39,40]

Ectopic ureters have long been a surgical disorder. Surgery remains the treatment of choice for extramural ectopic ureters. In these patients, the ureter must be relocated to the bladder. However, recent advances in minimally invasive technology have now afforded new options in the treatment of intramural ectopic ureters. Laser ablation of the tissue dividing the tunneling ectopic ureter from the urethra and the bladder has been shown to be effective in correcting intramural ectopic ureters. With surgery and laser ablation, the problem remains that the urethral sphincter muscle may be compromised by either the ectopic ureter itself or with the correction procedure. Some patients require medical management for sphincter incompetence or urethral collagen injections to help maintain continence.

Urethral sphincter mechanism incompetence

USMI is the most common cause of incontinence in middle-aged female dogs. The sphincter is a muscular segment in the proximal urethra that holds urine in the bladder. The sphincter is under control of the sympathetic nervous system, but estrogen influence is also important in maintaining normal function. Sphincter incompetence often follows an ovariohysterectomy and therefore is known as spaying incontinence or hormone-responsive incontinence. It is estimated that up to 20% of spayed female dogs are affected.[41] Large breed dogs seem to be at increased risk as are boxers, giant schnauzers, Dobermans, Wei-

maraners, German shepherds, and rottweilers.[42] A few cases are actually congenital and are associated with poor development of the urethral sphincter muscle. These patients may show signs as early as a few months of age. USMI is rare in males and appears to be unrelated to castration. A few female cats have been identified with the problem.[43]

Owners frequently report puddles of urine where the patient has been resting or sleeping. The amount of urine varies widely and may range from a few drops up to a large volume. Patients with sphincter incompetence typically do not show signs when they are completely awake or moving around. The urine is generally concentrated. No odor or blood should be noted when examining the urine.

Physical exam findings are largely unremarkable but may include a small to large pool of urine after sleeping or lying down. The perineum may be urine soaked and there may be perivulvar dermatitis or evidence of saliva staining.

Urethral sphincter incompetence may be confirmed with a urethral pressure profile. A normal sphincter will result in a focal pressure spike on the profile. In patients with sphincter incompetence, this pressure spike is greatly reduced or absent. The equipment to perform profile studies is only available in some referral hospitals; therefore, the diagnosis is often made on the patient's clinical history.

Several medical therapies are available for patients with sphincter incompetence. Various alpha-adrenergic agonists (phenylpropanolamine, ephedrine, or pseudoephedrine) are commonly used for their ability to increase urethral smooth muscle tone. Phenylpropanolamine is effective in approximately 85–90% of female dogs with USMI.[44,45] Estrogens (diethylstilbestrol [DES] and estriol) are commonly used in the treatment of the disease because of their ability to increase urethral closure pressure. Estrogens also increase the density and responsiveness of alpha-adrenergic receptors. Estrogen therapy alone is effective in approximately 50–65% of patients.[46] Because estrogens increase the number of adrenergic receptors, females that are refractory to a single medication may respond better to combination therapy. Patients that fail to respond to combination therapy should ideally have a pressure profile performed.

Cystoscopic injections of bulking agents have been investigated in patients with refractory incontinence. Collagen is injected into the periurethral tissue, which narrows the lumen, allowing for more effective urethral sphincter closure. Approximately 75–93% of dogs improve with this type of procedure.[47] Repeated injections are required in some patients months to years down the line.

Protein-losing nephropathy

PLNs comprise a variety of disorders affecting the microscopic subunits of the kidney, the nephrons. The glomerulus, renal tubule, and interstitium are components of the nephron that are most commonly affected. In a normal kidney, serum proteins are readily reabsorbed from urine as it passes through the nephron. In patients with PLN, serum proteins leak into the urine, indicating either an insufficiency of absorption or impaired filtration. Albumin is the predominant protein in the urine of dogs and cats with proteinuria. Severe or prolonged PLNs may lead to CKD in dogs. PLNs are rare in cats. Amyloidosis and glomerulonephritis are the two most commonly recognized PLN disorders.

Glomerulonephritis

Glomerulonephritis is characterized by inflammation of the glomeruli and often involves the deposition of immune complexes within the glomerular capillary walls. The deposition of immune complexes leads to proliferation and thickening of the glomerulus and eventual glomerular cell death. Proteinuria predominants early in the disease process, but patients may progress to CKD if sufficient numbers of glomeruli are lost. The immune complexes in glomerulonephritis are thought to be produced as a result of chronic inflammation, chronic infection, or neoplasia. An underlying cause is not always identified in patients with the disease. Hereditable forms of glomerulonephritis exist, which suggests genetic aberrations as an underlying cause in some patients. The age range for patients with glomerulonephritis is quite wide, but most patients tend to be over the age of 7 years.[43] Doberman pinschers, Samoyeds, rottweilers, greyhounds, Bernese mountain dogs, English cocker spaniels, and soft-coated wheaten terriers are at an increased risk.[48]

Amyloidosis

Amyloidosis can be a systemic disease, but has a predilection for the kidney and liver. In renal amyloidosis, beta-pleated sheets of amyloid A protein are deposited in the kidney. Amyloid is thought to be deposited as a result of chronic inflammation, chronic infection, or neoplasia, but hereditary forms of the disease also exist. Greater than 85% of patients are 7 years of age or older.[49] Females are affected more often than males. Beagles, Walker hounds, collies, and English foxhounds are at increased risk.[49,50] In cats, Abyssinians, Siamese, and Oriental shorthairs have a predisposition to the disease.[51] With the acquired form of the disease, amyloid is primarily deposited in the glomerulus and leads to profound proteinuria. In patients with heritable amyloidosis, Chinese shar-peis and Abyssinians, amyloid is deposited primarily in the interstitium. The heritable disease manifests at a younger age and as CKD, but proteinuria is typically lacking.[52]

A number of complications may arise in patients with chronic PLN. Weight loss can be gradual in patients with moderate proteinuria or may be dramatic in patients with severe disease. Hypertension is also commonly identified and may result in retinal detachment and sudden blindness in patients with PLN. Blood clots, or thromboembolic disease, rank as the most severe and life-threatening complication of glomerulonephritis. Blood clots to the brain or lungs are a common cause of death in patients with PLNs. Fluid retention in the tissues, or edema, often occurs in patients when the albumin is less than 1.5 g/dL. Pitting edema is readily recognized in the distal limb and on the ventral abdomen.

Physical exam findings in patients with PLN are often unremarkable in the early stages. In more advanced cases, evidence of muscle wasting and weight loss may be noted. Many patients have a dull or thin hair coat. Retinal hemorrhage and focal to complete retinal detachments can be seen on an ophthalmic examination. In severely affected patients, pale mucous membranes, pitting edema, or ascites may be noted. Poor profusion of the limbs may be observed in patients with thromboembolic disease.

Urinary neoplasia

The most common tumor affecting the urinary tract of dogs and cats is transitional cell carcinoma (TCC, as it is more commonly known).[53] TCCs tend to arise from the bladder neck (trigone) or the urethra. Squamous cell carcinomas and leiomyosarcomas have been also identified but are exceedingly rare compared to TCC.[54] Genetics and exposure to pesticides and insecticides have been associated with increased risk of tumor development.[55] Scottish terriers, West Highland white terriers, Shetland sheepdogs, beagles, and dachshunds have a known genetic predisposition.[56] Middle-aged male cats are predisposed to TCC.

Stranguria, pollakiuria, and hematuria are the most common symptoms of patients with bladder and urethral tumors. Most patients have to urinate more frequently or, in rare cases, patients may present with oliguria or anuria if the tumor obstructs the outflow of urine.

Physical exam findings may be minimal or may reveal a large distended bladder. A rectal exam should always be performed in patients that are straining to urinate or have blood in their urine. A rectal exam may reveal a thickened irregular urethra. Enlarged sublumbar lymph nodes may also be palpable dorsal to the bladder.

The most common tumor affecting the prostate is prostatic adenocarcinoma.[57] TCCs have also been known to develop within the prostate. Prostatic tumors may occur in both intact and castrated male dogs. Castration does not prevent the development of prostatic carcinomas and may actually increase the risk.[58] Prostatic adenocarcinomas are virtually unheard of in cats. Most patients are older than 10 years of age at the time of diagnosis.[57] Although bladder and prostate cancers are malignant, they typically do not spread until late in the disease. Metastatic sites include sublumbar lymph nodes, lumbar vertebrae, and lungs.[59]

Clinical signs of patients with prostatic tumors are similar to patients with TCCs. Stranguria, hematuria, and pollakiuria predominate. Physical exam findings often include a large, firm prostate. The prostate is typically asymmetric or irregular. However, a normal-sized prostate does not exclude a carcinoma. Sublumbar lymphadenopathy may also be palpable dorsal to the bladder.

Kidney tumors are exceedingly rare in both dogs and cats. However, most renal tumors are malignant when they do develop. Lymphoma is the most common kidney tumor in cats, and a large percentage of affected cats are feline leukemia virus (FeLV) positive.[60] Renal carcinomas and adenocarcinomas are the most common tumors in dogs.[61] Male dogs are slightly more likely to be affected. A genetic predisposition is known particularly in German shepherds.[62] Tumors tend to be bilateral in cats and in German shepherds.

Clinical signs for patients with kidney tumors include weight loss, anorexia, and vomiting. Hematuria may occur but is uncommon. Physical exam findings may include a large kidney on abdominal palpation. The kidney tends to be irregular in carcinoma or adenocarcinomas and is more likely to be smooth in the case of lymphoma. Skin nodules are common in German shepherds with kidney tumors.[62]

SECTION 4 URINARY DIAGNOSTICS AND THERAPEUTIC IMPLICATIONS

Urinalysis

A urinalysis is an essential component to the workup of a patient with suspected disease involving the urinary system or in any patient that is systemically sick from any cause. Not only is a urinalysis invaluable in helping to determine the underlying cause of azotemia (e.g., prerenal vs. renal), but there are also cases where the only useful diagnostic clues are provided by the urinalysis (e.g., proteinuria and glucosuria without hyperglycemia).

A fresh (within 3 h of collection), nonrefrigerated urine sample should ideally be used for analysis. Crystals can form with refrigeration, and casts and cellular elements degenerate rapidly at room temperature. If analysis will be delayed, the urine should be refrigerated and allowed to return to room temperature prior to completing the urinalysis.

Collection methods

Urine can be collected by one of three possible methods: cystocentesis, urinary catheterization, or by free catch. It is very important to always specify the method of collection as this may affect the interpretation of the results. In general cystocentesis is the preferred method of collection because there are fewer confounding factors to take into account when interpreting the results. However, there are some exceptions to this general rule. For instance, a free-catch sample may be preferable to a sample collected by cystocentesis or catheterization in cases where hematuria is being investigated or if a TCC of the bladder is suspected. A midstream free-catch sample is also preferable if there is a contraindication for performing a cystocentesis. In some cases, it is useful to compare urinalysis results from samples collected first by free catch and then by cystocentesis (e.g., when trying to localize the origin of hematuria, pyuria, or proteinuria within the urogenital tracts).

Free catch

When collecting a free-catch urine sample, a midstream sample is preferable; there is less bacterial contamination from normal urogenital flora. Samples collected into a sterile container from the midstream may still have false-positive urine culture results due to contamination from external hairs on the prepuce or vulva. Urine samples brought in by owners are rarely suitable for urine culture and obtaining a free-catch midstream urine sample from a cat can be challenging. The use of a litter pan with nonabsorbent litter or a litter box specifically designed to capture urine (e.g., Smart Cat Box™) may be helpful for collecting urine for a urinalysis when culture is not required.

Urinary catheterization

Collection of urine by urethral catheterization is straightforward in most male dogs, but heavy sedation is typically required in cats and in female dogs, making this an impractical collection method in many cases. Catheterization to collect a urinary sample is also appropriate if the patency of the urethra needs to be assessed. The risk of creating a UTI from catheterization is higher in female dogs compared with male dogs, and hematuria can occur if the proper technique is not followed. These factors may need to be accounted for when interpreting the results of a urinalysis. It is also good practice to discard the first few milliliters of urine when urine is collected by catheterization as this may be contaminated by debris carried into the bladder by the catheter. See Chapter 14 for more information on urinary catheterization techniques.

Cystocentesis

Collection of urine by cystocentesis is considered the gold standard when a urine culture is required to rule out a UTI. Cystocentesis samples can be collected in most awake feline and canine patients provided there are no clear contraindications. Absolute contraindications for performing a cystocentesis include a suspected coagulopathy, a pyoderma involving the ventral caudal abdominal skin, a suspected devitalized bladder wall secondary to prolonged urethral obstruction, and an unco-operative patient that cannot be manually restrained for the procedure. See Chapter 14 for more information on urinary cystocentesis techniques.

Components of a urinalysis

There are three components to a urinalysis: physical examination, chemical (dipstick) analysis, and sediment evaluation.

Gross examination of urine

Normal urine is yellow due to the presence of urochrome pigments. Normal urine should also be clear and transparent. Cloudy urine indicates turbidity from increased cells, crystals, protein, lipid (cats especially), sperm, and/or mucus. Dilute urine is often pale yellow. However, urine color should never be used in place of a urine specific gravity (USG) for the assessment of urine concentration. Discolored (e.g., red, orange, or blue) urine can be attributed to a variety of endogenous or exogenous pigments or compounds. For example, bilirubin can impart an orange to green color to urine; increased RBCs or pigmenturia from the abnormal presence of hemoglobin or myoglobin in the urine will impart a red color to urine. In addition, certain drugs (e.g., mitoxantrone chemotherapy, sulfonamides) or dietary constituents (e.g., beets) can also discolor urine. When abnormal urine color is reported, a thorough history of the pet's diet, medications, and environment should be gathered. In addition, inspection of the color of the patient's serum and the supernatant of their urine after centrifugation may be helpful for investigating the underlying cause, especially when trying to differentiate pigmenturia from true hematuria as the cause of red-colored urine. If hematuria is responsible, RBCs will settle out in spun urine, leaving a clear supernatant. The serum of the patient (spun hematocrit or blood tube) will also be clear and transparent. If pigmenturia is the cause of the discoloration, the urine supernatant will remain discolored. The serum will be discolored if hemoglobinuria is the causative agent but not if myoglobinuria is responsible.

Urine has a normal mild odor that is imparted by the presence of volatile fatty acids. Common causes of abnormal odor include ketonuria (sweet odor), very concentrated urine, or infected urine.

USG, performed preferably on the supernatant of centrifuged urine, is used to assess the concentrating ability of the kidneys and is measured with a refractometer. The USG can range from 1.001 to 1.080, but specific gravities >1.030 (dogs) and >1.035 (cats) are indicative of adequate tubular function in a dehydrated or concurrently azotemic animal. Storage of urine does not affect measurement of the USG. It is important to realize that because the USG varies with many nonrenal factors (diet, water intake, extrarenal diseases), there is no true "normal" USG for dogs. To determine the clinical significance of a USG, it is important to consider whether a USG is appropriate for a given patient by taking into account their hydration status, history of fluid losses (vomiting, diarrhea, polyuria, burns, etc.), prior treatments (e.g., diuretics, steroids, fluid therapy), suspected disease processes,

and assessment of their biochemical renal parameters (BUN and creatinine).

Based on the USG, urine can be categorized as isosthenuric or hyposthenuric. *Isosthenuric* urine has a concentration that is similar to that of plasma (USG of 1.008–1.015). The presence of persistent isosthenuria may be suggestive of primary CKD, Cushing's disease, diabetes mellitus, or hypercalcemia. *Hyposthenuric* urine has a concentration less than that of plasma, resulting in a specific gravity of <1.008. The presence of hyposthenuria does not distinguish between causes of PU and PD. Hyposthenuria can be the result of central diabetes insipidus, nephrogenic diabetes insipidus, medullary washout, and psychogenic PD. However, hyposthenuria eliminates CKD because hyposthenuria requires functional kidneys to create extremely dilute urine.

It must be stressed that normal cats and dogs can have a USG that is isosthenuric or hyposthenuric, so without a reliable history of PU/PD, this finding should not be overinterpreted.

Chemical analysis: dipstick

Urine dipstick analysis is a convenient method of assessing several biochemical aspects of urine. Dipstick analysis can be done on a fresh unspun urine sample. If the urine is turbid or bloody, then the urine should be centrifuged and the supernatant should be used for dipstick analysis.

Urine pH

The urine pH dipstick pad can measure urine in the 5–9 pH range. The pH of normal cat and dog urine is typically within the 5.5–7.5 range. However, urine pH can be affected by diet, disease processes, and medications, so it cannot be interpreted in isolation. Causes of acidic urine (pH < 5.5) can include a meat-based diet, metabolic or respiratory acidosis, catabolic state, and administration of acidifying drugs (potassium phosphate, ammonium chloride, etc.). Causes of alkaline urine (pH > 7.5) include old stored urine, a UTI caused by urease-producing bacteria, exclusive consumption of a vegetarian diet, metabolic or respiratory alkalosis, and medications (acetozolamide, bicarbonate). Urine pH can be important if the patient has uroliths since the pH can influence the solubility of various types of urinary crystals and therefore can influence their detection in the urine sediment analysis.

Urine glucose

The regent test strip on the urine dipstick is specific for glucose.

The test pad provides a semiquantitative assessment of the glucose concentration in the urine above a concentration of 80 mg/dL. Normal urine should not have any detectable glucose. Glucosuria can occur with concurrent hyperglycemia when the renal threshold for glucose (dogs about 180 mg/dL and cats about 300 mg/dL) is exceeded. This can occur with diabetes mellitus, stress or excitement in cats, or following IV dextrose administration. Glucosuria that occurs with concurrent normoglycemia can be caused by a renal tubular defect secondary to severe acute tubular necrosis from renal ischemia, pyelonephritis, nephrotoxins, or from a renal tubular metabolic defect such as Fanconi's syndrome.

Urine ketones

The urine from normal dogs and cats should be negative for ketones. Ketone bodies are formed when there is increased fatty acid catabolism as a result of a shift in energy production. This occurs most commonly with diabetic ketoacidosis. However, starvation, high protein or low carbohydrate diets, and disorders associated with hypoglycemia may also lead to increased ketones in the urine.

Urine bilirubin

The urine from normal cats should always be negative for bilirubin, while small amounts of bilirubin in dogs may be considered normal. Biliruburia may occur whenever there is either excessive formation of bilirubin (e.g., immune-mediated hemolytic anemia [IMHA]) or impaired hepatobiliary excretion of bilirubin (e.g., acute liver failure or biliary obstruction). Bilirubinuria usually occurs before clinical evidence of icterus is noted. When there is excessive formation or impaired hepatobiliary excretion of bilirubin, bilirubin is readily filtered by the glomerulus and the renal tubular threshold for reabsorption is easily overwhelmed, leading to increased amounts in the urine.

Urobilinogen

This test is of questionable clinical value. In theory, a negative result on the dipstick could reflect complete biliary obstruction. In reality, the reagent strip cannot detect an absence of urobilinogen. Increased amounts of urobilinogen can be seen with liver disease or hemolytic anemia; however, the correlation is poor.

Occult blood

The urine from normal dogs and cats should be negative for blood, but a false positive can result from sample collection. Hematuria may occur with hemorrhage from sampling trauma, reproductive tract disease, or diseases of the urinary tract. Increased RBCs are expected on the sediment examination for cases with true hematuria. Most urine dipsticks have a test pad labeled occult blood that can detect between 5 and 20 RBC/mL of urine. Large numbers of intact RBCs will cause a homogenous color change on the blood reagent test pad. Results for occult blood may be described in semiquantitative terms based on the degree of color change using some urine dipsticks.

Hemoglobinuria can also lead to positive reaction for occult blood on the dipstick. Hemoglobinuria can occur if intact RBCs hemolyze in the urine (e.g., in dilute urine with a USG < 1.008 and in alkaline urine), or if hemoglobin levels in the blood are elevated (e.g., IMHA, zinc toxicosis, genetic disorders, infectious agents, hypophosphatemia).

Myoglobinuria that occurs with trauma (e.g., crush injury), toxins, or ischemic injury of muscles (rhabdomyolysis) can also lead to a positive reaction for occult blood on the dipstick. To distinguish hematuria from hemoglobinuria or myoglobinuria, inspect the supernatant after centrifuging the urine sample and evaluate the color of serum after centrifugation of a microhematocrit tube (see earlier section).

False-positive reactions for occult blood or hemoglobin may occur if the sample is contaminated with oxidizing agents (e.g., disinfectants, if urine is collected from a table or floor). False-negative reactions may occur if RBCs have settled to the bottom of a urine sample and only the unspun supernatant is analyzed. In this situation, a disparity between the dipstick and sediment evaluation is expected. The opposite disparate reaction, with a positive occult blood dipstick and a negative sediment analysis, can occur if RBCs are lysed in dilute (USG < 1.008) or alkaline urine.

Protein

The dipstick reagent pad that detects protein is semiquantitative and only detects albumin. Changes in the color of the pad correspond to estimated protein concentrations, and results are reported as trace (5–20 mg/dL), 1+ (30 mg/dL), 2+ (100 mg/dL), 3+ (300 mg/dL), or 4+ (1000 mg/dL). Very alkaline or highly concentrated urine may cause false-positive results. The reagent test pad cannot detect globulins or Bence Jones proteins seen in some cases of lymphoma and multiple myeloma. Pigmenturia can interfere with the reagent pad and with the estimation of protein concentrations.

The significance of proteinuria for all qualitative and semiquantitative tests must always be interpreted in light of the USG and the urine sediment findings. If the urine sediment is inactive (i.e., there are no signs of inflammation or infection), then a positive dipstick result for proteinuria should be confirmed with a sulfosalicylic acid (SSA) turbidimetric test or confirmed and quantified with a urine protein creatinine ratio (UPC). Regardless of the level of proteinuria detected, protein loss at any level is always more significant in the presence of dilute urine.

Leukocytes

Analysis for the detection of WBCs in the urine, also known as pyuria, is more reliable on a sediment evaluation than as a color change on a reagent test pad. Significant numbers of WBCs in the urine indicate active inflammatory disease somewhere in the urinary tract or possibly in the genital tract. The urine dipstick reagent pad has a very low sensitivity in dogs and therefore a high rate of false-negative results. A positive result is indicative of pyuria in dogs, but a negative result does not rule out pyuria. In cats, the test has low specificity (i.e., a high rate of false positives), so it is not considered diagnostically useful.

Nitrites

The nitrites test is not suitable for use in small animal patients. Nitrites are produced by bacteria in urine. However, this test strip is not considered very sensitive in cats and dogs for detecting UTIs.

Dipstick USG

This method is not very useful because the highest value typically detected is between 1.025 and 1.030, which is below the

USG cutoff point for adequate renal concentrating ability in dogs and in cats. Even with less concentrated urine samples, the test is still not very accurate in dogs and in cats.

Urine sediment examination

Urine sediment examination is always done on a centrifuged urine sample. A standardized volume of urine should be centrifuged at a low speed (1000–1500 rpm) for 5 min. The supernatant is then decanted off and the remaining sediment is resuspended in 0.5 mL of the spun urine. A drop of sediment is then pipetted onto a clean microscope slide and a coverslip applied. Examination of unstained urine samples is preferable; however, one drop of a commercial sediment stain (e.g., Sedi-Stain®) can also be added to a drop of resuspended urine sediment to enhance contrast. Microscopic evaluation at low and high power is indicated for both unstained and stained samples. Cellular elements are quantified by counting the number per high power field. The method of urine collection should be noted as this will influence the interpretation of the sediment findings.

Cellular elements

RBCs

Normal urine contains very few RBCs (0–5 RBCs/hpf) and increased numbers indicate hematuria. Hematuria may be microscopic or macroscopic and can be caused by urinary (e.g., trauma, urolithiasis, neoplasia, inflammatory disease, parasites, idiopathic renal hemorrhage) and nonurinary diseases (e.g., coagulopathy).

In some cases, comparison of the urine sediment findings from samples collected by free catch and by cystocentesis may be helpful for localizing the source of bleeding within the urinary tract. Iatrogenic hematuria may result from cystocentesis, and if suspected, this should be accounted for when interpreting the results. Resubmission of a free-catch sample a few days later can clarify if the hematuria is from the cystocentesis or not.

White blood cells

Low numbers of WBCs (<5/hpf) in the urine sediment are normal. Increased numbers (>5/hpf) in a cystocentesis sample is indicative of inflammation from either an infection or sterile inflammatory process within the urinary tract. For free-catch samples, pyuria can indicate inflammation anywhere in the urinary tract as well as in the genital tract (e.g., vagina, vulva, or prepuce). Pyuria in a patient with clinical signs compatible with lower urinary tract inflammation (e.g., stranguria, pollakiuria, hematuria, dysuria), or systemic signs suggestive of upper urinary tract inflammation (anorexia, fever, lethargy, vomiting, PU), should prompt a culture of the urine. In addition, for patients with medical or anatomical conditions known to predispose them to UTIs (e.g., patients with diabetes mellitus or hyperadrenocorticism, patients with spinal injuries, or patients on long-term corticosteroids therapy), a urine culture may be warranted even in the absence of pyuria on the urine sediment.

Epithelial cells

It is normal to see occasional small epithelial cells in the sediment of a urine sample. Squamous cells in a free-catch urine sample most often are insignificant and result from normal sloughing of uroepithelial cells from the distal urethra or genital tract. Increased numbers of epithelial cells can be seen in association with infection, inflammation, irritation, and neoplasia of the urinary or urogenital tract.

Increased numbers of transitional epithelial cells can originate from the urothelium of the renal pelvis, ureters, urinary bladder, or proximal urethra. Low numbers are acceptable, but high numbers indicate mucosal disruption from inflammation or neoplasia. Transitional cells are very reactive and can display atypical features, making it difficult to distinguish inflammation from malignancy. Because of this, urine cytology is not considered ideal for confirming the diagnosis of TCC of the urinary bladder. If an increased number of transitional cells are seen in the urine sediment, then imaging (e.g., ultrasound or contrast cystourethrogram) of the urinary tract is indicated.

A veterinary bladder tumor antigen test (VBTA) can also be used as a possible screening test for TCCs. However, this test is not highly specific for TCC and can be positive in dogs with non-neoplastic disorders of the urinary tract.

Sperm

Sperm are commonly seen in the urine of intact male dogs and cats.

Bacteria

Normal urine is sterile. However, >10⁴ rods and >10⁵ cocci must be present per milliliter in order to be microscopically visible. So the microscopic absence of bacteria on a sediment evaluation does not rule out a UTI. Any bacteria seen on a sample collected by cystocentesis is significant, but bacteriuria seen in the sediment of a sample collected by free catch or catheterization is more difficult to interpret because the bacteria can represent normal flora. To confirm a suspicion of bacteriuria, it is advisable to stain an air-dried sample of the urine sediment with either a Gram or modified Wright's stain. Both of these staining techniques are superior for detecting bacteriuria compared to microscopic examination of an unstained urine sediment sample. If a UTI is suspected, urine should be collected by cystocentesis for culture and sensitivity unless there are clear contraindications to avoid a cystocentesis.

Microbes other than bacteria

Yeast and fungi are occasionally seen in the urine sediment examination, especially in samples collected by free catch. These usually represent contaminants (from the stain or from the skin, if the sample was collected by free catch). However, if an animal is immunosuppressed or has been on long-term antibiotics, then the presence of yeast or fungi could be significant. Fungal organisms can also be identified in the urinary bladder of patients with systemic mycoses (e.g., blastomycosis or aspergillosis). An enzyme immunoassay (EIA) for detection of blastomyces dermatitidis galactomannan antigen in body fluids, including urine, has been used for rapid diagnosis of blastomycosis in humans, and this test is also now currently used to aid in the early diagnosis of blastomycosis in dogs.

Casts

Casts are cylindrical molds of the renal tubules composed of aggregations of matrix mucoprotein and varying cell types and numbers. Small numbers of hyaline or granular casts seen on low power (one to two per low power field [lpf]) are normal. Increased numbers of casts, referred to as cylinduria, can be seen with diseases affecting the kidneys (e.g., pyelonephritis, ischemic damage to the kidneys associated with hypovolemic shock). The different types of casts that can be seen in the urine sediment include hyaline, cellular (epithelial, white cell, or red cell), granular, waxy, and fatty casts. The significance of each type of cast is outlined below. Monitoring for casts is indicated for patients receiving a potentially nephrotoxic drug, as detection of casts can provide the earliest evidence of drug-induced tubular injury. All types of casts degenerate with urine storage, so sediment analysis of fresh urine samples is essential if casts are to be detected.

Hyaline casts

These are the most common type of cast and are composed primarily of Tamm–Horsfall mucoproteins (THMs) that are secreted by tubular epithelial cells. Small numbers may be seen with fever, dehydration, or heavy exercise. They are also common with renal diseases associated with proteinuria. Hyaline casts are transparent and can be easily missed in an unstained urine sample. Using Sedi-Stain will make them appear pink and more visible.

Given the ubiquitous presence of Tamm–Horsfall protein, other cast types are formed via the inclusion or adhesion of other elements to the hyaline base.

Cellular casts

These casts can contain epithelial cells, RBCs, or WBCs and are always abnormal. Epithelial cell casts signify severe tubular disease from toxins or hypoxia. This cast is formed by inclusion or adhesion of desquamated epithelial cells from the tubule lining. RBC casts indicate tubular hemorrhage. The presence of RBCs within casts is always pathological and is strongly indicative of glomerulonephritis or vasculitis from various causes. They can also be associated with renal infarction. WBC casts suggest inflammation. They are seen most commonly in patients with acute bacterial pyelonephritis but can be seen with other forms of interstitial nephritis. Bacterial casts are also occasionally seen in patients with pyelonephritis. These should be seen in association with loose bacteria, WBCs, and WBC casts.

Granular casts

These casts contain debris associated with tubular cell necrosis and degeneration; increased numbers indicate tubular injury from hypoxia or toxins. Their appearance is generally more cigar shaped and of a higher refractive index than hyaline casts.

Waxy casts

Waxy casts may represent the final stage of degeneration of granular casts and are most often seen with very severe and long-standing renal disease. While cylindrical, waxy casts possess a higher refractive index than granular casts; they are also more rigid, demonstrating sharp edges, fractures, and broken-off ends.

Fatty casts

These are a type of granular cast with increased lipid inclusions; they are most often seen in patients with nephrotic syndrome and diabetes mellitus. They can be normal in cats.

Urine crystals

Crystals can form in the urine when the composition (e.g., pH, USG, mineral composition) of the urine favors oversaturation of certain minerals. Visualization of urine crystals in the sediment examination will also depend on the urine pH and temperature. Significance of crystalluria depends on the type of crystal and other clinical findings (Table 10.4.1).

Caution should be used when interpreting the significance of crystals seen in stored urine as they may be artifacts of delayed processing. Caution must also be used in interpreting the significance of some types of crystals (e.g., struvite, amorphous, and calcium oxalate) that can be found in the urine from normal patients without signs of lower urinary tract disease. Overinterpreting the importance of crystals in this setting commonly leads to inappropriate use of diets formulated for preventing crystalluria and uroliths formation.

Miscellaneous sediment findings

Contaminants such as plant grains or pollens, starch granules (from surgical gloves), and cat litter can occasionally be seen in the sediment. This is especially true from cases where the urine was collected by free catch.

Lipiduria

Increased lipid droplets can be normal in urine, especially in cats. However, increased fat droplets can also been seen in the urine of patients with diabetes mellitus or nephrotic syndrome.

Complete blood count and serum biochemistry profile

Complete blood count

Hematology is mainly used to assess for evidence of anemia, dehydration, and inflammation in patients with diseases that primarily or secondarily involve the kidneys or that cause hematuria.

A complete blood count (CBC) will allow assessment of the degree of anemia in patients with CKD or in patients with severe hematuria. A nonregenerative, normocytic, normochromic anemia is common in patients with moderate to severe CKD (IRIS stage III or IV). The pathogenesis of this anemia is multifactorial and may be exacerbated by concurrent illness.

Table 10.4.1   Urine crystal types, characteristics, and significance

Crystal type	Characteristics and significance
Bilirubin	"Red or yellow elongated spicules"; low numbers may be normal in a dog, but if there are high numbers or if seen in urine from a cat, they signify liver disease or hemolysis.
Struvite	"Prism or coffin lid" crystals; form in alkaline urine, most often seen in normal dogs but also may be present with concurrent urolithiasis in association with a urease-producing bacterial UTI. In cats, they may also be normal but can be associated with urolithiasis.
Calcium oxalate dihydrate	"Envelope-shaped" crystals; can be normal in dogs and cats, but if there is support for ARF and large numbers are present, ethylene glycol should be considered.
Calcium oxalate monohydrate	"Picket fence" or "dumbbell"-shaped crystals; their presence is usually associated with ethylene glycol toxicity.
Ammonium urate	"Thorn apple shape"; they can form in any pH but usually form in alkaline urine. Often found in Dalmatian dogs and in some English bulldogs. Concurrent urolithiasis may or may not be present. Urates also occur in animals with severe liver insufficiency (e.g., portosystemic shunts, liver failure).
Cystine	"Hexagon" crystals; forms in acidic urine and is never a normal finding. Its presence indicates that the kidneys are not reabsorbing certain amino acids properly due to an error in metabolism. Documented in many canine breeds, but the Newfoundland, English bulldog, and dachshund are predisposed. Also reported in cats.
Amorphous	Aggregates of crystalline material without any particular shape generally have no clinical significance unless they are xanthine crystals that occur following administration of allopurinol for urate urolithiasis.
Cholesterol	Rare crystal type in animals and has been seen in normal dogs.
Drug crystals	The most common drug crystal is the sulfonamide crystal, which forms in acidic urine. Other drugs that can form crystals in urine include radiographic contrast dyes, ampicillin, and primidone.

Source: http://ahdc.vet.cornell.edu/clinpath/modules/ua-rout/crystsed.htm.

The principal cause of the anemia is erythropoietin deficiency resulting from irreversible kidney damage. Other factors that contribute to the anemia include decreased RBC life span due to constant exposure to uremic toxins, circulating inhibitors of erythropoiesis caused by uremia, decreased erythropoiesis from iron deficiency or nutritional abnormalities, hemorrhage from uremic gastritis, or increased bleeding tendency due to uremic thrombopathy.

Alternatively, a CBC can permit detection of polycythemia that can occur as a result of a paraneoplastic syndrome associated with excessive erythropoietin secretion by some renal neoplasms (e.g., lymphoma, fibroma, or renal carcinoma) or can occur as an appropriate response to sustained renal hypoxia (e.g., unilateral renal artery thrombosis).

A leukocytosis with or without a left shift, plus or minus toxic change, can be seen with infections of the kidneys (e.g., bacterial or fungal pyelonephritis) or the prostate (e.g., acute or chronic prostatitis). An inflammatory leukogram may also be seen with a uroabdomen or neoplasms of the urogenital tract. Infections of the lower urinary tract (i.e., the bladder and urethra) do not commonly cause abnormalities on the CBC except in rare cases (e.g., emphysematous cystitis with rupture).

Thrombocytopenia may be seen in septic animals, in patients with certain infections that may involve the kidney (e.g., leptospirosis), and in animals with prostatitis or renal neoplasms. A

CBC is also important for ruling out idiopathic or secondary immune-mediated thrombocytopenia as the cause of hematuria in a patient.

Serum biochemistry profile

A serum biochemistry profile can be used to assess the degree of azotemia, hypoalbuminemia, as well as electrolyte disturbances that can occur with diseases that affect the kidneys.

Elevations in serum urea and creatinine concentrations (azotemia) are used clinically to assess renal GFR. Azotemia of renal origin only provides a crude estimate of GFR because blood work abnormalities do not begin to occur until >75% of the nephrons are lost or injured. This is especially true early in the course of kidney disease when large changes in GFR cause only minimal increases in the concentrations of urea and creatinine. In contrast, small changes in GFR can create large increases in the concentrations of urea and creatinine late in the course of renal failure.

Urea is considered a crude estimate of GFR for several reasons. First, production of urea by the liver and subsequent excretion by the kidneys does not occur at a constant rate. Second, some urea is reabsorbed by the renal tubules after filtration has already occurred. Finally, the serum urea concentration is affected by too many nonrenal factors. For example, levels may be increased postprandially, following a GI bleed, with a high protein diet, in states of increased protein catabolism (e.g., fever, starvation, septicemia) and following administration of some catabolic drugs (e.g., steroids). Decreased serum urea can be seen with a low protein diet, liver insufficiency (failure or portosystemic shunt), or following administration of anabolic steroids that decrease protein catabolism.

Serum creatinine concentrations provide a better crude index of GFR because it is produced at a constant rate from the degradation of phosphocreatine in muscle; it is freely filtered by the glomerulus; it is not reabsorbed by the renal tubules; and it is affected by fewer nonrenal factors. Muscle wasting and muscle necrosis can affect serum creatinine values, but diet does not affect serum creatinine. As a biochemical indicator of GFR, it has an advantage over urea in that it is not affected by the renal tubular flow rate.

Another limitation for using elevations in urea and creatinine to assess GFR is that they cannot distinguish between prerenal, renal, and postrenal causes of azotemia. The magnitude of increase in urea and creatinine concentrations cannot predict acute versus chronic disease, progressive versus nonprogressive disease, or the cause of the underlying renal problem.

Assessment of the severity of renal disease and the localization of the underlying cause for azotemia should ideally always be done by evaluating the USG prior to fluid therapy and must take into account any clinical signs of dehydration. A history of fluid losses from vomiting, diarrhea, and severe PU, and physical examination findings such as sunken eyes, exaggerated skin tent, prolonged capillary refill time, tachycardia, or poor peripheral pulses provide evidence of possible dehydration or hypovolemia. Urine should ideally be collected prior to the administration of drugs that may induce diuresis because the resulting dilute USG can delay attempts to localize the cause of azotemia and possibly delay the diagnosis of renal disease.

By using information about the hydration status and the USG, it is often possible to determine the underlying cause of azotemia in a patient. See Table 10.4.2 for criteria on the classification of azotemia as prerenal, renal, or postrenal. There are a few important exceptions to the general rules. Cats with renal failure can

have urine specific gravities >1.045, and some animals with glomerular disease and renal azotemia may have USGs > 1.035 (dogs) or >1.040 (cats). In addition, animals with other causes of PU/PD may have a reduced USG (<1.030 dogs and <1.035 cats) but may be azotemic from prerenal causes.

Interpretation of serum urea/creatinine concentrations

Renal azotemia occurs when the total GFR of the kidneys is reduced to <25% of normal. However, azotemia is a relatively crude measure of renal GFR and is fairly insensitive for the detection of early renal disease. Trends in serial BUN and creatinine values are important in monitoring renal function.

With *prerenal azotemia*, the azotemia is usually a consequence of reduced renal perfusion (e.g., severe dehydration and hypovolemia). Other less common causes of prerenal azotemia include GI fluid loss, high protein diets, extensive tissue necrosis, and the administration of some drugs (e.g., glucocorticoids). If azotemia is entirely prerenal in origin, then the kidney function is completely normal; however, prerenal azotemia maybe superimposed on renal or postrenal azotemia. The key feature of prerenal azotemia is that the degree of azotemia will be only mild to moderate (creatinine < 4 mg/dL, BUN < 80 mg/dL), and the concurrent USG should be >1.030 in dogs and >1.035 in cats. If the USG is greater than these minimums in a cat or dog that is dehydrated, then it is suggestive of adequate kidney function. If prerenal azotemia is severe and is not corrected in a timely fashion, then decreased renal perfusion may give rise to renal ischemia and, ultimately, renal azotemia.

With *renal azotemia*, the azotemia results from ARF and or CKD. Prerenal or postrenal azotemia may exist simultaneously. The key feature of renal azotemia is that it is accompanied by a USG that is <1.030 in a dog or <1.035 in a cat, although the degree of azotemia can be variable. It is not uncommon for the USG to be in the isosthenuric range (1.007–1.015), but it does not drop below 1.007. An exception to the rule includes any patient with a disease that impairs the ability of the kidney to concentrate urine (leading to PU/PD) and

Table 10.4.2 Localization of azotemia

Clinical feature	Prerenal azotemia	Renal azotemia	Postrenal azotemia
Azotemia	Mild to moderate Possible evidence of dehydration on physical examination	Mild to marked	Mild to marked
Urine specific gravity	>1.030 dogs >1.035 cats	<1.030 dogs <1.035 cats Often 1.007–1.015	Variable
Physical signs of urinary tract obstruction and/or signs of urinary tract rupture	Absent	Absent	Present
Response to fluid therapy	Azotemia resolves in 1–2 days	Partial or no resolution of azotemia	Complete, partial to no resolution of azotemia

is associated with prerenal azotemia (e.g., diabetes mellitus, hypoadrenocorticism).

With *postrenal azotemia*, the azotemia occurs when there is interference with excretion of urine from the body as a result of either an obstruction in the excretory pathway that affects both kidneys or a tear or rupture of the excretory pathway (uroabdomen). The magnitude of postrenal azotemia can vary, but typically, the values are markedly elevated. If the cause of postrenal azotemia is not corrected, renal damage can result. Typically, clinical findings include a distended turgid bladder, unproductive stranguria, hydronephrosis, or fluid-filled abdomen with a history of recent trauma.

Electrolyte abnormalities with urinary diseases

Because of the kidneys' central role in water balance and electrolyte homeostasis, electrolyte abnormalities are not uncommon with diseases that affect the kidneys. Electrolyte abnormalities may result from GI signs associated with uremia (vomiting and diarrhea), from the increased loss of electrolytes in the urine of patients with renal disease that have severe PU/PD, or from anuria that results in decreased renal excretion of electrolytes.

Hyperkalemia, hypokalemia, hypercalcemia, hypocalcemia, and hyperphosphatemia are all common electrolyte abnormalities seen with different disorders that affect the kidneys.

Hyperkalemia may be seen with ARF, uroabdomen, urethral obstruction from a tumor, uroliths, or protein mucus plugs. Hyperkalemia can also be seen in patients with chronic renal failure. It is important to remember that moderate to severe hyperkalemia can lead to life-threatening cardiac arrhythmias.

Hypokalemia is a relatively common abnormality with CKD, especially in cats (10–30% incidence). Hypokalemia results from inadequate intake and increased renal loss (PU). Hypokalemia can result in muscle weakness (stiff gait, ventroflexion of the neck), decreased renal responsiveness to ADH, and possibly progression of renal injury, especially in cats. Hypokalemia is also common in patients with postobstructive diuresis following correction of a urethral obstruction.

Hyperphosphatemia is another abnormality that can be seen on the biochemistry panel for patients with prerenal, renal, and or postrenal azotemia. The elevation in the serum phosphorous concentration typically correlates well with the degree of azotemia. The importance of hyperphosphatemia is that it helps initiate development and progression of secondary renal hyperparathyroidism and may predispose a patient to metastatic calcification of soft tissues when the product of the serum total calcium and phosphorus is greater than 60.

Severe hypocalcemia, characterized by low ionized calcium, can be seen with acute renal failure secondary to ethylene glycol toxicity. Mild hypocalcemia, typically with normal ionized calcium, is also common in cats and in dogs with moderate to severe CKD. Hypocalcemia can also occur in cats with complete urethral obstructions, and in this setting, hypocalcemia may exacerbate the cardiac effects of hyperkalemia. The etiology of the hypocalcemia in cats with a urethral obstruction is not entirely known, but a lack of adaption to acute hyperphosphatemia may contribute.

Mild hypercalcemia can be seen with prerenal azotemia resulting from dehydration and is also recognized in a small proportion of cats and dogs with CKD. Hypercalcemia seen with CKD is typically characterized by an elevation in the total calcium but not ionized calcium. Severe hypercalcemia from other causes (e.g., cancer, granulomatous disease, hypervitaminosis D or primary hyperparathyroidism) can also lead to acute or chronic renal failure or can predispose a patient to calcium-based uroliths.

Other biochemical abnormalities

Hypoalbuminemia, hypercholesterolemia, and possibly elevation of triglycerides are serum biochemical abnormalities that can be seen in patients with glomerular disease. When these biochemical changes are accompanied by peripheral edema or body cavity effusions, nephrotic syndrome exists.

Mild to severe metabolic acidosis is common with ARF or CKD. A low bicarbonate concentration on the serum biochemistry panel is expected with metabolic acidosis. The metabolic acidosis associated with renal failure results from the limited ability of the failing kidney to secrete excess hydrogen ions, decreased tubular bicarbonate reclamation, and disordered renal ammonia production in the surviving nephrons. Chronic acidosis can promote nausea, anorexia, vomiting, weight loss, and protein malnutrition, all of which can be detrimental for the patient.

Proteinuria

Proteinuria refers to any type of protein (e.g., albumin, globulins, Bence Jones proteins) detected in the urine. Proteinuria, when it occurs, can be classified as prerenal, renal, or postrenal based on the underlying cause. Proteinuria may also be classified as physiological or pathological. Quantification of proteinuria is indicated for suspected glomerular disease.

Prerenal proteinuria

Prerenal proteinuria can occur with strenuous exercise, seizures, or a fever. The mechanism responsible for physiological proteinuria is not completely understood; however, transient renal vasoconstriction, ischemia, and congestion may play a role. Other causes of prerenal proteinuria occur when pathological disease states release proteins small enough to be filtered by the glomerulus (e.g., hemoglobin, myoglobin, immunoglobulin light chains). IMHA, rhabdomyolysis, and dysproteinemias associated with either lymphoma or plasma cell neoplasia are examples of disease states that can lead to such pathological prerenal proteinuria. In such cases, proteinuria results when the amount of the low molecular weight proteins filtered by the glomeruli overwhelms the reabsorptive capacity of the proximal tubules.

Postrenal proteinuria

Postrenal proteinuria most frequently occurs in association with lower urogenital tract inflammation or hemorrhage. The urine sediment findings usually show evidence of underlying inflammation (e.g., pyuria, hematuria, bacteriuria, and increased numbers of transitional epithelial cells). A urine culture may be required to conclusively rule out a UTI as a possible cause of postrenal proteinuria.

Renal proteinuria

Renal proteinuria most commonly results from one of two major mechanisms. The first and most important is a disruption of the glomerular filtration barrier, which results in an increased amount of protein in the renal filtrate. The second is impaired reabsorption of filtered plasma proteins by the proximal renal tubular epithelial cells as a result of tubulointerstitial disease. In some cases, tubulointerstitial proteinuria may be accompanied by normoglycemic glucosuria and increased fractional excretion of electrolytes. Renal tumors and pyelonephritis are other causes of renal proteinuria.

In healthy animals, properties of the glomerulus are important for restricting the filtration of albumin, blood cells, and other large proteins on the basis of size, charge, and shape. Disease states that involve or target the glomeruli (e.g., glomerulonephritis, amyloidosis) can alter the size and or charge selectivity of the glomerular filtration barrier and can lead to proteinuria. Such injury can occur with immune-mediated injury that directly or indirectly targets the glomerular filtration barrier or with vascular injury or inflammation that leads to secondary damage to the glomerulus (e.g., systemic hypertension). The hallmark of glomerular disease is proteinuria in the face of an "inactive" urine sediment (lack of inflammatory changes) and lack of evidence of prerenal sources of proteinuria. Renal proteinuria that is moderate to severe is almost always from glomerular disease.

In a healthy patient, the renal tubules will almost completely reabsorb any smaller proteins that are filtered by the glomeruli. This reabsorption occurs through an active process termed endocytosis. When the rate of endocytosis is exceeded, excess protein will not be resorbed by the tubule and will subsequently be lost in the urine. Tubular proteinuria may occur with excessive production of small-molecular-weight proteins like Bence Jones proteins or with damage to tubular epithelial cells (e.g., nephrotoxic damage, chronic tubulointerstitial disease). The magnitude of proteinuria is usually mild with tubular proteinuria (<1 g/day), and the proteins lost are typically composed of only low molecular weight proteins (polypeptides and amino acids).

As a result of the mechanisms discussed, only a very small amount of protein is normally present in urine of normal dogs and cats. Albumin is the predominate protein that is lost in diseases that affect the glomerulus and lead to proteinuria.

Detection of protein in urine

Detection of proteinuria can be done by one of four possible mechanisms: two semiquantitative methods, the urine dipstick analysis and the SSA turbidimetric test; and two quantitative methods, the UP:C ratio and the measurement of 24-h urine protein excretion. Regardless of which method is used, urine protein detection or concentration must *always* be interpreted in light of the urine sediment and the concentration of the urine as measured by the USG. The more dilute the urine, the more potentially significant the proteinuria (e.g., 1+ protein with a 1.020 USG is potentially much more significant than 1+ protein with a 1.045 USG). The urine sediment (ideally with urine culture results) can be useful for determining the underlying cause of the proteinuria (e.g., inflammatory disease vs. glomerular disease).

The two semiquantitative methods used to detect proteinuria, the urine dipstick analysis and the SSA turbidimetric test, are both subject to false-negative and false-positive results. These tests are best viewed as screening tests, and if they indicate the presence of renal proteinuria/albuminuria, then further testing to quantify the amount of urine protein excretion should be pursued. Many laboratories use the SSA turbidimetric test to confirm positive reactions for protein on a urine dipstick test. For feline urine samples, both the urine dipstick and the SSA test perform poorly as screening tests for the detection of proteinuria and appear to be of minimal diagnostic value because of an unacceptably high number of false-positive results. On the basis of these data, detection of albumin in the urine of feline patients should always be performed with a higher quality assay. The species-specific microalbuminuria ELISA test (e.g., E.R.D.-HealthScreen Urine test) enables detection of low concentrations of albumin in urine, also referred to as microalbuminuria. Microalbuminuria is defined as urine albumin between 1 and 30 mg/dL. These concentrations cannot be routinely detected using the urine dipstick method.

Proteinuria detected by the use of the urine dipstick or SSA screening tests (or both) is often confirmed and quantitated by the use of either a UP:C ratio or an immunoassay for albuminuria. Both the UP:C and urine albumin:creatinine ratios preformed on spot urine samples have been shown to accurately reflect the quantity of protein or albumin, respectively, that is excreted in the urine over a 24-h period. Given the reliability of the tests, it has eliminated the previous requirement to collect urine for 24 h in order to quantify proteinuria.

The UP:C ratio can also be multiplied by 20 to give the milligram per kilogram of protein that is being lost in the urine per day. Dogs and cats are considered to be negative for proteinuria when the UP:C is <0.2. If the UP:C ratio is between 0.2 and 0.4 for a dog and between 0.2 and 0.3 for a cat, the patient is considered to have borderline proteinuria. If the UP:C ratio is ≥0.5 and ≥0.4 for dogs and cats, respectively, and pre- and postrenal causes of proteinuria have been ruled out, then the patient is considered to have overt proteinuria that is consistent with either glomerular or tubulointerstitial renal disease. A UP:C ratio >2.0 in either a cat or a dog, again provided prerenal and postrenal causes have been ruled out, is strongly suggestive of glomerular disease. Proteinuria that is believed to be a result of glomerular disease, determined to be persistent on three or more occasions 2 weeks or longer apart, is considered highly significant and warrants further investigation for the underlying cause.

In these patients, nonspecific treatments for glomerular disease are indicated if no underlying cause is found. Severe proteinuria (UPC > 4–5) determined to be of glomerular origin warrants immediate investigation for an underlying cause and nonspecific treatments if no underlying cause is found.

In the past, it has been recommended that urine be collected by cystocentesis for the determination of the UP:C ratio in order to avoid inaccurate results because of postrenal diseases such as urethral tumors or vaginitis. However, results of a recent study indicate that dogs with inactive urine sediment can also be correctly classified with proteinuria according to the IRIS staging system when urine samples are collected by free catch.

It has been reported that UP:C ratio measurements on the same urine using different methodologies (dry vs. wet chemistries) may not be comparable. So, if measurements are being done serially in the same patient for monitoring purposes, it is advisable to use the same lab and test each time. For patients with confirmed proteinuria resulting from glomerular disease, any change in the magnitude of proteinuria assessed by serial measurements of a UP:C ratio must be interpreted in light of the patient's serum creatinine concentration. This is important because proteinuria may decrease with progressive renal disease as the number of functional nephrons decreases. Decreasing proteinuria in the face of stable serum creatinine suggests improving renal function, whereas decreasing proteinuria in the face of increasing serum creatinine suggests disease progression.

Special procedures such as immunoelectrophoresis and protein electrophoresis are available to confirm Bence Jones proteinuria with multiple myeloma. Urine protein electrophoresis can also be used to distinguish tubular and glomerular proteinuria if required.

Significance of proteinuria

The complications of moderate to severe proteinuria associated with glomerular disease may include hypoalbuminemia, edema, ascites, hypercholesterolemia, hypertension, and hypercoagulability. Preliminary evidence in dogs and in cats suggests that proteinuria can cause glomerular and tubulointerstitial damage and can result in progressive nephron loss in patients with preexisting renal disease. In cats with naturally occurring CKD, mild proteinuria (UP:C > 0.43) has been shown to be a negative prognostic indicator for survival. Proteinuria has also been associated with an increased risk of mortality attributable to all causes in cats. In dogs with naturally occurring CKD, the relative risk of uremic crises and risk of mortality was approximately three times greater in dogs with UP:Cs greater than 1.0 compared with dogs with UP:Cs less than 1.0.

Blood pressure

Hypertension refers to a sustained increased in systemic arterial BP. Hypertension can be classified as either primary or secondary. The term idiopathic hypertension is preferred for primary hypertension that occurs in the absence of an identifiable cause. Secondary hypertension exists when hypertension can be attrib-

Table 10.4.3 Diseases or conditions associated with systemic hypertension

Hypertension	
Dogs	Cats
Chronic kidney disease	Chronic kidney disease
Acute kidney disease	
Hyperadrenocorticism	
Idiopathic	Idiopathic
Iatrogenic	Iatrogenic
Diabetes mellitus	Diabetes mellitus
Obesity	Obesity
Primary hyperaldosteronism	Primary hyperaldosteronism
Pheochromocytoma	Pheochromocytoma
Hypothyroidism	Hyperthyroidism

uted to a clinical disease, condition, or medication (exogenous glucocorticoids, mineralocorticoids, and phenylpropanolamine) (see Table 10.4.3). Secondary hypertension is the most common cause of high BP in dogs and in cats. A diagnostic workup including a CBC, serum biochemistry profile, urinalysis, imaging, and possibly testing for certain endocrine disorders is often required to establish if there is an underlying cause for the hypertension. Only after this is done, and no underlying cause is identified, can it be concluded that the patient has idiopathic hypertension.

Sustained increased systemic arterial blood pressure (SBP) results in injury to other tissues; this is commonly referred to as end-organ damage. The kidney, eyes, heart, and brain are considered the organs most at risk for severe injury from sustained hypertension.

As far as the kidney is concerned, sustained increases in SBP affects the glomerular capillary beds leading to injury and possibly the loss of nephrons; this is typically manifested as glomerular atrophy, proliferative glomerulonephritis, and glomerulosclerosis. In a patient with preexisting kidney disease, this damage will enhance the decline in renal function and may lead to proteinuria.

Routine measurement of BP should be a part of the physical examination for all geriatric patients. Disorders that are commonly associated with systemic hypertension (including CKD) are much more prevalent in this population and systemic hypertension can be clinically silent. BP should also be measured on a regular basis in any patient, regardless of their age, that has a disease(s) known to potentially cause hypertension (e.g., kidney disease, diabetes mellitus). Measurement of BP is also indicated in any cat or dog with clinical signs or physical examination findings consistent with hypertensive end-organ damage (e.g., epistaxis, deranged mentation, sudden blindness) and in any patient prescribed a medication that is known to affect BP.

In addition to the variability associated with BP instrumentation, the personality of the pet and the pet's tolerance of handling and restraint, there is also some variance in BP with respect to breed, body condition score (lean vs. obese), age, and health status of the patient.

It has been recommended to categorize hypertension based on the patient's risk of developing subsequent end-organ damage. If the BP is <150/95 mmHg, then there is minimal risk for developing end-organ damage and can therefore be classified as mild. Antihypertensive therapy is not recommended for a patient with mild hypertension. Risk for end-organ damage is still considered mild if the BP is 150–159/95–99 mmHg. Close monitoring is recommended, but antihypertensive medication is not necessarily indicated. If the BP is between 160–179/100–119 mmHg, then there is a moderate risk for end-organ damage. Most animals in this category, particularly those with evidence of end-organ damage or secondary hypertension, are candidates for antihypertensive therapy. If the BP is >180/120 mmHg, hypertension is considered severe and antihypertensive therapy is always indicated because the risk of end-organ damage is very high. Underlying diseases that may be causing secondary hypertension should be identified and treated whenever possible while continuing to monitor BP in any animal with a BP > 160/100 mmHg.

Incidence and implication of hypertension associated with renal disease

Systemic hypertension is common in dogs and in cats with renal disease. It has been reported to occur in 60–69% of cats with CKD[1,2] and in 31 to 93% of dogs with CKD.[3–5] Hypertension may be present at any stage of CKD. Serum creatinine concentrations do not directly correlate to BP. Therefore, hypertensive cats and dogs with CKD may have marked hypertension despite normal to mildly elevated BUN and creatinine.

Possible mechanisms involved in renal disease associated hypertension include increased vascular responsiveness to noradrenaline, increased cardiac output, increased peripheral vascular resistance, renal secondary hyperparathyroidism, and increased activity of the renin–angiotensin–aldosterone system.

Once hypertension has developed, it accelerates injury to the kidneys, resulting in a vicious cycle of glomerulosclerosis and further loss of nephrons. Increased intrarenal vascular resistance as a result of glomerulosclerosis may further exacerbate the development of hypertension associated with renal disease.

Dogs with renal failure and high systolic BP have been reported to be more likely to develop a uremic crisis, to die, or to undergo continued decline in renal function. In one study, dogs with more severe hypertension had significantly lower GFRs, higher UP : C ratios, and higher renal lesion scores than dogs with less severe hypertension.

Measurement of blood pressure

Measurement of SBP can be accomplished directly by intra-arterial catheterization or indirectly by devices that incorporate a compressive cuff. In the clinical setting, indirect devices are most commonly utilized.

When an indirect BP measurement device is used in a feline or canine patient, it should have been designed and validated for use in that species. A standard protocol should always be followed to help ensure accuracy of results and to allow for reliable comparison of serial measurements in the same patient. Having one or two technicians do all the measurements also helps ensure accuracy. These individuals should be properly trained on how to use the device and should be skilled at low stress restraint and handling of animals. Measurements should be done in a quiet room and should only be taken after the pet has had 10–15 min to acclimatize to their new surroundings since stress and anxiety can produce falsely elevated readings ("the white coat effect"). The patient should be restrained in a comfortable position in either lateral or sternal recumbency. The cuff location will need to be determined on an individual patient basis. If the cuff is placed on the forelimb, it should be at the level of the radius. If it is placed on the hind limb, the cuff should be placed proximal to the hock. If the tail is used, the cuff is placed near the base of the tail.

An appropriately sized cuff should cover approximately 40% of the circumference of the limb or the tail. The cuff size, site of the cuff placement, and the patient's stress level should be noted in the medical record for future reference. The cuff, despite its location on the limb or tail, should be at or near the level of their right atrium. This may involve elevating the limb during measurement if the patient is sitting down. The cuff needs to be snugly wrapped around the limb or tail and the sphygmomanometer attached. A series of three to seven consecutive measurements should be taken, and the individual values for the diastolic, mean, and systolic pressures should be averaged. In most cases, the first measurement may need to be discarded. Measurements that are widely disparate are unlikely to be reliable. If the measurements do not seem accurate, the procedure should be repeated later the same day when the animal is less stressed or on another occasion. For some patients, having their owner present may have a calming effect and may facilitate acquisition of the measurements, but in other cases, the exact opposite is true. When using a Doppler device, only the systolic BP should be recorded. Recent evidence, particularly in cats, suggests that systolic BP is the most important determinant of hypertensive tissue damage. Using this device, 5–10 readings are typically recorded and an average systolic BP is calculated. The fur will need to be clipped at the site of application of the Doppler crystal and ultrasound gel applied to the appropriate site. The Doppler crystal is placed over the palmar or plantar artery distal to the cuff and proximal to the metacarpal or metatarsal pad on the caudal aspect of the foot.

The normal BP reference ranges for *dogs* are as follows, based on an average of five studies using an *oscillometric* device for the measurement of the BP:

140 mmHg systolic; 100 mmHg mean, and 80 mmHg diastolic

The normal BP reference range for *cats* is as follows, based on an average of four studies using a *Doppler* device for the measurement of the BP:

140 mmHg systolic

Urine culture

Bacterial UTIs are quite common in dogs; it is estimated that 14% of all dogs will develop at least one UTI during their lifetime. In contrast, the incidence of bacterial UTIs in cats is quite low, especially relative to the increased incidence of lower urinary tract signs. Older cats (>10 years of age) are much more likely than younger cats to develop a UTI. Most UTIs in dogs and cats are caused by a single pathogen (75%); polymicrobial infections with two (18%) or three (6%) uropathogens are less common. Normal aerobic bacterial flora of the skin and colon cause most UTIs, and the route of infection is usually ascending from the perineum, vagina, or prepuce. Hematogenous infection (spread by blood) and direct extension from penetrating wounds are less common routes of infection. *E. coli* is the most common bacterial isolate of UTIs in dogs and cats. Other common bacterial isolates include coagulase-positive *Staphylococcus* species, *Klebsiella pneumoniae*, *Pseudomonas aeruginosa*, *Enterobacter* species, and *Proteus mirabilis*. Anaerobic, viral, parasitic, and fungal UTIs are very rare.

Patients with any of the following conditions are predisposed to develop a UTI: anatomic abnormalities involving the urinary system (e.g., "pelvic bladder," USMI), spinal disorders causing urine retention, urolithiasis, neoplasia, previous urinary tract catheterization, patients on immunosuppressive drugs, or patients that have certain endocrinopathies (diabetes mellitus, hyperadrenocorticism). Even in the absence of clinical signs suggestive of a UTI, a urine culture may be warranted in these patients.

Most UTIs involve the lower urinary tract. Most animals with lower UTIs will present for pollakiuria, hematuria, and dysuria, but these patients lack systemic signs of illness. Findings on the urine sediment examination generally support the suspicion of a UTI, including pyuria, hematuria, proteinuria, and bacteriuria.

UTIs that involve the upper urinary tract often result in nonspecific systemic signs including partial or complete anorexia, vomiting, weight loss, fever, depression, and possibly abdominal pain. The presence of casts (especially WBC casts or rarely bacterial casts) is reliable evidence of renal inflammation, but they are not commonly seen with pyelonephritis. Other laboratory findings may include neutrophilic leukocytosis with or without a left shift or a nonregenerative anemia if the infection is chronic. Prerenal or renal azotemia may be seen with pyelonephritis but is not expected with simple cystitis. Findings on the urine sediment that are consistent with inflammation such as pyuria, proteinuria, hematuria, or bacteriuria are also common.

When evaluating the significance of bacteriuria seen on urine sediment examination, the method of collection of the urine sample must always be taken into account. Cystocentesis is the gold standard method for urine collection when a urine culture is indicated. A cystocentesis is preferred over other methods of urine collection because there is decreased contamination from the lower urinary outflow tract, skin, or external environmental sources. If the urine sample is collected by cystocentesis, then any bacterial growth on culture should be considered significant. However, for some patients with lower urinary tract disease, collection of a sample by cystocentesis may be difficult, and it may be necessary to collect urine for culture by catheterization or from the less desirable midstream free-catch voided sample. In those cases, ideally, the external genitalia of the patient should be cleaned and the perivulvular fur clipped prior to collection to lessen the chances of contamination of the urine sample. Urinary catheterization in male dogs can typically be done without sedation. However, sedation is typically required in female dogs and cats. Sterile lubrication and a sterile catheter should always be used and the procedure should be performed aseptically.

Urine must be collected into a sterile container if it is to be used for culture. Care must be taken to collect, preserve, and transport the urine sample in a sealed container to avoid contamination, proliferation or death of bacteria. Processing of the urine for culture should begin as soon as possible since death of some fastidious bacteria may occur within an hour of collection. If the urine cannot be cultured immediately, the samples should be refrigerated at 4°C. Samples can be stored for 6–12 h if processing is delayed. Freezing of urine samples should be avoided because this can destroy bacteria. If a *Mycoplasma* or *Ureaplasma* infection is a concern, special culture media is required (consult your local laboratory).

In some cases, tissue biopsies from the urinary tract (bladder mucosa or renal biopsies) collected under aseptic conditions may be cultured, and positive cultures of any bacteria are indicative of a UTI regardless of the number of bacteria present. For patients with urolithiasis, it is recommended that a bladder mucosal biopsy as well as the center of an aseptically retrieved urolith be cultured for bacteria. This is important even in cases where a prior urine culture has been negative.

Types of urine cultures

There are basically two types of urine cultures: quantitative and qualitative.

A *quantitative urine culture* is performed by inoculation of MacConkey (gram-negative) and/or blood agar plates. Following incubation, individual colonies are identified on the basis of colony morphology, Gram staining, and standard biochemical reactions. The number of bacteria (colony-forming units per milliliter of urine) is estimated in order to allow differentiation of uropathogens from possible contaminants. The collection method needs to be accounted for when interpreting quantitative urine culture: $>10^3$ organisms/mL for cystocentesis or catheterization samples is significant. The threshold for samples collected by free catch is higher with $>10^5$ organisms/mL urine being significant. The definition of significant bacteriuria based on quantitative urine cultures is lower for cats because cats seem to be more resistant to UTIs than dogs.

A *qualitative urine culture* involves isolating and identifying bacteria in urine; it does not include quantifying bacterial numbers. After 48 h, the growth of bacteria is recorded as either positive or negative only.

False-positive bacteriuria or culture results

Although detection of bacteria on the sediment examination of fresh urine should prompt consideration of a UTI, this is best verified by a urine culture. A false-positive urine sediment finding of bacteriuria with a subsequent negative culture may be explained by the misidentification of debris or small crystals that can resemble bacterial organisms. Bacterial contamination during sampling (e.g., needle penetrates a loop of intestine during cystocentesis) or before analysis (e.g., sample is contaminated during transfer to culture media) can also result in a finding of bacteriuria and a false-positive culture result.

False-negative bacteriuria or culture results

False-negative cultures can result from iatrogenic bactericidal events during collection, storage (e.g., prolonged refrigeration), or transport (e.g., heating or freezing). Appropriate sample handling is imperative when samples are shipped for processing. Antibiotic use before urine collection may also inhibit bacterial growth. Therefore, urine should be collected for culture *before* antimicrobial therapy is started. If the patient is currently being treated with an antimicrobial drug that is suspected of being ineffective, the drug should be discontinued for approximately 3–5 days before a sample for culture and sensitivity is collected.

Commercially available urine culture collection tubes containing a preservative, when combined with refrigeration, may be used to preserve specimens for up to 72h if shipping to a laboratory is to be delayed. There are also commercially available blood agar and MacConkey agar plates that can be inoculated and incubated for 24h if the urine sample cannot be shipped immediately. When using in-house culture media, a calibrated bacteriologic loop or microliter mechanical pipette is used to transfer exactly 0.01 or 0.001 mL of urine to the culture plates. The urine is streaked over the plates using conventional methods. Blood agar supports growth of most aerobic uropathogens and MacConkey agar provides information that aids in the identification of bacteria.

In-house urine culture and susceptibility kits have recently become available (IndicatoRx*®). These kits can only identify bacteria as one of the primary gram-negative uropathogens (e.g., *E. coli*, *Klebsiella*, *Enterobacter* spp., and *Proteus* spp.). Antimicrobial sensitivity is predicted based on typical resistance patterns for each isolate. These kits are limited in their inability to identify more unusual bacteria that may be causing a urinary infection.

Antimicrobial sensitivity

When treating a UTI, choosing an antimicrobial agent is based on bacterial susceptibility testing whenever possible.

There are two basic methods for determining the antimicrobial sensitivity for different uropathogens. The first and more commonly used is the *Kirby–Bauer* or *disk diffusion method*. Paper disks impregnated with different antimicrobial drugs at particular serum concentrations are placed on the agar plate with a monofilm of the bacterial isolate. After inoculation and incubation at 38°C for 18–24h, antimicrobial susceptibility is estimated by measuring zones of inhibition of bacterial growth surrounding each disk. Zones of inhibition are then interpreted in light of established standards, and susceptibility is recorded as resistant, susceptible, or intermediate. The biggest drawback with this method is that the concentration of an antimicrobial (except nitrofurantoin) in paper disks is comparable to the typical serum concentration of the drug. Drugs that are found to be resistant by the agar disk diffusion method may *still* be effective in the urinary tract if the antimicrobial is excreted in higher concentrations in the urine (e.g., ampicillin, cephalexin). Because of differences in the ability of various antimicrobials to diffuse through agar, the antimicrobial disk surrounded by the largest zone of inhibition is not necessarily the drug most likely to be effective.

The second method for determining antimicrobial sensitivity for uropathogens is the *minimum inhibitory concentration (MIC) method*. Uropathogens are inoculated and incubated in wells containing serial twofold dilutions of antimicrobial drugs at concentrations achievable in tissues and urine. MIC is defined as the lowest antimicrobial concentration (or highest dilution) that allows no visible bacterial growth of the isolate. Determination of the MIC for a pathogen with respect to a specific antimicrobial is currently considered the gold standard technique for determining antimicrobial sensitivity and resistance patterns. If the urinary concentration of an antibiotic is four times the MIC for the infecting bacteria, then the drug will be at least 90% effective. If the urinary concentration is less than four times the MIC, then the drug will be minimally effective and should be considered resistant.

Follow-up and therapeutic urine cultures

Culture of urine at strategic times during antimicrobial therapy (so-called "therapeutic urine cultures") is an effective method of assessing therapeutic success.

The potential benefits of therapeutic urine cultures include verification of proper antimicrobial administration by the owner, early detection of bacterial resistance to the antibiotic chosen, and timely detection of a persistent infection. Negative therapeutic culture results during antibiotic administration are consistent with successful eradication of infection. Persistence of clinical signs should prompt further evaluation of the patient (e.g., radiographic and ultrasonographic imaging, cystoscopy) for concomitant nonbacterial disorders.

Culture results that remain unchanged (i.e., the same bacteria exhibiting susceptibility to the current antimicrobial drug) during appropriate antimicrobial therapy indicate that the antimicrobial drug is not reaching the site of infection. Incomplete or infrequent administration of the antibiotic and unwillingness of patients to accept medications are a common cause for inadequate tissue delivery of an apparently effective medication. In some situations, antimicrobial administration is sufficient, but intestinal absorption is impaired. In these patients, consideration should be given to other concurrent medications that may be interfering with the oral bioavailability of the antibiotic. Antacids containing aluminum, magnesium, and calcium can decrease oral absorption of some antibiotics (e.g., tetracyclines).

For patients with recurrent infections (e.g., a relapse, a reinfection, or a persistent infection), response to antimicrobial therapy should be considered effective only if a properly collected urine culture is negative for growth while the patient is on the antimicrobial. Relying on urine sediment findings to determine if a UTI has been eradicated is unwise because low numbers of bacteria can be missed on a urine sediment evaluation. If hematuria, pyuria, and proteinuria are detected on a urinalysis despite initiation of antimicrobial therapy, a therapeutic urine culture should be performed.

For a simple cystitis where no major predisposing factors are detected, follow-up should include a urinalysis and possibly a urine culture 3–5 days after the patient has completed the course of antibiotics. For complicated UTIs and pyelonephritis, it is ideal to repeat the urine culture 3–5 days after initiating therapy, 5–7 days after finishing antibiotics, and again 30–60 days following completion of therapy. It is also important that any underlying defects in host defenses be identified and treated in patients with recurrent or complicated UTIs.

Fungal urinary tract infections

Fungal UTIs (funguria) are rare, but *Candida albicans*, disseminated *Cryptococcus*, blastomycosis, histoplasmosis, or aspergillosis may colonize the urinary tract.

Candida infections have been reported in cats and dogs that are either immunosuppressed (immunosuppressive medications, diabetes mellitus) or that have been on long-term broad-spectrum antibiotic therapy. These infections may be symptomatic or asymptomatic.

Because free-catch urine samples will frequently contain fungal contaminants, diagnosis of a fungal UTI relies on the isolation of the organism from a cystocentesis sample and a positive fungal culture.

If a systemic mycosis is suspected, the urine sample must be sent to a laboratory equipped to handle such pathogens.

Conclusion

Collection of urine by cystocentesis is ideal if a bacterial UTI is suspected. A quantitative urine culture is preferable whenever possible. Treatment of UTIs should be based on the result of bacterial sensitivity findings from a properly collected and processed urine sample.

SECTION 5 URINARY TRACT BIOPSY TECHNIQUES

Aspiration biopsy

Percutaneous fine needle aspiration (FNA) with or without ultrasound guidance is widely used to establish a cytological diagnosis, to determine a prognosis, and to plan clinical management of abdominal malignancies in small animals. Advantages over biopsy include technical ease, rapid turnaround time for cytology versus histology results, and reduced incidence of clinical complications. Although cytological evaluation of lesions within the urinary system is not always diagnostic, the information obtained can be used to either direct further diagnostics (e.g., culture or biopsy), prevent ineffective surgical intervention (e.g., detect metastatic neoplasia), or differentiate between two diagnoses (e.g., abscess vs. cyst; lymphoma vs. feline infectious peritonitis [FIP]).

FNA cytology has been used primarily to diagnose inflammatory or neoplastic disorders of the kidney, urinary bladder, and prostate, but other focal lesions elsewhere in the urinary tract can also sometimes be aspirated for the purposes of establishing a diagnosis.

FNA of the kidneys to obtain cells for cytological evaluation is a simple, rapid, and relatively inexpensive procedure with a low incidence of complications. Renal FNA is most useful when evaluating solitary or multifocal renal masses, diffuse renomegaly without hydronephrosis, or when investigating a diffuse renal echotextural change detected on ultrasound.

Renal cytology is most useful when lymphoma, carcinoma, metastatic or disseminated neoplasia, FIP, abscess, fungal infection, or a cyst is considered likely. Ultrasound-guided pyelocentesis can be performed to collect urine for culture if infectious pyelonephritis is suspected. Renal cytology is not useful in the diagnosis of most congenital (polycystic kidney disease) and hereditary anomalies (e.g., dysplasia). It is also unlikely to be helpful in cases of suspected renal amyloidosis, glomerulonephritis, chronic or acute interstitial nephritis, or for the investigation of diseases involving the renal vasculature (infarcts, hemorrhages). FNA of the kidneys is not recommended when there is evidence of urinary obstruction/hydronephrosis and is very unlikely to be helpful when evaluating the cause of small or atrophied kidneys.

For disorders of the urinary bladder, FNA may be used to collect a urine sample (cystocentesis) directly from the bladder for culture or cytology and for sampling masses that involve the bladder wall. For disorders of the prostate, FNA cytology can be used to differentiate between prostatic neoplasia and BPH, for the temporary drainage of a prostatic or paraprostatic cyst, and for interventional drainage and ablation (using alcohol or tea tree oil) of prostatic cysts and abscesses.

FNA of the kidney, bladder, prostate, or of any discrete mass within the urinary system can be done with or without negative pressure (suction). In most cases, ultrasound guidance will be needed and is preferred because it allows the architecture of the urinary tract to be evaluated; it permits identification of some contraindications for biopsy (e.g., renal or prostatic abscess, hydronephrosis); it allows more accurate guidance of the needle into a focal lesion and helps avoid inadvertent aspiration of the renal medulla in the case of a kidney aspirate or of the vasculature supplying the urinary tract. Percutaneous blind aspiration of the kidney can be done with manual kidney immobilization in cats and is also sometimes possible in dogs with unilateral or bilateral renomegaly. This technique is best reserved for cases with diffuse lesions that result in renomegaly because focal lesions may be missed. With blind FNA, there is an increased risk of inadvertent puncture or laceration of major blood vessels.

Regardless of which technique is used, multiple aspirations in different areas of the kidney, prostate, or a mass are recommended to maximize cellular yield and diagnostic potential and to differentiate between primary and secondary inflammations. For focal or discrete masses, aspiration of both the central and peripheral areas is recommended; frequently, the center of a mass may consist of necrotic debris or inflammatory cells, resulting in a nondiagnostic sample. Pronounced inflammation incited by a tumor may actually mask an underlying neoplastic process.

Once the mass or structure (e.g., kidney) being aspirated has been entered, negative pressure (suction) is applied with an attached syringe and the needle is moved in and out rapidly 15–20 times, being careful not to go deeper with each pass of the needle. Suction should be kept constant during sampling and released before removing the needle from the lesion. FNA without suction can also be performed by just using a needle without a syringe attached or by using a fine needle capillary technique (also known as Zajelda's technique) to help reduce blood contamination.

It should be noted that many renal lesions and some tumors of the urinary tract exfoliate poorly, limiting a cytological diagnosis. As such, obtaining a sample of adequate cellularity can be an issue. Negative results do not exclude disease. Also, renal tissue is highly vascular, so significant blood contamination can occur. Adequate patient restraint and a nonaspiration technique can reduce blood contamination.

One serious complication or controversy with both FNA and needle biopsy of any intra-abdominal tumor is the risk of seeding the tumor along the needle tract. Needle-tract implantation after a FNA of adenocarcinomas and TCCs of the kidney has been reported in people, and there are rare reports of this following percutaneous ultrasound-guided FNA in dogs with TCC of the bladder, urethra, or prostate. Without rigorous follow-up, the incidence of tumor implantation along the needle tract with FNA and/or biopsy may be underestimated in our patients as they may die before metastasis becomes apparent. However, seeding of tumors has also been reported following surgical resection of a TCC of the urinary bladder in a dog, so this complication is not isolated to FNA or biopsy. Because this is a rare complication, the estimated risk of seeding a tumor along a needle tract is only 0.009% in people; many clinicians still advocate common use of this technique for diagnostic purposes. The use of larger bore needles (>1-mm outer diameter), an increased number of needle passes, and certain tumor types (prostatic carcinoma) may be associated with a higher incidence of this complication.

Biopsy

Renal biopsy, regardless of the method by which it is preformed, is indicated only when the results are likely to alter patient management by providing either an accurate histological diagnosis, by aiding in prognostication, or by facilitating decisions regarding response to therapy after renal transplantation.

Patients whose management is most likely to be altered by the results of a renal biopsy include those with glomerular disease (PLN), renal neoplasia, or ARF. Renal biopsy is very unlikely to benefit patients with suspected end-stage renal disease. All patients must undergo renal imaging with ultrasound and/or CT prior to biopsy to avoid biopsying patients with clear contraindications (e.g., small atrophied kidneys or those with obstructive ureteroliths or nephroliths). Also, renal biopsy should only be performed after extensive evaluation of the patient to rule out any contraindications for biopsy (e.g., severe anemia, clotting disorders). This involves collection of information on the patient's minimum database (i.e., complete history, physical examination findings, routine blood work, and urinalysis findings) as well as measurement of systemic BP and assessment of a coagulation profile (prothrombin time [PT] and partial thromboplastin time [PTT]).

There are several methods by which renal biopsy can be performed. Regardless of the method used, only the renal cortex should be biopsied; biopsy of the renal medulla should be avoided due to the greater risk of hemorrhage from laceration of vessels and because it is also associated with an increased risk of creating large areas of infarction and fibrosis.

Percutaneous renal core biopsy is typically done with the patient anesthetized or heavily sedated and ideally is performed using ultrasound or CT guidance. Laparoscopic or keyhole surgical renal biopsies through a flank incision are alternative methods by which a core renal biopsy can be obtained. Surgical biopsy, through a laparotomy incision, can be used to obtain a wedge biopsy of the kidney. Surgical biopsy is the preferred method in canine patients weighing <5 kg where the risk of complications is greater. This is also the most suitable method if the patient is undergoing a laparotomy for other reasons.

Absolute contraindications for renal biopsy include an uncontrolled coagulation disorder or severe anemia, uncontrolled hypertension (which will increase the likelihood of severe hemorrhage), extensive pyelonephritis, renal or perirenal abscess or multiple large renal cysts, and small end-stage kidneys from suspected CKD and hydronephrosis.

Relative contraindications for renal biopsy include unilateral renal neoplasia due to the risk of biopsy-induced metastasis and a patient with a solitary kidney if the procedure is deemed to pose substantial risk (e.g., decreased renal function) that would outweigh the value of the information obtained from the biopsy.

Complications associated with renal biopsy can be classified as minor (gross hematuria, silent hematoma), major (clinically evident hematoma, requiring embolization or transfusion, iatrogenic infection), and catastrophic (requiring surgery, loss of parenchymal functional mass, unintended perforated or trauma to another abdominal organ, and death). The overall incidence of complications varies. The skill of the person(s) performing the biopsy, the thoroughness of patient screening for contraindications, and the appropriate selection of patients that will benefit from a biopsy are the factors most likely to affect the complication rate.

Microscopic hematuria is an expected finding after renal biopsy; this is typically self-limiting and is expected to resolve within 48–72 h of biopsy. Macroscopic hematuria is less common but in veterinary studies is seen in 1–4% of dogs and cats following renal biopsy. Hematuria that persists longer than 24 h after the procedure warrants evaluation of the kidneys and biopsy site. Severe hemorrhage that requires transfusion support can occur if there is accidental laceration of the renal vasculature or another vascular organ, and in one study this was the most common reported complication occurring in 9.9% and 16.9% of dogs and cats, respectively.

Renal core needle biopsies

Ultrasound-guided renal core biopsy is the method of choice in dogs that weigh >5 kg and for all cats with no contraindications for renal biopsy. Blind percutaneous core biopsy of the kidneys should be avoided.

In dogs with bilateral kidney disease, the right kidney is preferred over the left kidney for renal biopsy because it is more stable (the caudate lobe of the liver provides resistance to movement during the biopsy procedure). However, in some cases, the left kidney will be biopsied because it is more accessible. This is often the case in deep-chested dogs where the right kidney is located more cranially under the rib cage. In cats, both kidneys are located more caudally in the abdomen, so either kidney can typically be localized and immobilized for renal biopsy.

All patients should be heavily sedated or anesthetized for renal biopsy. Failure to adequately immobilize the patient increases the likelihood of a serious complication. In addition, having the patient anesthetized during the procedure has been associated with procurement of better quality biopsy samples. For biopsy of the right kidney, the patient is placed in left lateral recumbency, and for biopsy of the left kidney, the patient is placed in right lateral recumbency. Clip and surgically prepare the skin overlying the biopsy site. Once the site of entry for the biopsy needle is determined using ultrasound, a small stab incision is made through the skin with a scalpel blade. Only the renal cortex should be biopsied; the medulla should never be biopsied due to the risk of severe hemorrhage. Using ultrasound, the normal renal cortex can easily be differentiated from the medulla. However, identification may be more difficult in severely diseased kidneys. The tip of the needle is guided toward the renal capsule at either the cranial or caudal pole of the kidney and is inserted through the renal capsule with the needle parallel to the long axis of the kidney before activation of the needle throw. Penetration through the capsule before activation of the spring-loaded needle prevents sliding of the needle along the capsule and reduces the risk of tearing the renal capsule. The needle must be kept in a shallow position just below the renal capsule within the renal cortex. Penetrating too deeply beyond the renal capsule will reduce the amount of renal cortex biopsied and increases the risk of entering the medulla. Ideally, at least two quality biopsy samples should be obtained. After each biopsy, digital pressure should be applied to the kidney transabdominally for 5 min to minimize hemorrhage. Ultrasound should be used to monitor for any active hemorrhage at the biopsy site postprocedure.

False-negative biopsies are usually due to an insufficient amount of tissue, sampling of a necrotic area, the presence of blood contamination, or simply missing the lesion. Unsatisfactory biopsies in cases of suspected neoplasia are more common with smaller tumors because of the increased difficulty in targeting these tumors; however, large tumors with large necrotic centers can also result in false-negative results.

Equipment

A disposable spring-loaded biopsy needle (E-Z Core Single Action Biopsy Devise®, Products group International, Inc., Lyons, CO) is preferred. They are available in various sizes (14, 16, 18, and 20 ga.) and various lengths (6, 9, or 15 cm). Automatic spring-loaded biopsy guns (e.g., Bard Biopsy®, C. R. Bard, Inc., Murray Hill, NJ) that use disposable needles of the appropriate gauge and length are also available. These are less suitable for renal biopsies because there is less control over the depth of the biopsy. Manual trucut needles can also be used but are less than ideal due to the greater risk of trauma associated with sample collection. Resterilized needles are not recommended because they dull quickly.

CT-guided renal biopsy

If an ultrasound-guided biopsy fails to yield a useful sample, a CT-guided biopsy can be attempted or a surgical biopsy of the kidney can be performed. Advantages of CT guidance over ultrasound are that gas and other structures do not obscure visibility; there is excellent spatial resolution; there is better needle visualization; and it is easier to avoid necrotic areas. The disadvantages of CT guidance are higher cost, exposure to radiation, and lack of real-time monitoring during actual needle insertion.

Keyhole renal biopsy

Laparoscopic (see below) and keyhole renal biopsies are two alternative methods by which a percutaneous needle renal biopsy can be performed, and both allow direct visualization of the kidney for biopsy. A keyhole renal biopsy can be used if ultrasound or CT is not available. Access to the kidney that will be biopsied is made through an ipsilateral paralumbar incision. The incision must be large enough to allow insertion of the index finger to help immobilize the kidney against the epaxial musculature. The biopsy needle is inserted through the body wall through a separate small stab incision. The tip of the needle is guided into and positioned at the surface of the kidney or stabbed just through the capsule. It is important to make sure the angle is such that the needle will pass only through the renal cortex. Closure of the incision through the abdominal wall is routine.

Cystoscopic biopsies

Cystoscopy allows visualization of the vestibule, urethra, urinary bladder, and the ureteral openings. Compared with a traditional cystotomy, the magnified images seen with cystoscopy have the potential to be more revealing and superior for localizing small lesions. Cystoscopy is also less invasive than surgery but both require general anesthesia. In addition to allowing visualization and biopsy of lesions within the lower urinary tract, cystoscopy has many other applications. These include resection of masses (e.g., obstructive polyps), removal of uroliths using stone baskets or laser lithotripsy, and investigation of causes of incontinence, and allows for injection of bulking agents submucosally within the proximal urethra for the treatment of urinary incontinence.

Cystoscopy is best used in conjunction with other diagnostic tests. A urinalysis and other noninvasive imaging should be performed prior to cystoscopy to avoid artifacts from contamination or minor trauma to the lower urinary tract associated with cystoscopy. The main disadvantage of cystoscopy is the need for general anesthesia and cost of the equipment; however, the procedure is typically quick and minimally invasive. Potential complications of cystoscopy include iatrogenic infection, urethral or bladder trauma causing hemorrhage, or perforation. Proper technique and selection of equipment appropriate to the patient are the best ways to minimize the risk of injury. Biopsies obtained using a cystoscopic approach are small and this may be an important limitation. Antibiotics and analgesia are required post cystoscopy.

Laparoscopic biopsy

Laparoscopy is an endoscopic procedure performed under sterile conditions using a rigid endoscope inserted through an access port cannula. Direct visualization and inspection of the kidneys and the serosal surface of the bladder is possible after the establishment of a pneumoperitoneum. Direct visualization also permits precise control when performing a renal biopsy. Laparoscopic biopsy is less invasive and when done by an experienced operator can be performed more quickly than surgical renal biopsies. They can also reduce intraoperative and anesthetic-related patient morbidity. If indicated, other abdominal organs can also be inspected and biopsied, which is an advantage over percutaneous renal biopsies. Postbiopsy hemorrhage can be monitored for and better appreciated with laparoscopy when compared with ultrasound or CT. Direct pressure can be applied with a laparoscope or laparoscopic tools if hemorrhage is seen.

Laparoscopy has also been used to assist in the removal of uroliths and foreign bodies from within the urinary system in dogs and people, respectively. Candidates for laparoscopic-assisted cystoscopy include dogs with calculi too large to be expelled by urohydropropulsion and those unlikely to resolve by medical dissolution. This technique minimizes injury to tissues caused by traditional open cystotomy and laparotomy. A variety of surgical instruments such as bladder spoons, calculi baskets, and forceps to grasp and extract calculi can be used with this technique. Another use of laparoscopic-assisted cystoscopy would be to examine and obtain biopsies of bladder masses in male dogs. This would be an alternative to doing a traditional cystotomy by open laparotomy or cystoscopy by the use of a long flexible endoscope. In female dogs, bladder masses are usually biopsied via transurethral cystoscopy (see below). If this technique is used for urolith removal, an imaging procedure such as radiography or urethrocystoscopy should be performed after the procedure to ensure complete removal of all uroliths.

Contraindications for laparoscopy include peritonitis, extensive abdominal adhesions, hernias, obesity, coagulopathies, and operator inexperience. Complications of laparoscopy include the creation of air emboli, pneumothorax, subcutaneous emphysema, the introduction of gas into a hollow viscus, damage to internal organs from the introduction of the Verress needle or trocar, and cardiac arrest in addition to the complications already outlined for renal biopsy.

Surgical biopsies

Surgical biopsy of the kidney may be the preferred method in dogs that are small (<5 kg) or in animals that either have isolated areas in the kidney that need to be avoided during the biopsy procedure (e.g., large cysts) or are undergoing laparotomy for another reason. Likewise, surgical biopsy may be safer in some animals that have other factors that make biopsy risky.

Surgical wedge biopsy specimens are larger and therefore should be superior in quality to needle biopsy samples. A surgical biopsy of the kidney can be obtained through a paracostal incision, if only one kidney needs to be examined and biopsied, or through a cranial midline abdominal incision if other intra-abdominal organs or if both kidneys need to be examined and biopsied. A wedge-shaped incision is made through the capsule and into the cortex. A monofilament absorbable suture material (e.g., 4-0 PDS) in a simple continuous pattern is used to close the defect in the renal capsule. The wedge biopsy specimen can be cut with a scalpel blade into multiple slices for submission for light, electron, and immunofluorescence microscopy.

Surgical biopsies of a bladder mass can also be performed after an open laparotomy and cystostomy. This has the disadvantage of being more invasive than other procedures discussed but can allow for complete and possibly curative excision of a mass in some circumstances, which is unlikely with the other biopsy techniques described. A surgical biopsy may also permit better hemostasis and allows biopsy of other organs in the abdomen if indicated for diagnosis or staging of a tumor (e.g., excisional biopsy of draining lymph nodes).

Traumatic urinary catheterization

Catheter biopsy of the lower urinary tract in dogs is an established technique. Sedation is required to place the urinary catheter in a female dog and is recommended for most patients undergoing this procedure.

Biopsies of bladder and urethral mucosal lesions may be obtained by placing the side holes of a urinary catheter against the lesion, applying suction using a syringe to draw tissue into the catheter, and then withdrawing the catheter while maintaining suction. Ultrasound guidance enables real-time accurate determination of biopsy catheter position. The tissue fragments obtained are usually large enough for histological examination.

This technique is simple, minimally invasive, and requires no specialized equipment. Tissue fragments greater than 2 mm are placed in formalin and are submitted for histological examination; smaller samples can be smeared or squashed on microscope slides and stained for cytology. Once the biopsy is obtained, the lesion can be observed ultrasonographically for signs of hemorrhage. Technical pitfalls encountered with this technique include limited size of the biopsy specimen and difficulty in accurately placing the catheter so that the side holes lie against the lesion. Surgical biopsy may be required if a traumatic biopsy is nondiagnostic. Other disadvantages of this technique compared to surgical biopsy include the inability to obtain submucosal tissue or biopsy extraluminal lesions, such as enlarged regional lymph nodes. However, compared to ultrasound-guided needle aspiration, the catheter biopsy technique offers several advantages. First, it is less invasive than a surgical biopsy and there is limited potential for either perforation of the bladder wall or peritoneal hemorrhage. Second, there is no potential for tumor seeding along a biopsy tract as has been described with FNAs of urinary tract neoplasms in dogs and humans.

Sample handling

Smears for cytology need to be prepared immediately and gentle technique is very important especially in renal aspiration biopsy cases. If the smears are not made rapidly, clots will form and possibly obscure tumor cells and compromise the diagnosis. Concurrent submission of a CBC taken in a conscious patient just prior to renal aspiration may permit the cytologist to better differentiate between peripheral blood contamination of the sample and true inflammation.

Impression smears from biopsy specimens can be made for cytological evaluation. This can aid in the rapid diagnosis of infectious agents or neoplasia. It is always advisable to contact the intended analyzing laboratory prior to collection for optimal sample preparation technique recommendations. Also, renal biopsies should always be sent to a pathologist with expertise in nephropathology. Light microscopy alone (± a small sample for culture) may be sufficient for patients with suspected ARF, but glomerular disease specimens should be evaluated by light, electron, and immunofluorescent microscopy. One sample, or a piece of a wedge biopsy, should be fixed in formalin for light microscopy; another sample or piece of a wedge biopsy should be fixed in 4% formalin plus 1% glutaraldehyde in sodium phosphate buffer for electron microscopy; and the final piece should be either frozen or immersed in Michel's solution for immunofluorescence microscopy.

Postbiopsy nursing care

All patients undergoing renal biopsy should be kept quiet and observed in the hospital for 24 h after the procedure, as most complications occur within this time period. Close monitoring of mucus membrane color, capillary refill time, BP, and serial hematocrits and total solids can assist in identifying complications. Intravenous fluids should also be administered postbiopsy

to induce a diuresis and to flush out any blood clots that form within the kidney to reduce the chance of a clot obstructing the renal pelvis or ureter.

SECTION 6 URINARY IMAGING

There are many different options for imaging the urinary tract. The best option for each patient depends on the goals of the study, the differential diagnoses, the portion of the urinary tract under consideration, and the patient's status.

Radiology

Basic radiographs can give information as to whether or not radiodense stones are present in the urinary tract (although not all urinary stones are visible on radiographs), the relative size of the kidneys and bladder, and the presence of free abdominal fluid (evidenced by loss of serosal detail). Basic radiographs (noncontrast) of the abdomen are extremely dependent upon good technique. The presence of stool in the colon can make it difficult to see the urinary tract and radiopaque material in the feces can be mistaken for stones. Therefore, an enema may be recommended prior to routine radiographs. The patient should be properly positioned, which may include the use of sedation, tape, sandbags, or physical restraint. The appropriate settings for the particular radiographic system should be used. In general, two orthogonal views are recommended (conventionally, right lateral and ventrodorsal [VD]). The entire abdomen (from at least the 10th rib to the caudalmost aspect of the animal) should be included in the radiograph. When looking for stones (especially in male cats), it is important to include the entire caudal aspect of the patient because stones may be present in the penis. Visualization of the bladder can be improved in obese animals by pressing on the bladder area with a large wooden spoon or by placing a belly wrap (such as a few layers of vet wrap around the middle of the abdomen). Oblique views may be necessary to look for small bladder stones superimposed on the vertebral column (Figure 10.6.1).

Contrast radiology

Sometimes, basic radiographs are not sensitive enough to detect problems in the urinary tract. In these situations, contrast radiographs are needed. These procedures are more sensitive for finding radiolucent stones, ectopic ureters, tears in the urinary tract, and tumors. Most of these procedures will be performed in stable patients as part of a thorough workup of urinary tract issues. However, sometimes, these procedures need to be done in less stable patients, such as those recently hit by cars. In those cases, the veterinarian will decide how to change the procedures. In all contrast procedures, adequate patient preparation will greatly increase the diagnostic utility. This involves withholding food for 12–24 h and a cleansing enema prior to the radiographs. Survey radiographs should always be taken initially to establish

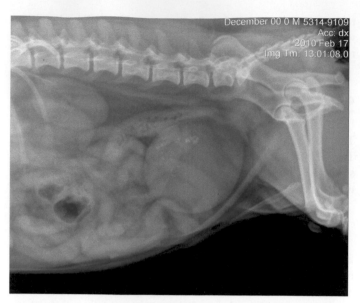

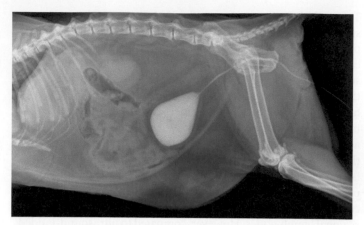

Figure 10.6.2 A lateral abdominal view of a positive contrast cystourethrogram in a cat with a history of urinary obstruction. No obvious obstruction is apparent, but the bladder wall is thickened. Image courtesy of Dr. Ale Aguirre.

Figure 10.6.1 Lateral radiograph of a shih tzu with a large distended bladder. Multiple calculi are visible in the bladder. Image courtesy of Dr. Ale Aguirre.

optimal positioning and radiographic technique. In procedures involving a urinary catheter, the urine should be evacuated prior to introducing the contrast.

Excretory urography

Excretory urography is used to look for ectopic ureters and tumors and to evaluate kidney function. This is the *only* contrast procedure that evaluates kidney function and structure. It is also the only contrast procedure that requires IV contrast. The contrast is excreted quickly, so it is important to have the proper technique and positioning determined prior to injecting contrast. Contrast (600–880 mg/kg of iodine) is injected quickly IV.[1] The patient should be monitored for anaphylactic reactions, including increased heart rate, breathing difficulties, and hives; if these signs are seen, discontinue injecting the contrast and alert the veterinarian immediately. Perivascular leakage of contrast generally only causes localized swelling. An IV catheter should ideally be used to limit such a complication. Lateral and VD views are taken at 1, 5, 15, and 30 min. If there is significant renal compromise, later views may be needed to give the kidneys enough time to take up contrast. A belly band or spoon may be used to improve visualization of the ureters. If fluoroscopy is available, it may be used to visualize the ureteral openings but must be performed within 3–5 min of giving contrast. If visualization of the ureters is difficult, oblique views may be required to prevent superimposition of the bladder over the ureters. Removing the urine from the bladder (via urinary catheterization) and injecting air into the bladder can also help visualize the ureteral openings.

Cystography

Unlike excretory urography, cystography requires that the contrast be given directly into the bladder rather than IV. Cystogra-

phy is used only to visualize the bladder; the urethra cannot be evaluated because the urinary catheter is present. These procedures generally require heavy sedation and/or anesthesia since urinary catheterization can be painful and difficult to perform (especially in male cats and female dogs). A urinary catheter is sterilely placed and survey radiographs are taken. Once the positioning and technique are determined, 3.5–13.1 mL/kg of aquaeous contrast is injected so that the bladder is completely distended.[2] The urinary catheter is then left in place (a Foley catheter may be considered to prevent accidental removal of the urinary catheter). The syringe should remain connected to the urinary catheter so that contrast material does not leak out onto the fur. If the contrast leaks out, make sure to clean it up completely as it can soak into the fur, making interpretation of the radiographs difficult. Lateral, VD, right and left oblique radiographs are taken. Occasionally, there will be some retrograde contrast taken up by the ureters. In order to visualize the urethra, cystourethrography is performed. The easiest method is to simply remove the urinary catheter, to express the bladder, and to take radiographs while there is still contrast within the urethra. The preferable method is to place a Foley catheter into the distal urethra (inserted only about 1–2 in.), to inject the contrast, and then to take radiographs. Only 10–15 mL of contrast is bolused at a time with this method.[3] A Foley catheter is mandatory to make sure the contrast does not leak out around the catheter. Pulling the hind legs cranially can make it easier to visualize the penile urethra in male patients (Figure 10.6.2).

Double contrast cystography utilizes the difference between the contrast medium and air to visualize bladder wall thickening, stones, and tumors. Again, a urinary catheter is placed into the bladder. Contrast medium is injected (0.5–1.0 mL per cat, 1–3 mL per dog <12 kg, 3–6 mL per dog >12 kg), and the patient is rolled so that the contrast fully coats the bladder wall.[2] While palpating the bladder, air or carbon dioxide is injected into the urinary catheter to fill the bladder. Carbon dioxide is preferred because of the reduced risk of an air embolism, but carbon dioxide is not always available. Four views of the abdomen are taken (VD, right lateral, right oblique, and left oblique).

Miscellaneous contrast procedures

Occasionally, the vagina needs to be evaluated for abnormalities. In this case, a foley catheter is placed into the vestibule and inflated. The vulva should be held closed (forceps can be used) and contrast is injected in 20–30 mL boluses.[3] Radiographs should be taken immediately. Therefore, inject the contrast while the patient is in lateral recumbency, take the radiograph, reposition the patient in VD, and immediately take another radiograph. Oblique views are usually not necessary.

Ultrasound

Abdominal ultrasound is a useful tool for identifying structural problems of the upper and lower urinary tract including stones, tumors, changes in kidney architecture such as pyelectasia (dilation of the renal pelvis), and evaluating for the presence of obstructions. However, it is not useful for visualizing the urethra due to its pelvic position. Typically, the patient is placed in dorsal recumbency when imaging the urinary tract, although left and right lateral recumbencies may also be used based on ultrasonographer's preference and patient anatomy. The hair is clipped on the abdomen prior to performing the ultrasound. If possible, restricting a patient's urination will help to ensure adequate urine in the bladder, which facilitates imaging of the urinary bladder. Ultrasound can also assist with cystocentesis by allowing visualization of the bladder.

Editor's Note: Ultrasonography performed by veterinary technicians is a controversial topic in some circles of veterinary medicine. By including this material, I, Linda Merrill, risk offending some in the profession. Nonetheless, I am a firm believer in the ever-evolving scope of practice for veterinary technicians. I believe the veterinary technician specialist is in a unique position to explore this area of advanced technical skills without straying into the area of diagnosis. I encourage continuing education for all interested parties. This text will not discuss ultrasound techniques in detail, but selected findings in urinary tract ultrasonography will be summarized.

Renal imaging

Ultrasongraphically, the kidney is composed of (from exterior to interior) the capsule, renal cortex, medulla, and the hilar region consisting of the renal sinus and the peripelvic fat. The hilar region of the renal pelvis contains the collecting system (renal pelvis and ureters) and the renal vessels. Ultrasound allows for imaging of the renal shape, architecture, and measurement of renal size. Abnormalities of size include small or large kidneys and complete agenesis (lack of a kidney). Abnormalities of shape include renal masses, renal cysts (abscess, hematoma, granuloma, cystic neoplasia), and dilated ureters (see Figures 10.6.3 and 10.6.4). In addition, changes to the structure or echogenicity of the kidneys may reveal renal infarcts, pyelectasia, increased cortical echogenicity (e.g., glomerulonephritis, amyloidosis, CKD), and decreased cortical echogenicity (e.g., necrosis, infil-

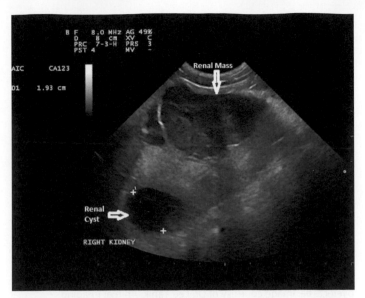

Figure 10.6.3 Sagittal view of the right kidney with a renal mass and a smaller renal cyst (+marks, 1.93 cm). Image courtesy of Dr. Lee Yanik, Animal Imaging Consultants.

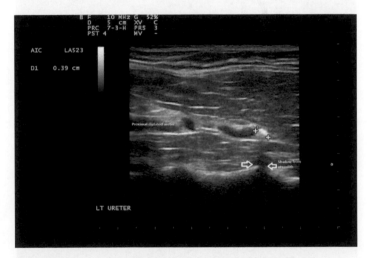

Figure 10.6.4 Sagittal view of the left ureter, which is dilated proximal to an ureterolith (+marks, 0.39 cm). The urolith casts a typical shadow. Image courtesy of Dr. Lee Yanik, Animal Imaging Consultants.

trative disease), which can result in alterations in the corticomedullary ratio (see Figure 10.6.5). Finally, renal or ureteral calculi and fluid in the perirenal, retroperitoneal, or subcapsular space can be observed.

Both kidneys must be examined in three planes: dorsal long axis, sagittal long axis, and transverse. Images of the renal pelvis, lateral to the pelvis, medial to the pelvis, cranial to the pelvis, and caudal to the pelvis should be obtained. Also, at least two planes of any lesion seen should be imaged.

Urinary bladder

Ultrasound evaluation of the urinary bladder allows for visualization of the bladder wall and of the contents of the bladder.

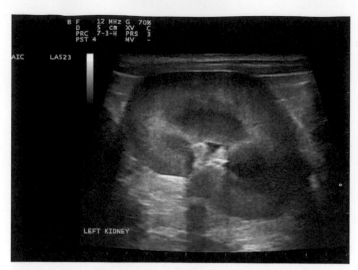

Figure 10.6.5 A sagittal view of the left kidney demonstrating pyelectasia. Image courtesy of Dr. Lee Yanik, Animal Imaging Consultants.

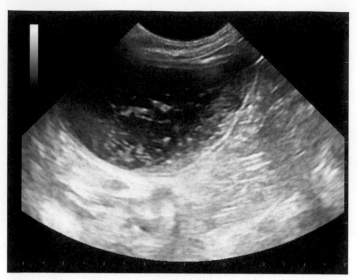

Figure 10.6.7 A sagittal ultrasound image of a cat's urinary bladder showing suspended and gravity-dependent "sludge." Image courtesy of Dr. Ale Aguirre.

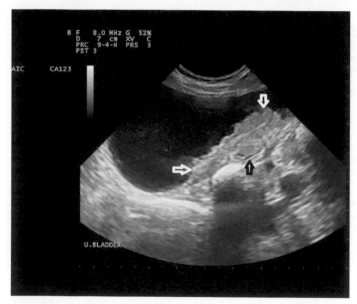

Figure 10.6.6 A sagittal view of a urinary bladder with a transitional cell carcinoma arising from the bladder wall (edges marked by three arrows). Image courtesy of Dr. Lee Yanik, Animal Imaging Consultants.

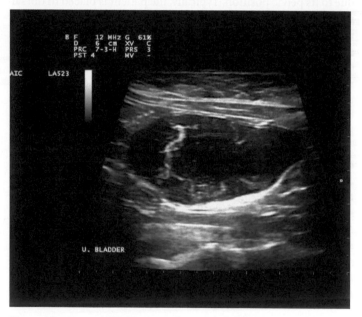

Figure 10.6.8 A sagittal image of the urinary bladder showing suspended material. Image courtesy of Dr. Lee Yanik, Animal Imaging Consultants.

Bladder wall imaging and measurement allows for evaluation of bladder wall thickness (e.g., increased in cystitis), the layering of the bladder wall, and the identification of bladder polyps and bladder masses (size, shape, and location) (see Figure 10.6.6). Imaging of the contents of the bladder can identify bladder calculi, urinary sediment, crystalline material, and hematuria (see Figures 10.6.7–10.6.9). Although difficult to image, patent urachal diverticula, ectopic ureters, and ureteroceles can be observed in some patients.

The urinary bladder is ideal for imaging, but a sufficient quantity of urine must be in the bladder in order to be accurately assessed. A complete scan of the urinary bladder includes the following views: at least three images in the sagittal plane—one

each of the trigone, to the right of center and to the left of center; And at least three images in the transverse plane—one each of the trigone, middle, and of the fundus of the bladder. If calculi are suspected, include an image made in the standing position. Include at least two planes of any lesion seen.

Prostate and caudal abdomen

In the male dog, evaluation of the prostate may also be indicated. This allows for observation of the size, shape, and architecture of the lobes of the prostate. However, their location in the pelvic canal and the reproductive status of the patient can make imaging

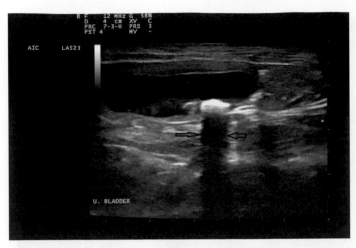

Figure 10.6.9 A sagittal image of the urinary bladder with a large calculus. Note the shadow cast by the stone (black arrows). Image courtesy of Dr. Lee Yanik, Animal Imaging Consultants.

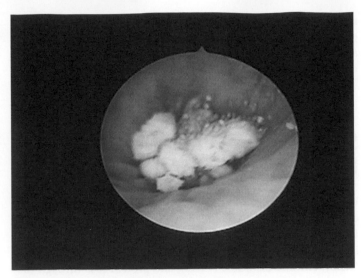

Figure 10.6.11 A cystoscopic view of calcium oxalate calculi in the apex of bladder. Image courtesy of Dr. Ale Aguirre.

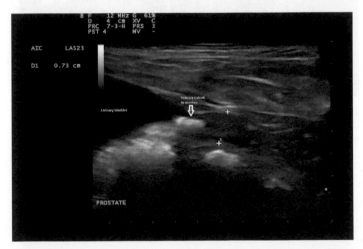

Figure 10.6.10 A sagittal image of the proximal urethra and prostate (+marks, 0.73 cm) with a urinary calculi in the urethra, just proximal to the prostate (arrow). Image courtesy of Dr. Lee Yanik, Animal Imaging Consultants.

challenging. Both sagittal and transverse images should be viewed (Figure 10.6.10).

Routine scanning of the caudal abdomen may also aid in the assessment of lymph nodes, ascites, and hernias, to name a few conditions.

Cystoscopy and vaginoscopy

Cystoscopy is an endoscopic examination of the lower urinary tract. It is used to directly visualize the urethra, bladder, and the openings of the ureters. This can aid in the diagnosis of ectopic ureters, bladder diverticuli, stones in the bladder and urethera, and tumors. The scope cannot be introduced into the ureters unless the dog is very large or the ureters are extremely dilated. A rigid cystoscope is used in female dogs, and the size of the scope is determined by the size of the dog and by what scope is available. In male dogs, a flexible scope can be used, but it has

to be of sufficient length and of small enough diameter to be introduced safely. Cystoscopy requires general anesthesia but tends not to be a painful procedure. The vulvar or penile area is shaved and sterilely prepped. Since this is a sterile procedure, the cystoscope should be gas sterilized prior to use and it should be handled sterilely throughout the procedure. Cold fluids (0.9% saline) should be attached to the influx port. An extension set needs to be attached to the efflux port and the other end placed in a bucket or other receptacle to catch urine. The camera is attached to the cystoscope, as is the light source. The veterinarian will introduce the cystoscope while keeping another hand clamped around the vulva or penis to prevent leakage. The fluids help with visualization of the bladder and dilation of the urethra. Cold saline helps to control bleeding, which may occur secondarily to the introduction of the cystoscope. Biopsies of abnormal tissues can be performed using the cystoscope as long as it contains a biopsy port. In this procedure, the sterile biopsy instrument is introduced through the port, manipulated to the area of interest, and a biopsy sample taken. The cystoscope can also be used to inject collagen into the urethra to treat urinary incontinence. The patient may have some blood in the urine for a day after the procedure and may have some perivulvar irritation due to the prepping (Figure 10.6.11).

Computed tomography

CT is used for evaluating the urinary tract in some referral institutions. Some studies have shown it to be the preferred technique for finding ectopic ureters.[4] CT can also be used for diagnosing tumors and stones of the urinary tract. Anesthesia or heavy sedation is needed in order to prevent patient motion artifact. The patient is placed in sternal recumbency in the machine and the CT scan is performed. Intravenous iodinated contrast can be used to help visualize structures but at half the dose (400 mg iodine/kg) as that used for excretory urography.[5] If the dog is 40 lb or more, two catheters should be placed. The contrast is rapidly excreted, so it should be injected quickly and the CT performed immediately. Make sure that the patient is completely anesthetized prior to injecting the contrast. A drop in BP following injection of the contrast is normal (see Figure 10.6.12 and Table 10.6.1).

SECTION 7 RENAL AND URINARY DISEASE PHARMACOLOGY

Urinary problems are broadly separated into upper (renal disease) and lower (remainder of the urinary tract) disorders. Renal disease is defined as any condition resulting in a decrease in function or injury to the kidneys. It includes acute disorders (ARF), chronic disorders (CKD), and protein loss through the kidneys (PLN). Lower tract disorders involve a decrease in function or injury to the ureters, urinary bladder, or urethra. Medical management targets the disease process (e.g., antibiotics to treat a bacterial pyelonephritis causing ARF) or a complication of the disease process (e.g., hypertension secondary to a PLN).

For any medication to be effective, the drug needs to be delivered to the site of action (e.g., the pelvis of the kidney with bacterial pyelonephritis), in an active form and in an appropriate concentration. For patients with ARF, renal blood flow can be reduced, which decreases the ability of certain drugs (e.g., thiazide diuretics) to reach the kidneys.[1] Situations that negatively impact the ability of drugs to work at the site of action include a change in pH (e.g., metabolic acidosis), protein content in the

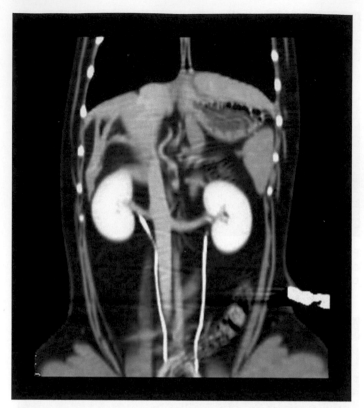

Figure 10.6.12 A CT scan of a dog's abdomen. The kidneys and ureters are enhanced following the administration of intravenous contrast. Image courtesy of Dr Ale Aguirre.

Table 10.6.1 Comparison of modalities when imaging the urinary tract

Procedure	Structures visualized	Sedation indicated	Contrast route	Dose	Contrast media
Basic radiographs	Entire abdomen	No	No	NA	
Excretory urogram	Kidneys, bladder, ureters, urethra	No	IV	600–880 mg iodine/kg	Iodinated contrast media
Cystogram	Bladder	Yes	Urinary catheter	3.5–13.1 mL/kg	Iodinated contrast media—diluted 100 mg iodine/mL
Cystourethrogram	Bladder, urethra	Yes	Urinary catheter	10–15 mL boluses	Iodinated contrast media—diluted 100 mg iodine/mL
Double contrast cystogram	Bladder	Yes	Urinary catheter	0.5–1.0 mL per cat; 1–3 mL per dog <12 kg; 3–6 mL per dog >12 kg	Iodinated contrast media—diluted 400 mg iodine/mL
Vaginourethrogram	Vagina, distal urethra	Yes	Urinary catheter	20–30 mL boluses	Iodinated contrast media—diluted 100 mg iodine/mL
Abdominal ultrasound	Entire abdomen	Possibly	No	NA	NA
CT scan	Entire abdomen	Yes—anesthesia	IV	1.4 mL/lb	Iodinated contrast media

NA, not applicable.

renal tubules (e.g., with PLN), or concurrent medications (e.g., nonsteroidals). In cases of noneffective drug therapy or refractory disorders, the therapy can be modified by increasing the dose, by changing how the drug is administered (e.g., given IV or as a constant rate infusion), or by adding additional and/or more effective drugs.[1] In patients with PLN resulting in nephrotic syndrome, diuretic dose increases of two- to threefold or decreasing the dosing interval may increase responsiveness.[1]

At a minimum, the goal with any medication is to "do no harm." In the case of ARF, CKD, and PLN, certain medications at standard or, in some cases, any dosage can exacerbate the underlying disease process.

Table 10.7.1 lists medications that are potential nephrotoxins. Table 10.7.2 lists medications commonly used in the treatment of patients with renal disease that may require modification of dosage depending on the type and degree of renal impairment.

IRIS has proposed a staging system for dogs and cats with CKD. The staging system is based on serum creatinine (two or more measurements, over several weeks) (see Table 10.3.1). Substaging by level of proteinuria and BP is also utilized to further classify the severity of kidney disease (see Tables 10.7.3 and 10.7.7 below). Table 10.7.3 is useful for modifying drug dosages in those patients with reduced kidney function.[2] A more precise alternative is to make adjustments based on drug

Table 10.7.1 Potential nephrotoxic medications in dogs and cats

Class	Examples
Antifungals/antivirals	Amphotericin B
	Acyclovir
	Foscarnet
Antimicrobials	Aminoglycosides (e.g., Amikacin)
	Aztreonam
	Carbapenems
	Cephalosporins
	Fluoroquinolones
	Nafcillin
	Penicillins
	Polymyxin
	Rifampin
	Sulfonamides
	Tetracyclines
	Tobramycin
	Vancomycin
Antiprotozoals	Trimethoprim–sulfamethoxazole
	Sulfadiazine
	Thiacetarsamide
	Pentamidine
	Dapsone
Immunosuppressants/chemotherapeutics	Azathioprine
	Cyclosporine
	Bisphosphonates
	Carboplatin
	Cisplatin
	Doxorubicin
	Interleukin-2
	Methotrexate

Class	Examples
Miscellaneous	Angiotensin-converting enzyme inhibitors (ACEIs)
	Allopurinol
	Apomorphine
	Calcium, EDTA
	Cimetidine
	Dextran 40
	Mannitol
	Non-steroidal anti-inflammatory drugs
	Penicillamine
	Streptokinase
	Thiacetarsemide
	Thiazide diuretics
	Cholecalciferol
	Methoxyflurane
	Lipid-lowering agents
	Lithium
	Phosphorus-containing urinary acidifiers
	Tricyclic antidepressants

Source: Complied from Langston C. Acute uremia. In: *Textbook of Veterinary Internal Medicine*, 7th edition, eds. SE Ettinger, EC Feldman, p. 1972. Canada: St. Louis, MO: W.B. Saunders; 2010; Polzin DJ. Chronic kidney disease. In: *Textbook of Veterinary Internal Medicine*, 7th edition, eds. SE Ettinger, EC Feldman, p. 1972. Canada: St. Louis, MO: W.B. Saunders; 2010; Stokes JE. Diagnostic approach to acute azotemia. In: *Kirk's Current Veterinary Therapy*, 14th edition, eds. JD Bonagura, DC Twedt, p. 856. St. Louis, MO: Saunders Elsevier; 2009.

Table 10.7.2 Medications that may need dosage alterations in patients with decreased renal function and medications that do not need dosage alterations in patients with decreased renal function

Drug	Route	Standard dose	Modified dosage based on IRIS staging			
			Stage I	Stage II	Stage III	Stage IV
Amikacin	IV	15–30 mg/kg q24h	11–22 mg/kg q24h[a]	7.5–15 mg/kg q24h[a]	3.75–7.5 mg/kg q24h[a]	3.75–7.5 mg/kg q24h-EOD[a]
Amoxicillin	IV, PO	10–20 mg/kg q24h	NA	NA	10–20 mg/kg q24h	10 mg/kg q24h
Ampicillin	IV	10–20 mg/kg q8–12h	NA	10–20 mg/kg q12h	10–20 mg/kg q12–24h	10 mg/kg IV q24h
Atenolol	PO	0.25 mg/kg q12–24h	NA	0.19 mg/kg q12–24h	0.125 mg/kg q12–24h	0.06 mg/kg q24h
Azithromycin	PO	5–10 mg/kg q24h	NA	NA	NA	NA
Benazepril	PO	0.25–0.5 mg/kg q12–24h	NA	NA	0.2–0.3 mg/kg q24h	0.125 mg/kg q24h
Cefazolin	IV	10–30 mg/kg q8h	NA	7.5–22.5 mg/kg q8h	5–15 mg/kg q12h	5–15 mg/kg q24h
Ceftriaxone	IV	15–20 mg/kg q12–24h	N.A	NA	12–16 mg/kg q24h[b]	7.5–10 mg/kg q24h[b]
Diltiazem	IV, PO	0.5–1.5 mg/kg q8h	NA	NA	NA	NA
Doxycycline	IV, PO	5–10 mg/kg q12h	NA	NA	NA	NA
Enalapril	PO	0.5 mg/kg q12–24h	NA	0.375–0.5 mg/kg q12–24h	0.25–0.375 mg/kg q12–24h	0.25 mg/kg q24h
Enrofloxacin	IV, IM, PO	2.5–5 mg/kg q12h	NA	1.25–2.5 mg/kg q12h	1.25–2.5 mg/kg q24h	0.825–1.65 mg/kg q24h
Famotidine	IV, PO	0.5–1 mg/kg q12–24h	NA	0.5 mg/kg q24h	0.5 mg/kg q24h	0.5 mg/kg q24h
Fluconazole	PO	5–10 mg/kg q12–24h	NA	5–10 mg/kg q24h	5–10 mg/kg q24-EOD	5–10 mg/kg qEOD-ETD
Imipenem	IV	5–10 mg/kg q8h	5.75 mg/kg q8h	2.5–5 mg/kg q8h	2.5–5 mg/kg q8–12h	1.25–2.5 mg/kg q12–24h
Ketoconazole	PO	5–10 mg/kg q12h	NA	NA	NA	NA
Metoclopramide	IV, PO	0.2–0.4 mg/kg q8h	NA	0.15–0.3 mg/kg q8h	0.1–0.2 mg/kg q8h	0.1–0.2 mg/kg q8h
Mirtazapine	PO	3.75 mg per cat q24h	NA	1.88 mg per cat q48h	1.88 mg per cat q48h	1.88 mg per cat q48h
Metronidazole	IV, PO	10–15 mg/kg q8–24h	NA	NA	NA	5–12.5 mg/kg q8–24h
Ondansetron	PO	0.1–1 mg/kg 12–24h	NA	NA	0.05–0.5 mg/kg q12–24h	0.025–0.25 mg/kg q12–24h
Prazosin	PO	1–4 mg per dog q12–24h	NA	NA	1–2 mg / dog q12–24h	0.75–1.5 mg / dog q12–24h
Propranolol	PO	0.1–0.2 mg/kg q8h	NA	NA	NA	0.08–0.16 mg/kg q8h

Table 10.7.2 *(Continued)*

Drug	Route	Standard dose	Modified dosage based on IRIS staging			
			Stage I	Stage II	Stage III	Stage IV
Ranitidine	IV, PO	0.5–2 mg/kg q8–12 h	NA	0.25–1 mg/kg q8–12 h	0.25–1 mg/kg q12–24 h	0.25 mg/kg q24 h-EOD
Spironolactone	PO	1–2 mg/kg q12 h	1 mg/kg q12 h	0.5 mg/kg q24 h	0.25 mg/kg q24 h	C.I.
Tramadol	PO	1–4 mg/kg q8–12 h	1–4 mg/kg q12 h	0.5–2 mg/kg q12 h	0.5–1 mg/kg q8–12 h	0.5–1 mg/kg q12–24 h
Vancomycin	IV	10–20 mg/kg q6–12 h	10 mg/kg q12 h[a]	5 mg/kg q12–24 h[a]	1.25–2.5 mg/kg q12–24 h[a]	1.25–2.5 mg/ kg q24 h-EOD[a]

[a] Preferable to monitor serum levels.
[b] Reduce further with hepatic insufficiency.
IRIS, International Renal Interest Society; NA, no adjustment required; PO, by mouth; IV, intravenous; EOD, every other day; ETD, every third day; C.I., Contraindicated.
Source: Compiled from Karriker M. Drug dosing in renal failure and the dialysis patient. In: *Proceedings of the Advanced Renal Therapies Symposium*, pp. 8–12. New York; 2006; Plumb DC. *Plumb's Veterinary Drug Handbook*, 6th edition. Ames, IA: Blackwell; 2008; Cowgill LD, Kallet AJ. Systemic hypertension. In: *Current Veterinary Therapy IX, Small Animal Practice*, ed. RW Kirk, p. 360. Philadelphia, PA: W.B. Saunders; 1986.

Table 10.7.3 International Renal Interest Society (IRIS) chronic kidney disease (CKD) substaging system based on urine protein to creatinine ratio

Substage	Dog	Cat
Non-proteinuric (NP)	<0.2	<0.2
Borderline proteinuric (BP)	0.2–0.5	0.2–0.4
Proteinuric (P)	>0.5	>0.4

Source: http://www.iris-kidney.com/pdf/IRIS2009_Staging_CKD.pdf.

clearance.[2] Drug clearance may be estimated by measuring GFR. The drug dosage is adjusted by the percentage reduction in GFR (the ratio of the patient's GFR to normal GFR). This percentage is used to adjust dosing regimens by increasing the dosing interval (best for drugs with a wide therapeutic range and long plasma half-life) or by decreasing the dosage (best for drugs with a narrow therapeutic range and a short plasma half-life).[2]

Fluid therapy and correction of electrolyte imbalances

Fluid therapy is commonly indicated in patients with ARF and decompensated CKD, and in certain patients with PLN. Administering fluids permits correction of dehydration, electrolyte and acid–base disorders, and initiates diuresis.[3] Initial calculations for fluid replacement is based on the presence and degree of dehydration (Table 10.7.4).

Besides the physical examination assessment for dehydration, laboratory and diagnostic tests (hematocrit, total protein, urine output, and central venous pressure) can aid in determining a

patient's hydration status. The fluid deficit is then calculated using the following formula:

$$\text{Percentage dehydrated} \times \text{body wt (kg)} = \text{fluid deficit in liters.}$$

The calculated fluid deficit is given intravenously, often rapidly, over 4–6 h. Following treatment for dehydration and repeating a physical examination to ensure replacement fluid needs, an hourly fluid rate is calculated based on maintenance requirements (40–60 mL/kg/day) and on an estimation of ongoing losses through PU, vomiting, and diarrhea. Replacement fluid choices include 0.9% NaCl, lactated Ringer's solution (LRS), Normosol-R (Norm), and Plasma-Lyte 56. In patients with mild hypernatremia or cardiac insufficiency where there is a concern for impending congestive heart failure, a low sodium fluid type, such as 0.45% NaCl/2.5% dextrose or half-strength LRS in 2.5% dextrose, can be utilized. It is important to closely monitor for signs of over- or underhydration in any patient on IV fluids. These include changes in body weight, decreased urine output, the development of tachypnea, tachycardia, coughing, clear nasal discharge, chemosis, or increased bronchovesicular sounds with or without pulmonary crackles. A progressive elevation in central venous pressure can also be an indication of overhydration. Following correction for dehydration, an appropriate urine output is 1–2 mL/kg/h.[1] For patients requiring maintenance fluid administration as part of their long-term therapy, fluids containing lower sodium content are recommended. Examples include Normosol-M, Plasma-Lyte 56, 0.45% NaCl/2.5% dextrose, and half-strength LRS in 2.5% dextrose.

Potassium

Potassium is one of the main electrolytes that is frequently managed with fluid therapy. Patients with renal disease can be

Table 10.7.4   Assessment of hydration status based on physical examination

Hydration status	Clinical signs			
	Skin	Eyes	Mucous membranes	Heart rate
<5%: Normal hydration	Turgor < 2 s	Moist, normal position	Moist, pink, CRT < 2 s	Normal for species
6–8%: Mild dehydration	Turgor > 3 s, inelastic and leathery; twist disappears immediately	Duller than normal, sunken	Tacky to dry, CRT < 2 s	Normal to possibly increased
8–10%: Moderate dehydration	Turgor > 3 s, inelastic and leathery; twist disappears slowly	Duller than normal, sunken	Tacky to dry, CRT normal to increased	Heart rate increased
10–12%: Severe dehydration	Turgor remains, no elasticity; twist remains	Dry, deeply sunken	Dry, cyanotic, CRT prolonged or absent	Heart rate increased, pulse weak
12–15%: Shock	Death is imminent			

CRT, capillary refill time.
Source: Jack CM, Watson PM. *Veterinary Technician's Daily Reference Guide*, 2nd edition, p. 360. Ames, IA: Blackwell Publishing; 2008.

hyperkalemic, normokalemic, or hypokalemic. Marked hyperkalemia is a life-threatening emergency that can result in death by inducing multiple types of arrhythmias. ECG changes may include peaked T waves, bracycardia, prolonged PR intervals, flattened and then absent P waves, widened QRS complexes, and ultimately, if the hyperkalemia is severe enough, ventricular fibrillation and atrial standstill.[1]

Initial therapy for patients with electrocardiographic abnormalities due to hyperkalemia usually entails the administration of calcium gluconate IV. Although calcium gluconate blocks the pathological effects of hyperkalemia on the heart, it does not lower serum potassium.[4] Short-term lowering of the serum potassium can be accomplished with sodium bicarbonate, dextrose injections in nondiabetic patients, and/or regular insulin combined with dextrose injections (see Table 10.7.5). Sodium bicarbonate is beneficial for the treatment of moderate hyperkalemia and metabolic acidosis. A standard mEq/kg dosing can be utilized for the treatment of hyperkalemia (see Table 10.7.5) or a dose can be determined by calculating the bicarbonate deficit. The bicarbonate deficit is determined by the following equation:

$$0.3 \times \text{body wt (kg)} \times \text{base deficit} = \text{bicarbonate deficit}$$

and

$$20 - \text{serum bicarbonate or total } CO_2 \text{ concentration}$$
$$= \text{bicarbonate deficit.}$$

Usually in patients with severe acidosis, one-fourth to one-third of the deficit is administered IV, either over a few hours or as a bolus with fluids. The balance of the deficit is given over an additional 4–6 h.[3,4] The acid–base status is then reevaluated to see if additional bicarbonate therapy is warranted.

Potassium chloride (KCl) is a common fluid additive that is used in the treatment of hypokalemia or to maintain normokalemia in patients receiving IV fluids. The dosing of KCl is ideally based on serum potassium levels, but the infusion rate should not exceed 0.5 mEg/kg/h (Table 10.7.6).[5]

When patients are receiving maintenance fluids, a total of 20–30 mEq KCl per liter of fluid is typically sufficient.[3]

Calcium and phosphorus

In patients with moderate to severe ARF and/or CKD, hyperphosphatemia is a common finding. When the product of calcium × phosphorus is greater than 60–70, soft tissue and renal mineralization develops, which results in progression of CKD. The first step in lowering mild to moderate hyperphosphatemia is restriction of dietary phosphorus, which may be accomplished with most diets designed for cats and dogs with kidney disease[3] (see Table 10.9.1). When dietary therapy is not successful in maintaining a serum phosphorus less than 6 mg/dL (or reducing the calcium phosphorus product to less than 60–70), then phosphate-binding agents or medical management for hyperparathyroidism may be administered (see Table 10.7.5). This is particularly important in patients with severe CKD or ARF. Phosphate-binding agents should be administered with food to reduce GI upset and to maximize binding of phosphorus in the diet.[6] Liquids or encapsulated preparations are preferable to tablets since they mix better with ingesta; however, tablets may be crushed for better efficacy.[3] Some authors state magnesium-based binders (aluminum hydroxide/magnesium hydroxide [Maalox®]) should be avoided.[6] Of the calcium-based phosphate binders, calcium carbonate is more likely to cause hypercalcemia and should be used with caution in patients with preexisting hypercalcemia.[3] In patients with persistent hyperphosphatemia, calcium- and aluminum-based agents can be utilized concurrently.[7] In cats and dogs with a phosphorus level less than 6 mg/dL, calcitriol may be used to suppress renal secondary hyperparathyroidism (see Table 10.7.5).[8]

Table 10.7.5 Drugs used in the management of acute renal failure and chronic kidney disease

Drug	Standard dose	Adverse effect
Therapies to treat hyperkalemia		
Calcium gluconate 10% solution	0.5–1.0 mL/kg IV slow bolus	Arrhythmias
Sodium bicarbonate	0.5–2 mEq/kg IV slow bolus	Hypernatremia, hypokalemia, decreased ionized calcium
Dextrose	0.1–0.5 g/kg IV or 1–2 mL/kg 25% solution	Hyperglycemia, hyperosmolality
Regular insulin/dextrose	0.25–0.5 U/kg insulin with 1–2 g dextrose per unit insulin given, IV	Hypoglycemia
Therapies to treat nausea/vomiting		
Cimetidine (Tagamet®)	5.0 mg/kg PO, IM, IV q6–8 h	Altered drug metabolism
Ranitidine (Zantac®)	0.5–2 mg/kg PO, IV q12 h	Rare, agranulocytosis, vomiting
Famotidine (Pepcid®)	0.5–1 mg/kg PO, IV, SC, IM q12–24 h	Bradycardia (IV), agranulocytosis, vomiting
Misoprostol (Cytotec®)	1–5 µg/kg PO q6–8 h	GI upset, uterine contraction
Sucralfate (Carafate®)	0.25–1 gram PO q8–12 h	Constipation (d)
Aminopentamide hydrogen sulfate (Centrine®)	0.1–0.4 mg SC, IM q8–12 h	Dry mouth, dry eyes, blurred vision, urinary hesitancy/retention
Metoclopramide (Reglan®)	0.2–0.4 mg/kg PO, SC, IM q8 h	Anorexia, vomiting, depression, mydriasis, neurological signs
Chlorpromazine (Thorazine®)	0.2–0.4 mg/kg SC, IM q8 h (d); 0.5 mg/kg IV, IM, SC q6–8 h (c)	CNS depression, vomiting, diarrhea, anorexia, paradoxical excitement (c)
Dolasetron mesylate (Anzemet®)	0.6–1 mg/kg PO q12 h	Dose related ECG interval prolongation
Ondansetron (Zofran®)	0.6–1 mg/kg PO, IV q12 h (d); 0.1–0.15 mg/kg slow IV q6–12 h	Constipation, extrapyramidal clinical signs, arrhythmias, hypotension
Maropitant citrate (Cerenia®)	1 mg/kg SC q24h, 2 mg/kg PO q24 h (d); extra label use at same dose (c)	Swelling/pain at injection site, diarrhea, anorexia
Therapies to manage hyperphosphatemia/hyperparathyroidism		
Aluminum hydroxide (Amphogel®, Alu-caps®)	30–90 mg/kg/day PO	GI upset, constipation, aluminum toxicity with advanced CKD
Aluminum hydroxide/magnesium hydroxide (Maalox®)	30–90 mg/kg/day PO	GI upset, constipation, aluminum toxicity with advanced CKD
Aluminum carbonate (Basalgel®)	30–90 mg/kg/day PO	GI upset, constipation, aluminum toxicity with advanced CKD
Calcium acetate (PhosLo®)	60–90 mg/kg/day PO	Hypercalcemia
Calcium citrate (Citracal®)	60–90 mg/kg/day PO	Hypercalcemia
Calcium carbonate	90–150 mg/kg/day PO	Hypercalcemia
Sevelamer (Renagel®)	25–40 mg/kg PO q12 h	Potentially GI upset
Lanthanum carbonate (Fosrenol®)	30–90 mg/kg per day	Potentially GI upset
Epakitin®	1 gm/5 kg PO q12 h with a meal	Hypercalcemia
Calcitriol (Rocaltrol®)	If creatinine 2–3 and P < 6 mg/dL = 2.5–3.5 ng/kg/day PO If creatinine >3 and P < 6 mg/dL, obtain PTH level = 3.5 ng/kg/day PO	Hypercalcemia (particular concern with calcium-based P binders, e.g., calcium carbonate)

(Continued)

Table 10.7.5   (*Continued*)

Drug	Standard dose	Adverse effect
Therapies to stimulate appetite		
Diazepam	0.05 to 0.15 mg/kg IV (c)	Avoid PO administration due to behavioral changes, hepatic failure
Oxazepam (Serax®)	0.25–0.5 mg/kg PO q12–24 h	Sedation, ataxia
Cyproheptadine (Periactin®)	0.2 mg/kg PO q12h (d), 0.35–1 mg/kg PO q12 h (c)	Sedation, mucous membranes dryness, paradoxical agitation (c)
Mirtazapine (Remeron®)	3.75 mg PO q24 (c)	Increased vocalization and affection
Assorted therapies		
Sodium bicarbonate	8–12 mg/kg PO q8–12 h (d) 1 mEq/cat PO q8–12 h (c)	Hypernatremia, hypokalemia, decreased ionized calcium
Potassium citrate (Cytra K Liquid®)	35 mg/kg PO q8h	Metabolic alkalosis, decreased ionized calcium, hyperkalemia
Potassium gluconate	2 mEq per 4.5 kg PO q12h	Hyperkalemia
Azodyl®	If <2.3 kg, 1 cap PO q24 h; If 2.3–4.5 kg, 1 cap PO q12 h; If >4.5 kg, 2 cap AM, 1 cap PM PO	Possible vomiting and diarrhea
Rubenal®	If 8–12 kg, 0.5 tab PO q12 h; If 13–25 kg, 1 tab PO q12 h; If 26–45 kg, 2 tab PO q12 h; If >45 kg, 3 tab PO q12 h	None listed
Essential fatty acids/omega fish oil (Dermapet Eicosaderm® and OFA plus EZ-C caps®; F.A. caps; Omega EFA capsules®)	Due to the unique composition of each product, see actual label directions	If contains vitamin A the acute toxicosis may result

CKD, chronic kidney disease; c, cat; d, dog; creat, creatinine; P, phosphorus; PO, by mouth; SC, subcutaneous; IM, intramuscular; IV, intravenous; h, hour; d, day; BW, body weight.
Source: Modified from Lane IF. Treatment of urinary disorders. In: *Small Animal Clinical Pharmacology Therapeutics*, ed. DM Booth. Philadelphia, PA: Saunders; 2001.

Table 10.7.6   Potassium supplementation based on serum potassium concentrations

Serum potassium concentration (mEq/L)	Recommended concentration in fluid (mEq/L)
3.5–5.5	20
3.0–3.5	30
2.5–3.0	40
2.0–2.5	60
<2.0	80

Metabolic acidosis

As kidney function in patients with CKD deteriorates or in patients with ARF, additional complications frequently develop. Metabolic acidosis can result from an inability to excrete acids via the kidneys. In addition to causing progressive renal damage, metabolic acidosis may also cause inappetence, vomiting, and weight loss. Patients with a total serum TCO_2 of less than 15–17 mmol/L should receive oral alkalization therapy (see Table 10.7.5). Those with total serum TCO_2 of less than 10–12 mmol/L should be administered parenteral alkalization therapy (see Table 10.7.5).[3] A 1 mEq/mL bicarbonate solution can be made from household baking soda (5 or 6 tablespoons of baking soda to 1 L of water = 1 mEq/mL).[7] Other therapies include potassium citrate, calcium carbonate, or acetate (see Table 10.7.5).[7] In addition to metabolic acidosis, patients with kidney failure will commonly be inappetent due to a multitude of other causes including dehydration, uremia, anemia, lingual and gastric ulceration, electrolyte abnormalities, and possible effects of the medications being administered.

Inappetence

Therapy for inappetence involves correction of any underlying complications (if possible), withdrawal of certain medications (if appropriate), optimizing administration of food (including introducing new diets slowly, in small amounts, and in a quiet, low stress environment), administration of appetite stimulants, and, in certain cases, use of enteric feeding tubes.[3] Gastric ulceration can be treated with a histamine (H2) blocker, a synthetic prostaglandin analogue (misoprostol), and/or a mucosal protectant (sucralfate) (see Table 10.7.5). As with other medications, any H2 blocker excreted via the kidneys requires a dose reduction with kidney failure. Cimetidine inhibits the metabolism of certain drugs (e.g., calcium channel blockers) and should be avoided in certain combinations. Since sucralfate is most effective in an acidic gastric environment, it should be administered 30 min prior to antacid medications.[3] A number of appetite stimulants have been tried in patients with kidney failure. None of these medications appear to have long-lasting benefits but, in certain cases, do provide short-term benefits. They appear to work best in combination with other therapies and dietary manipulations to improve appetite. The newest appetite stimulant to be evaluated is mirtazapine (Remeron®). This medication avoids the sedation side effect noted with the benzodiazepines,[9,10] is more cost-effective, and may be more effective than cyproheptadine. Mirtazapine is an antidepressant that antagonizes alpha-2 adrenergic and serotonin 5-HT2 receptors. It is given once daily in nonazotemic patients and every other day in azotemic patients (see Tables 10.7.2 and 10.7.5).[9,10]

Hypertension

Hypertension is a common complication of renal disease in cats and dogs and has been reported in more than 60% of these patients.[16] IRIS has established normal and grades of hypertension in both cats and dogs (see Table 10.7.7). Renal diets are designed to slow the progression of CKD and to help manage hyperphosphatemia. These diets are also designed to be moderately restricted in sodium and are the first step in the management of mild systemic hypertension.[3] For patients with repeatable moderate to severe hypertension (>160–200 mmHg), pharmacological therapy is indicated. This is particularly important if there is evidence of hypertensive damage to the eyes (e.g., retinal detachment), brain (e.g., seizures), or heart (e.g., left ventricular hypertrophy). Antihypertensive therapy is often based on the underlying etiology, the potential risk versus benefits for the patient, and the clinician's preference.[3] Table 10.7.8 lists medications that have been used to treat hypertension. Hypertensive cats with concurrent tachycardia may benefit from a beta blocker (e.g., atenolol); however, dogs with ARF or CKD appear to have minimal benefit from beta blockers or diuretics (e.g., furosemide).[11,12]

Table 10.7.7 Normal blood pressure ranges and stages of hypertension in dogs and cats

Blood pressure stage	Systolic	Diastolic	Potential adaptation[a]
Normal	120	80	None
Minimal risk	<150	<95	<10 mmHg above RR
Low risk	150–159	95–99	10–20 mmHg above RR
Moderate risk	160–179	100–119	20–40 mmHg above RR
Severe risk	≥180	≥120	≥40 mmHg above RR

[a] Although not widely available currently, it is ideal to use normal blood pressure ranges determined for specific breeds and to compare measurements to the upper limits of the normal range. Certain breeds (e.g., sight hounds) have a higher reference range.
RR, reference range.
Source: Modified from IRIS. *Staging of CKD.* http://www.iris-kidney.com/education/en/education06.shtml; 2009.

Angiotensin-converting enzyme inhibitors (ACEIs) have been shown to reduce proteinuria in dogs and in cats with PLN, to slow the progression of CKD in dogs and potentially in cats, and are helpful in controlling hypertension in cats and dogs.[13–15] One of the proposed mechanisms by which ACEI slows the progression of CKD is by reducing glomerular hypertension. However, excessive reduction in renal perfusion and GFRs, especially with preexisting CKD, may cause ARF. To avoid this complication, ACEIs are started at a low dosage and are slowly increased, while monitoring BP, BUN, and creatinine concentration.[3] The active metabolite of benazepril is eliminated principally via biliary excretion in cats, compared to renal excretion for enalapril. Therefore, benazepril does not require dose reduction for moderate CKD.[14] Newer medications that result in angiotensin receptor blockage (e.g., losartan) are being evaluated for the treatment of hypertension.

Calcium channel blockers (e.g., amlodipine, nifedipine) are commonly used in the treatment of hypertension in dogs and in cats. They reduce BP by peripheral vasodilation and are effective in cats with once-daily therapy.[16] Unlike ACEI, calcium channel blockers may improve renal perfusion and GFR; in addition, they contain cytoprotective qualities that may benefit patients with ARF or CKD.[3] Amlodipine results in an approximately a threefold increase in renin–angiotensin–aldosterone system activation, which is blunted by concurrent use of an ACEI.[17] Hydralazine is a direct-acting smooth muscle relaxant that is similar to calcium channel blockers. It induces peripheral vasodilation, thereby reducing BP. In renal transplantation cats with hypertension, hydralazine has been shown to reduce BP and the frequency of neurological complications.[18] A beta blocker (e.g., atenolol) may be needed if reflex tachycardia develops. For patients with severe and/or life-threatening hypertension, nitroprusside, a potent intravenous vasodilator of both

Table 10.7.8 Medications used in the treatment of hypertension in dogs and cats

Drug	Standard dose	Adverse effect
Furosemide (Lasix®)	2.5–5 mg/kg PO, IV, IM q 12–24 h	Fluid and electrolyte abnormalities, prerenal azotemia, ototoxicity
Spironolactone (Aldactone®)	1–2 mg/kg PO q 12 h (c)	Mild fluid and electrolyte abnormalities, azotemia, acidosis
Propranolol (Inderal®)	2.5–5 mg/cat PO 8–12 h (c)	Bronchoconstriction, hypotension, bradycardia, congestive heart failure
Atenolol (Tenormin®)	2 mg/kg/day (c), 0.25–2 mg/kg/day (d)	Bronchoconstriction, hypotension, bradycardia, congestive heart failure
Enalapril (Vasotec®)	0.25 mg/kg PO q 24 h to 0.5 mg/kg PO q 12 h	Hypotension, decreased renal perfusion, hyperkalemia, GI upset, rarely myelosuppression, seizures
Benazepril (Lotensin®)	0.25–0.5 mg/kg PO q 12–24 h	Hypotension, decreased renal perfusion, hyperkalemia, GI upset, rarely myelosuppression, seizures
Amlodipine (Norvasc®)	0.625–1.25 mg/cat PO q 12–24 h (c); 0.05–0.25 up to 1 mg/kg PO q 24 h (d)	Hypotension, cardiac arrhythmias, GI upset
Hydralazine (Apresoline®)	0.5–2 mg/kg PO q 8–12 h (d); 2.5 mg/cat PO q 12–24 h (c)	Hypotension, reflex tachycardia, sodium/water retention, GI upset
Nitroprusside sodium (Nitropress®)	1–2 mcg/kg/min (d); 0.5 mcg/kg/min (c)	Hypotension, nausea

c, cats; d, dogs; PO, by mouth; IM, intramuscular; IV, intravenous.

Table 10.7.9 Antimicrobial agent-specific factors that influence selection for urinary infections

1. Easy to administer
2. Associated with few, if any, adverse effects
3. Affordability
4. Able to attain urine concentrations (e.g., prostatitis) that exceed the bacterial minimum inhibitory concentration (MIC) by ≥4-fold
5. Unlikely to adversely affect gastrointestinal flora

arteries and veins, may be considered.[19] In all patients receiving antihypertensives, serial monitoring of BP and renal and cardiac function is critical to ensure the hypertension is controlled and to avoid potentially serious complications.

Antimicrobials

Antimicrobials are commonly used in the therapy of urinary disorders in dogs and in cats. The choice of an antimicrobial agent is based on many patient factors including the type, sensitivity, and anatomic site of the infection, the presence or absence of clinical signs, neuter status, concurrent disorders, imaging study results (e.g., presence of urinary bladder stones), and reoccurrence or persistence of the infection. Table 10.7.9

lists five antimicrobial agent factors that influence selection. Bacterial infections of the urogenital system are far more common than fungal or viral infections and can be confined to one site or to multiple sites.[20] Except for a simple, first-time UTI in middle-aged female dogs, it is best to determine antibiotic therapy based on bacterial identification and antimicrobial sensitivity. Urine for culture is best obtained by cystocentesis prior to antimicrobial therapy (or after antibiotics have been discontinued for 3–5 days), although sterile catheterization can provide valid results. The collected urine needs to be transported in a sterile container and processed as rapidly as possible to avoid bacterial proliferation, contamination, or bacterial death.[20] If laboratory processing of the urine sample is delayed by greater than 30 min, then the sample should be refrigerated at 4°C.[20]

In certain circumstances, antimicrobial therapy needs to be initiated empirically before urine culture and sensitivity results are available. For these patients, the initial antimicrobials chosen are based on common isolates that cause UTIs in dogs and cats, such as *E. coli*, *Staphylococcus* spp., *Streptococcus* spp., and *Enterococcus* spp.[20] A broad-spectrum antibiotic with excellent urine concentration should be administered, such as amoxicillin, cephalexin, or trimethoprim–sulfamethoxazole (see Table 10.7.10). For *uncomplicated UTIs*, these first-line antimicrobials should be chosen rather than second-line drugs, such as amoxicillin–clavulanic acid (Clavamox®), fluoroquinolones (e.g., Baytril®), or extended-release cephalosporins (e.g., cefovecin). Empiric use of

Table 10.7.10   Antimicrobial agents commonly used in urinary conditions

Drug	Administration route	Standard dose	Adverse effect
Amikacin	IV	15–30 mg/kg q 24 h	Nephrotoxicity, ototoxicity, neuromuscular blockade
Amoxicillin	PO, IV	10–20 mg/kg q 24 h	Anorexia, vomiting, diarrhea
Ampicillin	IV	10–20 mg/kg q 8–12 h	Hypersensitivity reactions (fever, bone marrow disorders)
Amoxicillin–clavulanic acid (Clavamox)	PO	12.5–13.75 mg/kg q 12 h	Anorexia, vomiting, diarrhea, hypersensitivity reactions
Cefazolin	IV	10–30 mg/kg q 8 h	Hypersensitivity reactions (fever, bone marrow disorders)
Cefovecin (Convenia®)	SC	8 mg/kg q 14 d	Hypersensitivity reactions (fever, bone marrow disorders), injection site pain
Ceftriaxone (Rocephin®)	IM, IV	15–50 mg/kg q 12 h	Hypersensitivity reactions (fever, bone marrow disorders)
Cephalexin	PO	30–40 mg/kg q 8 h	Salivation, tachypnea, excitability, nephrotoxicity, hypersensitivity reactions
Chloramphenicol	PO	45–60 mg/kg q 8 h	Dose-related, reversible bone marrow suppression, aplastic anemia (human)
Clindamycin	PO, SC, IM	5–11 mg/kg q 12 h	Vomiting, diarrhea, esophageal injuries
Doxycycline	PO, IV	5–10 mg/kg q 12 h	Vomiting, esophageal injuries (stricture)
Enrofloxacin	PO, IM, IV	2.5–5 mg/kg q 12 h	Vomiting, anorexia, ocular toxicity causing blindness, potential cartilage abnormalities
Gentamicin	SC, IM, IV	6–8 mg/kg q 24 h	Nephrotoxicity, ototoxicity, neuromuscular blockade
Nitrofurantoin	PO	4–5 mg/kg q 6–8 h	Vomiting, hepatopathy
Imipenem–cilastatin sodium	SC, IV	5–10 mg/kg q 8 h	Vomiting, anorexia, diarrhea, CNS toxicity, hypersensitivity
Penicillin G	IM, IV	25,000–40,000 U/kg q 12–24 h	Hypersensitivity reactions (fever, bone marrow disorders)
Tetracycline	PO	16 mg/kg q 8 h	Vomiting, anorexia, diarrhea, discoloration to teeth in young animals
Trimethoprim/sulfadiazine	PO	30 mg/kg q 24 h	Keratoconjunctivitis sicca, acute hepatitis, hypothyroidism, acute hypersensitivity
Vancomycin	IV	10–20 mg/kg q 6–12 h	Nephrotoxicity, ototoxicity

PO, by mouth; SC, subcutaneous; IM, intramuscular; IV, intravenous; h, hour; d, day; BW, body weight; CNS, central nervous system.

these second-line antimicrobials is discouraged, due to the rapid development of resistance and the inherent resistance of gram-positive organism to fluoroquinolones in particular.[20] Uncomplicated UTIs are usually treated with a 10- or 14-day course of antibiotics with resolution of clinical signs within 2 days.[20]

In contrast to uncomplicated UTIs, *complicated UTIs* are often treated for a longer duration and potentially with different antimicrobials. Most cats, intact dogs, and cats or dogs with polypoid cystitis, emphysematous cystitis, magnesium ammonium phosphate (struvite) urolithiasis, or pyelonephritis are considered to have complicated UTIs. Medical issues that may increase

the risk for infection can include CKD, endogenous or exogenous hyperadrenocorticism, and diabetes mellitus. These patients are treated with a 4- to 6-week course of antimicrobials based on urine culture and sensitivity results.[20] Intact male dogs with UTIs are assumed to have prostatitis and are treated with antimicrobials based on urine, prostatic wash, prostatic brush, or needle aspirate culture results. It these cases, it is very important that the antibiotic be able to penetrate the physiological barrier of the prostate. Examples of such antibiotics include fluoroquinolones, trimethoprim-sulfonamide, or chloramphenicol.[21] In addition to a longer course of antibiotics, some cases of polypoid cystitis may require surgery to remove the deep-seated bacterial infection.[20] Emphysematous cystitis (an accumulation of gas within the urinary bladder wall and lumen secondary to gas fermenting bacteria) most commonly develops in dogs and in cats with diabetes mellitus and often requires long-term antibiotics to eradicate the infection. In dogs, greater than 90% of magnesium ammonium phosphate uroliths are induced by urease-producing bacteria, such as *Staphylococcus* spp. *or Proteus* spp., and can be dissolved with a combination of long-term antibiotics and dietary therapy. For acute pyelonephritis, parental antibiotics, fluid therapy, and supportive care are often needed until the patient is eating and drinking on its own.[20] Following hospitalization for chronic pyelonephritis, the antibiotic should be continued for up to 6–8 weeks.[20]

In addition to antimicrobials, several ancillary therapies have been advocated for UTIs. These therapies are most commonly used in the prevention, rather than the treatment, of UTIs. They include urinary antiseptics (e.g., methenamine), which decrease the hospitability of urine for most bacteria pathogens without harming the patient. Cranberry juice has also been used to prevent UTIs by inhibiting the attachment of bacteria in the urinary mucosa; however, the benefit in dogs and in cats is currently unknown. An important component in the treatment of a complicated or recurrent UTI is ensuring eradication of the infection during therapy. This is accomplished by submitting urine cultures while on antibiotics, and again 5–7 days postcompletion of antibiotics.

Urinary incontinence

Urinary incontinence is an involuntary escape of urine during the storing phase of the urinary cycle.[22] One of the first steps in differentiating diseases that cause urinary incontinence is to estimate the size of the urinary bladder following voiding. In patients with overflow incontinence due to lower motor neuron or upper motor neuron disorders, the urinary bladder is still large even after voiding. In contrast, the urinary bladder is typically small after urinating with USMI ("spay incontinence"), detrusor hyperspasticity, and ectopic ureter(s).[22] Therapy is determined based on the underlying condition and can include both medications and surgery. For patients with lower motor neuron disease, treatment involves manual bladder expression three to four times daily and, in some cases, medications to stimulate bladder contractility (e.g., bethanechol) (see Table 10.7.11 for dosing

Table 10.7.11 Medications used in the therapy of urinary incontinence

Drug	Administration route	Standard dose	Adverse effect
Bethanechol	PO	5–25 mg (total dose) q 8 h	Vomiting, diarrhea, salivation, anorexia, bradycardia, arrhythmias, hypotension
Baclofen	PO	1–2 mg/kg q 8 h	Sedation, weakness, pruritus, salivation
Phenoxybenzamine	PO	0.25 mg/kg q 12–24 h	Hypotension, hypertension, miosis, increased IOP and heart rate
Prazosin	PO	1 mg per 15 kg of BW q 12–24 h	Hypotension, lethargy, dizziness, vomiting, diarrhea
Diazepam	PO	0.2 mg/kg or 2–10 mg total dose q 8 h	Sedation, excitement, irritability, weakness, depression
Dantrolene	PO	1–5 mg/kg q 8–12 h	Hepatotoxicity, weakness, sedation, dizziness, vomiting, constipation
Phenylpropanolamine	PO	1.0–1.5 mg/kg q 8–12 h	Restless; increased heart rate, BP, IOP; hepatic glycogenolysis
Diethylstilbestrol (DES)	PO	0.1–1 mg q 24 h × 3–5 d; then 1 mg/wk	Bone marrow suppression, alopecia, behavior changes, signs consistent of estrus
Testosterone cypionate	IM	2.2 mg/kg q 4–8 weeks	Prostate enlargement
Imipramine	PO	5–15 mg q12h	Sedation, seizures, constipation, vomiting, tachycardia, bone marrow suppression
Flavoxate	PO	100–200 mg (total dose) q 6–8 h	Weakness
Oxybutynin	PO	2–5 mg (total dose) q 8–12 h	Diarrhea, constipation, urine retention, hypersalivation, sedation
Propantheline bromide	PO	7.5–30 mg (total dose) from q 8 to 24 h	Dry mouth and eyes, urinary hesitancy, elevated heart rate, constipation

PO, by mouth; IM, intramuscular; h, hour; d, day; BW, body weight; IOP, intraocular pressure; BP, blood pressure.

information).[8] Since manual bladder expression is difficult in patients with upper motor neuron disease, treatment with baclofen, a skeletal muscle relaxant, is utilized. The patient may still need to be aseptically catheterized three to four times daily.[22] Patients with urge incontinence due to detrusor hyperreflexia are treated with smooth muscle relaxants (flavoxate, oxybutynin, dicylomine, and propantheline bromide).

Patients with USMI are treated with medication to increase urethral tone (e.g., phenylpropanolamine, DES, testosterone cypionate or methytestosterone [in male dogs], and, less frequently, imipramine) (see Table 10.7.11 for dosing information[8]). Cases of USMI that are nonresponsive to medical therapy have been successfully treated with either surgery (colposuspension, urethral imbrication) and/or minimally invasive procedures (urethral submucosa collagen injection, urethral artificial sphincter).[22]

SECTION 8 ANESTHETIC AND ANALGESIC CONSIDERATIONS

Patients with urinary tract disorders, and more specifically renal diseases, can have impaired metabolism and excretion abilities, putting them an increased risk for adverse events when administered certain medications and anesthetics. In particular, patients with existing renal impairments may experience advancement of their disease when administered certain analgesics and anesthetics. Patients with urinary tract diseases often require the administration of anesthesia for diagnostic and treatment procedures, making it important for nursing staff to understand how anesthetics can affect the renal patient. In addition, many urinary tract disorders are painful or cause discomfort, and patients may benefit from analgesic intervention. Proper drug selection and monitoring can help to mitigate potential adverse effects and can increase the quality of life.

Anesthesia

Patients with urinary tract disorders can present with several factors that can increase their risk for anesthetic-related complications. Patients with urethral and ureteral obstruction or renal insufficiency will have impaired excretory ability. Drugs primarily metabolized or eliminated by the urinary system should be avoided or administered at lower doses to avoid prolonged effects or toxicity. Patients with chronic renal disease often suffer from a chronic state of hypovolemia due to dehydration, and when severe, anesthesia should be postponed if possible until this can be corrected with fluid administration. Electrolyte and acid–base disturbances such as metabolic acidosis, hypokalemia, and hyperkalemia are common and can predispose patients to life-threatening arrhythmias or can potentiate nephrotoxicity. Patients with PLNs can suffer from a decrease

in serum proteins, which can make them sensitive to toxicity when administered drugs that are highly protein bound. Anemia secondary to CKD can impair the body's ability to deliver oxygen to tissues, and these patients are often hypothermic, which in turn can contribute to prolonged anesthetic recoveries and coagulation abnormalities. Correction of severe systemic derangements should always be attempted when possible before administering anesthesia to any patient.

Many anesthetics are well-known for their hypotensive effects. This is due to peripheral vasodilation, myocardial depression, and other factors. Anesthetic-induced hypotension can be detrimental to any patient in part due to its effect on renal function. The decreased renal perfusion caused by hypotension can induce renal tissue ischemia and can exacerbate patients already affected with existing renal dysfunction. Fluid administration prior to and during anesthesia can help to combat the physiological changes associated with anesthesia. Identifying hypotension is one of the first steps in mitigating its harmful effects. Serial BP measurement should be performed during anesthesia on patients with renal disease, and abnormalities in BP should be addressed promptly to avoid prolonged hypotension. BP under anesthesia can be measured indirectly by the Doppler or oscillometric methods, and directly by arterial catheterization. Direct arterial blood pressure measurement (DABP) by arterial catheterization should be considered in critically ill or high risk patients. DABP has the advantage of giving continuous readings even during times of severe hypotension, arrhythmia, and other extreme hemodynamic events. There are several methods of addressing anesthetic hypotension, and the method chosen is based on a number of factors including the volume status of the patient, product availability, and veterinarian preference. Common methods include the administration of crystalloid solutions, synthetic colloids, blood products, and synthetic inotropic medications. Care must be taken not to volume overload these patients, especially those at risk for hypervolemia, such as those with concurrent cardiac disease. Monitoring of central venous pressure in high risk patients can assist the anesthetist in preventing volume overload.

Most inhalant agents can cause a dose-dependent vasodilation, which can lead to hypotension. A common strategy used to prevent hypotension is by the use of multimodal pharmaceuticals in the form of premedications, local and regional anesthetics, induction agents, and continuous infusions of drugs, which can allow for lower inhalant flow rates. Induction agents and other medications should be chosen and dosed carefully to prevent overdose in renal patients. Drugs that are mainly or partially excreted by the kidney include ketamine (in cats), propofol, and thiopental. Drugs that are highly protein bound include propofol, diazepam, midazolam, and acepromazine and should be used with caution in patients with decreased serum proteins. Dose adjustments may be required when administering these induction agents to patients with urinary disorders that can affect the excretory function of the kidneys. Total intravenous anesthesia (TIVA) is becoming more widely used in small animal practice and can be used as an alternative to inhalant anesthesia in critically ill or high risk animals when the risks of hypotension are a concern.

Pain management

Patients with disorders of the urinary tract can experience pain from mild to severe. The pain from these disorders can also be acute, chronic, or a combination of both. Patients with urinary calculi, urinary neoplasia, and idiopathic cystitis can experience acute or chronic discomfort from inflammation in the urinary bladder causing pollakiuria, hematuria, and stranguria. Patients with CKD can suffer from painful uremic ulcers of the oral mucous membranes or the GI tract, which can cause discomfort and poor appetite. Recognition and resolution of pain and discomfort can play an integral role in restoring the quality of life for these patients. As previously described, many pharmaceuticals can be harmful to patients with renal dysfunction and dose adjustments should be considered in patients with diminished excretory function.

Opioids are commonly used analgesics in veterinary medicine. These drugs are excreted in the urine and may cause prolonged effects in patients with renal dysfunction. They are still considered a mainstay for the inpatient treatment of pain in renal patients when dosed and administered appropriately. It has been shown that dogs as well as cats can attain therapeutic plasma levels of buprenorphine by transmucosal administration, and this is often dispensed for the treatment of moderate pain in veterinary patients. Fentanyl transdermal patches are often used for moderate to severe pain in dogs and cats, but controversy exists about the reliability of absorption in animals, making it imperative to monitor them for breakthrough pain.

NSAIDs are widely used by veterinarians for their anti-inflammatory and analgesic effects. NSAIDs in some cases can cause alterations in renal blood flow, which can lead to ARF. This can be potentiated by the administration of NSAIDs to patients with hypovolemia and hypotension. Cats appear to be particularly sensitive to the renal effects of NSAIDs. It is generally accepted that NSAIDs should not be administered to patients with existing renal disease, hypotension, or dehydration. When these drugs are used in at-risk patients, appropriate fluid therapy to maintain renal perfusion and close monitoring of renal parameters is essential.

Local and regional anesthetic and analgesic techniques can be used to treat or prevent pain, can reduce or eliminate inhalant requirements in patients, and can provide lasting analgesia postanesthesia. Common techniques described for urinary patients include incisional blocks, bladder and urethral infusions, topical applications, and epidural administration. Careful calculation of local anesthetic drugs is important to prevent toxic levels of drugs in sensitive animals (especially cats). Some animals experience urinary retention after epidural administration of morphine, which can be detrimental to patients with certain urinary disorders. Careful monitoring of epidural patients including bladder expression or urinary catheter placement may be required in some patients.

SECTION 9 NUTRITIONAL CONSIDERATIONS

Chronic kidney disease

Dietary therapy is an integral component in the treatment of patients with CKD and should be used in conjunction with appropriate medical therapy. Diets for patients with CKD should provide adequate nutrition while ameliorating disturbances in electrolyte, acid–base, vitamin, mineral, and hydration status. Appropriate dietary therapy for canine and feline CKD can improve quality of life and increase survival time.[1-3] Commercial diets formulated for CKD patients are usually restricted in protein, phosphorous, and sodium; enhanced in levels of fatty acids, antioxidants, B vitamins, and soluble fiber; are either neutral or slightly alkalinizing; and are calorie dense. Additionally, diets designed for feline CKD patients often have increased potassium supplementation. Of these dietary components, only protein, phosphorous, fatty acids, and antioxidants have been extensively studied in canine and feline CKD patients.

Caloric intake

The first dietary goal for CKD patients is to provide sufficient caloric intake. Patients with CKD are often anorexic secondary to their renal disease but are thought to have caloric requirements similar to those of healthy dogs and cats. The energy requirements for a patient with CKD can be calculated as follows:[4]

$$\text{Dogs}: 132 \times \text{body wt (kg)}^{0.75} = \text{kilocalories per day}$$

and

$$\text{Cats}: 50 - 60 \times \text{body wt (kg)} = \text{kilocalories per day}.$$

Maintenance energy requirements will vary among individuals, and these calculations only provide a starting point. Energy requirements should also be estimated based on the approximate caloric intake of the pet when it was healthy, as well as serial evaluation of body weight and body condition scores.

It is preferable that the caloric requirements of a CKD patient are met with a renal-specific diet. Clients can be given small portions (e.g., one can and a small portion of kibble) of several types of "renal" diets to offer to their pet. This will help improve the chances of finding a palatable option for the CKD patient and in turn will help improve compliance. Feeding strategies to help stimulate appetite (e.g., warming food) should be used to improve compliance. Additionally, introducing a diet when systemic clinical signs such as vomiting are controlled is preferable. Examples of commercially available diets for CKD are included in the Table 10.9.1.

Protein

Diets designed for CKD patients should have controlled protein restriction. It is not certain if protein restriction actually slows

Table 10.9.1 Selected commercial diets for patients with chronic kidney disease

Canine	Feline
Royal Canin Veterinary Diet Canine Renal Low Protein (LP)	Royal Canin Veterinary Diet Feline Renal Low Protein (LP)
Royal Canin Veterinary Diet Canine Renal Medium Protein (MP)	
Royal Canin Veterinary Diet Canine-Reduced Protein	Royal Canin Veterinary Diet Feline-Reduced Protein
Hill's Prescription Diet Canine k/d	Hill's Prescription Diet Feline k/d
Iams Veterinary Formulas Canine Renal Early Stage[a]	Iams Veterinary Formulas Feline Multi-Stage Renal
Purina Veterinary Diets Canine NF	Purina Veterinary Diets Feline NF

[a] Only available in dry kibble.

the progression of renal injury in dogs and cats with CKD.[5,6] Excess protein intake in CKD patients leads to an increase in nitrogenous waste and uremic toxin production and in subsequent worsening of associated clinical signs.[7] However, excessive protein restriction is detrimental to the patient. Appropriate protein restriction will stabilize or reduce the degree of azotemia while avoiding signs of protein malnutrition such as alterations in body weight or tissue mass, anemia, and serum hypoalbuminemia. If signs of protein malnutrition are evident, the dietary protein should be increased to the point where these abnormalities resolve.

Phosphorous

Hyperphosphatemia is a common finding in dogs and cats with CKD. Phosphate retention is an important factor in the progression of CKD and has been associated with decreased survival in dogs and in cats.[3,8-11] Additionally, phosphorous retention is associated with the development of renal secondary hyperparathyroidism. Dietary phosphorous restriction is recommended as the first step in controlling serum phosphorous levels. Protein is a major source of phosphorous; hence, protein-restricted diets are usually phosphorous restricted as well. Dietary phosphorous restriction alone may be sufficient to normalize phosphorous levels as well as to decrease PTH levels.[12] If dietary therapy alone does not normalize phosphorous levels after 2–4 weeks, the addition of phosphate binders is recommended.

Potassium

Hypokalemia is a common finding in cats with CKD but is rare in dogs with CKD. Serum potassium levels likely underestimate total body potassium depletion. Hypokalemia can lead to progression of renal decline as well as muscle weakness. Some diets for feline CKD patients include potassium supplementation, but additional potassium supplementation (e.g., oral potassium gluconate) may be required. However, some cats with CKD are hyperkalemic, and the decision for potassium supplementation should be based on initial serum potassium levels. Hypokalemia

is more common in cats with earlier stages of CKD, with hyperkalemia becoming more frequently observed with the progression of CKD to an oliguric or anuric state.[9]

Sodium

Dietary sodium restriction in CKD patients is controversial. Sodium levels affect circulating volume and sodium retention as a consequence of CKD can theoretically be linked to hypertension. Increased dietary sodium has not been shown to affect BP in dogs or in cats with CKD.[13-16] In one study of cats with naturally occurring CKD, sodium restriction was associated with hypokalemia.[16] However, another study showed that increased dietary sodium chloride promoted the progression of feline CKD.[15] Current recommendations suggest that normal dietary sodium content (or mild sodium restriction) is appropriate for cats and dogs with CKD.

Fatty acids and antioxidants

Omega-3 polyunsaturated fatty acids (PUFAs) and antioxidants are common components to some diets designed for CKD patients. Omega-3 PUFA supplementation can preserve renal function, decrease renal inflammation, and lower BP. Cats offered a renal diet with added PUFAs had an increased survival compared with cats offered renal diets without PUFA supplementation.[17] Omega-3 PUFA supplementation was protective to kidney tissue in dogs with induced renal failure.[18] The ideal quantity or ratio of omega-3 to 6 PUFAs has not yet been determined. Antioxidant therapy (e.g., vitamin E) may be beneficial in reducing oxidative stress associated with renal disease, but extensive studies evaluating their efficacy have not been performed in veterinary medicine.

Acid–base

Metabolic acidosis is a common consequence of CKD, especially in later stages of the disease.[19] Diets designed for patients with CKD are neutral to slightly alkalinizing. Oral alkalinizing agents (e.g., potassium citrate, sodium bicarbonate) may be needed in patients with marked metabolic acidosis, and treatment should be based on serum bicarbonate or total CO_2 levels.

Water intake

Dehydration results from PU secondary to CKD, and patients may fail to consume adequate amounts of water. To help prevent chronic dehydration, adequate fresh water should be available. Additionally, feeding moist or canned diets, adding water to food, offering flavored water, and using water drinking fountains can promote dietary water intake.

Feeding tubes

Ensuring adequate caloric intake in patients with CKD can be challenging. Esophagostomy (E), percutaneous endoscopic gastrostomy (PEG), or surgically placed gastrostomy (G) tubes can be utilized to supplement nutritional requirements in the partially or completely anorexic animal. These feeding tubes can also be used to supplement fluid intake in these patients. Gastrostomy tubes (either PEG or G-tubes) may be easier to maintain on a long-term basis when compared with E-tubes.[4] One canine study showed that approximately half of the dogs in the study maintained or increased their body weight after tube placement, but stomal site infections were common. Other complications include accidental removal of the feeding tube and displacement of the tube into the abdominal cavity causing peritonitis. The study concluded that G-tubes were safe and effective in improving caloric intake in dogs with CKD.[20]

Evidence supporting the use of renal diets

The benefits of renal diets for dogs and cats with CKD have been demonstrated in double-blinded randomized controlled clinical trials (RCCTs). Compared to maintenance diets, renal diets in both studies were restricted in protein, phosphorous, and sodium and were supplemented with PUFAs.[1,2] In a canine double-blinded RCCT, dogs with stage II–III CRI were fed either a renal or a maintenance diet. Dogs fed a renal diet had fewer episodes of uremic crises and clinical signs, slower progression of CKD, higher quality of life perceived by owners, and reduced risk of death compared to dogs fed a maintenance diet. The median survival time for dogs fed the renal diet was 594 days compared to 188 days for dogs fed the maintenance diet.[1]

In a feline double-blinded RCCT, cats with stage II–III CRI were fed either a renal diet or a maintenance diet. The cats fed the renal diet had a reduced risk of uremic crises and death compared to the cats fed the maintenance diet.[2] In a nonrandomized feline study, cats fed a renal diet had a median survival time of 633 days compared to 264 days for cats that consumed their regular diet. Cats fed the renal diet also had reduced urea, phosphorus, and PTH levels compared to the cats fed their regular diet.[3] A retrospective study revealed that cats fed a renal diet had a median survival time of 16 months compared to 7 months for cats fed a conventional maintenance diet.[17]

A common clinical question remains: At what stage should a renal diet be introduced to a patient with CKD? Current evidence shows that protein-restricted diets are indicated in dogs with stage III and IV CKD, as well as in cats with midstage II–IV CKD. While evidence does not support or refute protein restriction in stage II CKD, the other benefits of commercial renal diets likely warrant their use in this group of patients. For example, if a patient in stage II CKD is hyperphosphatemic, dietary phosphorous restriction may be achieved with a low protein diet. Stage I CKD patients with proteinuria and suspected glomerular disease likely benefit from protein-restricted diets as well. Current evidence supports phosphorous restriction in dogs with stage II–IV CKD and is considered appropriate for cats with stage II–IV CKD. Dietary supplementation with omega-3 PUFAs should be considered in dogs and cats with stage II–IV CKD, as well as stage I patients with proteinuria.

Urolithiasis

Urolith formation occurs when the urine becomes supersaturated with calculogenic crystalloid substances. Dietary therapy for the treatment and prevention of urolithiasis focuses on promoting undersaturation of the urine with calculogenic crystalloids as well as on increasing their solubility. This can be achieved by altering urine pH to increase the urine solubility of calculogenic crystalloids and by decreasing the saturation of calculogenic crystalloids. In the case of struvite or urate uroliths, dietary manipulation can help dissolve the uroliths. Specific dietary therapy can also help prevent the recurrence of many types of uroliths (Tables 10.9.2 and 10.9.3).

Dietary water intake

Decreased urine volume can be a risk factor for the development of several urinary tract disorders, including urolithiasis. Therefore, along with specific dietary considerations listed below, increasing dietary water intake is recommended for the treatment and prevention of urolithiasis.[21] Increased water intake is also beneficial for patients with CKD and FIC. Increasing the water intake will increase urine volume and therefore will decrease the relative saturation of urinary calculogenic substances. Additionally, increased water intake will facilitate shorter transit time of calculogenic crystalloids in the urinary tract and will increase the frequency of voiding. USG can be measured periodically to determine if the desired increase in water intake has been achieved. A USG <1.020 in dogs and <1.025 in cats is preferable.

Dietary water intake can be increased by feeding canned food, by adding water to dry food, by using pet drinking fountains, and by offering flavored water. Bouillon cubes with onion powder must be avoided for flavoring water as the onion powder can cause Heinz body anemia in cats. Adding sodium chloride to the diet is another potential strategy to increase water intake, but this is controversial. Increased sodium intake may lead to impaired renal tubular absorption of calcium and subsequent

Table 10.9.2 Selected commercial diets for the treatment and prevention of canine uroliths

Canine urolith diets	Dissolution	Prevention
Struvite	Hill's Prescription Diet Canine s/d	Hill's Prescription Diet Canine c/d[a]
	Royal Canin Veterinary Diet Urinary SO	Royal Canin Veterinary Diet Canine Urinary SO
		Royal Canin Veterinary Diet Canine Preventative
Calcium oxalate	NA	Hill's Prescription Diet Canine u/d
		Royal Canin Veterinary Diet Urinary SO
Urate	Hill's Prescription Diet u/d	Hill's Prescription Diet u/d
	Royal Canin Veterinary Diet Urinary UC Low Purine	Royal Canin Veterinary Diet Urinary UC Low Purine

[a] Canine struvite uroliths are usually infection induced; dietary modification for prevention is usually not required.
NA, not applicable.

Table 10.9.3 Selected commercial diets for the treatment and prevention of feline uroliths

Feline urolith diets	Dissolution	Prevention
Struvite	Hill's Prescription Diet Feline s/d	Hill's Prescription Diet Feline c/d Multicare
		Iams Veterinary Formula Urinary-S-low pH/S
	Purina Veterinary Diet UR st/ox	Purina Veterinary Diets UR st/ox
	Royal Canin Veterinary Diet Feline Dissolution	Royal Canin Veterinary Diet Feline Preventative
		Royal Canin Veterinary Diet Urinary SO
Calcium oxalate	NA	Hill's Prescription Diet Feline c/d Multicare
		Iams Veterinary Formula Urinary-O-Moderate pH/O
		Purina Veterinary Diets UR st/ox
		Royal Canin Veterinary Diet Feline Urinary SO

hypercalciuria. High dietary sodium levels increase water intake and urine volume, leading to decreased USG and decreased calcium oxalate saturation of the urine in healthy dogs and cats.[22,23] However, the effects of a high sodium diet have not been studied on patients at risk for the development of uroliths. At this time, supplemental dietary sodium chloride to stimulate water intake in dogs and cats prone to urolithiasis should be used cautiously. High sodium diets should not be used in patients with renal insufficiency or cardiac disease due to the potential for exacerbation of hypertension with these conditions.

Struvite uroliths

Struvite uroliths are composed of magnesium ammonium phosphate hexahydrate. They are one of the most common types of uroliths in cats and dogs. In dogs, struvite urolithiasis is usually accompanied by a urease-producing bacterial infection that causes an alkaline urine environment. *Staphylococcus* spp. and *Proteus* spp. are common urease-producing bacteria associated with UTI-induced struvite urolithiasis in dogs. Feline struvite uroliths are usually not infection-induced. The etiology of struvite urolithiasis is likely multifactorial and includes gender, breed, and dietary factors.

Dissolution diets can be effective in the treatment of struvite uroliths, combined with treatment for a UTI where appropriate. Prior to attempting a dissolution diet, owners should be cau-

tioned of the potential passage of uroliths into the urethra once they are small enough. This can lead to urinary obstruction and is of particular concern for males due to their relatively smaller urethral diameter when compared with females.

Struvite dissolution diets should be restricted in protein and calculogenic crystalloids (e.g., urea, phosphorous, magnesium). Additionally, these diets produce a more acidic urine environment that is less favorable for struvite crystal formation. A diet used to prevent struvite urolith formation should maintain a urine pH of <6.8. Water intake should be promoted. If struvite uroliths are treated with a dissolution diet, patients should be evaluated with abdominal radiographs and a urinalysis every 4 weeks. Once the urolith has dissolved, dietary therapy should be continued for another month to ensure dissolution of uroliths too small (<3 mm) to be detected radiographically. Struvite uroliths associated with UTIs take an average of 3 months to dissolve in dogs, while sterile struvite uroliths dissolve in an average of 30 days in cats.[24,25]

Dissolution of struvite uroliths is not always successful. The reasons for this include mixed composition of the urolith (e.g., struvite and calcium oxalate layers), poor owner compliance, and inappropriate control of an associated UTI in canine patients. A urinalysis and urine culture can be helpful in determining if a UTI is present. Additionally, the urinalysis should reveal a urine pH of <6.8 with appropriate dietary compliance. If a mixed urolith composition is suspected after unsuccessful attempts at medical dissolution, mechanical urolith removal (surgery, lithot-ripsy) should be performed, followed by urolith analysis.

Cats appear to have a low rate of struvite recurrence.[26] Prevention of struvite uroliths should include increasing water intake. Prescription diets may be required for additional prevention if recurrence is a concern. Urine pH should be maintained below 6.8, but excessive acidification of the urine (<6.29) may increase the risk of calcium oxalate urolithiasis.[27] Prescription diets helped decrease the risk of recurrence of feline struvite urethral plugs in one study.[28] Additionally, diets low in fat and high in fiber, calcium, phosphorous, magnesium, and chloride are associated with an increased risk of struvite urolithiasis in cats.[21]

There are no specific dietary recommendations for the prevention of infection-associated struvite urolithiasis; medical strategies to prevent UTIs should be sufficient. In the uncommon case of sterile struvite urolithiasis in dogs, dietary therapy may be used as a preventative measure. Similar measures that are recommended for the prevention of feline struvite recurrence can be considered for these dogs. Caution should be exercised as some canine struvite diets are very low in protein and may not be suitable to feed on a long-term basis.

Calcium oxalate uroliths

Calcuim oxalate uroliths are one of the most common types of uroliths in dogs and cats.[29] Similar to struvite urolithiasis, the etiology of calcium oxalate urolithiasis is multifactorial. Factors in the development of calcium oxalate uroliths include sex, breed, hereditary factors, environment, and diet.[29–31]

Interestingly, struvite uroliths were the most common feline uroliths until the mid-1990s when the predominance shifted to calcium oxalate uroliths.[29–31] It is thought that this shift may be related to the development of acidifying diets used to decrease the risk of struvite urolithiasis.[21] With the increased awareness of acidifying diets being linked to the development of calcium oxalate uroliths, diets are being formulated to produce a less acidic urine (e.g., pH of 6.3–6.7).[30] Feline upper urinary tract uroliths (e.g., ureteroliths) are almost exclusively composed of calcium oxalate, but struvite uroliths increase in proportion in the lower urinary tract.[30,32] Similar to cats, calcium oxalate uroliths are becoming the most common urolith type in dogs.[29,33] This increase in calcium oxalate urolithiasis is likely multifactorial but may be related to diets that are acidifying and/or contain a high level of minerals.[33]

Calcium oxalate uroliths cannot be medically dissolved. Instead, these uroliths should be removed via voiding urohydropulsion or surgery. However, dietary modification can be an important factor in the prevention of calcium oxalate urolithiasis. Another important factor to consider when reducing the risk of calcium oxalate urolithiasis is the management of metabolic conditions that result in hypercalcemia.

Diets for preventing calcium oxalate uroliths should be nonacidifying and high in moisture.[21] Dogs and cats fed a canned diet have a lower risk of calcium oxalate urolithiasis.[34,35] Calcium oxalate uroliths can form in variable urine pHs, but acidic urine decreases the concentration of urinary inhibitors of calcium oxalate and increases calcium excretion in the urine.[21,36,37] Most pet foods are low in oxalic acid, and dietary oxalate precursors such as green leafy vegetables should be avoided. There are no studies to support severe dietary restriction of calcium in these patients. Moderate levels of calcium are desirable as calcium binds oxalate in the intestines and inhibits its absorption.[35] Phosphorous should not be restricted excessively because this will activate vitamin D and increase the absorption of calcium from the GI tract. Excess dietary phosphorous may complex with calcium to form insoluble calcium phosphate salts.

Potassium citrate is a component of some diets designed to reduce the risk of calcium oxalate urolithiasis. Citric acid inhibits formation of calcium oxalate complexes in the urine. Additionally, citrate helps alkalinize the urine. Potassium may decrease calcium excretion in the urine. Magnesium is thought to be an inhibitor of calcium oxalate urolith formation. However, excess magnesium may be a risk factor for calcium oxalate urolith development as it can promote hypercalciuria.[21] As such, diets to prevent calcium oxalate urolithiasis should have a moderate magnesium content.

Some diets designed to prevent calcium oxalate urolithiasis are supplemented with sodium chloride. The potential benefit of additional dietary sodium chloride is increased thirst, leading to increased urinary volume and subsequent decreased concentration of calcium and oxalate in the urine. However, further studies examining high sodium diets in patients predisposed to calcium oxalate urolithiasis are needed. Therefore, caution should be used when adding sodium to diets.

Urate uroliths

Urate uroliths are composed of ammonium urate, uric acid, and uric acid salts. Urate uroliths are the third most common type of urolith in dogs and in cats, although the overall prevalence of urate uroliths is low. Dalmatians are predisposed to developing urate uroliths due to a defect in urate transport. Other breeds such as the English bulldog also appear to be affected, although the genetic defect has not been identified in this breed. Additionally, dogs with hepatic dysfunction such as portovascular anomalies are at risk for developing urate urolithiasis. The underlying etiology of feline urate urolithiasis is unknown, but some cases are associated with portovascular abnormalities.[30]

Some urate uroliths are amendable to dietary dissolution. Some commercial diets designed specifically for the treatment and prevention of canine urate uroliths are available. Diets designed for medical dissolution and prevention of urate uroliths promote alkaline urine. These diets have an ultralow protein content, and the dietary protein is composed of low purine protein sources (e.g., milk and egg-based proteins). Patients treated with a urate dissolution diet should have a urine pH of 7.0. Acidification of urine may promote precipitation of uric acid. Urine alkalizing agents such as potassium citrate can be added to the diet to promote alkaline urine. Due to the restricted protein level of these diets, they are not suitable for growing, pregnant, or lactating patients. Increasing water intake is also beneficial in the treatment and prevention of urate urolithiasis.

While there are no studies showing the efficacy of a urate dissolution diet in patients with hepatic dysfunction, these diets are likely effective for this purpose. Although Dalmatians have defective urate transport, not all Dalmatians are affected by urate uroliths. Therefore, prescription diets for the treatment and prevention of urate uroliths should only be used for affected Dalmatians. The low dietary taurine and/or carnitine content of urate prescription diets may be associated with dilated cardiomyopathy, especially in English bulldogs. Therefore, it may be more suitable to feed a low protein diet such as those formulated for CKD rather than an ultralow protein diet in this breed.[38]

There are no commercially available diets specifically for the treatment and prevention of feline urate uroliths. Medical dissolution protocols for feline urate uroliths have not been reported, but low protein diets combined with medical treatment (allopurinol) may lead to dissolution of urate uroliths in cats.[39] Low protein diets such as those designed for CKD patients are likely suitable for the prevention in affected cats.

Feline idiopathic cystitis

FIC, also known as feline lower urinary tract disease, is a disorder of young to middle-aged cats that results in clinical signs of pollakiuria, dysuria, and stranguria. The etiology of this syndrome is not fully understood, making treatment of the condition difficult. Increasing water intake may be beneficial for these cats. This can be achieved through the use of canned foods along with the other strategies listed above. The transition from dry to canned food should be performed gradually to increase the likelihood of the cat accepting the new diet and to reduce stress associated with the change. By increasing water intake, the USG is decreased, diluting potentially noxious substances present in the urine. Reducing environmental stress and increasing water intake were two of the multimodal environmental modification strategies that decreased the recurrence of FIC in one study.[40] A prospective diet trial showed that cats fed with canned food had an 11% recurrence rate of FIC compared to a 39% recurrence rate for cats fed dry food.[41] For cats with a history of urinary calculi, specific diet therapy to reduce calculogenic materials in the urine and alteration of urinary pH may be indicated. Recommendations for dietary treatment of and prevention of urinary calculi are outlined in Table 10.9.3.

Bibliography

Section 1

1. Evans HE, Cristensen GC. The urogenital system. In: *Miller's Anatomy of the Dog*, 3rd edition, ed. HE Evans, pp. 494–558. Philadelphia, PA: W.B. Saunders, 1993.
2. Verlander JW. Renal physiology. In: *Textbook of Veterinary Anatomy*, 2nd edition, ed. JG Cunningham, pp. 511–554. St. Louis, MO: W.B. Saunders; 1997.
3. Koeppen BM, Stanton BA. *Renal Physiology*, 3rd edition. St. Louis, MO: Mosby; 2001.

Section 2

1. Lunn KF. Managing the patient with polyuria and polydipsia. In: *Kirk's Current Veterinary Therapy XIV*, eds. JD Bonagura, DC Twedt, pp. 844–850. St. Louis, MO: Elsevier; 2009.

Section 3

1. Polzin DJ. Chronic kidney disease. In: *Textbook of Veterinary Internal Medicine*, Vol. 2, 7th edition, eds. SJ Ettinger, EC Feldman, p. 1990. St. Louis, MO: Saunders Elsevier; 2010.
2. Brown S. Evaluation of chronic renal disease: a staged approach. *Compendium Continuing Education for Veterinarians* 1999;21: 752–763.
3. Kellum JA, Levin NW, Bouman C, et al. Developing a consensus classification system for acute renal failure. *Current Opinion in Critical Care* 2002;8:509–514.
4. Langston C. Acute uremia. In: *Textbook of Veterinary Internal Medicine*, Vol. 2, 7th edition, eds. SJ Ettinger, EC Feldman, pp. 1970–1972. St. Louis, MO: Saunders Elsevier; 2010.
5. Rentko VT, Clark N, Ross LR, et al. Canine leptospirosis: a retrospective study of 17 cases. *Journal of Veterinary Internal Medicine* 1992;6:235–244.
6. Birnbaum N, Barr SC, Center SC, et al. Naturally acquired leptospirosis in 36 dogs: serological and clinicopathological features. *Journal of Small Animal Practice* 1998;39:231–236.
7. Dambach DM, Smith CA, Lewis RM, et al. Morphologic, immunohistochemical, and ultrastructural characterization of a distinctive renal lesion in dogs putatively associated with *Borrelia burgdorferi* infection: 49 cases (1987–1992). *Veterinary Pathology* 1997;34:85–96.
8. Hutton TA, Goldstein RE, Njaa BL, et al. Search for *Borrelia burgdorferi* in kidneys of dogs with suspected "Lyme nephritis". *Journal of Veterinary Internal Medicine* 2008;22(4):860–865.
9. Bartges JW, Blanco L. Bacterial urinary tract infection in cats. *Standards of Care: Emergency and Critical Care Medicine* 2001;3: 1–5.
10. Ling GV, Norris CR, Franti CE, et al. Interrelations of organism prevalence, specimen collection method, and host age, sex, and breed among 8354 canine urinary tract infections (1969–1995). *Journal of Veterinary Internal Medicine* 2001;15:341–347.
11. Barsanti JA. Genitourinary infections. In: *Infectious Diseases of the Dog and Cat*, 3rd edition, ed. CE Greene, p. 937. St. Louis, MO: Mosby; 2006.
12. Bartges JW. Urinary tract infections. In: *Textbook of Veterinary Internal Medicine*, Vol. 2, 6th edition, eds. SJ Ettinger, EC Nelson, p. 1806. St. Louis, MO: Mosby; 2005.
13. Yuri K, Nakata K, Katae H, et al. Distribution of uropathogenic virulence factors among *Escherichia coli* strains isolated from dogs and cats. *The Journal of Veterinary Medical Science* 1998;60(3): 287–290.
14. Bartges JW. Diagnosis of urinary tract infections. *Veterinary Clinics of North America. Small Animal Practice* 2004;34(4): 923–933.
15. Osborne CA, Lulich JP, Polzin DJ, et al. Medical dissolution and prevention of canine struvite urolithiasis. Twenty years of experience. *Veterinary Clinics of North America. Small Animal Practice* 1999;29:73–111.
16. Bartges JW, Osborne CA, Polzin DJ. Recurrent sterile struvite urocystolithiasis in three related cocker spaniels. *Journal of the American Animal Hospital Association* 1992;28:459–469.
17. Osborne CA, Lulich JP, Kruger JM, et al. Canine uroliths, feline uroliths, and feline urethral plugs from 1981 to 2007: perspectives

from the Minnesota Urolith Center. *Veterinary Clinics of North America. Small Animal Practice* 2009;39:183–197.

18. Ling GV. Urinary stone disease. In: *Lower Urinary Tract Diseases of Dogs and Cats*, ed. GV Ling, pp. 144–177. St. Louis, MO: Mosby; 1995.

19. Lulich JP, Osborne CA, Thumchai R, et al. Epidemiology of canine calcium oxalate uroliths. Identifying risk factors. *Veterinary Clinics of North America. Small Animal Practice* 1999;29:113–122.

20. Ling GV, Franti CE, Ruby AL, et al. Urolithiasis in dogs. II: breed prevalence, and interrelations of breed, sex, age, and mineral composition. *American Journal of Veterinary Research* 1998;59:630–642.

21. Menon M, Resnick MI. Urinary lithiasis: etiology, diagnosis, and medical management. In: *Campbell's Urology*, eds. AB Retik, ED Vaughan, Jr., pp. 3229–3305. Philadelphia, PA: Saunders; 2002.

22. Bartges JW, Osborne CA, Lulich JP, et al. Canine urate urolithiasis. Etiopathogenesis, diagnosis, and management. *Veterinary Clinics of North America. Small Animal Practice* 1999;29:161–191.

23. Bartges JW, Osborne CA, Lulich JP, et al. Prevalence of cystine and urate uroliths in bulldogs and urate uroliths in dalmations. *Journal of the American Veterinary Medical Association* 1994;204:1914–1918.

24. Bannasch D, Safra N, Young A, et al. Mutations in the SLC2A9 gene cause hyperuricosuria and hyperuricemia in the dog. *PLoS Genetics* 2008;4(11):e1000246. Epub November 7, 2008.

25. Bannasch DL, Ling GV, Bea J, et al. Inheritance of urinary calculi in the Dalmatian. *Journal of Veterinary Internal Medicine* 2004;18:483–487.

26. Kruger JM, Osborne CA. Etiopathogenesis of uric acid and ammonium urate uroliths in non-Dalmatian dogs. *Veterinary Clinics of North America. Small Animal Practice* 1986;16:87–126.

27. Osborne CA, Lulich JP, Bartges JW, et al. Drug-induced urolithiasis. *Veterinary Clinics of North America. Small Animal Practice* 1999;29:251–266.

28. Johnston SD, Kamolpatana K, Root-Kustritz MV, et al. Prostatic disorders in the dog. *Animal Reproduction Science* 2000;60-61:405–415.

29. Forrester DS, Roudebush P. Evidence-based management of feline lower urinary tract disease. *Veterinary Clinics of North America. Small Animal Practice* 2007;37:533–558.

30. Willeberg P. Epidemiology of naturally occurring feline urologic syndrome. *Veterinary Clinics of North America. Small Animal Practice* 1984;14:455–469.

31. Kruger JM, Osborne CA. The role of viruses in feline lower urinary tract disease. *Journal of Veterinary Internal Medicine* 1990;4:71–78.

32. Kruger JM, Osborne CA, Goyal SM, et al. Clinical evaluation of cats with lower urinary tract disease. *Journal of the American Veterinary Medical Association* 1991;199:211–216.

33. Cannon AB, Ruby AL, Westropp JL, et al. Evaluation of trends in urolith composition in cats: 5230 cases (1985–2004). *Journal of the American Veterinary Medical Association* 2007;231:570–576.

34. Kruger JM, Conway TS, Kaneene JB, et al. Randomized controlled trial of the efficacy of short-term amitriptyline administration for treatment of acute, nonobstructive idiopathic lower urinary tract disease in cats. *Journal of the American Veterinary Medical Association* 2003;222:749–758.

35. Osborne CA, Kruger JM, Lulich JP, et al. Prednisolone therapy of idiopathic feline lower urinary tract disease: a double-blind study. *Veterinary Clinics of North America. Small Animal Practice* 1996;26:563–569.

36. Hayes HM, Jr.. Breed associations of canine ectopic ureter: a study of 217 female cases. *Journal of Small Animal Practice* 1984;25:501–504.

37. Holt PE, Thrusfield MV, Moore AH. Breed predisposition to ureteral ectopia in bitches in the UK. *The Veterinary Record* 2000;146:561.

38. Holt PE, Gibbs C. Congenital urinary incontinence in cats: a review of 19 cases. *The Veterinary Record* 1992;130(20):437–442.

39. Cannizzo KL, McLoughlin MA, Mattoon JS, et al. Evaluation of transurethral cystoscopy and excretory urography for diagnosis of ectopic ureters in female dogs: 25 cases (1992–2000). *Journal of the American Veterinary Medical Association* 2003;223:475–481.

40. Samii VF, McLoughlin MA, Mattoon JS, et al. Digital fluoroscopic excretory urography, digital fluoroscopic urethrography, helical computed tomography, and cystoscopy in 24 dogs with suspected ureteral ectopia. *Journal of Veterinary Internal Medicine* 2004;218:271–281.

41. Arnold S, Arnold P, Hubler M, et al. Incontinentia urinae beider kastrierten Hündin: Häufigkeit und Rassedisposition. *Schweizer Archiv fur Tierheilkunde* 1989;131:259–263.

42. Holt PE, Thrusfield MV. Association in bitches between breed, size, neutering and docking, and acquired urinary incontinence due to incompetence of the urethral sphincter mechanism. *The Veterinary Record* 1993;133(8):177–180.

43. Center SA, Smith CA, Wilkinson E, et al. Clinicopathologic, renal immunofluorescent, and light microscopic features of glomerulonephritis in the dog: 41 cases. *Journal of the American Veterinary Medical Association* 1987;190(1):81–90.

44. Richter KP, Ling GV. Clinical response and urethral pressure profile changes after phenylpropanolamine in dogs with primary sphincter incompetence. *Journal of the American Veterinary Medical Association* 1985;187:605–611.

45. Scott L, Leddy M, Bernay F, et al. Evaluation of phenylpropanolamine in the treatment of urethral sphincter mechanism incompetence in the bitch. *Journal of Small Animal Practice* 2002;43:493–496.

46. Nendick PA, Clark WT. Medical therapy of urinary incontinence in ovariectomised bitches: a comparison of the effectiveness of diethylstilboestrol and pseudoephedrine. *Australian Veterinary Journal* 1987;64:117–118.

47. Arnold S, Hubler M, Lott-Stolz G, et al. Treatment of urinary incontinence in bitches by endoscopic injection of glutaraldehyde cross-linked collagen. *Journal of Small Animal Practice* 1996;37:163–168.

48. Grauer GF, DiBartola SP. Glomerular disease. In: *Textbook of Veterinary Internal Medicine*, Vol. 2, 5th edition, eds. SJ Ettinger, EC Nelson, p. 1669. St. Louis, MO: W.B. Saunders; 2000.

49. DiBartola SP, Tarr MJ, Parker AT, et al. Clinicopathologic findings in dogs with renal amyloidosis: 59 cases (1976–1986). *Journal of the American Veterinary Medical Association* 1989;195:358–364.

50. Mason NJ, Day MJ. Renal amyloidosis in related English foxhounds. *Journal of Small Animal Practice* 1996;37:255–260.

51. Chew DJ, DiBartola SP, Boyce JT, et al. Renal amyloidosis in related Abyssinian cats. *Journal of the American Veterinary Medical Association* 1982;181:139–142.

52. DiBartola SP, Tarr MJ, Webb DM, et al. Familial renal amyloidosis in Chinese shar-pei dogs. *Journal of the American Veterinary Medical Association* 1990;197:483–487.

53. Mutsaers AJ, Widmer WR, Knapp DW. Canine transitional cell carcinoma. *Journal of Veterinary Internal Medicine* 2003;17(2):136–144.

54. Norris AM, Laing EJ, Valli VE, et al. Canine bladder and urethral tumors: a retrospective study of 115 cases (1980–1985). *Journal of Veterinary Internal Medicine* 1992;6(3):145–153.

55. Raghavan M, Knapp DW, Dawson MH, et al. Topical flea and tick pesticides and the risk of transitional cell carcinoma of the urinary bladder in Scottish terriers. *Journal of the American Veterinary Medical Association* 2004;225(3):389–394.

56. Chun R, Garrett LD. Urogenital and mammary gland neoplasia. In: *Textbook of Veterinary Internal Medicine*, Vol. 2, 7th edition, eds. SJ Ettinger, EC Feldman, p. 2208. St. Louis, MO: Saunders Elsevier; 2010.

57. Bell FW, Klausner JS, Hayden DW, et al. Clinical and pathologic features of prostatic adenocarcinoma in sexually intact and castrated dogs: 31 cases (1970–1987). *Journal of the American Veterinary Medical Association* 1991;199(11):1623–1630.

58. Sorenmo KU, Goldschmidt M, Shofer F, et al. Immunohistochemical characterization of canine prostatic carcinoma and correlation with castration status and castration time. *Veterinary and Comparative Oncology* 2003;1(1):48–56.

59. Cornell KK, Bostwick DG, Cooley DM, et al. Clinical and pathologic aspects of spontaneous canine prostate carcinoma: a retrospective analysis of 76 cases. *The Prostate* 2000;45(2):173–183.

60. Henry CJ, Turnquist SE, Smith A, et al. Primary renal tumours in cats: 19 cases (1992–1998). *Journal of Feline Medicine and Surgery* 1999;1(3):165–170.

61. Bryan JN, Henry CJ, Turnquist SE, et al. Primary renal neoplasia of dogs. *Journal of Veterinary Internal Medicine* 2006;5: 1155–1160.

62. Moe L, Lium B. Hereditary multifocal renal cystadenocarcinomas and nodular dermatofibrosis in 51 German shepherd dogs. *Journal of Small Animal Practice* 1997;38(11):498–505.

63. Ward MP. Seasonality of canine leptospirosis in the United States and Canada and its association with rainfall. *Preventive Veterinary Medicine* 2002;56:203–213.

64. Holt PE. Surgical management of congenital urethral sphincter mechanism incompetence in eight female cats and a bitch. *Veterinary Surgery* 1993;22(2):98–104.

65. Barth A, Reichler IM, Hubler M, et al. Evaluation of long-term effects if endoscopic injection of collagen into the urethral submucosa for treatment of urethral sphincter incompetence in female dogs: 40 cases (1993–2000). *Journal of the American Veterinary Medical Association* 2005;226:73–76.

Section 4

1. Kobayashi DL, Peterson ME, Graves TK, Lesser M, Nichols CE. Hypertension in cats with chronic renal failure or hyperthyroidism. *Journal of Veterinary Internal Medicine* 1990;4:58–62.

2. Green HW. Feline systemic hypertension: diagnosis and treatment. Proceedings of the NAVC conference, January 19 to 23, 2008, Orlando, pp. 213–215.

3. Cortadellas O, Del Palacio MJ, Bayón A, Albert A, Talavera J. Systemic hypertension in dogs with leishmaniasis: prevalence and clinical consequences. *Journal of Veterinary Internal Medicine* 2006;20:941–947.

4. Jacob F, Polzin DJ, Osborne CA, Neaton JD, Lekcharoensuk C, Allen TA, Kirk CA, Swanson LL. Association between initial systolic blood pressure and risk of developing a uremic crisis or of dying in dogs with chronic renal failure. *Journal of the American Veterinary Medical Association* 2003;222:322–329.

5. Cowgill LD, Kallet AJ. Systemic hypertension. In: *Current Veterinary Therapy IX*, ed. RW Kirk, pp. 360–364. Toronto: W.B. Saunders; 1986.

6. Reine NJ, Langston CE. Urinalysis interpretation: how to squeeze out the maximum information from a small sample. *Clinical Techniques in Small Animal Practice* 2005;20:2–10.

7. Brobst D. Urinalysis and associated laboratory procedures. *Veterinary Clinics of North America. Small Animal Practice* 1989;19: 929–949.

8. Swenson CL, Boisvert AM, Kruger JM, Gibbons-Burgener SN. Evaluation of modified Wright-staining of urine sediment as a method for accurate detection of bacteriuria in dogs. *Journal of the American Veterinary Medical Association* 2004;224:1282–1289.

9. Osborne CA, Sevens JB (eds.). Biochemical analysis of urine: indications, methods, interpretation. In: *Urinalysis: A Clinical Guide to Compassionate Patient Care*, pp. 45–150. Shawnee Mission, KS: Veterinary Learning Systems; 1999.

10. DiBartola SP. Clinical approach and laboratory evaluation of renal disease. In: *Textbook of Veterinary Internal Medicine: Disease of the Dog and the Cat*, 7th edition, eds. SJ Ettinger, EC Feldman, pp. 1955–1969. St. Louis, MO: Elsevier Saunders; 2010.

11. Stockham SL, Scott MA. Urinary system. In: *Fundamentals of Veterinary Clinical Pathology*, eds. SL Stockham, MA Scott, pp. 277–336. Ames, IA: Iowa State Press; 2002.

12. Waldrop JE. Urinary electrolytes, solutes, and osmolality. *Veterinary Clinics of North America. Small Animal Practice* 2008;38: 503–512.

13. DiBartola SP. Renal disease: clinical approach and laboratory evaluation. In: *Textbook of Veterinary Internal Medicine: Disease of the Dog and the Cat*, 6th edition, eds. SJ Ettinger, EC Feldman, pp. 1716–1730. St. Louis, MO: Elsevier Saunders; 2010.

14. Crow SE, Allen DP, Murphy CJ, Culbertson R. Concurrent renal adenocarcinoma and polycythemia in a dog. *Journal of the American Animal Hospital Association* 1995;31:29–33.

15. Gorse MJ. Polycythemia associated with renal fibrosarcoma in a dog. *Journal of the American Veterinary Medical Association* 1988;192:793–794.

16. Peterson ME, Zanjani ED. Inappropriate erythropoietin production from a renal carcinoma in a dog with polycythemia. *Journal of the American Veterinary Medical Association* 1981;179: 995–996.

17. Snead EC. A case of bilateral renal lymphosarcoma with secondary polycythaemia and paraneoplastic syndromes of hypoglycaemia and uveitis in an English Springer spaniel. *Veterinary and Comparative Oncology* 2005;3(3):139–144.

18. Nelson RW, Hager D, Zanjani ED. Renal lymphosarcoma with inappropriate erythropoietin production in a dog. *Journal of the American Veterinary Medical Association* 1983;182:1396–1397.

19. Bryan JN, Henry CJ, Turnquist SE, Tyler JW, Liptak JM, Rizzo SA, Sfiligoi G, Steinberg SJ, Smith AN, Jackson T. Primary renal neoplasia of dogs. *Journal of Veterinary Internal Medicine* 2006;20(5): 1155–1160.

20. Madewell BR, Wilson DW, Hornof WJ, Gregory CR. Leukemoid blood response and bone infarcts in a dog with renal tubular adenocarcinoma. *Journal of the American Veterinary Medical Association* 1990;197(12):1623–1625.

21. Jepson RE, Brodbelt D, Vallance C, Syme HM, Elliot J. Evaluation of predictors of the development of azotemia in cats. *Journal of Veterinary Internal Medicine* 2009;23:806–813.

22. Polzin DJ, Osborne CA, Ross S. Chronic kidney disease. In: *Textbook of Veterinary Internal Medicine: Disease of the Dog and*

the Cat, 6th edition, eds. SJ Ettinger, EC Feldman, pp. 1756–1785. St. Louis, MO: Elsevier Saunders; 2005.

23. Battaglia L, Petterino C, Zappulli V, Castagnaro M. Hypoglycemia as a paraneoplastic syndrome associated with renal adenocarcinoma in a dog. *Veterinary Research Communications* 2005;29(8): 671–675.

24. Grauer GF. Measurement, interpretation, and implications of proteinuria and albuminuria. *Veterinary Clinics of North America. Small Animal Practice* 2007;37:283–295.

25. Elliott J, Syme HM. Proteinuria in chronic kidney disease in cats—prognostic marker or therapeutic target? *Journal of Veterinary Internal Medicine* 2006;20:1052–1053.

26. Syme HM. Proteinuria in cats. Prognostic marker or mediator? *Journal of Feline Medicine and Surgery* 2009;11:211–218.

27. Lyon SD, Sanderson MW, Vaden SL, Lappin MR, Jensen WA, Grauer GF. Comparison of urine dipstick, sulfosalicylic acid, urine protein-to-creatinine ratio, and species-specific ELISA methods for detection of albumin in urine samples of cats and dogs. *Journal of the American Veterinary Medical Association* 2010;236: 874–879.

28. Beatrice L, Nizi F, Callegari D, Paltrinieri S, Zini E, D'Ippolito P, Zatelli A. Comparison of urine protein-to-creatinine ratio in urine samples collected by cystocentesis versus free catch in dogs. *Journal of the American Veterinary Medical Association* 2010;236: 1221–1224.

29. Jacob F, Polzin DJ, Osborne CA, Neaton JD, Kirk CA, Allen TA, Swanson LL. Evaluation of the association between initial proteinuria and morbidity rate or death in dogs with naturally occurring chronic renal failure. *Journal of the American Veterinary Medical Association* 2005;226:393–400.

30. Brown S, Atkins C, Bagley R, Carr A, Cowgill L, Davidson M, Egner B, Elliott J, Henik R, Labato M, Littman M, Polzin D, Ross L, Snyder P, Stepien R. Guidelines for the identification, evaluation, and management of systemic hypertension in dogs and cats. *Journal of Veterinary Internal Medicine* 2007;21:542–558.

31. Acierno MJ, Labato MA. Hypertension in renal disease: diagnosis and treatment. *Clinical Techniques in Small Animal Practice* 2005;20:23–30.

32. Henik RA. Systemic hypertension and its management. *Veterinary Clinics of North America. Small Animal Practice* 1997;27: 1355–1372.

33. Henik RA. Diagnosis and treatment of feline systemic hypertension. *Compendium* 1997;19:163–178.

34. Finco DR. Association of systemic hypertension with renal injury in dogs with induced renal failure. *Journal of Veterinary Internal Medicine* 2004;18:289–294.

35. Ling GV, Norris CR, Franti CE, Eisele PH, Johnson DL, Ruby AL, Jang SS. Interrelations of organism prevalence, specimen collection method, and host age, sex, and breed among 8354 canine urinary tract infections (1969–1995). *Journal of Veterinary Internal Medicine* 2001;15:341–347.

36. Bartges JW. Diagnosis of urinary tract infections. *Veterinary Clinics of North America. Small Animal Practice* 2004;34:923–933.

37. Torres SM, Diaz SF, Nogueira SA, Jessen C, Polzin DJ, Gilbert SM, Horne KL. Frequency of urinary tract infection among dogs with pruritic disorders receiving long-term glucocorticoid treatment. *Journal of the American Veterinary Medical Association* 2005;227(2): 239–243.

38. Lulich JP, Osborne CA. Urine culture as a test for cure: why, when, and how? *Veterinary Clinics of North America. Small Animal Practice* 2004;34:1027–1041.

39. Hamaide AJ, Martinez SA, Hauptman J, Walker RD. Prospective comparison of four sampling methods (cystocentesis, bladder mucosal swab, bladder mucosal biopsy, and urolith culture) to identify urinary tract infections in dogs with urolithiasis. *Journal of the American Animal Hospital Association* 1998;34:423–430.

Section 5

1. Borjesson DL. Renal cytology. *Veterinary Clinics of North America. Small Animal Practice* 2003;33:119–134.

2. Cannizzo KL, McLoughlin MA, Chew DJ, DiBartola SP. Uroendoscopy. Evaluation of the lower urinary tract. *Veterinary Clinics of North America. Small Animal Practice* 2001;31: 789–807.

3. Rawlings CA. Diagnostic rigid endoscopy: otoscopy, rhinoscopy, and cystoscopy. *Veterinary Clinics of North America. Small Animal Practice* 2009;39:849–868.

4. Richter KP. Laparoscopy in dogs and cats. *Veterinary Clinics of North America. Small Animal Practice* 2001;31:707–727.

5. Grauer GF, Twedt DC, Mero KN. Evaluation of laparoscopy for obtaining renal biopsy specimens from dogs and cats. *Journal of the American Veterinary Medical Association* 1983;183:677–679.

6. Vaden SL, Levine JF, Lees GE, Groman RP, Grauer GF, Forrester SD. Renal biopsy: a retrospective study of methods and complications in 283 dogs and 65 cats. *Journal of Veterinary Internal Medicine* 2005;19:794–801.

7. Vaden SL. Renal biopsy of dogs and cats. *Clinical Techniques in Small Animal Practice* 2005;20:11–22.

8. Nash AS, Boyd JS, Minto AW, Wright NG. Renal biopsy in the normal cat: examination of the effects of repeated needle biopsy. *Research in Veterinary Science* 1986;40:112–117.

9. Nash AS, Boyd JS, Minto AW, Wright NG. Renal biopsy in the normal cat: an examination of the effects of a single needle biopsy. *Research in Veterinary Science* 1983;34:347–356.

10. Nyland TG, Wallack ST, Wisner ER. Needle-tract implantation following us-guided fine-needle aspiration biopsy of transitional cell carcinoma of the bladder, urethra, and prostate. *Veterinary Radiology & Ultrasound* 2002;43:50–53.

11. Lamb CR, Trower ND, Gregory SP. Ultrasound-guided catheter biopsy of the lower urinary tract: technique and results in 12 dogs. *Journal of Small Animal Practice* 1996;37:413–416.

12. Bussadori C, Bigliardi E, D'Agnolo G, Borgarelli M, Santilli RA. The percutaneous drainage of prostatic abscesses in the dog. *La Radiologia Medica* 1999;98:391–394.

13. Kawakami E, Washizu M, Hirano T, Sakuma M, Takano M, Hori T, Tsutsui T. Treatment of prostatic abscesses by aspiration of the purulent matter and injection of tea tree oil into the cavities in dogs. *The Journal of Veterinary Medical Science* 2006;68: 1215–1217.

14. Boland LE, Hardie RJ, Gregory SP, Lamb CR. Ultrasound-guided percutaneous drainage as the primary treatment for prostatic abscesses and cysts in dogs. *Journal of the American Animal Hospital Association* 2003;39:151–159.

15. Anderson WI, Dunham BM, King JM, Scott DW. Presumptive subcutaneous surgical transplantation of a urinary bladder transitional cell carcinoma in a dog. *The Cornell Veterinarian* 1989;79: 263–266.

16. Volpe A, Kachura JR, Geddie WR, Evans AJ, Gharajeh A, Saravanan A, Jewett MA. Techniques, safety and accuracy of sampling of renal tumors by fine needle aspiration and core biopsy. *The Journal of Urology* 2007;178:379–386.

17. Rawlings CA, Mahaffey MB, Barsanti JA, Canalis C. Use of laparoscopic-assisted cystoscopy for removal of urinary calculi in dogs. *Journal of the American Veterinary Medical Association* 2003;222(6):759–761. 737.

18. Hager DA, Nyland T, Fisher P. Ultrasound-guided biopsy of the canine liver, kidney and prostate. *Veterinary Radiology & Ultrasound* 1985;26:82–88.

Section 6

1. Feeney DA, Johnston GR. Chapter 42: the kidneys and ureters. In: *Textbook of Veterinary Diagnostic Radiology*, 4th edition, ed. DE Thrall, pp. 556–570. Philadelphia, PA: W.B. Saunders; 2002.

2. Park RD, Wrigley RH. Chapter 43: the urinary bladder. In: *Textbook of Veterinary Diagnostic Radiology*, 4th edition, ed. DE Thrall, pp. 571–587. Philadelphia, PA: W.B. Saunders; 2002.

3. Pechman J. Chapter 44: the urethra. In: *Textbook of Veterinary Diagnostic Radiology*, 4th edition, ed. DE Thrall, pp. 588–592. Philadelphia, PA: W.B. Saunders; 2002.

4. Samii VF, McLoughlin MA, Mattoon JS, et al. Digital fluoroscopic excretory urography, digital fluoroscopic urethrography, helical computed tomography, and cystoscopy in 24 dogs with suspected ureteral ectopia. *Journal of Veterinary Internal Medicine* 2004;18:271–281.

5. Samii VF. Urinary tract imaging. In: *Waltham/OSU Symposium, Diseases of the Urinary Tract*, pp. 15–17. Trenton, NJ: Veterinary Learning Systems; 2003.

Section 7

1. Booth DM. Drugs affecting the kidneys and urination. In: *Small Animal Clinical Pharmacology Therapeutics*, ed. DM Booth, pp. 515–527. Philadelphia, PA: W.B. Saunders; 2001.

2. Polzin DJ. Chronic kidney disease. In: *Textbook of Veterinary Internal Medicine*, 7th edition, eds. SE Ettinger, EC Feldman, p. 1972. St. Louis, MO: Saunders Elsevier; 2010.

3. Lane IF. Treatment of urinary disorders. In: *Small Animal Clinical Pharmacology Therapeutics*, ed. DM Booth, pp. 528–552. Philadelphia, PA: W.B. Saunders; 2001.

4. Willard MD. Treatment of hyperkalemia. In: *Current Veterinary Therapy IX, Small Animal Practice*, ed. RW Kirk, p. 94. Philadelphia, PA: W.B. Saunders; 1996.

5. Devey JJ. Crystalloid and colloid fluid therapy. In: *Textbook of Veterinary Internal Medicine*, 7th edition, eds. SE Ettinger, EC Feldman, p. 494. St. Louis, MO: Saunders Elsevier; 2010.

6. Chew DJ, Dibartola SP, Nagode LA, Starkey RJ. Phosphorus restriction in the treatment of chronic renal failure. In: *Current Veterinary Therapy XI, Small Animal Practice*, eds. RW Kirk, JD Bonagura, p. 853. Philadelphia, PA: W.B. Saunders; 1992.

7. Polzin DJ, Osborne CA. Diseases of the urinary tract. In: *Handbook of Small Animal Therapeutics*, ed. LE Davis, p. 933. New York: Churchill-Livingstone; 1985.

8. Plumb DC. *Plumb's Veterinary Drug Handbook*, 6th edition, Ames, IA: Blackwell; 2008.

9. Quimby JM, Gustafson DL, Samber BJ, et al. The pharmacokinetics of mirtazapine in healthy cats. Abstract in the American College of Veterinary Medicine (ACVIM) 2009 forum, abstract 282.Montreal, Canada; 2009.

10. Quimby JM, Gustafson DL, Samber BJ, Lunn KF. The pharmacokinetics of mirtazapine in cats with chronic kidney disease. Abstract in the American College of Veterinary Medicine (ACVIM) 2010 forum, abstract 315. Anaheim, CA, USA, 2010.

11. Henik RA, Stepien RL, Wenholz LJ, Dolson MK. Efficacy of atenolol as a single antihypertensive agent in hyperthyroid cats. *Journal of Feline Medicine and Surgery* 2008;10(6):577–582.

12. Ross LA. Hypertension and chronic renal failure. *Seminars in Veterinary Medicine and Surgery (Small Animal)* 1992;7:221.

13. King JN, Gunn-Moore DA, Tasker S, et al. Tolerability and efficacy of benazepril in cats with chronic kidney disease. *Journal of Veterinary Internal Medicine* 2006;20(5):1054–1064.

14. King JN, Strehlaw G, Wernsing J, Brown SA. Effect of renal insufficiency on the pharmacokinetics and pharmacodynamics of benazepril in cats. *Journal of Veterinary Pharmacology and Therapeutics* 2002;25(5):371–378.

15. Lefebvre HP, Brown SA, Chetboul V, et al. Angiotensin-converting enzyme inhibitors in veterinary medicine. *Current Pharmaceutical Design* 2007;13(13):1347–1361.

16. Henik RA, Snyder PS, Volk LM. Treatment of systemic hypertension in cats with amlodipine besylate. *Journal of the American Animal Hospital Association* 1997;33(3):226–234.

17. Atkins CE, Rausch WP, Gardner SY, et al. The effect of amlodipine and the combination of amlodipine and enalapril on the renin-angiotensin-aldosterone system in the dog. *Journal of Veterinary Pharmacology and Therapeutics* 2007;30(5):394–400.

18. Kyles AE, Gregory CR, Wooldrige JD, et al. Management of hypertension controls postoperative neurologic disorders after renal transplantation in cats. *Veterinary Surgery* 1999;28(6):436–441.

19. Bond BR. Nitroglycerin. In: *Small Animal Critical Care Medicine*, eds. DC Silverstein, K Hopper, p. 179. St. Louis, MO: Saunders Elsevier; 2009.

20. Pressler B, Bartges JW. Urinary tract infections. In: *Textbook of Veterinary Internal Medicine*, 7th edition, eds. SE Ettinger, EC Feldman, pp. 2036–2047. St. Louis, MO: Saunders Elsevier; 2010.

21. Francey T. Prostatic diseases. In: *Textbook of Veterinary Internal Medicine*, 7th edition, eds. SE Ettinger, EC Feldman, pp. 2055–2056. St. Louis, MO: Saunders Elsevier; 2010.

22. Labato MA, Acierno MJ. Micturition disorders and urinary incontinence. In: *Textbook of Veterinary Internal Medicine*, 7th edition, eds. SE Ettinger, EC Feldman, pp. 160–164. St. Louis, MO: Saunders Elsevier; 2010.

23. Polzin DJ. Linkage between stage of chronic kidney disease and treatment recommendations. Proceedings of the Advanced Renal Therapies Symposium, March 3, 2006.

24. Chew DJ, Dibartola SP, Crisp MS. Peritoneal dialysis. In: *Fluid Therapy in Small Animal Practice*, ed. SP Dibartola, p. 554. Philadelphia, PA: W.B. Saunders; 1992a.

25. Polzin DJ. Classification of acute and chronic kidney disease. Proceedings of the Advanced Renal Therapies Symposium, New York, March 2006.

26. Stokes JE. Diagnostic approach to acute azotemia. In: *Kirk's Current Veterinary Therapy*, 14th edition, eds. JD Bonagura, DC Twedt, p. 856. St. Louis, MO: Saunders Elsevier; 2009.

27. Langston C. Acute uremia. In: *Textbook of Veterinary Internal Medicine*, 7th edition, eds. SE Ettinger, EC Feldman, p. 1972. St. Louis, MO: Saunders Elsevier; 2010.

28. Karriker M. Drug dosing in renal failure and the dialysis patient. In: *Proceedings of the Advanced Renal Therapies Symposium*, pp. 8–12. New York; 2006.

29. IRIS. 2009 Staging of CKD. http://www.iris-kidney.com/education/en/education06.shtml (accessed September 28, 2010).

30. Cowgill LD, Kallet AJ. Systemic hypertension. In: *Current Veterinary Therapy IX, Small Animal Practice*, ed. RW Kirk, p. 360. Philadelphia, PA: W.B. Saunders; 1986.

Section 8

1. Bulger RE, Nagle RB, Dobyan DC. Acute tubular necrosis in the rat kidney following sustained hypotension: physiologic and morphologic observations. *Laboratory Investigation* 1977;Oct;37(4): 411–422.
2. Davies G, Kingswood C, Street M. Pharmacokinetics of opioids in renal dysfunction. *Clinical Pharmacokinetics* 1996;Dec;31(6): 410–422.
3. Harris RJ. Cyclooxygenase-2 inhibition and renal physiology. *The American Journal of Cardiology* 2002;89(6):10D–17D.
4. Hikasa Y, Okuyama K, Kakuta T, et al. Anesthetic potency and cardiopulmonary effects of sevoflurane in goats: comparison with isoflurane and halothane. *Canadian Journal of Veterinary Research* 1998;62(4):299–306.
5. Muir WW, Weise AJ, March PA. Effects of morphine, lidocaine, ketamine, and morphine-lidocaine-ketamine drug combination on minimum alveolar concentration in dogs anesthetized with isoflurane. *American Journal of Veterinary Research* 2003;64(9): 1155–1160.
6. Sun H, Frassetto L, Benet LZ. Effects of renal failure on drug transport and metabolism. *Pharmacology & Therapeutics* 2006; 109(1-2):1–11.

Section 9

1. Jacob F, Polzin DJ, Osborne CA, et al. Clinical evaluation of dietary modification for treatment of spontaneous chronic renal failure in dogs. *Journal of the American Veterinary Medical Association* 2002;220(8):1163–1170.
2. Ross SJ, Osborne CA, Kirk CA, Lowry SR, Koehler LA, Polzin DJ. Clinical evaluation of dietary modification for treatment of spontaneous chronic kidney disease in cats. *Journal of the American Veterinary Medical Association* 2006;229(6):949–957.
3. Elliott J, Rawlings JM, Markwell PJ, Barber PJ. Survival of cats with naturally occurring chronic renal failure: effect of dietary management. *Journal of Small Animal Practice* 2000;41(6):235–242.
4. Elliott DA. Gastrostomy tube feeding in kidney disease. In: *Kirk's Current Veterinary Therapy XIV*, eds. JD Bonagura, DC Twedt, pp. 906–910. St. Louis, MO: Saunders Elsevier; 2009.
5. Adams LG, Polzin DJ, Osborne CA, O'Brien TD, Hostetter TH. Influence of dietary protein/calorie intake on renal morphology and function in cats with 5/6 nephrectomy. *Laboratory Investigation* 1994;70(3):347–357.
6. Brown SA, Finco DR, Crowell WA, Navar LG. Dietary protein intake and the glomerular adaptations to partial nephrectomy in dogs. *The Journal of Nutrition* 1991;121(11 Suppl):S125–S127.
7. Leibetseder JL, Neufeld KW. Effects of medium protein diets in dogs with chronic renal failure. *The Journal of Nutrition* 1991; 121(11 Suppl):S145–S149.
8. Brown SA, Crowell WA, Barsanti JA, White JV, Finco DR. Beneficial effects of dietary mineral restriction in dogs with marked reduction of functional renal mass. *Journal of the American Society of Nephrology* 1991;1(10):1169–1179.
9. King JN, Tasker S, Gunn-Moore DA, Strehlau G. BENRIC (benazepril in renal insufficiency in cats) study group. Prognostic factors in cats with chronic kidney disease. *Journal of Veterinary Internal Medicine* 2007;21(5):906–916.
10. Boyd LM, Langston C, Thompson K, Zivin K, Imanishi M. Survival in cats with naturally occurring chronic kidney disease (2000–2002). *Journal of Veterinary Internal Medicine* 2008;22(5): 1111–1117.
11. Finco DR, Brown SA, Crowell WA, Groves CA, Duncan JR, Barsanti JA. Effects of phosphorus/calcium-restricted and phosphorus/calcium-replete 32% protein diets in dogs with chronic renal failure. *American Journal of Veterinary Research* 1992;53(1):157–163.
12. Barber PJ, Rawlings JM, Markwell PJ, Elliott J. Effect of dietary phosphate restriction on renal secondary hyperparathyroidism in the cat. *Journal of Small Animal Practice* 1999;40(2):62–70.
13. Greco DS, Lees GE, Dzendzel GS, Komkov A, Carter AB. Effect of dietary sodium intake on glomerular filtration rate in partially nephrectomized dogs. *American Journal of Veterinary Research* 1994;55(1):152–159.
14. Greco DS, Lees GE, Dzendzel G, Carter AB. Effects of dietary sodium intake on blood pressure measurements in partially nephrectomized dogs. *American Journal of Veterinary Research* 1994;55(1):160–165.
15. Kirk CA, Jewell DE, Lowry SR. Effects of sodium chloride on selected parameters in cats. *Veterinary Therapeutics* 2006;7(4): 333–346.
16. Buranakarl C, Mathur S, Brown SA. Effects of dietary sodium chloride intake on renal function and blood pressure in cats with normal and reduced renal function. *American Journal of Veterinary Research* 2004;65(5):620–627.
17. Plantinga EA, Everts H, Kastelein AM, Beynen AC. Retrospective study of the survival of cats with acquired chronic renal insufficiency offered different commercial diets. *The Veterinary Record* 2005;157(7):185–187.
18. Brown SA, Brown CA, Crowell WA, et al. Beneficial effects of chronic administration of dietary omega-3 polyunsaturated fatty acids in dogs with renal insufficiency. *The Journal of Laboratory and Clinical Medicine* 1998;131(5):447–455.
19. Elliott J, Syme HM, Reubens E, Markwell PJ. Assessment of acid-base status of cats with naturally occurring chronic renal failure. *Journal of Small Animal Practice* 2003;44(2):65–70.
20. Elliott DA, Riel DL, Rogers QR. Complications and outcomes associated with use of gastrostomy tubes for nutritional management of dogs with renal failure: 56 cases (1994–1999). *Journal of the American Veterinary Medical Association* 2000;217(9): 1337–1342.
21. Lekcharoensuk C, Osborne CA, Lulich JP, et al. Association between dietary factors and calcium oxalate and magnesium ammonium phosphate urolithiasis in cats. *Journal of the American Veterinary Medical Association* 2001;219(9):1228–1237.
22. Stevenson AE, Hynds WK, Markwell PJ. The relative effects of supplemental dietary calcium and oxalate on urine composition and calcium oxalate relative supersaturation in healthy adult dogs. *Research in Veterinary Science* 2003;75(1):33–41.
23. Hawthorne AJ, Markwell PJ. Dietary sodium promotes increased water intake and urine volume in cats. *The Journal of Nutrition* 2004;134(8 Suppl):2128S–2129S.
24. Osborne CA, Lulich JP, Forrester D, Albasan H. Paradigm changes in the role of nutrition for the management of canine and feline urolithiasis. *Veterinary Clinics of North America. Small Animal Practice* 2009;39(1):127–141.
25. Houston DM, Rinkardt NE, Hilton J. Evaluation of the efficacy of a commercial diet in the dissolution of feline struvite bladder uroliths. *Veterinary Therapeutics* 2004;5(3):187–201.
26. Albasan H, Osborne CA, Lulich JP, et al. Rate and frequency of recurrence of uroliths after an initial ammonium urate, calcium

oxalate, or struvite urolith in cats. *Journal of the American Veterinary Medical Association* 2009;235(12):1450–1455.

27. Markwell PJ, Buffington CT, Smith BH. The effect of diet on lower urinary tract diseases in cats. *The Journal of Nutrition* 1998;128(12 Suppl):2753S–2757S.

28. Lekcharoensuk C, Osborne CA, Lulich JP. Evaluation of trends in frequency of urethrostomy for treatment of urethral obstruction in cats. *Journal of the American Veterinary Medical Association* 2002;221(4):502–505.

29. Osborne CA, Lulich JP, Kruger JM, Ulrich LK, Koehler LA. Analysis of 451,891 canine uroliths, feline uroliths, and feline urethral plugs from 1981 to 2007: perspectives from the Minnesota urolith center. *Veterinary Clinics of North America. Small Animal Practice* 2009;39(1):183–197.

30. Cannon AB, Westropp JL, Ruby AL, Kass PH. Evaluation of trends in urolith composition in cats: 5230 cases (1985–2004). *Journal of the American Veterinary Medical Association* 2007;231(4):570–576.

31. Houston DM, Moore AE, Favrin MG, Hoff B. Feline urethral plugs and bladder uroliths: a review of 5484 submissions 1998–2003. *The Canadian Veterinary Journal* 2003;44(12):974–977.

32. Kyles AE, Hardie EM, Wooden BG, et al. Clinical, clinicopathologic, radiographic, and ultrasonographic abnormalities in cats with ureteral calculi: 163 cases (1984–2002). *Journal of the American Veterinary Medical Association* 2005;226(6):932–936.

33. Low WW, Uhl JM, Kass PH, Ruby AL, Westropp JL. Evaluation of trends in urolith composition and characteristics of dogs with urolithiasis: 25,499 cases (1985–2006). *Journal of the American Veterinary Medical Association* 2010;236(2):193–200.

34. Lekcharoensuk C, Osborne CA, Lulich JP, et al. Associations between dietary factors in canned food and formation of calcium oxalate uroliths in dogs. *American Journal of Veterinary Research* 2002;63(2):163–169.

35. Lulich JP, Osborne CA, Thumchai R, et al. Epidemiology of canine calcium oxalate uroliths. Identifying risk factors. *Veterinary Clinics of North America. Small Animal Practice* 1999;29(1):113–122. xi.

36. Hess B, Nakagawa Y, Parks JH, Coe FL. Molecular abnormality of Tamm–Horsfall glycoprotein in calcium oxalate nephrolithiasis. *American Journal of Physiology. Renal Physiology* 1991;260(4):F569–F578.

37. Lekcharoensuk C, Osborne CA, Lulich JP, et al. Associations between dry dietary factors and canine calcium oxalate uroliths. *American Journal of Veterinary Research* 2002;63(3):330–337.

38. McCue J, Langston C, Palma D, Gisselman K. Urate urolithiasis. *Compendium on Continuing Education for the Practicing Veterinarian* 2009;31(10):468–475.

39. Bartges J, Kirk C. Nutrition and urolithiasis. Proceedings from the 25th Annual American College of Veterinary Internal Medicine Forum, Seattle WA, 2007.

40. Buffington CA, Westropp JL, Chew DJ, Bolus RR. Clinical evaluation of multimodal environmental modification (MEMO) in the management of cats with idiopathic cystitis. *Journal of Feline Medicine and Surgery* 2006;8(4):261–268.

41. Markwell PJ, Buffington CA, Chew DJ, et al. Clinical evaluation of commercially available urinary acidification diets in the management of idiopathic cystitis in cats. *Journal of the American Veterinary Medical Association* 1999;214(3):361–365.

Chapter 11 Infectious Diseases

Editors: Jennifer Garcia and Meri Hall

SECTION 1 INFECTIOUS BACTERIAL DISEASES

Bartonella

Bartonella spp. are hemotropic gram-negative bacterium that are known to infect many mammals, including dogs, cats, and humans. *Bartonella* is a zoonotic organism responsible for cat scratch disease (CSD) and other disorders in humans.

Pathogenesis and transmission

Six of the *Bartonella* spp. that are known to infect humans have been isolated from cats and dogs.[1] Cats are the main reservoir host for *Bartonella henselae* and *Bartonella quintana*, but they may likely host other bartonella species as well.[2] Although dogs can be infected with *Bartonella*, their role as a reservoir host is unknown at this time.

The *Bartonella* bacterium is most commonly known to be transmitted by fleas, but other vectors have been implicated, such as ticks and biting lice. Serology testing has shown that a large number of clinically normal cats are positive for exposure to a *Bartonella* spp.

Clinical signs

Bartonella has been associated with several disease processes including endocarditis, uveitis, stomatitis, lymphadenopathy, and neurological and urinary disorders in cats.[3] The high

Small Animal Internal Medicine for Veterinary Technicians and Nurses, First Edition. Edited by Linda Merrill.
© 2012 John Wiley & Sons, Inc. Published 2012 by John Wiley & Sons, Inc.

prevalence rate in healthy cats makes proving *Bartonella*-associated illness difficult. There are a small number of documented cases of clinical manifestations of *Bartonella* spp. in dogs. Cases of infectious endocarditis, meningoencephalitis, granulomatous hepatitis, and cutaneous vasculitis have been attributed to *Bartonella* infection.[4]

Diagnostic testing

There are several testing modalities available for the detection of *Bartonella* in dogs and in cats including blood culture, and polymerase chain reaction (PCR) testing. Proving bartonellosis as cause for clinical illness in cats is difficult due to the large number of clinically healthy cats that test positive for exposure. In contrast, detection of antibodies against *Bartonella* in dogs may provide strong evidence of active infection due to the low seroprevalence in dogs within endemic regions.[4] Clinical manifestation may best be supported by detection of the organism via histology at the site of infection.

Pharmacology and treatment

There are many antibiotics that are effective against *Bartonella* spp. *in vitro*, but studies showed elimination of bacteremia in some patients but not in others.[2] Much of the treatment recommendations have been extrapolated from human literature. Commonly used antibiotics include doxycycline, azithromycin, enrofloxacin, rifampin, and amoxicillin/clavulanate. Resistance to doxycycline may be of concern in canine patients, but doxycycline is considered an appropriate first choice in feline patients with clinical bartonellosis.[2] Resistant cases may respond to combination therapy. Longer-term therapy is often recommended (4–6 weeks). Treatment is only recommended in patients with confirmed or highly suspect cases of *Bartonella*-associated disease and should be considered in patients with immunocompromised owners.

Prevention

Bartonella is transmitted to pets through an arthropod vector. Prevention is primarily achieved through vigorous flea control, although many cats have already been exposed at the time of adoption. This organism has zoonotic potential, especially to immunocompromised people. Pet owners and veterinary personnel should be advised to avoid bites, scratches, and contact with flea excrement. Wounds should be immediately washed with soap and water.

Lyme borreliosis

Borreliosis is a tick-borne bacterial disease caused by the spirochete *Borrelia burgdorferi*. The disease is also known as Lyme disease, named for Lyme, Connecticut, where the disease was first described. Borreliosis is primarily a disease of humans and dogs, although cats can be affected. In the United States, most of the reported cases of Lyme disease occur in the Northeastern and Eastern states and the West Coast.

Pathogenesis and transmission

B. burgdorferi is transmitted by *Ixodes* ticks that acquire the infection by feeding on an infected reservoir host (usually rodents). Transmission requires at least 48 h of tick attachment, during which the organism multiplies in the gut of the tick, migrates into the hemolymph, and travels to the salivary glands to be transmitted in the tick saliva to a new host while the tick feeds. Organisms then migrate from the site of tick attachment to infect other tissues, particularly connective tissue and synovium (thin layer of tissue that lines the joint space), to establish a persistent infection. The host's immune response to the organism appears to be responsible for many of the clinical signs.

Clinical signs

Most dogs are asymptomatic. The most often noted well-characterized clinical manifestation of canine borreliosis is polyarthritis. Clinical signs include fever, anorexia, lethargy, lymphadenomegaly, stiff gait, shifting leg lameness, and joint swelling. Lameness is usually first manifested in the limb closest to the site of tick attachment (oligoarthropathy). Lyme disease has also been associated with a progressive renal disease in dogs and in humans. In dogs with presumed Lyme nephropathy, the clinical signs are those of renal insufficiency (vomiting, anorexia, polyuria/polydipsia, weight loss) and protein-losing nephropathy (peripheral edema, ascites). Labrador and golden retrievers appear to be predisposed to Lyme nephropathy. Neurological disease (neuroborreliosis) is well documented in humans; in dogs, seizures and behavior changes have been attributed to *Borrelia* infection, but the association is poorly documented. Likewise, cardiac arrhythmias have been noted in dogs with evidence of exposure to *Borrelia*, but causality is unclear. Dogs exposed to *Borrelia* do not develop the characteristic cutaneous "bull's-eye" lesion (erythema chronicum migrans [ECM]) at the site of the tick bite seen in humans.

Diagnostic testing

Borreliosis should be considered as a differential for any dog in a Lyme endemic region with shifting leg lameness or progressive nonresponsive renal disease. Animals diagnosed with tick-borne disease have probably been exposed to multiple tick-borne agents, so the possibility of coinfection with other organisms should always be considered.

Laboratory findings

In animals with polyarthritis, the complete blood count (CBC), serum chemistry profile, and urinalysis are expected to be normal; therefore, if thrombocytopenia, leukopenia, anemia, hyperglobulinemia, hypoalbuminemia, or elevated liver enzymes are noted, another cause should be sought because these changes are *not* consistent with a diagnosis of borreliosis. In dogs with presumptive Lyme nephropathy, elevated serum creatinine, blood urea nitrogen (BUN), phosphorus, and cholesterol, hypoalbuminemia, proteinuria, glucosuria, hematuria, and renal casts (cylinduria) are found.

Imaging

There are no imaging findings specific for borreliosis, but imaging studies are useful for ruling out other diseases causing similar clinical signs. In patients with polyarthritis, radiographs may show joint effusion and help characterize the arthritis as nonerosive (consistent with Lyme polyarthritis) versus erosive.

In patients with nephropathy, abdominal ultrasound may help to rule in/rule out other causes of renal failure.

Other diagnostic tests

Specific diagnostic tests for borreliosis detect *Borrelia* antigen (PCR) or detect *Borrelia*-specific antibody (indirect fluorescent antibody [IFA], enzyme-linked immunosorbent assay [ELISA], Western blot). Demonstration of the organism provides definitive diagnosis of infection (culture, cytology, or histopathology with silver or immunohistochemical stains). PCR can be performed on fluid or tissue samples: Samples of synovium or skin from the region of the tick bite are more likely to contain organisms, so are preferred samples for analysis. Serology is often used to make a clinical diagnosis of borreliosis, but no serologic technique can distinguish exposure versus infection. Tests that identify antibody directed against the C6 peptide of the *Borrelia* organism, which is expressed only when the organism is transmitted to the dog via a tick bite, are able to distinguish natural exposure versus vaccination. This includes the point-of-care SNAP4DX® test used by many small animal practices as a screening test for tick-borne disease agents and heartworm. Arthrocentesis and joint fluid analysis and culture should be performed in patients with polyarthritis. Joint fluid typically shows increased cell counts, predominantly neutrophils. Cultures provide definitive diagnosis if positive but require several weeks to complete and may be negative in the face of active infection because of low organism numbers. Cerebrospinal fluid (CSF) from patients suspected to have neuroborreliosis may be normal or may show mild mononuclear pleocytosis and mild increases in protein. Differential *Borrelia* antibody concentration between CSF and serum may provide better evidence of neuroborreliosis. A presumptive diagnosis of borreliosis may be made if the patient has a history of potential exposure, is seropositive for anti-C6 peptide antibody, has clinical signs consistent with Lyme borreliosis, other differentials have been ruled out, and a rapid response to appropriate antibiotic treatment is observed.

Pharmacology and treatment

Borreliosis is treated with antimicrobials. Doxycycline (10 mg/kg PO q 24 h for a minimum of 4 weeks) is used most commonly because of its effectiveness, relative safety, and reasonable cost. Doxycycline also has the added benefit of being effective for coinfection with some other tick-borne agents. Amoxicillin,

ceftriaxone, erythromycin, and azithromycin are also effective. Ceftriaxone and azithromycin are used to treat humans with refractory disease. Clinical improvement of acute arthritis is often evident within 24–48 h of initiating antibiotic therapy (potentially longer if the patient is treated later in the infection). It is uncertain if treatment completely clears the organism from treated animals and relapse can occur after antibiotics are discontinued. Some treated dogs remain *Borrelia* positive by PCR or culture of tick attachment sites but do not have recurrence of clinical signs. Patients with Lyme nephropathy should be treated intensively for renal failure in addition to antibiotic therapy. The prognosis for patients with Lyme nephropathy is grave. For asymptomatic dogs that are seropositive for *Borrelia*, current recommendations are *not* to treat with antibiotics but to monitor them two to four times per year for proteinuria.

Prevention

Borrelia bacterins and subunit (OspA antigen) vaccines are commercially available for dogs but their use is much debated. Studies of vaccine effectiveness have indicated some protection against clinical illness in seronegative dogs. There are significant concerns about use of a vaccine to stimulate an immune response to *Borrelia* bacterial antigens when much of the clinical illness associated with borreliosis is due to the patient's immune response against the organism in joints or immune-complex disease in the kidneys; that is, vaccination may make the patient worse. If a vaccine is used, it has been recommended that puppies are vaccinated early before exposure (9–12 weeks of age with a second dose 2–4 weeks later). Immunity with vaccination is short-lived and yearly revaccination would be required. It is unclear if bacterins or subunit vaccines are the better choice. Discussion on vaccination can also be found in Chapter 12.

Control of tick exposure by avoiding tick-infested areas and routine use of tick-control products to treat individual animals and to treat premises are important components of borreliosis control. If attached ticks are found on the animal, prompt removal may minimize transmission of *Borrelia* organisms from the tick (which requires 48–72 h of tick attachment). Ticks should be removed carefully to ensure removal of the head and mouthparts and to avoid crushing the tick to prevent exposure to hemolymph. Most pet supply companies market special instruments designed to safely remove attached ticks.

Nutritional considerations

Patients with renal dysfunction should be fed appropriate renal diet formulations that are restricted in protein and sodium content.

Anesthetic and analgesia considerations

Anesthetized patients with borreliosis should be monitored for cardiac arrhythmias, though the association with cardiac abnormalities is weak. Lameness usually responds rapidly to antibiotic treatment, but additional analgesic medication can be beneficial.

Non-steroidal anti-inflammatory drugs are preferred to corticosteroids. The use of anti-inflammatory/analgesic medications can complicate the interpretation of clinical response to antibiotics.

Canine brucellosis

Brucellosis is a significant cause of reproductive loss and infertility in animals as well a potential zoonotic disease of humans. The causative agent is an intracellular, gram-negative coccobacillus or rod-shaped bacteria from the family Brucellaceae. Various species exist, each primarily infecting and being maintained by a limited number of reservoir hosts. For the canid species, *Brucella canis* is of main concern, although *Brucella abortus*, *Brucella melitensis*, and *Brucella suis* have been isolated from dogs.

Pathogenesis and transmission

The route of infection is mainly by ingestion and via contact with the genital, oronasal, and conjunctival mucosa. Transmission through broken skin may also occur. Postabortion fetuses, fluids, placentas, and vaginal discharge from infected females either during heat, breeding, or postwhelp are common infective materials, all containing very high numbers of the brucella bacteria. Postabortion shedding can occur for 4–6 weeks. Once infection occurs, bacteremia usually ensues within 3 weeks. The intracellular bacteria eventually localize within the reproductive (steroid-dependent) tissues such as the prostate and epididymis of the male and the uterus of the female.[5] Asymptomatic carriers, especially of the male species, often propagate the disease. The male prostate and epididymides serve as excellent reservoirs from which the bacteria can spread. Significant shedding can occur in the semen of dogs for up to 2 months after infection with intermittent shedding of smaller numbers occurring for years after. Other excretions such as urine, feces, saliva, milk, and oral and nasal secretions can contain bacteria. A common route of transmission from dog to dog is venereal, hence the need to do serologic testing of both the male and female prior to mating.

Clinical signs

Clinical signs of the disease are variable and it is unusual for dogs to appear seriously ill. Many infections are asymptomatic. Reproductive failure in a male or female dog should prompt testing for *B. canis*. Lymphadenitis is typical and can be regional, based on the infection site, or generalized. Clinical signs such as lethargy, inappetance, weight loss, and poor performance may be noted. Occasionally, diskospondylitis, uveitis, endophthalmitis,[6] pyogranulomatous dermatitis, endocarditis, and meningoencephalitis have been reported. By far, the most common sign in healthy appearing females is abortion and stillbirths occurring between 45 and 60 days of gestation. Some pups delivered alive, fade and die in a short period due to infection with the bacteria. A copious brown to gray green mucoid discharge for 1–6 weeks classically follows an abortion. Early embryonic death at 2–3 weeks of pregnancy may occur (typically venereal infection). This is often misdiagnosed as conception failure.[7]

In male dogs, epididymitis, scrotal edema, and orchitis occur as the hallmark signs. Morphological abnormalities, agglutination, and reduced viability of spermatozoa may be noted. Prolonged infections often lead to unilateral or bilateral atrophy of the testes. Males often become infertile.

Diagnostic testing

Bacterial isolation of *B. canis* will give a definitive diagnosis of the disease. Early in the course of the disease (before the body has had time to react), this is the preferred method. The ideal media for testing is blood agar, although the bacteria will grow on most common aerobic media. Bacterial growth is quite slow, leading to overgrowth by contaminant bacteria and false-negative results.

Serologic evaluation will provide a presumptive diagnosis of *B. canis*. Serologic tests vary in sensitivity and specificity, leading to false negatives and positives, depending on the stage of the disease and the test conducted.[7] The use of a combination of tests or repetitive testing will assist with drawing a definitive conclusion (Table 11.1.1).

Currently, the common protocol for serologic testing is to use a rapid slide agglutination test (RSAT) with or without 2-mercaptoethanol (2-ME) for initial screening. This test is rapid, is commercially available (D-Tec CB, Synbiotics, San Diego, CA), can be performed on site, and is sensitive. Results give a high percentage of false positives even with the addition of the 2-ME, but false negatives are rare. Hence, one can screen out negative animals and do further testing on positive animals. The confirmatory test for the RSAT test is the agar gel immunodiffusion (AGID) using cell wall antigen or cytoplasmic antigen from *B. canis*. The use of cytoplasmic antigen appears the most specific. Laboratories currently qualified to conduct the AGID testing include Cornell University, the University of Florida, and the Tifton Veterinary Diagnostic and Investigational Laboratory in Georgia.[5]

In a breeding kennel, any animals testing positive must be eliminated either by neutering and removal or euthanasia. Euthanasia is recommended due to the zoonotic potential of the disease.[8] Transmission to humans appears low and is of greatest significance to young people and immunosuppressed individuals. All animals should test negative prior to entering a breeding kennel or prior to mating to prevent the spread of the disease.

Pharmacology and treatment

Brucella's intracellular nature makes treatment challenging, if not impossible. The bacteria remains sequestered within immune cells with episodic bacteremia. Combinations of antibiotics over prolonged periods have proved most successful with relapse common after treatment. Combinations found successful are tetracyclines (tetracycline HCl, chlortetracycline, doxycycline, minocycline) and dihydrostreptomycin. Gentamicin has been used in place of dihydrostreptomycin.[5] Recent evidence has shown that enrofloxacin is an alternative option, potentially a

Table 11.1.1 Serologic tests for *Brucella canis* in the dog

Serologic test	Antigen	Time frame for positive results	Comments
2-ME-RCAT	Cell wall	8–12 weeks after infection to 3 months after the animal is abacteremic	Very sensitive; false-positive results are common; few (1%) false-negative results are reported; easy and fast
2-ME-TAT	Cell wall	10–12 weeks after infection to 3 months after the animal is abacteremic	Semiquantitative; false-positive results are possible
AGID test	Cell wall	12 weeks after infection to 4 months after the animal is abacteremic	Test procedure is complex; more specific than 2-ME-RCAT
AGID test	Cytoplasmic	12 weeks after infection to 36 months after the animal is abacteremic	Most specific serologic test but not sensitive, detects chronic cases when other tests give negative results
ELISA	Cell wall	Unknown (expect time to be similar to that observed with the TAT)	Very specific, less sensitive than TAT, limited availability
ELISA	Cytoplasmic	Unknown (expect time to be similar to that observed with AGID-cytoplasmic)	Very sensitive and specific, detects chronic infection, limited availability

RCAT, card slide agglutination test; 2-ME, 2-mercaptoethanol; TAT, tube agglutination test; AGID, agar gel immunodiffusion; ELISA, enzyme-linked immunosorbent assay.
Source: Adapted from Johnston SD, Root-Kustritz MV, Olson PN. *Canine and Feline Theriogenology.* Philadelphia, PA: W.B. Saunders; 2001.

single treatment drug but probably best as a partner antibiotic to one of the above-listed drugs.[6,7,9]

Prevention

Currently, there is no vaccine available; testing dogs and bitches prior to mating remains the best preventative. Since it is a zoonotic disease, people should wear standard personnel protective equipment, especially when handling aborted materials and infected or suspected infected canines to help prevent human infection.

Ehrlichiosis

Ehrlichiosis is a bacterial disease caused by obligate intracellular gram-negative coccobacilli that infect circulating monocytes and granulocytes in vertebrate hosts. Ehrlichiosis primarily affects dogs; cats are affected rarely. The causative organisms of canine monocytic ehrlichiosis (CME), the major ehrlichial disease of dogs, include *Ehrlichia canis*, *Ehrlichia chaffeensis*, *Ehrlichia ruminantium*, and *Neorickettsia risticii*, of which *E. canis* is the most common and the most pathogenic. Canine granulocytic ehrlichiosis (CGE) is associated with *Ehrlichia ewingii*. *Ehrlichia* are transmitted by ticks. *E. canis* can also be transmitted via blood transfusion and is one of the agents that should be considered in screening potential blood donors.

Pathogenesis and transmission

Ticks acquire the infection by feeding on a bacteremic vertebrate host and transmit the infection during subsequent feeding. During a 1- to 3-week incubation period, the inoculated organisms multiply in mononuclear cells and disseminate throughout

the body, where they may subsequently be associated with a multitude of clinical signs related to which tissues are affected. Clinical illness occurs in three phases: acute, subclinical, and chronic. In the acute phase, dogs are often febrile and anorectic. Nasal discharge, lymphadenomegaly, and evidence of vasculitis (petechiation, edema) may be present. Thrombocytopenia, mild anemia, and leukopenia are often present. The acute phase lasts for 2–4 weeks in untreated dogs, after which clinical signs resolve as dogs enter the subclinical phase, which may last for months to years. In this phase, dogs are still infected but are clinically normal, although mild thrombocytopenia usually persists. Immunocompetent dogs may clear the infection in this phase; otherwise, dogs may remain lifelong carriers or may enter the chronic phase, which can be associated with severe disease, especially in young dogs and in German shepherds.

Clinical signs

In acute CME, clinical signs may be nonspecific signs of inflammatory disease (fever, anorexia, lethargy, lymphadenomegaly). More severely affected dogs may develop petechiation/ecchymosis, neurological abnormalities, muscle pain, peripheral edema, or dyspnea. Clinical signs may be severe and can include weight loss and debilitation, anterior uveitis, overt bleeding, neurological abnormalities, polyuria/polydipsia due to renal insufficiency, and secondary infections as a result of bone marrow suppression. Fever is common in both the acute and chronic phases. CGE is generally manifested as polyarthritis.

Diagnostic testing

Ehrlichiosis should be considered as a differential for any dog with thrombocytopenia, uveitis, vasculitis, polyarthritis, unexplained fever, or hemorrhagic disease. Because animals with tick-borne disease have potentially been exposed to multiple tick-borne agents, the possibility of coinfection with other organisms should always be considered when a tick-borne disease like ehrlichiosis is diagnosed.

Laboratory findings

Thrombocytopenia and mild anemia are the most consistent CBC abnormalities in animals with monocytic ehrlichiosis and are present in over 80% of affected dogs. Thrombocytopenia often precedes the onset of clinical illness and persists through the subclinical phase of the disease. The white blood cell (WBC) count is variable and may show leukopenia or leukocytosis. Lymphocytosis may be seen. Some patients have pancytopenia. Serum biochemical abnormalities may include hyperglobulinemia, hypoalbuminemia, and elevated liver enzymes (alanine aminotransferase [ALT], alkaline phosphatase [ALP]). Elevated BUN and creatinine may be present in patients with interstitial inflammation of the kidney associated with chronic ehrlichiosis. A urinalysis may show proteinuria and/or hematuria. Hyperglobulinemic patients further evaluated by protein electrophoresis usually have a polyclonal gammopathy, but a monoclonal pattern is sometimes seen. E. canis is an important differential for monoclonal gammopathy; in this regard, the disease can mimic plasma cell tumors/multiple myeloma. Patients undergoing bone marrow aspiration for further evaluation of cytopenias may show plasmacytosis, which again must be distinguished from multiple myeloma as a cause. CSF from patients with neurological manifestations of ehrlichiosis may show increased protein concentration and mononuclear pleocytosis.

Imaging

Imaging studies are frequently done in animals with ehrlichiosis before a diagnosis is made as part of the overall assessment and diagnostic evaluation of patients with thrombocytopenia, fever, musculoskeletal pain, or respiratory signs. However, there are no imaging findings characteristic of ehrlichiosis. Lymphadenomegaly and/or splenomegaly may be present due to lymphoid and plasma cell hyperplasia in response to infection or splenic sequestration of red blood cells and platelets. Interstitial to alveolar lung patterns may be evident on thoracic radiographs as a result of vasculitis or hemorrhage. In animals with joint involvement, radiographs may show evidence of joint effusion and soft tissue swelling. Although nonspecific for ehrlichiosis, imaging studies are useful for ruling out other diseases causing similar clinical signs.

Other diagnostic tests

Definitive diagnosis is made by demonstrating the presence of the organism in an animal with compatible clinical signs. Intracellular Ehrlichia morulae may be observed on peripheral blood smears or buffy coat smears, but morulae are generally present in low numbers during the initial phase of infection, so cytology is not sensitive for identifying infection. Collection of samples from a peripheral capillary bed such as an ear margin can increase the likelihood of demonstrating morulae. Culture of the organism is not used clinically because of low sensitivity and relatively high cost. Clinical diagnosis is generally based upon serology (detection of antibody to Ehrlichia spp. by IFA at a commercial laboratory or point-of-care SNAP4DX test) or PCR (detection of Ehrlichia-specific DNA). A presumptive diagnosis of ehrlichiosis may be made if compatible clinical signs are present in a seropositive dog, but positive serology is not a definitive test. Dogs may be seropositive because of cross-reaction among some other tick-borne agents or because of exposure or subclinical infection with Ehrlichia. Dogs with ehrlichiosis can be seronegative so a negative serology does not rule out the disease. PCR detects organism-specific DNA in blood, CSF, joint fluid, aqueous fluid, and tissues and therefore documents infection, not just exposure. PCR becomes negative quickly with antibiotic treatment, so samples for PCR should be collected before treatment is initiated. Many commercial laboratories offer tick-borne disease panels, which include tests for multiple tick-borne agents; most include testing for E. canis.

Pharmacology and treatment

Ehrlichiosis is treated with antimicrobials. Doxycycline (10 mg/kg PO q 24 h for 4 weeks) is used most commonly because of its effectiveness, relative safety, and reasonable cost.[10] Chloramphenicol (20 mg/kg PO q 8 h for 4 weeks) is also effective and may be used instead of tetracyclines to avoid yellowing of erupting teeth in young dogs but is generally not used because of the risk of serious side effects in humans exposed to the drug and because potential side effects in animals (thrombocytopenia, anemia, pancytopenia) parallel the abnormalities already present in ehrlichiosis patients. Enrofloxacin is not effective in eradicating Ehrlichia. In resistant infections, imidocarb (5 mg/kg IM, repeat administration in 15 days) may be effective. Clinical improvement is rapid following initiation of treatment. Fever is expected to resolve, and platelet counts begin to rise within 24–48 h concurrent with general improvement in the attitude and activity of the patient. Platelet counts usually normalize in the first 2 weeks of treatment. If patients fail to show improvement in the first few days, the accuracy of the diagnosis should be reevaluated. It is uncertain if treatment completely eliminates the organism as treated animals may remain seropositive, but treated animals can be considered clear of infection if clinicopathologic abnormalities (thrombocytopenia, hyperglobulinemia, anemia, leukopenia) have resolved.

In addition to antimicrobial therapy, some patients will require supportive care with intravenous fluid therapy and potentially blood transfusions for anemia. Glucocorticoids at immunosuppressive doses (prednisone or prednisolone 1–2 mg/kg PO q 12 h for 7–14 days depending on response then attempt to taper) may be necessary to treat severe thrombocytopenia where secondary immune-mediated destruction is believed to contribute to the platelet loss. Infection with Ehrlichia does not confer permanent immunity and dogs can be reinfected after successful treatment. Reinfection is likely in dogs maintained in endemic areas.

Prevention

No vaccines are available for protection against ehrlichiosis. Prevention centers on control of tick exposure by avoiding tick-infested areas and by the routine use of tick-control products to treat individual animals and to treat premises. If attached ticks are found on the animal, prompt removal may minimize transmission of tick-borne pathogens. Ticks should be removed carefully to ensure removal of the head and mouthparts and to avoid crushing to prevent exposure to hemolymph. A number of devices designed for the safe removal of attached ticks are available from pet supply companies. Ehrlichiosis is a reportable disease in some states of the United States, but reporting requirements vary; reporting regulations for a given practice area should be verified to ensure compliance.

Nutritional considerations

Patients with renal dysfunction should be fed appropriate renal diet formulations that are restricted in protein and sodium content until organ function normalizes.

Anesthetic and analgesia considerations

Renal dysfunction, vasculitis, anemia, and clotting abnormalities put ehrlichiosis patients at increased risk of anesthetic and surgical complications.

Helicobacter-associated disease

Helicobacter species are gram-negative, urease-positive, microaerophilic, spiral-shaped, flagellated, motile bacteria related to Campylobacter and Arcanobacter.[11,12] Most are 4 to 8 μm long and 1 to 2 μm in diameter.[13] Helicobacter organisms have been found in the gastric mucous layer, closely adhered to the gastric epithelial or parietal cells, or invading gastric mucosa.[14] Helicobacter felis, Helicobacter bizzozeronii, Helicobacter salomonis, Flexispira rappini, and Helicobacter heilmannii have been recovered from the stomachs of dogs, and H. felis, Helicobacter pametensis, Helicobacter pylori, and H. heilmannii have been found in the stomachs of cats. Additionally, nongastric species of Helicobacter have been isolated from the intestines and livers of small animals.[11]

Over 30 organisms characteristic of Helicobacter, not all pathogenic, are known, and each varies in its preferred animal host and in the type and degree of disease that it causes. Collectively, these organisms are known as gastric Helicobacter-like organisms (GHLOs).[11] H. pylori has been acknowledged for its role in chronic gastritis, gastroduodenal ulcers, and neoplasia in humans.[15,16] However, it is a mistake to apply directly what is known about H. pylori infection in humans to other species. Gastric spiral bacteria have been documented in monkeys, foxes, and pigs, and have been associated with gastritis in cats, dogs, ferrets, and cheetahs.[14] The clinical significance of Helicobacter spp. in cats and dogs is still controversial, and there is no evidence that Helicobacter infection in cats and dogs leads to gastric ulceration or neoplasia.[12] Pets have been implicated in the zoonotic transmission of H. heilmannii and H. felis to a small number of humans with gastritis.[17]

Although it has been speculated that H. pylori could have zoonotic potential, no correlation between pet ownership and human H. pylori infection has been shown.[16]

The prevalence of GHLOs is very high in cats and dogs, but infection appears to be asymptomatic in most. Up to 100% of clinically healthy pet cats and dogs are infected with a GHLO and gastric biopsies in 57–76% of cats and in 61–95% of dogs with chronic vomiting revealed GHLOs.[11,13] (see Figure 11.1.1). Living conditions may be important to transmission since shelter or colony animals show higher prevalence than pets,[11] and Helicobacter spp. may be cultured from the feces of children in underdeveloped countries.[14] This is consistent with a proposed fecal–oral route of transmission. Oral–oral transmission is also hypothesized, although the exact route of transmission is unclear.

Pathogenesis and transmission

H. pylori causes chronic superficial gastritis in humans by the disruption of the gastric mucosal barrier, secretion of cytotoxins, increased gastrin production, and the production of inflammatory cytokines. However, GHLOs are not thought to interfere with gastric acid production in animals.[13] The urease produced by Helicobacter species breaks down urea into ammonia, which is directly toxic to epithelial cells, and bicarbonate ions, providing a buffer that allows the bacteria to survive the low pH gastric environment.[16] In cats and dogs, inflammation and glandular degeneration does not always accompany Helicobacter infection, and studies have found no correlation between the number of organisms found and the degree of inflammation.

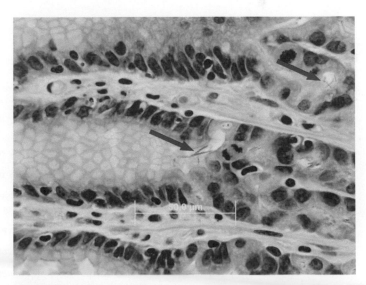

Figure 11.1.1 Spiral GHLO organisms in the gastric mucosa of a clinically healthy cat (red arrows). Hematoxylin and eosin stain, ×100 magnification. Courtesy of Dr. A. Gal, University of Illinois at Urbana-Champaign.

Demonstrating a clear relationship between GHLO colonization and gastric inflammation in cats and dogs has been difficult. Coinfection with multiple GHLO species also makes assigning species pathogenicity difficult.[11]

Clinical signs

Most humans and animals infected with GHLOs are asymptomatic. Clinical signs most commonly reported in dogs and in cats are chronic vomiting and diarrhea, although inappetence, weight loss, fever, and polyphagia may also be seen.[14] Belching, lip smacking, repeated swallowing, and regurgitation have been reported as well.[13]

Diagnostic testing

Testing for GHLO organisms in cats and dogs may be invasive (requiring gastric or duodenal biopsy samples) or noninvasive. The only way to confirm the presence of *Helicobacter* in veterinary patients is through direct observation using invasive methods. A common approach in human medicine is to use an invasive technique for initial diagnosis and a noninvasive technique to document eradication.[14,16] The techniques described differ in how sensitive to and specific for *Helicobacter* infection they are[16] (see Table 11.1.2).

Laboratory findings

There are no abnormalities on routine CBC, serum chemistry, urinalysis, or fecal evaluation that are characteristic of helicobacteriosis; results are often normal or may show evidence of dehydration or other consequences of vomiting (electrolyte disturbance, acid–base abnormality).

Circulating antibodies against *Helicobacter* spp. may be detected using ELISA test kits. IgG test kits designed for humans may not identify animals infected with a GHLO since they are designed to detect antibodies against *H. pylori*, which is rarely found in animal patients.[13]

Stool antigen ELISA tests to detect active infection are also available, but their accuracy may be compromised by gastrointestinal (GI) bleeding.[16]

The PCR of GHLO DNA from a biopsy sample, gastric juice, or dental plaque provides a diagnosis and identification of the particular species. This method is superior to histology and rapid urease testing when colonization density is low, but PCR availability may be limited.[11]

Urea breath and blood tests indirectly measure the ammonia produced by the action of the enzyme urease, which is expressed by *Helicobacter* organisms. A special urea substrate labeled with a carbon isotope is ingested by the patient, and the carbon dioxide containing the labeled carbon is released and can be measured either in the patient's blood or in exhaled air. The urea breath test is the preferred method to assess for eradication of the bacteria since it detects active infection by *Helicobacter* spp. However, false-negative results are possible if colonization levels are low or if the patient has been treated with proton pump inhibitors or histamine receptor antagonists, which decrease the urease activity of *Helicobacter* spp.[13,16]

Imaging

Abdominal imaging studies (radiographs, ultrasound) are frequently performed in assessing patients with a clinical problem of vomiting and are useful to rule out other causes of these clinical signs, but helicobacteriosis does not generally result in imaging abnormalities.

Biopsy techniques

Gastric biopsy via endoscopy or laparotomy remains the standard technique for the diagnosis of helicobacteriosis in small animal patients. Histopathology of gastric biopsy samples stained

Table 11.1.2 Methods used to diagnose *Helicobacter* infections

Method	Sensitivity	Specificity	Invasiveness	Notes
Bacterial culture	Up to 90%	100%	Biopsy required	Sensitivity varies with laboratory expertise
Rapid urease test	88–100%	88–100%	Biopsy required	Commercial assays available
Histology	>90%	100%	Biopsy required	
PCR	High	High	May use biopsy specimen, gastric juice, or dental plaque	Sensitivity varies with the primers used
Urea breath test	>95%	>95%	Noninvasive	May be done on blood or breath
Stool antigen test	>92%	>92%	Noninvasive	
Antibody ELISA	60–100%	60–100%	Noninvasive	Commercial assays available

Modified from Flatland B. *Helicobacter* infection in humans and animals. *The Compendium on Continuing Education for the Practicing Veterinarian* 2002;24:688–696.

with special silver, Giemsa, or toluidine blue stains allows the observation of *Helicobacter* spp. and the evaluation of the degree of inflammation or lymphoid follicle hyperplasia in gastric tissue. Distribution of the organism in the stomach may be patchy, so biopsy samples must be obtained from the gastric antrum, corpus, and cardia. Additionally, the distribution of GHLO in cats appears to be predominantly in the antrum of the stomach, while in dogs the distribution seems to be in the fundus and body.[13] Cytology by Diff-Quik® or Gram stain of a touch prep or brush cytology specimen offers a simple, rapid diagnostic test for GHLO, but it does not allow the extent of inflammation to be assessed.[11]

Bacterial culture of organisms retrieved by biopsy is difficult, requiring special culturing media and conditions,[17] but it is the only way to determine sensitivity to specific antibiotics, and it is considered the gold standard of the invasive diagnostic tests.[16]

Electron microscopy may be used to identify certain *Helicobacter* spp. based on their morphology, but caution must be used since organisms may lose their typical *in vivo* morphologies when cultured.[11]

Commercially available rapid urease tests detect the breakdown of urea into ammonia by the urease produced by *Helicobacter* spp. in a biopsy sample (see Figure 11.1.2). Though diagnosis of active infection may be obtained in about an hour, false-positive readings may result from other urease-producing bacteria in the sample or from contamination with blood from an ulcer. False-negative readings may result when bacterial numbers are low.[16]

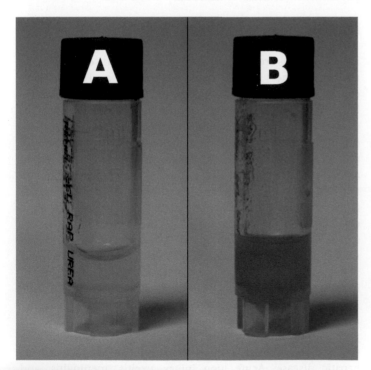

Figure 11.1.2 A commercially available rapid urease test (A) prior to exposure to urease-producing bacteria and (B) after. The urease produced by the *Helicobacter* organisms hydrolyzes urea to ammonia, raising the pH and changing the color of the phenol red in the medium from yellow to pink.

Pharmacology and treatments

Asymptomatic humans with *H. pylori* infection are generally not treated and, likewise, it is recommended that treatment for GHLO infection in pets be restricted to those with obvious clinical signs and histological evidence of infection only when no other cause for gastritis can be found.[13,16]

Helicobacter can be difficult to eradicate in dogs and cats, and reinfection or recrudescence after treatment is possible. Although numerous protocols have been described, combination therapies consisting of an antisecretory drug such as an H2 antagonist or a proton pump inhibitor and two different classes of antibiotic for 2–4 weeks seem to be effective and minimize drug side effects and the potential for antibiotic resistance. Commonly recommended antibiotic combinations include metronidazole with amoxicillin, tetracycline or clarithromycin, or amoxicillin with clarithromycin[17-19] (see Table 11.1.3). The optimal duration of treatment is unclear and treatment may not eradicate the bacteria. Eradication should be confirmed 4–8 weeks after the end of treatment.[14,16]

Nutritional considerations

Patients that are vomiting or are inappetent should receive nutritional support to maintain caloric intake. Small-volume feedings of fat- and protein-restricted diets may be better tolerated until secondary gastric discomfort and dysmotility are resolved.

Leptospirosis

Leptospirosis is a bacterial disease of humans and wild and domestic animals caused by *Leptospira interrogans* and *Leptospira kirschneri*. *Leptospira* are aerobic gram-negative spirochetes.

There are over 200 subtypes (serovars) of *Leptospira* that are pathogenic; these serovars are associated with host animals that act as reservoirs of infection. There are at least eight serovars (*L. interrogans*: Autumnalis, Bataviae, Bratislava, Canicola, Hardjo, Icterohaemorrhagiae, Pomona; *L. kirschneri*: Grippotyphosa) infectious to dogs and cats. Individual serovars have particular reservoir hosts that develop asymptomatic or mild infections but remain carriers, shedding the organism and maintaining it in the environment (Autumnalis—mouse; Bataviae—dog, mouse, rat; Bratislava—rat, pig, horse; Canicola—dog; Grippotyphosa—opossum, raccoon, skunk; Hardjo—cow; Icterohaemorrhagiae—rat; Pomona—cow, opossum, pig, skunk).

Pathogenesis and transmission

Animals may become infected by direct transmission of the spirochete (direct contact with infected urine or blood, ingestion of infected tissues, bite wound, and venereal or placental transfer). More commonly, animals become infected by indirect

Table 11.1.3 Sample protocols for treatment of *Helicobacter* infections

Protocols	Drug	Drug type	Dose	Route	Frequency	Notes
Protocol 1	Amoxicillin	Antibacterial	20 mg/kg	PO	q 12 h	
	Metronidazole	Antibacterial	10–20 mg/kg	PO	q 12 h	62.5 mg total in cats
	Famotidine	Antisecretory	0.5 mg/kg	PO	q 12 h	
	Bismuth subcitrate	Coating agent	6 mg/kg	PO	q 12 h	
Protocol 2	Tetracycline	Antibacterial	22 mg/kg	PO	q 8 h	
	Metronidazole	Antibacterial	10–20 mg/kg	PO	q 12 h	62.5 mg total in cats
	Ranitidine	Antisecretory	1–2 mg/kg	PO, IV	q 12 h	3.5 mg/kg in cats, PO
	Bismuth subsalicylate	Coating agent	0.5–1.0 mg/kg	PO	q 12 h	Use with caution in cats.
Protocol 3	Clarithromycin	Antibacterial	7.5–10.0 mg/kg	PO	q 12 h	
	Omeprazole	Proton pump inhibitor	0.5–1.0 mg/kg	PO	q 24 h	

Modified from Happonen I, Linden J, Westermarck E. Effect of triple therapy on eradication of canine gastric helicobacters and gastric disease. *Journal of Small Animal Practice* 2000;41:1–6; Fox JG. Enteric bacterial infections. In: *Infectious Diseases of the Dog and Cat*, 3rd edition, ed. CE Greene, pp. 343–351. St. Louis, MO: W.B. Saunders; 2006; Lieb MS, Duncan RB. Gastric *Helicobacter* spp. and chronic vomiting in dogs. In: *Kirk's Current Veterinary Therapy XIV*, 14th edition, eds. JD Bonagura, DC Twedt, pp. 492–497. St. Louis, MO: W.B. Saunders; 2009.

transmission (exposure to water, soil, food, or fomites contaminated by infected urine). Leptospires enter the body by penetrating mucous membranes or through abraded or water-softened skin, enter the bloodstream, and multiply and spread rapidly; this leptospiremic phase lasts 7–10 days during which the organism can spread widely to tissues throughout the body. The kidney, liver, spleen, central nervous system (CNS), eyes, and genital tract are common sites impacted by disseminated infection. The resulting clinical signs depend on which tissues are affected and the severity of the tissue damage. Leptospires penetrate and proliferate in renal tubular cells where they can cause acute injury and acute or chronic renal failure. *Leptospira* persist in the renal tubules of animals surviving the infection despite neutralizing antibody production and clearing of the leptospiremia by the host. These chronically infected carrier animals may then shed the bacteria for months to years postinfection. After shedding into the environment, the organisms can survive for weeks to months in contaminated water and moist soils. Risk factors for leptospirosis include outdoor activities, exposure to wildlife or livestock (maintenance hosts), and exposure to moist environments or standing water. Flooding is associated with sudden increases in disease rates. Leptospirosis is a zoonotic disease: Humans are susceptible to infection by a number of different serovars and become infected by direct or indirect transmission from animal reservoirs. Most human infections are asymptomatic or associated with a mild, flu-like illness, but severe disease, including renal failure, liver dysfunction, meningitis, respiratory failure, bleeding diatheses, and death can occur. Risk factors for human leptospirosis include contact with domestic animals (veterinary personnel, farm workers, and slaughterhouse personnel), exposure to potentially contaminated environments (forestry workers, participants in water sports, fishery or rice field workers), and exposure to wild rodent populations (residents of unsanitary urban areas).

Clinical signs

Most infections are subclinical. Typical clinical disease is usually a subacute illness in adult dogs (4–7 years of age) and is more common in hounds, working dogs, and herding breeds, perhaps because of greater exposure related to outdoor activities or contact with reservoir host animals. Younger dogs are more susceptible to severe disease and leptospirosis can sometimes present as a septicemic condition in more susceptible young animals. Cats can become infected but do not become ill and do not become renal carriers. Clinical signs depend on which tissues are affected, and the clinical picture is variable. In acute diseases, nonspecific signs are those of systemic illness (fever, anorexia, lethargy, vomiting, dehydration, and generalized muscle pain) and are consistent with many infectious or inflammatory diseases. Therefore, leptospirosis may not be suspected in these patients unless more specific signs of renal or hepatic injury develop, or if uveitis develops concurrently with enlargement and pain of the kidneys and/or the liver, oliguria/anuria or polyuria/polydipsia, vomiting, and icterus. The classical presentation of leptospirosis is that of acute inflammatory renal or hepatic disease. Acute lung injury, uveitis, meningitis, and abortion/infertility have been reported less frequently. Severe vasculitis, coagulopathy, or disseminated intravascular coagulation (DIC) occurs in some cases. Physical examination findings may include fever, dehydration, injected mucous membranes, icterus, petechial and ecchymotic hemorrhages, conjunctivitis, uveitis, abdominal pain (liver or kidney swelling), muscle pain, or increased lung sounds.

Diagnostic testing

Leptospirosis should be considered as a differential for any dog with acute or chronic renal disease, uveitis, vasculitis, unexplained fever, or hemorrhagic disease.

Laboratory findings

A CBC will usually show an inflammatory leukogram, often with a left shift, and mild thrombocytopenia is present in about one-third of the cases. A serum biochemical profile will show azotemia and hyperphosphatemia in patients with renal involvement and elevated ALT, ALP, and bilirubin in patients with hepatic infection. Hypoalbuminemia may be seen in association with severe hepatic injury or vasculitis. Electrolyte abnormalities (hyponatremia, hypochloremia, and hypokalemia) and metabolic acidosis may be seen. A urinalysis may show glucosuria, proteinuria, granular casts, and isosthenuria due to renal injury or marked bilirubinuria in patients with hepatic disease.

Imaging

Thoracic radiographs may be abnormal in patients with respiratory involvement or vasculitis: Unstructured interstitial, nodular, or patchy alveolar lung patterns may be present. Abdominal imaging may show enlargement of the liver, spleen, and/or kidneys; abdominal ultrasonography may reveal accumulation of fluid around the kidneys and a renal "medullary rim sign" (hyperechoic ring) in cases of renal infection.

Other diagnostic tests

Specific tests for leptospirosis include serology to identify *Leptospira*-specific antibody (the microscopic agglutination test [MAT]) and tests to demonstrate the presence of the organism (PCR, dark-field microscopy, bacterial culture, IFA, and histopathology). The MAT has been widely used as a diagnostic tool for leptospirosis but may be positive due to recent vaccination (within 3 months) rather than infection and may give a false negative result in early phases of infection. Also, with the MAT, there is significant cross-reaction among serovars, which precludes accurate identification of the infecting serovar by this technique. A MAT titer of greater than 1:800 in an unvaccinated animal (>1:3200 in a vaccinated animal) or a fourfold increase of the titer in a convalescent sample (2–4 weeks from the first titer) is considered diagnostic of leptospirosis in animals with compatible clinical signs.

Dark-field microscopy and bacterial culture (leptospires are difficult to grow in culture) are rarely used because of low sensitivity and frequent false-negative results.

PCR assays are sensitive and specific for identifying the presence of the organism. PCR may be run on serum or urine, but urine is the preferred sample. PCR may be positive early in infection before an increase in specific antibody can be detected by MAT but does not distinguish which serovars are present.

Fluorescent antibody (FA) techniques are not commonly used but can identify organisms in fluid or tissue samples and thereby improve the sensitivity of histopathology, which otherwise shows nonspecific changes not limited to leptospirosis.

Because of the zoonotic potential of this infection, all samples from patients with suspected or confirmed leptospirosis should be clearly labeled as such to alert laboratory personnel and others who may handle the samples.

Pharmacology and treatment

Leptospirosis is treated with antimicrobials to eliminate the infecting leptospire bacteria. General treatment of dehydration and electrolyte imbalance and treatment of associated renal failure, hepatic failure, or DIC may also be necessary. Penicillins (penicillin sodium 20,000 IU/kg IV q 4 h) or aminopenicillins (ampicillin 22 mg/kg IV or PO q 8 h or amoxicillin 22 mg/kg PO q 8 h) are used during the initial phase of treatment to clear the leptospiremia. In patients with suspected leptospirosis, immediate initiation of penicillin or aminopenicillin administration is advisable while confirmatory test results are pending. Doxycycline (5 mg/kg PO q 12 h for 2 weeks) is used subsequently to eliminate bacteria from tissues and to prevent renal shedding. About 75–85% of treated patients survive but may have persistent renal or liver dysfunction. CBC and serum chemistry values should be monitored to assess progression or response to therapy and to evaluate for residual liver or renal dysfunction.

Prevention

Vaccination with available *Leptospira* bacterins or subunit vaccines, which help prevent clinical disease and prevent establishment of the carrier state in exposed animals, is recommended for animals at risk. The duration of immunity provided by these products varies from 6 to 13 months, and vaccines differ in which serovars are included. Vaccine-induced immunity is serovar specific. Whole-cell bacterin vaccines have been associated with frequent adverse reactions, which can be minimized by using subunit vaccines or by pretreating with diphenhydramine (2 mg/kg IM) and glucocorticoids (dexamethasone 0.2 mg/kg IM). More information may be found in Chapter 12.

Because leptospirosis can be transmitted from infected animals to humans and other animals, protective measures should be taken when handling leptospirosis patients, their bedding, or laboratory samples to prevent exposure of people and other animals to the disease. Leptospirosis patients or suspects should be isolated from other patients and, if moved, should be transported by gurney or carrier, which can be easily disinfected. The organism is susceptible to bleach and other disinfectants as well as detergents. Urine containment to prevent exposure of personnel and other animals may be achieved by confining the patient to a cage that is easily cleaned and that has complete dividing walls that prevent leakage/run-off of urine to adjacent surfaces. Patients that cannot be managed by complete cage confinement may be transported to a designated area away from access by other animals (designated run or walk area) with urine being captured (disinfectable bowl or disposable container) by an appropriately garbed/gloved attendant. It is important to consider that urine on paws or on the hair coat may cause contamination of surfaces in contact with patients being walked or otherwise repositioned in the hospital environment. Hoses should not be used to clean cages of infected animals because they generate aerosols that can spread the bacteria to people and other animals and distribute the organisms to various surfaces within the facility. Goggles, masks, and gloves are useful in preventing exposure via mucous membranes (eyes, nose, and mouth) and skin contact. Owners should be advised of the zoonotic potential of *Leptospira*. Leptospirosis is a reportable disease in many states of the United States, but reporting requirements vary; reporting regulations for a given practice area should be verified to ensure compliance.

Nutritional considerations

Patients with renal or hepatic dysfunction should receive appropriate diet formulations that are restricted in protein and sodium content until organ function normalizes. In patients with renal or hepatic dysfunction that does not resolve, dietary modifications may be permanent.

Anesthetic and analgesia considerations

Organ dysfunction (kidney, liver, and lung), vasculitis, and clotting abnormalities put leptospirosis patients at increased risk of anesthetic and surgical complications. Additionally, infected patients are a source of disease exposure to personnel handling them, and surgeons would be at particular risk of potential direct exposure to infected tissues.

Methicillin-resistant *Staphylococcus aureus*

There has been an increased incidence of reports of both human- and veterinary-related cases of MRSA in the last several years. The moniker, MRSA, is often used to describe several different types of bacterial infections that are resistant to multiple antibiotics. Other names, such as oxicillin-resistant *Staphylococcus aureus* (ORSA), may be more appropriate in specific instances, but the bulk of the literature is devoted to MRSA.[42]

Anatomy and pathology

All of the numerous species of staphylococci are gram-positive facultative anaerobes that colonize the skin, mucous membranes, and urinary or GI tract in healthy people. In people, up to 60% are colonized with *S. aureus*, but only 1.5% are colonized with MRSA in the nasal passages. In people, there are two location-associated infection models, hospital or health care associated (MRSA-HA) or community associated (MRSA-CA). A newly emerging threat, livestock associated (MRSA-LA), appears to be associated with pig farming.[41] Veterinarians and veterinary technicians appear to be at an increased risk of colonization with MRSA compared with the general public. Livestock veterinarians are at an even higher risk of being carriers.[40]

Virulence varies as many of the strains possess superantigenic toxins or virulence factors, making them even more dangerous. MRSA infections have been isolated from cats, dogs, horses, and several other animal species. Infections are potential zoonoses and owners must be made aware of this (in writing recommended) and given appropriate precautions.

Clinical signs

MRSA can cause lesions on the skin and soft tissues, osteomyelitis, endocarditis, sepsis, pneumonia, or necrotizing fasciitis. The most common lesions associated with MRSA in pet dogs and cats are wound infections and pyoderma. Other reports included otitis and urinary tract infections.

Diagnostic testing

Appropriate samples should be collected as soon as infection is suspected in an animal. If a skin lesion is identified, swabs should be made and submitted for culture and susceptibility testing. Other options for testing include urine culture, blood culture, and airway secretions. It is essential to contact the laboratory used by the clinic before submitting samples to assure the correct testing is available.

Pharmacology and treatment

Topical therapy is the treatment of choice when a skin wound is present. There are several topical treatments that are effective. Mupirocin is a topical antibiotic that is commonly used for the treatment of MRSA. Honey has been reported to be effective against several strains of antibiotic-resistant bacterial infections when applied topically and is very cost-effective. Covering the wound will help minimize spread.

Systemic antimicrobial drugs are recommended for infections that are not limited to the skin alone. These can be used in conjunction with topical treatment if skin lesions are involved as well. Systemic antibiotics should be chosen based on culture and susceptibility results. In general, MRSA infections are resistant *in vivo* (regardless of what the culture and susceptability shows) to B-lactam antimicrobials, and rapid resistance seems to develop to fluoroquinolones. Therefore, these two classes of antibiotics should be avoided if possible. Vancomycin should be reserved only for human use to minimize the risk of developing a vancomycin-resistant strain.

Prevention

Hand washing is essential after handling any animal and can be very helpful in halting the spread of disease. A thorough cleaning of all areas of contact with the infected animal should be done as soon as the area is clear. Barrier clothing (gloves, gowns, and booties) should be used when handling the animal in the clinic.

Ideally, a designated exam room will be assigned for potential infectious diseases and very limited contact with health-care personnel would occur. This room, along with all affected areas, can then be cleaned thoroughly between animals as MRSA can survive in the environment for weeks. Most topical disinfectants will be effective against MRSA.

Infections are usually spread via direct contact and fomites. Dogs and cats should not be allowed to sleep in the same bed as an infected human and vice versa. Most small animal cases are transmitted from owner to pet. Most pig-related cases are transferred from pig to human.

Surveillance should be part of every veterinary hospital and can vary from a highly sophisticated multitier surveillance system to a simple surface swab C&S done monthly. MRSA organisms are increasingly emerging as infections of great concern in both veterinary and human medicine, and infection control measures will assist in limiting the morbidity and mortality in veterinary medicine.

Client education

It is imperative that clients be informed about the transmission and prevention of MRSA. Frequent hand washing along with washing of pet beds/blankets in hot soapy water cannot be overemphasized. Client communication regarding prevention of MRSA must be documented in the medical record. Ideally, a client information sheet will be either created or downloaded and given to each client. Once the client has received this information, it should be documented in the medical record.

Role of the veterinary technician

The veterinary technician is essential in the consistent implementation of established hospital policies, particularly regarding infectious disease. Technicians can encourage others to follow policy guidelines by simplifying the process. The creation of easy-to-follow, simplified, laminated guidelines to hang on cages will go a long way toward encouraging compliance.

Mycobacterial disease

Mycobacterial diseases are caused by bacteria from the order *Actinomycetales* family Mycobacteriaceae. The pathogenic mycobacteria are found in the genus *Mycobacterium*. This genus includes numerous species of saprophytic microorganisms found in water and soil, along with the pathogenic *Mycobacterium* spp. and other pathogenic bacteria. The *Mycobacterium* spp. are morphologically similar, non-spore-forming, nonmotile, aerobic bacteria that are 0.6–1.0 × 1.0–10.0 μm in size.[20] They are classified by their growth in culture, whether they produce granulomatous disease with or without dissemination and if they produce tubercles.[21] Mycobacteria can be diagnosed by needle aspirates, crush preparations of biopsy material, and histology. The organisms are slender rods located within macrophages that stain negatively with Diff-Quick or Giemsa stains. Cultures should also be submitted to determine if the lesions are actually caused by slow-growing bacteria. When submitting suspected samples to a laboratory, microbiology laboratory personnel should be alerted as cultures may present a potential danger for laboratory personnel if the plates are mishandled. Molecular diagnostic techniques such as PCR may give a more definitive diagnosis.

Granulomas are the primary lesions caused by *Mycobacterium* spp. The bacteria survive and replicate within host cells. Mycobacteria are resistant to pH changes, heat, and routine disinfection. The minimum criteria for pasteurization and heat disinfection were developed to kill mycobacteria. They are susceptible to 5% phenol, direct sunlight, and 5% sodium hypochlorite (household bleach) after a contact time of 15 min at room temperature.[21]

Difficult to grow mycobacteria

Difficult to grow *Mycobacterium* spp. requires very controlled techniques to culture.

Mycobacterium Lepraemurium

Mycobacterium lepraemurium is a mycobacteria that is thought to be the cause of feline leprosy. It was first documented during the 1960s in Australia and in New Zealand. It has since been documented in England, Canada, France, the Netherlands and the United States. Bites from infected rats are thought to be the source of infection for cats; however, infection of cutaneous wounds via contaminated soil is also thought to be a cause.[22] Research has revealed that there are several organisms that cause a leprosy syndrome. It appears to be more common in certain geographic regions such as temperate coastal locations, port cities, and inland tropical areas.

Typically, young (under 5 years of age) male cats are infected. The syndrome begins as focal granulomas that are raised, fleshy, painless lesions. They develop rapidly and may ulcerate and rupture. Regional lymph nodes may become involved. Normally, the lesions are found on the limbs and head of infected cats. Some cats develop the lesions on the tongue and nose. It is common for the lesions to occur in only one region of the body, but in some cases, the lesions are found in multiple locations. The organisms can be seen on cytology and range from 2 to 4 μm and do not stain with hematoxylin. *M. lepraemurium* infections can be confirmed by PCR.[21]

Mycobacterium Leprae, Mycobacterium Malmoense, and Mycobacterium Haemophilum

Infections of older cats (older than 9 years) are thought to be caused by *M. leprae*, *M. malmoense*, and *M. haemophilum*. Some infected cats are presented with localized lesions that become widespread and others have generalized lesions from the beginning. Renal disease is commonly seen. Most infected cats are from semirural or rural areas. The causative agent may be a saprophyte that can be found in soil or stagnant water. Cats may become affected after trauma or bites from arthropods. The compromised immune status of older cats may play a part in their inability to fend off infection. Infection is susceptible to antimycobacterial therapy.[23]

Mycobacterium Visibilis

In western Canada and the northwestern United States (Oregon and Idaho), a multisystemic granulomatous mycobacteriosis has been reported. It is caused by *M. visibilis*.[21] Rather than localized, cutaneous lesions, it is characterized by diffuse generalized disease that is disseminated to multiple organs. The bacteria are capable of intracellular survival and the histological findings are dependent upon the immune status of the host. In immunocompromised animals, lesions have minimum lymphoid cells and plasma cells.

Pharmacology and treatment

Due to the slow-growing nature of the organism, determination of drug susceptibility is not possible. Treatment options include surgical removal of the lesions and empirical antimicrobial therapy. The use of surgical removal alone may be beneficial if the numbers of lesions are low. Medical treatment with a combination of drugs may give the best results. Treatment with clofazimine, rifampin, or clarithromycin for at least 2 months after the lesions disappear is the recommended drug protocol.[21]

Care should be taken when working with infected animals. Strict isolation protocols should be adhered to due to the zoonotic potential. Gloves and masks should be worn when working with animals with active lesions.

Canine leproid granuloma syndrome

Canine leproid granuloma syndrome is common in Australia and has been documented in dogs of New Zealand, Brazil, Zimbabwe, Florida, and California. Short-coated breeds are highly affected. Boxer and boxer crosses account for nearly 50% of all reported cases.[21] The causal organism has not been identified, but many of the affected dogs generally have lesions in regions of the body where bites from vectors are seen. This includes the head and particularly the dorsal pinna of the ears. The skin lesions are single or multiple nodules that are circumscribed. The nodules are hard and painless and large lesions may ulcerate. The lesions are subcutaneous and do not involve lymph nodes, internal organs, or nerves. The lesions can be irritating and may cause disfigurement, especially when secondary infection is involved.

Diagnosis is made by the location of the lesions in an at-risk breed. Needle aspirate smears stained with Diff-Quick reveal numerous macrophages, variable lymphocytes and plasma cells, and low numbers of neutrophils. Negative staining medium length bacilli can be seen extracellularly or within the macrophages. The lesions consist of pyogranulomas composed of giant cells, epithelioid macrophages, and scattered small lymphocytes, plasma cells, and neutrophils. Cultures can serve to exclude other mycobacteria as the causal organism. Care must be taken when obtaining samples as saprophytic mycobacteria can be easily cultured from dirt present on the skin of dogs. PCR may be used to confirm diagnosis.

Many cases resolve within 1–3 months with no treatment. Surgical removal or the use of antimicrobials known to have an effect against other mycobacterial diseases may be beneficial. Treatment should continue until lesions have reduced in size (4–8 weeks), but ideally until the lesions are gone.

Slow-growing mycobacteria

Slow-growing *Mycobacterium* spp. can take more than 7 days to months for growth to appear on culture. These include *Mycobacterium tuberculosis* and *Mycobacterium avium* complexes.

M. Tuberculosis, Mycobacterium Microti, M. Avium, Mycobacterium Bovis

M. tuberculosis is a highly pathogenic, slow-growing mycobacterium that can survive in the environment for 1–2 weeks. It is the primary agent for human tuberculosis.[20] The transmission of infection of *M. tuberculosis* to dogs and cats is from humans via respiratory secretions. Cats are more resistant to *M. tuberculosis* than are dogs.

M. avium and *M. bovis* affect cattle. Dogs and cats are not the reservoir hosts for *M. tuberculosis* or *M. bovis*, but they are susceptible to infections caused by both.

M. microti has been identified in cats who hunt; it is also called vole bacillus. It is significant in that cats do not get the infection from people.

M. Bovis

The portal of entry for *M. bovis* is through the GI tract. Dogs and cats acquire *M. bovis* infections from ingestion of contaminated milk or contaminated carcasses. *M. bovis* has been identified in White-tailed deer in Michigan and badgers in the United Kingdom and in Ireland.[20] The significance of wildlife for the spread of *M. bovis* to cattle, cats, and dogs has not been established. Dogs usually excrete the organism from the respiratory tract, and cats via feces. Outside of the host, the organism can survive from 4 days in the summer and up to 28 days in the winter. On farms where the infected cows have been removed, subclinically infected dogs and cats may act as reservoirs for the disease.

M. Avium

M. avium organisms survive for at least 2 years in coastal plains, acidic swamp areas, municipal water supplies, dairy products, and soil. *M. avium* has been identified in deer and in rabbits.

Clinical signs

In dogs and cats, tuberculosis is frequently a subclinical disease. If clinical signs occur, they will reflect the site of infection. If the site of infection is the respiratory system, then bronchopneumonia, lymphadenomegaly, weight loss, anorexia, fever, and a harsh, nonproductive cough may be seen. Hypersalivation, tonsillar enlargement, and ulcerated, chronically draining oropharyngeal lesions may also be evident. If the disease is disseminated from the respiratory system, then pleural or pericardial effusion with dyspnea and cyanosis may be seen. If the primary lesions are in the GI tract, then weight loss, vomiting, diarrhea, and anemia may be seen. Abdominal effusion and enlarged mesenteric lymph nodes are common. GI dissemination results in generalized lymphadenomegaly, fever, anorexia, and weight loss. Sudden death may also occur.

Cats with *M. bovis* infections have developed choroiditis and retinal detachments. In some cases, CNS signs and granulomatous uveitis has occurred. Dogs with *M. avium* infections have extensive granulomatous disease of the mesenteric lymph nodes, liver, bowel, and spleen. Vomiting, diarrhea, fever, hematochezia, lethargy, and weight loss have been observed but may be intermittent.

Diagnostic testing

Laboratory findings are nonspecific and may include moderate leukocytosis and a nonregenerative anemia. Hyperglobulinemia and hypercalcemia are frequently reported with normal to reduced serum albumin levels. Organisms may be seen in leukocytes on blood and bone marrow smears, buffy coat smears, or in urine. In *M. avium* infections, dogs may have increased liver enzymes. Radiographs may reveal visible masses in various organ systems. Metastatic lesions are seen as miliary densities. Tissue aspirates or impression smears should be submitted for cytology. Skin testing is diagnostic for tuberculosis in dogs, but this test is unreliable in cats.[22] Serologic testing is available when skin testing is inconclusive. The standard for diagnosis continues to be bacterial isolation; however, organisms may fail to grow in culture and if they do, may take months to do so.[21]

Pharmacology and treatment

Treatment should be based on cytology or histology diagnosis. No single-agent therapy should be given as drug resistance can occur. Enrofloxacin, doxycycline, and azithromycin have been used for the treatment of the slow-growing mycobacterial disease.

Care should be taken when working with infected animals. Strict isolation protocols should be adhered to due to the zoonotic potential. Personal protective equipment should be worn when working with animals with active lesions.

Fast-growing mycobacteria

Rapid-growing mycobacteria typically will grow within 7 days on cultures. They are free-living saprophytes that can be easily isolated from dirt and water. They include *Mycobacterium smegmatis* and *Mycobacterium thermoresistibile*.

The fast-growing *Mycobacterium* spp. produce mycobacterial panniculitis, pyogranulomatous pneumonia, and disseminated systemic disease. Mycobacterial panniculitis is more common in cats than in dogs. Typically, a penetrating injury allows entry by the mycobacteria. The causative organism has been found in temperate regions of Australia, Finland, Germany, Japan, Canada and the United States.[21]

Infections in cats typically start in the inguinal region and may spread to the subcutaneous tissues of the abdominal wall and perineum. Common injuries such as vehicular trauma and fight wounds that are exposed to dirt or contaminated water can give rise to infection by the fast-growing *Mycobacterium* spp. Early infections can resemble abscesses from cat fights but do not have the typical odor or purulent discharge. Punctate fistulae appear and gradually increase in size and may involve the entire ventral surface of the affected animal, and they may develop a nonhealing wound.[21] Cats typically have a disease that is localized to the skin with the disease rarely developing systemic infections. They may become lethargic, inappetant, febrile, and have weight loss.

Infection in dogs should be suspected with chronic nonhealing wounds that are unresponsive to antimicrobial therapy. The lesions appear as firm to fluctuant subcutaneous swellings that ulcerate, drain, and spread with new lesions at the edge of older lesions.[21] These lesions are typically nonpruritic or painful. Some animals may present with lameness, pain, or fever. Both dogs and cats with pyogranulomatous pneumonia present with fever, inappetance, dyspnea, and cough.

Diagnostic testing

Diagnosis is made by cytology and culture of the discharge or tissue. When preparing the site for sample collection, the skin should be carefully disinfected with 70% ethanol to prevent sample contamination with saprophytic mycobacteria. Fluid obtained by aspiration should be placed immediately into a commercially available mycobacteria culture bottle. For suspected cases of mycobacterial pneumonia, bronchoalveolar lavage specimens, deep bronchial washings or ultrasound-guided transthoracic fine needle aspirates give the best results. Cytology samples should be stained with Diff-Quick stain and typically reveal pyogranulomatous inflammation. Generally, visualizing the organisms is possible.[21]

Pharmacology and treatment

The treatment for mycobacterial panniculitis is dependent on disease severity and on how quickly a diagnosis can be made. Empirical therapy with oral antimicrobials should be initiated until *in vitro* susceptibility data are available. In the United States, clarithromycin is the initial drug of choice since mycobacterial organisms susceptible to this drug are commonly found.[21] In many cases, treatment with antimicrobials is sufficient, but in severe cases, surgical resection is required. Antimicrobial therapy should continue for a minimum of 3–12 months or 1–2 months past clinical resolution of affected tissues.[21]

Mycoplasmal diseases

Mycoplasmas are gram-negative, nonacid fast, aerobic, or facultative anaerobic bacteria that lack cell walls. Mycoplasmal disease and mycoplasmosis are terms pertaining to infections with microorganisms in the genus *Mycoplasma*. Mycoplasmal pathogens can be further categorized into hemotropic mycoplasmas (hemoplasmas) and nonhemotropic mycoplasmas.

Pathogenesis and transmission

Hemotropic mycoplasmas were previously called *Haemobartonella* and eperythrozoon until research in the late 1990s showed that they more closely resembled mycoplasmas.[24] Hemotropic mycoplasmas are epicellular parasites of erythrocytes and can trigger hemolytic anemia of varying severity in infected animals. *Mycoplasma haemofelis*, *Candidatus* (temporary taxonomic term for a noncultivable bacterium), *Mycoplasma haemominutum*, and *Candidatus Mycoplasma turicensis* are the three main hemotrophic mycoplasmal species of cats, while *Mycoplasma haemocanis*, and *Candidatus Mycoplasma haematoparvum* are the main species affecting dogs. Infection in cats is thought to be transmitted by fleas and by the administration of contaminated blood products. Transmission from an infected queen to her offspring via an unknown nonarthropod vector route also occurs. Hemotropic mycoplasmosis is more frequent in cats that are male, live outdoors, are unvaccinated, or have concurrent infections with feline leukemia virus (FeLV) and/or feline immunodeficiency virus (FIV).[25] A role for cat bites as a mode of transmission has been suggested. Transmission in dogs occurs via the brown dog tick (*Rhipicephalus sanguineus*), intravenous or oral administration of infected blood, and possibly *in utero*. Most infections are asymptomatic. Clinical disease is usually restricted to dogs that are immunosuppressed, splenectomized, or have splenic disease.[26]

Many nonhemotropic mycoplasmas are commensals on various mucosal surfaces such as the respiratory tract, urogenital tract, conjunctiva, and colon. These bacteria have also been isolated from the musculoskeletal system, abscesses, and organ parenchyma, probably secondary to spread from mucosal surfaces where the organisms are part of the normal flora. They may therefore cause or contribute to systemic disease in animals that are severely ill due to other disorders, such as immunosuppression.[27]

Clinical signs

Clinical signs of hemotropic mycoplasmosis vary with the degree of anemia, and some animals may be asymptomatic. Coinfection with *Candidatus Mycoplasma haemominutum* may increase the severity of anemia. Lethargy, anorexia, and weight loss are often the primary presenting complaints. Tachycardia, tachypnea, pale mucous membranes, and weakness may be observed. A heart murmur and splenomegaly may also be noted upon physical examination. Jaundice is an inconsistent finding. Fever may be present in the acute phase, but patients may also be normothermic or hypothermic.[28]

Respiratory, joint, genitourinary and GI disease, and cat abscesses have been attributed to nonhemotropic mycoplasma infection. The clinical signs of nonhemotropic mycoplasmosis vary depending on what tissues or organs are affected.

Diagnostic testing

Laboratory

Hemotropic mycoplasmas cause anemia, which can be determined from a packed cell volume or CBC. *M. haemofelis* is the most pathogenic of the feline hemoplasmas and may be identified as coccoid, rod-shaped, or circular organisms in an epicellular location on red blood cells: The organism can be demonstrated on blood smears approximately 50% of the time during the acute phase of infection. Blood smears must be made and evaluated soon after collection of the sample because ethylenediaminetriacetic acid (EDTA) can cause the bacterium to detach from the erythrocytes. Many Romanowsky-type stains can be used, and samples should be taken before antibiotic therapy is initiated. The individual examining the blood smears needs to be able to differentiate these organisms from artifact (stain precipitation), basophilic stippling, Howell–Jolly bodies, and other erythrocyte parasites. The anemia associated with hemotropic mycoplasmosis is regenerative unless there is concurrent infection with FeLV.[29] Spherocytosis and erythrophagocytosis may also be identified. Cats with hemotropic mycoplasmosis should be tested for retrovirus infection: About half of cats with *M. haemofelis*-associated disease are FeLV positive, and immunosuppression associated with retroviral infection may predispose to *Mycoplasma* infection and to more severe clinical disease.

PCR can be a useful diagnostic tool in the evaluation of blood samples or of samples from other body systems. Although this diagnostic tool is more sensitive than blood smears, false negatives may occur in asymptomatic carriers or cats treated with antibiotics due to low numbers of organisms. A positive mycoplasma PCR from other samples (such as from a bronchoalveolar lavage) is difficult to interpret since mycoplasmas are natural commensals of many mucosal surfaces (upper respiratory tract, distal urogenital tract) and their role as a primary pathogen versus an opportunistic invader or contaminated sample is not entirely understood.[30] Bacterial cultures for identification of nonhemotropic mycoplasma can be performed in specialty laboratories, but special transport and growth media (Amies or modified Stuart transport medium, Hayflick medium) and growth conditions are required.[27]

Imaging

Splenomegaly may be evident on abdominal radiographs in cats with hemotropic mycoplasmosis. Dogs with clinical signs due to hemoplasmas may have no spleen due to a prior splenectomy.[31]

Pharmacology and treatment

Susceptibility testing is often unavailable, but mycoplasmas are typically susceptible to tetracyclines, fluoroquinolones, macrolides, and chloramphenicol. Doxycycline is the treatment of choice and is administered at 10 mg/kg PO q 24 h or 5 mg/kg PO q 12 h for 3 weeks. Enrofloxacin may be an alternative choice and can be given at 10 mg/kg PO q 24 h; however, doses of >5 mg/kg can cause retinal damage in cats. None of these antibiotics have been shown to reliably clear the infection,[32] so persistence of a chronic carrier state is likely.

In patients with hemotropic mycoplasmosis, removal of parasitized red blood cells by the reticuloendothelial cells may occur.

Prednisone given at 1–2 mg/kg PO q 12 h is thought to decrease the amount of erythrophagocytosis. Transfusions can be given when deemed necessary. Terminal patients may be hypoglycemic and may require glucose supplementation.[31]

Nutritional considerations

Patients with mycoplasmal infections may be anorectic due to fever, nausea, or systemic illness, and some patients develop GI upset and anorexia related to administration of antibiotics used to treat mycoplasmosis. Nutritional support through highly palatable diets, syringe feeding, or placement of feeding tubes should be provided as needed for inappetant patients.

Anesthetic and analgesic considerations

Mycoplasmosis is not expected to impact anesthesia beyond consideration of anemia and fever. These patients may have underlying disease conditions that may impact the choice of anesthetic agents. Hemotropic mycoplasmosis is not considered to be a painful condition, but analgesic medications may be indicated for patients with musculoskeletal (joint) disease or abscesses associated with nonhemotropic mycoplasmosis.

Plague

Plague is a bacterial disease caused by infection with the gram-negative coccobacillus *Yersinia pestis*. Plague is a zoonotic disease that has been associated with a high number of human deaths throughout history and is classified as a category A bioterrorism agent. *Y. pestis* is widely distributed worldwide except in Australia and occurs in certain regions where its vectors (fleas), animal reservoirs (rodents), and suitable environmental conditions (semiarid to arid) coexist. In the United States, *Y. pestis* is typically found in the western United States, in a region between the Pacific Ocean and the Rocky Mountains, with sporadic outbreaks extending the region of occurrence temporarily into Colorado, Oklahoma, Texas, and Kansas. In cats, the disease occurs more frequently in the summer, although cases may occur at other times of the year as well.

Pathogenesis and transmission

Y. pestis is maintained in the environment by chronically infected rodent reservoir hosts and the fleas that parasitize these rodents (dog and cat fleas are inefficient vectors for plague). Fleas acquire the organism by ingesting blood from a bacteremic rodent host, after which the organism may be cleared by the flea or it may survive and replicate in the gut of the flea. At a subsequent feeding, it is then regurgitated by the flea into the bite wound to transmit the infection to a new animal host. Less commonly, *Y. pestis* can be transmitted via contact with mucous membranes or broken skin, or via inhalation of droplets of respiratory secretions from animals with the respiratory (pneumonic) form of plague. Cats and dogs become infected by ingesting infected rodents or rabbits or potentially by being bitten by infected rodent fleas. Dogs and other canines are less susceptible to plague than are wild and domestic cats.

Clinical signs

In cats, there are three distinct clinical forms of the disease: bubonic, septicemic, and pneumonic plague. Fever is a consistent finding in all forms, although moribund cats may be hypothermic. Other signs include anorexia, weight loss, vomiting, diarrhea, ocular discharge, and oral ulceration; neurological signs may also occur. The most common form is bubonic plague. This form develops from inoculation of *Y. pestis* via the bite of an infected flea or by ingestion of infected tissues (mucous membrane contact). Bacteria are phagocytized by mononuclear cells at the site of exposure (flea bite) then replicate within these cells. The infected cells travel to regional lymph nodes where bacteria continue to replicate and trigger inflammation causing the lymph nodes to enlarge, forming a bubo (the term used to indicate a swollen lymph node in bubonic plague cases). In cats, buboes typically occur on the head and neck with marked submandibular and cervical lymphadenomegaly. These lymph nodes go on to necrose and form abscesses, which may open and drain. If the bubonic form of plague is not treated, the infection may spread hematogenously or via the lymphatics to manifest as septicemic plague. Hematogenous spread of *Y. pestis* can develop with or without the bubonic form and can result in dissemination of infection to any organ or tissue in the body. In cats, the lungs are most commonly affected. Clinical signs of septicemic plague are those of septic shock (fever or hypothermia, tachycardia, hypotension, and DIC) typically progressing to death within 24–48 h after the development of bacteremia. The pneumonic form of plague is the form that carries the highest mortality rate and the poorest prognosis. In cats, the pneumonic form, if it occurs, is usually secondary to the hematogenous or lymphatic spread of *Y. pestis*. In animals with bubonic or septicemic plague, however, primary pneumonic plague can occur via droplet transmission (rarely occurs in cats).

Dogs are more resistant to *Y. pestis* infection and most infections are asymptomatic. Some dogs develop mild disease with transient fever and anorexia, and rarely, lymphadenomegaly.

Diagnostic testing

Animals suspected of having plague are often treated presumptively before a definitive diagnosis is obtained: It is important to collect samples for diagnostic testing then to initiate therapy, as rapid treatment can decrease the mortality rate associated with this disease. Plague is often suspected and treatment initiated based on geographic location (likelihood), clinical signs, and some diagnostic evidence (such as cytology).

Laboratory

Cats with septicemic plague may show marked leukocytosis and thrombocytopenia. Elevated fibrinogen degradation products (FDPs), decreased fibrinogen levels, and prolonged clotting times may be present in cats with DIC. Elevated liver enzymes and hyperbilirubinemia may be seen in cats with hepatic involvement. Definitive diagnosis is based on demonstrating the organism or demonstrating a specific serologic response to the organism. Diagnosis can be attempted from cytology of tissues. Cytology of blood smears or fine needle aspirate samples of affected lymph nodes (buboes) or affected tissues may show gram-negative bacteria, which may be present in large numbers in infected tissues.

FA testing on impression smears of exudates or aspirate samples can be done to confirm the presence of the organism. Serologic testing can be done, but paired acute and convalescent titers 2–3 weeks apart are required. A fourfold rise in titers is needed to make a diagnosis. Serology is often negative early in the infection. High titers can persist for over 1 year in cats surviving infection, but infection does not confer immunity to reinfection. The organism can also be identified by bacteriologic culture of blood, exudate, or tissue samples collected before initiation of treatment. Because of the significant zoonotic potential of the organism, culture should only be performed by specialized laboratories. Caution should be exercised to avoid contact with exudate or infected tissues when obtaining and preparing diagnostic samples.

Imaging

Cats with pneumonic plague show pulmonary changes consistent with interstitial pneumonia or area of necrosis and abscess formation on thoracic radiographs.

Biopsy techniques

Fresh tissue from biopsy of lymph nodes or postmortem sampling of lung, liver, and spleen can be submitted for culture and FA testing. Tissues should be kept moist with sterile nonbacteriostatic saline (i.e., a moistened sterile cotton ball or sterile gauze in a collection tube with the sample). Tissue can be frozen for transit times exceeding 24 h. Formalin or other preservatives should *not* be used.

Treatment and pharmacology

Patients with suspected plague should be hospitalized in isolation facilities for the first 3 days of antibiotic treatment, and all personnel should exercise extreme caution when handling infected animals or diagnostic samples. At-home treatment is inadvisable due to the risk of human exposure. Aminoglycosides are the most effective antibiotics for *Y. pestis*. Enrofloxacin is an acceptable alternative for patients with renal disease. Tetracyclines or chloramphenicol may be used to treat the bubonic form and for prophylaxis. Often, a combination of medications (aminoglycoside and doxycycline) is used. Penicillins are *not* efficacious. Injectable antibiotics are preferred for the first 3 days of treatment to avoid contact with oral secretions and to reduce the risk of bite injury to hospital personnel. Infected cats should be treated for a minimum of 21 days or until at least 3 days past the resolution of buboes and pneumonic changes. If the bubonic form is present, buboes/abscesses should be lanced and flushed with a chlorhexidine solution. In addition to instituting antimicrobial therapy for *Y. pestis*, affected animals and their environment should be treated to eradicate fleas, which may harbor infection.

Prevention

All caretakers should wear surgical masks, eyewear, and disposable hospital gowns during the initial three days of antibiotic treatment. The pneumonic form is of particular danger to others as inhalation of infected droplets may initiate pneumonic plague in veterinary staff or in others exposed to the patient. The infectious droplets can be generated via coughing, sneezing, or during lancing of the abscesses. If a patient has pneumonic plague, it is essential that everyone in the hospital is aware of the risk of droplet or airborne spread. Humans should seek medical attention immediately in the face of known exposure (bite, scratch, and contact with fluid) or acute onset of febrile illness. The incubation period for bubonic plague in people is 2–6 days; the incubation for pneumonic plague is much shorter at 1–2 days. Most human fatalities are related to delayed antimicrobial therapy.

Nutritional considerations

The cat's nutritional status should be monitored closely. If prolonged anorexia is present, a feeding program (consisting of pharmacological and/or feeding techniques) to manage the inappetent patient should be initiated.

SECTION 2 FUNGAL DISEASES

Infectious fungal disease

Systemic fungal infections are infections that enter from a single port of entry and are then disseminated throughout the body. The clinical signs are dependent upon the organ(s) involved but typically are cough, exercise intolerance, dyspnea, weight loss, fever, and lymphadenopathy. The most common point of entry is the respiratory system. If the GI system is the point of entry, then severe diarrhea and weight loss may be noted.

Accurate diagnosis involves demonstrating the presence of the organism in tissue by means of culture, histopathology, or molecular techniques. When submitting suspected systemic fungal samples to a laboratory, microbiology laboratory personnel should be alerted to the suspected causative agent. Serology may be used to support the diagnosis, but most assays determine the presence of antibody and may only indicate prior exposure and not an active infection.

Histoplasmosis

Histoplasmosis is a systemic fungal infection that originates in the lungs, or potentially the GI tract, and disseminates to the lymph system, bone marrow, eyes, liver, and other organs. The causative agent is the fungus *Histoplasma capsulatum*. When cultured at 25°C, the colonies grow in 7–10 days.[1] In nature, it is a soil saprophyte that can survive a wide range of temperatures. Additional information on histoplasmosis can be found in Chapter 8.

Most cases in the United States occur with geographic distribution following the Mississippi, Missouri and Ohio rivers in the central states.[1]

Pathogenesis and transmission

Histoplasmosis is an infectious agent but not a contagious disease, as it is spread from the environment but not from animal to animal. Infection usually occurs by a respiratory route after the animal inhales infective conidiophores. In dogs, ingestion of the conidia also occurs. The incubation period in dogs is 12–16 days, and lymphatic dissemination to the lungs, GI system, eyes, adrenal glands, bone marrow, spleen, and liver can occur. Cats may be more susceptible to infection than dogs. In cats, the incubation period is 12–16 days, and lymphatic dissemination to the lungs, eyes, liver, and bone marrow can occur. Animals younger than 4 years of age are at an increased risk.

Clinical signs

Feline histoplasmosis occurs most frequently in cats under 4 years of age. There is no breed or sex predilection. The disease is usually nonspecific with clinical findings of great variety due to the multisystemic nature of the infection. Common clinical signs range from weight loss, pale mucous membranes, anorexia, depression, and fever. In about half of the animals affected, tachypnea, dyspnea, or abnormal lung sounds are noted, but coughing is uncommon. In approximately a third of infected animals, lymphadenopathy, hepatomegaly, or splenomegaly is present. Ocular involvement may result in abnormal retinal pigment, retinal edema, anterior uveitis, optic neuritis, granulomatous chorioretinitis, or panophthalmitis. Lameness may occur with fungal osteomyelitis. Multiple small nodules that ulcerate and drain are less commonly noted than with cats infected with blastomycosis. The only common GI sign is anorexia. Oral and lingual ulceration are typically not observed, although cats with hepatic involvement occasionally are jaundiced. Subclinical infection is common.

Canine histoplasmosis also is most commonly seen in dogs less than 4 years of age. Male dogs are affected more frequently than females, with Brittany spaniels and Weimaraners overrepresented.[1] GI signs are more common than respiratory signs in dogs. Early in the disease, large intestinal diarrhea with mucus and fresh blood is common. As the disease progresses, voluminous small intestinal diarrhea associated with protein-losing enteropathy, malabsorption, or both may be seen.

Common clinical signs range from severe weight loss, anorexia, depression, and fever. In less than half of the animals affected, abnormal lung sounds with or without tachypnea, dyspnea, or coughing are seen. In rare cases, pleural effusion may be noted. Occasionally, infected animals show lymphadenopathy, hepatomegaly, or splenomegaly.

Diagnostic testing

Cytology from affected tissues reveals pyogranulomatous inflammation. Intracellular yeast cells 2–4 μm in diameter with a basophilic center and light halo may be noted. In cats, cytology from lymph node aspiration, bone marrow aspiration, bronchoalveolar wash, or transtracheal wash may yield the organism. In dogs, cytology from biopsies and/or aspirations from the liver, lymph nodes, spleen, bone marrow, rectal scrapings, bronchoalveolar wash, or transtracheal wash will typically reveal organisms. Buffy coat smears, pleural or peritoneal effusion cytology, lytic bone lesion aspirates and impression smears or aspirates of skin lesions may also yield organisms.

CBC results commonly show a normocytic-normochromic nonregenerative anemia. Neutrophilia and monocytosis are often seen. In cats, some affected animals will demonstrate a neutropenia or pancytopenia or both. *Histoplasma* organisms are occasionally seen in monocytes or neutorphils. In approximately 50% of affected dogs and 33% of affected cats, thrombocytopenia will occur.

The most consistent blood chemistry abnormality reported is hypoalbuminemia. In cases with hepatic involvement, increases in ALP, total bilirubin, serum ALT, and serum aspartate aminotransferase (AST) may be seen. Hypercalcemia is more common in cats than in dogs.

Samples submitted for culture include bone marrow aspirates, lymph nodes and nodal aspirates, lung, spleen, liver and/or skin nodules, and rectal scrapings from dogs. When submitting samples to a laboratory, microbiology laboratory personnel should be alerted because a culture of *H. capsulatum* does present a potential danger for laboratory personnel if the plates are mishandled.

Serology is an ineffective method of diagnosis as false negatives early in the disease are common[1] and antibody titers are not useful as an assessment tool posttreatment. Antigen testing is now available.

Radiographs of the thorax often reveal a linear or diffuse interstitial pattern.

Pharmacology and treatment

Pulmonary histiomycosis can be a self-limiting disease because it is inapparent and may be confined to the respiratory tract without disseminating to other organs. Antifungal treatment with amphotericin B, ketoconazole, or itraconazole is recommended due to the potential for chronic systemic dissemination. Patients with systemic findings indicative of disseminated histomycosis usually die without treatment.[1] Dogs with GI involvement should be fed a highly digestible diet. Nonspecific therapy for diarrhea should be instituted until clinical signs resolve. Treatment with antifungals for 1-month postclinical signs is recommended. Any animal receiving azole antifungals should be monitored on a monthly schedule with a complete physical examination, including ocular examination and blood work to evaluate liver function.

Aspergillosis

Aspergillosis can be seen as either a localized or a systemic fungal infection.

Localized aspergillosis

The causative agent of the localized form is the fungus *Aspergillus fumigates*. It is more common in dogs than in cats. Localized aspergillosis is typically seen as a sinonasal infection. It may occur as a primary infection or may be secondary to nasal trauma, the presence of a foreign body, or neoplasia. Localized aspergillosis occurs most frequently in young to middle-aged dogs, with German shepherds and rottweilers most commonly affected. It can disseminate to other organs.

Pathogenesis and transmission

Aspergillus spp. is considered normal flora in many animals. When present in the soil, the spores are introduced through broken skin or on the surface of the nasal passages. The mold then develops into plaques within the nasal passages.

Clinical signs

Clinical signs of anorexia, sneezing, facial pain, and copious mucoid to hemorrhagic nasal discharge and crusting have been reported. The colonization can result in the destruction and necrosis of the nasal turbinates and is often accompanied by frontal sinus osteomyelitis. Life-threatening epistaxis can occur with erosion of the nasal vasculature. In severe cases, the cribriform plate, palatine bones, and orbit can become involved. Erosion of the cribriform plate may result in fungal meningoencephalitis and seizures.

Diagnostic testing

Diagnosis is made by direct observation of invasive fungal plaques on the nasal mucosa. A culture positive for aspergillosis from affected tissues supports the diagnosis. Biopsy of affected tissue and a positive histopathologic evaluation is confirmatory. In older dogs with confirmed aspergillosis, a high suspicion of neoplasia as the primary condition must be considered.

Radiography will demonstrate a loss of fine nasal turbinate detail and fluid density in nasal passages. Radiology or computed tomography (CT) is best performed prior to rhinoscopic evaluation to avoid artifacts from tissue manipulation and lavage.

Pharmacology and treatment

Treatment options for sinonasal aspergillosis include surgical removal of the lesions and systemic and topical antifungals. Oral ketoconazole, thiabendazole, fluconazole, and itraconazole and topical enilconazole (compounded) and clotrimazole have been used with fair results. Improved results are seen with intranasal application of enilconazole or clotrimazole. For this procedure, the animal is anesthetized and the medication of choice is instilled via catheterization into the nasal passages.[2]

Disseminated aspergillosis

Disseminated aspergillosis is most commonly diagnosed in animals that are terminally ill from the disease. The disseminated form involves multiple organ systems and the causative agents are *Aspergillus terreus*, *Aspergillus deflectus*, and *Aspergillus flavipes*. German shepherds that are between 2 and 8 years are overrepresented. There appears to be a genetic predisposition to the disseminated form, and dysfunctional mucosal immunity is involved.[2] Affected cats typically have concurrent immunosuppressive diseases and are less than 2 years of age.

Transmission and pathogenesis

In primary infections, aspergillus spores are aerosolized and then inhaled when animals dig in infected soil. It then may disseminate throughout the body.

Clinical signs

The clinical signs are nonspecific and are dependent upon the organ system(s) involved. The most common signs include weight loss, pyrexia, lethargy, anorexia, bone pain, paraparesis, draining sinus tracts, and muscle wasting. Ocular signs of uveitis, endophthalmitis, and chorioretinitis have been reported. Mycotic granulomas of the liver, spleen, intervertebral disks, pancreas, kidneys, lymph nodes, prostate, brain, myocardium, uterus, and thyroid glands have also been seen.

Diagnostics

In addition to the diagnostics for localized aspergillus, serum antibody testing is available, but false negatives may occur.

Pharmacology and treatment

Turbinectomy and rhinotomy have been used, along with systemic and topical antifungal therapy, to surgically treat aspergillosis. Ketoconazole, itraconazole, and fluconazole systemically and clotrimazole topically have been used to medically treat. The prognosis for recovery is poor even with appropriate antifungal therapy and supportive care.

Coccidioidomycosis

Coccidioidomycosis is a systemic fungal infection that originates in the lungs and disseminates to the lymph system, skin, eyes, bones, and other organs. It is commonly referred to as "valley fever" or "valley rheumatism,"[1] and it is found in the southwestern United States, western Mexico, and Central and South America. Young, male, medium to large breed, outdoor dogs are at an increased risk of infection.

The two causative agents are the fungus *Coccidioides immitis* and *Coccidioides posadasii*. In nature, it is a soil saprophyte but the organism can rarely be cultured from the environment.

Pathogenesis and transmission

Routes of infection are inhalation or cutaneous contamination. Coccidioidomycosis can be spread by direct inoculation of body fluids. In tissue, *C. immitis* transforms into a spherule, which undergoes endosporulation and ruptures at maturity. Under correct conditions, such as under bandages, the organism can revert to mycelia form.

Clinical signs

The severity of clinical disease is dependent on the immunocompetence of the host. It can range from subclinical to multisystem dissemination.

Common clinical signs are nonspecific and include severe weight loss, anorexia, cough, fever, lethargy, cervical or head pain, and chronic lameness. Lymphatic dissemination can involve the CNS, eye, pericardium, myocardium, prostate gland, liver, or spleen.

Diagnostic testing

Serologic testing in the early stages of the disease (2–5 weeks) shows increased IgM levels. At 8–10 weeks, complement fixation (CF) testing shows the presence of IgG antibodies. A specific and sensitive PCR has been developed and is the recommended test.

CBC results commonly show a mature neutrophilic leukocytosis, mild anemia, or monocytosis. The most consistent blood chemistry abnormalities reported are hypoalbuminemia and hyperglobulinemia.

Histopathology and serology are currently the best options for diagnosis of coccidiomycosis. Cytology may not yield the infective organism. Cultures may pose a threat to laboratory personnel, who should be alerted to the suspected causative organisms.

Radiography may demonstrate pulmonary and/or skeletal lesions. Coccidioidomycosis is a reportable disease in humans and is a serious biohazard due to the highly infectious nature of *Coccidioides* sp.

Pharmacology and treatment

Treatment with antifungal medication (amphotericin B, ketoconazole, itraconazole, or fluconazole), alone or in combination, for dogs with clinical signs of pulmonary disease is highly recommended and is thought to reduce the potential for dissemination. Treatment is recommended to be continued for a minimum of 4–6 months past clinical signs along with reduced or resolved serologic findings.[3]

Cryptococcosis

Cryptococcosis is a systemic fungal infection that originates in the nasal cavity, paranasal tissue, or lungs and then may disseminate to the CNS, skin, or eyes. The most common causative agents are *Cryptococcus neoformans* and *Cryptococcus gattii*. The subspecies that most commonly causes disease is *Cryptococcus neoformans* var. *neoformans*, which is associated with pigeon droppings. In infected tissue, the organism is a variable-sized yeast. In nature, it is found in areas where pigeons often gather or roost. The *Cryptococcus* organism in the desiccated state can survive up to 2 years in the environment.

It is found worldwide, and the enzootic areas are in the southeastern and southwestern United States and the east coast of Australia. Cats are more commonly infected with cryptococcosis than are dogs.

Pathogenesis and transmission

Infections occur from the inhalation of the yeast from the environment. Infected animals may become asymptomatic carriers. Dissemination can occur by direct extension from the nasal cavity through the cribriform plate to the CNS or to the soft tissue. Dissemination can go to any organ system, but the skin, CNS, and eyes are the most commonly affected.

Clinical signs

The severity of clinical disease is determined by the immune response. An association with FeLV and FIV infections in cats has been reported, as has chronic glucocorticoid use as a predisposing factor in dogs and in cats.[1]

In cats, the clinical signs are usually nasopharyngeal, cutaneous, ocular, upper respiratory, or CNS involvement. The lungs are not normally affected. Typically, sneezing, snuffling, and mucopurulent nasal discharge (either unilateral or bilateral) are reported. Nonspecific generalized clinical signs include depression, anorexia, and weight loss. Soft tissue masses or lesions within the nasal cavity are seen in 70% of cases with respiratory signs.[1] Skin lesions include papules or nodules that may ulcerate and drain. Lymphadenopathy, lameness secondary to osteomyelitis, and renal failure are common. Ocular involvement can include granulomatous chorioretinitis, retinal detachment, panophthalmitis, optic neuritis, and blindness. In cases with invasion through the cribriform plate, the forebrain is most commonly affected due to its close proximity. CNS signs include depression, seizures, circling, blindness, ataxia, cranial nerve deficits, paresis, head pressing, and behavior changes. Cats with concurrent FeLV or FIV infection may be more likely to develop neurological or ophthalmic signs.

Canine cryptococcosis is typically seen in dogs less than 4 years of age. The clinical findings typically seen in dogs include CNS, upper respiratory system, ocular, or cutaneous lesions. Common, nonspecific clinical signs are depression and anorexia. The brain is affected in the majority of dogs with CNS involvement, but the spinal cord may be affected as well. In dogs with CNS involvement, clinical signs include mental depression, vestibular syndrome, ataxia, cranial nerve deficits, seizures, paresis, blindness, hypermetria, and cervical pain. Subcutaneous lesions with ulcerative tracts are often seen on the head, nail beds, and mucous membranes of the mouth and feet. Occasionally, lesions within the ear canals are seen and direct extension into the CNS may occur (Table 11.2.1).

Diagnostic testing

In animals with cryptococcosis, CBC and blood chemistry results are usually normal. Occasionally, a mild nonregenerative anemia with mature neutrophilia or neutrophilia with a left shift may be noted.

Due to the high incidence of CNS involvement, CSF taps or culture and cytology should be considered. In approximately 90% of dogs with CNS involvement, the organisms are visualized.

On thoracic radiographs, nodular infiltrates, pleural effusion, an interstitial pattern, and tracheobronchial lymphadenopathy are occasionally seen. Nasal radiographs may demonstrate bone destruction in the nasal passages and frontal sinuses with soft tissue density.

Nasal swabs, aspirates, subretinal or vitreal aspirates, exudates from cutaneous lesions, and CSF often reveal the organism. Cytology is the easiest and quickest method of identifying cryptococcal organisms.

Serology for the detection of cryptococcal antigen is useful, noninvasive, and should be considered early in the diagnostic process. CSF is the best sample to submit for serologic testing for animals with neurological signs, whereas serum is preferred for upper respiratory or cutaneous signs alone. The preferred test is for the capsular antigen, not antibodies. Most infected animals do not have a humoral response, so antibody titers are not useful diagnostically.

Pharmacology and treatment

Treatment with amphotericin B used alone or in conjunction with itraconazole and fluconazole has proven to be effective in treating cryptococcal infections (see Tables 11.2.2 and 11.2.3). Resolution of clinical signs is the most effective means of monitoring a patient, but serial serologic testing can be of benefit. The prognosis for cats with non-CNS involvement is good. The prognosis for dogs with any form of the disease or cats with CNS involvement is guarded.

Blastomycosis

Blastomycosis is a systemic fungal disease caused by infection with the organism *Blastomyces dermatitidis*. The disease is most common in dogs, especially in young sporting breeds, but can also affect cats. There are marked regional differences in the rate of occurrence of blastomycosis: The disease is endemic in the Ohio and Mississippi River valleys, the southern Great Lakes region, and the mid-Atlantic states.

Pathogenesis and transmission

B. dermatitidis is a dimorphic fungus that exists in the environment in a saprophytic mycelial phase, which produces spores that are inhaled or, less commonly, inoculated by puncture to establish infection in the animal. At body temperature, the fungus transforms into a yeast form, replicates at the site of introduction (usually the lungs), and then may disseminate to other tissues via lymphatics and the bloodstream. The lymph

Table 11.2.1 System involvement in canine cryptococcosis

System involved	Percent of dogs affected (%)
Upper respiratory	50
Integument	10–20
Ocular involvement	20–40
CNS involvement	50–80

Source: Nelson RW, Couto CG (eds.). *Small Animal Internal Medicine*, 4th edition. St. Louis, MO: Elsevier Mosby; 2009.

Table 11.2.2 Antifungal drugs of choice for dogs

Drugs of choice for dogs	Dose	Comments
Amphotericin B—regular	0.25 mg/kg IV as test dose, then 0.5 mg/kg IV up to three times a week 0.05–0.8 mg/kg SQ two to three times weekly	Can be used in combination with fluconazole, flucytosine, itraconazole, or ketoconazole. BUN or creatinine should be monitored prior to each treatment.
Amphotericin B—liposomal or lipid complex	0.5 mg/kg IV as test dose, then 1.0 mg/kg IV three to five times a week	Can be used in combination with fluconazole, flucytosine, itraconazole, or ketoconazole. BUN or creatinine should be monitored prior to each treatment.
Fluconazole	5 mg/kg PO q12–24 h	
Flucytosine	50 mg/kg PO TID	Can be used in combination with amphotericin B
Ketoconazole	10 mg/kg PO q12–24 h	Azole antifungals have been shown to be successful as monotherapy.
Itraconazole	5 mg/kg PO BID for 4 days, then 5–10 mg/kg PO q24 h	Itraconazole is the treatment of choice.

Source: Plumb DC. *Plumbs Veterinary Drug Handbook*, 6th edition. Ames, IA: Blackwell Publishing; 2008; Nelson RW, Couto CG (eds.). *Small Animal Internal Medicine*, 4th edition. St. Louis, MO: Elsevier Mosby; 2009.

Table 11.2.3 Antifungal drugs of choice for cats

Drugs of choice for cats	Dose	Comments
Amphotericin B—regular	0.25 mg/kg IV every other day to three times a week 0.05–0.8 mg/kg SQ two to three times weekly	Can be used in combination with fluconazole, flucytosine, itraconazole, or ketoconazole BUN or creatinine should be monitored prior to each treatment.
Amphotericin B—liposomal or lipid complex	0.5 mg/kg IV as test dose, then 1.0 mg/kg IV three to five times a week	Can be used in combination with fluconazole, flucytosine, itraconazole, or ketoconazole BUN or creatinine should be monitored prior to each treatment.
Fluconazole	50 mg PO q12–24 h	Azole antifungals have been shown to be successful as monotherapy.
Flucytosine	50 mg/kg PO TID	Can be used in combination with amphotericin B
Ketoconazole	10 mg/kg PO q12–24 h	
Itraconazole	50–100 mg/cat PO once daily (may be divided into twice-daily dosing)	3 months or more

Source: DC Plumb. *Plumbs Veterinary Drug Handbook*, 6th edition. Ames, IA: Blackwell Publishing; 2008; Nelson RW, Couto CG. *Small Animal Internal Medicine*, 4th edition. St. Louis, MO: Elsevier Mosby; 2009.

nodes, eyes, skin, and bone are common sites affected by disseminated infection. *Blastomyces* incites a severe suppurative to pyogranulomatous inflammatory response that contributes to the tissue injury and dysfunction in blastomycosis. The disease is not considered to be contagious between individuals, although infection with the tissue yeast phase can be transferred by accidental inoculation with a contaminated needle in the process of sampling infected tissues.

Clinical signs

Unlike other systemic fungal diseases such as histoplasmosis, subclinical infection with *Blastomyces* appears to be uncommon. Although relatively few animals, in areas where the organism is endemic and exposure rates are high, acquire blastomycosis, the reasons for differences in susceptibility to infection are uncertain. In dogs, males are more commonly affected than females, and sporting breeds and hounds are at an increased risk. Other risk factors for dogs include living in proximity to a body of water and living near an excavation site. Small breed dogs are less commonly affected. Most cases occur in young adult dogs of 2–4 years of age, although all ages and breeds can be affected. Clinical signs of blastomycosis reflect which tissues are affected. Because most animals become infected via inhalation of infective spores, respiratory signs are common. Increased respiratory rate and dyspnea may arise because infection and inflammation of pulmonary parenchymal tissue impair oxygen diffusion to the bloodstream, causing hypoxemia. In addition, peribronchial lymph node enlargement may cause extramural compression of the distal trachea and mainstem bronchi, which triggers coughing and may impair ventilation.

Physical examination often reveals increased respiratory rate and effort, harsh lung sounds, and, potentially, cyanosis of mucous membranes. Many dogs have oozing or crusted solitary skin lesions, which usually result from systemic dissemination of fungus from a respiratory infection rather than from cutaneous inoculation. Fever is present in about 50% of clinical cases, and many dogs have generalized lymphadenomegaly. Other findings, consistent with a diagnosis of disseminated blastomycosis, include ocular disease (uveitis, chorioretinitis, glaucoma, vitreal hemorrhage) and lameness (fungal osteomyelitis, joint infection). Inflammatory lesions of the testes or prostate, neurological abnormalities due to CNS involvement, and sneezing or nasal discharge due to nasal infection are less commonly identified. Kidney and urinary bladder infections are uncommon and GI involvement is extremely rare. Generally, extrapulmonary lesions, including skin lesions, should be considered to be manifestations of infection that has disseminated from a primary pulmonary infection (Table 11.2.4).

Diagnostic testing

Laboratory findings

There are no particular clinicopathologic abnormalities that are characteristic of blastomycosis. On a CBC, leukocytosis reflecting a significant inflammatory response to infection is usually present. Mild thrombocytopenia occurs in some cases. Mild elevations of ALT may be present, indicating reactive hepatopathy secondary to systemic inflammation or effects of hypoxemia on liver cells, and hypoalbuminemia may be seen. A minority of patients have hypercalcemia related to the granulomatous inflammation seen with systemic fungal infections. Otherwise, serum biochemical values and urinalysis are usually normal. Pulse oximetry or arterial blood gas analysis will often show hypoxemia of varying degrees depending on the severity of

Table 11.2.4 Frequency of clinical signs—canine blastomycosis

Clinical sign	Percent of dogs affected (%)
Pulmonary signs	65–85
Diffuse lymphadenopathy	40–60
Cutaneous signs	30–50
Ocular involvement	20–50
Febrile	40
Lameness	25
Reproductive system involvement	5–10
Nervous system involvement	<5

Source: Modified from Taboda J, Grooters AM. Systemic mycoses. In: Textbook of Veterinary Internal Medicine, 6th edition, eds. SJ Ettinger, EC Feldman, pp. 671–690. St. Louis, MO: Elsevier Saunders; 2005.

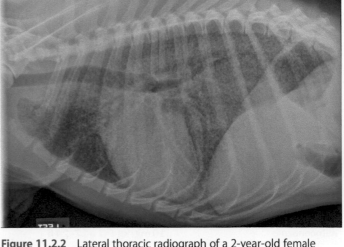

Figure 11.2.2 Lateral thoracic radiograph of a 2-year-old female German shorthaired pointer with fatal blastomycosis showing a diffuse miliary lung pattern.

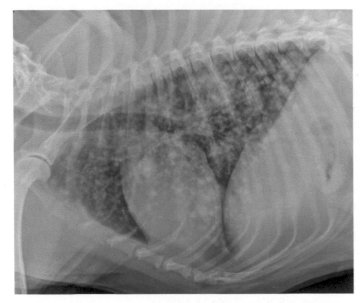

Figure 11.2.1 Lateral thoracic radiograph of a 4-year-old male golden retriever with pulmonary blastomycosis. A diffuse nodular lung pattern with nodules of varying size is present.

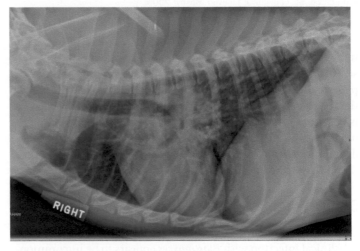

Figure 11.2.3 Lateral thoracic radiograph of a 2.5-year-old male basset hound with pulmonary blastomycosis showing severely enlarged tracheobronchial lymph nodes displacing mainstem bronchi and prominent bronchial pattern.

pulmonary involvement. Arterial blood gas analysis is the test of choice for initial evaluation of respiratory function and for monitoring disease progression and response to treatment in pulmonary cases.

Imaging

Thoracic radiographs are usually abnormal. Diffuse nodular interstitial changes are considered a classical finding in blastomycosis (Figure 11.2.1), but other lung patterns, focal solitary lesions, and pleural effusion are sometimes seen (Figure 11.2.2). Tracheobronchial lymph node enlargement is common and may be severe, causing compression of the carina and mainstem bronchi (Figure 11.2.3). Thoracic radiographs should be obtained

in all cases of suspected blastomycosis because some animals will have lung abnormalities but no respiratory signs. In animals with bone involvement, bone lesions are usually solitary and occur in the limbs; radiographically the lesions are lytic with periosteal proliferation and swelling of adjacent soft tissues.

Other diagnostic tests

Serology is not diagnostic but may provide supportive evidence of exposure to the organism. Some patients with active blastomycosis are seronegative.

An enzyme immunoassay (EIA) for the detection of Blastomyces antigen is available commercially (MiraVista Diagnostics—http://www.miravistalabs.com) and is a useful test for infection in animals in which the organism cannot be demonstrated cytologically. Urine is the preferred sample for Blastomyces EIA, but any fluid (serum, CSF, pleural fluid) can be tested. EDTA interferes with the assay, and blood collected into an EDTA tube should not be used; heparin is an acceptable substitute anticoagulant.

Biopsy techniques

Samples of affected tissues should be obtained for cytological evaluation. Fine needle aspiration of enlarged lymph nodes or other affected peripheral tissues, lung aspiration, arthrocentesis, impression smears of cutaneous lesions, smears of sputum, vitreal aspirates, and transtracheal wash or bronchoalveolar lavage fluid can provide suitable samples for cytology. A definitive diagnosis of blastomycosis is made by demonstrating the organism in infected tissues. *Blastomyces* appears in tissue samples as a thick-walled broad-based budding yeast with associated suppurative to pyogranulomatous inflammation (Figures 11.2.4 and 11.2.5). Sometimes, the organism is difficult to dem-

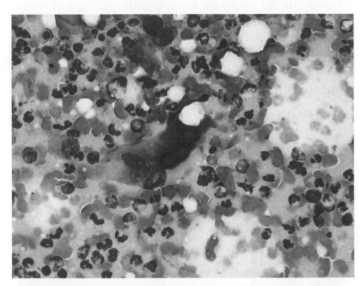

Figure 11.2.4 Fine needle aspirate cytology showing three deep-staining thick-walled yeast (tissue) forms of *Blastomyces* organisms in a background of pyogranulomatous inflammation.

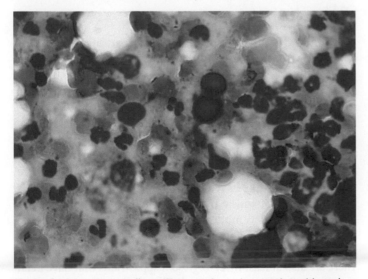

Figure 11.2.5 Fine needle aspirate cytology showing broad-based budding yeast form of *Blastomyces*.

onstrate because of low numbers of yeasts or overriding intensity of the inflammatory response, but a finding of pyogranulomatous inflammation should raise concern about blastomycosis or another systemic fungal infection as a potential underlying cause. Impression smears of cutaneous lesions and vitreal centesis of infected eyes are more likely to yield organisms than sampling of other sites.

Pharmacology and treatment

Animals with clinical blastomycosis do not recover without treatment. Blastomycosis is generally treated with long-term oral administration of itraconazole (dog: 5 mg/kg PO q 24 h; cat: 5 mg/kg PO q 12 h) or fluconazole (dog and cat: 2.5–5.0 mg/kg PO q 12–24 h). Fluconazole is preferred for patients with ocular, CNS, or genitourinary involvement because it crosses the physiological barriers between the blood and brain, eye, and prostate and is excreted in the urine. Treatment should be continued for a minimum of 3 months or until resolution of any evidence of active disease. Patients should be monitored for hepatotoxicity, which may occur with the azole antifungal drugs. Respiratory lesions on thoracic radiographs may persist indefinitely and may represent scarring of lung tissue rather than active infection; if thoracic lesions remain unchanged over 3 consecutive months while on treatment, disease may be considered inactive. Antifungal treatment is expensive because of the relative cost of the drugs and the long duration of administration, especially for the larger breed dogs which are typically affected, in addition to the treatment costs of patient monitoring (serial radiographs, blood work, +/– arterial blood gas, fine needle aspirate cytology). Fluconazole often works out to be less expensive than itraconazole. Pharmacies differ significantly in their pricing for these antifungal drugs, so checking multiple sources to get the best pricing for the client is recommended. Additionally, although generic formulations of itraconazole are available and are much less expensive than the proprietary Sporanox®, some generics have been found to have reduced bioavailability, which may lead to treatment failure. Ketoconazole (dog: 5–15 mg/kg PO q 12 h) may be considered as a less expensive alternative to other antifungal drugs but is less effective against *Blastomyces* and is associated with more frequent and more severe GI side effects and hepatotoxicity. Amphotericin B is an injectable fungicidal drug with good efficacy against *Blastomyces* but is nephrotoxic and requires careful monitoring of renal function. Amphotericin is generally administered via every-other-day dosing as an intravenous infusion of 0.25–0.5 mg/kg q 48 h to a target cumulative dose of 8–10 mg/kg if used as a single agent (4–5 mg/kg if used in conjunction with oral azole antifungals). Drug-associated fever during administration is common. Lipid-complexed formulations of amphotericin (Abelcet®, AmBisome®, Amphocil®) are available that are less nephrotoxic but are more expensive and require higher doses (2–3 mg/kg q 48 h to a cumulative dose of 24–27 mg/kg). Treatment with amphotericin B or, preferably, a lipid-complexed formulation of the drug is recommended for patients with severe disease or for those not responding adequately to oral antifungal agents.

In addition to antifungal drugs, other treatments for respiratory and ocular disease are often necessary. Patients with respiratory dysfunction will often require continuous supplemental oxygen for 4–8 days until respiratory function improves. Bronchodilators may help in some cases. Additional treatment for uveitis (topical corticosteroids and miotics) or secondary glaucoma (carbonic anhydrase inhibitors) may be indicated. Treatment is successful in about three-quarters of the cases. Patients that do not survive are usually those with severe respiratory involvement. Patients that survive the first week of treatment often survive and ultimately respond well to antifungal therapy, but recurrence is common, occurring in about one-fifth of treated patients, generally within the first few months after stopping antifungal drug administration.

Prevention

There are currently no vaccines available for immunization against blastomycosis, but development of an effective vaccine is actively being researched.

Nutritional considerations

Animals with blastomycosis often have increased caloric requirements because of fever and increased work of breathing. However, many are inappetant, and animals with pulmonary involvement may find it difficult to interrupt their breathing efforts in order to eat. Additionally, GI function and motility may be adversely affected by hypoxemia in some patients. Diets that are calorie dense and highly palatable are ideal, and frequent feedings of small volume may be better tolerated. Bulky diets or large meals should be avoided because gastric distension with food may restrict breathing by pressing on the diaphragm.

Anesthetic and analgesia considerations

Virtually all animals with blastomycosis have respiratory involvement, and though the severity of respiratory dysfunction varies from nonclinical to severe, the presence of respiratory disease should be addressed in assessing patient risk for anesthesia. In patients ultimately requiring surgical procedures such as enucleation of an infected glaucomatous eye (frequent in patients with severe ocular involvement) or lung lobectomy (uncommon), surgery should be postponed until the patient has begun antifungal treatment and is stable with good respiratory function.

SECTION 3 PROTOZOAL DISEASES

Protozoal diseases

Protozoans are single-cell organisms that are classified based on their mode of locomotion. The classifications are flagellates (*Giardia* spp., *Leishmania* spp.), coccidian (*Toxoplasma*, *Neospora* spp.), amoeba, ciliates, microspora, and piroplasmia. They range in size from 10 to 52 μm but can grow up to 1 mm. The protozoans typically cause GI tract disease, polysystemic disease, or both.

Amebiasis

Entamoeba histolytica is a parasitic amoeba that predominately infects people and nonhuman primates. The occurance in the United States has declined, but it is still problematic in tropical areas in the world. The trophozoites inhabit the colon lumen and rarely disseminate to other organs. Cysts passed in human feces are infective and transmission is through fecal oral ingestion. Amebiasis is a disease that is transmissible to pets but is seldom transmitted from pets to people. The trophozoites damage the intestine by attaching to the cells where they secrete enzymes that disrupt the intracellular connections.

Usually, the infections are asymptomatic, but signs of severe ulcerative colitis may be seen. Extraintestinal amebiasis is unknown in cats and rare in dogs. Clinical signs in humans refer to the affected tissue.

Diagnosis

Diagnosis of amebiasis in dogs and cats requires identification of trophozoites in the feces or tissues. It is not possible to detect the trophozoites in fecal floatation; however, direct smears of fresh feces will reveal the slow-moving motility of the trophozoite. There is an ELISA-based antigen test that has been shown to be species specific for dogs. The best diagnostic test available is tissue biopsy and histopathology.[1]

Treatment and prevention

If clinical signs are present, metronidazole and furazolidone can be used to eliminate the organism. The only prevention is cleanliness and removal of fecal material from the environment.

Babesiosis

Babesia spp. are piroplasmia, intracellular parasites of erythrocytes. *Babesia canis* has a piriform shape and exists singly or paired within erythrocytes. It is approximately 2.4 × 5.0 μm in size, whereas *Babesia gibsoni* has a pleomorphic shape and exists singly within erythrocytes. It is small in comparison to *B. canis*, measuring approximately 1.0 × 3.2 μm. Babesisosis is transmitted through ticks, blood transfusions, and dog bites. Both have distribution in the United States, Japan, Australia, Africa, Asia, and Europe. *B. canis* is also found in South America. Three strains of *B. canis* spp. have been identified. *Babesia canis rossi* is highly pathogenic and is transmitted by *Haemaphysalis leachi*; *Babesia canis canis* is moderately pathogenic and is transmitted by *Dermacenter reticulates*; and *Babesia canis vogeli* is the least pathogenic and is transmitted by *R. sanguineus* (brown dog tick). There are also at least three *B. gibsoni* spp. strains that have been identified: *California*, *Asia*, and *Theileria annae*, which is a *B. gibsoni*-like organism). In the United States, *B. canis vogeli* is the most common species found in dogs. There is a possibility that dog bites may be a route of transmission of *B. gibsoni*. There are several *Babesia* spp. found in cats throughout the world: in India, *Babesia cati*; in Africa, Europe and South Asia, *Babesia felis*; in South America and Africa, *Babesia herpailuri*; and in Israel, *Babesia canis presentii*. None of these strains have been recognized in America.

Transmission is through ticks, blood transfusions, and dog bites. The organism replicates intracellularly and results in intravascular hemolytic anemia. Immune-mediated reactions to the parasite or against self-antigens worsen the anemia. A positive Coombs test is possible. The severity of the anemia depends on the patient's immune status, species, and strain of *Babesia* spp. The incubation period is from days to weeks.

Clinical signs

Chronic and subclinical infections are possible. Clinical signs of acute infection can include anemia, fever, tachycardia, tachypnea, hypoxia, depression, anorexia, and weakness. Some animals will have jaundice, petechiation, azotemia, and hepatosplenomegaly. In acute infections, DIC, metabolic acidosis, and renal disease have been seen.

In chronic disease, clinical signs include weight loss, anorexia, ascites, GI signs, CNS disease, edema, and clinical evidence of cardiopulmonary disease. In cases of chronic disease, glucocorticoid use or splenectomy may activate the disease.

Diagnosis

Hematology may reveal a regenerative anemia or thrombocytopenia. Blood chemistries commonly show hyperbilirubinemia, azotemia, and metabolic acidosis. Common findings on urinalysis include bilirubinuria, hemoglobinuria, and renal casts.

Presumptive diagnosis is based on history, physical examination, hematology, blood chemistry, urinalysis, and serology. Immunofluorescent assays for *B. canis* and *B. gibsoni* are available. False negatives can result in peracute conditions or in immunosuppressed animals. Currently, there is no definitive cutoff for positive results, but increasing titers over a 2- to 3-week period is consistent with recent or active infection. Many dogs will be seropositive but have a subclinical infection. PCR testing is available, but it does not always correlate with clinical illness. *Babesia* spp. organisms can be demonstrated in erythrocytes using Wright's stain or Giemsa stain. *B. canis* is typically found as paired, piriform bodies measuring $2.4 \times 5.0 \mu m$. *B. gibsoni* is found as single, annular bodies $1.0 \times 3.2 \mu m$.

Treatment and prevention

In the United States, the only drug approved for use in the treatment of *Babesia* spp. is imidocarb dipropionate. It appears to be more effective against *B. canis* than *B. gibsoni*. Azithromycin, atovaquone, clindamycin hydrochloride, doxycycline, or metronidazole has been effective in reducing the parasite load and may lessen disease if imidocarb dipropionate is not available.[2] In pre-

viously affected dogs, avoid immunosuppressive drugs and splenectomy. The best prevention is to control ticks.

Giardia

Giardia spp. is one of the most common protozoal organisms infecting the GI tract of dogs and cats. The organisms are flagellates that replicate in the GI tract of multiple warm-blooded animal species. The average size of the trophozoite is $15 \times 10 \mu m$, and the cysts are on average $10 \times 8 \mu m$ in size. Transmission of *Giardia* spp. is by fecal oral ingestion of the trophozoite or cyst form. Although both the trophozite and cysts are infectious, typically gastric secretions kill the trophozoites. The fecal shedding period is variable. Many cases are associated with overcrowded and unsanitary conditions.[1]

The cyst form can survive for months outside of a host in wet, cold conditions. Giardia has a direct life cycle, and once the cyst is ingested, the trophozoites mature in the GI system. Pathogenic mechanisms of the trophozoites include disruption of normal flora, inhibition of normal enterocyte enzymatic function, induction of motility disorders, and blunting of microvilli. *Giardia* spp. can cause disease in animals of any species or age. In animals with immunodeficiency, clinical disease is more common.[1]

Clinical signs typically are vomiting, small bowel diarrhea, or inappetence. Fever is uncommon with *Giardia* spp. More information is available in Chapter 8.

Diagnosis

Diagnosis is made by documentation of oocysts, cysts, or trophozoites. Zinc sulfate centrifugation is the floatation solution of choice for *Giardia* spp., as sugar solution is hypertonic and will distort the cysts. Trophozoites may be noted on direct smears. To aid in visualizing the internal structure of protozoa, a stain such as Lugol's solution, acid methyl green, or methylene blue can be used. Antigens of *Giardia* spp. can be detected using ELISA tests; however, it is possible to have a false negative because there are some *Giardia* spp. that are canine specific, and the antigens used to create the ELISA test kits are not species specific. *Giardia* spp. live chronically in the intestinal tract and may not be a significant finding for the cause of disease.

Treatment and prevention

Treatment of giardiasis includes metronidazole and fenbendazole. Commonly, animals are infected after swimming in lakes and ponds. The best prevention is to avoid water that is infected.

Trichomoniasis

Trichomonads are highly motile flagellates similar in size to *Giradia* spp. that are spindle to pear shaped and only exist as trophozoites. They have an undulating membrane, which is a characteristic feature. Trichomonads divide by binary fission and are transmitted directly by fecal oral ingestion. It is not uncommon to have a coinfection with *Giardia* spp. and *Tritrichomonas foetus*. Due to the similar appearance of *Trichomona* and *Giardia*, misdiagnosis of trichomoniasis as infection with *Giardia* is common.[1] Overcrowding appears to increase the risk for infection. Cats with *T. foetus* infection range in age from 3 months to 13 years. Infections are seen in both purebred cats and cats from shelter environments.

The infection is characterized by large bowel diarrhea, semiformed to cow pie in consistency. When animals with trichomoniasis are administered antimicrobial drugs, the diarrhea improves.

Diagnosis

Observation of trophozoites in feces is diagnostic of infection. In contrast to *Giardia*, *T. foetus* has a single nucleus with an undulating cell membrane. Trichomonads will not survive refrigeration. Feces may be cultured for *T. foetus*, but a PCR test is available, which is superior to fecal culture.

Treatment and prevention

Treatment with ronidazole may be effective; however, neurological side effects are a potential concern. Clinical signs may resolve spontaneously but may take months.[2]

Leishmaniasis

Leishmania spp. are flagellates that cause visceral, arthritis, cutaneous, and mucocutaneous disease in mammals. Rodents and dogs are the primary reservoirs, with humans and cats as incidental hosts. The prime vector of *Leishmania* spp. is the sandfly. In 2000, *Leishmania donovani* was confirmed in dogs in a Foxhound kennel in New York. Since that time, *L. donovani* or *Leishmania* spp. infection has been confirmed in 30 other foxhound kennels in 20 states and in Ontario, Canada. It appears that Foxhounds are the predominant canid infected with *Leishmania* spp. The vector for *Leishmania* spp. in North America has not been identified but appears to be dog to dog.[1] *Leishmania* spp. has been transmitted by blood transfusion, shared needles, fighting, congenital transmission, and breeding. In transmission by the sandfly, flagellated promastigotes develop in the sandfly and are injected when the sandfly feeds. Macrophages engulf the promastigotes, which then loses the flagella and become amastigotes. The amastigotes multiply by binary fussion, rupture the macrophage, and are spread throughout the body. The incubation period for *Leishmania* spp. ranges from 1 month to 7 years. The formation of amastigotes (nonflagellates) causes cutaneous lesions to develop.

Clinical signs

Infection by the intracellular organism induces an extreme immune response. The proliferation of macrophages, histiocytes, and lymphocytes in lymphoreticular organs is seen, and commonly the immune-complex formation results in glomerulo-nephritis and polyarthritis. Generally, dogs develop visceral leishmaniasis and may have subclinical disease for months or years. Cats are usually subclincally infected. The cutaneous lesions that develop are characterized by hyperkeratosis, scaling, thickening, mucocutaneous ulcers, and intradermal nodules on the muzzle, pinnae, and footpads.

Common clinical signs include weight loss even with normal to increased appetite, polyuria, polydipsia, muscle wasting, depression, vomiting, diarrhea, cough, epistaxis, sneezing, and melena. On physical examination, splenomegaly, lymphadenopathy, facial alopecia, fever, rhinitis, dermatitis, increased lung sounds, jaundice, swollen painful joints, uveitis, and conjunctivitis are commonly seen. CBC results may reveal leukocytosis with a left shift, lymphopenia, and thrombocytopenia. Blood chemistry results typically reveal hyperglobulinemia, hypoalbuminemia, increased liver enzymes, and azotemia. Urinalysis typically reveals proteinuria. The hyperglobulinemia is usually polyclonal. Some dogs develop a neutrophilic polyarthritis and some dogs may develop bone lesions.

Diagnosis

Diagnosis is made by demonstration of amastigotes ($2.5 \times 5.0\,\mu m \times 1.5$–$2.0\,\mu m$) in lymph node aspirates, bone marrow aspirates, and skin impression smears using Wright's or Giemsa stain. The organism can also be identified by histopathologic or immunoperoxidase evaluation of skin, organ biopsy, or PCR. Antibody testing can be used as IgG titers develop 14–28 days after infection and decline 45–80 days posttreatment.

Treatment and prevention

Dogs are unlikely to eliminate the infection spontaneously, and *Leishmania* spp. cannot be eliminated with drugs. It has been reported that allopurinol, antimony, and liposomal amphotericin B have some activity against *Leishmania* spp.,[1] but the prognosis is variable and most cases are recurrent. A poor prognosis is indicated if concurrent renal insufficiency is present.

The only prevention is to avoid vectors, typically infected sandflies. In enzootic areas, house animals indoors during the night and control sandflies. All potential blood donors and breeders from enzootic areas should be serologically screened. Dogs act as a reservoir for the organism and are a primary zoonotic risk.

Toxoplasmosis

Toxoplasma gondii is a coccidian protozoa that is the most prevalent parasite that infects vertebrates.[1] The only host to complete the coccidian life cycle is the cat, which passes environmentally resistant oocysts in the feces. Dogs can pass oocysts after ingestion of feline feces. The average oocyst measures $10 \times 12\,\mu m$. Sporozoites develop in the oocysts after 1–5 days of exposure to oxygen, high environmental temperature, and humidity. Tachyzoites disseminate in the blood or lymphatic system during active infection and cause cell destruction via rapid intracellular replication. Bradyzoites are the slowly dividing persistent tissue stage that form in the extraintestinal tissues of infected hosts as immune responses attenuate tachyzoite replication. Tissue cysts form readily in muscle, CNS, and visceral organs. Infection can occur after ingestion of any of the life stages, or it can occur transplacentally. Most cats are not coprophagic and are usually infected by ingestion of the bradyzoite during carnivorous feeding. Oocysts are shed in the feces from 3–21 days. Sporulated oocysts can survive for months to years and are resistant to most disinfectants. Bradyzoites may persist in tissues for the life of the host. Approximately 30–40% of cats and 20% of dogs are seropositive. Many dogs diagnosed prior to 1988 with toxoplasmosis were based on histological evaluation and were actually *Neospora caninum*.

Clinical signs

Clinical disease with the GI phase is rare. Only 10–20% of experimentally inoculated cats develop self-limiting small bowel diarrhea after primary oral inoculation.[1] Detection of *T. gondii* oocysts in feces is rarely reported in naturally exposed cats with diarrhea.

In dogs and cats, following primary infection, death may occur from an overwhelming intracellular replication of tachyzoites causing cellular necrosis (*T. gondii* does not produce any toxins). There are no percentages available on the number of animals that die due to this process. *T. gondii* spreads to other organs by the bloodstream or the lymphatic system. This spread of disease leads to hepatic, pulmonary, CNS, and pancreatic tissue involvement. The skeletal muscle, lungs, liver, brain, and eyes are common sites of replication and chronic infection. Transplacental or lactationally affected kittens develop the most severe signs of extraintestinal infection and usually die of pulmonary or hepatic disease. Common clinical signs with disseminated toxoplasmosis include depression, anorexia, fever, then hypothermia, peritoneal effusion, jaundice, and dyspnea.

Chronic toxoplasmosis can occur in both dogs and cats. Clinical findings in cats with toxoplasmosis include anterior or posterior uveitis, fever, muscle hyperesthesia, weight loss, anorexia, respiratory tract disease, vomiting, abdominal effusion, splenomegaly, ataxia, circling, twitching, tremors, seizures, blindness, icterus, lens luxation, diarrhea, and pancreatitis. Chronic toxoplasmosis in immunosuppressed animals can cause bradyzoites in tissue to replicate and disseminate as tachyzoites. This has been documented in cats with FeLV, FIV, FIP, and renal transplantation. *T. gondii* may be a common infectious cause of uveitis in cats, based on *T. gondii*-specific aqueous humor antibody and PCR studies. Transplacental or lactationally infected kittens commonly develop ocular disease and organ dysfunction. Toxoplasmosis has been found to be the cause of fading kittens and stillbirths.

In dogs, infections are typically respiratory, GI, or neuromuscular. The clinical signs are similar to feline toxoplasmosis with fever, vomiting, diarrhea, dyspnea, and jaundice noted. Toxoplasmosis occurs most frequently in immunosuppressed animals. Neurological signs are dependent on location of the primary lesions and include ataxia, seizures, tremors, paresis, cranial nerve deficits, and paralysis. Animals with myositis have weakness, stiff gait, and muscle wasting. Rapid progression to tetraparesis and paralysis with lower motor neuron dysfunction can occur. In some dogs, myocardial infection resulting in ventricular arrhythmias may occur. In polysystemic disease, dyspnea, vomiting, and diarrhea may occur. In some dogs, retinitis, anterior uveitis, iridocyclitis, and optic neuritis may occur, but these are less common than in the cat.

Diagnosis

In some animals, routine laboratory data may be abnormal. The most common hematologic findings are a nonregenerative anemia, neutrophilic leukocytosis, lymphocytosis, monocytosis, neutropenia, and eosinophila. Urinalysis may reveal proteniuria and bilirubinuria. Blood chemistry may show increases in serum proteins, bilirubin concentration, creatinine kinase, ALT, ALP, and lipase.

Pulmonary toxoplasmosis commonly causes diffuse interstitial to alveolar patterns with pleural effusion.

There may be protein present in the CSF with higher than normal cell counts. Rarely are bradyzoites or tachyzoites detected in tissues, effusions, CSF, or bronchoalveolar lavage.

The presence of oocysts in the feces is not conclusive of toxoplasmosis, as *Hammondia* and *Besnoitia* infections have similar oocysts.

The most accurate diagnosis of toxoplasmosis is DNA detection by PCR, but DNA can be detected in animals that do not have an active infection.[2]

Treatment and prevention

Treatment of toxoplasmosis consists of supportive care and appropriate antibiotic therapy. Fluid therapy and nutritional support may be required for the hospitalized patient dependent upon the severity of the clinical signs. Antibiotics successfully used for the treatment of clinical toxoplasmosis include clindamycin hydrochloride, trimethoprim-sulfonamide, and azithromycin. In animals with uveitis, treatment with topical, oral, or parenteral glucocorticoids is recommended to avoid secondary glaucoma and lens luxation.

The most common route for humans to acquire toxoplasmosis is from ingesting sporulated oocysts, tissue cysts, or transplacentally. Humans should avoid eating undercooked meats or ingesting sporulated oocysts on vegetables. Cats generally only shed oocysts for days to several weeks after primary inoculation, so routine contact with individual cats is not a common cause of toxoplasmosis infection in humans. Repeat oocyst shedding is rare and cats usually do not allow feces to remain on their coat or skin long enough to have oocysts sporulate.

Neosporosis

N. caninum is a coccidian that has been confused with *T. gondii* in the past due to similar morphology. The tachyzoites can measure from 5–7 μm × 1–5 μm depending on the stage of division. The tissue cysts can measure up to 100 μm in diameter and can be found in neural cells and occasionally in the muscle. The sexual cycle is completed in the GI tract of dogs; oocysts are then passed in the feces, and the sporozoites develop within 24 h of passage. The shedding of oocysts may continue for months in dogs. The two other life stages are tachyzoites (fast dividing stage) and tissue cysts containing hundreds of bradyzoites (slow dividing). The route of infection in dogs is by ingestion of bradyzoites but not by tachyzoites. Infection has been documented after ingestion of infected bovine placental tissue and other intermediate hosts. Transplacental transmission is well documented, and there is increased risk for pups whose dam previously delivered infected offspring.[3] There have been no reports of clinical disease in naturally infected domestic cats; however, N. caninum has been reported in nondomestic felids. Glucocorticoid administration my activate bradyzoites in tissue, causing clinical disease.[1]

Clinical signs

The primary clinical illness reported is neuromuscular. The most common clinical presentation is puppies younger than 6 months of age that are congenitally infected. These puppies develop an ascending paralysis with hyperextension of the hind limbs. In many cases, muscle atrophy can occur. Multifocal CNS disease and polymyositis alone or in combination can be noted. Hyperesthesia, incontinence, dysphagia, and respiratory muscle paralysis are the clinical signs of myositis. Clinical signs may be seen beginning at 3–9 weeks of age. Neonatal death is common. In dogs over 6 months of age, regional or generalized myositis and CNS manifestation are common.[3] The clinical signs include behavior changes, head tilt, seizures, blindness, Horner's syndrome, and trigeminal neuropathy. Systemic signs of fever, dyspnea, cough, myocarditis, megaesophagus, and vomiting have been noted.

In experimentally infected cats, the infection is more severe for prenatal and neonatal kittens. Subclinical disease has been found in adult cats, but the disease is more severe when the cats were immunosuppressed with glucocorticoids. The predominant lesions are hepatitis, encephalomyelitis, and polymysitis. Antibodies to N. caninum have been reported in domestic cats, but natural clinical infections have not been documented.[4]

The disease tends to be most severe in congenitally infected pups, but dogs up to 15 years of age have been infected. It is uncertain in older animals if the clinical signs are from an acute, primary infection or from chronic infection. Clinical findings of myocarditis, dysphagia, ulcerative dermatitis, pneumonia, and hepatitis can occur in some dogs. Tissue cysts that are intact are not usually associated with inflammation as are ruptured cysts. The intracellular replication of N. caninum causes the disease. CNS infection usually causes mononuclear cell infiltrates. It is believed that there is an immune-mediated component to the pathogenesis of the disease. If not treated, it is fatal in most dogs. The prognosis for animals with severe neurological involvement is grave.[1]

Diagnosis

There are no specific hematologic or biochemical findings. Commonly, increases in creatine kinase (CK) and AST are found.

In CSF, increased protein concentrations (20–50 mg/dL) and mild mixed inflammatory cell pleocytosis (10–50 cells/dL) consisting of monocytes, lymphocytes, neutrophils, and, occasionally, eosinophils can be found.

Thoracic radiographs can reveal interstitial and alveolar patterns.

Tachyzoites are rarely identified. Oocysts may be detected in feces after flotation or by PCR. N. caninum is differentiated from T. gondii by electron microscopy, immunohistochemistry, and PCR.[1]

Demonstration of the organism in CSF or tissues gives a definitive diagnosis. Presumptive diagnosis can be made by clinical signs, positive serology, or the presence of antibodies in the CSF. Detection of serum antibodies to N. caninum by IFA or ELISA confirms the diagnosis.

Treatment and prevention

Trimethoprim, macrolides, tetracyclines, and lincosamides have been used to treat canine neosporosis. If one pup from the litter has been diagnosed with neosporosis, all pups in the litter should be placed on treatment. Once a dam has been known to harbor the organism, successive litters and litters from their progeny may be affected. This must be taken into consideration when planning the breeding of Neospora-infected females.[3]

Cytauxzoonosis

Cytauxzoon felis is a piroplasmia organism that can infect cats in southeastern, south central, and mid-Atlantic regions of the United States. It is transmitted to cats through a tick bite. The organisms are 1–2 μm in size and appear as round bodies or oval "safety pin" forms. Bobcats are usually subclinically affected and are likely the natural host of the organism. C. felis has been passed experimentally from infected bobcats to domestic cats by Dermacentor variabilis (American dog tick).

The incubation period is from 5 to 20 days. Infected macrophages line the lumen of veins; as merozoites are released from infected macrophages, they infect erythrocytes. Obstruction of blood flow through tissues by mononuclear infiltrates and hemolytic anemia creates the clinical signs. Clinical signs rapidly progress and usually, in less than a week's duration, leads to death.

Clinical signs

Clinical signs of fever (103°–107°F/39.4°–41.6°C), dyspnea, depression, jaundice, anorexia, dark urine, lethargy, dehydration, and pale mucous membranes have been observed. In many cases, the patient's temperature will go from febrile to subnormal as the disease progresses. Respiratory distress may be noted in some animals. In terminally ill cats, hypothermia, coma and recumbency are common clinical findings. Late in the disease, parasitized erythrocytes may be observed. After the temperature peak, cats usually die within 2–3 days.[1]

Cytauxzoonosis should be suspected in any cat permitted to go outdoors in tick-infested areas that develops a high fever, depression, anemia, or jaundice. Cats typically present with regenerative anemia and neutrophilic leukocytosis. The anemia is typically mild with regard to the amount of icterus. With some animals, thrombocytopenia is occasionally found. It is uncommon to find hemoglobinemia, hemoglobinuria, bilirubinemia, or bilirubinuria.

Diagnosis

Diagnosis is based on demonstration of the piroplasms on blood smears stained with Wright's or Giemsa stain. The number of parasites will increase as the disease progresses. Thoracic radiographs may show a bronchointerstitial pulmonary pattern. Infected macrophages may be detected in the bone marrow, spleen, liver, or lymph node aspirates. PCR may be used, but serologic testing is not available.

Treatment and prevention

Treatment consists of supportive care including fluid therapy and blood transfusion if indicated. Imidocarb dipropionate, diminazene, parvaquone, buparvaquine, or thiacetarsemide have been used with some success. If none of these drugs are available, enrofloxacin, azithromycin, and atovaquone have been used but have had little success.[1]

The best prevention is to control ticks in the area. Cats living in an enzootic area should be kept indoors during periods of tick activity.

Hepatozoonosis

Hepatozoonosis is an arthropod-borne protozoal infection. *Hepatozoon canis* is the predominant agent in South America, Asia, Africa, or Europe, and *Hepatozoon americanum* is the predominant agent in the United States, specifically in the Gulf Coast region. Ticks serve as both definitive host and principal vector of hepatozoon organisms. *H. canis* is transmitted primarily by *R. sanguineus*, the brown dog tick, and may result in asymptomatic infections or clinical disease of variable severity. Clinical disease is most commonly seen in animals with diminished immune response such as young puppies and immunosuppressed dogs (by medications or concurrent disease). *H. americanum* is more pathogenic than *H. canis*, generally causing severe clinical signs in most dogs that become infected, and will be the focus of this discussion.

The definitive host and principal vector for *H. americanum* is the Gulf Coast tick, *Ambylomma maculatum*, and the distribution of *H. americanum* parallels the distribution of *A. maculatum*. *H. americanum* has been identified in Texas, Oklahoma, Louisiana, Mississippi, Alabama, Georgia, and Florida. However, the range of the vector tick is expanding northward, so the occurrence of *H. americanum*-associated disease may expand accordingly.

Anatomy and physiology

H. americanum is primarily transmitted through ingestion of an infected tick, *A. maculatum*. Dogs do *not* become infected with *H. americanum* after being bitten by a tick. This ingestion can occur during normal grooming or by the consumption of small mammals that carry this tick or its various life stages. When the tick is ingested, the infective organism is released in the intestines to infect phagocytic cells and endothelial cells and then disseminate to other tissues, especially muscle (skeletal and cardiac). Once it has reached the target organs (muscle), it forms mucopolysaccharide concentric layers to form an "onion skin" cyst (Figure 11.3.1).

The cyst itself causes no clinical symptoms since it is protected from the host's immune system by its mucopolysaccharide layers. As the organism matures, new, immature stages (merozoites) are released into the muscle. Inflammatory cells will travel to the site of the rupture and often incite a marked pyogranulomatous inflammatory response.

H. americanum life cycle

1. Dog ingests the infected tick.

2. Sporozoites are released into the GI tract and penetrate the wall of the gut.

3. Sporozoites travel to skeletal and cardiac muscle via blood or lymph vessels and affect monocytes as a cyst

4. Concentric layers of mucopolysaccharide material surround the cyst forming an onion skin appearance

5. Cysts either remain dormant or undergo merogany and form meronts that contain large numbers of merozoites

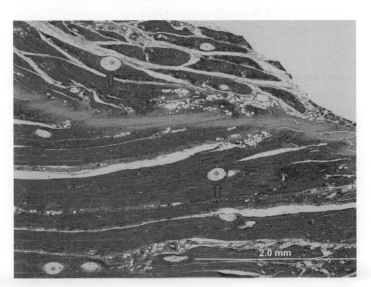

Figure 11.3.1 Myocytes contain clear onion skin cysts (arrow), which contain zoites. Image courtesy of Dr. Kuldeep Singh, Clinical Assistant Professor, Pathobiology, University of Illinois.

6. Meronts rupture and release merozoites causing inflammation and attract phagocytes that ingest the merozoites.

7. Merozoites circle until ingested by another tick to continue the cycle as gamots in WBCs or travel to other tissues to continue asexual reproduction.

8. The zygote matures into an oocyst within the tick gut until it is ingested by another dog.

Clinical signs

H. americanum infection causes severe, debilitating, and fatal disease. Common clinical signs include an intermittent fever, generalized muscle atrophy, weakness, muscle stiffness, and cachexia. Cachexia, which is secondary to the increased caloric needs of chronic states of inflammation, may even be seen in patients with a normal appetite. Hyperesthesia, ocular discharge, and keratoconjunctivitis sicca (KCS) may also be noted. The disease may wax and wane as the amount of inflammation in muscle varies with the life cycle phases of the organism. Untreated chronic infections can lead to glomerulonephritis, and amyloidal deposits in organs may cause death within 12 months.

Diagnostic testing

Laboratory

Dogs infected with *H. americanum* can have a neutrophilia, ranging from mild to severe. A normocytic, normochromic anemia is a common clinical pathologic finding as well. Serum biochemical testing can yield hypoglycemia if the sample is not processed correctly (resulting from postcollection glucose metabolism occurring as a result of large numbers of circulating WBCs). Elevated ALP, hypoalbuminemia, and azotemia can be seen in patients with renal compromise as a result of amyloidosis and glomerulonephritis. Proteinuria may be present due to secondary glomerular disease caused by chronic inflammation and immune-complex deposition or amyloidosis.

The diagnosis of *H. americanum* is typically made via organism identification by cytology. The organism can be identified in a blood smear (in the neutrophils or monocytes), but it should be noted that the identification of *H. americanum* is difficult due to a low number of neutrophils or monocytes being affected (typically less than 0.1%). Buffy coat smears may increase the chances for diagnosis by this procedure. The histopathologic diagnosis can be made on muscle biopsies and will reveal the presence of onion skin cysts within the striated muscle. An ELISA for serum antibodies exists, but it is not commercially available. The most reliable diagnostic test is PCR performed on whole blood in EDTA (Auburn University), which distinguishes hepatozoonosis from other protozoal infections.

Imaging

Periosteal bony changes have been identified in dogs with *H. americanum*, and because of this, survey radiographs are often taken of long bones and the pelvis to evaluate for characteristic periosteal proliferative changes. These radiographic changes are not evident in all affected dogs, so the absence of bony lesions does not rule out hepatozoonosis. It is speculated that the bony proliferative changes are due to the attachment of affected (and inflamed) skeletal muscle to the bone.

Biopsy technique

A diagnosis can be made via demonstrating any life stage of *H. americanum* in muscle biopsy samples with or without pyogranulomatous inflammation. The rate of false-negative results with a muscle biopsy is much less than with analysis of a blood smear due to the high number of organisms present in muscles of infected dogs (Figures 11.3.2 and 11.3.3).

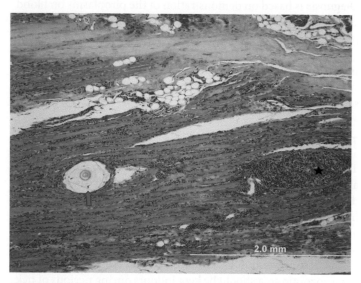

Figure 11.3.2 Focally, a myocyte contains an onion cyst (arrow); also note a pyogranuloma (star). Image courtesy of Dr. Kuldeep Singh, Clinical Assistant Professor, Pathobiology, University of Illinois.

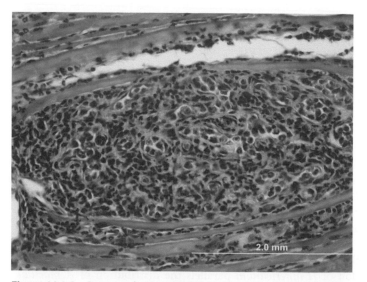

Figure 11.3.3 Pyogranuloma containing numerous neutrophils and macrophages with intracytoplasmic parasites. Image courtesy of Dr. Kuldeep Singh, Clinical Assistant Professor, Pathobiology, University of Illinois.

Treatments and pharmacology

Some cysts will remain dormant and have been found on biopsy up to 10 years after infection. The cysts are difficult to destroy and will rupture at unpredictable intervals, creating a disease that is difficult, if not impossible, to eradicate.

Treatment of hepatozoonosis usually leads to rapid resolution of clinical signs but does not eradicate the *H. americanum* organisms from the host. Hepatozoonosis is treated with a combination of antimicrobial drugs, typically trimethoprim-sulfonamide, clindamycin, and pyrimethamine, typically for 2 weeks. This combination controls acute disease, but, as the organism changes and matures, new organisms are released into the muscle and many dogs experience a relapse of clinical signs. Addition of the anticoccidial drug decoquinate (10–20 mg/kg orally BID for 2 years) to the standard triple protocol reduces recurrence of clinical disease and improves survival. In addition to the specific treatment recommendations, dehydration support is often needed.

Prevention of hepatozoonosis should begin with adequate vector control and client education.

Analgesia considerations

Non-steroidal anti-inflammatory medications can be given to provide pain relief and to reduce fever. Glucocorticoids should be avoided in these patients.

Nutritional considerations

Dogs with *H. americanum* are often cachexic. These dogs should have their food intake monitored and adjusted to ensure that it is sufficient. For animals experiencing decreased appetite, feeding a food that is calorically dense will allow for smaller meals while still maintaining adequate calories. Many puppy and recovery diets are calorically dense enough to help maintain body condition with the added bonus of being highly palatable.

SECTION 4 INFECTIOUS VIRAL DISEASES

Canine and feline herpesvirus

Canine herpesvirus (CHV) and feline herpesvirus (FHV) are enveloped, double-stranded DNA viruses that belong to the family Herpesviridae.

Canine

Pathogenesis and transmission

CHV is transmitted through direct contact with the respiratory or genital secretions of an infected dog. In addition, *in utero* transmission may occur and transplacental exposure results in some of the most serious CVH infections. Neonates can also be infected with CHV through direct contact with the genital or respiratory secretions of the dam or another infected dog.

Clinical signs

Most genitally infected adult dogs remain asymptomatic, but some infections may result in mild clinical illness, such as vaginal hyperemia or genital vesicular lesions. Adult respiratory infections of CHV may cause mild upper respiratory or ocular symptoms, but the extent of clinical illness in adult patients is still unknown. CHV has also been associated with infectious tracheobronchitis or the "kennel cough" syndrome.

Transplacental infection may result in late-term abortion, stillborn, or mummified puppies. Infected puppies that reach full term usually develop systemic infection in the first 9 days after birth.[1] Puppies exposed at less than 2 weeks of age are more likely to develop fatal infections than older puppies. Infection causes multiorgan hemorrhage and necrosis. The commonly affected organs are the lungs, spleen, kidneys, and liver. Puppies with severe systemic infection usually present as "poor doers," which is why it is commonly referred to as "fading puppy syndrome." Clinical signs include poor weight gain, lethargy, dyspnea, abdominal pain, inappetance, oculonasal discharge, and persistent vocalization. These signs develop into mucous membrane petechiation and erythematous rash with subcutaneous edema of the ventrum. Pups eventually develop neurological signs leading to seizures and loss of consciousness before death. Death most often occurs rapidly within 24–48 h of the onset of clinical signs. Systemic disease from herpesvirus has a high mortality rate in puppies less than 3 weeks of age likely due to their immature immune system and impaired ability to thermoregulate. Puppies that survive mild clinical symptoms often suffer renal damage and lifelong neurological symptoms, such as ataxia and blindness. Due to the fact that the virus can remain latent in the nerve ganglia, surviving patients can be chronic carriers of the virus and recrudescent illness can occur during times of stress or corticosteroid administration.[2]

Clinical signs of recrudescent disease in otherwise healthy adult patients can include mild upper respiratory symptoms or vesicular lesions of the genital mucosa.

Diagnostic testing

Diagnosis of CHV in sick neonates is usually made by clinical history, physical exam, and often by gross examination of the internal organs at necropsy. Litters of puppies that die rapidly within 1–3 weeks of age and have characteristic hemorrhagic and necrotic renal lesions should be highly suspect of CHV, but histological analysis of affected organs can assist in supporting the diagnosis. Serum chemistries and CBC may reveal thrombocytopenia or marked increases in ALT, but these abnormalities are nonspecific.[1] Definitive diagnosis is made by the detection of viral DNA in affected tissues. Multiple modalities are available, such as cell cultures, immunohistochemical techniques, and PCR. Serologic testing only indicates exposure but does not prove active infection.[1]

Pharmacology and treatment

Treatment of infected neonates is supportive care and is often disappointing. Thermal support may be helpful because the virus replicates poorly at higher temperatures. Some texts describe the intraperitoneal administration of serum collected from bitches that have recently lost a litter to CHV. Antibodies in the sera may decrease mortality in affected litters. Antiviral medications are available, but there is no information on their effectiveness in puppies with CHV. Patients suspected of having CHV should be strictly isolated from other patients using proper isolation practices and disinfection techniques to prevent the spread of disease to other patients.

Prevention

Prevention is usually aimed at protecting gravid females and neonates from exposure to CHV. Latent CHV infection is common among the canine population, which makes it difficult to know which animals could transmit the virus. Females never before exposed to CHV are at very high risk of infecting their puppies if exposed during pregnancy. Proper husbandry techniques are the best way to reduce the risk of exposure to these patients. Fetuses are most susceptible to CHV infection during the last 3 weeks of gestation and during the first 3 weeks after birth. During this time, gravid females and new litters should be strictly isolated from other dogs. Subsequent litters from an infected bitch are unlikely to develop serious clinical illness. Anecdotally, keeping neonates warm until their ability to thermoregulate is fully developed may assist in reducing the severity of infection if exposed but will not prevent or eliminate infection. CHV is stable in the environment for 3 h at 37°C and is readily killed by commercial disinfectants, so routine disinfection of housing facilities and equipment will help to reduce environmental and fomite causes for exposure. A vaccine is available in Europe, but it is unlikely that a vaccine will be developed for use in the United States.

Feline

Pathogenesis and transmission

FHV is an important cause of upper respiratory disease in cats. Cats become infected with FHV through direct contact with the oronasal or conjunctival secretions of an infected cat actively shedding the virus. Infection is common in shelters and in cattery environments. Transplacental infection has not been proven, but neonates are commonly infected by the queen at a very early age, before vaccination. Most patients infected with FHV become lifelong latent carriers[3] and recrudescent illness is common.

Clinical signs

Clinical signs of acute infection in kittens and adults include sneezing, conjunctivitis, and serous oculonasal discharge that usually last about 10–14 days. Signs are usually more severe in young kittens, which may be attributed to an immature immune system. Atypical acute infection can manifest with dermal ulcerations, oral ulceration, pneumonia, systemic disease, and acute death. Chronic active infections can present with chronic sneezing and rhinitis, and/or chronic ulcerative keratitis. There are several other disorders that have been seen in patients with FHV such as corneal sequestration, neurological disorders, eosinophilic keratitis, and uveitis, but a causal association has not yet been proven. Recrudescent disease usually occurs during times of stress or glucocorticoid administration.[3] Some causes of reactivation can include moving to a new environment and parturition.

Diagnostic testing

Diagnosis of FHV is similar to CHV. A detailed history should be obtained in patients presenting with upper respiratory or ocular symptoms. Owners should be asked about recent contact with other cats, past history of similar symptoms, or administration of immunosuppressive medications because these can help to support a diagnosis of FHV. A history of thick or opaque oculonasal discharge, inappetance, lethargy, or dyspnea can indicate more severe infection or concurrent infection and can assist the veterinarian in choosing appropriate therapy. There are several laboratory techniques for identifying patients infected with FHV. Virus isolation of infected tissues can be used to confirm infection but is not often performed in the clinical setting. PCR of conjunctival and pharyngeal swabs is becoming more widely performed, but a positive result can indicate latent infection and does not prove the cause of clinical symptoms.[4]

Treatment

There is no specific treatment for FHV. Treatment of active FHV infection is usually aimed at treating or preventing secondary infection. Concurrent infection with other respiratory pathogens such as mycoplasma, *Staphylococcus* spp., *Bordetella bronchiseptica*, *Escherichia coli*, and others is not uncommon and appropriate antimicrobial therapy should be aimed to control these pathogens when suspected. Fluid and nutritional support is indicated when infection is severe enough to cause dehydration or inappetance. Poor appetite can be caused by the inability of the cat to smell its food due to nasal crusting. Nasal crusts should be gently moistened and removed carefully to prevent ulceration of the planum and this may help to restore the patient's appetite. Warming of the food and administration of appetite stimulants can be used to encourage the patient to eat. Feeding tube placement for supplemental enteral nutrition may be needed in severe cases. Nebulization with saline can be used to moisten dry airways. Nasal and periocular ulcerations should be treated with topical ointments to eliminate or prevent local dermal infections. Conjunctivitis and corneal ulceration should be treated with appropriate topical antibiotics to prevent secondary ocular infection. Severe or refractory corneal disease such as herpes keratitis can be treated with topical antiviral agents, but they must be applied frequently (every 2–4 h) and may cause local irritation. The benefit of oral antiviral medication such as famcyclovir is currently being investigated. Oral administration of the amino acid l-lysine is very safe and may reduce spontaneous shedding of virus in latently infected cats.[5] Strict isolation and good disinfection practices should be employed when housing patients with suspected FHV to prevent transmission to other patients.

Prevention

Avoiding exposure is the best way to prevent infection of cats with FHV. Because exposure is common in shelter and cattery environments, measures should be taken to avoid cat-to-cat contact in these environments. Symptomatic cats should be promptly isolated from other cats, and all cats should be housed in single enclosures unless they originate from the same household. New cats should be quarantined for at least 2 weeks before being housed near other cats. Pet owners should be educated about the potential for FHV infection when adopting a new cat, and the same quarantine procedure should be exercised in the home environment if they have existing cats. Like CHV, FHV is stable in the environment for 3 h at 37°C and is easily inactivated by commercial disinfectants. Proper disinfection of cages, treatment tables, and equipment should prevent infection of cats from the environment. Kittens are often infected by the queen at an early age. Early weaning (4 weeks of age) and isolation of litters from infected queens can help to prevent serious infection until vaccination can be instituted. Besides exposure prevention, vaccination is the mainstay of disease prevention. The American Association of Feline Practitioners recommends vaccinating kittens as early as 6 weeks of age, and at 3- to 4-week intervals until 16 weeks of age.[6] Adult cats with unknown vaccination history should be immunized with two doses, administered 3–4 weeks apart. The initial vaccination series in adults and kittens should be followed with a booster 1 year later, and then every 3 years. An additional booster should be considered before exposure to a high risk situation such as a cattery or shelter. Vaccination may protect against disease but not against infection and viral latency. Please see Chapter 12 for additional information.

Influenza

Influenza viruses are caused by RNA viruses of the Orthomyxoviridae family.[7] There are three genera that contain the influenza viruses: influenza virus A, influenza virus B, and influenza virus C. The structure is similar for all influenza viruses, with enveloped virus particles that are either filamentous or spherical in shape, that range in size from 80 to 120 nm in diameter.[8] Viruses can only replicate in living cells. They affect all species of birds and mammals but are usually host specific. Transmission of the influenza virus interspecies is a concern due to the emergence of novel endemic influenza strains and reverse transmission.[9]

The subtypes of the virus are labeled for the hemagglutinin (HA) and neuraminidase (NA) proteins of the virus. HA (H) codes the hemagglutinin glycoprotein and NA (N) codes the neuraminidase enzyme. There are 16 different H antigens and nine different N antigens at this time.[7] Each subtype has mutated into a variety of strains that are pathogenic to either one or multiple species.

Influenza A

There is only one species of the influenza virus A, but there are many strains of influenza A. Wild aquatic birds are the natural hosts for a great many of the influenza A viruses. They can be the most virulent of the influenza types. The H5N1 strain, also known as avian flu, has been transmitted to domestic and wild felids that were fed uncooked chickens with the virus. The H3N8 strain was originally an equine influenza, which crossed species in the last decade to create canine influenza.

Influenza B

There is only one species of the influenza virus B. Humans are the host for the vast majority of the influenza B viruses. It has been shown that the ferret[10] and seal[11] can be susceptible to influenza B viruses. This species mutates at a slower rate than influenza A and has only one influenza B serotype.[12]

Influenza C

Influenza virus C also has only one species, but unlike influenza virus B, it does infect humans, dogs and pigs. Influenza C is less common but can cause both severe illness and local epidemics.[13]

Pathogenesis and transmission

Transmission of the virus is by direct contact, aerosolization, and fomites, and the duration of transmission is 5–7 days postinfection. In seasonal human flu outbreaks, the strains of influenza that are seen change from year to year. Influenza viruses are capable of surviving cold weather. They can survive in the environment for 24–48 h on hard, nonporous material, 15 min on paper and 5 min on the skin. In mucous, the virus has been shown to survive for 17 days.[14]

Clinical signs

Clinical signs for all of the influenza viruses can appear 1–2 days postinfection and may include fever, cough, nasal discharge, lethargy, dehydration, pain, reddened eyes, and, occasionally, diarrhea.

Diagnostic testing

Hematology may reveal moderate lymphopenia, normal leukogram, and hemoconcentration. Thoracic radiographs may reveal a bilateral, caudodorsal alveolar pattern to the lungs.

Pharmacology and treatment

Treatment options are primarily supportive care, rest, and nutritional support. Antiviral drugs such as oseltamivir (Tamiflu) or zanamivir (Relenza) may be beneficial to halt the spread of the disease. Many owners do not realize an animal has been affected until secondary bacterial infections, such as pneumonia, occur.

Effective reduction of the transmission is through minimizing human/animal contact when owners are ill and includes frequent hand washing and covering coughs and sneezes. Influenza viruses can be inactivated by sunlight, disinfectants, and detergents.[15] Thoroughly sanitizing surfaces with quaternary ammonium compounds or diluted bleach is indicated.

H1N1

In the spring of 2009, an influenza strain underwent an antigenic shift and evolved to have genes from four influenza strains. The A/H1N1 strain was officially declared to be a pandemic by the World Health Organization in July 2009. This strain emerged in Mexico and the United States. It contained genes from North American swine influenza, North American avian influenza, human influenza viruses and swine influenza viruses found in Europe and in Asia.[16] During the pandemic, there were several confirmed cases of H1N1 in cats, dogs, and ferrets. All but one of the infected companion animals was in close contact with humans, who were confirmed to have H1N1. The one case, in which there was no confirmation of human illness, was a cat who was adopted within 24 h of placement in a shelter. It is thought to have come in contact with an asymptomatic carrier.[16] A reverse zoonotic situation occurred.

Diagnostic testing

Hematology may reveal a normal CBC. If secondary bacterial infection is present, a tracheal wash or bronchoalveolar lavage may be indicated. Diagnosis of A/H1N1 is made by clinical signs, detailed history (including any illness in the family), and PCR to confirm H1N1. PCR is available utilizing nasal swabs or repiratory tissue samples. It is unclear at this time if this strain of H1N1 will continue to cause disease or if it will mutate again. As of June 2010, the Center for Disease Control stated that there is little 2009 A/H1N1 currently circulating in the United States. The Department of Health and Human Services urges continued vigilance and preventative measures.[17]

Papillomas

Papillomas appear as whitish or gray pedunculated masses that are often referred to as warts. They are common in the dog and rare in cats. Caused by species-specific viruses that are fairly stable in the environment, the virus can survive for over 2 months at 4–8°C and for 6h at 37°C.[18] The virus is a non-enveloped double-stranded DNA virus from the family Papillomaviridae. Papillomaviruses can be transmitted by direct and indirect contacts; the infection occurs in damaged skin.

Canine oral papillomavirus

Canine oral papillomavirus (COPV) is closely related to papillomaviruses that affect other species, including humans. The virus infects basal layer cells of the epithelium of the conjunctiva, oral cavity, skin, penis, and vulva. Cell-mediated immune response causes the T-cell infiltration. Increased mitotic activity in the cells produces the characteristic warts. Young dogs younger than 1 year of age and immunocompromised animals are affected more frequently than older animals.[18] Cutaneous inverted papillomas are cup-shaped lesions also caused by a papillomavirus. They occur on the ventral abdomen and groin of young dogs.

Clinical signs

The appearance of warts is the primary clinical sign. Typically, the warts appear in the oral cavity or other epithelial sites. The warts develop 4–8 weeks postinfection and typically regress within 4–8 weeks after appearance. The impact on function is usually minimal unless the warts are located in places that result in dysphagia or respiratory obstruction.

Diagnostic testing

Diagnosis is usually based on the appearance of the characteristic warts. Immunohistochemical techniques, electron microscopy, or PCR-based analysis can document the viral antigen.

Pharmacology and treatment

Treatment is usually not warranted unless the lesions compromise eating or respirations, in which case removal of the warts may be indicated. Currently, there is no preventative vaccine available for dogs. Generally, dogs that have recovered from COPV are immune to reinfection.[19]

Feline papillomavirus

Feline papillomavirus has been confirmed in the domestic cat, bobcat, snow leopard, clouded leopard, Florida panther, and Asian lion. The lesions are typically located in the oral cavity with the tongue being most commonly involved. The papillomavirus has been shown to be involved with the development of feline tumors.[20] Introduced through lesions or abrasions of the skin, hyperplasia develops and the lesions become evident in 4–6 weeks postinfection. Most reported cases have been in animals 6–13 years old.[19] Immunocompromised animals appear to be at higher risk.

Clinical signs

In cats, the oral papillomas are small, light-pink oval lesions localized on the ventral surface of the tongue. Cutaneous papillomas are slightly raised plaques and do not have the appearance of warts. They are located on the abdomen, neck, head, and dorsal thorax. Solitary cutaneous warts are typically not caused by papillomavirus.

Diagnostic testing

Diagnosis is achieved by full-thickness biopsy processed for immunohistochemistry, electron microscopy, or histopathologic methods.

Pharmacology and treatment

Treatment is usually not warranted, although removal of the lesions is curative. Currently, there is no preventative vaccine available and, as with canine papillomas, spontaneous regression is expected.

SECTION 5 INFECTIOUS DISEASE TESTING

Interest in early detection of disease has increased based in part on society's expectations of increased levels of medical care.

Laboratory tests have varying levels of specificity and sensitivity. Analytic sensitivity is defined as the minimum detectable amount that can be measured, whereas diagnostic sensitivity is the proportion of positive results from known infected animals. Analytic specificity is defined as whether a substance will cross-react with another substance, and diagnostic specificity is the proportion of negatives from known uninfected animals. A test with high specificity has few false-positive results and a test with high sensitivity has few false-negatives.

Infectious agents, infectious antigens, or antibodies to the agent can be detected in cells, tissues, feces, and body fluids. There are several diagnostic methods currently available for diagnosing infectious diseases. The testing methodology is dependent upon the suspected infectious agent itself as well as on the site of infection. Cytology, bacterial culture, histology, immunohistochemistry, nucleic acid-based testing such as PCR, organism isolation, and serological testing have been used to diagnose disease. Proper sample handling will help maximize diagnostic yield.

Sample collection

When collecting samples for laboratory analysis, the collection method must adequately preserve the sample, preclude contamination, and be representative of the infection. Sample collection containers must be sterile. Appropriate sample collection devices can include swabs or containers. Specific devices may be needed depending on the type of sample submitted. For example, anaerobic bacterial cultures should be submitted in a special vial to prevent sample exposure to oxygen. Culture vials with various growth media are available. Submission of the appropriate sample using proper handling precautions will help ensure most accurate diagnostic results. Some bacterial culture samples can be refrigerated for a short period prior to submission. Samples for serology and PCR that are expected to arrive at the laboratory within 24–36 h should be promptly refrigerated. If the samples are expected to arrive long term (2–4 days), check with the reference laboratory for handling instructions. In some instances, the samples should be frozen and shipped on wet ice (Table 11.5.1).

Serology

Serology is the measure of specific antibodies in serum or other body fluids. Common methodologies for detecting antibodies include complement fixation, hemagglutination inhibition, serum neutralization, agglutination assays, agar gel immunodiffusion,

Table 11.5.1 Appropriate sample selection

Sample selection for diagnosis of disease		
Organ system or clinical sign	Sample collection *in vivo*	Samples collected at necropsy
Central nervous system[a]	Serum, whole blood, feces, cerebrospinal fluid	Brain sections
Gastrointestinal tract	Serum, whole blood, feces, vomitus	Small intestine sections, mesenteric lymph nodes, intestinal contents
Genitourinary tract	Serum, whole blood, urine, urogenital swabs, vaginal mucus	Kidney, liver, spleen, fetal lung, and placental tissue
Respiratory and ocular	Serum; whole blood; transtracheal wash; conjunctival scrapings; nasal, ocular, and pharyngeal swabs	Bronchiolar lymph nodes and selected tissue
Skin and mucous membranes	Serum, whole blood, scraping of lesions, vesicle fluid	Regional lymph nodes and selected tissues
Blood dyscrasias, hematologic abnormalities, immunosuppression	Serum, whole blood, bone marrow	Lymph nodes and selected tissues

[a] Handle animals with neurological signs with caution due to the possibility of rabies.
Source: Modified from Greene CE. *Infectious Diseases of the Dog and Cat*, 3rd edition, p. 3. St. Louis, MO: Elsevier Saunders; 2006.

immunofluorescence assay, direct fluorescent antibody, enzyme linked immunosorbent assay, and Western blot immunoassay.

Antibody detection depends on the immune systems response. Once exposed to foreign antigens, the immune system produces serum antibodies. This is known as a humoral response.

Complement fixation, hemagglutination inhibition, serum neutralization, and agglutination assays can be used as nonspecific antibody detection tests. Specific antibody assays can be performed to detect IgM, IgG, IgA, and IgE. The first antibody produced by the immune response is IgM. After days to weeks, IgG and IgA are produced.

IFA, Western blot immunoassays, and ELISA technology are usually adapted to detect specific IgM, IgG, or IgA. Comparison of IgM, IgG, and IgA titers can be supportive of recent or active infection.

Serologic testing does have limitations. Some serologic tests cannot distinguish between antibodies produced in response to vaccination from those in response to infection. Examples are feline coronavirus, FIV, calicivirus, and canine distemper. Additionally, detection of antibodies does not always correlate with active clinical disease but may instead be present due to subclinical disease or a carrier state.

The timing of testing is important for disease detection. Testing of puppies and kittens should not be performed until 8–12 weeks of age due to the presence and possible interference of maternal antibodies. False negatives can occur in animals of any age during the acute phase of disease, prior to a detectable antibody response being mounted. It is recommended to repeat the test in 2–3 weeks to assess seroconversion. A fourfold increase in the antibody titer is suggestive of active infection. Due to interassay variation, it is preferable to analyze both samples at the same time and in the same laboratory.

PCR

Polymerase chain reaction (PCR) testing is used to detect genetic material of microbial organisms and can be performed on a variety of samples including fluid and tissues. During this process, a minute quantity of microbial DNA is amplified until it can be detected. PCR testing can be used to diagnose infections that have low microbial shedding, low antibody titers, or low antigen levels. When diagnosing an RNA virus, reverse transcriptase (RT) is added to the PCR method. Reverse transcriptase polymerase chain reaction (RT-PCR) can also be used to detect the presence of RNA produced by a DNA virus. Because RNA degrades in living animals quickly compared to DNA, detection of either messenger or ribosomal RNA using RT-PCR may be more indicative than PCR for active infection.[1] False positives can occur with PCR testing due to contaminated samples or reagents, nonspecific primers, inactive nucleic acid, or immunization. False negatives can be obtained from inactivation of nucleic acid, nucleases, desiccation, heating, or formalin fixation. Advantages of PCR include its high sensitivity and lack of false-positive results due to the presence of vaccination-induced or maternal antibodies.[1]

Culture and sensitivity

Samples for culture may require special collection and handling. If possible, culture samples should be acquired prior to antimicrobial therapy. Except in systemic fungal or bacterial infections requiring blood culture, culture samples should be taken directly from the site of infection. Cleaning the surface of skin lesions will aid in removing potential contamination from the environment or normal flora.

Collection of blood for bacterial cultures requires special preparation. Best practice techniques have not been established for veterinary patients, but guidelines for human medicine may be followed. When collecting blood for culture, the site must first be clipped and aseptically prepared with 2% chlorhexidine solution followed by 70% alcohol. Sterile gloves should be worn. Blood should be collected using a syringe and needle; collection of blood from intravenous catheters is not recommended. The top of the blood culture vial should be disinfected (e.g., 70% alcohol) prior to transferring 1–9 mL of blood into the culture medium with a new needle. Adequate sample volume may help increase diagnostic yield; however, patient size may preclude collection of large volumes of blood. Collection of three or more blood cultures from separate sites over 1–3 h may increase diagnostic yield. Samples may be incubated at 37°C prior to transport to the laboratory. Positive culture of the same organism from more than one culture vial is likely representative of a true bacteremia.

Voided urine samples often have bacterial contamination from the lower urogenital tract and are not suitable for culture. If a urinary catheter is in place already, urine culture samples can be obtained from the catheter. Otherwise, urine samples for culture are best obtained by percutaneous cystocentesis.[2] Samples may be refrigerated for up to 8 h prior to culture. Special preservation systems should be used for longer storage.

Tissue samples, such as a surgical biopsy, can be submitted for culture. A storage container that prevents sample desiccation of the sample should be used. Both swabs and tissue samples of the lesions should be submitted for culture. Any fluid (e.g., pus) present with the lesion should also be submitted for culture. Tissue samples submitted for culture should not be fixed or preserved. Samples may be refrigerated for 8–12 h if immediate culture is not performed.

Culture samples can be tested for antimicrobial sensitivity or susceptibility. Results can help guide antimicrobial choices. Two common methods of determining bacterial antimicrobial sensitivity are agar diffusion and minimum inhibitory concentration (MIC). The MIC shows the lowest concentration of an antimicrobial that inhibits bacterial growth. In the agar diffusion method, disks impregnated with various antimicrobials are placed directly on an agar plate containing a pure culture of the bacterial specimen grown. If the bacteria are susceptible to a particular antimicrobial, growth around that disk will be inhibited (Table 11.5.2).

Each diagnostic laboratory has information available on how samples should be collected and submitted. Care must be taken

Table 11.5.2   Sample collection and processing techniques

Sample collection and processing		
Test	Sample	Collection and processing
Culture—bacterial and fungal	Body fluids; tissue; fine needle aspirates; nail clippings; feces; transtracheal wash; conjunctival scrapings; nasal, ocular and pharyngeal swabs	Collect aseptically to prevent contamination. Use appropriate swab and suitable transport medium
Cytology	Feces or body fluids	Collect fresh; do not fix or freeze. Make impressions on clean, dry microscope slide and air dry. Fix in alcohol.
Direct fluorescent antibody (FA)	Tissue	Fix in Michel's fixative for antibody testing by direct FA
	Tissue impressions	Make impressions on clean, dry microscope slide and air dry. Fix in acetone.
Electron microscopy	Tissue	Collect aseptically to prevent contamination. Cut into 1×2 mm sections. Fix in 2–4% glutaraldehyde (at 10× volume) for 24 h at 20°C
Enzyme-linked immunosorbent assay (ELISA) for antigen	Whole blood, tissue biopsy, feces, swabs	Collect aseptically to prevent contamination. Store at ≤10°C to prevent inactivation. Do not freeze or fix.
Histology	Tissue	Collect aseptically to prevent contamination. Cut into 5-mm sections and fix in 10% buffered formalin (at 10× volume)
Immunohistochemistry	Tissue	Collect aseptically to prevent contamination. Cut into 5-mm sections and fix in 10% buffered formalin (at 10× volume)
Nucleic acid-based testing	Whole blood, tissue biopsy, feces, swabs	Collect aseptically to prevent contamination. Store at ≤10°C to prevent inactivation. Do not freeze or fix.
Organism isolation	Whole blood, tissue biopsy, feces, swabs	Collect aseptically to prevent contamination. Store at ≤10°C to prevent inactivation. Do not freeze or fix.
Serology	Cerebrospinal fluid, serum, synovial fluid	Collect aseptically to prevent contamination. Handle gently to prevent hemolysis. Centrifuge and pipette serum into clean, sterile tube. Paired samples (10–14 days preferred)

Modified from Greene CE. *Infectious Diseases of the Dog and Cat*, 3rd edition, p. 4. St. Louis, MO: Elsevier Saunders; 2006.

Table 11.5.3   Veterinary diagnostic laboratories

Antech Diagnostics Many regional locations	800-745-4725 800-872-1001 http://www.antechdiagnostics.com
Idexx Laboratories Many regional locations	800-444-4210 888-433-9987 http://www.idexx.com
Mira Vista Diagnostics Indianapolis, IN	866-647-2847 http://www.miravistalabs.com
American Association of Veterinary Laboratory Diagnosticians	See http://www.aavld.org for a current listing of accredited laboratories by state

Note: See the Appendix for a complete listing of accredited laboratories by state.

to ensure that the sample is handled according to the diagnostic laboratory specifications.

Diagnostic laboratories

There are several commercial diagnostic laboratories and accredited veterinary diagnostic laboratories that perform diagnostic testing. For a complete listing of state-accredited veterinary laboratories, please refer to the Appendix and Table 11.5.3.

Laboratory testing selection

As mentioned earlier, the testing methodology is dependent upon the infectious agent, the site of infection, the sensitivity and specificity of the test, and the needs of the patient and the client. See Table 11.5.4 for recommendations on testing options.

Table 11.5.4 Laboratory testing for infectious disease

Laboratory testing for infectious disease			
Infectious agent	Type of organism	Test methodology	Sample
Anaplasmosis	Rickettsial	Cytology	Blood smears, bone marrow smears
		ELISA	Serum
		Fluorescent antibody	Serum
		PCR	Whole blood
		Protein electrophoresis	Serum
Aspergillosis	Fungal	Agar gel immunodiffusion	Serum
		Complement fixation	Serum
		Culture	Tissue or exudates
		ELISA	Blood or serum
Blastomycosis	Fungal	Agar gel immunodiffusion	Serum
		Culture	Tissue or fluid aspirates
		Cytology	Tissue or fluid aspirates
		Complement fixation	Serum
		ELISA	Serum, body fluids
		Histology	Tissue biopsy
Babesiosis	Protozoal	Complement fixation	Serum
		Cytology	Blood smear
		Fluorescent antibody	Serum
		PCR	Whole blood, ticks
Botulism	Bacterial	Toxin analysis	Blood, serum, feces, intestinal contents
Brucellosis	Bacterial	Agar gel immunodiffusion	Serum
		Culture	Blood, tissue, feces, testicles, placenta, semen, genital swab
		Fluorescent antibody	Serum
		PCR	Blood, tissue, feces, testicles, placenta, semen, genital swab
		Slide agglutination test	Serum
		Tube agglutination test	Serum
Campylobacter	Bacterial	Culture	Gastric biopsy, feces
		Histological	Intestine, colon, lymph node, lung, spleen
		PCR	Gastric biopsy, feces
Candidiasis	Fungal	Culture	Blood or tissue
Canine bartonellosis	Bacterial	Culture	Blood
		Fluorescent antibody	Serum
		PCR	Blood
Canine calicivirus	Viral	Viral inclusion	Oropharyngeal swab, fecal swab, trachea, lung, kidney, intestine

Table 11.5.4 *(Continued)*

Laboratory testing for infectious disease			
Infectious agent	**Type of organism**	**Test methodology**	**Sample**
Canine coronavirus *In vivo*	Viral	ELISA	Feces
		Electron microscopy	Feces
		Fluorescent antibody	Serum
		Immunoprecipitation test	Serum
		PCR	Feces
		Viral inclusion	Feces
		Viral neutralization	Serum
Canine coronavirus Postmortem	Viral	ELISA	Intestine
		Fluorescent antibody	Intestine
		Histology	Intestine
		Viral inclusion	Intestine
Canine distemper *In vivo*	Viral	Fluorescent antibody	Blood, buffy coat smear, conjunctival scraping, CSF, transtracheal wash
		PCR	Serum, blood, urine, CSF
		Viral neutralization	Serum, CSF
Canine distemper Postmortem	Viral	Fluorescent antibody	Tissue, conjunctival smear
		Histology	Tissue
		Immunohistochemistry	Tissue
		PCR	Tissue
		Viral inclusion	Tissue
		Viral neutralization	Tissue
Canine herpesvirus infection *In vivo*	Viral	Fluorescent antibody	Nasal swab, vaginal swab
		Immunoprecipitation test	Serum
		Viral inclusion	Serum
		Viral neutralization	Nasal swab, vaginal swab
Canine herpesvirus Postmortem	Viral	Fluorescent antibody	Brain, lymph node, liver, adrenal, kidney, spleen, lung
		PCR	Puppy/fetus tissue
		Viral inclusion	Lung, liver, kidney, CNS
Canine influenza	Viral	ELISA	Nasal swab, tissue
		Hemagglutination inhibition	Nasal swab, tissue
		PCR	Nasal swab, tissue
Canine papillomavirus	Viral	Electron microscopy	Tissue
		Histology	Tissue
Canine parainfluenza	Viral	Fluorescent antibody	Respiratory wash or tissue
		Hemagglutination inhibition	Serum or CSF
		Viral inclusion	Transtracheal wash, oropharyngeal swab, CSF
		Viral inclusion	Serum

(Continued)

Table 11.5.4 *(Continued)*

Laboratory testing for infectious disease			
Infectious agent	Type of organism	Test methodology	Sample
Canine parvovirus	Viral	ELISA	Serum, feces
		Electron microscopy	Feces, intestinal mucosa
		Fluorescent antibody	Feces, intestinal mucosa
		Hemagglutination	Feces, intestinal mucosa
		Hemagglutination inhibition	Serum, feces
		PCR	Serum, feces
Canine rotavirus *In vivo*	Viral	ELISA	Feces
		Fluorescent antibody	Feces
		Latex agglutination	Feces
		Viral inclusion	Feces
Canine rotavirus Postmortem	Viral	Electron microscopy	Intestine
		Fluorescent antibody	Intestine
Chlamydial infection	Bacterial	Complement fixation	Serum
		Culture	Nasal and ocular swabs
		ELISA	Nasal and ocular swabs, serum
		Fluorescent antibody	Conjunctival or tissue smear, serum
		Immunohistochemistry	Tissue
		PCR	Blood or tissue
Clostridium perfringens	Bacterial	Culture	Feces or intestine
		ELISA	Feces or intestine
		Latex agglutination	Feces or intestine
		PCR	Feces or intestine
		Reverse passive latex agglutination	Feces or intestine
Coccidiosis	Protozoal	Oocyst flotation	Feces
Coccidioidomycosis	Fungal	Agar gel immunodiffusion	Serum
		Complement fixation	Serum
		Culture	Fluid aspirate, tissue
		Cytology	Tissue
		Fluorescent antibody	Serum
Cryptococcosis	Fungal	Culture	Fluid aspirate or tissue
		Cytology	Fluid aspirate smear or tissue
		ELISA	Serum or CSF
		Fluorescent antibody	Tissue
		Latex agglutination	Serum, CSF
Cryptosporidiosis	Protozoal	ELISA	Feces
		Fluorescent antibody	Feces
		Oocyst floatation	Feces
		PCR	Feces or intestine

Table 11.5.4 *(Continued)*

	Laboratory testing for infectious disease		
Infectious agent	Type of organism	Test methodology	Sample
Cytauxzoonosis	Protozoal	Cytology	Blood smear, bone marrow
Ehrlichiosis	Rickettsial	Cytology	Blood smears, bone marrow smears
		ELISA	Serum
		Fluorescent antibody	Serum
		PCR	Whole blood
		Protein electrophoresis	Serum
Feline bartonellosis	Bacterial	Culture	Blood
		Fluorescent antibody	Serum
		PCR	Blood
Feline calicivirus *In vivo*	Viral	Electron microscopy	Oropharyngeal swab, intestinal and fecal swab
		Fluorescent antibody	Serum, oropharyngeal swab, intestinal and fecal swab
		Viral inclusion	Oropharyngeal swab, intestinal and fecal swab
		Viral neutralization	Serum
Feline calicivirus Postmortem	Viral	PCR	Trachea, lung, kidney, intestine
		Viral inclusion	Trachea, lung, kidney, intestine
Feline foamy virus (syncytium-forming)	Viral	Titer	Serum
Feline immunodeficiency virus	Viral	ELISA	Serum, whole blood
		Immunoblot	Serum, whole blood
		Indirect fluorescent antibody	Serum, whole blood
		PCR	Whole blood, bone marrow, lymphoid tissue
Feline infectious peritonitis *In vivo*	Viral	ELISA	Serum
		Fluorescent antibody	Serum
		Protein electrophoresis	Serum
Feline infectious peritonitis Postmortem	Viral	Fluorescent antibody	Tissue
		Histology	Tissue
		Immunohistochemistry	Tissue, CSF, lymphoid tissue, effusion fluid
Feline leukemia virus *In vivo*	Viral	ELISA	Serum or whole blood
		Fluorescent antibody	Blood smear, buffy coat or bone marrow smear
		PCR	Lymphoid tissue or bone marrow
		Rapid immunomigration	Blood or serum
		Viral inclusion	Blood or serum
Feline leukemia virus Postmortem	Viral	Fluorescent antibody	Blood or tissue or bone marrow
		PCR	Lymphoid tissue or bone marrow

(Continued)

Table 11.5.4 (*Continued*)

Laboratory testing for infectious disease			
Infectious agent	Type of organism	Test methodology	Sample
Feline Lyme borreliosis *In vivo*	Bacterial	ELISA	Serum
		Fluorescent antibody	Serum
		Immunoblot	Serum
		PCR	Body fluid, blood, tissue
Feline Lyme borreliosis Postmortem	Bacterial	Fluorescent antibody	Tissue
		Immunohistochemistry	Tissue
Feline panleukopenia *In vivo*	Viral	ELISA	Feces, serum
		Electron microscopy	Feces
		Fluorescent antibody	Serum
		Hemagglutination inhibition	Serum
		PCR	Feces
		Viral inclusion	Feces
		Viral neutralization	Serum
Feline panleukopenia Postmortem	Viral	Electron microscopy	Tissue
		Histology	Tissue
		Immunohistochemistry	Tissue
		PCR	Tissue
		Viral inclusion	Tissue
Feline papillomavirus	Viral	Fluorescent antibody	Skin biopsy
		Histology	Skin biopsy
		Immunohistochemistry	Skin biopsy
Feline rotavirus *In vivo*	Viral	ELISA	Feces
		Fluorescent antibody	Feces
		Latex agglutination	Feces
		Viral inclusion	Feces
Feline rotavirus Postmortem	Viral	Electron microscopy	Intestine
		Fluorescent antibody	Intestine
Giardia	Protozoal	ELISA	Feces
		Fecal flotation	Feces
		Fecal smears	Feces
		Fluorescent antibody	Feces
Helicobacter	Bacterial	Culture	Gastric biopsy, feces
		Histological	Intestine, colon, lymph node, lung, spleen
		PCR	Gastric biopsy, feces
Hemobartonella	Parasite	Cytology	Blood smear
		Fluorescent antibody	Blood smear
		PCR	Serum, whole blood
Hepatozoonosis	Protozoal	Cytology	Blood smear
		Histology	Muscle biopsy, tissues

Table 11.5.4 *(Continued)*

Laboratory testing for infectious disease			
Infectious agent	Type of organism	Test methodology	Sample
Infectious canine hepatitis *In vivo*	Viral	Complement fixation	Serum
		Fluorescent antibody	Serum
		Hemagglutination inhibition	Serum
		Histology	Tissue
		Immunohistochemistry	Liver tissue
		PCR	Blood, urine, liver
		Viral inclusion	Oropharyngeal swab, urine, feces
		Viral neutralization	Serum
Infectious canine hepatitis Postmortem	Viral	Cytology	Liver tissue
		Fluorescent antibody	Spleen, liver, brain
		Histology	Tissue
		Immunohistochemistry	Liver tissue
Leishmaniasis	Protozoal	Cytology	Lymph node aspirate
		ELISA	Serum
		Fluorescent antibody	Serum or dried blood spots
		PCR	Blood, tissue
		Western blot	Serum
Leptospirosis	Bacterial	Culture	Serum, urine
		Fluorescent antibody	Tissue or body fluids
		Histology	Kidney, placenta, urine, fetal fluid
		Immunohistochemistry	Tissue
		Latex agglutination	Serum
		Microscopic agglutination	Serum
		PCR	Kidney or urine
Canine Lyme borreliosis *In vivo*	Bacterial	ELISA	Serum
		Fluorescent antibody	Serum
		Immunoblot	Serum
		PCR	Serum
Canine Lyme borreliosis Postmortem	Bacterial	Fluorescent antibody	Tissue
		Immunohistochemistry	Tissue
Mycobacteriosis	Bacterial	Culture	Exudates or tissue
		Histology	Tissue
Mycoplasmal infection	Parasite	Culture	Nasal swab, transtracheal wash
		PCR	Serum or swab
Neorickettsiosis	Rickettsial	Cytology	Blood smears, bone marrow smears
		ELISA	Serum
		Fluorescent antibody	Serum
		PCR	Whole blood
		Protein electrophoresis	Serum

(Continued)

Table 11.5.4 (*Continued*)

Laboratory testing for infectious disease			
Infectious agent	Type of organism	Test methodology	Sample
Neosporosis	Protozoal	ELISA	Serum
		Fluorescent antibody	Tissue biopsy
		Indirect fluorescent antibody	Serum
		Immunohistochemistry	Tissue
		PCR	Tissue
Nocordiosis	Bacterial	Culture	Pleural, pericardial nor peritoneal fluid
Plague	Bacterial	Culture	Blood, swab, fluid, tissue
		Fluorescent antibody	Blood, swab, fluid, tissue
		Hemagglutination	Serum
		PCR	Body fluids or tissue
Pneumocystosis	Fungal	Cytology	Lung aspirates, sputum
		Fluorescent antibody	Lung aspirates, sputum
Rabies *In vivo* Vaccination titers	Viral	Fluorescent antibody viral neutralization	Serum
		Rapid fluorescent focus inhibition test	Serum
		Viral inclusion	CSF
Rabies Postmortem	Viral	Fluorescent antibody	Brain
		Histology	Brain
		Immunohistochemistry	Brain
Rhinotracheitis virus *In vivo*	Viral	ELISA	Serum, whole blood
		Electron microscopy	Serum, whole blood
		Fluorescent antibody	Serum, whole blood
		Immunohistochemistry	Tissue
		PCR	Tissue
		Viral inclusion	Tissue, respiratory wash, feces, oropharyngeal swabs, conjunctival smears, CSF, whole blood, body fluids
		Viral neutralization	Serum, whole blood
Rhinotracheitis virus Postmortem	Viral	PCR	Trachea, lung, kidney, intestine
		Viral inclusion	Trachea, lung, kidney, intestine
Rocky Mountain spotted fever	Rickettsial	Fluorescent antibody	Serum
		Latex agglutination	Serum
		PCR	Serum
Salmonellosis	Bacterial	Culture	Feces, fecal swab, blood, intestinal lymph node
		Immunohistochemistry	Intestine, colon, lung, lymph node, spleen
		PCR	Intestine, colon, lung, lymph node, spleen

Table 11.5.4 (*Continued*)

Infectious agent	Type of organism	Test methodology	Sample
		Laboratory testing for infectious disease	
Sporotrichosis	Bacterial	Culture	Lymphatic exudate
		Cytology	Lymphatic exudate
Toxoplasmosis	Protozoal	Complement fixation	Serum
		ELISA	Serum
		Fluorescent antibody	Serum
		Hemagglutination	Serum
		Histology	Tissue biopsy
		Immunohistochemistry	Tissue biopsy
		Indirect fluorescent antibody	Serum
		Oocyst flotation	Feces
		PCR	Tissue or body fluids
Trichomoniasis	Protozoal	Fecal flotation	Feces
		Fecal smears	Feces
		PCR	Feces
Trypanosomiasis	Protozoal	Cytology	Blood smear
		Fluorescent antibody	Serum
Tularemia	Bacterial	Culture	Exudate or swab
		Microagglutination	Serum
		PCR	Swab or exudate

Source: Modified from Greene CE, et al. *Infectious Diseases of the Dog and Cat*, 3rd edition, p. 4, St. Louis, MO: Elsevier Saunders; 2006.

Disease prevention and control in the small animal hospital

An ounce of prevention is worth a pound of cure.

Benjamin Franklin

It is always better to prevent the spread of disease than to treat disease. One of the best ways to prevent any disease is to avoid exposure. Since it is impossible for anything to live in a vacuum or a bubble, veterinary personnel should be aware of the mode of transmission for individual diseases. Awareness of disease prevention and of the modes of transmission allows us to provide education to clients and staff. This in turn helps to prevent the spread of disease. The modes of transmission for viruses, bacteria, and fungus include aerosolization, GI (fecal/oral), vectors, fomites, and direct contact.

Standard (universal) precautions

Human health-care workers in the 1980s adopted universal precautions to avoid contact with bodily fluids when treating patients.

The premise was that all patients are potentially infectious and are treated as such until proven otherwise. These precautions were expanded and are now known as standard precautions. The practice of standard precautions should be used in the veterinary setting to aid in the prevention of disease transmission.

Client education precautions

Each time an animal is presented to the veterinary hospital, the vaccine status of the patient should be verified with the client and the vaccine status should be documented in the medical record. Clients should be educated regarding the benefits of core vaccines (unless vaccination is not recommended due to health concerns) and on any vaccines recommended for the area or the patient's individual risk factors. In addition, client education regarding control of ectoparasites (e.g., fleas and ticks) and endoparasites is indicated. All hospitalized patients should be checked for ectoparasites prior to admission to the hospital and, if these parasites are found, should be treated accordingly. A parasite prevention program including semiannual fecal parasite examinations and the use of preventative treatments appropriate to the region should be discussed with the clients.

Examination precautions

Front desk staff should be trained to recognize the presenting complaints for infectious diseases. Patients with clinical signs associated with infectious disease (e.g., vomiting, diarrhea, coughing, or sneezing) should be immediately placed into isolation if possible, otherwise, directly into a designated examination room upon arrival at the veterinary facility. This will decrease the potential for direct or indirect pathogen transmission to healthy animals in the waiting room and will alert the staff to a possible infectious patient on the premises.

A thorough patient history is a key component in identifying an infection. Information including travel history and exposure to other animals (especially those with similar clinical signs) may alert veterinary staff to the presence of a potentially infectious disease.

Movement of a potentially infectious patient within the hospital should be restricted. These potentially infectious patients should not be removed from the isolation room or designated examination room (unless the patient is in an emergency situation) until it is determined the patient is noninfectious. It is important that there is a limited amount of contact with the staff with these patients to stop the potential spread of these diseases to other patients. Any staff interacting with these patients should limit their contact with other patients for the rest of their shift. Effective hand washing and the use of personal protective equipment (PPE) help limit the spread of infectious organisms. Depending on the clinical signs, necessary protective clothing may include barrier gowns, gloves, masks, booties, and eye protection.

For effective disinfection and removal of the infectious agent, each and every room, equipment, surface, or item with any patient contact should be thoroughly disinfected before use and, if possible, taken out of use for 12–24 h.

Any laboratory samples submitted from these animals should be clearly marked to prevent potential contamination of other personnel and patients. All outer containers should be sprayed with a disinfectant prior to being taken from the room to the laboratory area. Gloves should be worn and hands should be washed after removing the gloves. Care must be taken to not touch door handles, equipment, or other animals with soiled hands or gloves. All trash from a suspected infectious patient should be double bagged, and the outer bag should be sprayed with the appropriate disinfectant prior to disposal.

Hospital precautions

When hospitalizing patients with transmissible infectious diseases, staff should be aware that aerosolization of pathogens, contamination of surfaces, and fomites are potential means of disease transmission. Aerosolized particles can travel up to 20 ft and microorganisms can survive in the environment for hours to months. For this reason, traffic flow around infectious patients should be limited. Cleanliness is imperative to prevent the spread of disease. All floors, cages, food bowls, and bedding should be thoroughly cleaned and disinfected daily. Individual cages should be disinfected after each use. All walls, cages, and equipment should be thoroughly cleaned and disinfected at least weekly. Examination tables should be sanitized between patients. Any food bowls used for infectious patients should be disinfected in the isolation area and used only for that patient during their hospitalization.

In addition to cleaning procedures, consideration should be given to reduce the spread of infectious agents throughout the hospital. Hospitalized patients should not be moved from cage to cage unless absolutely required. Disposable shoe covers and footbaths with the appropriate disinfection agent should be used to prevent staff from carrying the microorganism throughout the hospital. All laundry in the veterinary hospital should be washed in hot water with the addition of an appropriate chemical agent; alternatively, the laundry can be soaked in the agent prior to washing.

There are some organisms that can survive for months in the environment. Disinfection is the process of destroying all living tissue. Sanitization reduces the number of infective organisms to a level where they are considered safe from a public health standpoint.[3] Disinfecting and sanitizing agents may be physical processes or chemical substances. Heat, either dry or steam, and light are examples of physical disinfection or sanitization processes. Chemical disinfection or sanitization agents are divided into eight main categories. There are several cleaning agents commercially available within each category. Some agents can be used for both sanitizing and disinfecting, depending on the concentration and/or contact time (Table 11.5.5).

Removal of gross organic material is needed prior to sanitizing or disinfecting surfaces. Not every agent is effective against every microorganism that causes disease. In addition, some agents must be used at specific concentrations and contact times to be effective against certain microorganisms. Always check the product label for concentration, application method, and contact time. Cleaning and disinfecting protocols should be reviewed on an annual basis or if there is an outbreak of disease in the veterinary hospital.

Table 11.5.6 provides examples of some common microorganisms of importance to veterinary medicine.[4–7]

Table 11.5.5 Chemical agents by category

Chemical agent	Concentration	Presence of organic material
Alcohols	50–95% Ethanol, isopropyl	Ineffective
Aldehydes	Formaldehyde Glutaraldehyde	Some effect
Halogens	1:30 (sodium hypochlorite bleach)	Ineffective
	Iodine	May be reduced
	Iodophor (betadine) 1–10% (1:9)	May be reduced
Oxidizing agents	5–20% Hydrogen peroxide Peracetic acid	Some effect
Phenolics	Pine-Sol (5% solution)	Effective
Quaternary ammonium	Roccal® D-256® Benzalkonium chloride	Not effective against nonenveloped viruses
Biguanides	Chlorhexidine (0.78%)	Ineffective

Source: Greene CE (ed). *Infectious Diseases of the Dog and Cat*, 3rd edition, St. Louis, MO: Saunders Elsevier; 2006.

Table 11.5.6 Common microorganisms in veterinary medicine and their modes of transmission, survivability, and recommended disinfectants

Microorganism	Mode of transmission	Environmental temperature	Time of survival	Disinfecting agent	Contact time to disinfect
Feline rhinotracheitis virus	Aerosol	4°C/39.2°F	154 days	Heat[a] 56°C/132.8°F	4–5 min
		25°C/77°F	33 days	70% Alcohol	10 min
		37°C/98.6°F	3 h	Sodium hypochlorite[b]	10 min
				100% Iodine	10 min
				Phenol	10 min
				0.5% Quat[c]	10 min
				Formaldehyde	10 min
				Glutaraldehyde	10 min
				0.78% Big[d]	10 min
Canine herpesvirus	Direct contact	4°C/39.2°F	48 h	Heat-56°C/132.8°F	4–5 min
	Fomites	37°C/98.6°F	48 h		
Canine distemper virus	Aerosol	−65°C/−85°F	7 years	Heat—60°C/140°F	30 min
	Body fluids	4°C/39.2°F	7–8 weeks	Formaldehyde	120 min
	Transplacental	25°C/77°F	3 h	0.2% Quats	30 min
Canine parvovirus	Fecal/oral	25°C/77°F Very stable in the environment	3 months or more	Heat—56°C/132.8°F	15 min
				Sodium hypochlorite	15 min
Feline panleukopenia virus	Fecal/oral	Very stable in the environment	3 months or more	0.05% Phenol	Rapid
				Sodium hypochlorite	10 min
				Formaldehyde	10 min
				Glutaraldehyde	10 min
				0.78% Big	10 min
Infectious canine hepatitis	Fecal/oral	4°C/39.2°F	2 months	Heat- 60°C/140°F	30 min
		25°C/77°F	14 days	Ultraviolet	120 min
		37°C/98.6°F	6 h	Formaldehyde	24 h
				Sodium hypochlorite	10 min
				100% Iodine	10 min
				Phenol	10 min
Feline calicivirus	Aerosol	7°C–20°C/ 44.6°F–68°F	10 days	Heat—50°C/122°F	30 min
				Phenol (at 50%)	10 min
				Sodium hypochlorite	10 min
				Formaldehyde	10 min
				Glutaraldehyde	10 min
Canine and feline rotavirus	Fecal/oral	24°C/75.2°F	2 days	Heat—60°C/140°F	30 min
		37°C/98.6°F	19 h	70% Alcohol	25 min
				Formaldehyde	56 min
Chlamydia	Aerosol	0°C/32°F	24 h	Heat—60°C/140°F	15 min
	Ocular discharge	25°C/77°F	7 days	0.5% Quats	10 min

(Continued)

Table 11.5.6 (*Continued*)

Microorganism	Mode of transmission	Environmental temperature	Time of survival	Disinfecting agent	Contact time to disinfect
Mycoplasma	Aerosol	28°C/82.4°F	21 days	Heat—55°C/131°F	15 min
				1% Phenol	<5 min
				Formaldehyde	<5 min
Gram + staphylococci	Direct contact Aerosol	4°C/39.2°F	Several months	Heat—60°C/140°F	30 min
				1% Phenol	15 min
Brucella	Direct contact	25°C/77°F	3 months	Heat—60°C/140°F	15 min
				1% Phenol	15 min
Salmonella	Fecal/oral	25°C/77°F	12–14 weeks	Heat—60°C/140°F	20 min
Clostridium spores		Very resistant in the environment		Heat—120°C/248°F	10 min
				5% Phenol	10–12 h
Leptospira	Direct contact Urine	0–25°C/32–77°F		Heat—50°C/122°F	10 min
				Iodine	10 min
Toxoplasma cysts	Fecal/oral	4°C/39.2°F	68 days	Heat—56°C/132.8°F	10–15 min
				Freeze	
Isospora	Fecal/oral	25°C/77°F	24 h	Heat—50°C/122°F	4 h
Canine influenza H3N8	Aerosol	Surfaces	48 h	Sodium hypochlorite	10 min
	Fomites	Clothing	24 h	Quats	10 min
		Hands	12 h		
Canine infectious Tracheobronchitis	Aerosol Fomites	28°C/82.4°F	21 days	Heat—55°C/131°F	15 min
				1% Phenol	<5 min
				Formaldehyde	<5 min
				0.78% Big	10 min
Influenza H1N1	Aerosol	Paper/cloth	8–12 h	Sodium hypochlorite	10 min
	Fomites	Surfaces Wet areas	24–48 h Up to 72 h	Quats	10 min
Methicillin-resistant *Staphylococcus aureus*	Direct contact	4°C/39.2°F	Several months	Heat—60°C/140°F	30 min
				1% Phenol	15 min
				Sodium hypochlorite	15 min
				Quats	15 min
Methicillin-resistant *Staphylococcus intermedius*	Direct contact	4°C/39.2°F	Several months	Heat—60°C/140°F	30 min
				1% Phenol	15 min
				Sodium hypochlorite	15 min
				Quats	15 min

[a] Heat—dry or steam.
[b] Sodium hypochlorite—household bleach.
[c] Quats—quaternary ammoniums.
[d] Big—biguanides.

Immunocompromised patients

Good nursing care is imperative for the prevention of nosocomial infections for all hospitalized patients. Postoperative patients may have a lowered immune system and may be more susceptible to bacterial infections. Care should be taken to ensure that these animals are kept clean and dry. If a postoperative patient is unable to shift its weight, such as dogs with intravertebral disk disease, the patient's cage should be well padded and the patient turned every few hours to prevent decubital ulcers (a potential source of infection).

Care must be taken when immunocompromised patients are hospitalized to reduce the risk of exposure to infectious diseases. If possible, dedicated examination rooms should be used for animals with immunocompromised status, such as patients receiving chemotherapy. Hospital staff should wear gowns and gloves to protect immunocompromised patients from normal flora carried by personnel. Protocols for minimizing contact between patients is optimal for providing protection to all patients.

Protocols and training

Each facility should create an isolation protocol and it should be reviewed frequently to ensure that there are no "breaks" in the system. New staff should be thoroughly trained on the isolation protocols before working with any infectious patient. It is recommended that the isolation protocol be posted outside and inside of the isolation area to aid the staff in adhering to the procedures. Dedicated equipment, the use of PPE such as disposable gowns and gloves, and the use of disposable supplies within the isolation area is recommended. No other equipment should be stored within this area. If equipment cannot be dedicated for isolation, it must be cleaned and disinfected prior to returning it to general use.

The individual technician bears the responsibility to prevent disease transmission not only to the patients but also to their coworkers. Judicious hand washing or the use of hand sanitizers, consuming food and beverages only in approved areas, appropriate animal restraint techniques (to reduce bites and scratches), and prompt attention to personal health will limit the transmission of infectious disease.

Conclusion

Good client education is imperative to prevent the spread of disease and is every veterinary team member's responsibility. Clients who have animals with infectious diseases should be given direction on disinfection and how to prevent the spread of disease to their other pets or future pets. If an animal has a zoonotic disease, it is very important that those clients are given information on how to reduce their own risk of acquiring the disease. Special attention to clients whose animals are undergoing chemotherapy or are immunocompromised is imperative. It is heartbreaking when animals become ill due to preventable circumstances (Table 11.5.7).

Table 11.5.7   Recommended standard precautions

Precaution	Action
Individual	
Hand hygiene	Frequent hand washing or use of alcohol based gels; use gloves appropriately
Personal protective equipment	Gowns, lab coats, eye protection, masks appropriately utilized
Personal health	Current personal immunizations; stay home when ill, seek prompt medical attention
Employer	
Safety committee	Provide ongoing training, monitor for compliance of policies
Ill worker policy	Enforce ill worker policy, send ill employees home
Food and beverage	Prevent ingestion, limit food and beverages to appropriate areas
Animals	
Isolation procedures	Both in hospital and in isolation protocols in place
Restraint	Proper restraint techniques and appropriate use of anesthesia/sedatives to prevent bites/scratches
Client education	
Vaccination	Current on all core and recommended vaccines
Flea and tick control	Educate and recommend
Internal parasites	Check fecal samples q 6 months, recommend year-round preventatives if appropriate
Facilities	
Clean and disinfect	All patient contact items daily and as needed
Isolation decontamination	Exam rooms, hospital and isolation areas, barriers and procedures

Modified from Ehnert K. Zoonotic disease problems. In: *Textbook of Veterinary Internal Medicine*, eds. SJ Ettinger, EC Feldman, Table 222-2. Saunders Elsevier; 2010.

Bibliography

Section 1

1. Breitschwerdt EB. Canine bartonellosis. *Clinician's Brief* 2010;epub July 2010:13–17.

2. Brunt J, Kordick DL, Kudrak S, et al. American Association of Feline Practitioners 2006 Panel report on diagnosis, treatment, and prevention of Bartonella spp. infections. *Journal of Feline Medicine and Surgery* 2006;Aug;8(4):213–226.

3. Guptill-Yoran L. Feline bartonellosis. In: *Infectious Diseases of the Dog and Cat*, 3rd edition, ed. CE Greene, pp. 511–518. Philadelphia, PA: Saunders; 2006.

4. Breitschwerdt EB, Chomel BB. Canine bartonellosis. In: *Infectious Diseases of the Dog and Cat*, 3rd edition, ed. CE Greene, pp. 518–524. Philadelphia, PA: Saunders; 2006.

5. Hollett RB. Canine brucellosis: outbreaks and compliance. *Theriogenology* 2006;66:575–587.

6. Ledbetter EC, Landry MP, Stolkol T. *Brucella canis* endophthalmitis in 3 dogs: clinical features, diagnosis, and treatment. *Veterinary Ophthalmology* 2009;12(3):183–191.

7. Wanke MM. Canine brucellosis. *Animal Reproduction Science* 2004;82–83:195–207.

8. Marley MS, Rynders PE. Theriogenology question of the month. *JAVMA* 2007;231(6):867–869.

9. Wanke MM, Delpino MV, Baldi PC. Use of enrofloxacin in the treatment of canine brucellosis in a dog kennel (clinical trial). *Theriogenology* 2006;66(6–7):1573–1578.

10. Neer TM, Breitschwerdt EB, Greene RT, Lappin MR. Consensus statement on ehrlichial disease of small animals from the infectious disease study group of the ACVIM. *Journal of Veterinary Internal Medicine* 2002;16:309–315.

11. Neiger R, Simpson KW. Helicobacter infection in dogs and cats: facts and fiction. *Journal of Veterinary Internal Medicine* 2000; 14:125–133.

12. Simpson KW, Neiger R, DeNovo R, et al. The relationship of *Helicobacter* spp. infection to gastric disease in dogs and cats. *Journal of Veterinary Internal Medicine* 2000;14:223–227.

13. Simpson J. Helicobacter infection in dogs and cats: to treat or not to treat? *In Practice* 2005;27:204–207.

14. Jenkins CC, Bassett JR. *Helicobacter* infection. *The Compendium on Continuing Education for the Practicing Veterinarian* 1997;19: 267–279.

15. Warren JR, Marshall B. Unidentified curved bacilli on gastric epithelium in active chronic gastritis. *Lancet* 1983;1:1273–1275.

16. Flatland B. Helicobacter infection in humans and animals. *The Compendium on Continuing Education for the Practicing Veterinarian* 2002;24:688–696.

17. Fox JG. Enteric bacterial infections. In: *Infectious Diseases of the Dog and Cat*, 3rd edition, ed. CE Greene, pp. 343–351. St. Louis, MO: W.B. Saunders; 2006.

18. Happonen I, Linden J, Westermarck E. Effect of triple therapy on eradication of canine gastric helicobacters and gastric disease. *Journal of Small Animal Practice* 2000;41:1–6.

19. Lieb MS, Duncan RB. Gastric *Helicobacter* spp. and chronic vomiting in dogs. In: *Kirk's Current Veterinary Therapy XIV*, 14th edition, eds. JD Bonagura, DC Twedt, pp. 492–497. St. Louis, MO: W.B. Saunders; 2009.

20. *Pathogenesis of Bacterial Infections in Animals*, 4th edition, eds. CL Gyles, JF Prescott, G Songer, CO Thoen. Ames, IA: Wiley-Blackwell; 2010.

21. *Infectious Diseases of the Dog and Cat*, 3rd edition, eds. CE Greene, pp. 439–436. St. Louis, MO: Saunders Elsevier; 2006.

22. *Textbook of Veterinary Internal Medicine*, 7th edition, eds. S Ettinger, E Feldman. St. Louis, MO: Elsevier Saunders; 2010.

23. *Textbook of Veterinary Internal Medicine*, 6th edition, eds. S Ettinger, E Feldman. St. Louis, MO: Elsevier Saunders; 2000.

24. Neimark H, Johansson KE, Rikihisa Y, et al. Proposal to transfer some members of the genera *Haemobartonella* and eperythrozoon to the genus *Mycoplasma* with descriptions of "Candidatus Mycoplasma haemofelis," "Candidatus Mycoplasma haemomuris," and "Candidatus Mycoplasma wenyonii." *International Journal of Systematic and Evolutionary Biology* 2001;51 (Part 3):891–899.

25. Sykes JE, Terry JC, Lindsay LL, et al. Prevalences of various hemoplasma species among cats in the United States with possible hemoplasmosis. *Journal of the American Veterinary Medical Association* 2008;232:372–379.

26. Chalker VJ. Canine mycoplasmas. *Research in Veterinary Science* 2005;79:1–8.

27. Greene CE. Mycoplasmal, ureaplasmal, and L-form infections. In: *Infectious Diseases of the Dog and Cat*, 3rd edition, ed. CE Greene, pp. 260–265. St. Louis, MO: Elsevier; 2006.

28. *Small Animal Internal Medicine*, 4th edition, eds. R Nelson, CG Couto. St. Louis, MO: Elsevier Mosby; 2009.

29. *Saunders Manual of Small Animal Practice*, eds. SJ Birchard, RG Sherding, et al. Philadelphia, PA: W.B. Saunders; 1994.

30. Chandler JC, Lappin MR. Mycoplasmal respiratory infections in small animals: 17 cases (1988–1999). *Journal of the American Animal Hospital Association.* 2002;38:111–119.

31. Harvey JW. Hemotrophic mycoplasmosis (hemobartonellosis). In: *Infectious Diseases of the Dog and Cat*, 3rd edition, ed. CE Greene, pp. 252–260. St. Louis, MO: Elsevier; 2006.

32. Sykes JE. Feline hemotropic mycoplasmas. *Journal of Veterinary Emergency and Critical Care* 2010;20:62–69. 6. 6.

33. Fritz CL. Emerging tick-borne diseases. *Veterinary Clinics of North America Small Animal Practice* 2009;39(2):265–278.

34. Bowman D, Little SE, Lorentzen L, et al. Prevalence and geographic distribution of *Dirofilaria immitis*, *Borrelia burgdorferi*, *Ehrlichia canis* and *Anaplasma phagocytophilum* in dogs in the United States: results of a national clinic-based serologic survey. *Veterinary Parasitology* 2009;160(1–2):138–148.

35. Littman MP, Goldstein RE, Labato MA, Lappin MR, Moore GE. ACVIM small animal consensus statement on Lyme disease in dogs: diagnosis, treatment and prevention. *Journal of Veterinary Internal Medicine* 2006;20(2):422–434.

36. Whitney EAS, Ailes E, Myers LM, et al. Prevalence of and risk factors for serum antibodies against *Leptospira* serovars in US veterinarians. *Journal of the American Veterinary Medical Association* 2009;234(7):938–944.

37. Stokes JE, Kaneene JB, Schall WD, et al. Prevalence of serum antibodies against six Leptospira serovars in healthy dogs. *Journal of the American Veterinary Medical Association* 2007;230(11): 1657–1664.

38. Van De Maele I, Claus A, Haesebrouck F, Daminet S. Leptospirosis in dogs: a review with emphasis on clinical aspects. *Veterinary Record* 2008;163:409–413.

39. Guerra MA. Zoonosis update: leptospirosis. *Journal of the American Veterinary Medical Association* 2009;234(4):472–478.

40. Smith TC, Pearson N. The emergence of *Staphylococcus aureus* ST398. *Vector Borne and Zoonotic Diseases* 2011;Apr 11(4): 327–39. DOI: 10.1089/vbz.2010.0072.

41. Ippolito G, Leone S, Lauria F, et al. Methicillin-resistant *Staphylococcus aureus*: the superbug. *International Journal of Infectious Diseases* 2010;Oct;14 Suppl 4:S7-11. DOI: 101016/j.ijid.2010.05.003.

42. Cohn L, Middleton JR. A veterinary perspective on methicillin-resistant staphylococci. *JVECC* 2010;20(1):31–45.

43. *Plumbs Veterinary Drug Handbook*, 6th edition, ed. DC Plumb. Ames, IA: Blackwell Publishing; 2008.

44. VanSteenhouse JL, Taboada J, Dorfman MI. 42. *Haemobartonella felis* infection with atypical hematological abnormalities. *Journal of the American Animal Hospital Association*. 1995;31(2): 165–169.

45. *Textbook of Veterinary Internal Medicine*, 7th edition, eds. SJ Ettinger, EC Feldman, Vols. 1&2, p. 1105. St. Louis, MO: Saunders Elsevier; 2010.

Section 2

1. *Infectious Diseases of the Dog and Cat*, 3rd edition, ed. CE Greene. St. Louis, MO: Elsevier Saunders; 2006.

2. *Small Animal Internal Medicine*, 4th edition, eds. R Nelson, CG Couto. St. Louis, MO: Elsevier Mosby; 2009.

3. *Textbook of Veterinary Internal Medicine*, 6th edition, eds. S Ettinger, E Feldman. St. Louis, MO: Elsevier Saunders; 2000.

4. *Plumbs Veterinary Drug Handbook*, 6th edition, ed. DC Plumb. Ames, IA: Blackwell Publishing; 2008.

5. *Saunders Manual of Small Animal Practice*, eds. SJ Birchard, RG Sherding. Philadelphia, PA: W.B. Saunders; 1994.

6. *Small Animal Pediatrics, The First 12 Months of Life*, eds. ME Peterson, MA Kutzler. St. Louis, MO: Elsevier Saunders; 2011.

7. Baumgartner DJ, Steber D, Galzier R, et al. Geographic information system analysis of blastomycosis in norther Wisconsin: waterways and soils. *Medical Mycology* 2005;43(2):117–125.

8. Chen T, Legendre AM, Bass C, Odoi A. A case-control study of sporadic canine blastomycosis in Tennessee, USA. *Medical Mycology* 2008;46(8):843–852.

9. Crews LJ, Feeney DA, Jessen CR, Newman AB. Radiographic findings in dogs with pulmonary blastomycosis: 125 cases (1989–2006). *Journal of the American Veterinary Medical Association* 2008;232(2):215–221.

10. Kerl ME. Update on canine and feline fungal diseases. *Veterinary Clinics of North America Small Animal Practice* 2003;33(4):721–747.

11. Spector D, Legendre AM, Wheat J, et al. Antigen and antibody testing for the diagnosis of blastomycosis in dogs. *Journal of Veterinary Internal Medicine* 2008;22(4):839–843.

Section 3

1. Nelson R, Couto CG. *Small Animal Internal Medicine*, 4th edition, St. Louis, MO: Elsevier Mosby; 2009.

2. Ettinger S, Feldman E. *Textbook of Veterinary Internal Medicine*, 6th edition, St. Louis, MO: Elsevier Saunders; 2000.

3. Peterson M, Kutzler MA. *Small Animal Pediatrics, The First 12 Months of Life*. St. Louis, MO: Elsevier Saunders; 2010.

4. Greene CE. *Infectious Diseases of the Dog and Cat*, 3rd edition. St. Louis, MO: Elsevier Saunders; 2006.

5. Ettinger S, Feldman E. *Textbook of Veterinary Internal Medicine*, 7th edition, St. Louis, MO: Elsevier Saunders; 2010.

6. Plumb DC. *Plumbs Veterinary Drug Handbook*, 6th edition, Ames, IA: Blackwell Publishing; 2008.

7. Vaden SL, Knoll JS, Smith FWK, Tilley L. *Blackwell's Five-Minute Veterinary Consult: Laboratory Tests and Diagnostic Procedures Canine and Feline*. Ames, IA: Wiley-Blackwell; 2009.

8. Birchard SJ, Sherding RG. *Saunders Manual of Small Animal Practice*. Philadelphia, PA: W.B. Saunders; 1994.

9. Bonagura JD. *Kirk's Current Veterinary Therapy XIII. Small Animal Practice*, pp. 310–313. Philadelphia, PA: W.B. Saunders; 2000.

Section 4

1. Greene CE, Carmichael LE. Canine herpesvirus infection. In: *Infectious Diseases of the Dog and Cat*, 3rd edition, ed. CE Greene, pp. 47–53. Philadelphia, PA: Saunders; 2006.

2. Ledbetter EC, Kim SG, Dubovi EJ, Bicalho RC. Experimental reactivation of latent canine herpesvirus-1 and induction of recurrent ocular disease in adult dogs. *Veterinary Microbiology* 2009;Jul 2;138(1–2):98–105.

3. Gaskell RM, Dawson S, Radford A. Feline respiratory disease. In: *Infectious Diseases of the Dog and Cat*, 3rd edition, ed. CE Greene, pp. 145–154. Philadelphia, PA: Saunders; 2006.

4. European Advisory Board on Cat Diseases. *ABCD Guidelines on Feline Herpesvirus*, Panel Report; 2006.

5. Maggs DJ, Nasisse MP, Kass PH. Efficacy of oral supplementation with L-lysine in cats latently infected with feline herpesvirus. *American Journal of Veterinary Research* 2003;Jan;64(1):37–42.

6. American Association of Feline Practitioners. *The 2006 American Association of Feline Practitioners Feline Vaccine Advisory Panel Report*; 2006.

7. Urban MA. Influenza: viral infections: Merck manual home edition. http://www.merck.com/mmhe/sec17/ch198/ch198d.html (accessed July 27, 2010).

8. International Committee on Taxonomy of Viruses. The universal virus database, version 4: influenza A. http://www.ncbi.nlm.nih.gov/ICTVdb/ICTVdB/00.046.0.01.htm (accessed July 27, 2010).

9. Spnseller BA, Trujillo JD, Jergens A, et al. *Apparent Reverse Zoonotic transmission of Pandemic H1N1 Influenza Virus Infection in Domestic Cats: Clinical Diagnoses and Disease*, ACVIM Forum, June 9–12, 2010.

10. Jakeman KJ, Tisdale M, Russell S, Leone A, Sweet C. Efficacy of 2'-deoxy-2'-fluororibosides against influenza A and B viruses in ferrets. *Antimicrobial Agents and Chemotherapy* 1994;38(8):1864–1867. http://www.ncbi.nlm.nih.gov/pubmed/7986023 (accessed July 27, 2010).

11. Osterhaus A, Rimmelzwaan G, Martina B, Bestebroer T, Fouchier R. Influenza B virus in seals. *Science* 2000;288(5468):1051–1053. http://dx.doi.org/10.1126%2Fscience.288.5468.1051 (accessed July 27, 2010).

12. Nobusawa E, Sato K. Comparison of the mutation rates of human influenza A and B viruses. *Journal of Virology* 2006;80(7):3675–3678. http://dx.doi.org/10.1128%2FJVI.80.7.3675-3678.2006 (accessed July 27, 2010).

13. Taubenberger JK, Morens DM. The pathology of influenza virus infections. *Annual Review of Pathology* 2008;3:499–522. http://www.pubmedcentral.nih.gov/articlerender.fcgi?tool=pmcentrez&artid=2504709 (accessed July 27, 2010).

14. Weber TP, Stilianakis NI. Inactivation of influenza A viruses in the environment and modes of transmission: a critical review. *The Journal of Infection* 2008;57(5):361–373. http://dx.doi.org/10.1016%2Fj.jinf.2008.08.013 (accessed July 27, 2010).

15. Suarez D, Spackman E, Senne D, Bulaga L, Welsch A, Froberg K. The effect of various disinfectants on detection of avian influenza virus by real time RT-PCR. *Avian Diseases* 2003;47(3 Suppl): 1091–1095. http://dx.doi.org/10.1637%2F0005-2086-47.s3.1091 (accessed July 27, 2010).

16. Schrenzel MD, Tucker TA, Stalis IH, et al. Letter Pandemic (H1N1) 2009 virus in 3 wildlife species, San Diego, California, USA. *Emerging Infectious Disease Journal* 2011;17(4).

17. CDC H1N1 flu, http://www.cdc.gov/h1n1flu/ (accessed July 27, 2010).

18. Peterson ME, Kutzler MA. *Small Animal Pediatrics, The First 12 Months of Life*. St. Louis, MO: Elsevier Saunders; 2011.

19. Ettinger S, Feldman E. *Textbook of Veterinary Internal Medicine*, 6th edition, St. Louis, MO: Elsevier Saunders; 2000.

20. Greene CE. *Infectious Diseases of the Dog and Cat*, 3rd edition, St. Louis, MO: Elsevier Saunders; 2006.

Section 5

1. Greene CE. *Infectious Diseases of the Dog and Cat*, 3rd edition, p. 3. St. Louis, MO: Elsevier Saunders; 2006.

2. Vaden SL, Knoll JS, Smith FWK, Tilley L. *Blackwell's Five-minute Veterinary Consult: Laboratory Tests and Diagnostic Procedures Canine and Feline*. Ames, IA: Wiley-Blackwell; 2009.

3. Dvorak G. Disinfection 101. http://www.cfsph.iastate.edu/BRM/resources/Disinfectants/Disinfection101Feb2005.pdf (accessed January 14, 2009).

4. Crawford C. 2009. Canine influenza: frequently asked questions from veterinarians, University of Florida. http://www.vetmed.ufl.edu/ college/pr/documents/CanineinfluenzaFAQ.Veterinarians_000.pdf (accessed July 29, 2010).

5. Cleaning to reduce the risk of H1N1 flu virus—Guidelines for cleaning, janitorial and maintenance staff. http://www.enichols. com/downloads/cleaning_to_reduce_the_risk_of_h1n1_flu_ virus.pdf (accessed July 29, 2010).

6. Healthcare-associated infections (HAI). http://www.cdc.gov/ ncidod/dhqp/ar_MRSA.html (accessed July 29, 2010).

7. Greene CE (ed.). *Infectious Diseases of the Dog and Cat*. Philadelphia, PA: W.B. Saunders; 1990.

8. *Textbook of Veterinary Internal Medicine*, 6th edition, eds. S Ettinger, E Feldman. St. Louis, MO: Elsevier Saunders; 2000.

9. *Plumbs Veterinary Drug Handbook*, ed. DC Plumb, 6th edition. Ames, IA: Blackwell Publishing; 2008.

10. *Small Animal Internal Medicine*, 4th edition, eds. R Nelson, CG Couto. St. Louis, MO: Elsevier Mosby; 2009.

11. *Saunders Manual of Small Animal Practice*, eds. SJ Birchard, RG Sherding. Philadelphia, PA: W.B. Saunders; 1994.

12. *Small Animal Pediatrics, The First 12 Months of Life*, eds. ME Peterson, MA Kutzler. St. Louis, MO: Elsevier Saunders; 2011.

13. Crawford C, Rada KA. *Canine Influenza*. http://www. sheltermedicine.com/shelter-health-portal/information-sheets/ canine-influenza (accessed March 5, 2012).

Chapter 12 Vaccine, Vaccination, and Immunology

Editors: Shauna Blois and Linda Merrill

SECTION 1 THE IMMUNE RESPONSE AND CANCER IMMUNOTHERAPY

The immune response in an individual represents a collective and coordinated response to the introduction of foreign substances or cellular changes such as cancer. The immune response is mediated by the cells and molecules of the immune system.[1] The two primary components of the immune system are the innate (nonspecific, typically rapid) and adaptive (highly specific but slower developing) immune responses.[2]

Innate and adaptive immune response

Innate immunity is the immunity that one is born with—physical and chemical barriers such as intact skin, stomach acids, mucus, lysozyme in tears, body temperature, phagocytic cells (neutrophils and macrophages), natural killer (NK) cells, and cytokines. The innate immune system lacks any form of memory,

so its response is the same regardless of the cellular trigger—inflammation. The complex set of reactions caused by inflammation increases blood flow, allowing for the accumulation of phagocytic cells and enzymes triggered by the presence of invaders at the site.[3]

Like the skin, the mucosal epithelia of the gastrointestinal and respiratory tracts serve as a barrier between the internal and external environment. Defense against microbes that enter through these routes is provided by the mucosal immune system, which is one of the effector arms of the adaptive immune response. High levels of immunoglobulin (Ig antibody), specifically IgA, are present in the mucosal tissue. IgA's function is to bind to the microbe, making it too large to enter the host.[1] The mucosal immune system plays a role with both innate and adaptive functions.

Adaptive immunity represents the response of the body to a specific antigen. An antigen is a substance that is capable of activating the immune system and stimulating the formation of antibodies or cell-mediated immunity. Adaptive immunity is mediated by lymphocytes and stimulated by exposure to molecules recognized as foreign or nonself. Such antigens include infectious agents, foreign material, and malignant or transformed cells. Nonself molecules differ from self-molecules (which are the body's own tolerated antigenic substances).[1] The separate arms of the immune system are linked by the ability of the innate response to stimulate and influence the nature of the adaptive response.[2]

Humoral and cell-mediated immunity

Humoral immunity and cell-mediated immunity are two types of adaptive immune responses that function in different ways against microbes and other agents such as cancerous cells. Humoral immunity acts against extracellular foreign antigens, mediated by antibodies in serum produced by B lymphocytes (bone marrow-derived cells) which bind and direct the elimination of these antigens.[1] As it relates to oncology, one example of humoral immunity is the elimination of premalignant cells that express nonself antigens. Cell-mediated immunity is the primary adaptive immune response against intracellular pathogens as well as tumor antigens, mediated by T lymphocytes, which are cells that have matured in the thymus.[1] T lymphocytes can either be directly cytotoxic or can moderate cell destruction by a host of complicated mechanisms.[3]

There are five types of tumor antigens recognized by T cells: (1) differentiation antigens (antigens associated with specific stages in the development of a cell type, i.e., those normally present in a fetal cell but not in an adult cell); (2) mutated forms of normal proteins; (3) normal proteins produced in excessive quantities; (4) cancer/testes antigens (tumor antigens with gene expression restricted to male germ cells); and (5) tumors induced by viruses that produce viral antigens (e.g., oncogenic virus such as feline leukemia).[3]

Cell-mediated immunity involving T cells and natural killer (NK) cells are likely the most important components of the immune response mediating the bodies' resistance to cancer. The immune system is capable under certain circumstances, via both innate and adaptive responses, of recognizing and eliminating tumor cells. The NK cells of the innate response kill tumor cells by direct lytic mechanisms. NK cells can also be stimulated by cytokines, which are cell-signaling proteins that mediate inflammatory and immune responses. In the adaptive response, lymphocytes, specifically T cells, are continually surveying the body for cancerous or abnormal cells and eliminating them—this is the concept of immunosurveillance. As it relates to cancer development, the immune system ideally functions by recognizing and eliminating the transformed cells before they grow into tumors. Tumor cells are detected due to the expression of antigens that are identified as foreign.[1] However, as there are many cases of cancer in otherwise immunocompetent patients, the cancer cells develop complex ways to avoid being detected, either by evading or overcoming host defenses.[1,2]

One of the major mechanisms of immunotherapy "works" by using biologically active proteins to alter the specific and nonspecific immune responses of the patient.[4] In cancer immunotherapy, the body is stimulated with agents that can either make them hypersensitive to the presence of abnormal/cancer cells or remove the immune tolerance so that nonself/cancerous antigens can be recognized and subsequently attacked.[1]

Immunomodulation

The first attempts at modulating the immune system occurred in the late 1800s, when a surgeon named William Coley noticed that patients that had cancer and developed secondary bacterial infections often lived longer than those that did not get infected. He developed the first bacterial "vaccine," referred to as "Coley's toxins" using killed cultures of *Serratia marcescens* and *Streptococcus pyogenes*. His goal was to induce sepsis and associated pyrexia to cause tumor regression. This treatment led to many complete and durable tumor remissions in patients with inoperable bone and soft tissue sarcomas; however, the development of frequent side effects and the lack of support from other physicians led to the technique falling out of favor.[5]

There is evidence for the immune system playing a major part in the treatment of cancer. Specific examples include the presence of tumor-specific cytotoxic T cells within tumor or draining lymph nodes, as well as the presence of monocytic, lymphocytic and plasmacytic infiltrate in tumors. Reports of spontaneous remissions in patients who have cancer and do not have treatment, the increased incidence of some types of cancers in immunosuppressed patients, and documentation of cancer remissions in patients treated with immunomodulators also lend support to the role of the immune system in cancer treatment.[2]

It is possible to stimulate the immune system to kill tumor cells using a number of methods. In review, active immunity is immunity in which the individual plays an active role in the response; in passive immunity, the recipient receives immune cells or their products. Vaccination with tumor cells or antigens can enhance active immune responses, while passive immunity can be established by administering antitumor antibodies or activated T cells.[1]

It is proposed that the ideal cancer immunotherapy agent should have high specificity (able to differentiate between cancer and normal cells), high sensitivity (potency to kill small or large numbers of malignant cells), and durability (able to prevent tumor recurrence).[2] As with most other forms of cancer treatment, immunotherapy appears to work best in the presence of minimal residual disease. Minimal residual disease refers to the malignant cells that remain after surgical removal or other local tumor treatment. These residual cells are not clinically evident but can promote a relapse or recurrence of disease. Therefore, immunotherapy is likely most appropriate as an adjuvant treatment combined with local tumor control such as surgery and/or radiation therapy.[2]

Cancer vaccines

Adaptive immunity can alter an individual's immune system so that it can remember a pathogen previously encountered, differentiate self from nonself, and respond more quickly to repeated exposure to the pathogen. The goal in creating a cancer vaccine is to cause an immune response that results in regression of the tumor and/or the metastases, or to protect against disease progression. Because of the slower speed of adaptive immunity, the clinical response may take up to several months or more to appear while the immune response becomes fully functional.[2]

In veterinary medicine, the canine melanoma vaccine Oncept™ by Merial is the most frequently discussed cancer vaccine and was approved for use by the Food and Drug Administration (FDA) in 2007. The vaccine uses xenogeneic (different species, in this case human) deoxyribonucleic acid (DNA) expressing the human tyrosinase gene. This tyrosinase protein (encoded by the DNA) is found on normal and cancerous melanocytes. The protein produced from the human tyrosinase gene is different enough from the canine tyrosinase protein that it will stimulate an immune response, but similar enough to canine melanoma cells that the immune system targets the cancerous cells that contain the tyrosinase protein.[6]

Cytokine immunotherapy

Cytokine immunotherapy refers to the administration of cytokines to stimulate antitumor immune responses. Cytokines are produced by many different cell types such as mononuclear macrophages, activated mast cells, dendritic cells, bone marrow stromal cells, and leukocytes. Interleukins and interferons are examples of cytokines used in cancer immunotherapy.[1]

Interleukins are proteins released from lymphocytes or macrophages that can, among other more complex mechanisms, promote lymphocyte, monocyte, and macrophage proliferation, activate NK cells, or mediate inflammation.[1,7] Interleukin-2 (IL-2) is a cytokine that can induce a number of anticancer activities in the innate and adaptive arms of the immune response such as activation of cytotoxic T cells and augmentation of NK cell function.[7] Side effects associated with IV administration of IL-2, such as vascular leak syndrome, necessitated exploring other delivery options.[8] Inhalational therapy was explored as a method of maximizing drug exposure to the lungs while minimizing systemic toxicities. Liposomal formulations are used in this setting to increase the retention time of active drug in the lungs. Inhalational therapy with both free IL-2 and IL-2 liposomes has been investigated, with IL-2 liposomes showing greater activity in the treatment of pulmonary metastases.[7]

IL-12 is another cytokine being investigated in veterinary medicine. It has both immunostimulatory and antiangiogenic potential, meaning it can slow tumor growth by reducing the ability of the tumor to form new blood vessels. IL-12 may be a useful adjuvant therapy in the treatment of localized tumors such as subcutaneous hemangiosarcoma.[5]

Interferons are cytokines with antiviral, antiproliferative, and immunomodulatory effects. Recombinant feline interferon-ω (omega), available by special FDA permission from England, has been used in the treatment of a number of different cancers, including feline fibrosarcoma, as well as in the treatment of retroviral infections (feline leukemia virus [FeLV]/feline immunodeficiency virus [FIV]) associated with tumor development.[9]

Interferon-ω works by inhibiting the growth of tumor cells, inducing apoptosis, activating NK cells and by a number of other complicated mechanisms.[9] There are no published studies on efficacy at the time of publication.

Summary

Immunotherapy is an exciting field that is expanding as new tools in molecular biology are developed and a better understanding of ways to modulate the immune system are discovered.[2] The veterinary profession is in a unique position to complement human medicine as many dog and cat tumors are comparable to human cancers in how they behave biologically. In addition, these tumors may in fact be caused by the same etiologic factors, as our pets share our environment, drink the same water we do, breathe the same air we do, and in many cases, eat the same food as us. Another advantage to studying cancer in pets—specifically, the development and treatment of the disease—stems from the fact that dogs and cats live a compressed life span as compared to our own. We are then able to witness treatment successes and failures within a shorter period of time. This may help get successful therapies, such as anticancer vaccines, into human clinical trials faster than waiting the 20 or 30 years it might otherwise take to monitor for side effects and effectiveness in human clinical trials. Although immunotherapy may never be a single-agent therapy, it will likely play a supporting role alongside treatments such as surgery, radiation, and chemotherapy.

SECTION 2 LABORATORY DIAGNOSTICS IN IMMUNOLOGY

Serology

Antinuclear antibody test

The antinuclear antibody (ANA) test detects antibodies (either anti-IgG or anti-IgM) that react with nuclear components of cells by the use of a fluorescence microscope (optical microscope using the phenomena of fluorescence and phosphorescence) or an enzyme-linked immunosorbent assay (ELISA).

Indications

The ANA test is used as an adjunctive test to support a diagnosis of systemic lupus erythematosus (SLE). The test is species specific. The results are reported as a positive or negative titer. Positive titers are reported as a ratio, for example, 1:20. Positive tests may also be reported with the pattern of nuclear staining observed (homogenous, peripheral, speckled, or nucleolar). A positive titer (>1:80) with concurrent clinical disease and specific laboratory findings is supportive but not definitive for the diagnosis of SLE, but SLE should not be diagnosed or excluded based upon this single test result.[1]

Limitations

False positives may be caused by inflammation, infection, or neoplastic disease. Previous corticosteroid therapy may cause a false-negative test result.

Coombs test

The direct Coombs test detects antibody and complement bound onto the surface of erythrocyte antigens.

Indications

The Coombs test is used in anemic animals suspected of immune-mediated hemolytic anemia (IMHA) that have a negative saline agglutination test. The saline agglutination test is the first choice in these patients (see Chapter 7 for more information). The results are reported as negative or positive; positive results also indicate the dilution at which the test became negative. The Coombs test is performed by incubating species-specific antibodies against IgG, IgM, and C3 (the third component of complement) with the patient's erythrocytes at both 37 and 4°C. The presence of hemolysis and agglutination at various antibody dilutions indicates a positive result. The Coombs test is usually performed at several dilutions of antiglobulin sera (e.g., 1:2, 1:4, 1:8) to help decrease the possibility of a false-negative result due to a prozone effect. The prozone effect occurs in the presence of excessive antibody. Dilution allows for an appropriate ratio of red cell antigen to antiglobulin, permitting agglutination.[2]

Limitations

False positives can occur and can be the result of nonspecific coating of erythrocytes, *in vitro* complement binding, and previous blood transfusion. False negatives may occur and can be the result of levels of antibody that are too low, prior use of corticosteroids or laboratory processing issues. The reported sensitivity of the test is about 60%.[3] An indirect Coombs test is available but is less sensitive than the direct Coombs, so it is rarely utilized.

Miscellaneous testing

Lymphocyte proliferation/blastogenesis

Lymphocyte proliferation/blastogenesis is a functional test of lymphocyte responsiveness. There are multiple modalities used for this test and they are specific to T cells and B cells. The testing procedure starts with culture and stimulation of lymphocytes with antigen or mitogen (protein to encourage cell division). Flow cytometry, colorimetric assay, polymerase chain reaction (PCR), or ELISA are utilized to measure response.

Neutrophil bacterial killing assay

The neutrophil bacterial killing assay, also called the neutrophil function test, tests the ability of neutrophils to phagocytize bacteria and to generate an oxidative burst (the rapid release of reactive oxygen species). Flow cytometry is used to enumerate the percentage of neutrophils with normal function.

Immunophenotyping

Immunophenotyping detects cellular proteins in fresh or fixed tissue or in cellular suspensions. Commonly, this test uses antibodies to detect the presence of cellular epitopes (the part of an antigen that is recognized by the immune system), allowing for the classification of cell types. Immunophenotyping can be used to detect populations of leukocytes to aid in the diagnosis of immunodeficiencies. Additionally, immunophenotyping can aid in the detection of clonal expansion of malignant cell populations. Detection of specific cell markers (e.g. cluster of differentiation [CD] antigens) can aid in the diagnosis of such malignancies as leukemias, lymphosarcomas, and histiocytic sarcomas. Flow cytometry can be used for immunophenotyping, and tissue can be stained with labeled antibodies (immunohistochemistry). Panels of multiple antibodies may be used when performing immunophenotyping, as this documents the presence and proportion of various cellular populations of interest.

Rheumatoid factor

Rheumatoid factor (RF) is a nonsensitive and nonspecific antigen/antibody test of questionable value. A positive RF may be found in patients with rheumatoid arthritis, as well as some cases of SLE.

Immunologic testing modalities and techniques

Enzyme-linked immunosorbent assay

Also referred to as an enzyme immunoassay (EIA), the ELISA is an immunoassay test used to detect a specific antigen or antibody in a sample. Blood, urine, saliva, feces, or other samples may be used depending on the specific test. To perform an antigen ELISA, a sample containing an unknown amount of antigen is applied to a surface (e.g., a membrane or sample well). The surface contains an antibody to allow for the antigen within the sample to bind to the surface. A specific antibody is then applied and binds to the antigen in the sample. An enzyme is linked to this antibody, either directly or via a secondary antibody. The enzyme is typically a chromogenic substance that undergoes a color change after the addition of a substrate. An ELISA to detect the presence of antibody in a sample uses a similar procedure.[4] Originally performed at reference laboratories, this modality is now commonly run in-house. A point-of-care example of ELISA testing is the Snap® FeLV/FIV/feline heartworm (FHW) test, which detects the presence of FeLV, heartworm antigen, and FIV antibody.

Immunofluorescent antibody assay

Also called an indirect fluorescent antibody assay, this immunoassay detects the presence of a specific antibody in a variety of biological samples such as blood, bone marrow, and tissue. The immunofluorescent antibody assay (IFA) tests for a specific antigen using a fluorescent dye-tagged viral antibody (direct) or using a primary antibody that binds directly to the antigen and a secondary fluorescent dye-tagged antibody that binds to the primary antigen (indirect). An example of this testing modality is the FeLV IFA.

Radioimmunoassay (RIA)

This is a nuclear medicine test for a specific virus or antigen using a radioactive tagged element (e.g., iodine) combined with the antigen. The radioactive antigen is combined with a known quantity of the specific antibody. The sample, containing an unknown quantity of antigen, is then added. The sample antigen competes with the radiolabeled antigen for antibody binding sites. The bound antigen is removed from the sample and a gamma counter is used to measure the radioactivity of remaining free antigen in the sample. This is then compared to known standards, allowing the amount of antigen in the original sample to be quantified. An example of this modality is antiacetylcholine receptor antibody testing (myasthenia gravis).

Polymerase chain reaction

This modality tests for a specific microorganism using two nucleic acid primers (short DNA fragments) that are complimentary to (react with) the target portion of the DNA (genome) of the organism. A polymerase (enzyme) then amplifies (reproduces) by means of a chain reaction involving thermal cycling (alternating heating and cooling) of the DNA. By the addition of an additional step to this process (reverse transcriptase), RNA is converted into DNA and therefore can be detected. The number of tests available using this modality has dramatically increased recently, but there is minimal laboratory standardization of assays and the validation data for an individual test may not yet be available. For more information on PCR testing and the database of American Association of Veterinary Laboratory Diagnosticians (AAVLD) accredited and affiliated laboratories and PCR tests available, please refer to the Web site http:// pcr.sdstate.org. The specificity of PCR testing can be very high but is dependent on the primers used.[5] Care must be taken during collection to help prevent false positives from contamination. The predictive value of a positive test (probability that a test positive animal is diseased) can be very low. This is due to a variety of factors including the detection of DNA or RNA from both live and dead organisms, the detection of *modified live virus* (MLV) vaccine, or the presence of the organism in healthy animals.

Western blot

This test is also called immunoblotting and involves separating the proteins by gel electrophoresis, immobilizing the proteins on membranes, and then using specific antibodies to detect the target protein of interest. This technique was developed after earlier work by Professor Sir Southern and is a play on the name of his work, which was called Southern blot (there are also techniques called Northern blot and Eastern blot). An example of this test is the FIV Western blot test, which is the confirmatory test for FIV.

Biopsy techniques

Fine needle cytology collection

Needle aspirations, also known as needle biopsies, utilize a needle as the "biopsy" instrument to collect cells for cytological analysis. The goal of needle aspiration is to reach a diagnosis without the need for surgical biopsy.

Indications

Needle aspirations can aid in the diagnosis of lymphadenomegaly, organomegaly, and masses.[6]

Limitations

The limitations of needle aspirations are that the technique cannot characterize tissue architecture, cannot distinguish between a lipoma and SQ fat, may result in a nondiagnostic sample as certain cells do not readily exfoliate, and may not be able to distinguish between lymph node hyperplasia and lymphoma.

Advantages and disadvantages

The advantages of this technique are the relative ease of collection, minimal tissue trauma, usually no need for sedation, and a fast turnaround time.

The disadvantages include a low number of cells for analysis, the possibility of seeding tumor cells along the needle track, and the increased possibility of collecting a nonrepresentative sample.

Potential complications

Complications are uncommon. Hemorrhage and sharp trauma to surrounding tissues or organs are of concern if biopsying thoracic or abdominal masses. Degranulation of mast cell tumor (MCT) is a possibility, and pretreating with diphenhydramine may be indicated if MCT is suspected.

Contraindications

A coagulation disorder may be a contraindication. Note that normal coagulation profile and buccal mucosal bleeding time (BMBT) results do not eliminate the risk of hemorrhage.

Patient preparation

Coagulation tests should be considered prior to aspiration of internal organs, particularly the liver or spleen. For superficial aspirates, such as a dermal mass or a lymph node, the site may or may not be clipped and cleaned prior to aspiration. Site preparation consisting of clipping and a surgical prep of the area should be preformed prior to aspiration of the internal organs.

Restraint

Manual restraint usually is sufficient for superficial aspirates. Sedation or anesthesia may be required for the aspiration of internal organs. Some clinicians choose to avoid opioids such as hydromorphone prior to lung aspiration due to the increased panting that this drug can cause.

Patient monitoring

For superficial masses, monitor for hemorrhage postprocedure; apply gauze and digital pressure if needed. Monitor the patient postaspiration of MCTs for possible release of histamine and the resultant systemic reaction. Monitor patients postaspiration of the thoracic cavity for signs of hemorrhage or pneumothorax, (e.g., dyspnea, tachycardia, respiratory distress, cyanosis, or decreasing lung sounds). Monitor patients postaspiration of the abdomen for signs of hemorrhage (e.g., increasing heart or respiratory rate, pale mucus membranes, decreasing blood pressure, or increasing effusion).

Techniques

Needle aspiration may be blind or guided. In blind aspiration, when possible, the nondominant hand stabilizes the tissue of interest, for example, a lymph node. If the tissue is too small to be stabilized with the fingers, then the nondominant hand and fingers may simply rest on the skin surface, possibly providing some surface tension by holding the skin on either side.

Guided aspirations are real-time aspirates; usually ultrasound guided in nature, although other imaging techniques (e.g., fluoroscopy) may be utilized. Guided aspirations allow the clinician to visualize needle placement in the tissue to be sampled and to adjust the position in order to optimize collection location.

The size of the needle selected is determined by the size and type of tissue to be evaluated and the clinician preference. Typically, a 25- or 22-ga. needle is utilized. Needle length is selected based on the location or depth of the tissue to be sampled.

There are two basic techniques that may be utilized during a needle aspiration. There can be minor variations on these procedures, and often the selection of one method over another will be dependent on the clinician's or the technician's preference. The two basic techniques for needle aspiration are outlined below:

1. *Fenestration* is the repeated insertion of the needle into the desired tissue. Usually, fenestration is performed with the needle only, but if the tissue in question is in the thorax or abdomen, then a syringe may be placed on the needle to prevent air from entering the cavity. During fenestration, the needle is held by the dominant hand and inserted into the tissue. Once into the tissue, a rapid up-and-down motion is utilized and, if the tissue is large enough in size, the angle of insertion may be altered slightly. The needle is kept under the skin or surface of the organ and typically moved four to eight times. The term "needle aspiration" is somewhat of a misnomer for this technique since no actual aspiration occurs. The disadvantage of this method is the possibility of a low number of cells collected. The advantage is the small amount of cellular disruption.

2. *True needle aspiration* is the insertion of the needle into the desired tissue and then applying negative pressure to the syringe, often 2–4 mL of negative pressure is applied two to three times. The size of the syringe is typically 6–12 mL. The use of a syringe "gun" helps to stabilize the syringe during

the aspiration process. The disadvantage of this method is the increased incidence of cellular disruption. The advantage is the possibility of an increased number of cells for analysis and little needle movement in sensitive areas or when near critical structures.

Splenic cytology

Indications

Aspiration of the spleen is indicated when splenomegaly or splenic nodules are present and as part of disease staging (e.g., MCTs).

Limitations

The spleen is a large, vascular organ; therefore, samples may not be representative of focal disease and may have hemodilution artifact.

The advantages and disadvantages are similar to those listed for needle aspirations.

Potential complications

Some degree of hemorrhage is almost always noted postsampling. Seeding of the abdomen with neoplastic cells is a possibility.

Contraindications

Splenic aspiration is contraindicated in patients with hemoabdomen, if the splenic lesions are cystic in nature, and in patients with coagulation disorders.

Patient preparation

Clipping and surgical preparation of the skin is indicated. Cooperative patients may not require sedation or anesthesia. If sedation or anesthesia is used, the selection of drugs that do not cause splenic congestion is imperative. Avoid the use of acepromazine.

Restraint

Manual restraint is usually sufficient for cooperative patients. Typically, patients are restrained in right lateral or ventral recumbency, but this is dependent on the location of the spleen, the location of any nodules, if present, and the clinician's preference.

Patient monitoring

Monitor the patient postaspiration for any signs of hemorrhage. Utilization of ultrasound to monitor the abdomen for any indication of hemorrhage is helpful. Hematocrits, pre- and postprocedure, and as indicated by the results and the clinical signs of the patient, are indicated.

Techniques

The ultrasound-guided fenestration collection method is the preferred method for splenic needle aspiration. A syringe should be attached during the collection process to prevent air from entering the abdominal cavity. The syringe may or may not contain any air and is a matter of clinician preference. The spleen is a highly vascular organ and hemodilution from excessive tissue trauma, cystic lesions, or splenic engorgement will affect sample quality.

Lymph node cytology collection

Lymph node aspiration is indicated when lymph node enlargement is present and as part of the staging process in certain diseases such as neoplasia.[7]

As stated earlier, the cytology from a lymph node aspiration may not be able to distinguish between hyperplasia and lymphoma; in some cases, a lymph node biopsy may be needed.

The advantages, disadvantages, potential complications, contraindications, patient preparation, and restraint are similar to those listed for fine needle aspirations.

Techniques

Either collection method (fenestration or aspiration) may be utilized for lymph nodes, but the fenestration method is preferred.[8] Lymph node cells readily exfoliate and are relatively fragile, so care must be used to minimize trauma during the collection process.

Slide preparation techniques

To expel the contents in the needle, detach the syringe, aspirate some air into the syringe, and reattach to the needle. Expel the contents of the needle onto one end of the slide. Typically, no visible material is noted in the needle hub, but visible material can be observed on the slide after expulsion.

The pull technique is preferred for preparing cytology slides. Place a second slide onto the sample, overlapping either parallel or perpendicular to the sample. Usually, no additional pressure is needed to flatten and expand the sample. The slides are gently, horizontally pulled apart to make two slides. The bottom slide is usually superior in preparation to the top slide.

Alternate techniques may be used based on sample characteristics (solid, liquid) and include the push (similar to blood smears and suitable for fluids), starfish (for spreading very thick material), squash (see below), slant (often used for bone marrow samples), and concentrating techniques.

In addition to the pull technique, the squash preparation is the most commonly used technique for thicker material. The material is expressed onto the end of the first slide. A second slide is placed on top, either perpendicular or parallel to the first slide. When the weight of the second slide is not enough to spread out the material, slight pressure may be applied to the slides to spread out the material. Excessive pressure must be avoided so as not to disrupt the integrity of the cells. A pull technique is used to smear the material for cytological interpretation.

If the material is a very thin fluid, prepare as if making a blood slide except toward the end of the smear; stop and lift the top slide to leave a concentrated line of fluid. Alternately, if a large amount of fluid is obtained from an aspirate, the sample may be placed in an EDTA collection tube. The sample can then be centrifuged to concentrate the cellular material. Once centrifuged, most of the supernatant can be discarded, and the pellet remaining at the bottom of the tube can be resuspended in a small amount of remaining fluid. Slides can then be prepared from this sample.

All slides should be air-dried before enclosing in the slide holder. Avoid too rapid or too slow air-drying techniques. Never submit slides for cytology in the same container as samples in formalin.

Bone marrow collection

See diagnostic techniques in the nursing chapter.

SECTION 3 IMMUNOSUPPRESSIVE MEDICATIONS

Immunosuppressive medications are used for the treatment of immune-mediated diseases as well as for immunosuppression following graft or transplant surgery.

Corticosteroids

Corticosteroids are the standard and most commonly used medication for the treatment of immune-mediated diseases. They carry a wide range of adverse effects and contraindications. Doses range from lower physiological and anti-inflammatory doses to higher immunosuppressive doses. Corticosteroids suppress the immune system by decreasing the numbers of circulating T cells and suppressing complement activity. They also decrease the migration of neutrophils, macrophages, and monocytes, thus decreasing phagocytosis and antigen processing.

Corticosteroids can have a wide range of effects, both positive and negative, upon each organ system within the body. These include an increase in blood pressure by causing vasoconstriction, as well as by increasing blood volume. There is an increased risk of acquired infections due to their suppressive effects on the immune system. The secretion of gastric acid, pepsin, and trypsin is increased within the gastrointestinal tract. For this reason, the administration of an H2-receptor antagonist (e.g., famotidine or cimetidine) to potentially decrease possible gastric upset and ulceration may be recommended. Adipose tissue is redistributed from the limbs to the trunk, which contributes to the potbellied appearance and muscle wasting that can be seen with the long-term use of corticosteroids. Gluconeogenesis and lipogenesis is increased and plasma levels of triglycerides and cholesterol are elevated, which can lead to markedly lipemic serum, even in a fasted patient.

Corticosteroid therapy may cause increased activity of alkaline phosphatase (ALP) and, to a lesser extent, alanine aminotransferase (ALT) and gamma-glutamyl transpeptidase (GGT). Corticosteroid administration may increase potassium and calcium excretion and can also increase sodium and chloride reabsorption. However, hypokalemia and hyperkalemia are uncommon unless there is concurrent administration of medications that compound electrolyte imbalances (e.g., diuretics). In the central nervous system (CNS), corticosteroids may lower the seizure threshold, stimulate appetite, and change the patient's behavior (negatively or positively).

The endocrine system is the most profoundly affected by corticosteroids. At higher doses and with chronic use corticosteroids, suppress the release of adrenocorticotropic hormone (ACTH) and, in turn, decrease the amount of endogenous cortisol released during times of stress. When long-term corticosteroids are discontinued suddenly, iatrogenic hypoadrenocorticism can occur as a result of diminished levels of endogenous corticosteroid production. Antidiuretic hormone (ADH) production and function is decreased, resulting in diuresis and the polyuric, polydipsic effects that are often seen with corticosteroid administration. The negative effects of the follicle-stimulating hormone (FSH) will cause hair loss and poor hair regrowth. High doses of corticosteroids have been associated with reduced thyroid-stimulating hormone (TSH) levels as well as altered metabolism of T3 and T4. Corticosteroids can cause insulin resistance by inhibiting insulin binding to the insulin receptors. Diabetic patients treated with corticosteroids require close monitoring as well as increased insulin dosing. Nondiabetic patients on long-term corticosteroid therapy should be monitored for the development of diabetes mellitus, which is rare but has been reported.[1]

The administration of corticosteroids is contraindicated in the face of bacterial, viral, or fungal infections. Some of the most common adverse effects of corticosteroid administration are polyuria, polydipsia, polyphagia, and panting. With longer use of anti-inflammatory and immunosuppressive doses, poor hair coat, weight gain, and a potbellied appearance are common. Other adverse effects may include vomiting, diarrhea, elevated liver enzyme activity, gastric ulceration, and worsening or activation of diabetes mellitus. Adverse effects in cats are typically less pronounced.

When patients are treated with corticosteroids at either anti-inflammatory or immunosuppressive doses, instructions should be followed explicitly to prevent the relapse of immune-mediated disease or iatrogenic hypoadrenocorticism. Clients should also be instructed to discontinue any non-steroidal anti-inflammatory medications prior to the start of corticosteroid administration, as concurrent use has high potential to cause gastrointestinal ulceration and perforation (Table 12.3.1). While there is no clinical evidence, the typically washout period prior to starting corticosteroids in a patient that has received non-steroidal anti-inflammatory drugs (NSAIDs) ranges from 5 to 10 days, depending on clinician preference and on the patient's need for corticosteroids.

Prednisone/prednisolone/dexamethasone/ dexamethasone sodium phosphate

Either short- or intermediate-acting corticosteroids are typically chosen for immunosuppression. Prednisone and dexametha-

Table 12.3.1 Drug interactions with corticosteroids

Drug	Interactions
Amphotericin B	Hypokalemia
Anticholinesterase drugs	Muscle weakness in myasthenia gravis patients
Aspirin	Reduced salicylate blood levels
Cyclophosphamide	Inhibited hepatic metabolism of cyclophosphamide
Cyclosporine	Increased blood levels of corticosteroids and cyclosporine
Digoxin	Increased risk for cardiac arrhythmia as a result of hypokalemia
Furosemide/ thiazides	Hypokalemia
Ephedrine	Increased metabolism of corticosteroids
Insulin	Increased insulin requirements
Ketoconazole	Decreased metabolism of corticosteroids
Mitotane	Decreased metabolism of corticosteroids
NSAIDs	Increased risk of gastrointestinal ulceration
Phenobarbital/ phenytoin/rifampin	Increased metabolism of corticosteroids
Vaccines	Decreased immune response may occur.

Source: Plumb D. *Plumb's Veterinary Drug Handbook*, 6th edition, pp. 88–90, 234–240, 248–249, 265–269, 427–429, 526–527, 639–640, 755–762. Ames, IA: Blackwell.

sone are the most commonly administered oral corticosteroids. Prednisone and prednisolone have 1–4 times the anti-inflammatory activity than hydrocortisone (cortisol), while dexamethasone has 7–30 times the activity. Prednisone/prednisolone may have some mineralocorticoid activity, while dexamethasone has none. Dexamethasone has the longest duration of activity (with greater than 48 h), while prednisone and prednisolone have lesser activity (at about 12–36 h). Patients with liver failure and perhaps cats are unable to absorb or convert prednisone to prednisolone (active form) efficiently, and therefore the use of prednisolone is indicated. Immunosuppressive doses of prednisone/prednisolone can range from 2 to 4 mg/kg/day orally. Dexamethasone is typically administered as an intravenous or subcutaneous injection and is often used when oral medication cannot be given. An immunosuppressive dose of dexamethasone is 0.25 mg/kg/day.

Immunosuppresives

Azathioprine (Imuran®)

Azathioprine is an immunosuppressive medication primarily used to treat immune-mediated disease. This medication is for use in dogs only, as severe bone marrow suppression can result in feline patients. Azathioprine inhibits RNA and DNA synthesis and mitosis, and primarily affects cellular immunity. It is absorbed in the gastrointestinal tract, metabolized by the liver, and excreted by the kidneys. It is contraindicated in pregnant and nursing dogs as it has teratogenic and mutagenic properties and can be found in milk. The principal adverse effects of this medication may include bone marrow suppression (resulting in neutropenia, thrombocytopenia, and/or anemia), gastrointestinal upset, acute pancreatitis, and hepatoxicity. Increased toxicity has been seen when given with angiotensin-converting enzyme (ACE) inhibitors, aminosalicylates, trimethoprimsulfa, and cyclophosphamide.

The reported time to onset of azathioprine activity is variable and may range from 1 to 5 weeks. As a result, azathioprine is usually not used as a primary single-agent immunosuppressive medication but as an adjunct to other treatments (often in conjunction with prednisone) or when other immunosuppressives cannot be continued. The use of azathioprine in conjunction with a corticosteroid can allow for a more rapid tapering of the corticosteroid. Azathioprine is dosed at 2 mg/kg orally every 24 h with tapering doses for long-term use. An increased dose of 1–5 mg/kg has been used in conjunction with other medications to prevent transplant rejection. Serial monitoring of complete blood count (CBC) and serum biochemical panels are needed. Patients should be monitored closely for evidence of liver toxicity or pancreatitis (which may manifest as jaundice, lethargy, vomiting, diarrhea, or inappetence).

Cyclosporine (Atopica®, Neoral®, Sandimmune®, Cyclosporine-A®), optimmune (topical), and tacrolimus (Tacrolimus®, Protopic®)

Cyclosporine has been used in the prevention of allograft rejection in transplant patients and to treat immune-mediated diseases in small animals. Cyclosporine primarily inhibits T-helper cell activity but also has an effect of T-suppressor cells. Additionally, cyclosporine appears to have broader anti-inflammatory and antipuritic properties, making it an effective treatment for atopy. Cyclosporine is primarily metabolized by the liver and excreted into the bile. It is contraindicated for use in dogs with malignancies, in dogs and cats with renal or liver disease, and in pregnant or nursing patients as it can cause adverse fetal effects and can be found in the milk. The adverse effects of cyclosporine are primarily gastrointestinal, which may include vomiting, anorexia, and diarrhea, which typically occur within the first week of therapy. Uncommon adverse effects include gingival hyperplasia, hypertrichosis, excessive shedding, and papillomatosis.

Opportunistic infections may occur due to immunosuppression induced by cyclosporine. With extremely high blood levels (>3000 ng/mL), nephrotoxicity and hepatoxicity are possible. Cyclosporine administration has been associated with the development of neoplasia in humans and in dogs[2] (Table 12.3.2).

The dosing of cyclosporine is varied depending on the form chosen. The Neoral/Atopica or modified forms have a higher bioavailability in small animals and are recommended for use over Sandimmune. Cyclosporine should be administered on an empty stomach; liquid forms have limited palatability, so they may need to be mixed with juices/broths for administration.

Dosing for Neoral, Atopica, and modified forms of cyclosporine for immunosuppression ranges from 5 to 10 mg/kg orally twice

Table 12.3.2 Drug interactions with cyclosporine

Drugs causing increased cyclosporine levels	Drugs causing decreased cyclosporine levels	Other interactions with cyclosporine
Allopurinol/amiodarone	Nafcillin	Increased digoxin levels
Ketoconazole/fluconazole	Rifampin	Increased methotrexate levels
Bromocriptine	Phenobarbital	Increased hyperkalemia when used with spironolactone
Calcium channel blockers	Phenytoin	Decreased effectiveness of vaccination
Cimetidine	St. Johns wort	Increased nephrotoxicity with nephrotoxic drugs
Cisapride		
Danazol		
Digoxin		
Macrolide antibiotics		
Corticosteroids		
Losartan		
Metoclopramide		
Omeprazole		
Sertraline		
Grapefruit juice[a]		

[a] Grapefruit juice is a nonpharmaceutical that can also increase cyclosporine levels in small animals.
Source: Plumb D. *Plumb's Veterinary Drug Handbook*, 6th edition, pp. 88–90, 234–240, 248–249, 265–269, 427–429, 526–527, 639–640, 755–762. Blackwell.

daily in dogs and from 1 to 4 mg/kg orally once to twice daily in cats. Therapeutic drug monitoring may be used to guide dosing (see below). Topical cyclosporine ophthalmic ointment (Optimmune®) is used as a treatment of keratoconjunctivitis sicca, an immune-mediated disease of the lacrimal ducts.

Because oral absorption of cyclosporine can vary among patients, measuring cyclosporine trough levels is recommended. Therapeutic drug monitoring ensures the dose administered is achieving therapeutic levels (usually 300–500 ng/mL)[3] while not reaching toxic levels. A trough level can be measured 72 h after starting treatment and is performed on blood obtained immediately before the next dose is due. Routine monitoring of drug levels (e.g., every 2–4 weeks) is likely not necessary once the effective dose is achieved but is recommended if treatment efficacy is poor or if adverse effects are suspected. Serial CBC and serum biochemical panels should also be performed at least every 3 months or in accordance to guidelines for the disease being treated.

Tacrolimus is closely related to cyclosporine, and the two drugs share a similar mechanism of action. Topical tacrolimus has been successfully used in the treatment of atopic dermatitis, perianal fistulae, and anal furunculosis.

Less commonly used immunosuppressives

Cyclophosphamide (Cytoxan®)

Cyclophosphamide is an immunosuppressive and antineoplastic medication used for the treatment of immune-mediated disorders. It is an alkylating agent that interferes with DNA and RNA synthesis. Cyclophosphamide has been used for the management of various immune-mediated disorders but is not recommended for the treatment of IMHA due to its reported lack of efficacy.[1,3–5] Cyclophosphamide is metabolized by the liver and excreted in the urine. It is contraindicated in pregnant and nursing patients due to its possible teratogenic effects. Adverse effects with this medication include myelosuppression, anorexia, vomiting, diarrhea, alopecia, and sterile, hemorrhagic cystitis (in up to 30% of dogs treated long term with cyclophosphamide).[4] (Table 12.3.3).

The recommended dosage range for cyclophosphamide is quite variable and the dosing regimens vary depending on the disease treated. An example dosage regimen for the treatment of immune-mediated thrombocytopenia (IMT) is 50 mg/m² given once a day for 3–4 days then followed by tapering doses. For erosive arthritis/rheumatoid arthritis/polyarthritis, the dose is based on the weight of the patient. In patients weighing less than 10 kg, the dose is 2.5 mg/kg; for patients weighing 10–35 kg, the dose is 2 mg/kg, and if the patient is greater than 35 kg, the dose is 1.5 mg/kg; all doses are given for 4 consecutive days per week. For polymyositis, 1 mg/kg given orally once daily for 4 days, then off for three is recommended. Feline patients typically receive 2.5 mg/kg once daily for 4 days a week for 3 weeks, or 50 mg/m² given 4 days/week.

Table 12.3.3 Drug interactions with cyclophosphamide

Interactions causing increased myelosuppression	Interaction causing decreased cyclophosphamide metabolism	Other drug interactions
Allopurinol	Chloramphenicol	Barbiturates—increased metabolism of cyclophosphamide
Thiazide diuretics	Phenothiazine	Cardiotoxic drugs—increased cardiotoxicity
	Potassium iodide	
	Vitamin A	

Source: Plumb D. *Plumb's Veterinary Drug Handbook*, 6th edition, pp. 88–90, 234–240, 248–249, 265–269, 427–429, 526–527, 639–640, 755–762. Blackwell.

Danazol

Danazol is an androgen, anabolic steroid that is uncommonly used for immunosuppression in dogs and cats. Danazol may have a synergistic affect when used with corticosteroids and has been used to reduce the amount of corticosteroids needed for the treatment of immune-mediated diseases. The efficacy of danazol as an adjunctive agent with glucocorticoids in cases of IMHA and IMT is questionable. Danazol suppresses the immune system by binding antibodies and reducing Fc receptor-mediated phagocytosis. It is primarily metabolized by the liver and absorbed by the gastrointestinal tract. The adverse effects of danazol may include cardiac impairment, renal damage, weight gain, lethargy, edema, alopecia, and rarely, hepatotoxicity.

Danazol is contraindicated in patients with cardiac, renal, or hepatic disease, or during pregnancy due to fetal abnormalities and fetal risk. Pregnant people should avoid handling this medication. Danazol may also decrease thyroxin levels and may cause increased liver enzyme activity. Concurrent use of danazol and cyclosporine may increase blood levels of cyclosporine. Danazol administration may increase insulin requirements in diabetic patients. Canine patients start with a loading dosage of 10 mg/kg/day then decrease to a maintenance dose of 5 mg/kg once to three times a day. Cats are dosed at 5 mg/kg given twice daily; however, some dose recommendations have been found to be as high as 10–15 mg/kg once daily. It is very important to monitor these patients for any adverse effects, which include signs of hepatotoxicity (e.g., jaundice, melena, vomiting).

Novel immunosuppressive medications

Mycophenolate mofetil (MMF)

Mycophenolate is used in human medicine for the treatment of immune-mediated diseases and as part of a multidrug treatment regimen to prevent rejection in transplantation medicine. There is limited experience with mycophenolate in veterinary patients; potential applications include the treatment of IMHA, myasthenia gravis, pemphigus, glomerulonephropathy, and the prevention of transplant rejection. Mycophenolate suppresses the immune system by inhibiting proliferation of T and B cells, decreasing B cell formation of antibodies, and limiting leukocyte deployment to sites of inflammation.

The use and handling of mycophenolate is contraindicated in nursing and pregnant people due to possible fetal malformations, so clear, thorough client communication is important with this medication. Mycophenolate may cause drug interactions with acyclovir, antacids, aspirin, iron, and vaccines. Adverse effects of mycophenolate are primarily gastrointestinal (vomiting, diarrhea), especially with the sodium enteric-coated tablets versus the capsules.[4] The dosing ranges from 12 to 39 mg/kg/day and varies with the diseases being treated. Serial monitoring of the CBCs, renal and liver function, and electrolytes should be performed when using mycophenolate.

Immunomodulating medications

Leflunomide

Leflunomide is used as a primary immunosuppressive medication or as adjunct therapy with other immunosuppressive medications and is a part of some transplant rejection protocols. It inhibits T-cell production and autoantibody secretion by B cells. It is metabolized by the gastrointestinal mucosa and liver and is excreted in urine. Leflunomide is contraindicated in pregnant animals due to its teratogenic effects. The primary adverse effects of leflunomide are related to the gastrointestinal tract and include vomiting and decreased appetite. Uncommon and severe adverse effects such as lymphopenia and anemia have also been observed (Table 12.3.4).

Table 12.3.4 Drug interactions with leflunomide

Drug	Interaction
Charcoal (activated)	Increased elimination of leflunomide/decrease of drug concentration
Cholestyramine	Increased elimination of leflunomide
Hepatotoxic agents	Increased risk liver toxicity
Methotrexate	Increased adverse effects of methotrexate/increased ALT
Phenytoin	Increased phenytoin levels
Rifampin	Increased leflunomide levels

Source: Plumb D. *Plumb's Veterinary Drug Handbook*, 6th edition, pp. 88–90, 234–240, 248–249, 265–269, 427–429, 526–527, 639–640, 755–762. Blackwell.

Patients treated with leflunomide should be monitored with serial CBC and serum biochemical testing. Dosing recommendations in canines is 4–6 mg/kg orally every 24 h for immune-mediated diseases and transplant protocols, and 2–4 mg/kg orally every 24 h for canine systemic and cutaneous reactive histiocytosis. Dosing can be adjusted to reach target trough levels of 10 mcg/mL for the treatment of immune-mediated diseases and a 20 mcg/mL target range for transplant rejection protocols. Dosing guidelines for cats is 10 mg orally every 24 h, decreased to twice weekly when used with methotrexate for the treatment of erosive arthritis.

Human intravenous immunoglobulin

Human intravenous immunoglobulin (hIVIG) is used in small animals for the short-term treatment of immune-mediated diseases, primarily IMHA and IMT; however, little research material is available. It contains IgG and small amounts of IgM, IgA, CD4, CD8, and human leukocyte antigen molecules. IVIG inhibits Fc-mediated phagocytosis of erythrocytes, interferes with complement, suppresses antibody production, and binds to canine lymphocytes. Studies have reported no known adverse effects, either during the infusion or within a 6-month period after treatment.[6] A single infusion (0.5 g/kg) is usually administered in conjunction with other immunosuppressive therapies. Clinical trials of dogs with IMT have shown that IVIG treatment significantly reduced platelet count recovery time and duration of hospitalization times.[6]

Conclusion

Client compliance is important to the successful use of any of these mediations, and extensive, complete client instruction, both oral and written, is indicated. Inappropriate adjustment or discontinuation of immunosuppressive medications can lead to overdose, increased incidence of adverse effects, relapse of immune-mediated diseases, or transplant rejection. In addition to dosing guidelines, clients should also be informed of their pets increased susceptibility to infection as well as decreased healing time during the immunosuppressive period.

SECTION 4 VACCINES AND VACCINATION

Vaccination strategies

Vaccination is an effective strategy to help prevent canine and feline infectious diseases. Recently, vaccine recommendations have become more refined for the individual dog or cat depending on individual lifestyle. Prior to vaccinating an animal, veterinary staff must determine if it is appropriate to vaccinate an animal and, if so, what infectious agents the animal should be vaccinated against. The vaccine recommendations in this chapter are based on the guidelines published by the American Animal

Hospital Association (AAHA) and the American Association of Feline Practitioners (AAFP) in 2006.[1,2] Veterinary technicians are encouraged to consult the most current vaccination guidelines published by these groups.

Vaccine technology

There are several vaccine types available. The most common vaccines are *modified live* and *killed products*.

Modified live virus vaccines

The MLV vaccines contain a pathogen that has been rendered noninfective. Attenuation of the pathogen causes minimal changes to the antigens. Because MLV vaccines contain a live but attenuated pathogen, there is the rare potential for these pathogens to revert to virulence and/or to cause vaccine-induced illness. Additionally, MLV vaccines may become inactivated over time or with improper storage. MLV vaccines are able to replicate within the host, amplifying the antigenic mass that was initially administered and producing a strong immune response after one dose. These vaccines do not require an adjuvant and can stimulate humoral, cell-mediated, and mucosal immunity. Both injectable and topical forms of MLV vaccines may be available.[3]

Killed vaccines

Killed vaccines are comprised of a pathogen or part of a pathogen that has been completely inactivated. Because these products are killed, the antigenic mass that is initially administered is unable to replicate, and at least two doses are needed for maximal immune system stimulation. Killed vaccines primarily induce humoral immunity with little cellular or mucosal immunity. These vaccines are stable in storage. Killed vaccines are usually administered via injection and frequently require an adjuvant.[3]

Vaccine-induced sarcoma in cats

There is some concern about a possible link between the inflammatory responses induced by adjuvanted vaccines and the development of vaccine-associated sarcomas in cats. Adjuvants are compounds that cause inflammation, increasing the immune response to vaccine antigens. Adjuvants can be metals (such as aluminum), oil emulsions, microbial components (such as lipopolysaccharide), or mammalian proteins (such as complement protein derivatives).[4] Aluminum has been identified as a foreign object in the macrophages of the vaccine-induced sarcoma.[5] Following vaccine administration, a local inflammatory and granulomatous process may be noted. This reaction to chronic inflammation is thought to be the precursor to tumor development in cats affected by vaccine-associated sarcomas. This process is estimated to take anywhere from 3 months to 3 years. Neoplasia of mesenchymal origin, of which fibrosarcoma is a subcategory, has been associated with sites of previous vaccines. The fibrosarcoma associated with vaccine adminis-

tration does differ, on a molecular level, from noninjection site fibrosarcoma.

The majority of vaccine-induced fibrosarcomas are surrounded by a fibrous capsule and infiltrated by lymphocytes and macrophages. Even though encapsulated, these sarcomas are highly invasive and very aggressive. While fibrosarcoma is the most common type of vaccine-induced sarcoma, other subcategories have been reported. Aggressive surgery, radiation therapy, chemotherapy, or a combination of these protocols is required for the treatment of these tumors. Even with these treatment(s), local metastasis is common. The ability to obtain wide surgical margins can be difficult when the tumor is located on the trunk of the animal. Therefore, the current vaccine location recommendations are for administration on a limb, as distally as possible. It is recommended that certain vaccines always be administered in specific limbs (e.g., feline leukemia vaccine in the left hind, rabies vaccine in the right hind). This may help identify the causative vaccine if a vaccine-associated sarcoma develops.

A multicenter study examining the association of vaccines with sarcomas did not find a higher risk of sarcoma development in cats receiving adjuvanted vaccines.[6] However, nonadjuvanted vaccines were not used frequently in this study. The exact causative agent or agents have yet to be proven, but adjuvants in rabies and leukemia vaccines have an apparent causal relationship. While a direct causal relationship has not been specifically demonstrated between postvaccination inflammatory responses and sarcoma development, the Feline Advisory Panel recommends that less inflammatory (i.e., nonadjuvanted) vaccine products are used when possible.[2]

Recombinant vaccines

Recombinant vaccines are a third type of vaccine product and are becoming more common. Recombinant vaccines can be formed using several different methods. *Live vector vaccines* are developed by identifying the protective antigens of a pathogenic organism. The genes encoding these antigens are then inserted into another nonpathogenic organism that serves as the vector. After vaccination, the nonpathogenic vector introduces these genes into the host. The antigenic proteins are expressed in the host and induce an immune response. Because only protective antigens from the pathogen are used, the pathogen cannot revert back to a virulent state nor can it cause infection in immunosuppressed animals. Examples of live vector vaccines include a recombinant canine distemper virus (CDV) vaccine, which uses a canarypox vector.

Similar to live vector vaccines, *subunit vaccines* contain the portion of a pathogen that contains the protective antigens rather than the entire pathogen. An example of a subunit vaccine is the *Borrelia burgdorferi* vaccine that contains the outer surface membrane protein OspA.[3]

Investigational vaccines

Vaccine technology is constantly evolving, and some vaccine types that are currently being investigated are *gene deleted* and *nucleic acid* vaccines. Gene deleted vaccines can be either live or killed products. To produce these vaccines, a gene that is not responsible for conferring protection against the organism is either altered or deleted. DNA vaccines isolate the genetic material that codes for the protective antigens of an organism. The DNA is inserted into a bacterial plasmid where it replicates within the bacteria. After replication, the DNA is purified from the bacteria and directly inserted into the host.[3]

Vaccine labels

Vaccine label directions contain information regarding route and dose volume, as well as recommended revaccination intervals. The dose and route of administration on the label should be followed closely as these reflect the testing performed to evaluate the vaccine's safety and efficacy. The label also indicates recommended revaccination intervals, and these may differ from the current published canine and feline vaccine guidelines. Rabies vaccines should be administered according to regional laws. In general, these laws state to vaccinate against rabies every 1 or 3 years. Veterinarians do have some discretion over the extralabel use of nonrabies vaccines, provided this use meets the current recommended standard of practice. For example, some vaccine manufacturers recommend annual revaccination of dogs against distemper, parvovirus, and adenovirus-2. However, studies have shown a duration of immunity for these vaccines of up to 7 years after giving an MLV vaccine to an adult dog.[1,7] Similarly, immunity after vaccination of adult cats against feline panleukopenia, herpesvirus-1, and calicivirus lasts 3–7 years or more.[8,9] After the initial series and 1-year booster are completed, current guidelines suggest that revaccination intervals of every 3 years is sufficient.[1,2]

Serologic testing

Overvaccination is a concern for many pet owners and veterinary professionals. Vaccine titer measurement is performed by some veterinary clinics and may be a useful complement to vaccine protocols. However, vaccine titers have limitations, and interpretation of titer results can be confusing.

Serum titers can be used to demonstrate the duration of immunity (measured by the presence of serum antibody) to a previous vaccination or infection. Vaccination induces both a humoral and a cell-mediated immune response. However, serum titer levels only measure the humoral response induced by a vaccine. Therefore, titers may be useful to measure protection against pathogens that replicate extracellularly (i.e., pathogens that are eliminated from the body primarily via humoral immunity). Examples of such pathogens include canine parvovirus (CPV), distemper virus, and adenovirus; as well as feline panleukopenia virus, herpesvirus-1, and calicivirus. A positive titer does not ensure that an animal is protected, while a negative titer does not equate lack of protection. If a veterinary clinic chooses to add vaccine titer measurements to their health-care protocols,

it is important to choose tests that are validated. Such tests have established "protective" titer levels correlated with protection from disease in challenge studies.[3,10] Due to the limitations of vaccine titers, they are not routinely recommended in place of vaccination.

Rabies antibody titers may be required prior to importing an animal into a rabies-free region (e.g., Hawaii or the United Kingdom). An adequate serum titer must be proven after rabies vaccination as part of these import–export laws, and specific details vary depending on the region involved.

Vaccine information in medical records

A patient's medical record should include information about any vaccine administered. Vaccination details recorded should include the date of vaccination, the name of the person administering the vaccine, vaccination site and route of administration, and the vaccine name and manufacturer, lot number, and expiration date. Most vaccine vials have peel-off labels to affix to the medical record to facilitate this documentation. Additionally, the benefits and risks of each vaccine should be discussed with the client, and a notation in the medical record of this discussion and the client's informed consent for vaccine administration should be documented. Benefits of vaccination include control of infectious disease at the level of the individual and the pet population. Additionally, vaccination also benefits public health (e.g., rabies vaccination limits human exposure to this zoonotic disease). Potential drawbacks include that no vaccine is 100% protective and the potential risks that vaccination may induce (e.g., hypersensitivity reactions and vaccine-associated sarcomas). Given the potential benefits and risks, vaccination should be considered a medical decision based on the individual pet's lifestyle and potential exposure to pathogens.

Considerations when developing vaccine protocols

Vaccine protocols for individual animals are based on that individual's risk factors and its exposure to infectious disease. Risk factors to consider include age, indoor only versus outdoor access, group housing or shelters, regional disease prevalence, and travel of the pet. For example, young animals are generally more susceptible to infections. Outdoor cats have potential exposure to various infections such as feline leukemia compared to the solitary indoor cat. Group housing arrangements may increase the risk for upper respiratory infections such as herpesvirus-1 and calicivirus for cats and *Bordetella bronchiseptica* and parainfluenza virus for dogs. Some infections such as leptospirosis are more prevalent in certain regions, and a thorough knowledge of travel is important when making decisions about vaccinations.[1,2]

It is preferable that only healthy animals are vaccinated. A thorough client interview and physical examination can help determine a pet's health status. Vaccines should be delayed for any pet with an acute illness until this condition has been resolved or appropriately managed. Animals with chronic stable conditions such as diabetes mellitus can be safely vaccinated provided that the animal is receiving appropriate diagnostic and therapeutic care. Patients receiving immunosuppressive therapy (e.g., chemotherapy and high dose corticosteroids) may not mount an effective immune response to a vaccine. Low to moderate doses of corticosteroids given for a short period did not interfere with vaccine response in puppies in one study.[11] However; it is recommended that vaccination should be delayed until after immunosuppressive therapy concludes in these patients, if possible.

Vaccine-induced sarcoma is one reason to individualize vaccine recommendations in cats. Currently, the benefit of immunization with a core vaccine outweighs the risk of development of a vaccine-induced sarcoma.

The literature regarding the link between vaccination and immune-mediated disease is mixed. While one study showed an association between recent vaccination and IMHA, this study did not prove a causal relationship.[12] Additionally, no studies have definitively documented the risks of vaccination in patients with a history of immune-mediated disease. Common opinion is that animals with previous immune-mediated diseases should have limited stimulation of the immune system, including vaccination. The advantages and disadvantages of vaccination should be discussed with the owners of these patients on an individual basis. Vaccines should be limited based on an individual patient's risk of exposure to infectious agents. However, owners and veterinary clinics are advised to follow their area's rabies vaccination guidelines. Some areas will not allow a medical waiver and titer measurements in lieu of current rabies vaccination status. Veterinary professionals are encouraged to contact their regional veterinary and public health resources for specific information regarding rabies laws.

Core versus noncore vaccines (lifestyle vaccines)

Designation of vaccines into *core* and *noncore* categories has helped to design individual vaccine protocols. Core vaccines are those that protect against diseases with high rates of morbidity and mortality, diseases with a significant public health risk, diseases that are common, and/or diseases that are easily transmissible. Core vaccines are recommended for all dogs or cats.

Noncore vaccines, also referred to as lifestyle vaccines, protect against infections that produce mild or self-limiting disease, diseases that are not easily transmissible, and/or diseases that have a low prevalence. Additionally, noncore vaccines may have limited efficacy or may interfere with screening tests for diseases. Noncore vaccines are best given only to those pets that have risk factors for exposure to a particular infection.

A third category of vaccines includes those that are *not generally recommended*. This category includes vaccines with unknown benefit, vaccines that target diseases with low prevalence, or vaccines against diseases that are considered low risk to pets.

Vaccine products and recommendations are continually evolving. Veterinary technicians can be instrumental in ensuring that clinical vaccine practices remain up-to-date with the most current recommendations. By tailoring vaccine protocols based on an individual pet's risk factors, veterinary health professionals will help promote preventative health care. Technicians are encouraged to refer to the guidelines published by the AAHA (http://www.aahanet.org) and the AAFP (http://www.catvets.com) for the most up-to-date canine and feline vaccination recommendations.[1,2] However, these guidelines are not meant to be used as vaccine standards but rather as a starting point when developing individual vaccine protocols.

Canine vaccines

In many practices, canine core vaccines are administered as a monovalent rabies product and a multivalent CDV, CPV, and canine adenovirus (CAV)-2 product. To help standardize vaccination sites, practices will often use the right hind limb for the rabies vaccination ("R"abies in the "R"ight) with the multivalent CDV, CPV, and CAV-2 product usually in the left hind limb. Each vaccine product should be administered in a different location, as distal on the limb as possible. Giving each vaccine product in a different site will help identify which vaccine produces a local reaction (e.g., granuloma) if one occurs.

Core canine vaccines

Rabies

Rabies is an enveloped RNA virus of the Rhabdoviridae family affecting all warm-blooded animals including humans and is found almost worldwide. Some island and peninsular countries remain rabies free through stringent import regulations. Wildlife is the major reservoir for the disease, although domesticated animals can be another disease vector. Transmission is usually through contact with infected saliva introduced by a bite wound. Other routes of transmission include exposure of an open wound to infected saliva or neural tissue or ingestion of infected tissue. After ascending to the central nervous tissue, the rabies virus replicates, then spreads to the salivary glands or other tissues. The incubation period is highly variable. Animals typically begin to show clinical signs several days to weeks after infection, although longer incubation periods up to 6 months have been reported. Rabies virus produces a rapidly progressive encephalopathy and death.[13]

The animal may become infectious prior to displaying clinical signs. Outside of the host, the virus is relatively sensitive to sunlight and to most disinfectants but may remain viable in a carcass or tissues for several days. Rabies is a fatal disease that is capable of infecting all mammals (including humans), and because of its zoonotic potential, treatment should not be attempted. Canine, feline, and wildlife rabies vaccination programs are an important aspect of controlling this disease. Clinical disease is divided into three stages, but not all animals will exhibit all three distinct stages. Behavioral changes may be noted in the initial (prodromal) stage, which usually lasts 1–3 days. On physical examination, fever, dilated pupils, and slow corneal and palpebral reflex may be noted. Progression of clinical disease can include signs related to forebrain lesions, such as unpredictable aggression, hyperresponsiveness to stimuli, muscle twitching and weakness, dysphagia, and ptyalism. This stage may be referred to as the "furious" stage and can last 1–7 days. The paralytic or "dumb" phase of infection is usually apparent 2–4 days after the initial clinical signs. It is characterized by progressive paresis, paralysis, and coma, eventually resulting in respiratory arrest and death. Rabies is diagnosed on necropsy, following the procedures recommended or required by the state or federal government. Rabies submission recommendations usually involve decapitation and refrigeration of the head (never freeze the tissue). Using appropriate biosafety procedures, the head is transported to the state or federal veterinary laboratory. Laboratories should be contacted prior to submission of a rabies suspect.

Incidence of rabies in domestic animals and humans has decreased over the previous decades. In 2008, there were 294 cases of feline rabies and 75 cases of canine rabies reported in the United States. During that same year, 15 cases of rabies were reported in domestic animals in Canada and 31 cases of canine rabies were reported in Mexico.[14] Approximately 3% of the reported cases of canine and feline rabies in the United States from 1997 to 2001 had a previous history of rabies vaccination, including 0.5% of dogs and cats in which rabies vaccination was considered current.[15] There are approximately three cases of human rabies reported in the United States each year, with fewer cases in Canada. Most human cases are attributable to bats.[16,17]

Rabies vaccination protocols may vary depending on regional laws. The initial rabies vaccine is administered as early as 12 weeks of age depending on local regulations. A second rabies vaccine is given 1 year following the initial vaccination. Subsequent revaccinations are given every 1–3 years, depending on the product used and the regional laws. Rabies vaccination products are typically killed virus products.

Canine distemper virus

Canine distemper is an enveloped RNA virus of the Paramyxoviridae family that can infect dogs, wolves, coyotes, fox, weasels, minks, skunks, badgers, ferrets, lions, leopards, tigers, and seals.[41] Young animals are most susceptible, but all ages can be infected. The incubation period is typically 1–2 weeks but can be as long as 4–5 weeks. Viral shedding occurs by 7 days postinfection and can be transmitted for 60–90 days. Transmission is predominately by aerosolization of respiratory exudates, but the virus can be isolated in other body tissues and secretions including urine. Transplacental transmission is possible. Although distemper is found worldwide, it is well controlled in most of North America due to widespread vaccination. However, this infection still exists and is highly contagious. The virus is not durable at room temperature and is inactivated by most disinfectants. It can persist for several weeks in cold moist environments.

Manifestations of the disease are dependent on the virus strain and body system involved but can include gastrointestinal, respiratory, and neurological signs. Clinical signs can be mild and nonspecific in nature (e.g., fever and leukopenia), making early diagnosis challenging. Upper respiratory signs of coughing and mucopurulent nasal and ocular discharges are noted commonly and may progress to dyspnea and pneumonia. Diarrhea, dehydration, anorexia, and vomiting may occur if the gastrointestinal system is infected. The eyes, skin, teeth enamel, or the neurological system may also be affected. This infection can be highly fatal.

The diagnosis of distemper is often made presumptively on the basis of a poor vaccine history and compatible clinical signs. Persistent lymphopenia may be present on the CBC. Immunologic testing (IFA and immunohistochemistry) and serology are available, but false-negative results are possible; PCR testing cannot distinguish between vaccination and field strains of CDV.

Treatment is supportive depending on the systems affected. Secondary bacterial pneumonia infections are common and should be treated with the appropriate antimicrobial therapy and nebulization. Vomiting and diarrhea can be seen with systemic cases of CDV and may require antiemetics, fluid therapy, and electrolyte monitoring. Antiepileptic drugs may be necessary to control seizures. Some dogs that recover from canine distemper may develop neurological disease such as seizures, optic neuritis, or mycolonus later in life. Nursing care includes strict isolation procedures to prevent viral transmission, pain assessment, facial hygiene, nebulization and coupage, and nutritional support. Monitoring of the patient's temperature, hydration level, electrolytes, lung sounds, and nutritional intake are indicated.

MLV or recombinant vaccines are recommended for the control of canine distemper. CDV is often found as part of a multivalent vaccine including modified live vaccines against CPV and CAV-2 (+/−canine parainfluenza virus [CPiV]) and is abbreviated as "D" in distemper, hepatitis, parvovirus, parainfluenza (DHPP) (or DA$_2$PP or DAP). Puppies are initially administered three vaccines, 3–4 weeks apart, between the ages of 6 and 16 weeks. The third vaccine in the initial series should be administered at 14–16 weeks of age. Dogs >16 weeks of age with no previous vaccine history are initially administered two vaccines, 3–4 weeks apart. Revaccination occurs 1 year after the initial series. Although some vaccine manufacturers recommend subsequent revaccination for CDV annually, the duration of immunity studies show protection for 4–9 years; current AAHA guidelines state that revaccination every 3 years is adequate.[7] The recombinant canarypox-vectored CDV vaccine is combined with modified live CAV-2, parainfluenza virus, and CPV. The recombinant CDV vaccine may be less affected by the presence of maternal antibodies compared to MLV CDV vaccines.[18]

Distemper may occur rarely in previously vaccinated dogs. Purported reasons for this include immunosuppression at the time of vaccination, infection prior to vaccination, or improper vaccine handling or administration. Rarely, distemper may be attributable to the MLV vaccine itself. Signs of encephalitis may develop within 3 weeks of vaccination using a modified live vaccine. Other systemic signs, such as gastrointestinal or respiratory signs, are not present.

Canine parvovirus

CPV is a small, nonenveloped DNA virus that is a member of the family Parvoviridae and can be found worldwide. Canine parvovirus subtype 2 (CPV-2) is the most common cause of parvovirus infection in dogs. Natural infections have been reported in domestic dogs, coyotes, foxes, and wolves. Experimental infections have been produced in ferrets, cats, and mink. Puppies under 6 months old are most likely to have severe disease. Rottweilers, Dobermans, pit bulls, and mixes of these breeds may be especially vulnerable. This virus is resistant to most disinfectants and can survive in the environment for months to years. A 1:30 dilution of sodium hypochlorite (household bleach) with a minimum contact time of 10 min is required for disinfection. For surfaces where it is difficult to maintain the contact time or are sensitive to sodium hypochlorite, steam cleaning has been shown to be effective.[58]

Transmission of parvovirus is primarily through exposure to contaminated feces via the oronasal route. The incubation period is 3–14 days. The virus replicates in the lymphoid tissue. Viral shedding can occur 3–4 days after exposure and can continue intermittently for up to 2 weeks. Clinical signs are usually noted 5–7 days after exposure to the virus; therefore, dogs can begin shedding the virus prior to showing signs of illness. Clinical signs can vary from mild to severe and may include fever, lethargy, anorexia, vomiting, and diarrhea, leading to dehydration and possibly death in severe cases. Gram-negative sepsis, due to bacterial translocation, or disseminated intravascular coagulation (DIC) may occur. Myocarditis can develop in pups younger than 8 weeks of age. Young dogs appear to be most prone to severe, life-threatening infection.[3]

Suspicion of parvoviral enteritis may be based on the presence of foul smelling, hemorrhagic diarrhea. Laboratory diagnosis can be achieved with in-house fecal ELISA CPV antigen tests. False positives have been noted postvaccination (see below), and false-negative tests may occur due to intermittent or low numbers of viral shedding or timing of testing (either early or late in the disease). Marked leukopenia observed on the CBC is highly indicative of parvovirus infection and will help to determine prognosis and therapeutic options. Without treatment, the prognosis for parvovirus infection is poor. Survival rates are high when supportive treatment is instituted quickly and aggressively. During treatment, full isolation procedures must be utilized. Supportive care may include fluid therapy to address dehydration and electrolyte imbalances, broad-spectrum antibiotics for secondary bacterial infections due to compromised intestinal integrity, and antiemetics to prevent ongoing emesis. The addition of colloids, plasma and/or red blood cells may be warranted in severe cases. Nursing care includes strict isolation procedures to prevent virus transmission and opportunistic bacterial infections, and nutritional support (either enteral or parenteral). Close monitoring of the patient's temperature, electrolytes, blood glucose, protein levels, red blood cell count/hematocrit, and white blood cell counts are warranted. Care must be taken to ensure that intravenous catheters are protected from environmental or gastrointestinal contamination. More information can be found in Chapter 8.

Modified live parvovirus vaccines should be used to prevent parvovirus as the killed products are susceptible to maternal antibody interference in dogs up to 18 weeks of age. Vaccine recommendations are similar to those outlined above in the canine distemper section. Briefly, puppies are given three doses, 3–4 weeks apart, between 6 and 16 weeks of age. Dogs >16 weeks of age with no vaccine history should be given two doses initially, 3–4 weeks apart. All puppies should be revaccinated 1 year later, then at intervals of 3 years. Similar to distemper vaccines, many parvovirus vaccine products are labeled for annual revaccination, but duration of immunity studies show 4–9 years of protection after an MLV vaccine.[7] CPV is typically found as part of a multivalent vaccine and is often abbreviated as "P" in DHPP (or DA$_2$PP, DAP). The effects of recent vaccination on testing for parvovirus are controversial. Recent vaccination may cause a false-positive result using fecal ELISA tests, although a recent abstract reported that dogs vaccinated 3–7 days before testing produced negative fecal ELISA test results.[20]

Canine adenovirus

CAVs are nonenveloped DNA viruses of the family Adenoviridae. CAV-1 is found worldwide and is the causative agent of infectious canine hepatitis (ICH) affecting dogs, wolves, coyotes, bears, and foxes. CAV-1 is moderately resistant and can survive for months under ideal conditions. Resistant to most household disinfectants, the use of a 1:30 bleach or quaternary ammonium solution with 10 min of contact time or steam cleaning will inactivate the virus.

Infection with CAV-1 is uncommon. It manifests as a multisystemic disease that primarily affects the kidneys and liver. The incubation period is 4–9 days during which time the virus replicates in the tonsils and associated lymph nodes. Transmission is through oronasal exposure to infected body secretions, primarily feces and urine. Recovered animals can shed virus for up to 6 months. Clinical signs include fever, tachypnea, tachycardia, lethargy, and depression in the early stages of the disease followed by hepatomegaly, abdominal pain, anorexia, and tonsillar enlargement. Hepatic failure from hepatocellular necrosis is common. Coagulopathies secondary to liver failure may occur. Neurological signs related to hepatic encephalopathy or coagulopathy may be noted and include seizures and disorientation.

Diagnosis of CAV-1 infection is based on compatible clinical signs and laboratory findings. Increased ALT and serum ALP may be seen dependent upon the amount of hepatic necrosis.[21] Leukopenia, neutropenia, lymphopenia, and thrombocytopenia are usually present on a CBC. Confirmatory diagnosis is through detection of rising antibody titers.

Treatment is primarily supportive. Severely affected dogs should be maintained on intravenous fluid therapy. Treatment of hepatic encephalopathy and/or hypoglycemia may be indicated based on the clinical picture. Care must be taken during venipuncture or when placing the intravenous catheter as hypocoagulability secondary to liver failure may be present. Nursing care includes strict isolation procedures to prevent transmission of the virus, pain assessment, and nutritional support. Monitoring of the patient's temperature, hydration level, hematocrit, coagulation status, and nutritional intake are indicated. Severe CAV-1 infections can be fatal; dogs with less severe disease often show improvement within 7 days of initiation of supportive care.

Infection with CAV-2 causes mild, self-limiting respiratory signs. CAV-1 vaccines have been associated with adverse effects including corneal edema ("blue eye") and uveitis. Therefore, it is recommended to vaccinate dogs against adenovirus infections using a CAV-2 product, which is cross protective against CAV-1. CAV-2 MLV parenteral vaccines induce a more effective immune response and are recommended over killed or MLV topical products. Recommendations for vaccinating against CAV-1 are similar to those outlined above in the section "Canine Distemper Virus." Briefly, puppies receive three doses initially, 3–4 weeks apart between the ages of 6 and 16 weeks. Dogs >16 weeks with no vaccine history should receive two doses, 3–4 weeks apart. Revaccination after the initial series should be performed 1 year later, then every 3 years. While some vaccine manufacturers may recommend annual revaccination, challenge studies have shown that CAV-2 MLV vaccines induce protection against CAV-1 for at least 7 years.[22] CAV-2 is typically found as part of a multivalent vaccine and is often abbreviated as "H" in DHPP or as "A_2" in DA_2PP.

Noncore canine vaccines

Leptospirosis

Leptospires are helical bacteria of the family Leptospiraceae. They are approximately $0.1\,\mu m$ wide $\times$ 6–20 μm long.[23] Leptospira interrogans can cause renal and/or hepatic disease and are typically found in water. Most mammals are susceptible to leptospirosis infection. Natural hosts do not show clinical disease but instead shed the infection for months to years. Infection of incidental hosts results in clinical disease. Clinical signs are usually nonspecific and can include anorexia, vomiting, and severe weakness. Dogs are the reservoir host for L. interrogans serovars Canicola and Bataviae (and possibly serovar Bratislava), but many serovars can infect dogs[23] (Table 12.4.1).

Table 12.4.1 *Leptospira* spp. serovars and hosts

Genomospecies	Serovar	Known primary reservoir host	Incidental domestic hosts	Wild animal hosts	Serovar included in vaccine?
Leptospira interrogans	Autumnalis	Mouse	Cow, dog, human	Opossum, rat, raccoon	No
L. interrogans	Bataviae	Dog, rat, mouse	Cat, cow, human	Armadillo, hedgehog, shrew, vole	No
L. interrogans	Bratislava	Rat, pig, horse	Cow, dog, horse human	Fox, hedgehog, mouse, opossum, raccoon, skunk, vole, weasel	No
L. interrogans	Canicola	Dog	Cat, cow, horse, human, pig	Armadillo, hedgehog, raccoon, rat, skunk, vole	Yes—bivalent and quadrivalent product
Leptospira kirschneri	Grippotyphosa	Vole, opossum, skunk, raccoon	Cat, cow, dog, goat, human, pig, rabbit, sheep	Bobcat, fox, hedgehog, mouse, muskrat, rat, shrew, squirrel, weasel	Yes—quadrivalent product only
L. interrogans	Hardjo	Cow	Dog, horse, human, pig, sheep		No
L. interrogans	Icterohemorrhagica	Rat	Cat, cow, dog, horse, human, pig	Ape, civet, fox, hedgehog, mouse, muskrat, opossum, skunk, woodchuck	Yes—bivalent and quadrivalent product
L. interrogans	Pomona	Skunk, opossum, pig, cow	Cat, cow, dog, gerbil, goat, human, pig, rabbit, sheep	Civet, fox, deer, hedgehog, mouse, sea lion, vole, wolf, woodchuck	Yes—quadrivalent product only

Source: Greene CE, Sykes JE, Brown CA, Hartmann K. Leptospirosis In: *Infectious Diseases of the Dog and Cat*, 3rd edition, ed. CE Greene, pp. 402–416. St. Louis, MO: Saunders Elsevier; 2006; Rentko VT, Clark N, Ross LA, Schelling SH. Canine leptospirosis. A retrospective study of 17 cases. *J Vet Intern Med* 1992;6(4):235–244.

The bacteria are transmitted by direct contact with infected urine, placental transfer, bite wounds, or ingestion of infected tissue. Indirect contact with contaminated water, soil, bedding, or food can also cause infection. The bacteria can live for several months in moist soil. Leptospires enter the body through the mucous membranes of the eyes, nose, mouth, or scratched skin. They replicate in the kidney, spleen, liver, eyes, genital tract, or the CNS.[24]

Dogs may be vaccinated against leptospirosis if they are at high risk, depending on lifestyle, geographic location, and season. Male dogs of working and herding breeds were at greater risk for infection of leptospirosis than other dogs in one study.[25] Additionally, dogs in urban areas are at higher risk than dogs in rural areas, presumably due to the urbanization of previously rural areas and a greater opportunity for dogs to be exposed to wildlife reservoirs in some of these areas[26,27] (see Chapter 11 for more details on this disease).

A bivalent leptospirosis killed bacterin vaccine was introduced in the 1970s and provided protection against the serovars Canicola and Icterohemorrhagica. This led to a decrease in infection by these serovars and an overall decrease in the incidence of leptospirosis. However, leptospirosis began to reemerge in the 1990s, and infections with unusual serovars were demonstrated.[59] A quadrivalent leptospirosis bacterin vaccine containing serovars Grippotyphosa, Canicola, Icterohemorrhagica, and Pomona was introduced. Serovar prevalence varies geographically, and the vaccine is not considered cross protective against other serovars that can infect dogs. The most commonly reported serovars infecting dogs in North America in recent years include Grippotyphosa, Pomona, Autumnalis, and Bratislava.[19,25,28–30]

The leptospirosis killed bacterin vaccine is given in an initial series of two vaccines, 2–4 weeks apart. This is repeated annually if the dog is still considered to be at risk for exposure. Dogs should be >12 weeks of age prior to vaccination. The duration of immunity against serovars Canicola and Icterohemorrhagica has been shown to be approximately 1 year; similar duration of immunity is assumed for serovars Grippotyphosa and Pomona. One challenge study identified *Leptospira* organisms in the blood 27 and 56 weeks after vaccination with a bivalent bacterin product, showing some decline in sterile immunity over time.[31] Revaccination at intervals of every 6–9 months may be indicated for dogs that are at exceptionally high risk of infection. Veterinarians and technicians should be aware of anecdotal reports of a higher incidence of acute hypersensitivity reactions after this vaccine is administered, especially toy breeds and puppies. Subunit vaccines have been developed to help reduce the antigenicity of the leptospirosis bacterin vaccine.[3] A recent study using a purified multivalent leptospirosis subunit bacterin vaccine did not demonstrate a higher rate of vaccine reactions with this product compared with other vaccines.[32]

Canine infectious respiratory disease complex

CIRDC is a disease complex found worldwide involving the oral cavity, nasal passages, sinuses, upper airway, and/or lower airway of dogs. CIRDC is a clinical disease syndrome with multiple infectious etiologies also known as infectious tracheobronchitis, canine respiratory complex disease, or "kennel cough." Infection with a single or multiple causative agents may occur. Causative agents associated with CIRDC include CAV-1, CAV-2, CPiV, canine reovirus-1, 2, and 3, canine herpesvirus, canine influenza virus (CIV), CDV, *Mycoplasma* spp., and *Streptococcus zooepidemicus*. These infectious agents may also be opportunistic, secondary pathogens to the primary infection.

B. Bronchiseptica

B. bronchiseptica is a small, motile, gram-negative, aerobic coccobacilli agent considered to be part of the infectious tracheobronchitis complex. It may infect the respiratory tract alone or as a coinfection with other pathogens of CIRDC. *B. bronchiseptica* is highly contagious and is transmitted through aerosol or direct contact. There is frequently a history of exposure to other dogs and is therefore often referred to as kennel cough. Dogs may continue to shed the bacteria for up to 14 weeks postresolution of clinical signs. Environmental factors such as host immune response, stress, contact rate, duration of exposure, and crowding play a role in susceptibility to infection. Young, unvaccinated, and the immunocompromised individual are most susceptible. *Bordetella* can survive in the environment for weeks but is susceptible to inactivation by common disinfectants.

Clinical signs develop approximately 3–5 days after exposure and include a dry, hacking cough that may persist for up to 3 weeks. The cough is occasionally productive. Other signs may include fever, lethargy, ocular and/or nasal discharge, and inappetence. Severe cases can progress to pneumonia.

Mild cases of the disease are self-limiting and do not warrant antimicrobial therapy. In cases where secondary bacterial infections or pulmonary parenchymal involvement are suspected, antimicrobial therapy should be used. Antitussives and bronchodilators have been used to treat *B. bronchiseptica* infections. Antitussive therapy is not recommended in cases that are complicated with bacterial pneumonia and/or when a productive cough is present.[21] Nebulization therapy with saline or antimicrobials have been shown to be of some benefit for animals with excessive accumulations of secretions or those with secondary bacterial infections. Nebulization with mucolytic agents has been shown to be irritating and induce bronchospasm and is therefore not recommended. Supportive care is directed at maintaining fluid and nutritional intake. The majority of cases are mild and are treated on an outpatient basis. If hospitalization is indicated during treatment, full isolation procedures must be utilized. Close monitoring of the patient's temperature, hydration status, lung sounds, and nutritional status is indicated. See Chapter 6 for more information.

B. bronchiseptica vaccines are available as mono- and multivalent (with CPiV ± CAV-2) products. Vaccination does not completely eliminate the risk of CIRDC because several infectious components of this complex are not included in the vaccine. Vaccination should be considered for dogs exposed to other dogs (e.g., kennels, dog shows, day care) or in group housing environments (e.g., shelters).

Parenteral and intranasal *B. bronchiseptica* vaccines are available. Parenteral products include a single-agent *B. bronchiseptica* killed bacterin vaccine and a single-agent *B. bronchiseptica* cell wall antigen extract. Additionally, a MLV parenteral CPiV vaccine is available. A topical intranasal product combining *B. bronchiseptica* live avirulent bacteria and an MLV CPiV vaccine is also available. Combination *B. bronchiseptica* and CPiV vaccines are often administered due to the potential of many infectious agents contributing to this infectious complex.

The parenteral *B. bronchiseptica* vaccine requires that two vaccines are initially given, 2–4 weeks apart. Immunity is expected within several days after the second dose, and the vaccine should be administered at least 1 week before anticipated exposure. The intranasal *B. bronchiseptica* and CPiV vaccine is initially administered as two doses, given 2–4 weeks apart. However, a single dose can induce protective immunity 72 h after vaccination.[33] Some parenteral vaccines are labeled for puppies as young as 6–8 weeks, while the intranasal vaccine may be administered in dogs as young as 3–4 weeks of age. However, administering a *B. bronchiseptica* vaccine is generally not indicated in such young dogs except for those in kennels with high rates of infection. Dogs considered to be at low to moderate risk of exposure should be revaccinated every 12 months. Dogs at high risk of exposure (e.g., frequently kenneled or at dog shows) should be revaccinated every 6 months.

Both the parenteral and intranasal vaccines likely result in decreased severity of coughing after exposure to *B. bronchiseptica*. However, a recent study showed that an intranasal *B. bronchiseptica* vaccine resulted in less shedding and less severe cough after challenge with live *B. bronchiseptica* when compared to a parenteral vaccine.[34] Intranasal vaccines may cause transient (3–10 days) mild coughing and/or sneezing after administration in a small subset of dogs.

B. bronchiseptica is a potential zoonosis that may cause respiratory signs in humans. Risk of transmission is considered low but may be a concern for immunosuppressed humans.

Borreliosis (Lyme disease)

B. burgdorferi is a spirochete bacteria transmitted by *Ixodes* spp. ticks and is the causative agent of Lyme disease. Approximately 95% of dogs exposed to *B. burgdorferi* do not show clinical signs of disease. Clinically affected dogs may show signs of fever, anorexia, acute or chronic renal failure, or lameness secondary to polyarthritis. Routine administration of this vaccine is controversial due to the low percentage of exposed dogs that show clinical signs, and also because the efficacy and duration of immunity conferred by the vaccine is unknown.[35] See Chapter 11 for more details on this disease.

Vaccination against *B. burgdorferi* may be warranted if a dog lives in an endemic area and if tick exposure is high. However, the best prophylaxis for *B. burgdorferi* infection is likely tick prevention. Two types of vaccines against *B. burgdorferi* exist: a killed bacterin product and a recombinant outer surface protein (Osp) A vaccine. Both vaccines induce antibody production against OspA, generating anti-OspA antibodies which are ingested when an infected tick bites an immunized dog. The anti-OspA antibodies kill *B. burgdorferi* in the tick's midgut, and the tick fails to transmit the spirochetes to the dog. The initial vaccine may be given to dogs as young as 9–12 weeks of age if warranted, followed by a second vaccine 3–4 weeks later. Subsequently, annual revaccination is recommended for at-risk dogs and is usually administered prior to the onset of the region's tick season.

Canine influenza virus

Canine influenza is usually caused by influenza A virus and results in respiratory disease. In January 2004, an outbreak of a respiratory virus was evident in racing greyhounds at a track in Florida with similar outbreaks occurring in other states later that year. PCR and gene sequencing determined the virus to be closely related to equine influenza A (H3N8) virus. It was named *A/canine/Florida/43/2004 (canine/FL/04)*.[36] Research conducted at the University of Florida concluded that CIV was in the racing greyhound population as early as 1999.[37] Since the initial outbreaks of CIV, nongreyhound dogs have been reported to be affected in the United States and in the United Kingdom. CIV is considered to be enzootic in New York, Pennsylvania, Florida, and Colorado. The pathogenesis is still being investigated, but it is most likely similar to other influenza A viruses.

Canine influenza is highly contagious and spread through respiratory secretions. Transmission may occur through dog-to-dog contact or aerosolized droplets via sneezing and coughing. The virus can survive in the environment for up to 48 h, and as a result, fomites can also transmit the infection. The incubation period is 2–5 days, with peak viral shedding occurring during this time.[37] Dogs begin to shed the virus prior to showing clinical signs.

Approximately 20% of infected dogs are asymptomatic. Affected dogs exhibit a mild cough persisting over 10 days and a low grade fever. Some dogs may have a dry hacking cough and are mistaken for cases of *B. bronchiseptica*. Secondary bacterial infections may occur and progress to bronchopneumonia. Illness with fever and cough is self-limiting, and dogs recover within 3 weeks. A more severe but less common form of the infection is associated with tachypnea, dyspnea, fever (>104°F or 40°C), purulent nasal discharge, depression, anorexia, and moist cough. Thoracic radiographs may reveal lung lobe consolidation and pleural effusion. The severe form of canine influenza can result in bronchopneumonia, hemorrhage within the respiratory tract, and acute death.[36]

The CBC is usually normal. PCR of nasal swabs or respiratory tissue is best performed at the peak of viral shedding, approximately 2–3 days after infection, but this may occur prior to the onset of clinical signs. Serological testing for virus-specific antibodies is available through the University of Florida College of Veterinary Medicine or Cornell Animal Health Diagnostic Center. The presence of antibody is indicative of viral exposure but not necessarily infection. Antibody levels may not be detected early in the course of disease. Therefore, it is recommended that paired serum samples are performed. A fourfold rise in titer indicates active infection.[38,39] There have been no published reports on the effect of the available vaccine on serological testing.[40] If secondary bacterial infection is suspected, a transtracheal wash or bronchoalveolar lavage for cytology and culture and sensitivity is recommended.

Treatment is primarily supportive care. Most cases of mild CIV are self-limiting and do not require any treatment. Nonproductive coughs may be treated with antitussives. Saline nebulization and coupage may be beneficial with dogs having lower airway involvement.[41] In dogs with productive cough, lower respiratory involvement, or systemic illness, antimicrobials should be utilized based on culture and sensitivity of the secondary bacterial infection. Supplemental oxygen, intravenous fluid therapy, and nutritional support may be required in more severe cases.[41] Antiviral agents such as oseltamivir (Tamiflu®) are not recommended as the dose, efficacy, and safety of this medication are unknown in dogs. In March 2006, the FDA published a final rule prohibiting the extra label use of adamantine, oseltamivir, and zanamivir in poultry to retain the efficacy of these drugs for the treatment of influenza infections in humans.[42]

Prevention of CIV can be achieved by vaccination and by limiting susceptible dogs' exposure. A killed canine influenza H3N8 virus vaccine is available in the United States. Vaccination reduces the severity of clinical signs and decreases shedding but does not prevent infection. The initial vaccination requires two doses 2–4 weeks apart, followed by annual revaccination. Vaccination is indicated for healthy dogs >6 weeks of age at risk of exposure to canine influenza, such as those in group housing.[40] The risk of infection in household pets is very low and routine vaccination is not recommended.

Canine influenza suspects must be isolated from other dogs. If affected dogs require hospitalization, barrier precautions including disposable clothing should be used when handling these dogs. Proper isolation procedures are essential to avoid transmission of this infection. The virus is killed by routine disinfectants, such as quaternary ammoniums or diluted bleach. Any surface contacted by the infected dog must be appropriately disinfected.

Canine vaccines not generally recommended

Giardia lamblia

G. lamblia is a protozoal infection that can result in diarrhea. A killed vaccine is available but is generally not recommended due to unknown benefit, low risk, and low prevalence. The Giardia vaccine does decrease oocyst shedding, but evidence showing protection against infection or development of clinical signs is lacking. Additionally, diarrhea and other clinical signs caused by G. lamblia are usually controlled with routine medication. Finally, most animals are at low risk of exposure to infection with G. lamblia.

Canine measles

The canine measles vaccine has been used in puppies with a maternal antibody level that is not protective but interferes with MLV distemper vaccination. The vaccine can cause acquired immune responses and is not recommended. If maternal antibody against distemper virus is suspected to interfere with an MLV distemper vaccination, a recombinant CDV vaccine should be used as an alternative. The canine measles vaccine should not be given to dogs >12 weeks of age.

Canine coronavirus

Canine coronavirus may produce subclinical infections or mild, self-limiting diarrhea in young dogs. The prevalence of coronavirus infection in dogs is unknown, and vaccine efficacy is questionable. Therefore, vaccination against canine coronavirus is not recommended. See Chapter 8 for more information.

Rattlesnake vaccine

A vaccine designed to protect against envenomation by the Western diamondback rattlesnake (Crotalus atrox) and other pit vipers has recently become available for use. The vaccine does not offer complete protection from the effects of envenomation but reportedly slows the onset and decreases the severity of clinical signs. The efficacy of this vaccine is currently unknown.

Canine adenovirus-1

CAV-1 causes infectious hepatitis. The CAV-1 vaccine is associated with adverse effects including uveitis and corneal edema. Vaccination against CAV-2 is safer and provides cross protection against CAV-1.

Porphyromonas dental vaccine

The Porphyromonas denticanis-gulae-salivosa bacterin vaccine is designed to help reduce bone loss caused by pathogens commonly associated with periodontal disease. Some veterinary dentists advocate using this vaccine as part of a complete dental care plan to help decrease the risk of periodontal disease, especially in at-risk dogs. However, large clinical trials are needed prior to recommending this vaccine for all dogs as its efficacy, duration of immunity, potency, and risks have not yet been fully evaluated.

Feline vaccines

In practice today, the current standard of care for the feline core vaccines is the administration of rabies as a univalent product and feline parvovirus (FPV), feline calicivirus (FCV), and feline herpesvirus type 1 (FHV-1) as a multivalent product. To help standardize vaccination sites, the AAFP and the Academy of Feline Medicine recommend the right hind limb for the rabies vaccination ("R"abies in the "R"ight) with the multivalent product administered intranasally or by injection in the right forelimb. The noncore feline leukemia product should be administered in the left hind leg ("L"eukemia in the "L"eft). Each vaccine product should be administered in a different location, as distal on the limb as possible. Giving each vaccine product in a different site will help identify which vaccine produces a local reaction if one occurs.

Core vaccines

Feline rabies

As noted with canine rabies, feline rabies immunization is an important aspect of public health. In fact, during 2000–2008, more cats than dogs were reported rabid in the United States. The majority of these cases were associated with the epizootic of rabies among raccoons in the eastern United States. The large number of rabid cats compared with other domestic animals might be attributed to a lower vaccination rate among cats because of less stringent cat vaccination laws; fewer confinement or leash laws for cats; and the nocturnal activity patterns of cats, placing them at greater risk for exposure to infected raccoons, skunks, foxes, and bats.[43] Rabies infection in feral cat colonies remains a concern. Cats are naturally, highly resistant to rabies virus infection.[44]

Vaccination with a killed rabies vaccine is highly preventative, although rabies in vaccinated animals can occur.[15] The vaccine is available as canarypox recombinant, nonadjuvanted vaccine or as an inactivated 1- or 3-year adjuvanted vaccine. Initial vaccination for kittens is a single dose at 8–12 weeks of age. Revaccination intervals are subject to local laws and regulations and the manufacturer's vaccine recommendations. All cats, including indoor only cats, should continue to receive rabies vaccination throughout their lives. This recommendation is based on the zoonotic potential of the disease, chance of escape and/or interaction with wildlife, and the reported incidences of bats entering houses or apartments. Discussion continues on the pros and cons of the use of the nonadjuvanted annual vaccine versus the adjuvanted triannual vaccine. The location recommendation for vaccine administration is the distal right hind leg.

Feline parvovirus (panleukopenia)

FPV is a resilient nonenveloped DNA virus found worldwide that, among domestic cats, most commonly affects the young unvaccinated cat. FPV is very similar morphologically and antigenically to CPV.[45] The transmission of the disease is primarily through oronasal exposure to the infected host's secretions and excretions or via external parasites such as fleas, although fomites such as bowls, bedding, litter pans, and veterinary personnel can also play a role. The incubation period is reported as 2–14 days. The virus is actively shed during the acute phase of the disease and can persist in the feces for up to 6 weeks postinfection.[46] A carrier state is not observed in cats that have recovered from parvovirus. The incubation period is 3–14 days, typically 5–7 days. FPV is a very stable virus that can persist in the environment for over 1 year. Inactivation of the virus can be achieved with bleach (sodium hypochlorite) in a 1:32 dilution or with glutaraldehyde; a 10-min contact time is recommended for both to be effective. The manifestations of the disease are systemic and enteric in nature. The virus most commonly replicates in the intestinal crypts, the bone marrow, and the lymphoid tissue. The most common clinical signs are vomiting, diarrhea, lethargy,

fever, abdominal pain, anorexia, and dehydration. FPV in the queen can result in abortion or, if the *in utero* kittens survive, in cerebellar hypoplasia. The immunosuppressive effects on the bone marrow lead to the name panleukopenia. The mortality rate in the unvaccinated is very high and without treatment is estimated at >95%. The clinical diagnosis is often presumptive based on the history, presenting symptoms, and vaccine status. Laboratory diagnosis is difficult but possible by virus culture of FPV in the feces of infected cats. Although not approved for this use, fecal ELISA tests for CPV antigen appear to detect FPV and can be used as a more rapid method for detecting FPV in feces.[47] Recently, a fecal PCR test has been developed. The prognosis is guarded, but with aggressive symptomatic treatment, recovery is possible. During treatment, full isolation procedures must be utilized. Supportive care usually consists of fluid therapy to address dehydration and electrolyte imbalances, broad-spectrum antibiotics for secondary bacterial infections due to compromised intestinal integrity, and antiemetics to prevent ongoing emesis. The addition of colloids, plasma, and/or red blood cells may be warranted in severe cases. Nursing care includes strict isolation procedures to prevent cross contamination, scrupulous patient hygiene to decrease the chance of opportunistic bacterial infections, and vigorous nutritional support (either enteral or parenteral). Close monitoring of the patient's temperature, electrolytes, blood glucose, protein levels, red blood cell count/hematocrit, and white blood cell counts are warranted. See Chapter 8 for more information.

FPV vaccination is not completely preventative but is effective in reducing clinical signs. Vaccines available for use are either MLV or inactivated, adjuvanted or nonadjuvanted, and injectable or intranasal forms. The MLV is preferred due to the reduced antigen quantities and to the fact that it is available in a nonadjuvanted form. Inactivated (killed) vaccine is warranted for use in pregnant queens, in kittens <4 weeks of age, and in immunocompromised felines. The intranasal form of the vaccine avoids the risks of vaccine-induced sarcoma and provides a more rapid onset of local mucosal immunity. Current recommendations for kittens are for three vaccines, starting at 6–8 weeks of age given every 3–4 weeks. The last vaccine should be administered after 16 weeks of age. Kittens older than 16 weeks and unvaccinated adults should initially receive two doses of FPV, 3–4 weeks apart, with at least one dose in the injectable form. All cats should receive a booster vaccine 1 year after the initial series. The adult booster vaccine schedule for FPV is still being debated. Most vaccine manufacturers recommend annual vaccination. The current veterinary recommendation is for triannual vaccination, although some argue protection is lifelong. In addition, some practitioners will recommend the triannual vaccine schedule only after an adequate vaccine titer has been shown. Typically, FPV is found in combination with feline herpesvirus, and FCV and may just be abbreviated as "P" in FVRCP. FPV is now an uncommon disease due to the widespread use of the vaccine. Nevertheless, veterinary personnel should be alert for this disease in feral or unvaccinated cats or in cats from overcrowded conditions. The location recommendation for vaccine administration is the distal right front leg.

Feline upper respiratory disease complex

Feline upper respiratory disease complex is a disease complex involving the mouth, nasal passages, sinuses, and/or upper airway of cats found most often in those kept in close confinement. Simultaneous infection with multiple causative agents often occurs. The predominant causative agents are thought to be feline herpesvirus and FCV. Other causes include *Chlamydophilia felis*, feline reovirus, *B. bronchiseptica*, *Pasteurella* spp., and mycoplasmas. These infectious agents may also be opportunistic, secondary pathogens to the viral infection.

Feline calicivirus

FCV is a nonenveloped RNA virus found worldwide that most commonly affects the young cat and those in multicat environments. FCV is one of two important viral causes of respiratory infection in cats that account for >50% of the cases. There are multiple subtypes of one serotype of FCV. The subtypes of FCV have varying levels of antigenic cross-reactivity, but they are closely related and are thought to induce some degree of cross protection.[48] In addition, studies have demonstrated that there has been an antigenic shift in clinically relevant subtypes isolated from naturally infected cats.[49] The transmission of the disease is through ingestion or inhalation of the infected host's secretions or excretions or through contact with contaminated fomites. The incubation period is usually 2–6 days but can range from 1 to 14 days. The duration of illness is typically 1–2 weeks. Recovered cats can be lifelong carriers of the disease in which the virus is shed continually from the oral cavity. FCV is a relatively stable virus that can persist in the environment for up to 4 weeks. Inactivation of the virus can be achieved with bleach (sodium hypochlorite) in a 1:32 dilution. The manifestations of the disease are generally upper respiratory in nature, although a rheumatic form of the illness exists. The virus most commonly replicates in the oropharyngeal tissues but progresses to replication in the epithelial tissues of the nose, mouth, and eyes. The most common clinical signs are sneezing, rhinitis, fever, conjunctivitis, and salivation. Lesions on the tongue, hard palate, and nose are often observed; these lesions usually present as superficial vesicles. Histologically, cats infected with FCV may show evidence of pneumonitis. Coinfection with FHV-1 and other feline upper respiratory diseases is common and can increase the severity of the symptoms. Infection with FCV alone is experimentally reported as mild and self-limiting, usually resolving in 10–14 days.[47] Kittens presenting with the rheumatic form typically present with fever, joint pain and swelling, and muscle soreness. The mortality rate for the respiratory form is relatively low. Recently, more virulent strains[50] have developed and with that, the emergence of virulent systemic feline calicivirus (VS-FCV). The mortality rate of the virulent strain is reported as up to 67%[51] and is higher in adult cats then in kittens. The clinical signs include limb and facial edema, icterus, blood in the feces, and nasal hemorrhage.

The clinical diagnosis of upper respiratory infection often suffices, without differentiation between the numerous causative agents. Laboratory diagnosis is possible by detection of FCV by viral culture, reverse transcriptase polymerase chain reaction (RT-PCR), or immunohistochemical stains of samples obtained from conjunctival scrapings, nasal discharge, or oral/respiratory collection. During treatment, full isolation procedures must be utilized. Supportive care usually consists of fluid therapy, broad-spectrum antibiotics for secondary bacterial infections, and nutritional support. Nursing care includes strict isolation procedures to prevent cross contamination, pain assessment, facial hygiene, and nutritional support. Monitoring of the patient's temperature, hydration level, lung sounds, and nutritional intake are indicated. FCV has also been found in cats with lymphocytic-plasmacytic gingivitis, although its exact role has not been determined.

FCV vaccination is not completely preventative but is effective in reducing clinical signs. Vaccines available for use are either MLV or inactivated, adjuvanted or nonadjuvanted, and injectable or intranasal forms. The vaccination schedule for FCV is the same as for FPV. FCV is often abbreviated as "C" in FVRCP.

Feline herpesvirus

FHV-1 is a double-strand, enveloped DNA virus found worldwide that most commonly affects cats in multicat environments. It is also known by its common name of rhinopneumonitis and is one of two important viral causes of respiratory infection in cats. The transmission of FHV-1 is primarily through direct contact with infected animals or their secretions/excretions. It is rarely contracted through aerosolization. The incubation period for FHV-1 is 2–17 days. The duration of illness is a bit longer than FCV at 2–4 weeks. Recovered cats can become intermittent carriers; they often typically shed the virus in response to stress or corticosteroid administration. FHV-1 can remain in the environment for 1 month, but it is not a hardy virus and is susceptible to most hospital disinfectants. Feline herpesvirus manifests as an upper respiratory disease, but it can have systemic effects including pneumonia, ocular disease, and dermatitis. The virus replicates in slightly below normal core temperatures,[52] so therefore the eyes, mouth, and upper respiratory tract are the most common locations. The clinical signs are varying degrees of conjunctivitis with discharge, sneezing, salivation, fever, anorexia, and rhinitis. In severely affected cats, herpetic keratitis, with or without a secondary bacterial infection, can lead to corneal ulceration and even corneal sequestration in some individuals. These cats may become the chronic carriers that intermittently have reoccurrence of keratitis and/or conjunctivitis. Another possible chronic condition is sinus and nasal cavity congestion due to the destruction of the nasal turbinates leading to secondary bacterial infection. Reactivation of the virus is often found after a stressor situation. At that time, the carrier may exhibit a mild reoccurrence of upper respiratory signs. The clinical diagnosis of upper respiratory infection often suffices, without differentiation between the numerous causative agents, although herpetic keratitis is pathognomonic. Laboratory diagnosis utilizing virus isolation of conjunctival, nasal, or pharyngeal swabs/scrapings or PCR testing is an option.

During treatment, full isolation procedures must be utilized. Supportive care usually consists of symptomatic treatment with fluid therapy, broad-spectrum antibiotics for secondary bacterial infections, ophthalmic antibiotics and antivirals (avoidance of ophthalmic corticosteroids is imperative), and nutritional support. In addition, supplementation with oral L-lysine may be beneficial in acute and chronic infections. Nursing care includes strict isolation procedures to prevent cross contamination, pain assessment, facial hygiene (with particular care and cleaning of the nose and eyes), and nutritional support. Humidification and an increased ambient temperature may be beneficial. Monitoring of the patient's temperature, hydration level, lung sounds, and nutritional intake are indicated.

FHV-1 vaccination is not completely preventative but is effective in reducing clinical signs. Vaccines available for use are either MLV or inactivated, adjuvanted or nonadjuvanted, and injectable or intranasal forms. The vaccination schedule for FHV-1 is the same as for FPV. FHV-1 is often abbreviated as "FVR" in FVRCP.

Noncore vaccines

Feline leukemia virus

FeLV is a retrovirus found in domestic cats worldwide. The virus encodes several major protein groups, including group-specific antigens (gag), of which p27 is the basis for most testing modalities. There are three known subgroups of the virus (A, B, and C). Recently, a fourth subtype has been identified, FeLV-T. While the subgroups vary in their clinical pathogenesis, laboratory determination is not readily available and therefore is not of a practicable significance. FeLV is shed in the saliva, urine, feces, and other secretions, passing horizontally among cats with close communal contact and vertically from queens to kittens either in utero or through the mother's milk. The virus is relatively fragile outside of the host, so transmission is generally through the oronasal route or bite wounds. Indirect transmission is not a known risk. Inactivation of the virus can be achieved with routine disinfectants and detergents. Older studies suggested that exposure to FeLV and the resultant anti-FeLV antibodies accumulated with age but that susceptibility to infection simultaneously decreased.[47] Even though recent studies have demonstrated natural infection in adult cats,[53] kittens remain the most susceptible to infection. Other reasons for susceptibility are multifold and include the fragility of the virus and the relatively large viral load needed to cause infection. This combination of reasons leads to an increase in infection for cats chronically exposed to infected cats actively shedding the virus. The initial or primary stage of infection is usually transient, although it may be pronounced in its presentation. The clinical signs include fever, diarrhea, and lymphadenopathy; lethargy and leukopenia may also be noted. The virus propagates in the lymphoid organs. The timeline for pathogenesis is unknown but is reported as weeks to months. Most cats in the early stage of infection can

mount an immune response, which clears the infection. As the infection progresses to secondary viremia, bone marrow involvement leads to the production of infected, circulating leukocytes and platelets. If the cat is viremic for greater than 16 weeks, or if there is bone marrow involvement, the virus will most likely become part of the host's DNA. The exact presentation for cats with secondary or persistent viremia varies based on subgroup and the host's immune system. They include lymphoma, nonregenerative anemia, leukopenia, and thrombocytopenia. The timeline for this phase is reported as months to years. Clinical diagnosis is through laboratory testing by PCR, IFA, or the ELISA method on whole blood, serum, plasma, tears, or saliva. It is recommended that the retroviral status be known on all cats. The preferred screening test, and the most commonly used test, is the ELISA, and it is the most accurate when run on plasma or serum samples. There is a reported increase of ELISA false-negative results when the test is run on tears or saliva. A positive ELISA test indicates circulating virus. However, a percentage of cats infected with FeLV are able to clear the virus, and therefore some cats may revert to negative. It is unclear at this time if this is a true conversion to negative status or if this is an inability to demonstrate the virus. Recent studies using PCR techniques suggest that cats are likely to remain infected for life.[54] Asymptomatic ELISA-positive cats should be tested using the IFA modality and/or retested in 1–3 months. IFA is the confirmatory test modality and represents antigen in the cytoplasm of infected blood cells. The IFA test is run on either whole blood or bone marrow smears at a reference laboratory. PCR testing is not yet standardized and currently is unvalidated. It is possible for cats with retroviruses to live normal lives for many years. Their eventual cause of death may or may not be caused by their retroviral status. The median survival after diagnosis was 2.4 years.[54] All healthy, positive cats should be on a biannual examination schedule and, minimally, annual laboratory evaluations (CBC, chemistries, urinalysis, and fecal parasite testing). Core vaccination using inactivated vaccines is preferred. Close monitoring of the cat's weight, body condition score (BCS) and oral health is indicated. During treatment, routine nosocomial precautions are indicated. Cats should be housed individually, but isolation is not indicated and is in fact contraindicated since this may expose the immunocompromised individual to other animals with infectious agents. Treatment with antiviral chemotherapy, most commonly interferon, and immune modulatory therapy are used, but the effectiveness of these treatments is variable. Supportive care consists of treating secondary infections, bone marrow disorders, neoplasia, or other manifestations of the disease. Nursing care includes attending to the patient's cleanliness and nutritional intake. Close monitoring of the patient's temperature, weight, blood counts, lymph nodes, and neurological status are indicated.

The efficacy of FeLV vaccines to challenge studies is still under debate; therefore, the protection provided from these vaccines is uncertain. Vaccines available for use are inactivated, adjuvanted and nonadjuvanted whole virus, viral subunits, or recombinants. The current recommendations by AAFP are that all cats be tested for FeLV prior to immunization. Only those adult cats at risk for or for potential exposure to FeLV are recommended to be vaccinated. It is highly recommended that all kittens receive vaccination, regardless of exposure factors, in order to provide some protection when at their most vulnerable. The location recommendation for vaccine administration is the distal left hind leg.

Chlamydia

C. felis is an intracellular bacterium occurring worldwide that affects cats, birds, and humans. This bacterium can play a role in feline upper respiratory disease complex. The transmission of the disease is primarily through contact with contaminated fomites, host secretions and excretions, or through aerosolization. The incubation period is 5–10 days. All age groups of cats are susceptible, but it is predominantly seen in young cats from 2 to 9 months of age. Young kittens (7–10 day old) are also vulnerable to neonatal conjunctivitis with symptoms persisting for some time. Once contracted, cats can be carriers for as long as 18 months postinfection. Episodes of shedding bacteria are often preceded by stressful events. The bacterium can be disinfected with household detergents. The primary clinical sign of this highly contagious disease is acute, severe conjunctivitis characterized by blepharospasm, conjunctival hyperemia, chemosis, and ocular discharge. Other less common conditions include abortion, polyarthritis, and feline pneumonitis (FPn). FPn is characterized by sneezing and coughing. Although mortality is not great, infected kittens and older cats may become severely debilitated. Because of its extreme infectivity, feline chlamydiosis constitutes a major problem in pet hospitals, clinics, and catteries. Laboratory diagnosis is through positive culture of excretions or secretions. During treatment, full isolation procedures must be utilized. Supportive care usually consists of fluid therapy to address dehydration and oral and/or ocular antibiotics. Nursing care includes strict isolation procedures to prevent cross contamination, facial hygiene particularly cleansing of ocular discharges, and nutritional support, if indicated. Close monitoring of the patient's temperature, lung sounds, hydration status and nutritional intake is indicated.

There is a reported high rate of adverse vaccine reaction and a low rate of disease complications. These two factors plus a vaccine that does not prevent, only lessens the course of the disease, warrants the noncore status of this vaccine. Additionally, the use of the vaccine does not prevent shedding of the organism. The vaccine may be used as part of a control regime for cats in multiple cat environments where confirmed clinical disease is present. The vaccine is available as a nonadjuvanted MLV and as an inactivated, adjuvanted injectable product. The initial dose can be administered as early as 9 weeks of age, with a booster vaccine administered 3–4 weeks later. Boosters, if indicated, are annual.

Bordetella

Bordetella spp. are small, motile, gram-negative, aerobic coccobacilli that can be found in conjunction with other pathogens in the feline upper respiratory disease complex or as the sole causa-

tive agent. In most cats, *Bordetella* spp. cause mild and self-limiting respiratory tract disease of approximately 10 days duration. Bronchopneumonia, often acute and fatal, can develop and is more prevalent in kittens. *B. bronchiseptica (Bb)* infection is unusual in cats, found mostly in catteries and in shelter situations. *Bb* infection presents, as with other upper respiratory diseases, as fever, sneezing, nasal discharge, submandibular lymphadenopathy, and rales. The characteristic cough noted in dogs is not as prevalent in cats. The mode of transmission is by direct contact with infected individuals (dog or cat) or through aerosolization. The incubation period is typically about 5 days. An asymptomatic carrier state is common with reemergence of symptoms often associated with times of stress. *Bb* is easily killed with most disinfectants. If a definitive diagnosis is indicated/pursued, it is through culture of oropharyngeal and nasal swabs, or sputum samples. During treatment, full isolation procedures must be utilized. The first line of treatment is with antibiotics—tetracycline derivatives, quinolones, or amoxicillin/clavulonic being the antibiotics of choice. Supportive care usually consists of fluid therapy to address dehydration, facial hygiene, and nutritional support if indicated. Nursing care includes strict isolation procedures to prevent cross contamination, scrupulous patient/facial hygiene, and nutritional support, if indicated. Close monitoring of the patient's temperature, hydration status, lung sounds, and nutritional status is indicated.

The vaccine is only recommended for cats with a likely, specific risk of infection. The vaccine is available as a nonadjuvanted MLV topical vaccine for intranasal administration. Parenteral administration will cause a severe local reaction and possible death. A single dose can be administered in cats as young as 8 weeks of age, followed by annual booster vaccination if indicated.

Feline immunodeficiency virus

FIV is a T-lymphotropic lentivirus that causes an acquired immunodeficiency syndrome (AIDS). It is found in domestic cats worldwide. FIV shares many characteristics with the human immunodeficiency virus, but it is a distinct virus that is not transmissible between cats and humans. Five known subtypes exist (A–E). FIV is shed in the saliva, and transmission is via bite wounds. Passing of the virus horizontally among cats with close, friendly communal contact is uncommon. The virus is relatively fragile outside of the host and indirect transmission is not a known risk. Inactivation of the virus can be achieved with routine disinfectants or detergents. The symptoms of the initial stage or acute phase of infection are fever, malaise, and diarrhea. The virus propagates in different cells of the immune system and/or in the CNS; the exact location of replication may be indicative of the eventual manifestation of the disease. A decrease in the lymphocyte count with inversion of the T-lymphocyte ratio is noted during viral propagation. Cell-mediated immunity is more profoundly affected than humoral immunity.[55] FIV produces a persistent, lifelong infection (carrier state). The disease is characterized by a relatively long latent period (asymptomatic phase) with a gradual decline in immune function (terminal phase). It is possible for cats with FIV to live normal lives for many years. Their eventual cause of death may or may not be caused by their viral status. Eventual opportunistic infections, myelosuppression, stomatitis, neoplasia, ocular inflammation, anemia, leucopenia, or neurological disease may be noted. The median survival after diagnosis is 4.9 years. Clinical diagnosis is through laboratory testing for antibodies performed using the ELISA method. Confirmatory testing by a second antibody test or Western blot is suggested. PCR testing is not yet standardized and currently is unvalidated. It is recommended that the retroviral status be known on all cats. Vaccination against FIV produces anti-FIV antibodies that cannot be distinguished from natural infection for at least 1 year. In addition, previously vaccinated queens will pass these antibodies via passive transfer onto their kittens in their colostrum. All healthy, positive cats should be on a biannual examination schedule and, minimally, annual laboratory evaluations (CBC, chemistries, urinalysis, and fecal parasite testing). Core vaccination using inactivated vaccines is preferred. Close monitoring of the cat's weight, BCS, and oral health is indicated. During treatment, routine nosocomial precautions are indicated. Cats should be housed individually, but isolation is not indicated and is in fact contraindicated since this may expose the immunocompromised individual to infectious agents. Treatment with antiviral chemotherapy, most commonly interferon, and immune modulatory therapy are used, but the effectiveness of these treatments is variable. Supportive care consists of treating opportunistic infections, stomatitis, anemia, or other manifestations of the disease. Nursing care includes attending to the patient's cleanliness and, especially in cases of stomatitis, to their nutritional intake. Close monitoring of the patients temperature, weight, blood counts, eyesight, and neurological status is indicated.

This vaccine has been shown to provide protection against subtype A and subtype D strains of FIV, but its protective value against all of the strains is unknown. Because cats vaccinated with FIV will exhibit a positive FIV test, some form of permanent identification is recommended. This vaccine is available as an adjuvanted, killed product. The initial vaccination schedule is a series of three vaccines as early as 8 weeks of age with subsequent doses every 2–3 weeks. Annual boosters are recommended only if warranted.

Feline vaccines not generally recommended

Giardia

Giardia spp. are protozoal agents found worldwide that can infect any mammal, including humans, dogs, and cats. The most common source for human infection is drinking contaminated water, not from contact with infected pets. Infection in children, puppies, and kittens is often subclinical and does not necessarily indicate treatment. This protozoa is extremely hardy in the environment and can persist for years in the cystic form.

Insufficient studies are available to support the role of this vaccine in preventing clinical disease. It may prevent shedding, but it does not prevent infection. Since the vaccine does not

prevent infection, a minimum duration of immunity based on challenge has not been reported. The vaccine is available as an adjuvanted, inactivated injectable vaccine licensed for use in dogs. It may be administered as early as 8 weeks of age, with a booster vaccine in 2–4 weeks. Boosters, if indicated, are annual according to the manufacturer.

Feline infectious peritonitis

Feline infectious peritonitis (FIP) is a positive-stranded RNA feline coronavirus. The virus is a transmissible gastroenteritis through the fecal–oral route. FIP eventually results in a fatal Arthus-type immune-mediated vasculitis.

At this time, proof is lacking that vaccination provides clinically relevant protection. In addition, only cats known to be feline coronavirus antibody negative at the time of vaccination are likely to develop some level of protection. Vaccination of coronavirus antibody-positive cats or exposure to cats with FIP is not recommended. The vaccine is a nonadjuvanted, MLV, topical product. Initial vaccine is as early as 16 weeks of age, with a booster vaccine in 3–4 weeks. Annual booster vaccine is recommended by the manufacturer.

Vaccinations and adverse reactions

As with any and all medications or drugs, the administration of vaccinations can result in adverse effects. Possible adverse effects include pain at the site of injection, fever, inappetence, and lethargy. There are many different reactions that can occur after exposure to a vaccination. They can range from minor (sensitivity and/or a small mass at the injection site) to more generalized reactions (urticaria, fever, lethargy) to the most severe with anaphylactic shock (vomiting, salivation, dyspnea, and incoordination) and death. In one study, mild to severe adverse effects within 3 days of vaccination were reported in 0.38% of dogs. The highest risk of adverse reactions was observed when multiple vaccine products were administered on the same visit, especially in young adult small dogs (<10 kg).[32] Most reactions were reported within 1 day of vaccination. Multivalent vaccine products did not pose a higher risk than monovalent products in this study. In another study, 0.52% of cats had adverse effects of varying severity within 30 days of vaccination. Similar to dogs, the highest risk was associated with cats receiving multiple vaccine products per visit, and most reactions occurred within 3 days of vaccination.[56]

Physiology of anaphylaxis

After the initial exposure to an antigen or hapten, IgE binds to mast cells (sensitization). When the sensitized animal is exposed to the allergen for the second time, the IgE antibodies on the mast cells react, causing the cells to release their chemical mediators (degranulation). The chemical mediators involved in this process include histamine, proteases, chemotactic factors, leukotrienes, prostaglandin D, and cytokines (tumor necrosis factor and interleukins). These chemical mediators cause the clinical signs associated with anaphylaxis.

Anaphylaxis is classified as a type I (immediate) hypersensitivity reaction that typically occurs within minutes to 1 h of exposure; however, the time to onset can be delayed. A late-stage (biphasic) response may reoccur hours to days later.

Anaphylactoid reactions or psuedoanaphylaxis are due to the direct degranulation of mast cells in the absence of IgE. These reactions present and are treated similarly as anaphylaxis but are not true allergic reactions. An anaphylactoid reaction does not require prior sensitization and can be observed after the administration of some drugs (e.g., certain radiocontrast agents).

Localized anaphylaxis

Localized anaphylaxis (also known as cutaneous anaphylaxis) is limited to the site of the antigen exposure, usually resulting in such clinical signs as urticaria or wheals (hives), pruritis, and erythema. If the site of exposure is the respiratory tract (inhaled), localized anaphylaxis can result in rhinitis or asthma. If the site of exposure is the gastrointestinal tract (swallowed), localized anaphylaxis can result in allergic gastroenteritis.

The treatment for localized anaphylaxis is antihistamine administration. Severe reactions may require corticosteroids, epinephrine, and/or oxygen therapy.

Systemic anaphylaxis (hypersensitivity reactions)

Systemic anaphylaxis is an acute, life-threatening, whole body, hypersensitivity response to an antigen (e.g., drugs, hormones, vaccines, iodinated contrast media, and venom) in a sensitized animal.[57] Anaphylaxis is also called anaphylactic shock, anaphylactoid reaction, severe allergic reaction, or hypersensitivity reaction.

The clinical signs may include urticaria, pruritis, facial edema, periocular swelling, angioedema (generalized permeability of the peripheral vasculature), hypotension, collapse, dyspnea (from bronchospasm), nausea, vomiting, and diarrhea. This can progress to respiratory arrest from upper airway obstruction or angioedema and cardiovascular collapse and death, possibly within 30 min of exposure to an antigen.

Immediate emergency care is needed during anaphylaxis. The administration of epinephrine is the first response with antihistamines and corticosteroids often used as adjuncts to therapy. Patients with anaphylaxis require close monitoring and may require resuscitation measures such as supplemental oxygen, airway management, and intravenous fluids.

Vaccine anaphylaxis

Anaphylaxis is among the most severe reactions that can be seen after vaccinating an animal. Since anaphylaxis can occur after exposure to any foreign antigen and it is not limited to vaccine exposure, diagnosing the offending antigen is problematic in some cases. Also, if more than one vaccine is administered at a time, it is difficult to identify which vaccine, and which component within the vaccine may be responsible for the reaction. The introduction of microbial agents, adjuvant, inactivators, preservatives, or other proteins in a vaccine product may cause an allergic reaction.

Previous vaccination reaction history

If the patient has a history of vaccine reaction, precautions should be taken with any future vaccination. If at all possible, further vaccinations should be avoided. Depending on local regulations, rabies titers may be acceptable in lieu of vaccination. If further vaccinations are required, the following guidelines are recommended.[3]

1. *Different Vaccination Manufacture.* Selection of a vaccine from a different manufacturer may decrease the possibility of a repeated vaccine reaction. If possible, avoid the same vaccine as used previously.

2. *Administer by an Alternate Route.* Avoid IM administration of a vaccine; administer by intranasal or subcutaneous route.

3. *Switch to an MLV Product.* Avoid adjuvanted inactivated products.

4. *Premedication.* Premedication with an antihistamine, such as diphenhydramine (Benadryl®), and a corticosteroid, such as prednisolone sodium succinate, can be given 30 min prior to vaccine administration.

5. *Observation.* Vaccinate early in the day; hospitalization of the patient for observation may be needed. The length of observation is dependent somewhat on the history, but typically 4–8 h is indicated.

6. *Only Administer One Vaccine at a Time.* Only single-agent products should be administered at each visit. A 2-week waiting period between all vaccines is advised.

Postvaccinal masses

A biopsy should be obtained from any vaccinate-associated mass as per the following guidelines from the American Veterinary Medical Association:

a. if the mass is present for >3 months,

b. if the mass is ≥2 cm in diameter, or

c. if the mass increases in size after 1 month.

Inadequate immune response to vaccination aka vaccine failure

If a vaccinated animal develops the disease for which it had been vaccinated against, there are a number of factors to investigate. Possible causes include host factors, vaccine factors, and human error (Table 12.4.2).

Client education after vaccination

Regardless of previous vaccination history, all clients should be educated about the possibility of adverse effects including the clinical signs of anaphylaxis, length of time to observe their pet postvaccine administration, and the possibility of postvaccinal mass formation. This education should include information on the site(s) of administration and recommendations on when to contact the veterinary team. In addition, the vaccination schedule for their pet should be reiterated.

Table 12.4.2   Factors causing inadequate immune response to vaccination

Host factors	Human error	Vaccine factors
Primary immunodeficiencies	Improper mixing of products	Rendered noninfectious/inactivated during handling
Maternal antibody interference	Exposed at the time of vaccination	Improper storage
Insufficient time between vaccination and disease exposure	Concurrent use of antimicrobials or immunosuppressive drugs	Vaccines not protecting 100% of population (biological variation)
Age—very young and very old	Simultaneous use of vaccine and antisera	Disinfectant used on needles and syringes
Pregnancy	Too frequent administration (<2-week intervals)	Different or wrong strain
Stress, concurrent illness	Delay between vaccines in initial series	Excessive attenuation
Pyrexia, hypothermia	Wrong route of administration	
Incubating disease at the time of vaccination	Omission of booster vaccination	
Immunosuppressive drugs—cytotoxic, glucocorticoids	Concurrent surgery or anesthesia	
Hormonal fluctuations	Excessive time between reconstitution and administration	
General debilitation, malnutrition	Not administering entire dose	
Overwhelming exposure	Disinfectant of skin (uncertain)	
Concurrent surgery or anesthesia (uncertain)		

Source: Greene C. *Infectious Disease of the Dog and Cat,* 2nd edition. St. Louis, MO: W.B. Saunders, 1999.

While reporting suspected vaccine reactions is voluntary, veterinarians and technicians are encouraged to do so. Suspected vaccine reactions should be reported to the manufacturer and the government regulating agency (e.g., United States Department of Agriculture). By reporting suspected reactions, veterinary staff can help maintain the safety and efficacy of vaccine products.

Vaccination adverse effects and anaphylactic reactions may occur, but they are uncommon. Client fears of a reaction should not outweigh the benefits from disease protection, both for the pet and the owner. The benefits of vaccinations *do* outweigh the vaccination risks.

Bibliography

Section 1

1. Abbas A, Lichtman A, Pillai S. *Infectious Cellular and Molecular Immunology,* 6th edition, pp. 4–7, 63, 346, 397, 410–415, 489, 500–502, 507–508. Philadelphia, PA: Saunders Elsevier; 2010.
2. Bergman PJ. Cancer immunotherapy. *Vet Clin North Am Small Anim.* 2010;40:507–508, 511–512.
3. Tizard I. *Veterinary Immunology an Introduction,* 8th edition, pp. 4–5, 394–395. St. Louis, MO: Saunders Elsevier; 2009.
4. Hampel V, Schwarz B, Kempf C, et al. Adjuvant immunotherapy of feline fibrosarcoma with recombinant feline interferon-ω. *J Vet Intern Med* 2007;21:1340–1341.
5. Biller B. Cancer immunotherapy for the veterinary patient. *Vet Clin North Am Small Anim* 2007;37(1137):1141–1142.
6. Bergman P, McKnight J, Novosad A, et al. Long term survival of dogs with advanced malignant melanoma after DNA vaccination with xenogeneic human tyrosinase: a phase I trial. *Clin Cancer Res* 2003;9:1284–1285.
7. Khanna C, Hasz D, Klausner J, et al. Aerosol delivery of interleukin 2 liposomes is nontoxic and biologically effective: canine studies. *Clin Cancer Res* 1996;2:721, 727.
8. Khanna C, Anderson P, Hasz D, et al. Interleukin-2 liposome inhalation therapy is safe and effective for dogs with spontaneous pulmonary metastases. *Cancer* 1997;79(7):1410, 1415.
9. de Mari K, Maynard L, Sanquer A, et al. Therapeutic effects of recombinant feline interferon-ω on feline leukemia virus (FeLV)-infected and FeLV/feline immunodeficiency virus (FIV)-coinfected symptomatic cats. *J Vet Intern Med* 2004;18:477.

Section 2

1. http://ahdc.vet.cornell.edu/sects/clinpath/test/immun/ana.cfm.
2. Wardrop KJ. The Coombs test in veterinary medicine: past, present, future. *Vet Clin Pathol* 2005;34(4):325–334.
3. Warman SM, Murray JK, Ridyard A, et al. Pattern of Coombs' test reactivity has diagnostic significance in dogs with immune-mediated haemolytic anaemia. *J Small Anim Pract* 2008;49:525–530.

4. Lappin MR. *ELISA Tests: Methods and Interpretation*. CVT XIII, pp. 8–11. Philadelphia, PA: W.B. Saunders; 2003.

5. Lappin MR. Laboratory diagnosis of infectious disease. In: *Textbook of Veterinary Internal Medicine*, 7th edition. St. Louis, MO: Saunders Elsevier; 2010.

6. Garrett L. *Fine-Needle Aspiration*, NAVC Clinician's Brief, June 2010, pp. 61–66.

7. Siedlecki CT. Lymph node aspiration and biopsy. In: *Textbook of Veterinary Internal Medicine*, 7th edition. St. Louis, MO: Saunders Elsevier; 2010.

8. Couto CG. Cytology. In: *Small Animal Internal Medicine*, 4th edition, eds. RW Nelson, CG Couto p. 1143. St. Louis, MO: Mosby Elsevier; 2009.

Section 3

1. Ettinger SJ Feldman EC. *Textbook of Veterinary Internal Medicine (Diseases of the Dog and Cat)*, 5th edition, Vol. 2, pp. 1793–1798, 1819–1823. Philadelphia, PA: Saunders; 2000.

2. Blackwood L, German AJ, Stell AJ, O'Neill T. Multicentric lymphoma in a dog after cyclosporine therapy. *J Small Anim Pract* 2004;45(5):259–262.

3. Al-Ghazlat S. Immunosuppressive therapy for canine immune mediated hemolytic anemia. *Compendium* 2009;31(1).

4. Plumb D. *Plumb's Veterinary Drug Handbook*, 6th edition, pp. 88–90, 234–240, 248–249, 265–269, 427–429, 526–527, 639–640, 755–762. Stockholm, WI: Blackwell; 2010.

5. Mason N, Duval D, Shofer FS, Giger U. Cyclophosphamide exerts no beneficial effect over prednisone alone in the initial treatment of acute immune-mediated hemolytic anemia in dogs: a randomized controlled clinical trial. *J Vet Intern Med* 2003;17(2):206–212.

6. Bianco D. A prospective, randomized, double-blinded, placebo-controlled study of human. *J Vet Intern Med* 2009;23:1071–1078.

7. Sharpe C. Standards of Care, Vol. 10, No. 10, Nov 2008, Immune Mediated Hemolytic Anemia on Lifelearn. http://www.vetlearn.com/ArticleDetails/tabid/106/ArticleID/3903/Default.aspx

8. Misseghers BS, Binnington AG, Mathews KA. Clinical observations of the treatment of canine perianal fistulas with topical tacrolimus in 10 dogs. *Can Vet J* 2000;41(8):623–627.

Section 4

1. Paul MA, Carmichael LE, Childers H, et al. 2006 AAHA canine vaccine guidelines. *J Am Anim Hosp Assoc* 2006;42(2):80–89.

2. Richards JR, Elston TH, Ford RB, et al. The 2006 American Association of Feline Practitioners feline vaccine advisory panel report. *J Am Vet Med Assoc* 2006;229(9):1405–1441.

3. Greene CE, Schultz RD. Immunoprophylaxis. In: *Infectious Diseases of the Dog and Cat*, 3rd edition, ed. CE Greene, pp. 1069–1119. St. Louis, MO: Saunders Elsevier; 2006.

4. Spickler AR, Roth JA. Adjuvants in veterinary vaccines: modes of action and adverse effects. *J Vet Intern Med* 2003;17(3):273–281.

5. Morrison WB, Starr RM. Report of the vaccine-associated feline sarcoma task force. *JAVMA* 2001;218 No. 5:697–702.

6. Kass PH, Spangler WL, Hendrick MJ, et al. Multicenter case-control study of risk factors associated with development of vaccine-associated sarcomas in cats. *J Am Vet Med Assoc* 2003;223(9):1283–1292.

7. Schultz RD, Thiel B, Mukhtar E, Sharp P, Larson LJ. Age and long-term protective immunity in dogs and cats. *J Comp Pathol* 2010;142 Suppl 1:S102–S108.

8. Lappin MR, Andrews J, Simpson D, Jensen WA. Use of serologic tests to predict resistance to feline herpesvirus 1, feline calicivirus, and feline parvovirus infection in cats. *J Am Vet Med Assoc* 2002;220(1):38–42.

9. Scott FW, Geissinger CM. Long-term immunity in cats vaccinated with an inactivated trivalent vaccine. *Am J Vet Res* 1999;60(5):652–658.

10. Moore GE, Glickman LT. A perspective on vaccine guidelines and titer tests for dogs. *J Am Vet Med Assoc* 2004;224(2):200–203.

11. Nara PL, Krakowka S, Powers TE. Effects of prednisolone on the development of immune responses to canine distemper virus in beagle pups. *Am J Vet Res* 1979;40(12):1742–1747.

12. Duval D, Giger U. Vaccine-associated immune-mediated hemolytic anemia in the dog. *J Vet Intern Med* 1996;10(5):290–295.

13. Warrell MJ, Warrell DA. Rabies and other lyssavirus diseases. *Lancet* 2004;363(9413):959–969.

14. Blanton JD, Robertson K, Palmer D, Rupprecht CE. Rabies surveillance in the United States during 2008. *J Am Vet Med Assoc* 2009;235(6):676–689.

15. Murray KO, Holmes KC, Hanlon CA. Rabies in vaccinated dogs and cats in the United States, 1997–2001. *J Am Vet Med Assoc* 2009;235(6):691–695.

16. Centers for Disease Control and Prevention (CDC). Human rabies—Kentucky/Indiana, 2009. *MMWR Morb Mortal Wkly Rep* 2010;59(13):393–396.

17. Centers for Disease Control and Prevention (CDC). Human rabies—Alberta, Canada, 2007. *MMWR Morb Mortal Wkly Rep* 2008;57(8):197–200.

18. Pardo MC, Bauman JE, Mackowiak M. Protection of dogs against canine distemper by vaccination with a canarypox virus recombinant expressing canine distemper virus fusion and hemagglutinin glycoproteins. *Am J Vet Res* 1997;58(8):833–836.

19. Goldstein RE, Lin RC, Langston CE, Scrivani PV, Erb HN, Barr SC. Influence of infecting serogroup on clinical features of leptospirosis in dogs. *J Vet Intern Med* 2006;20(3):489–494.

20. Schultz RD, Larson LJ, Lorentzen LP. Effects of modified live canine parvovirus vaccine on the snap ELISA antigen assay. *J Vet Emerg Crit Care* 2008;18(4):410.

21. Greene CE. Infectious canine hepatitis and canine acidophil cell hepatitis. In: *Infectious Diseases of the Dog and Cat*, 3rd edition, ed. CE Greene, pp. 41–47, 58. St. Louis, MO: Saunders Elsevier; 2006.

22. Schultz RD. Duration of immunity for canine and feline vaccines: a review. *Vet Microbiol* 2006;117(1):75–79.

23. Adler B, de la Pena Moctezuma A. Leptospira. In: *Pathogenesis of Bacterial Infections in Animals*, 4th edition, ed. CL Gyles, et al., pp. 527–541. Ames, IA: Wiley-Blackwell; 2010.

24. Greene CE, Sykes JE, Brown CA, Hartmann K. Leptospirosis. In: *Infectious Diseases of the Dog and Cat*, 3rd edition, ed. CE Greene, pp. 402–416. St. Louis, MO: Saunders Elsevier; 2006.

25. Ward MP, Glickman LT, Guptill LE. Prevalence of and risk factors for leptospirosis among dogs in the United States and Canada: 677 cases (1970–1998). *J Am Vet Med Assoc* 2002;220(1):53–58.

26. Alton GD, Berke O, Reid-Smith R, Ojkic D, Prescott JF. Increase in seroprevalence of canine leptospirosis and its risk factors, Ontario 1998–2006. *Can J Vet Res* 2009;73(3):167–175.

27. Ward MP, Guptill LF, Wu CC. Evaluation of environmental risk factors for leptospirosis in dogs: 36 cases (1997–2002). *J Am Vet Med Assoc* 2004;225(1):72–77.

28. Adin CA, Cowgill LD. Treatment and outcome of dogs with leptospirosis: 36 cases (1990–1998). *J Am Vet Med Assoc* 2000;216(3):371–375.

29. Prescott JF, McEwen B, Taylor J, Woods JP, Abrams-Ogg A, Wilcock B. Resurgence of leptospirosis in dogs in Ontario: recent findings. *Can Vet J* 2002;43(12):955–961.

30. Ribotta M, Fortin M, Higgins R, Beaudin S. Canine leptospirosis: Serology. *Can Vet J* 2000;41(6):494–495.

31. Klaasen HL, Molkenboer MJ, Vrijenhoek MP, Kaashoek MJ. Duration of immunity in dogs vaccinated against leptospirosis with a bivalent inactivated vaccine. *Vet Microbiol* 2003;95(1–2): 121–132.

32. Moore GE, Guptill LF, Ward MP, et al. Adverse events diagnosed within three days of vaccine administration in dogs. *J Am Vet Med Assoc* 2005;227(7):1102–1108.

33. Gore T, Headley M, Laris R, et al. Intranasal kennel cough vaccine protecting dogs from experimental *Bordetella bronchiseptica* challenge within 72 hours. *Vet Rec* 2005;156(15):482–483.

34. Davis R, Jayappa H, Abdelmagid OY, Armstrong R, Sweeney D, Lehr C. Comparison of the mucosal immune response in dogs vaccinated with either an intranasal avirulent live culture or a subcutaneous antigen extract vaccine of *Bordetella bronchiseptica*. *Vet Ther* 2007;8(1):32–40.

35. Littman MP, Goldstein RE, Labato MA, Lappin MR, Moore GE. ACVIM small animal consensus statement on lyme disease in dogs: Diagnosis, treatment, and prevention. *J Vet Intern Med* 2006;20(2):422–434.

36. Yoon K-J, Cooper VL, Schwartz KJ, et al. Influenza virus infection in racing greyhounds. *Emerg Infect Dis* 2005;11(12):1974–1976.

37. Hilling K, Hanel R. Canine Influenza. *Compendium: Cont Educ Vet* 2010;6:E1–E9. http://www.vetlearn.com/compendium/canine-influenza-ce (accessed July 28, 2010).

38. Crawford C, Rada KA, UC Davis Koret Shelter Medicine Program. Information: canine influenza. http://www.sheltermedicine.com/shelter-health-portal/information-sheets/canine-influenza (accessed July 28, 2010).

39. Cornell University College of Veterinary Medicine Animal Health Diagnostic Center. Appropriate samples for detecting presence of canine influenza virus. http://www.diaglab.vet.cornell.edu/issues/civ.asp (accessed July 28, 2010).

40. Intervet/Schering-Plough Animal Health. Canine influenza vaccine, H3N8. http://www.intervetusa.com/products/nobivac-canine-flu-h3n8/productdetails_130_121109.aspx (accessed July 28, 2010).

41. Crawford PC, Sellon RK. Chapter 216: Canine viral diseases. In: *Textbook of Veterinary Internal Medicine*, eds. SJ Ettinger, EC Feldman, pp. 958–970. St. Louis, MO: Saunders; 2010.

42. US Federal Food and Drug Administration. 21 CFR 530.41. http://www.accessdata.fda.gov/scripts/cdrh/cfdocs/cfcfr/CFRSearch.cfm?fr=530.41 (accessed July 28, 2010).

43. CDC-Human Rabies Prevention—United States. 2008 Recommendations of the Advisory Committee on Immunization Practices. Prepared by Manning SE, Rupprecht CE, Fishbein D, et al.

44. Ettinger SJ, Feldman EC. *Textbook of Veterinary Internal Medicine*, 5th edition, Vol. 1, pp. 449–450. St. Louis, MO: Saunders; 2000.

45. Truyen U, Gruenberg A, Chang SF, et al. Evolution of the feline-subgroup of parvovirus and control of canine host range in vivo. *J Virol* 1995;69:4702.

46. Kahn CM. *Merck Veterinary Manual*, 9th edition. Whitehouse Station, NJ: Merck & co; 2008. Online, last accessed 2/2011.

47. Ettinger SJ, Feldman EC. *Textbook of Veterinary Internal Medicine*. 6th edition, 653, 2004.

48. Ettinger SJ, Feldman EC. *Textbook of Veterinary Internal Medicine*, 7th edition, p. 946; 2010.

49. Lauritzen A, Jarrett O, Sabara M. Serological analysis of feline calicivirus isolates from the United States and United Kingdom. *Vet Microbiol* 1997;56:55.

50. Radford A, Coyne K, Dawson S, Porter C, Gaskell R. Feline calicivirus. *Vet Res* 2007;38(2):319–335. DOI: 10.1051/vetres:2006056. PMID 17296159.

51. Foley JE. Calicivirus: spectrum of disease. In: *Consultations in Feline Internal Medicine*, Vol. 5. ed. JR August, pp. 3–10. St. Louis, MO: Elsevier Saunders; 2005.

52. Lehmann R, Franchini M, Aubert A, et al. Vaccination of cats experimentally infected with feline immunodeficiency virus, using a recombinant feline leukemia virus vaccine. *J Am Vet Med Assoc* 1991;199:1446–1452.

53. Torres AN, Mathiason CK, Hoover EA. Re-examination of feline leukemia virus: host relationships using real-time PCR. *Virology* 2005;332:272–283.

54. Levy JK, Lorentzen L, Shields J, Lewis H. 2006. *Long term outcome of cats with natural FeLV and FIV infection*. 8th International Feline Retrovirus Research Symposium, Washington, DC.

55. Levy JK, Ritchey JW, Rottman JB, et al. Elevated interleukin-10-to-interleukin-12 ratio in feline immunodeficiency virus-infected cats predicts loss of type 1 immunity to *Toxoplasma gondii*. *J Infect Dis* 1998;178:503–511.

56. Moore GE, DeSantis-Kerr AC, Guptill LF, Glickman NW, Lewis HB, Glickman LT. Adverse events after vaccine administration in cats: 2560 cases (2002–2005). *J Am Vet Med Assoc* 2007;231(1): 94–100.

57. Waddell LS. Systemic anaphylaxis. In: *Textbook of Veterinary Internal Medicine*, eds. SJ Ettinger, EC Feldman, pp. 531–534. St. Louis, MO: Saunders; 2010.

58. *Infectious Diseases of the Dog and Cat*, 4th edition, ed. CE Greene, pp. 75 St. Louis, MO: Elsevier Saunders; 2012.

59. Rentko VT, Clark N, Ross LA, Schelling SH. Canine leptospirosis. A retrospective study of 17 cases. *J Vet Intern Med* 1992;6(4): 235–244.

Chapter 13 Pain and Its Management

Author: Barry Kipperman

Managing pain in our animal patients is one of the most important and challenging charges of all veterinary personnel. This responsibility is explicitly stated in the veterinarian's oath ("the relief of animal suffering")[1] and in the veterinary technician's code of ethics ("shall prevent and relieve the suffering of animals with competence and compassion").[2] It is hard to imagine there was a time just 50 years ago when infants and children were assumed not to require pain management. In fact, when this author was an intern 22 years ago, administration of analgesics to trauma patients was a rare and extraordinary event, the emphasis being placed on managing shock instead.

Our profession was slow to embrace pain management in animals due to a lack of experience with analgesics, fear of the side effects of opioids, concerns regarding the management of controlled substances, and the perceived rapid recovery of our patients from surgery in the absence of analgesics. The fact that dogs and cats could recover uneventfully from routine surgery lulled veterinary personnel into the presumption that there is no need to manage pain. This can be referred to as the "he didn't die did he?" phenomenon, in which the veterinary staff equates the animal's survival with a successful outcome. Although we'd all agree that survival is a desired outcome for our patients, survival does not necessarily presume a humane or expedient path.

Veterinary technician as pain management team leader

At many hospitals, it is assumed that the staff veterinarians are responsible for overseeing patient pain management and pain management protocols. In this paradigm, veterinary technicians or nurses are expected to administer analgesics to patients and to follow the orders of the veterinarian. Although this system provides a simple and straightforward hierarchy, a paradigm shift that empowers the veterinary technician to a far greater degree of involvement would improve management of pain in our patients. Let us examine the reasoning for this shift using the common example of an animal being admitted to the hospital for a surgical biopsy. Who admits the animal, observes its behaviors prior to anesthesia, scores the patient's pre-op pain status and anticipated pain levels, spends time assisting and managing this patient after its surgery, and speaks to the animal's caretaker after surgery? At most hospitals, the answer to most, if not all, of these questions is the veterinary technician. It has been stated that pain is the fifth "vital sign." Certainly, no one would question the ability of the veterinary technician to measure and record the four recognized vital signs of temperature, heart rate, respiratory rate, and capillary refill time. The recognition and monitoring of pain, the fifth vital sign, should become as standard as the other four signs.

A partnership between the veterinarian and the veterinary technician provides the patient with the best opportunity for adequate pain management. In this team approach, the veterinarian proposes a suitable analgesic protocol, and the veterinary technician administers the protocol and provides frequent and valued feedback to the veterinarian regarding whether the protocol is managing the patient as per expectations. This partnership requires a keen sense of trust and communication that may take time to develop.

The veterinary technician who is knowledgeable regarding the causes of pain and the available options to control it, and who is

Small Animal Internal Medicine for Veterinary Technicians and Nurses, First Edition. Edited by Linda Merrill.
© 2012 John Wiley & Sons, Inc. Published 2012 by John Wiley & Sons, Inc.

willing to advocate on his/her patient's behalf to prevent and relieve pain, can be a tremendous asset both to the veterinarian and to his/her patients.

What is pain?

Pain is an unpleasant sensation involving the peripheral and central nervous systems (CNS) that can range from mild to debilitating. Pain is usually caused by stimuli that can arise externally (bone marrow needle) or internally (inflamed pancreas). Pain is an adaptive response that allows us to modify behaviors or motions in order to preserve function. At its most mundane, this can mean limiting use of an affected limb due to soreness after a bone marrow aspiration. In the case of abdominal pain, altering posture or simply resting may allow the animal patient to better cope with recovery from an inflamed pancreas.

Pathophysiology of pain

The technician who understands how pain is perceived and elicited can better comprehend pain and is more apt to apply the concept of multimodality analgesia to control it.

Nociception

Nociception is the physiological process that results in the conscious perception of pain.[3]

Peripheral nociceptors

In skin, muscle and viscera, noxious stimuli are translated into electrical impulses by specialized nerve endings called nociceptors.[4] This involves the opening of sodium (Na^+) channels, which

in turn causes depolarization and development of action potentials. Nociceptors are unique in that repeated activation can result in either an enhanced response (sensitization) or a lessened response (habituation) to subsequent stimuli.[5] There are few interventions currently available that target the nociceptor, though active research to find receptor antagonists is ongoing (Figure 13.1).

Afferent nerve fibers

Signals generated by the activation of nociceptors are transmitted to the CNS by afferent fibers or axons.[3] Local anesthetics such as lidocaine and bupivicaine block the Na^+ channels and inhibit transmission of the painful signal to the CNS. Unfortunately, these drugs are nonselective and block painful as well as "normal" sensation. This lack of selectivity is well-known by anyone who's had a local administered at the dentist, or who's seen the Seinfeld episode where Kramer is assumed to be intellectually challenged due to his impaired speech after a visit to the dentist. The veterinary technician must take precautions to prevent the animal patient from harm when he/she is still desensitized from local anesthesia. For example, the animal receiving prolonged external heat applied to a numb limb would be at risk for thermal injury.

Dorsal horn neurons

Afferent nerve fibers synapse with dorsal horn neurons in the gray matter of the spinal cord. The signal here is mediated by excitatory and inhibitory neurotransmitters, particularly glutamate. Analgesic drugs that act at the dorsal horn include opioids, alpha-2 agonists, and non-steroidal anti-inflammatory drugs (NSAIDs). Dense populations of opioid receptors exist in this region.

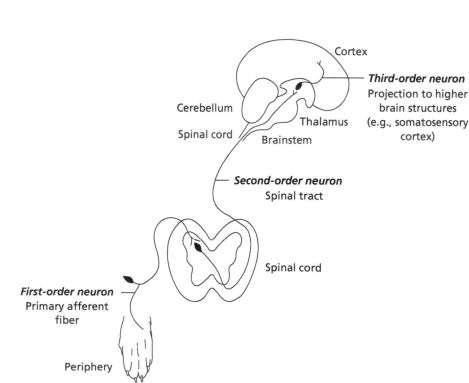

Figure 13.1 A simplified representation of nociceptive processing as a three-neuron chain. A noxious stimulus activates a primary afferent fiber that transmits the stimulus to the dorsal horn of the spinal cord. Here, a second neuron ascends in a spinal tract to the level of the thalamus. Finally, a tertiary neuron transmits the modified stimulus to higher brain centers for perception.

Source: Lamont LA, Tranquilli WJ, Grimm K. Physiology of pain. In: *Management of Pain*, in the series *Veterinary Clinics of North America, Small Animal Practice*, Vol. 30, No. 4, ed. KA Mathews, p. 705. Philadelphia, PA: W.B. Saunders; 2000, with permission.

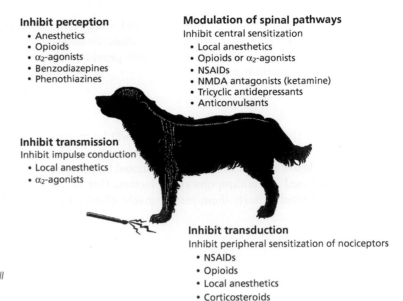

Inhibit perception
- Anesthetics
- Opioids
- α_2-agonists
- Benzodiazepines
- Phenothiazines

Modulation of spinal pathways
Inhibit central sensitization
- Local anesthetics
- Opioids or α_2-agonists
- NSAIDs
- NMDA antagonists (ketamine)
- Tricyclic antidepressants
- Anticonvulsants

Inhibit transmission
Inhibit impulse conduction
- Local anesthetics
- α_2-agonists

Inhibit transduction
Inhibit peripheral sensitization of nociceptors
- NSAIDs
- Opioids
- Local anesthetics
- Corticosteroids

Figure 13.2   Sites of action of the major classes of analgesics.

Source: Lamont LA, Tranquilli WJ, Grimm K. Physiology of pain. In: *Management of Pain*, in the series *Veterinary Clinics of North America, Small Animal Practice*, Vol. 30, No. 4, ed. KA Mathews, p. 722. Philadelphia, PA: W.B. Saunders; 2000, with permission.

Brain

The actual perception of a painful stimulus is believed to be mediated by neurons that synapse in the thalamus and cerebral cortex.[3] Opioids and alpha-2 agonists inhibit brain nociceptive pathways. Acepromazine and general anesthetics may modify the behavioral manifestations of pain by modifying consciousness, but these are not primary analgesic agents.

Descending pathways

These pathways can modulate sensory input and are located in the cerebral cortex and thalamus, the periaqueductal gray matter of the midbrain, the rostral brain stem, and the dorsal horn of the spinal cord.[6] Opioids play the most significant role in modulating these descending pathways (Figure 13.2).

Systemic responses to pain

It is well-known that pain can induce systemic changes that can significantly influence patient outcomes and response to therapy. Pain-induced reflex responses result in increased sympathetic tone, vasoconstriction, increased systemic vascular resistance, increased cardiac output, increased myocardial work, and increased secretion of stress hormones.[7,8] Stimulation of brainstem centers causes increased respiratory rate. Recognizing and mitigating these stress responses is an important component of any pain management protocol.

Types of pain

Painful stimuli can be categorized in many ways including physiological versus pathological, inflammatory or neuropathic, visceral, and acute or chronic. As these phrases will be found in any discussion of pain management as well as on the clinical floor, further clarification is warranted.

Acute pain

This is often a result of sudden onset of trauma (e.g., surgery, accidents) or inflammation (pancreatitis). The response to acute pain, such as rest, facilitates repair and healing.

Chronic pain

Chronic pain is arbitrarily defined as pain of greater than 3 months duration.[9] The most common causes include cancer, osteoarthritis, and postamputation phantom pain. Unlike acute pain, this form of pain is maladaptive (serves no useful purpose), can have a significant negative influence on patient quality of life, can be very difficult to discern as signs are often attributed to old age, and can be very difficult to treat. The old paradigm of "I know he seems painful, but the rest will do him good" is no longer an accepted reason to allow a patient to suffer the debilitating consequences of chronic pain. Pain scoring systems have difficulty in assessing this type of pain.

Visceral pain

Pain that arises from internal organs can sometimes remain untreated by the veterinary team as the perceived life-threatening aspects of these conditions withdraw attention from the concurrent pain. Distension of hollow organs, such as occurs with feline urethral obstruction and resultant bladder distension, gastrointestinal (GI) distension from ileus, obstruction or GDV syndrome, and inflammation such as pancreatitis, cause some of the most severe signs of pain in our patients.

Neuropathic pain

This type of pain results from insult to the nervous system. Human patients report burning sensations, allodynia, in which seemingly ordinary sensations cause pain, and exaggerated responsiveness to stimuli. Common examples include the dachshund with a herniated intervertebral disk and patients with amputated limbs (phantom pain).

Causes of pain

For purposes of this discussion, causes of pain will be categorized by whether the etiology is spontaneous or iatrogenic, and by the typical degree of pain commonly manifested by patients, or presumed based on anthropomorphic factors, that is, "If it hurts us, it probably hurts them just as much" (Tables 13.1 and 13.2).

General approach to pain control

Although our profession has made significant strides in acknowledging the role of pain in animals and the benefits of its management, all too often, animals in pain still do not receive any analgesics or receive therapy inappropriate relative to their degree of pain. Also, pain management in cats seems to be lagging compared to pain management in dogs. Common examples include lack of provision of analgesics to animals that sustain head trauma and cats given only a single dose of butorphanol after a declaw procedure.

Reasons veterinary personnel proclaim for withholding analgesics include the following.

Fear of Sedation. Therapeutic doses of opioids seldom result in profound sedation and weakness.

Interference in Ambulatory Status. Seldom will adequate analgesia result in loss of the ability to walk. In addition, it may be beneficial for the patient not to ambulate within the immediate postoperative period.

Interference in Mental Alertness. Stupor and obtundation are only noted in patients overdosed with medication. If using a constant rate infusion (CRI) administration, the potential effects of drug on mentation can be abolished by discontinuing administration for 20–30 min and then reassessing.

Cats Cannot or Will Not Tolerate the Drugs. Although cats are more sensitive to drug-related side effects, it is very rare that they will not tolerate a drug. With proper drug selection and dosing, most cats can and should be treated for pain.

Patient Does Not Appear to Exhibit Pain. Our ability to assess and treat pain should not be limited to general observation of patient demeanour. Many of our patients suffer in silence and we should not ignore them in return. Ask yourself, "Would I be in pain under the same conditions?"

General rules of thumb in managing pain

1. *Treat Early = Preemptive Analgesia.* Pain is far easier to prevent than to manage once signs manifest. Patients should never have to prove they are in pain to receive therapy. Therapy should be given prior to the painful procedure if at all possible. The classic example of this approach occurs when the pain is planned and iatrogenic in nature, being a result of surgery or other invasive procedure.

Table 13.1 Common causes of pain

Spontaneous		
Mild	**Moderate**	**Severe**
Lacerations	Osteoarthritis	Neuropathic, cervical disk, meningitis
Cystitis	Degenerative joint disease	Aortic thromboembolism, limb infarction
Wounds	Torsion—gastric dilatation–volvulus (GDV), spleen	Peritonitis, pancreatitis, sepsis
	Urethral obstruction	Large wounds (degloving, burns)
	Cancer	Polytrauma, fractures
	Trauma—head, thorax	Bone cancer

Source: Modified from Mathews K. Pain assessment and general approach to pain management. *Management of Pain. Veterinary Clinics of North America* 2000;30(4):735–736.

Table 13.2 Common causes of pain

Iatrogenic		
Mild	**Moderate**	**Severe**
Castration	Onychectomy/declaw	Thoracotomy
Ovariohysterectomy (OVH)	Amputation	Perianal surgery
Biopsies	Laparotomy	Extensive soft tissue surgery—sarcoma, mast cell tumor (MCT)
Laparoscopy	Radiation therapy	Ear ablation
Bone marrow	Chest tube	
IV and urinary catheters		

Source: Modified from Mathews K. Pain assessment and general approach to pain management. In management of pain. *Veterinary Clinics of North America* 2000;30(4):735–736.

2. *Treat Often.* Do not deny an uncomfortable patient analgesic therapy because the next dose is not yet due.

3. *Be Empathic.* Would you be asking for pain relief if you were the patient?

4. *Consider a Multimodal Approach.* Many of our patients have pain mediated through differing physiological pathways. It should therefore seem apparent that a "one-size-fits-all" approach, in which all patients receive a standard dose of analgesic, will seldom provide the most effective pain management. Combinations of drugs that influence these varied paths are often more successful than single agents.

5. *Adjust and Modify Medications until Pain Appears to be Relieved.* This is best put into practice when patients are monitored regularly and progress is communicated to the attending veterinarian.

Questions to consider

1. *How Painful Is the Condition or Surgery?* The more painful the anticipated procedure, the more compelling a multimodal, intravenous CRI and prolonged analgesic program (24 hour) become.

2. *Is the Patient Especially Anxious?* If so, sedative/anxiolytic medications should be considered prior to anesthetic recovery.

3. *Is This Patient a Suitable Candidate for Multimodal Analgesics?* For example, a patient with renal insufficiency may not be deemed a suitable candidate to receive NSAIDs.

4. *What Route of Administration Is Most Suitable?* For most patients in acute pain, intravenous administration of opioids is the preferred route. For severe pain, a CRI of analgesics provides the ability to best titrate doses to achieve relief, and avoids the pitfalls of intermittent boluses in which the patient rests for a few hours after a dose, and then seems restless and uncomfortable while waiting for the next scheduled dose. For chronic pain, oral administration is the most reasonable.

5. *Will the Timing of Administration Provide an Analgesic Effect?* Keep in mind that it may take at least 30–60 min to obtain adequate blood levels of analgesics, even after intravenous administration. Beginning analgesic therapy at the time of surgical induction may not provide your patient with maximal benefits.

6. *What Dose Should Be Utilized?* As a general rule, we can often manage with lower doses of individual drugs when using a multimodal approach, in the very debilitated and in geriatric patients. Conversely, high end doses may be advised in a young, anxious patient or when only a single analgesic is used.

7. *Does Pain End at Closing Time?* One of the major limitations our patients face in managing pain adequately is our proclivity to send patients home at 6 p.m. when the majority of hospitals close. Until it is proved that pain somehow resolves from 6 p.m.–8 a.m., giving the postoperative patient a subcutaneous injection of narcotic at 6 p.m. and telling the client he/she is managed for the night has no basis in physiology or fact. The duration of action of most opioids given parenterally is 2–8 h. This statement is simply our way of rationalizing what is convenient for the veterinarian and client, who naturally would like their pet to come home. If one is in doubt as to whether the patient's pain is apt to recur during the 14 h your hospital may be closed or have no one on site, then referral to an overnight facility should be advised so that appropriate monitoring and pain management can be continued.

8. *Is the Procedure Starting at a Time and with Adequate Staffing to Maximize Chances of a Positive, Pain-Free Outcome?* The later in the day you begin a painful procedure, the more compelling it becomes to inform the animal's caretaker that overnight observation for pain management is advised. On some occasions, our best-laid plans are interrupted by emergencies, and suddenly, a procedure planned to begin at noon is now being considered at 5 p.m. In this circumstance, the animal advocate will inform the client that unexpected emergencies arose, and it is no longer in Muffy's best interest to begin an elective procedure this late in the day. This requires swallowing pride and risking an upset client. This minimizes postprocedural complications at closing time or asking the client to transport an unconscious animal to the overnight emergency center for observation and unanticipated cost. One option is to offer to board the patient overnight at no charge and to apologize for the inconvenience.

How to be an analgesic advocate for your patient

Since our animal patients cannot ring for the nurse to increase their rate of narcotic CRI, the veterinary technician is in the most suitable position to detect when his/her patient is uncomfortable and to request a modification or initiation of analgesic therapy.[10] Each nurse should approach his/her patient as "mine," with a sense of ownership and accountability. Your task for that day is to do your best to care for the needs of that animal. Once this mindset is undertaken, it becomes clear that there is no greater need than managing pain and discomfort.

Despite the best of intentions, the attending veterinarian occasionally will not provide orders for analgesics in a painful patient. In these situations, a gentle reminder from the technician is all that should be necessary, and a "thanks for reminding me about that," the ideal response from the doctor. In practice, accomplishing this successfully requires more than good intentions; a willingness to speak up on your patient's behalf and checking egos at the door is required. An all too common refrain among technicians is that the veterinarian with the ability to prescribe analgesics ignores the request of the technician. In my experience, the manner that the technician uses to apprise the veterinarian can make the difference between relative ignorance of your request versus immediate evaluation and action.

Let us look at the following example: Max, a canine recovering from a biopsy, has already received narcotics, but you conclude pain persists based on noting the patient will not lie down, is panting excessively, and has a persistent tachycardia that was not present prior to the procedure. The blood pressure is normal, the packed cell volume is static, and the dog has an empty bladder.

Technician 1: "Dr. Kipperman, Max seems painful. We need to do something."

Technician 2: "Dr. Kipperman, I think Max needs more fentanyl. Can we increase his dose?"

Technician 3; "Dr. Kipperman, Max seems much more restless than before surgery, and he won't lie down. He's been out for a walk but is panting a lot, and his heart rate is 180/minute despite a normal blood pressure. Would you please evaluate him to see if you agree that we should consider modifying his medications?"

When I am interrupted by technician 1, I have received no evidence that he/she has performed a thorough evaluation of Max. I am apt to then ask the technician to assess vital signs and to get back to me, and Max's discomfort is prolonged in the meantime. Technician 2 has offered a solution for Max but has not clarified why he requires a dose adjustment. In other words, what signs are prompting the suggestion? I am far more apt to get to Max's cage because technician 3 has communicated concern and the results of her evaluation. In addition, she has respected the teamwork philosophy of managing Max's care. I might conclude that Max is either anxious or painful, and my response may be, "We can increase the fentanyl dose or we can add on an anxiolytic; was Max nervous or agitated before the procedure?"

In a busy hospital environment, most attending veterinarians may be involved with other procedures or appointments when you report your concerns. Technicians can and should exert significant influence on the analgesic protocol regarding the types, timing, route, and dose of analgesics administered to their patients. When you fail to motivate the veterinarian to assess your patient, you fail your patient as well.

Clinical signs and means of detection

One may ask, "Why is it important to detect signs of pain, when most of my patients are premedicated with analgesics prior to invasive procedures?" First, a solid preemptive strategy is certainly sound and will be emphasized repeatedly here, but the best-laid plans certainly do not abate spontaneous causes of pain. Second, as there is no one-size-fits-all approach that manages pain similarly in all patients, spotting when your patient is in pain allows the veterinary team to modify the protocol, thereby suiting the therapy to the individual patient.

As already discussed, it is in the animal's best interest for the veterinary technician to be the first responder in determining his/her patient's pain level as the technician typically spends more time cage side than any other member of the health-care team. By the time the veterinarian notices the patient is painful, you are probably playing catch-up.

Signs of pain can be divided into behavioral and physiological. Those of you who can recall the sound of a dog vocalizing after extubation know that "the squeaky dog gets the grease"; that is, vocal patients tend to receive far greater attention from nurses and doctors than patients suffering in silence. Clearly, rational consideration while you read this at home leads to the conclusion that all vocalizations are not an expression of pain, and silence is not necessarily an expression of comfort. Yet in the bustle of the treatment room, we tend to feel a need to "put out the fire" and often sedate the vocal patient, sometimes without consideration as to whether this is providing analgesia or addressing the root of the problem. Your patients will be far better served by a deliberate, rational response to these circumstances than by a "get the hammer out and stop this" mentality.

So how can we distinguish whether crying and vocalizing are expressions of pain? I consider the following guidelines:

- Anesthetic-induced dysphoria usually resolves within a few minutes after recovery (admittedly, this may feel like a few hours). Give these patients a little time before you run for the drugs.
- If the degree of patient vocalization is the same as before the procedure, it is seldom necessary to treat with additional analgesics. Anxiolytics may be appropriate.
- If the vocalization abates when the nurse gently speaks to or picks up the animal, this may be attention-getting behavior or a painful dog that was temporarily distracted. Further evaluation is warranted.
- If the vocalization abates after basic nursing needs are addressed such as voiding, clean bedding and warmth, then no additional treatment is considered.

In some instances, it is still impossible to discern whether your patient is vocalizing due to persistent pain, dysphoria, or anxiety. In these instances, consider an opioid trial; if the behavior resolves, one may conclude a response to the narcotic or time. If the behavior persists, consider a sedative, anxiolytic, narcotic antagonist, or benign neglect.

In cases where the cause of pain is iatrogenic, it is extremely helpful to assess the demeanor and vitals of your patient before the procedure. Is the patient anxious and vocal in its cage, or fearful and hiding? What is the heart rate and respiratory pattern? Ideally, the veterinary technician utilizes all the evidence available when assessing a patient for pain. This requires a keen knowledge of the patient and of causes of changes in physiological parameters. A continuous electrocardiogram (ECG) monitor is an underutilized, noninvasive means of assessing heart rate without disturbing the patient. In many small patients or those that sustained thoracic trauma or surgery, frequent manipulations to auscult heart rates may be detrimental. No single symptom is clearly diagnostic of pain in all patients, and each patient's treatment regimen should be individualized.

For example, a patient whose heart rate coming out of an invasive procedure is greater than baseline may initially be

Table 13.3 Clinical signs of pain

Physiological	Behavioral
Increase in heart rate from baseline (exclude anemia and hypotension)	Abnormal posture—hunched stance, unable to get comfortable or lie down, unwilling to stand/walk, pacing
Panting/tachypnea	Abnormal gait—stiff
Mydriasis	Abnormal movements—shaking, thrashing
Hypertension	Vocalizations (exclude dysphoria, anxiety)
	Aggressive
	Hiding

Source: Modified from Mathews K. Pain assessment and general approach to pain management. In management of pain. *Veterinary Clinics of North America* 2000;30(4):732–733.

attributed to pain once hypotension has been excluded by measuring blood pressure. If the procedure induced extensive bleeding and anemia has developed, the tachycardia may be due to acute anemia, and further administration of opioids may actually be detrimental. If your feline patient was hiding under a towel before the procedure, then post-op hiding may not be an indicator of pain. Alternatively, if the cat was vocal and seeking attention pre-op then hides and stares at the back of the cage, this change in behavior should be considered as a possible manifestation of pain (Table 13.3).

In essence, recognition of multiple clinical signs of pain should elicit therapeutic trials to attempt to improve/resolve said clinical signs. A tentative diagnosis of pain can only be accrued via a high level of suspicion, action, and serial monitoring of clinical signs by the veterinary technician.

Pain scoring systems

In an attempt to standardize documentation of pain and responses to therapy, varied pain scales have been reported in human and veterinary medicine.[10] The most commonly used types are visual analogue scales (VASs), which utilize both the observer's subjective assessments of patient behaviors combined with physiological parameters. The rationale for these systems is similar to those more commonly in use such as anesthetic monitoring forms; they provide a documented numerical scale by which patient level of pain and success or failure of any interventions can be monitored (Figures 13.3–13.5, Box 13.1).

In the clinical setting, these systems have not been fully embraced, possibly because these are better suited for managing acute pain and because the diverse causes and responses of patients make a standardized approach difficult to fit for all patients.

Analgesics

The number of analgesics available for use in animals is greater than ever before, providing the veterinary health-care team with a wide array of choices. As with anesthetics, this can seem overwhelming at first glance. It is useful to develop experience with at least one drug in each category listed below, and, ideally, more than one opioid to manage mild to severe signs of pain.

Opioids

Narcotic medications are the most potent and effective analgesics and are used with increasing frequency in managing pain. In most cases, these are utilized to manage acute pain inhospital until the patient can be sent home on oral analgesics. The most common side effects of opioids include sedation/dysphoria/excitement, panting/tachypnea, bradycardia, nausea, constipation/ileus, and urine retention. It has been my experience that dogs weighing greater than 80–100 lb are frequently overdosed and sedated with doses based on body weight. I usually treat giant dogs as 80–100 lb dogs and increase doses if necessary.

Opioid myths

Myth #1—*All narcotics cause CNS side effects in cats.*

The most common side effect of overnarcotization in cats is severe mydriasis and dysphoria. Buprenorphine and butorphanol very rarely cause these signs, while morphine and fentanyl will induce these clinical signs periodically.

Myth #2—*Narcotic administration cannot be given until hemodynamic stability has been achieved.*

Although slowing of the heart rate from opioids could confound interpretation of patient heart rate, profound bradycardia from routine doses of opioids is rare. Patients who have sustained head and vehicular trauma are in pain and require rapid relief.

Myth #3—*Interpreting patient recovery after receiving narcotics will be more difficult.*

With intermittent bolus administration, sedation can occur and may take hours to resolve. With continuous-rate-infusion administration of fentanyl, any sedation would be resolved 20 min after the CRI is discontinued.

Myth #4—*Morphine and hydromorphone cannot be used in cats.*

Morphine and hydromorphone have been reported to cause hyperthermia and may cause vomiting and ptyalism.[11,12] Although these drugs are used to manage pain in cats, I avoid these on the premise that alternate options are available devoid of these potentially serious side effects.

Myth #5—*The last narcotic administration before closing time will last until morning.*

There is no rational explanation for assuming that an injection of narcotic at discharge will provide adequate pain relief for

The CSU acute pain scale is intended primarily as a teaching tool and to guide observations of clinical patients. The scale has not been validated and should not be used as a definitive pain score. Use of the scale employs both an observational period and a hands-on evaluation of the patient. In general, the assessment begins with quiet observation of the patient in its cage at a relatively unobtrusive distance. Afterward, the patient as a whole (wound as well as the entire body) is approached to assess reaction to gentle palpation, indicators of muscle tension and heat, response to interaction, and so on.

1. The scale utilizes a generic 0–4 scale with quarter marks as its base along with a color scale as a visual cue for progression along the five-point scale.

2. Realistic artist's renderings of animals at various levels of pain add further visual cues. Additional drawings provide space for recording pain, warmth, and muscle tension; this allows documentation of specific areas of concern in the medical record. A further advantage of these drawings is that the observer is encouraged to assess the overall pain of the patient in addition to focusing on the primary lesion.

3. The scale includes psychological and behavioral signs of pain as well as palpation responses. Further, the scale uses body tension as an evaluation tool, a parameter not addressed in other scales.

4. There is a provision for nonassessment in the resting patient. To the authors' knowledge, this is the only scale that emphasizes the importance of delaying assessment in a sleeping patient while prompting the observer to recognize patients that may be inappropriately obtunded by medication or by a more serious health concern.

5. Advantages of this scale include ease of use with minimal interpretation required. Specific descriptors for individual behaviors are provided, which decreases interobserver variability. Additionally, a scale is provided for both the dog and the cat.

6. A disadvantage of this scale is a lack of validation by clinical studies comparing it to other scales. Further, its use is largely limited to and is intended for use in acute pain.

Source: Hellyer PW, Uhrig SR, Robinson NG, Colorado State University, Veterinary Medical Center; 2006, with permission.

the 14-h interval between 6 p.m. and the following morning. If your patient's discomfort is likely to persist after 6 p.m., overnight analgesic care should be advocated.

Opioid medications

1. *Butorphanol.* This drug is a partial agonist-antagonist. Butorphanol is used commonly but is falling out of favor as an analgesic due to its short duration of effect and its lack of efficacy in managing moderate–severe pain. Sedation is common at doses greater than 4 mg per patient. Its main utility is in combination with anxiolytics such as dexmedetomidine, or acepromazine as a sedative, or to minimize anxiety in patients with severe dyspnea. It is also used as an antitussive for at-home use.

2. *Buprenorphine.* This drug is one of the most widely used analgesics due to its minimal side-effect profile, prolonged duration of effect (6–8 h) relative to other opioids, and its effectiveness in both dogs and cats. Systemic uptake after oral dosing (transmucosal) in cats is almost 100%, allowing for at-home use; sedation is the most common side effect in this setting.[13] Recent literature has confirmed systemic absorption of the drug transmucosally in dogs as well.[14] A dose of 0.12 mg/kg in dogs given transmucosally induced a longer and more consistent duration of analgesia than did 0.02 mg/kg given IV or orally.[15] This drug is most useful in managing mild–moderate pain in dogs and mild–severe pain in cats. Peak effect occurs approximately 60 min after IV administration and 15 min after transmucosal adminis-

tration.[15] Duration of effect at doses (see Table 13.5) is estimated at 6–8 h in dogs and cats. The duration of effect at doses of 0.02–0.12 mg/kg in dogs has been reported to be 16–20 h.[15]

3. *Fentanyl.* This narcotic is a very potent mu-agonist, with a very short duration of effect (15–20 min). Parenteral use of this drug is commonly utilized at veterinary teaching hospitals and referral practices, and is slowly gaining acceptance in general practice. Due to its short half-life, CRI administration is necessary. Fentanyl is used to manage moderate–severe pain in dogs and cats. Dysphoria is uncommon in cats. Fentanyl is the most popular drug for CRI administration in veterinary medicine.

Once staff have developed familiarity with CRIs, it has been my experience that management of severe pain is more effective as steady blood concentrations of narcotic is provided, which can be titrated based on patient needs and monitoring, as opposed to intermittent dosing, in which patient comfort is often reported to wane hours after drug administration. At our facility, the drug is provided via a separate syringe pump from the IV fluids. Fluid volumes are negligible. Internet Web sites (http://www.vasg.org) are readily available that provide spreadsheets for rapid and easy calculations (Table 13.4).

4. *Hydromorphone.* This is a potent analgesic, used commonly in clinical practice. Tachypnea/panting and vomiting are common side effects in dogs. Ultrasonographers prefer alternate opioids as tachypnea can compromise the diagnostic

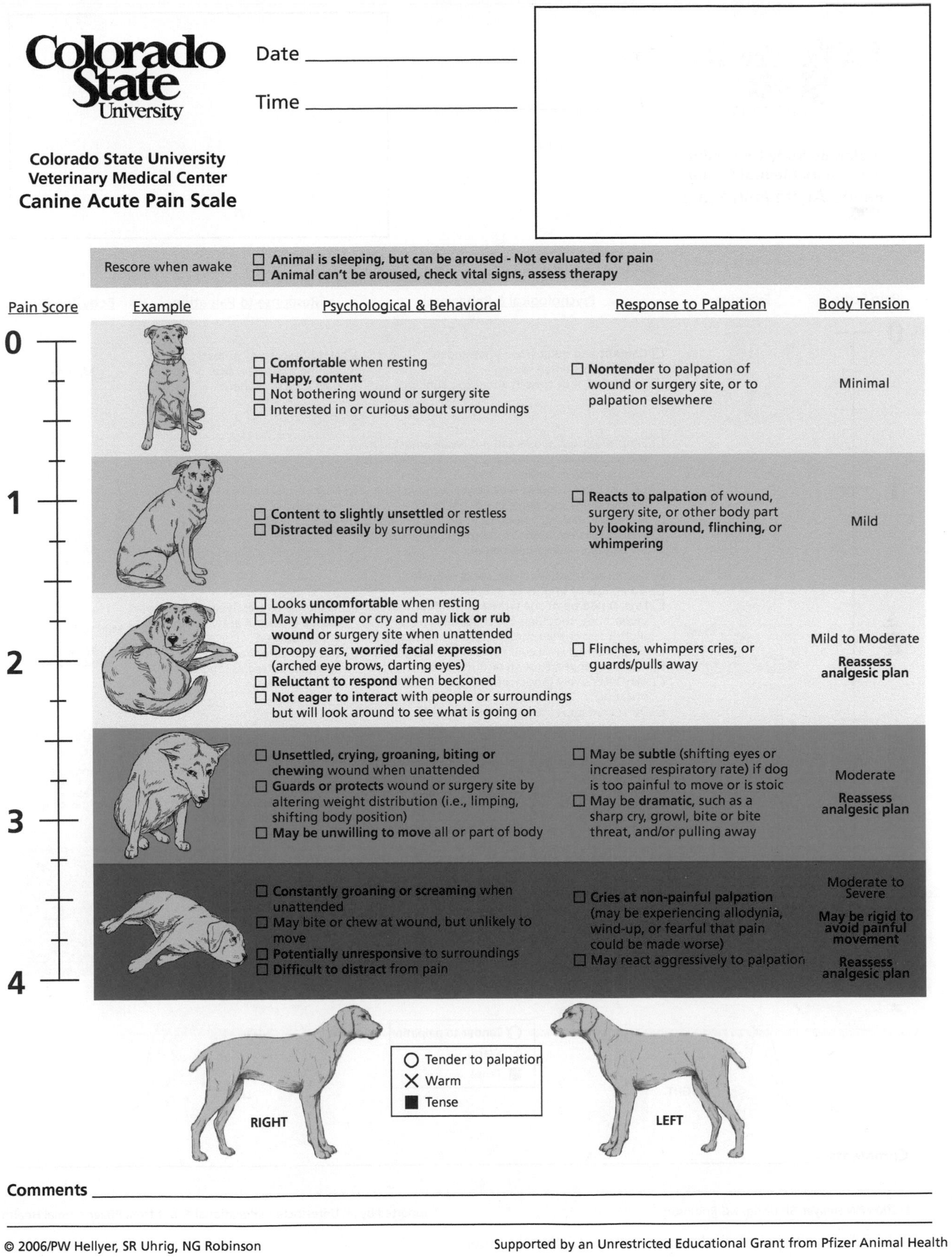

Figure 13.3   Canine acute pain scale. Image courtesy of Colorado State.

Colorado State University

Date _____

Time _____

**Colorado State University
Veterinary Medical Center
Canine Acute Pain Scale**

Rescore when awake	☐ Animal is sleeping, but can be aroused - Not evaluated for pain ☐ Animal can't be aroused, check vital signs, assess therapy

Pain Score	Example	Psychological & Behavioral	Response to Palpation	Body Tension
0		☐ **Comfortable** when resting ☐ **Happy, content** ☐ Not bothering wound or surgery site ☐ Interested in or curious about surroundings	☐ **Nontender** to palpation of wound or surgery site, or to palpation elsewhere	Minimal
1		☐ **Content to slightly unsettled** or restless ☐ **Distracted easily** by surroundings	☐ **Reacts to palpation** of wound, surgery site, or other body part by **looking around, flinching,** or **whimpering**	Mild
2		☐ Looks **uncomfortable** when resting ☐ May **whimper** or cry and may **lick or rub wound** or surgery site when unattended ☐ Droopy ears, **worried facial expression** (arched eye brows, darting eyes) ☐ **Reluctant to respond** when beckoned ☐ **Not eager to interact** with people or surroundings but will look around to see what is going on	☐ Flinches, whimpers cries, or guards/pulls away	Mild to Moderate **Reassess analgesic plan**
3		☐ **Unsettled, crying, groaning, biting or chewing** wound when unattended ☐ **Guards or protects** wound or surgery site by altering weight distribution (i.e., limping, shifting body position) ☐ **May be unwilling to move** all or part of body	☐ May be **subtle** (shifting eyes or increased respiratory rate) if dog is too painful to move or is stoic ☐ May be **dramatic**, such as a sharp cry, growl, bite or bite threat, and/or pulling away	Moderate **Reassess analgesic plan**
4		☐ **Constantly groaning or screaming** when unattended ☐ May bite or chew at wound, but unlikely to move ☐ **Potentially unresponsive** to surroundings ☐ **Difficult to distract** from pain	☐ **Cries at non-painful palpation** (may be experiencing allodynia, wind-up, or fearful that pain could be made worse) ☐ May react aggressively to palpation	Moderate to Severe **May be rigid to avoid painful movement** **Reassess analgesic plan**

RIGHT   LEFT

○ Tender to palpation
X Warm
■ Tense

Comments _____

© 2006/PW Hellyer, SR Uhrig, NG Robinson   Supported by an Unrestricted Educational Grant from Pfizer Animal Health

441

Colorado State University

Date _____

Time _____

Colorado State University Veterinary Medical Center
Feline Acute Pain Scale

Rescore when awake	☐ Animal is sleeping, but can be aroused - Not evaluated for pain ☐ Animal can't be aroused, check vital signs, assess therapy

Pain Score	Example	Psychological & Behavioral	Response to Palpation	Body Tension
0	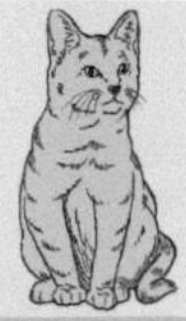	☐ **Content and quiet** when unattended ☐ **Comfortable** when resting ☐ Interested in or **curious** about surroundings	☐ **Not bothered** by palpation of wound or surgery site, or to palpation elsewhere	Minimal
1	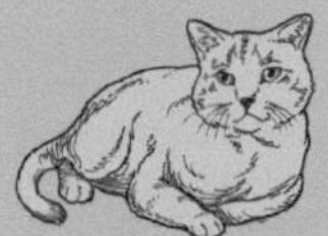	☐ **Signs are often subtle and not easily detected in the hospital setting;** more likely to be detected by the owner(s) at home ☐ Earliest signs at home may be <u>withdrawal from surroundings or change in normal routine</u> ☐ In the hospital, may be content or slightly unsettled ☐ **Less interested** in surroundings but will look around to see what is going on	☐ May or may not react to palpation of wound or surgery site	Mild
2	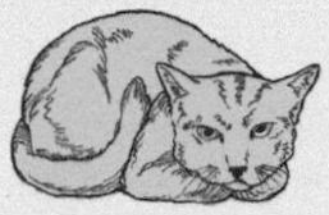	☐ Decreased responsiveness, **seeks solitude** ☐ **Quiet**, loss of brightness in eyes ☐ **Lays curled up or sits tucked up** (all four feet under body, shoulders hunched, head held slightly lower than shoulders, tail curled tightly around body) with eyes partially or mostly closed ☐ **Hair coat appears rough** or fluffed up ☐ May intensively groom an area that is painful or irritating ☐ Decreased appetite, **not interested in food**	☐ **Responds aggressively or tries to escape** if painful area is palpated or approached ☐ Tolerates attention, may even perk up when petted as long as painful area is avoided	Mild to Moderate **Reassess analgesic plan**
3	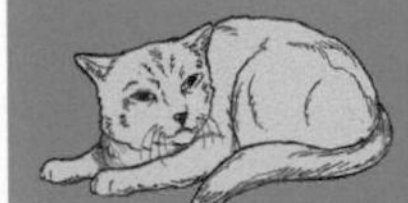	☐ Constantly **yowling, growling, or hissing** when unattended ☐ May bite or chew at wound, but **unlikely to move** if left alone	☐ **Growls or hisses at non-painful palpation** (may be experiencing allodynia, wind-up, or fearful that pain could be made worse) ☐ **Reacts aggressively** to palpation, **adamantly pulls away** to avoid any contact	Moderate **Reassess analgesic plan**
4	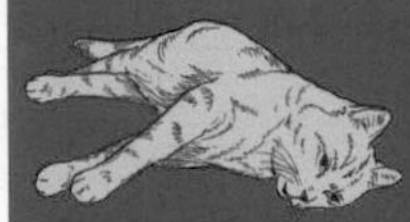	☐ Prostrate ☐ Potentially **unresponsive** to or unaware of surroundings, difficult to distract from pain ☐ Receptive to care (even mean or wild cats will be more tolerant of contact)	☐ **May not respond** to palpation ☐ **May be rigid** to avoid painful movement	Moderate to Severe May be rigid to avoid painful movement **Reassess analgesic plan**

RIGHT   ○ Tender to palpation   ✕ Warm   ■ Tense   **LEFT**

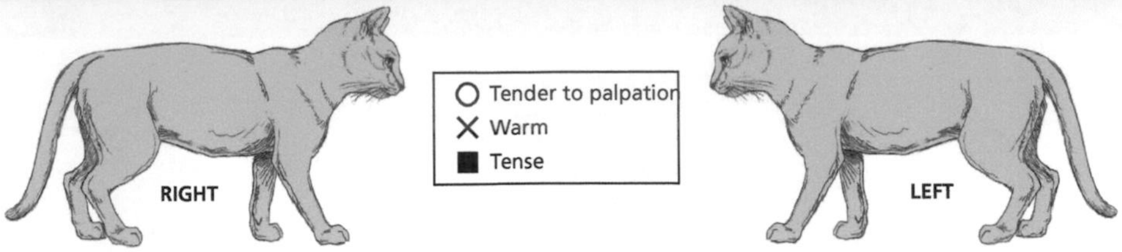

Comments _____

© 2006/PW Hellyer, SR Uhrig, NG Robinson   Supported by an Unrestricted Educational Grant from Pfizer Animal Health

Figure 13.4   Feline acute pain scale. Image courtesy of Colorado State.

SHORT FORM OF THE GLASGOW COMPOSITE PAIN SCALE

Dog's name _____

Hospital Number _____ **Date** / / **Time**

Surgery Yes/No (delete as appropriate)

Procedure or Condition _____

_____

In the sections below please circle the appropriate score in each list and sum these to give the total score.

A. Look at dog in Kennel

Is the dog?

(i)

Quiet	0
Crying or whimpering	1
Groaning	2
Screaming	3

(ii)

Ignoring any wound or painful area	0
Looking at wound or painful area	1
Licking wound or painful area	2
Rubbing wound or painful area	3
Chewing wound or painful area	4

In the case of spinal, pelvic or multiple limb fractures, or where assistance is required to aid locomotion do not carry out section **B** and proceed to **C** *Please tick if this is the case*☐ then proceed to C.

B. Put lead on dog and lead out of the kennel.

When the dog rises/walks is it?

(iii)

Normal	0
Lame	1
Slow or reluctant	2
Stiff	3
It refuses to move	4

C. If it has a wound or painful area including abdomen, apply gentle pressure 2 inches round the site.

Does it?

(iv)

Do nothing	0
Look round	1
Flinch	2
Growl or guard area	3
Snap	4
Cry	5

D. Overall

Is the dog?

(v)

Happy and content or happy and bouncy	0
Quiet	1
Indifferent or non-responsive to surroundings	2
Nervous or anxious or fearful	3
Depressed or non-responsive to stimulation	4

Is the dog?

(vi)

Comfortable	0
Unsettled	1
Restless	2
Hunched or tense	3
Rigid	4

Total Score (i+ii+iii+iv+v+vi) = _____

Figure 13.5 Short form of the Glasgow composite pain scale. Image courtesy of the University of Glasgow.

Note: The short-form Composite Measure Pain Score (CMPS-SF) can be applied quickly and reliably in a clinical setting and has been designed as a clinical decision-making tool, which was developed for dogs in acute pain. It includes 30 descriptor options within six behavioral categories, including mobility. Within each category, the descriptors are ranked numerically according to their associated pain severity, and the person carrying out the assessment chooses the descriptor within each category that best fits the dog's behavior/condition. It is important to carry out the assessment procedure as described on the questionnaire, following the protocol closely. The pain score is the sum of the rank scores. The maximum score for the six categories is 24, or 20 if mobility is impossible to assess. The total CMPS-SF score has been shown to be a useful indicator of analgesic requirement, and the recommended analgesic intervention level is 6/24 or 5/20.

value of studies. Hyperthermia in cats has already been noted above.

5. *Morphine.* This is an inexpensive, effective, and commonly used drug. Its systemic use has declined in recent years with the advent of alternate drugs. Morphine is used frequently via the epidural route.

6. *Morphine–Lidocaine–Ketamine (MLK) CRI.* A few years ago, a report documenting the use of an MLK cocktail garnered interest.[16] Adding 12 mg morphine, 150 mg lidocaine, and 30 mg ketamine in 500 mL fluids dripped at 10 mL/kg/h provides morphine at 4 µg/kg/min, lidocaine at 50 µg/kg/min, and ketamine at 10 µg/kg/min. Although benefits similar to those from narcotic CRIs are noted, at our hospital, this protocol has been replaced by fentanyl based on ease of use and simplicity (Table 13.5).

Alpha-2 agonists

This group of sedative-analgesics is most frequently used in clinical practice as a readily reversible sedative for procedures in young dogs and cats as a preanesthetic. At the time of this writing, available drugs include xylazine and dexmedetomidine. These are utilized as adjunct analgesics, usually in conjunction with opioids, and are presently approved for use in dogs only. These drugs are seldom used as a sole analgesic. Dexmedetomidine is most commonly used as a perioperative CRI in dogs deemed to benefit from mild to moderate sedation. The combination of opioid and dexmedetomidine CRI can be especially useful in exuberant and anxious dogs recovering from orthopedic and upper airway surgery. An IV bolus followed by a CRI is particularly effective. As side effects can include hypotension and bradycardia, the drug is contraindicated in patients who are not hemodynamically stable or in geriatric patients that may be more prone to hypotension. Blood pressure monitoring is advised. Reports discuss epidural administration, though this usage is not yet common in clinical practice[17] (Table 13.6).

NSAIDs

All non-steroidal anti-inflammatories are cyclooxygenase (COX) enzyme inhibitors, resulting in reduced synthesis of prostaglandins and their subsequent inflammatory mediators. Although much marketing literature has been devoted to selective advantages dependent on which COX enzyme is inhibited, clinical studies have not revealed any differences in efficacy or safety.[18] This group of drugs has been used to manage chronic pain for decades, and parenteral formulations of carprofen and meloxi-

Table 13.4　Advantages of CRIs for analgesia

Allows for rapid titration of drug dosages to achieve adequate analgesia or sedation

Less costly to client due to reduced number of injections

Reduces patient stress due to fewer injections

Allows for rapid discontinuation if dysphoria or excess sedation occurs

Improved pain control for patient due to steady blood levels of analgesic

Table 13.5　Opioid dosages

Drug	Indication	Dose	Route	Duration
Buprenorphine	Dog—mild to moderate pain	0.005–0.02 mg/kg or 0.02–0.12 mg/kg	IV, IM TM	6–8 h or 16–20 h
	Cat—all types pain	0.005–0.02 mg/kg	IV, IM, or TM	6–8 h or 16–20 h
Butorphanol	Dog and cat—mild pain	0.1–0.2 mg/kg	IV, IM or SC	2–4 h
	Sedative	0.2–0.25 mg/kg	As above	2–6 h
Fentanyl	Dog—moderate to severe pain	2 mcg/kg loading dose, then 2–5 mcg/kg/h as CRI	IV	Dose and CRI dependent
	Cat—moderate to severe pain	2–5 mcg/kg loading dose, then 2–5 mcg/kg/h as CRI	As above	Dose and CRI dependent
Hydromorphone	Dog—moderate to severe pain	0.05–0.2 mg/kg	IV, IM	3–6 h
	Cat—moderate to severe pain	0.02–0.05 mg/kg	As above	3–6 h
Morphine	Dog—moderate to severe pain	0.2–1.0 mg/kg	IV, IM, or SC	3–4 h
	Cat—moderate to severe pain	0.1–0.2 mg/kg	As above	3–4 h
Oxymorphone	Dogs-moderate to severe pain	0.05-0.2 mg/kg	IV, IM, or SC	4 h
	Cats-moderate to severe pain	0.05-0.1 mg/kg	IV, IM, or SC	4 h

Table 13.6   Alpha-2 agonist dosages

Drug	Indication	Dose	Route	Duration
Dexmedetomidine	Canine—sedative-analgesic	1–3 µg/kg loading dose, then 1–3 µg/kg/h as CRI	IV	Dose and CRI dependent

Table 13.7   NSAID dosages

Drug	Indication	Dose	Route	Duration (h)
Carprofen		4 mg/kg × 1 dose, then 2.2 mg/kg	SC, PO	12
Deracoxib		3–4 mg/kg	PO	24
Etodolac		10–15 mg/kg	PO	24
Meloxicam	Dog	0.2 mg/kg × 1 dose, then 0.1 mg/kg	IV, SC, PO	24
	Cat[a]	0.03 mg/kg as a single dose		[b]
Tepoxalin		20 mg/kg × 1 dose, then 10 mg/kg	PO	24
Firocoxib		5 mg/kg	PO	24
Piroxicam		0.3 mg/kg	PO	24

Note: All doses for dog only except meloxicam.
[a] Use of oral meloxicam in cats is not approved as no safe dose has been confirmed. The use of additional meloxicam or other NSAIDs is contraindicated. Do not use in cats with renal dysfunction.
[b] Repeated use in cats has been associated with acute renal failure and death.

cam in the last decade have prompted their utility in acute pain settings as well.

Side effects include GI signs from gastroduodenal ulcers and, rarely, GI perforation caused by local irritation and prostaglandin inhibition.[19] Renal ischemia and decline in renal function have seldom been documented in the literature, but clinical experience has been that patients with preexisting renal disease and/or hemodynamic compromise or decline under anesthesia are at higher risk for decline in renal function. Hepatotoxicity is a rare idiosyncratic side effect in dogs. Approved NSAIDs in dogs include carprofen, etodolac, meloxicam, deracoxib, firocoxib, and tepoxalin.

Because of their well-documented sensitivity due to prolonged half-lives of aspirin and acetaminophen, cats were typically excluded from consideration for treatment with NSAIDs until meloxicam was approved in this species a few years ago. Recent warnings from the manufacturer advise this to be used in cats as a single dose only, and not to use this in cats with any preexisting renal compromise or in patients that may develop hypotension.

NSAIDs have a lower margin of safety than opioids in the acute setting due to their potential for serious side effects. Relative contraindications for NSAID use include patients with preexisting renal disease, geriatric patients, and those in which hemodynamic instability or marked dehydration is anticipated. It may be prudent to wait 12–24 h after trauma before using this group of drugs as analgesics (Table 13.7).

Local anesthetics and epidural anesthetics

The safest and most underutilized class of drugs are those that are administered locally at the site of pain rather than systemically. They can be considered the "poor man's opioids." Although narcotics garner the most attention, local anesthetics should always be considered in a multimodality analgesic plan. These have a large safety profile, with systemic side effects of seizures and tremors seldom seen. The most commonly used local anesthetics include lidocaine and bupivacaine. Lidocaine has an onset of 1–10 min and a duration of 60–90 min. Bupivicaine has a more delayed onset (20 min) and longer duration of action (4–8 h). These can be used via the following techniques:

1. *Topical Application.* Lidocaine is available as a spray and as a gel. It can be used for catheter placement in the skin and nose and to aid in endotracheal intubation in cats. Cats are more sensitive to systemic side effects.

2. *Local Infiltration.* Used for soft tissue surgery, lacerations, biopsies, bone marrow aspiration, laparoscopy, and rib fractures. Varied forms of wound catheters can be utilized; these are surgically adhered in the region of the surgery site, and the drug is infused into the wound via the catheter.

3. *Epidural.* Administration of local anesthetics and/or opioids at the L7-S1 space are used to benefit patients undergoing painful procedures including perianal, tail, pelvic, and hind limb surgery. Urine retention is the most common side effect.

Table 13.8   Local anesthetics

Drug	Indication	Dose	Forms	Duration
Lidocaine 2%		4–5 mg/kg	Topical and injectable	60–90 min
Bupivacaine		1–2 mg/kg	Injectable	4–8 h
Intracavitary bupivacaine	Cats and small dogs	0.2 mL/kg of 0.5% bupivacaine + 0.01 meq/kg NaHCO$_3$[a]—dilute with saline to 3 mL		
	Large dogs	Same-dilute to total volume of 6–12 mL		

[a] Often diluted with NaHCO$_3$ to reduce patient discomfort.

4. *Intracavitary.* Instillation of bupivacaine with saline can provide local pain relief in patients with peritonitis, pancreatitis, in patients with chest tubes, and in those recovering from thoracotomy.

5. *Local Nerve Blocks.* Patients with rib fractures and those undergoing dental/orofacial and limb procedures all benefit from regional anesthesia (Table 13.8).

Tramadol

Tramadol is a synthetic codeine analogue with mild mu-agonist properties.[20] Its use has increased in the past few years as a result of not being a controlled substance, its wide safety profile, and limited options for at-home analgesic choices. The most common side effects are sedation and, rarely, dysphoria in cats. Doses are 3–10 mg/kg BID-TID in dogs and 1–5 mg/kg SID-BID in cats. It is likely a weak analgesic by itself and is best used for at-home management of acute or chronic pain in conjunction with other drugs.

Lidocaine and fentanyl patches

Lidocaine dermal patches are used in humans with neuropathic pain; limited use has been reported in veterinary medicine. These should be considered as adjunctive pain management in patients with cutaneous pain (burn and thermal injuries).

Fentanyl transdermal patches are available in varying strengths (25, 50, 75, 100 mcg) and have been used extensively in small animal patients. Side effects are minimal. These have fallen out of favor in the past few years due to their 12- to 24-h onset of action (must be placed the night before procedure) and reports of marked variability in blood levels between patients. If using these, it is better not to assume your patient is "covered" because the patch has been applied. These should be used as an adjunct with more conventional methods of analgesia as mentioned above.

Gabapentin

This is an anticonvulsant medication used in humans with chronic neuropathic pain. Its analgesic use has increased in recent years, likely due to the limited number of effective options available for management of chronic pain conditions. Reasonable indications include management of phantom limb pain, pelvic trauma, and intervertebral disk disease. The drug is available as 100, 300, 400, 600, and 800 mg strengths. The tablet is bitter tasting, which can make home compliance problematic if owners are unable to administer easily by hiding it in food or pill pockets. Starting doses in dogs are 10 mg/kg TID and the dose range is 5–25 mg/kg BID-TID. Doses in cats are 5 mg/kg BID. Sedation is a common side effect. This drug is usually used in conjunction with an NSAID and/or tramadol. Acute discontinuation is discouraged to avoid rebound pain. A recent study found no benefits in the acute setting when used in addition to standard protocols in dogs undergoing amputation.[21]

Amantadine

This is an oral N-methyl-D-aspartate (NMDA) antagonist, with actions similar to ketamine. It is available as 100 mg capsules or tablets and as 10 mg/mL syrup. Indications include refractory degenerative joint disease (DJD) and chronic cancer pain. Studies of efficacy are few. The starting dose is 3 mg/kg SID in dogs.

Pamidronate

This is a bisphosphonate drug that inhibits bone resorption and osteoclast activity. Clinical indications include management of bone cancer (osteosarcoma [OSA], multiple myeloma, bony metastases) and hypercalcemia of malignancy.

Nursing care as analgesic

Some of the safest and most cost-effective methods of providing relief from pain, stress, and discomfort in animal patients are empathic and thoughtful nursing care. Examples include but are not limited to the following.

Ensuring ability to void

It is not uncommon for large dogs to receive 500 mL to 2 L of fluids in the perioperative period. By the time these dogs are able to stand, they may manifest signs of anxiety or vocalizing. If these clinical signs are misperceived as pain and opioids are administered, this will only worsen the patient's problem by predisposing to urine retention. All dogs at our hospital receive a preanesthetic walk. Consider urinary catheterization and drainage (intermittent or indwelling) coming out of the operating room if your patient is expected to be nonambulatory all evening (pelvic fracture repair). Try walking the patient as a trial before providing additional analgesics if this seems reasonable. Give cats litter pans as soon as recovery justifies.

Consolidate cage visits

It is not uncommon for a critical patient to receive orders for multiple injections and serial monitoring of temperatures, Sp02, blood pressures, and so on. The inexperienced nurse may comply with treatment orders as written, entailing hourly visits to disturb the patient. The astute nurse will recognize that the patient is apt to receive little rest unless the doctor's orders are consolidated to minimize patient disturbance. This concept receives little attention but can go a long way in relieving patient stress.

Minimize needlesticks and probes

If it is anticipated your patient is to require multiple sets of labs, consider placing a central venous catheter in the saphenous or jugular vein under anesthesia to facilitate samplings and to minimize frequent venipunctures. Consider continuous temperature rectal probes to avoid serial thermometer insertions.

External stabilization

Apply bandages/splints expeditiously in patients with distal limb fractures. These measures can be as important as any systemic analgesic as anyone wearing a brace for tendonitis can attest to.

Soft and clean bedding

If your canine patient is intentionally sedated as a part of his/her analgesic protocol, involuntary urinations should be anticipated and checked for frequently.

Peace and quiet

It never ceases to amaze me how noisy our treatment rooms are. (I usually note this when not on duty.) Between electrocardiogram (ECG) monitors, beeping infusion pumps, dogs crying, phones ringing, and loud veterinary staff, many of our patients are probably wondering when they can get home. Patients on opioids are typically noise sensitive and may be startled easily. Although I used to be able to fall asleep on the subways in New York en route to my internship, now that I am older and wiser, peace and quiet suits me better. I suspect our patients feel the same.

Hot/cold packs

Reducing swelling and inflammation can be a useful adjunct in preventing swelling induced by trauma and surgery. We use a GameReady™ unit for this purpose.

Send some patients home

We have all seen the Labrador recovering from an anterior cruciate ligament (ACL) repair or a laryngeal tieback, who requires sedation every 2–3 h due to incessant barking and panting. There are some patients who will never rest in a hospital; once stable, these patients are simply better off at home. Do not allow any preconceived duration of stay or concern of personal credibility to get in the way of being a patient advocate. Typically, after discharge, these clients will tell me on the phone, "You know doctor, he slept for about 24 h after coming home. Is that normal?" While my ears may still be ringing from that particular dog's barking, I assure her that the rest will do him (and me) well.

Clinical examples

Bone marrow aspiration

This is considered to be a procedure inducing an acute, moderate degree of pain lasting a short duration. Many of these patients are systemically ill and debilitated and thus are at moderate-high risk for NSAID-related side effects.

Protocol:

– Buprenorphine IV 30–60 min prior to the procedure
– Local periosteal infiltration with lidocaine
– Cold packs at site if tolerated
– Tramadol as needed at home

Laparoscopy

This is a procedure deemed to induce a mild degree of transient, local discomfort at the trocar site/s and possibly from the induced abdominal insufflation. Patients may be young and healthy (laparoscopic ovariohysterectomy) or older and debilitated (ascites with carcinomatosis, feline infectious peritonitis [FIP]).

Protocol:

– Buprenorphine IV 30–60 min before anesthetic induction
– Local bupivacaine at trocar sites at the end of the procedure
– NSAID, buprenorphine, or tramadol for at-home use

Pancreatitis

Local peritonitis in dogs and cats with this disease can cause severe and profound pain, often refractory to routine analgesic protocols. Some of these patients are debilitated and in poor condition, suffering from systemic signs as well as local peritonitis, with resultant gastric distension/atony and recumbency. These patients can be some of the most challenging to manage as their pain can be severe and persistent.

Protocol:

– Fentanyl bolus and CRI IV at 3–5 µg/kg/h
– Alpha-2 agonists prn

- Orogastric suction prn to relieve significant gastric distension
- Instill bupivicaine into the abdomen if significant ascites present q 4–6 h (see Table 13.8 for protocol)
- Indwelling urine collection system to monitor urine output and to relieve bladder distension

Head and/or thoracic trauma

Small dogs and cats that sustain head trauma can be diagnosed with any/all of the following problems: reduced/dull mentation, oral/dental fractures, and ocular trauma/proptosed globes. In addition, rib fractures and pulmonary contusions may be confirmed as well. These patients are in severe and ongoing pain and are often denied proper analgesic therapy out of concern of causing or worsening patient obtundation or inability to ambulate. Veterinary personnel with experience with opioids are aware that these side effects are very rare at proper dosages.

Protocol:

- Stabilize hemodynamics via serial blood pressure monitoring and IV fluids.
- Fentanyl bolus 3 μg/kg IV, then 3-μg/kg/h CRI prior to radiographs
- External stabilization of any fractured limbs
- Local bupivicaine at the site of rib and oral/orbit fractures q 4–6 h
- No NSAIDs for 12–24 h minimum
- Ocular topical anesthetic (proparacaine) prn for ocular trauma

Conclusion

Managing pain in our patients is one of the most fundamental callings of our profession. The veterinary technician should be the designated leader of the hospital pain management team. The technician who can participate in designing analgesic protocols, anticipate and recognize pain and discomfort, communicate the relative success or failure of the plan to the veterinarian effectively, and is aware of options for modification including pharmacological and anxiety-relieving nursing care is a tremendous asset to his/her patients. You are the pain advocate for your animal patients who cannot speak for themselves.

Bibliography

1. AVMA-Veterinary Oath. Executive Board AVMA; 2010.
2. NAVTA-Veterinary Technician Code of Ethics. NAVTA Ethics Committee; 2007.
3. Lamont LA. Physiology of pain. In management of pain. *Vet Clin N Am* 2000;30(4):704–710.
4. Woolf CJ, Ma Q. Nociceptors-noxious stimuli detectors. *Neuron* 2007;55:353–364.
5. Pascoe P. Local and regional anaesthesia and analgesia. *Semin Vet Med Surg (Small Anim)* 1997;12:94–105.
6. Jessell TM, Kelly DD. Pain and analgesia. In: *Principles of Neural Science*, 3rd edition, eds. ER Kandel, JH Schwartz, TM Jessell, pp. 385–399. New York: Elsevier Science; 1991.
7. Thurmon JC, Tranquilli WJ, Benson GJ (eds.). Perioperative pain and distress. In: *Lumb and Jones Veterinary Anesthesia*, 3rd edition, pp. 40–60. Baltimore, MD: Lea &Febiger; 1996.
8. Wright EM, Jr., Woodson JF. Clinical assessment of pain in laboratory animals. In: *The Experimental Animal in Biologic Research*, eds. BE Rollin, ML Kesel, pp. 205–216. Boca Raton, FL: CRC Press; 1990.
9. Merskey HM. Classification of chronic pain syndromes{abstract}. *Pain Suppl* 1986;3:S217.
10. Shaffran N. Pain management: the veterinary technicians perspective. In update on management of pain. *Vet Clin N Am* 2008;38(6):1415–1427.
11. Clark WG, Cumby HR. Hyperthermic responses to central and peripheral injections of morphine sulphate in the cat. *Br J Pharmacol* 1978;63(1):65–71.
12. Posner LP, Gleed RD, Erb HN, et al. Post-anesthetic hyperthermia in cats. *Vet Anaesth Analg* 2007;34(1):40–47.
13. Robertson SA, Taylor PM, Sear JW. Systemic uptake of buprenorphine by cats after oral mucosal administration. *Vet Rec* 2003;152(22):675–678.
14. Abbo LA, Ko JC, Maxwell LK, et al. Pharmacokinetics of buprenorphine following intravenous and oral transmucosal administration in dogs. *Vet Ther* 2008;9:83–93.
15. Ko JC, Freeman LJ, Barletta M, et al. Efficacy of transmucosal and intravenous administration of buprenorphine before surgery for postoperative analgesia in dogs undergoing ovariohysterectomy. *JAVMA* 2011;238:318–327.
16. Muir WW, Wiese AJ, March PA. Effects of morphine, lidocaine, ketamine and morphine-lidocaine-ketamine combination on minimum alveolar concentration in dogs anesthetized with isoflurane. *Am J Vet Res* 2003;64:1155–1160.
17. Branson KR, Ko JC, Tranquilli WJ, et al. Duration of analgesia induced by epidurally administered morphine and medetomidine in dogs. *J Vet Pharmacol Ther* 1993;16:369–372.
18. Papich MG. An update on nonsteroidal anti-inflammatory drugs in small animals. *Vet Clin N Am* 2008;38(6):1246–1250.
19. Whittle BJ. Mechanisms underlying intestinal injury induced by anti-inflammatory COX inhibitors. *Eur J Pharamcol* 2004;500(1–3):427–443.
20. Gutstein HB, Akil H. Opioid analgesics. In: *Goodman and Gilman's The Pharmacological Basis of Therapeutics*, 10th edition, eds. JG Harman, LE Limbird, A Goodman Gilman, p. 569. New York: McGraw Hill; 2001.
21. Wagner AE, Mich PM, Uhrig SR, Hellyer PW. Clinical evaluation of perioperative administration of gabapentin as an adjunct for postoperative administration analgesia in dogs undergoing amputation of a forelimb. *JAVMA* 2010;236(7):751–756.

Chapter 14 Nursing

Editors: Marnin Forman and Linda Merrill

SECTION 1 OCCUPATIONAL HEALTH AND SAFETY

Making the work place safe

Occupational health and safety in veterinary hospitals is a topic not always routinely considered but one that is of utmost importance. Veterinary facilities and other facilities involved in animal care not only have the physical and chemical hazards, but workers also need to consider zoonotic hazards. It is not only the responsibility of the owners of the practice but also of the staff to ensure exposure to hazards is reduced as much as possible and to abide by governmental regulations. This section is intended to give an overview of common hazards and how to prevent them. Further information should be found through such sources as your local veterinary and veterinary technician associations, government health and safety divisions (e.g., Occupational Safety and Health Administration [OSHA] in the United States), the Centers for Disease Control, workers' health and safety organizations, and the World Health Organization (WHO).

Health and safety committees

Depending on the size of the facility, you may be required by law to form a health and safety committee. In Canada, the *Workers Compensation Act* requires employers to establish a committee in any workplace that regularly employs 20 or more workers[1]; this includes part-time as well as full-time staff. This may vary between countries and even local areas. The best way to find out is through your government's health and safety branch. The main focus of the committee is to identify and resolve health and safety problems in the workplace (Table 14.1.1).

Small Animal Internal Medicine for Veterinary Technicians and Nurses, First Edition. Edited by Linda Merrill.
© 2012 John Wiley & Sons, Inc. Published 2012 by John Wiley & Sons, Inc.

Table 14.1.1   Role of the joint health and safety committee

To promote safe work practices

To assist in creating a safe and healthy workplace

To recommend actions that will improve the effectiveness of the occupational health and safety program

To promote compliance with Workers' Compensation Board regulations

Adapted from the Workers' Compensation Board of BC, Joint Health and Safety Committee workbook, February 2000.

One of the main tasks for the committee is to provide information on hazards in the workplace and to develop and periodically review the written safety protocols.

Hazards in the workplace

Hazards can be split up into three general categories: physical, chemical, and biological. It is important for staff to be aware of how to identify these hazards, how to reduce or prevent exposure, and how to respond in the event of an accident.[2]

Physical hazards

Examples of physical hazards include slips and falls, animal-induced injuries (bites and scratches), needlestick injuries, machinery and equipment, ergonomic hazards, and ionizing radiation. Many of these hazards are preventable. Brightly colored kennel labels are examples of easy and useful tools to bring staff attention to possible hazards as well as reminders for preventative action (e.g., aggressive, chemotherapy patient, sedated patient, infectious patient).

First aid signs are important in identifying where the first aid kit is located. Eye wash station signs and spill kit signs for possible chemical injury to the eye or anesthetic gas or chemotherapy drug spills can all reduce the amount of time a situation takes to get under control and therefore possibly reducing injuries.

Wearing nonslip shoes and installing proper floor mats in wet areas of the hospital can cut down on the number of slips and falls. Posting a "Caution Wet Floor" or "Caution Slippery Floor" sign, whenever you wipe up a spill or when cleaning floors, is another technique to reduce slips and falls in the hospital. Always keep stairways clear of materials and do not use these as storage space, even if only on a temporary basis. General good housekeeping of all travel areas will also decrease obstructions and will thereby decrease accidents.

There are entire books and courses are dedicated to information on safe animal restraint techniques and animal behavior, and an in-depth discussion is beyond the scope of this text. Avoiding bite wounds and animal scratches is the responsibility of everyone on the veterinary health-care team, and open lines of communication between team members is the first step in the process.

One of the more common methods employed to circumvent a needlestick injury is to avoid recapping needles and to use a sharps container. Other methods to handle sharps are one-handed recapping, needleless adaptors, or using self-recapping needles. Client education on these safety techniques is also indicated whenever providing owners with recommendations for therapies requiring needles. Avoid injuries from other sharps by safely opening ampules, by removing scapel blades with the appropriate instrument, and by the safe handling of all sharp instrumentation.

There are many pieces of equipment in the veterinary hospital that pose a health or safety risk. Steam autoclaves are hot to the touch, and when opened, the steam can burn the skin or, if inhaled, the respiratory track. Gas autoclaves contain a toxic gas that cannot be seen and is odorless. Proper ventilation procedures must be strictly followed. Cage dryers and external heat support devices can be hot to the touch. Care should be exercised around pinch points on machinery, such as the ones that can occur on lift table joints. Overhead obstructions such as open cage doors, dental X-ray arms, and X-ray collimators need to be observed and avoided. Electrical equipment can pose a shock hazard and should be plugged into a grounded circuit. Surgical and therapy lasers can pose a threat to our eyesight and eye protection should be worn whenever it is in use. This goes for both the staff and the patients. Hearing protection is an often overlooked area of personal protective equipment. Not only are some of the machines we use a potential source of noise but the animals we work with can also raise quite the commotion.

Ergonomics is essential not only to your longevity as a worker but also in performing activities in your daily life. Veterinary technicians will lift thousands of patients in their career. No matter what size, it is up to you to ensure that correct lifting (bend at the knees, *not* the waist!) as well as restraint techniques are utilized each and every time. Several ergonomic guidelines for specific industries are published by OSHA (http://www.osha.gov/SLTC/ergonomics/guidelines.html).

Work-related musculoskeletal disorders (WMSDs) are a group of painful disorders affecting muscles, tendons, and nerves. Carpal tunnel syndrome, tendonitis, and thoracic outlet syndrome are all examples of WMSDs. Frequent and repetitive activities or awkward posture when performing activities can lead to any of these disorders, which may cause pain either during work or at rest.[3]

Radiation exposure is one of the easier hazards to protect against. Human and lab animal studies have shown that regular exposure to radiation can cause cancer and can mutate healthy genes,[4] therefore exposing not only yourself but any future offspring. Still, a surprising number of veterinary staff continue to lay the lead glove over their hand (exposing themselves to scatter radiation) instead of wearing it. Wearing, as well as properly maintaining, the lead gowns, gloves, and thyroid protectors are extremely important. This involves regularly imaging the protective equipment (every 6–12 months) to look for signs of tears or breakages in the lead. It is also important that the gowns themselves are stored correctly and are not folded to prevent the lead from being damaged. Routine use of personal dosimeters and regular monitoring of exposure through government health services is usually required. Health Canada's National Dosimetry Services keeps lifelong measurements of health workers' exposure to radiation. OSHA guidelines state an exposure level of 1¼ Rems per calendar quarter to a person's whole body, with different dose limits placed on the arms, hands, and skin. Positioning techniques in radiology, including the use of positioning devices such as sandbags and ropes, as well as the use of chemical restraint, all aid in protecting the health of the clinic staff. Much of the general safety information may be found on human radiology organization Web sites and also includes information for staff involved in procedures using MRI, computed tomography (CT), and fluoroscopy.

Chemical hazards

Chemical hazards include, but are not limited to, exposure to anesthetic gases, disinfectants, insecticides, and allergies to latex. In many countries, an employer is required to maintain up-to-date information on products in the form of a *material safety data sheet* (MSDS). These are available online or from the manufacturer.

Anesthetic gases

Occupational exposure to waste anesthetic gases has been linked to reproductive problems in women, and numerous animal studies have shown embryo lethal and teratogenic effects.[5] Regular maintenance of anesthetic machines, hoses, and scavenger system, as well as system leak checks is an easy way to help reduce exposure.

Disinfectants

As with any product, take note of warning labels and MSDS forms and use the product according to the manufacturer's instructions. This includes knowing what personal protective equipment should be worn, what to do if you come into contact with the product, how to clean up any spills, and if the product is flammable, explosive, poisonous, or reactive.

Latex allergies

Latex, as found in nature, is the milky substance that comes from a flowering plant. Natural latex rubber is made from the latex of the rubber tree (*Hevea brasiliensis*) and is in some veterinary products such as latex gloves and catheters. Latex allergies are a sensitivity reaction to certain proteins found in natural rubber. Workers who use latex gloves on a regular basis are at increased risk for developing sensitivities to these proteins. It is unknown how much exposure to these products will result in a latex sensitivity.

Latex allergies were first recognized in the 1970s, and between 1988 and 1996, the Food and Drug Administration (FDA) had over 1000 exposures and 15 deaths reported.[6] For more extensive information on latex allergies, please refer to your own government Web sites regarding health and safety. Sensitivity reactions can range from mild skin reactions (type IV reactions) to anaphylaxis (type I reactions). Skin reactions, also known as allergic

contact dermatitis, present in the form of rash, hives, redness, or itching. Type I reactions present as more severe respiratory symptoms including runny nose, sneezing, coughing, and asthmatic attacks. Respiratory signs may occur when gloves are donned or removed as the powder inside, to which the proteins have become attached, becomes airborne and is inhaled.[7]

The main way to protect against latex sensitivity is to use nonlatex gloves. Nitrile gloves are made of synthetic latex and do not contain the proteins responsible for latex sensitivity. If you must wear latex gloves on a regular basis, try to wear powderless gloves and refrain from using creams or lotions on your hands.[8]

Should you find out you are allergic to latex, it is imperative you let your employer, as well as any health-care providers, know to reduce your chances of exposure.

Biological hazards

Biohazardous material

Biohazards are infectious agents or hazardous biological materials that present a risk or potential risk to the health of humans, animals, or the environment. The risk can be direct, through infection, or indirect, through damage to the environment. Biohazardous materials include certain types of recombinant DNA; organisms and viruses infectious to humans, animals, or plants (e.g., parasites, viruses, bacteria, fungi, prions, rickettsia); and biologically active agents (i.e., toxins, allergens, venoms) that may cause disease in other living organisms or cause significant impact to the environment or community.[6]

Nosocomial infections and zoonosis

Nosocomial infections pertain to or originate in a hospital.[10] This is said of an infection not present or incubating prior to admittance to the hospital, but generally occurring 72 h after admitting. The term usually refers to patient disease, but hospital personnel may also acquire nosocomial infections (e.g., *methicillin-resistant Staphylococcus aureus* [MRSA]).

Zoonosis is a disease of animals transmissible to humans[10] (e.g., rabies).

Zoonotic and nosocomial infections are an inherent risk in veterinary facilities. They are not avoidable; however, their risk can be greatly reduced by a few simple steps:

1. *Wash Your Hands!* Washing hands in between patients, before eating or smoking, and after washroom use greatly reduces the chances of contacting an infection.

2. *Change Patient Bedding Daily.* This also includes disinfecting the kennel itself, *including* the roof of the kennel.

3. *Proper Management and Housing of Infected Animals.* Recognizing the clinical signs of infections is an important step in preventing infection from getting worse.

If you think you may have been exposed to a zoonotic disease, it is important to seek the advice of a medical professional as soon as possible. In some cases, you may be required to report exposure to your country of residence's Centers for Disease

Control; this may also be discussed at the time of your medical examination. Any hospital staff that are immunocompromised should speak to their personal medical doctor about any concerns and safety precautions. They may be advised to refrain from handling certain patients or to wear personal protective equipment when handling patients with certain infections. This is in particular true for staff with immunosuppressive disorders, on immunosuppressive medications, or whom have had their spleens removed.

There have been entire books written on the topic of zoonotic diseases, so this section is written more so to provide the reader with information on a few of the more common infections they may see in the hospital setting, as well as a list of other infections veterinary staff should be aware of.

Please refer to Chapter 11 for information on leptospirosis, MRSA, and other zoonotic diseases.

Salmonella and Clostridium difficile, infectious diarrheal disorders

Due to the popularity of raw food diets for dogs and cats, the risk of veterinary staff coming into contact with *Salmonella* is increased. Studies have shown an increase in the incidence of *Salmonella* in the feces of pets fed with raw food diets versus regular diets.[11] *Salmonella* is also reported to be much more prevalent in reptile species. Clinical signs include fever and diarrhea in dogs and in cats. In humans, *Salmonella* can cause acute gastroenteritis, with symptoms such as vomiting, diarrhea, and abdominal pain.[12]

C. difficile is one of the most common infections detected in human health-care facilities. It is a bacterium that causes infection of the colon producing watery diarrhea, nausea, and vomiting. It is more common among immunocompromised people, surgical patients, and patients on long-term antibiotic therapy. As with any nosocomial infection, diligence with regular hand washing, not eating in treatment areas of the hospital, and communicating to staff the possibility of an infected patient help keep exposure to a minimum.[13]

Chemotherapy safety

Chemotherapy is becoming more of a routine treatment in veterinary hospitals; however, many hospitals do not have the funds or the space to house the biological safety cabinets many human hospitals and larger veterinary facilities use to mix and prepare chemo drugs. There are numerous health risks associated with improper handling of chemotherapy drugs. All hospital personnel should be aware of the following procedures for handling and disposing of chemotherapeutic drugs:

1. *Potential Exposure to Self and the Environment.* Exposure is most often through inhalation of aerosolized particles, direct absorption through skin contact, indirect contact from unprotected hand-to-face contact, or accidental inges-

tion from eating/drinking or smoking via hand-to-mouth contact.

2. *The Safety Concerns and Proper Methods of Cleaning Up after Patients (Including Vomitus, Urine, and Stools) and Spills.* All patients receiving chemotherapy should be marked appropriately so that all hospital personnel are aware of the safety hazard. A written protocol for the proper disposal methods for used chemotherapy vials, expired drugs, and all chemotherapy equipment used should be followed (e.g., state and federal laws). The use of a separate, properly labeled chemotherapy waste disposal container is mandatory.

3. *Use of Proper Preparation and Administration Equipment for Chemotherapy.* This includes the use of fume hoods, vented needles, and a closed administration system (e.g., PhaSeal® system). The use of the proper type of equipment greatly reduces the chances of exposure.

Hospital staff members who are trying to conceive, are pregnant, breastfeeding, or are immunosuppressed should refrain from administering chemotherapy.

A written protocol for the safe handling of patients receiving chemotherapy should be outlined for each drug used in the hospital. Chemotherapy patients should be clearly identified. A different colored name tag/ID band and/or cage label will visually help hospital staff identify these patients and indicate the need to use extra precautions when handling. Another label indicating the drug given and the length and method of excretion is also recommended. Staff should be knowledgeable in the methods of how to clean up after a chemotherapy patient should they eliminate in their kennel or elsewhere in the hospital, how to clean their kennels, and the proper way to launder their bedding.

Storage and handling of chemotherapy drugs

In the written chemotherapy protocol, a section should outline the policies and procedures to safely handle chemotherapeutics from the time they arrive at the hospital (including inventory personnel), while stored at the hospital, and during and after use. The protocol should include the following steps:

1. Store chemotherapy drugs in a separate, secure, well-marked area.

2. Keep chemotherapy drugs away from areas of food or drink preparation and storage. Do not allow food or drink in areas utilized for chemotherapy.

3. Each open bottle should be separately stored in a ziplock bag and kept within the original container.

4. Reconstituted drugs need to be dated with the strength and expiry date marked on the bottle. Read and be familiar with drug inserts and the manufacturer's instructions with regard to storage and drug viability after reconstitution.

5. All personnel opening or unpacking boxes containing chemotherapy drugs should wear personnel protective equipment and the drugs should be labeled with chemotherapy or biohazard labels.

Recommended safety equipment

- Nitrile gloves—latex gloves do not provide adequate protection when handling chemotherapy drugs
- N 99 or N 100 particulate face mask—surgical masks do not provide protection against aerosolized particles
- Impermeable gown
- Safety goggles
- Nurse's cap

Chemotherapy spills

In the written protocol, a section should detail management of spills ("spill" includes drugs or fluids, e.g., urine and vomit) to assure the safe handling of chemotherapy drugs or contaminated eliminations. The safety procedures should include the following:

1. Immediately clear the area; postwarning signs on all entrances to the area.
2. Alert staff; designate a few people to be involved in the actual cleanup, those not involved should remain outside the area until the cleanup is completed.
3. Cleanup personnel should wear all appropriate safety gear (e.g., gown, gloves, mask, and goggles).
4. Use a spill kit (see Table 14.1.2).
5. Gently cover and absorb liquid spills with absorbent material; pick up solids (powder) with moistened absorbent material.
6. Use a scoop to pick up any sharp or broken objects. Clean the spill area three times using ordinary detergent and water.
7. All disposable spill items should be placed in biohazard. Nondisposable items should be washed in soap and water by staff wearing gloves and a gown.

Conclusion

Everyone from the veterinarians to the part-time kennel staff who help out every other weekend is responsible for his or her

Table 14.1.2   Chemotherapy spill kit

Safety clothing—gowns, masks, goggles, gloves

Absorbent material (e.g., paper towel, gauze, kitty litter)

Small scoop, spatula, or forceps to collect sharp objects

Two large plastic waste disposal bags, 4 mil or thicker
Puncture- and leak-resistant waste container for sharp or breakable objects and liquids

Warning sign

"Chemotherapy Safety and Administration" Tanya Crocker, RVT, VTS (SAIM), CWVS lecture series.

own safety and the safety of his or her coworkers. Regular training, revision of safety procedures, plain old hand washing and common sense will help keep your workplace productive and healthy.

Health and safety web sites

The United States Department of Labor, http://www.osha.gov
WorkSafe BC, http://www.worksafebc.com
American Latex Allergy Association Inc.,
http://www.latexallergyresources.org
Occupational Health and Safety for Healthcare in BC,
http://www.ohsah.bc.ca
Canadian Centre for Occupational Health and Safety,
http://www.ccohs.ca
The Centers for Disease Control has many handouts under National Institute for Occupational Health and Safety (NIOSH), http://www.cdc.gov/niosh
United Kingdom—Institution of Occupational Safety and Health, http://www.iosh.co.uk
Australia—Safe Work Australia, http://www.safeworkaustralia.gov.au
Europe—European Agency for Safety and Health at Work http://osha.europa.eu/en

SECTION 2 PHARMACOLOGICAL IMPLICATIONS IN INTERNAL MEDICINE

Drug calculations, compatibilities, dosing, and administration

For the hospitalized patient, the most common routes of medication administration are the oral, topical, and the injectable routes. When administering medications via the oral and injectable routes, the timing of the drug administration is dependent upon the uptake of the drug into the system.

Constant rate infusion

There are many injectable medications that are ultrashort in duration of action. In these situations, frequent administration still may not maintain effective serum concentrations and may lead to inaccurate dosages.

Constant rate infusion (CRI) is a method of injectable medication administration where a precisely calculated amount of a drug is administered at a constant rate. By administering drugs at a constant rate, the efficacy of the drug and the total daily dose may be reduced. A loading dose (LD) is administered before beginning a CRI for some medications that are ultrashort in duration, such as fentanyl citrate. Most CRI doses are recorded as micrograms per kilogram body weight per minute. As with any medication, calculation of the drug dose must be done accurately. The use of a syringe pump provides the most accurate dosing since the drug is not diluted prior to use. If a syringe pump is not available, accurate dosing can be achieved by combining the drug with a dilutant fluid (commonly 0.9% NaCl).

If a syringe pump is not utilized, then the following calculations are required:

Determine the length of time a fluid bag will last at the current rate of infusion by dividing the volume of fluid in the bag by the rate:

$$\text{Volume in fluid bag in mL} \times \frac{\text{per hour}}{\text{fluid administration rate}}$$
$$= \text{length of infusion in hours.}$$

For some medications, the dose is by the minute; to obtain the length of the infusion in minutes, multiply the number of hours the fluid bag will last by 60 to determine the number of minutes in each bag:

$$\text{Length of infusion in hours} \times \frac{60 \text{ min}}{\text{h}}$$
$$= \text{length of infusion in minutes.}$$

For other medications, the dose is by day (24 h); to obtain the length of the infusion in days, divide the number of hours the fluid bag will last by 24 h to determine the number of days in each bag:

$$\text{Length of infusion in hours} \times \frac{\text{day}}{24 \text{ h}}.$$
$$= \text{length of infusion in days.}$$

Then multiply the weight of the animal in kilogram by the dose:

$$\text{wt in kg} \times \frac{\text{mg}}{\text{kg}} = \text{dose in mg.}$$

Now you will need to figure the total amount of the drug to add to the fluid bag. The dosage may be in milligram, microgram, or international unit; the dosage units are the first number in the equation. All dosages will be by weight (kilograms). The final number in the dosage equation is the time and will be measured in minutes, hours, or by day.

For example, if the drug dose is in milligram per kilogram per hour, multiply the dose in milligram by the number of hours each liter bag will last. This is the total number of milligrams to place in the bag:

$$\text{Dose in mg} \times \text{length of infusion} = \frac{\text{mg}}{\text{L}}.$$

If the drug dose is in microgram per kilogram per minute, multiply the dose in microgram by the number of minutes each liter bag will last. Divide this number by 1000 to convert to milligrams (since most medications have concentrations of milligram per milliliter). This is the total number of micrograms to place in the bag.

$$\text{Dose in } \mu\text{g} \times \text{length of infusion in minutes}$$
$$\div \frac{\text{mg}}{1000 \, \mu\text{g}} = \text{Dose in mg.}$$

To ensure accurate dosing, the amount of the drug to be added should be removed from the base fluid.

Example: A 20-kg dog requires a metoclopramide CRI at a dose of 1 mg/kg/day. The fluid administration rate is 40 mL/h.

1. A 1-L bag of 0.9% NaCl will last 25 h:

$$1000 \text{ mL} \times \frac{\text{h}}{40 \text{ mL}} = 25 \text{ h.}$$

2. Number of days the 1-L bag of fluids will last 1.04 days:

$$25 \text{ h of infusion} \times \frac{1 \text{ day}}{24 \text{ h}} = 1.04 \text{ days.}$$

3. Metoclopramide required per 24 h = 20 mg:

$$20 \text{ kg} \times \frac{1 \text{ mg}}{\text{kg}} = 20 \frac{\text{mg}}{\text{day}}.$$

4. Metoclopramide required for 1 L of fluids = 20.8 mg:

$$20 \text{ mg} \times 1.04 \text{ days} = 20.8 \frac{\text{mg}}{\text{day}}.$$

5. Milliliters of metoclopramide required for 1 L =

$$20.8 \text{ mg} \times \frac{\text{mL}}{5 \text{ mg}} = 4.16 \text{ mL.}$$

See Table 14.2.1.

Drug compatibilities

Care must be taken to check drug compatibilities when administering multiple medications to a patient. Drug interactions can potentiate the effects, counteract the expected outcomes, or create toxic effects. Potential drug interactions in commonly used medications have been reported with cimetidine, sucralfate, ketoconazole, fluoroquinolones, metoclopramide, cisapride, furosemide, omeprazole, phenobarbital, and clomipramine.[1] These interactions may occur during intravenous administration, in the gastrointestinal (GI) system after oral dosing, at the target site, or during elimination in the hepatic and renal systems. With some medications, the timing of the administration must be separated to ensure effective uptake. Always use a current formulary to confirm the safe use of multiple medications.

Drug dosage adjustments in patients with heart, renal, and hepatic insufficiency or failure

Care must be taken to consult a drug formulary when administering any drug to a patient. Information regarding any known contraindications and adverse effects will be listed. Special attention must be given to animals with heart and renal or hepatic insufficiency or failure prior to administering any medications.[2]

Animals in heart failure have a decrease in cardiac output and may have preferential shunting of blood to the brain or heart

Table 14.2.1 Table of drugs commonly used in CRIs

Drug name and concentration	Indications	Constant rate infusion dose	Recommended diluant (D) and incompatibilities (I)	Comments
Atracurium besylate 10 mg/mL	Induction of respiratory muscle paralysis during mechanical ventilation	LD: 0.2–0.5 mg/kg CRI: 3–9 mcg/kg/min (dog) 0.37 mcg/kg/min (cat)	D: 5% dextrose, 0.9% NaCl I: Should not be mixed with other drugs	Start infusion 5 min after loading dose; must monitor respiratory and cardiovascular function
Butorphanol 10 mg/mL	Analgesia ± sedation	LD: 0.2 mg/kg CRI: 0.1 mg/kg/h	D: Any fluid I: Diazepam, pentobarbital	
Calcium gluconate 100 mg/mL	Hypocalcemia, hyperkalemic dysrhythmias, hypermagnesemia	CRI: 10 mg/kg/h	D: Any fluid I: Dobutamine, sodium bicarbonate, potassium phosphate	ECG should be monitored. CRI should be discontinued if bradycardia develops
Cimetidine 300 mg/2 mL	Treatment of gastric ulceration, metabolic alkalosis	LD: 2.5 mg/kg CRI: 0.5 mg/kg/h	D: Any fluid I: Pentobarbital, atropine	Too rapid of an infusion or use of a central vein may cause hypotension and arrhythmias
Cisplatin 1 mg/mL	Antineoplastic agent	CRI: 60–70 mg/m² over 2–6 h	D: 0.9% NaCl I: Metoclopramide	Should not be used in cats; saline diuresis should be provided to avoid nephrotoxicity
Diazepam 5 mg/mL	Anticonvulsant, sedative and skeletal muscle relaxant effects	LD: 5–10 mg CRI: 0.1–0.5 mg/kg/h; increase to effect	D: 5% dextrose, 0.9% NaCl I: Many drugs, cloudiness in admixture indicates precipitation and reduced potency	Adsorbs to plastic IV tubing resulting in unreliable dosing; does not adsorb into plastic syringes; should be protected from light. New CRI should be started every 4 h
Diltiazem 5 mg/mL	Hypertrophic cardiomyopathy and supraventricular tachycardias	LD: 0.2–0.4 mg/kg CRI: 0.2–0.5 mg/kg/h or 5–20 mcg/kg/min to effect	D: Any IV fluid I: None listed at this time	Loading dose is not always needed
Dobutamine 12.5 mg/mL	Useful in cardiogenic or septic shock to treat decreased cardiac contractibility	2–20 mcg/kg/min (dog) 1–15 mcg/kg/min (cat)	D: 5% Dextrose or 0.9% NaCl I: Alkaline solutions, sodium bicarbonate; mixing with other drugs should be avoided	Pink discoloration occurs with slight oxidation, but no loss of potency if used within 24 h; may cause focal facial seizures in cats
Dopamine 40 mg/mL	Low dose: improves renal blood flow, may play a role in treatment of oliguric renal failure Moderate dose: positive inotrope High dose: increases blood pressure	2–5 mcg/kg/min 5–10 mcg/kg/min 7–20 mcg/kg/min	D: 5% dextrose or 0.9% NaCl I: Sodium bicarbonate or alkalinizing solutions	Do not use if solution has a pink or violet color; stable in fluids for 24–48 h. Extravasation may cause necrosis; should be treated locally with 5–10 mg phentolamine in 10–15 mL saline
Epinephrine 1:1000 (1 mg/mL)	Used in cardiac arrest, hypotension, severe asthma and anaphylaxis	0.1–1.5 mcg/kg/min to effect	D: 5% dextrose, 0.9% NaCl I: Alkaline solutions, calcium containing solutions	Solution should be protected from light

(Continued)

Table 14.2.1   (Continued)

Drug name and concentration	Indications	Constant rate infusion dose	Recommended diluant (D) and incompatibilities (I)	Comments
Esmolol 10 mg/mL	Used in tachycardia or hypertension	LD: 500 mcg/kg over 1 minute CRI: 25–200 mcg/kg/min	D: 5% dextrose, 0.9% NaCl I: Sodium bicarbonate	Concurrent use of calcium channel blockers should be avoided
Ethanol 100% 1000 mg/mL	Treatment of ethylene glycol toxicity	LD: 0.6 g/kg CRI: 100 mg/kg/h	D: 0.9% NaCl to a 7% solution I: None listed at this time	7% solution is prepared by adding 7 mL 100% ethanol to 93 mL NaCl
Fentanyl citrate 0.05 mg/mL (50 mcg/mL)	Analgesia and sedation; may be used to facilitate mechanical ventilation	Dog: LD: 10–20 mcg/kg IV CRI: 0.3–0.7 mcg/kg/min Cat: LD: 2 mcg/kg CRI: 0.1–0.3 mcg/kg/min	D: 5% dextrose I: Mixing with other drugs should be avoided	Alternative dose: 1–5 mcg/kg/h
Furosemide 50 mg/mL	Promotes diuresis in oliguric renal failure, treats pulmonary edema in congestive heart failure (CHF), promotes calciuria in hypercalcemia	3–8 mcg/kg/min or 0.1–1 mg/kg/h to effect	D: Any IV fluid I: Acidic solutions; precipitates when combined with many drugs	Should be protected from light
Heparin 1000 U/mL	Activates antithrombin III, prevents thrombin and fibrin formation; used in DIC and thromboembolic disease	LD: 100–300 U/kg CRI: 10–50 U/kg/h (dog) 5–10 U/kg/h (cat)	D: Any IV fluid I: Any drugs that are unstable in an acidic environment	Adjust dose based on activated partial thromboplastin time
Hetastarch 6 g/100 mL	Synthetic colloid, used for its oncotic properties and as a volume expander	1–2 mL/kg/h		Do not use if brown in color or precipitate is present.
Hydrocortisone sodium phosphate 100-, 250-, or 500-mg vials	Treatment of Addisonian crisis and of adrenal insufficiency induced after adrenalectomy	0.625 mg/kg/h	D: Any IV fluid, should be diluted to 0.1–1.0 mg/mL I: Mixing with other drugs	Proper dilution volume should be used to avoid precipitation; do not use if discolored.
Insulin (regular) 100 U/mL	Lowers blood glucose, used in diabetic ketoacidotic patients and adjunctive treatment of hyperkalemia	1.1–2.2 U/kg/day	D: 0.9% NaCl I: Sodium bicarbonate; mixing with other drugs should be avoided	Binds to IV tubing; tubing should be flushed with insulin solution prior to IV infusion
Isoproterenol 0.2 mg/mL	Causes positive inotropy and chronotropy; also vasodilator and bronchodilator; used in advanced heart block	0.02–0.1 mcg/kg/min	D: 5% Dextrose or 0.9% NaCl; dilute to 1 mg in 500 mL	Causes peripheral vasodilation
Ketamine 100 mg/mL	May be used as an adjunct to opioid therapy to ease severe pain	1–3 mcg/kg/min	D: 5% dextrose or 0.9% NaCl I: Diazepam, barbiturates	Should be used with opioid or tranquilizers

Drug	Use	Dose	Dilution/Incompatibility	Notes
Lidocaine 20 mg/mL (2%)	Ventricular antiarrhythmic	Dog: LD: 2–4 mg/kg CRI: 50–100 mcg/kg/min Cat: LD: 0.25–0.75 mg/kg CRI: 10–20 mcg/kg/min	D: 5% Dextrose; 0.9% NaCl less preferred I: Alkaline solutions, mixing with other drugs should be avoided	Adsorption to polyvinyl chloride bags; stable in IV fluids for 24 h; cats are very sensitive (seizures)
Magnesium sulfate (parenteral) 4.06 meq/mL 50% (500 mg/mL)	Used as a source of magnesium in hypomagnesemia and refractory hypokalemia	Up to 1 mEq/kg/day	D: 5% dextrose diluted to <20% I: Many drugs, including those containing calcium, vitamin B complexes, sodium bicarbonate	Use with caution with impaired renal function, overdose causes bradycardia, muscle weakness; treat with calcium
Mannitol 25% (250 mg/mL)	Osmotic diuretic; has a role in treatment of oliguric renal failure, glaucoma, cerebral edema	0.5–1 g/kg/h for 2–6 h	D: 5% dextrose to 8%–10% solution I: Blood, strongly acidic or alkaline solutions; mixing with other drugs should be avoided	Warm to remove/prevent crystallization
Methylprednisolone sodium succinate 40 mg/mL	Treatment of head/spinal cord trauma	LD: 30 mg/kg followed by 15 mg/kg at 2 and 4 h CRI: 2–5 g/kg/h for 42 h, reducing dose gradually	D: 5% dextrose or 0.9% NaCl I: Normosol-R, Normosol-M,	Precipitation may occur; reconstituted solution should be used within 48 h
Metoclopramide 5 mg/mL	Antiemetic, gastrointestinal stimulant	1–2 mg/kg/day or 0.7–1.4 mcg/min or dog: 0.01–0.02 mg/kg/h Cat: 0.01 mg/kg/h	D: Any IV fluid without calcium I: Sodium bicarbonate; mixing with other drugs should be avoided	Should be protected from light
Midazolam 5 mg/mL	Anticonvulsant, sedative, similar to diazepam	Dog: LD: 0.1 mg/kg CRI: 0.35 mcg/kg/min	D: 5% dextrose or 0.9% NaCl I: Mixing with other drugs should be avoided	Does not adsorb to plastics
Morphine 15 mg/mL	Opiate agonist, used in treatment of acute pain	LD: 1–10 mg/kg CRI: 0.01–0.1 mg/kg/h	D: 5% dextrose; should be diluted to 0.1–1 mg/mL I: Mixing with other drugs should be avoided	Cats may exhibit CNS excitability; lower doses should be used in cats.
Norepinephrine 1 mg/mL	Potent adrenergic vasopressor; used for short-term blood pressure support	0.05–1.0 mcg/kg/min to effect	D: 5% dextrose or 0.9% NaCl I: Mixing with other drugs should be avoided	Extravasation should be treated with phentolamine; systolic pressure should not be raised by >40 mmHg
Nitroprusside 200 mcg/mL	Venous and arterial vasodilator; used in acute, congestive heart failure to treat fulminant pulmonary edema or systemic hypertension	Dog: 0.5–10 mcg/kg/min Cat: 0.1–0.3 mcg/kg/min Start low and increase slowly; blood pressure (BP) should be monitored.	D: 5% Dextrose; must use with infusion pump only I: Mixing with other drugs should be avoided	Use with extreme caution; should not be used in oliguric patients; must be shielded from light; overdose results in cyanide toxicity

(Continued)

Table 14.2.1   (Continued)

Drug name and concentration	Indications	Constant rate infusion dose	Recommended diluant (D) and incompatibilities (I)	Comments
Oxytocin 20 U/mL	Used for enhancement of uterine contractions at parturition	Dog: 5–10 U over 30 min Cat: 2–5 U over 30 min	D: 5% dextrose or 0.9% NaCl I: Mixing with other drugs should be avoided	Ensure normal glucose and calcium levels prior to use; use when cervix is open
Pancuronium 1 mg/mL	Neuromuscular blockade as an adjunct to anesthesia or mechanical ventilation	LD: 0–0.04–0.1 mg/kg CRI: 0.06–0.1 mg/kg/h	D: 5% dextrose or 0.9% NaCl By syringe pump I: Drug insert should be consulted	Cardiovascular and respiratory monitoring must be used
Pentobarbital 65 mg/mL	Used as an anticonvulsant and for chemical restraint during mechanical ventilation	LD: 3–30 mg/kg to effect CRI: 0.2–1 mg/kg/h	D: 5% dextrose or 0.9% NaCl I: Mixing with other drugs should be avoided	Respiratory activity should be monitored; ventilatory support may be required
Phenylephrine 100 mg/mL	Causes vasoconstriction via alpha-adrenergic effects; used to treat hypotension under anesthesia	1–3 mcg/kg/min	D: 5% dextrose or 0.9% NaCl I: Sodium bicarbonate	Extravasation injuries must be treated with phentolamine locally
Potassium chloride 2 mEq/mL	Used to treat serum potassium deficits	In IV fluids: 28–80 mEq/L	D: Any IV fluid I: Diazepam	IV administration should not exceed 0.5 mEq/kg/h
Potassium phosphate 3 mM/mL phosphorous, 4.4 mEq/mL potassium	Used in correction of hypophosphatemia	0.01–0.03 mM/kg/h for 6 hr or 0.03–0.12 mM/kg/h for diabetic ketoacidosis (DKA) patients	D: 0.9% NaCl I: Dobutamine, lactated Ringer's solution	50–75% of potassium supplied using KCl, the rest as KPO4; phosphorus levels checked every 12 h in DKA patients until >2.5 mg/dL
Procainamide 100 or 500 mg/mL	Antiarrhythmic, used in treatment of ventricular arrhythmias	Dog: LD 2–20 mg/kg over 5 min CRI: 20–50 mcg/kg/min Cat: LD: 1–2 mg/kg CRI: 10–20 mcg/kg/min	D: 0.9% NaCl I: Decomposes if mixed with dextrose	Light yellow (but not amber) discoloration does not affect potency; should not be used if dark yellow; stable in fluids for 24 h
Propofol 10 mg/mL	Short-acting hypnotic	0.05–0.2 mg/kg/min	D: 5% dextrose I: Should not be mixed with other drugs	Propofol supports bacterial growth; should be used with strict asepsis
Sodium bicarbonate 1 mEq/mL	Alkalinizing agent; used to treat metabolic acidosis; adjunctive therapy in hyperkalemic crisis	50% of calculated dose (based on deficit) IV over 4–6 hours	D: 5% dextrose or 0.9% NaCl I: Mixing with other drugs should be avoided	Deficit calculation: 0.3× kg body weight × base deficit
Verapamil 2.5 mg/mL	Calcium channel blocker; used for supraventricular tachyarrhythmias	LD: 0.05–0.15 mg/kg CRI: 2–10 mcg/kg/min	D: 5% dextrose or 0.9% NaCl I: Mixing with other drugs should be avoided	Loading dose not always used
Vitamin B complex (injectable)	Provides B complex supplementation	2–4 mL/L at maintenance fluid rate	D: Any IV fluid I: Sodium bicarbonate	Compatible with IV fluid and TPN solutions

Source: Silverstein DC, Hopper K. Small Animal Critical Care Medicine. St. Louis, MO: Elsevier Saunders; 2009; Ettinger S, Feldman E. Textbook of Veterinary Internal Medicine, 6th edition. St. Louis, MO: Elsevier Saunders; 2000.

muscle. Some drugs will enhance cardiac toxicity and clinical signs may be apparent. One example would be an increase in cardiac arrhythmias. In animals with shunting of blood to the brain, central nervous system (CNS) toxicity can be manifested by seizures or nausea. With heart failure, the decreased blood flow to the GI system can be manifested by GI edema resulting in erratic oral absorption.

Hepatic insufficiency can decrease drug metabolism, especially in cases of severe disease (e.g., portosystemic shunts and hepatic lipidosis). Common examples of drugs that may have decreased drug metabolism include metronidazole and diazepam. Many pharmacological compounds are metabolized by the liver and must be excreted through the biliary system. Care must be taken when using compounds whose modes of action target the liver. Animals with hypoalbuminemia can have an increase in the acute effects of drugs that are highly protein bound, such as non-steroidal anti-inflammatory drugs (NSAIDs) and benzodiazepines. For animals with ascites, the protein-bound drugs should be dosed on the total body weight including the ascites. With water and lipid-soluble drugs, the ideal body weight should be used. The estimated weight of the ascites should be subtracted from the weight of the animal prior to calculating the drug dose. Some animals with liver disease may have an increased sensitivity to CNS depressants. The dose of opioids should be reduced and the use of reversible agents is recommended. Avoid the use of or use decreased doses of benzodiazepines and barbiturates. If animals have hepatic encephalopathy, stored whole and packed blood should be avoided due to the increased ammonia concentration in stored red blood cell (RBC) products[3] (Table 14.2.2).

There are some drugs that are frequently associated with, or are suspected to cause, drug-associated liver disease, and their use should be carefully monitored or avoided in animals with known hepatic insufficiency[4] (Table 14.2.3).

Increased knowledge of canine genetics has led to the discovery of the MDR1 gene. This gene codes P-glycoprotein (P-gp) and is known as the multidrug resistance 1 gene. P-gp transports (or pumps) chemicals from inside the cell across membranes to outside the cell. P-gp is normally found in many locations including intestinal epithelial cells, brain capillary endothelial cells, biliary canalicular cells, and renal proximal tubular cells. If mutated, this gene results in a nonfunctional protein that alters CNS penetration, enhances oral absorption, and alters urinary and biliary excretion of some drugs. The failure to pump these drugs out of the brain can result in abnormal neurological signs.

The Washington State University Veterinary Clinical Pharmacology Laboratory (WSU-VCPL) has a test available to easily check for the MDR1 mutation, by submission of either a cheek swab or EDTA blood.[5] Certain breeds, primarily the herding breeds, are affected by the MDR1 gene mutation, although mixed breeds can be affected. The affected dogs in order of frequency of mutation include collie, long-haired whippet, Australian shepherd (standard and mini), McNab, Silken Windhound, English shepherd, Shetland sheepdog, German shepherd, Old English sheepdog, and Border collie. With testing, an individual dog can be identified as a normal animal (no gene mutation), a

Table 14.2.2 Drugs frequently associated with liver disease

Drug	Species
Acetaminophen	Cat and dog
Amoxicillin/ampicillin products	Cat and dog
Azathioprine	Dog
Azithromycin	Cat
Azole antifungals	Cat and dog
Cephalosporins	Dog
Cyclosporine	Cat and dog
Diazepam	Cat
Diethylstilbestrol	Dog
Enrofloxacin	Dog
Glucocorticoids	Dog (less commonly cat)
Lomustine	Dogs
Mebendazole	Dog
Megestrol acetate	Dog
Methimazole	Dog
Nonsteroidal anti-inflammatory drugs	Cat and dog
Oxibendazole	Dog
Phenobarbital	Cat and dog
Phenytoin	Dog
Primidone	Dog
Stanozolol	Cat
Sulfonamides	Dog
Tetracycline antibiotics	Cat and dog
Thacetarsemide	Cat and dog
Trimethoprim–sulfa combinations	Dog
Ormetoprim-sulfadiazine	Dog

Table adapted from Kirk's *Current Vet Therapy XIV*.

heterozygous animal (one normal and one mutated gene), or a homozygous animal (two mutated genes).

Some drugs have been shown to be pumped out of the brain by P-gp but, at this time, appear to be safely tolerated by dogs with the mutation; these drugs include cyclosporine, digoxin, and doxycycline.[5] Other drugs, reported to be pumped out of the brain by P-gp in humans, appear to be safely tolerated by dogs; these drugs include buprenorphine, fentanyl, and morphine. However, the use of these drugs should be carefully monitored in dogs with the mutation. Table 14.2.4 lists drugs shown to cause problems in dogs with the MDR1 gene mutation and the recommended dose titrations.

Table 14.2.3 Drugs known to be associated with liver disease

Drug	
Acarbose	Albendazole
Allopurinol	Amitraz
Amlodipine	Butorphanol
Clomipramine	Danazol
Desoxycorticosterone	Diethylcarbamazine
Enalapril	Ethanol
Etodolac	Febantel/praziquantel
Fenbendazole	Griseofulvin
Iron	Isoniazid
Ivermectins	Lufenuron
Lisinopril	Mabofloxacin
Marcrolide antibiotics	Meclofenamic acid
Metronidazole	Methotrexate
Mexiletine	Mibolerone
Mitotane	Ormetoprim
Rifampin	Tamoxifen
Terbinafine	Trilostane
Trovafloxacin	Valproic acid

Source: Table derived from Kirk's *Current Veterinary Therapy XIV.*

Table 14.2.4 Drugs with documented problems in dogs with MDR1 mutation

Drug	Suggested dosing for dogs with the MDR1 mutation
Acepromazine	Reduce dose by 25% in heterozygous dogs. Reduce dose by 30–50% for homozygous dogs.
Butorphanol	Reduce dose by 25% in heterozygous dogs. Reduce dose by 30–50% for homozygous dogs.
Doxorubicin	Reduce dose by 25–30% and monitor carefully.
Emodepside (Profender®)	Not recommended for use
Erythromycin	Not recommended for use
Ivermectin	Safe at 6 µg/kg (heartworm preventative dose) May cause toxicity in heterozygous dogs at 300–600 µg/kg Neurological toxicity in homozygous dogs at 300–600 µg/kg
Loperamide (Imodium™)	Avoid use
Milbemycin oxime (Interceptor®)	Safe at manufacturer's recommended dose for heartworm prevention. Doses at 10–20 × recommended doses toxic for animals with the mutation
Moxidectin	Safe at manufacturer's recommended dose for heartworm prevention. Doses at 10–20 × recommended doses toxic for animals with the mutation
Selamectin (Revolution®)	Safe at manufacturer's recommended dose for heartworm prevention. Doses at 10–20 × recommended doses toxic for animals with the mutation
Vinblastine	Reduce dose by 25–30% and monitor carefully.
Vincristine	Reduce dose by 25–30% and monitor carefully.

Derived from: WSU CVM Veterinary Clinical Pharmacology Lab, http://www.vetmed.wsu.depts-VCPL/drugs.aspx.

Other drugs are excreted via the renal system. Care must be taken to ensure that over dosing of patients with impaired renal filtration does not occur due to incomplete or slow elimination of these drugs. In patients with renal disease, there may be a decrease in the filtration of drugs eliminated primarily by the kidneys or a decrease in tubular secretions. Tubular secretions include potassium, ammonia, hydrogen ions and some drugs.

Some drugs should be used with caution in animals with one or more physiological diseases. A common loop diuretic, furosemide, needs to be used with caution in patients with impaired hepatic function and renal insufficiency or failure. In cases of hepatic function, caution must be taken as furosemide may cause hepatic coma (due to the possibility of electrolyte imbalances). Its use should be discontinued in patients with progressive renal disease especially if oliguria or increasing azotemia occurs. The serum half-life is prolonged in patients with renal failure.[6] See information in the pharmacology section of Chapter 10 for more information on specific drug dosages.

Oxygen therapy

Supplementation with oxygen is very important in the management of critical patients including systemic inflammatory response syndrome (SIRS), cardiopulmonary disease, sepsis, and head trauma. Hypoxemia occurs as a result of decreased oxygen content of inspired air, ventilation–perfusion mismatch, cardiac shunting, hypoventilation, diffusion impairment, and intrapulmonary shunting. Systemic illnesses also cause inadequate tissue oxygen delivery. Examples include anemia, metabolic and respiratory acidosis, or alkalosis.

The patient's arterial oxygen content (CaO_2) and cardiac output (Q) affects the delivery of oxygen to the tissues. To calculate arterial oxygen, utilize the following formula, where SaO_2 is the arterial oxygen saturation, reported from a pulse oximeter in percent. The PaO_2 is the partial pressure of arterial oxygen, reported from arterial blood gas as millimeters of mercury (mmHg).

$$CaO_2 = \left[1.34\left(mL\ O_2\Big/g\right) \times SaO_2 \times hemoglobin \right.$$
$$\left. \left(\frac{g}{dL}\right) + PaO_2\ mmHg \times 0.003(mL\ O_2/dL/mmHg)\right]$$

An example using this equation where the patient's $SaO_2 = 93\%$, the $PaO_2 = 90\,mmHg$, and the hemoglobin $= 14\,g/dL$ is as follows:

$$CaO_2 = \left[1.34\left(mL\ O_2\Big/g\right) \times 93\% \times 14 \right.$$
$$\left. \left(\frac{g}{dl}\right) + \left[90\ mmHg \times 0.003(mL\ O_2/dL/mmHg)\right]\right],$$

$$CaO_2 = 17.44\ mL\ O_2\Big/dL + 0.27\ mL\ O_2\Big/dL,$$

and

$$CaO_2 = 17.71\ mL\ O_2\Big/dL.$$

Normal CaO_2 is 17.5–18.0 mL O_2/dL.

Most arterial oxygen is carried while bound to hemoglobin. A very small fraction $(0.003 \times PaO_2)$ is carried unbound in the plasma. By providing supplemental oxygen, it is possible to increase the fractional concentration of the oxygen in the inspired gas (FiO_2) above 21%. When a patient's PaO_2 is below 70 mmHg or the SaO_2 on room air is less than 93%, oxygen supplementation should be provided.[3]

All methods of oxygen supplementation require humidification if used for more than a few hours. Oxygen supplementation may cause drying and dehydration of the nasal mucosa, impaired mucociliary clearance, epithelial degeneration of the respiratory tract, and increased risk of infection. Humidification is easily achieved by bubbling the oxygen through a container with sterile saline or distilled water and then delivering to the patient by noninvasive or invasive methods.

Noninvasive methods include flow-by oxygen, administration via face mask, oxygen hood, or use of an oxygen cage. Flow-by oxygen is the simplest technique used. An oxygen flow rate of 2–3 L/min held within 2 cm of a patient will provide an FiO_2 of 25–40%. Administration with a face mask at 8–12 L/min can provide an FiO_2 of 50–60%. The drawback for long-term administration by flow-by and administration with a face mask is that both require a staff member to ensure the oxygen is getting to the patient. Administration with an oxygen hood can be achieved with a rigid Elizabethan collar and clear plastic wrap. The plastic wrap is applied to the open end of the collar, with a small space so the hood can vent. Once the hood has been loaded with oxygen, flow rates of 0.5–1.0 L/min will deliver an FiO_2 of 30–40%.[3] Higher FiO_2 concentrations are possible with an oxygen cage. FiO_2 with an oxygen cage can be maintained up to 60%.

If oxygen therapy will be required for over 24 h, invasive methods of supplemental oxygen can be achieved by nasal or nasopharyngeal administration. Nasal catheters are simple to place, are tolerated well by most patients, and require minimal equipment. To place nasal catheters, anesthetize the nasal passage with topical 2% lidocaine or proparacaine. Use a 5- to 10-Fr red rubber catheter, with the tip pointing toward the eye; measure from the nose to the medial canthus of the eye. Mark the catheter with a permanent marker at the level of the nostril. Lubricate the tip of the catheter and insert gently into the ventral nostril to the line marked on the catheter. Secure the tube with suture or staples to the lateral maxilla or between the eyes. Flow rates of 50–150 mL/kg/min can provide 30–70% FiO_2 dependent upon the patient's size, respiration rate, and open mouth breathing. With nasopharyngeal placement, the tip of the catheter is placed at the ramus of the mandible. Care must be taken not to force the catheter into the turbinates as epistaxis can occur. An Elizabethan collar should be placed to prevent the patient from dislodging the catheter.

Hypercapnia is the primary stimulus for respiration. In patients with chronic hypercapnia, such as chronic obstructive pulmonary disease (COPD), administration of supplemental oxygen can result in severe hypoventilation and respiratory failure.[3] Some patients may require mechanical ventilation such as animals with myasthenia gravis, consolidated lung lobes, or when paralytic agents have been used. Pulmonary oxygen toxicity can occur with exposure to 100% oxygen. An FiO_2 of over 60% should not be administered for longer than 24–72 h to avoid pulmonary oxygen toxicity.[3]

Drug calculations

Some medications, such as chemotherapeutic agents, are often calculated on the basis of body surface area (BSA) in meter squared, rather than by a patient's weight. BSA is used because it is less affected by abnormal fat mass and is a better indicator of metabolic mass. Common equations used to calculate BSA are

$$Canine: \frac{10.1 \times (weight\ in\ grams)^{2/3}}{10,000}$$

and

$$Feline: \frac{10 \times (weight\ in\ grams)^{2/3}}{10,000}.$$

Another way to calculate the BSA is with this formula:

$$Canine\ and\ feline: \frac{(weight\ in\ kg)^{2/3}}{10}.$$

The chart below is an effective way to convert from kilogram body weight to meter squared surface area (Table 14.2.5).

Table 14.2.5 Conversion from kilogram body weight to meter squared surface area

Body surface area conversion chart (body weight in kilograms to meters squared)

Weight to body surface area conversion chart—dogs

kg	m²	kg	m²	kg	m²	kg	m²	kg	m²
0.5	0.064	10.0	0.469	20.0	0.744	30.0	0.975	40.0	1.181
1.0	0.101	11.0	0.500	21.0	0.759	31.0	0.997	41.0	1.201
2.0	0.160	12.0	0.529	22.0	0.785	32.0	1.018	42.0	1.220
3.0	0.210	13.0	0.553	23.0	0.817	33.0	1.029	43.0	1.240
4.0	0.255	14.0	0.581	24.0	0.840	34.0	1.060	44.0	1.259
5.0	0.295	15.0	0.608	25.0	0.864	35.0	1.081	45.0	1.278
6.0	0.333	16.0	0.641	26.0	0.886	36.0	1.101	46.0	1.297
7.0	0.370	17.0	0.668	27.0	0.909	37.0	1.121	47.0	1.302
8.0	0.404	18.0	0.694	28.0	0.931	38.0	1.142	48.0	1.334
9.0	0.437	19.0	0.719	29.0	0.953	39.0	1.162	49.0	1.352
								50.0	1.371

Weight to body surface area conversion chart—cats

kg	m²	kg	m²	kg	m²	kg	m²	kg	m²
0.1	0.022	1.4	0.125	3.6	0.235	5.8	0.323	8.0	0.400
0.2	0.034	1.6	0.137	3.8	0.244	6.0	0.330	8.2	0.407
0.3	0.045	1.8	0.148	4.0	0.252	6.2	0.337	8.4	0.413
0.4	0.054	2.0	0.159	4.2	0.260	6.4	0.345	8.6	0.420
0.5	0.063	2.2	0.169	4.4	0.269	6.6	0.352	8.8	0.426
0.6	0.071	2.4	0.179	4.6	0.277	6.8	0.360	9.0	0.433
0.7	0.079	2.6	0.189	4.8	0.285	7.0	0.366	9.2	0.439
0.8	0.086	2.8	0.199	5.0	0.292	7.2	0.373	9.4	0.445
0.9	0.093	3.0	0.208	5.2	0.300	7.4	0.380	9.6	0.452
1.0	0.100	3.2	0.217	5.4	0.307	7.6	0.387	9.8	0.458
1.2	0.113	3.4	0.226	5.6	0.315	7.8	0.393	10.0	0.464

Source: Derived from Formula found in Plumb DC. *Plumbs Veterinary Drug Handbook*, 7th edition. Ames, IA: Blackwell Publishing; 2011.

Client education

Veterinary technicians play a large part in client education when discharging patients from the hospital. When instructing clients on how to administer oral medications, care must be taken to ensure that the client is instructed on the time of the dosing with regard to other medications, if the medication must be administered on an empty stomach or with food and storage of the medications.

Care must also be taken to inform the client of any potential toxicities and monitoring of side effects (such as vomiting or diarrhea). If the medication has been shown to cause harmful effects to humans, this information must be relayed to the client. It is recommended to have client education handouts available on any drug that is being prescribed and dispensed from the clinic.

During discharge, many clients are overwhelmed with information. The use of a discharge form has been shown to increase client compliance with continued home care. A simple form can be created for use when discharging a patient that includes a description of what was found, treatments that were given, care at home instructions, and medication information. Information should include the name of the medication, when to start the

Table 14.2.6   Sample medication discharge form

Medications for "Dusty"					
Drug	What it is for	How much to give	When to give	When to start	Comments
Sucralfate	Gastrointestinal protectant	1 tablet in a slurry	5 a.m., 5 p.m.	Tomorrow morning	Give on an empty stomach, 1 h before and 2 h after food
Misoprostol	Gastrointestinal protectant	½ tablet	6 a.m., 6 p.m.	Tonight with a small meal	Give with food Women should wear gloves when handling

medication, what time to administer the medication, and any special handling issues (Table 14.2.6). When administering medications that can be given with food, it can be placed in a small meatball of canned food, pill pocket, or treat. The use of gelatin capsules can ease administration of medications that are bitter, such as tramadol. If possible, show the owner how to administer the medication during discharge. If a client feels comfortable administering the medications, client compliance will increase. For some pets, the use of a commercial pet piller would be beneficial.

The veterinary technician plays a very important role in the administration of medications. In the hospital setting this includes confirming that the proper patient is receiving the correct medication at the appropriate dosage at the prescribed time. It is imperative that the veterinary technician has a full understanding of and the ability to relay information on; the indications for use, pharmacokinetics, contraindications, precautions, safety issues, adverse effects, drug interactions, and monitoring parameters of the medications they encounter in practice.

SECTION 3 NUTRITIONAL SUPPORT

Nutritional support

Many hospitalized and critically ill dogs and cats are at risk of becoming severely malnourished because they lack an appetite or the ability to eat.

Decreased food intake can be caused by any number of factors ranging from primary medical problems (such as diabetic ketoacidosis, inflammatory bowel disease, pancreatitis, or liver or renal failure) to fear, anxiety, and untreated pain.[1]

Who is at risk?

Dogs and cats of any age or any physiological stage (i.e., life stage) may become malnourished from inadequate nutrient intake. Malnutrition is any disorder with inadequate or unbalanced nutrition that is associated with either nutritional deficiencies or excessive nutrient intake. Protein and energy

malnutrition can also result from diets that are inappropriate for the physiological status of the patient (i.e., low protein diet when increased protein is required, such as during gestation or lactation).[2]

Insufficient nutrient intake can cause impaired immunity, decreased resistance to infection, inability to withstand shock, surgery or the effects of drugs, decreased wound strength, muscular weakness, organ failure, and death.[1]

Nutrition goals

The minimum goals of nutritional support are to meet the patient's nutritional needs, and if possible, to prevent further deterioration. This can be done by providing protein, carbohydrate, fat, and other nutrients in a formula that can be utilized by the body with maximum efficiency, minimal adverse effects, and minimum discomfort.[3]

When the body uses exogenous (those provided outside of the body) rather than endogenous (those provided by the animals own body stores) nutrients, the breakdown of lean body mass is slowed down and the patient's response to therapy is optimized.[4] Increased protein breakdown in response to illness or injury depletes the body of functional protein stores, thereby affecting wound healing, immune and cellular functions, and cardiac and respiratory functions.[5]

When subjected to starvation, body tissues, except for the brain and bone, loses cell mass by varying degrees. Tumors and wounds may act as additional burdens and can further increase the patient's caloric and nutritional requirements.[3] Malnutrition from inappropriate diets and/or unwillingness or inability to eat can impair immune function and wound healing, decrease organ function, and affect the prognosis for recovery.

The magnitude of metabolic aberration is determined by the severity of the illness or injury and the associated tissue damage. Even with the initiation of adequate nutritional support, muscle wasting and negative nitrogen balance can occur.[5]

Guidelines for support

General guidelines for initiating nutritional support include the loss or anticipated loss of more than 10% of the body weight; anorexia for longer than 3 days; trauma; surgery (even including some elective surgeries); severe systemic infiltrative disease; and increased nutrient loss through diarrhea, vomiting, draining wounds, or burns associated with decreased serum albumin.[5] In the case of elective surgeries, just because we "elect" to have the surgery performed does not make it any less stressful. A nutritional assessment should be done on any animal who presents under these conditions and nutritional support provided when deemed necessary.

Other issues that must be considered include GI tract function, whether the patient can tolerate enteral nutrition (feedings administered via the intestinal tract) or parenteral nutrition (food administered intravenously, i.e., total or partial parenteral nutrition), the physical or chemical restraint risks required for placing a feeding tube or central line catheter, venous accessibility, whether the patient is at risk for pulmonary aspiration (e.g., megaesophagus), availability of skilled nursing care and equipment, and client cost.

Nutritional assessment

The cornerstones of nutritional assessment are obtaining a detailed patient history, conducting a complete physical examination, recording body weight and body condition score (BCS), and evaluating blood chemistry profiles.[4] The testing included in the blood chemistry profile depends on the patient's condition (Table 14.3.1).

The BCS used for healthy animals often do not apply to sick animals. When an animal is physiologically stressed, lean body mass is its preferred energy source; in contrast, healthy animals use stored body fat for energy. The result is increased catabolism of body protein.[1]

A patient may present with increased amounts of body fat but may be at serious risk of malnutrition-associated complications caused by protein catabolism. Careful palpation of skeletal muscles over bony prominences (e.g., the scapula, vertebrae, ischium, and occipital crest) can help identify any muscle wasting consistent with increased protein catabolism.[2] Another indicator of poor nutritional status is pitting edema of the lower extremities and ascites. These may reflect low serum protein levels secondary to malnutrition, likely in combination with intestinal or renal protein loss. Poor hair coat and skin condition can also result from inadequate food intake or micronutrient deficiencies.[2]

Calculating energy requirements

Caloric requirements are determined by body weight and activity level/lifestyle and can be estimated by using the resting energy requirements (RER) for healthy adults at rest in environmentally comfortable cages.[3] (See Table 14.3.5.) The RER has previously been multiplied by illness factors based on the patient gender, neutered status, and/or underlying condition; however, illness factors are now thought to lead to excessive calories and more complications rather than improve clinical outcome and are therefore discouraged.[6] It is important to remember the caloric requirement calculations provide only an estimate of a patient's needs and may be off by up to 25%. It is vitally important to closely monitor these patients for persistent undernutrition or overnutrition. Water requirements equal those for energy (1 mL = 1 kcal).[7] Patients that eat more than the calculated RER amounts should not be discouraged from doing so while recovering from surgery or trauma.

Routes of administration

Enteral feeding via the GI tract is generally the safest, most cost-effective, and most natural route for administering nutrients. Enteral feeding also has the ability to maintain the intestinal mucosa to help prevent bacterial translocation.[8] Voluntary oral intake is the preferred route for enteral nutrition; however, patients must be able to consume at least 85% of their calculated RERs for this method of feeding to be effective.[3,7] Technicians often need to devise ways to encourage patients to accept oral feedings (Table 14.3.2).

Table 14.3.2   Hints for increasing oral intake of food

- Hand-feed or pet the patient during feeding.
- Warm the food to slightly below body temperature; if microwaving, be sure food is stirred well before feeding. Always warm food in microwave-approved containers.
- Add warm water to dry food or make a slurry from canned foods by adding warm water.
- Use baby food meats as a top dressing; dogs may also like cat food used as a top dressing.
- Try various shapes and types of bowls. Shallow dishes for cats and brachycephalic dog breeds; plastic may have a strange smell to the animals.
- Use foods that have a strong smell or odor.
- Raise food (and water) bowls in patients with neck pain.
- Add appetite stimulants to "jump start" the feeding process (usually ineffective over the long term).

Table 14.3.1   Nutritional questions

- When was the last time your pet ate or drank? How much was offered? How much was consumed?
- What type of food is usually fed (canned, dry, table food, scraps)? How much and how often?
- What brand of food is usually fed? For how long?
- Have there been any recent changes in your pet's eating or drinking habits? If so, what changes and over what period of time?
- Have there been any recent changes in body condition (e.g., muscle loss, swollen abdomen, hair loss, or poor grooming)?
- Has your pet recently taken, or is it currently taking any medications? Were there any changes in your pet's condition while taking these medications? Is so, what?

Source: Abood SK. Nutritional assessment of the critical care patient. In: *Purina Nutrition Forum*. St. Louis, MO: Ralston Purina; 1997.

Source: Torrance AG. Intensive care nutritional support. In: *Manual of Companion Animal Nutrition and Feeding*, pp. 171–180. Ames, IA: Iowa State University Press; 1996.

If a patient is unwilling or unable to eat voluntarily, tube feeding should be strongly considered. Tube feeding, however, is somewhat limited by diet selections. In most instances, only liquid or highly blendarized gruel diets can be fed through the tube due to the smaller internal diameter size, but this is somewhat dependent upon the tube selected. In addition, tubes may become clogged, but flushing with water can prevent this from occuring.[2] Even with these limitations, tube feeding may be appropriate in some cases.

Parenteral nutrition

When enteral nutrition is not an option, as with severe GI disease resulting in intractable vomiting, when enteral nutrition could exacerbate a disease (e.g., necrotic hemorrhagic pancreatitis), or the animal's airway cannot be protected and aspiration pneumonia is a concern, parenteral nutrition is an option.[9]

Parenteral nutrition uses a modified solution with nutrients that can be absorbed by the cells without passing through the gastrointestinal tract (GIT) first. Parenteral solutions can be used alone or as a supplement to enteral feedings when insufficient caloric intake is seen. Using parenteral nutrition as the only means of calories (termed total parenteral nutrition [TPN]) is recommended only for patients that cannot be fed enterally. Drawbacks include higher administration expenses (including hospitalization fees) and difficulty in obtaining the sterile, properly prepared TPN solutions. Short-term (less than 24 h) use of TPN is usually not justified, and most animals will need support for greater than 5 days.[9]

TPN has several disadvantages. A dedicated central venous catheter is required, which requires close monitoring. Thrombophlebitis and sepsis are serious complications if strict aseptic technique is not followed.[10] Lack of nutrients in the intestinal lumen may lead to a breakdown of the bacterial barrier in the GIT, further increasing the incidence of sepsis. Lastly, a transitional period is necessary to wean the patient from parenteral to enteral feedings.[3]

Total parenteral solutions have very high osmolality (often greater than 800–1200 mOsm), and therefore a central venous catheter is required to prevent phlebitis. Partial parenteral solutions have lower osmolality and a peripheral catheter can be used. Partial parenteral solutions are diluted to decrease the osmolality, but this also dilutes the caloric content. Since both total and partial parenteral solutions are mostly fluid, administration rates of concurrent intravenous fluids must be adjusted to prevent fluid overload. Separation of the fluid line at connection points (even when out of the cage during walks) or line damage/breakage must be avoided to decrease the incidence of introducing bacteria to the solution[10] (Table 14.3.3).

Diets

Patients with stress starvation can be glucose intolerant, and if so, use glucose less efficiently as an energy source. Therefore, protein and fat are important sources of energy. Before evaluating the need for fat, protein, and carbohydrate, however, a good

Table 14.3.3 Practices that adversely affect nutritional status

- Failing to record weight daily
- Failing to observe, measure, and record amounts of food consumed
- Allowing diffusion of responsibility for patient care during staff rotation
- Prolonged administration of dextrose and electrolyte containing solution without providing additional nutritional support
- Delaying nutritional support until a patient reaches an advanced state
- Withholding food to conduct multiple diagnostic tests or procedures
- Failing to recognize and treat increased nutritional needs
- Failing to appreciate the role of nutrition in prevention and recovery from infection and placing unwarranted reliance on drugs
- Allowing surgery to be performed without verifying whether the patient is optimally nourished
- Providing inadequate nutritional support after surgery
- Failing to use laboratory tests to assess nutritional status

Source: Saker KE, Remillard R. Critical care nutrition and enteral-assisted feeding. In: *Small Animal Clinical Nutrition*, 5th edition, eds. MS Hand, CD Thatcher, RL Remillard, P Roudebush, BBJ Novotny, pp. 439–471. Marceline, MO: Walsworth Publishing; 2010.

Table 14.3.4 Recommended levels of protein, fat, and carbohydrate in critical care diets

Species	Protein % ME	Fat % ME	Carbohydrate % ME
Dogs	20–30	30–55	15–50
Cats	25–35	40–55	15–25

Source: Tennant B. Feeding the sick animal. In: *Manual of Companion Animal Nutrition and Feeding*, pp. 171–180. Ames, IA: Iowa State University Press; 1996.

diet strategy should address the animal's requirement for water and correct any preexisting fluid and acid–base deficits. After these needs have been satisfied, sufficient fat, carbohydrate and protein should be provided to meet the animal's energy requirements and to minimize the gluconeogenesis of amino acids[10] (Table 14.3.4).

Commercial pet foods are specifically designed to meet the dietary requirements of cats and dogs and contain ingredients (e.g., glutamine, taurine, carnitine) not usually found in liquid enteral or parenteral human diets. The principal difference between human and animal liquid diets is the extent that ingredients are subject to hydrolysis and the protein content. For example, most human enteral diets contain 14–17% protein, which is insufficient for both dogs and cats. In addition, arginine and methionine levels in human enteral diets tend to be too low, especially for cats.[10]

Pediatric or growth pet diets are often recommended because they are highly digestible, have high fat and protein contents, and are very palatable.[8] Meat-based baby foods contain 30–70% protein and 20–60% fat. However, because they are deficient in calcium, vitamin A, and thiamine, baby foods should not be used as the sole dietary source[5] (Table 14.3.5).

Rate of diet initiation

Because nutritional support is not an emergency procedure, the general guidelines are to start slowly.[8] Food intake should be gradually increased over a 2- to 3-day period until the estimated caloric intake is met.[10] If the patient shows discomfort, vomits, is nauseous, or becomes distressed, the diet and the route and rate of delivery need to be assessed.

In most cases, 50% of the RER, divided into multiple small meals, is offered on the first day. If this amount is well tolerated, then 100% of the RER can be fed on the second day. If the feedings are not well tolerated, the increases should be more gradual over the next 2–3 days. Smaller meals tend to be better tolerated because they do not cause overdistension of the stomach (and the subsequent delayed gastric emptying) or aggravate nausea, as can occur with larger meals.[2] For patients receiving assisted feedings (via nasoesophageal, esophageal, or gastrostomy tube), by delivering the food as a CRI (using a syringe pump), more food can be fed than if bolus feedings were utilized. This can significantly decrease the incidence of nausea because only small amounts of food are in the stomach at any given time.[11] This method is also much easier on the nursing staff than if frequent small bolus feedings are given every 2–4h.

When using CRI feedings, the animals must be monitored closely to ensure that the feeding tube does not become displaced, allowing food to enter the lungs.

Refeeding syndrome is an electrolyte disturbance that occurs in patients with depleted intracellular cations (e.g., potassium, phosphorus, magnesium, and calcium) and can be seen with malnutrition, starvation as with feline hepatic lipidosis, or prolonged diuresis as seen with uncontrolled diabetes or renal failure. This syndrome can be avoided by monitoring patients closely, introducing feedings slowly, monitoring electrolytes frequently (every 12–24h), and appropriately supplementing diets.[3]

Implementing feeding orders

Clear instructions listing the type and form (i.e., liquid, canned, or dry) of food to be offered, how much to give, and how often to feed are needed on each patient's treatment sheet. Technicians need to record the food that was offered, the technique used to feed the patient, the amount eaten, and the food that was offered (e.g., one-half can of slightly warmed Hill's ID* dog food offered by hand at 3:00 p.m., ate 100%). A flowchart can be used to record this information. One method of charting appetites is to draw a circle on the treatment sheet and to fill in the amount of food the patient consumed (e.g., filling in one-quarter of the circle if the patient ate one-fourth of the amount offered). If the patient refused to eat, the technician should record an R

Table 14.3.5   Example of enteral nutrition worksheet

Enteral nutrition worksheet

Client_____   Patient_____   Case #_____

Date _____   Body condition score_____/5

Actual body weight (kg) _____   Desired body weight (kg)_____

Resting energy requirements (RER) (wt in kg) 30 + 70 = kcal/day

   Patient's RER =_____ kcal/day

Product selected_____ which contains (complete as appropriate)

_____ kcal/mL

_____ kcal/can

_____ kcal/cup

Total volume to be administered/day based on kcal required/day (complete as appropriate)

   kcal/mL of selected diet =_____mL/day

   kcal/can of selected diet =_____cans/day

   kcal/cup of selected diet =_____mL/day

Administration schedule (differs for hepatic lipidosis)

   1/3 of total requirement on day 1 =_____ mL/day

   2/3 of total requirement on day 2 =_____ mL/day

   Total requirement on Day 3 =_____ mL/day

Feeding instructions (complete as appropriate)

   For liquid diets: Feed_____mL_____ times/day

   For canned diets: Feed_____cans_____ times/day

   For dry food diets: Feed_____cups_____ times/day

Feeding schedule

   Divide total daily volume into 4–6 feedings/day (depending on duration of anorexia and patient tolerance)

      Day 1 =_____ feedings/day

      Day 2 =_____ feedings/day

      Day 3 =_____ feedings/day

   Volume/feeding

      Day 1 =_____ mL/feeding

      Day 2 =_____ mL/feeding

      Day 3 =_____ mL/feeding

in the circle. The technician should also record whether the offered food, the amount offered or the technique differs from the instructions. Such record keeping provides veterinarians with an accurate measurement of food intake and technicians with feeding methods that have succeeded or failed on a per-

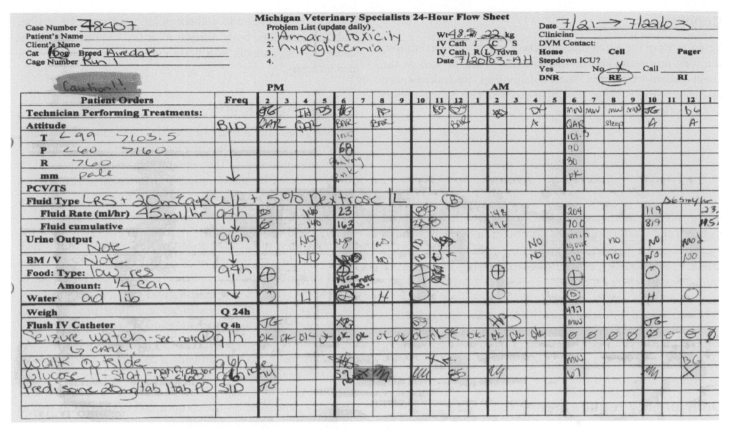

Figure 14.3.1   Sample nutritional administration flowchart.

Table 14.3.6   Sample diet transition—therapeutic diet (current diet) to maintenance diet (new diet)

Day 1–4	Day 5–8	Day 9–12	Day 13
¾ therapeutic diet	½ therapeutic diet	¼ therapeutic diet	100% maintenance diet
¼ maintenance diet	½ maintenance diet	¾ maintenance diet	

Source: Author.

patient basis. This is especially helpful during shift changes (Figure 14.3.1).

Diet transitions

Although diet transitions may occur while the patient is hospitalized, typically, this is done at some point following discharge from the hospital. One risk of transitioning to goal diet while a patient is hospitalized is the development of food aversions. Food aversion is the negative association of a certain diet with hospitalization and leads to the avoidance of the offered diet. The transition depends on the diet being fed, the condition of the patient, its response to therapy, and the owner's willingness. As with diet initiation, it is best to proceed slowly. For example, when shifting from a therapeutic, support diet (current diet in hospital) to a maintenance diet (new diet at home), each dietary change should represent an additional one-quarter of the current

diet every 3–4 days. For days 1–4, feed three-fourths of the therapeutic diet and one-fourth of the maintenance diet; days 5–8, feed one-half of the therapeutic diet and one-half of the maintenance diet; days 9–12, feed one-fourth of the therapeutic diet and three-fourths of the maintenance diet; day 13, feed 100% maintenance diet (i.e., transition phase of 12–16 days). If a problem develops at any stage, the owners should be instructed to return to the last diet combination that worked.

Technicians should supply owners with well-written, concise discharge instructions and a reasonable expectation of what the diet being fed can accomplish. Unfortunately, therapeutic or maintenance diets cannot "cure" inflammatory bowel disease, chronic renal failure, or diabetes mellitus, though they are often used to help control the clinical signs of these diseases or to slow their progression. It is very important that owners are fully educated and have reasonable expectations on the diet being fed (Table 14.3.6).

Conclusion

Being aware of the nutritional aspects of patient care can improve the long-term outcome of the patient's health as well as the client–patient–veterinary team relationship. Technicians can assume a primary role in providing excellent nutritional support to our patients.

Energy balance: weight loss versus weight gain

Energy balance is when an animal's intake is sufficient to meet its needs and when minimal changes occur in the energy stored by the body.[12,13] Positive energy balance happens when caloric intake exceeds energy expenditure. In growing and pregnant animals, excess energy is converted primarily to lean body tissue; in adult animals, excess energy is stored primarily as fat with only some increase in lean tissue.[12,13] A negative energy balance occurs when caloric intake is insufficient to meet energy expenditures; with this scenario, weight loss and a decreases in both fat and lean body stores can be seen.

Daily energy requirements

The daily energy requirement (DER) for dogs and cats depends on the amount of energy that the body expends on a daily basis.[12] Energy balance is achieved by matching input and output over a period of time. Even a small imbalance, maintained over a long period of time, can cause weight gain or weight loss dependent on the direction of the imbalance.

The principal mechanism for control of energy balance is thought to be via the regulation of intake, though some variation in output can be important.[13] The energy requirement of the animal and the energy density of the food will determine the quantity of food required on a daily basis. Regulation of intake is considered to be a negative feedback system, meaning that as weight increases, intake will decrease, and when weight decreases, intake will increase. Palatability can disrupt this feedback system. A highly palatable food can lead to excess intake over energy expenditure, and a poorly palatable food can lead to an insufficient intake to meet energy requirements.

Energy expenditure can be divided into three major areas: RER, voluntary muscular activity, and meal-induced thermogenesis.[12]

Resting energy requirements

RER, also called resting metabolic rate (RMR), accounts for the largest portion of an animal's energy expenditure, ~60–75% of the total daily intake.[12] RER is the amount of energy used in a nonfasted animal while resting quietly in a thermoneutral environment.[12–14] This represents the energy required to maintain homeostasis in all of the integrated systems of the body while at rest.[12] Factors influencing RER include sex, reproductive

status, thyroid gland and autonomic nervous system function, body composition, body surface area (BSA), and nutritional status.[12] As an animal's lean body mass or BSA increase, RER also increases.

Energy expenditure

Voluntary muscular activity, or exercise, is the most variable area of energy expenditure. Muscular activity uses ~30% of the total energy expenditures.[12] The amount of energy expended is directly affected by the duration and intensity of the activity, though the amount of energy used can also increase as weight increases.

Meal-induced thermogenesis is the heat produced following the intake of a meal.[12] The ingestion of nutrients causes heat production through the actions of digestion and absorption. The use of enzymes by the body allows these chemical reactions to occur at the relatively low temperatures found within the body. To achieve the same results in an industrial process would require much more extreme conditions of temperature, pH, or highly reactive ingredients.[15] When a meal containing a mixture of carbohydrates, fats, and proteins is consumed, thermogenesis uses ~10% of the ingested calories to digest, absorb, metabolize, and store these nutrients.[12] The final amount of calories used is ultimately dependent on the composition of the diet as well as the nutritional status of the animal.

Adaptive thermogenesis is the change in the RER secondary to environmental stresses. These stresses include changes in ambient temperature (both heat and cold), alterations in food intake, and emotional stress.[12] Thermogenesis allows the body to maintain the energy balance despite changes in caloric intake by being more or less efficient in energy use. Therefore, an animal can maintain its weight over short periods of time without a corresponding increase or decrease in food intake. Adaptive thermogenesis has been documented in laboratory animals and in humans but has not been documented in companion animals yet.[12]

RER can be affected by body composition, age, caloric intake, and hormonal status.[12] The RER naturally decreases as an animal ages and lean body tissue is lost. Changes in the RER can occur secondarily to decreased food intake. When caloric intake is decreased, hormones will cause an initial decrease in requirement to conserve body tissue.[12,15] If caloric restriction continues, RER will be readjusted and will not be corrected until levels of lean body tissue return to normal.

Persistent overeating can lead to an increase in energy expenditure in part due to the increase in lean body mass with weight gain, but also due to increased meal-induced thermogenesis.[12,15]

Reproductive status affects energy requirements with neutered animals having significantly lower estimated RER than intact animals. This is due to both a change in body composition (less lean body tissue) and also a decrease in activity levels.[12] Intact animals tend to be more active both during breeding season and in territorial disputes, which are usually not as much of a concern for a neutered animal.

Voluntary oral intake

Voluntary food intake is regulated by both internal physiological controls and external cues.[12] The animal also receives cues from the body in the form of physical signs. For example, the stomach contracts when it is empty, stimulating eating, or the stomach distends when full, inhibiting eating.[15] There are also numerous neural and hormonal mechanisms that provide direct stimulation or inhibition to eating. Glucagon and insulin would be examples of two of these hormones. Glucagon is a peptide produced in the intestines that causes a decrease in food intake. Insulin, on the other hand, is produced by the pancreas and stimulates hunger and increased food intake.[12] The administration of exogenous steroids can have the same effect as insulin on hunger and food intake.

External controls of food intake include stimuli such as diet palatability, food composition and food texture, and the timing and environment of meals.[12] Feeding a highly palatable diet is considered a primary environmental factor contributing to the overconsumption of food, which in turn leads to obesity. This can be seen with high fat diets, calorically dense diets, and foods that offer a variety of palatable flavors.[12] The animal eats more than is physiologically required because it tastes good, resulting in excess caloric intake and subsequent weight gain.

Both dogs and cats have definite taste and texture preferences. The majority of dogs prefer canned and semimoist foods over dry food, with beef being the preferred flavor and cooked meat preferred over raw.[12] Dogs also have a strong preference for sucrose, while cats have been shown to lack the taste receptors in their tongues to even detect sugars.[12,16] Dogs and cats can detect several specific amino acids that are only weakly bitter to people. These amino acids and peptides help to give foods their meaty and savory aromas. Dogs and cats also respond to selected nucleotides and fatty acids that appear to increase the meaty taste perception in foods. A nucleotide that accumulates in decomposing meat is distasteful to cats but not to dogs. This may help explain dogs' fascination with dead animals.[17] Both animals prefer warm food to cold food, with increasing palatability seen with increased fat levels in the diet.[12]

The timing of meals as well as the environment that they are offered in can affect eating behavior.[12] Dogs and cats rapidly become conditioned to receiving their meals at a specific time of day; this can be seen with both behavioral and physical signs. Activity will generally increase at anticipated mealtimes, and gastric secretions and motility increase in anticipation of eating. The number of animals being fed can also increase the amount of food consumed with each meal in dogs; this is a phenomenon called social facilitation.[12] This causes a moderate increase in interest in food and an increased rate of eating. The degree that this affects individual dogs can vary greatly. Social hierarchies between dogs can also affect the amount of food eaten, with subordinate dogs eating less in the presence of dominate dogs during mealtimes.[12]

The frequency of meals can affect both food intake and metabolic efficiency. With increased meal frequency, there is actually an increase in energy loss through increased thermogenesis. With smaller, more frequent meals, the body actually uses more energy to digest, absorb, and metabolize the food than when one or two larger meals are fed.[12]

Nutrient composition

The nutrient composition of the food can affect both the nutrient metabolism and the amount of food voluntarily eaten by the animal.[12] Most animals will decrease their intake of a high fat diet to compensate for energy needs, though the greater caloric density of the diet with increased palatability can still cause increased energy intake in some animals. The body is also metabolically more efficient at converting dietary fat to body fat for storage than it is at converting dietary carbohydrate or protein to body fat. Because of this, if an animal is eating calories of a high fat diet in excess of its requirements, it will gain more weight than if it were consuming the same number of calories of a high protein or high carbohydrate diet.

The addition of treats and table scraps to the diet can also override the satiety cues the body gives. These treats tend to be highly desirable and appealing, and even if full, the animals will not turn them down. This leads to an increase in energy intake and obesity because owners seldom will decrease the amount of "regular food" offered to the pet. Feeding a variety of new food types can also cause the same affect.[12]

Estimated energy requirements

Many formulas have been used to calculate the estimated energy requirements for animals. Dogs present a unique challenge in that their sizes have one of the widest ranges in the animal kingdom (from the 4-lb Chihuahua to the 200-lb Great Dane). Cats tend to have a smaller range of sizes, usually between 4 and 20 lb. Some references use allometric formulas, some linear equations, and still some use BSA. All of these formulas are helpful, but all still are only estimates of actual caloric needs. Numerous charts have also been devised that allow quick access to estimate energy needs (Table 14.3.7).

All of these formulas have been compared, and when calculated out, the results are within a reasonable distance of each other. Ultimately, all energy estimates will need to be adjusted based on the desired response from the animal (weight gain, weight maintenance, or weight loss). Variability between individual animals and environmental living conditions can result in a difference up or down of up to 25% of the calculated energy need.[12] In the end, all of these are estimates, and the actual animal will have to be periodically evaluated to determine if the amount being fed is sufficient to their individual energy requirements.

Certain life stages can result in increased energy needs. These would include growth, gestation, lactation, periods of strenuous physical work, and exposure to extreme environmental conditions.[12]

Table 14.3.7   Formula(s) for calculating MER in adult maintenance in kilocalories per day, using body weight (BW) in kilograms

Canine	Feline
Inactive $99 \times BW^{0.67}$ (1)	Inactive $60 \times BW$ (2,4)
Active $132 \times BW^{0.67}$ (1)	Moderately active $70 \times BW$ (4)
Very active $160 \times BW^{0.67}$ (1)	Highly active $80 \times BW$ (4)
Endurance/performance $300 \times BW^{0.67}$ (5)	Kitten 0–3 month $250 \times BW$ (4)
$<2\,kg$ (BER $70 \times BW^{0.75}$) $\times 1.3 - 2.0$ (5)	Kitten 3–5 months $130 \times BW$ (4)
$>2\,kg$ (BER [$30 \times BW$] $+ 70$) $\times 1.3 - 2.0$ (5)	$<2\,kg$ (BER $70 \times BW^{0.75}$) $\times 1.3 - 2.0$ (5)
$1500 \times BSA$ (3)	$>2\,kg$ (BER [$30 \times BW$] $+ 70$) $\times 1.3 - 2.0$ (6)

Source: Compiled from Case LP, Carey DP, Hirakawa DA, Daristotle L. Energy balance. In: *Canine and Feline Nutrition*, 2nd edition, pp. 75–88. St. Louis, MO: Mosby; 2000; Donoghue S. The underweight patient. In: *Manual of Companion Animal Nutrition and Feeding*, eds. N Kelly, J Wills, p. 103. Ames IA: Iowa State Press; 1996; Gross KL, Jewell DE, Yamka RM, et al. Macronutrients. In: *Small Animal Clinical Nutrition*, 5th edition, eds. MS Hand, CD Thatcher, RL Remillard, et al., pp. 50–88. Marceline, MO: Walsworth Publishing; 2010; Simpson JW, Anderson RS, Markwell PJ. Anorexia, enteral and parenteral feeding. In: *Clinical Nutrition of the Dog and Cat*, p. 107. Cambridge, MA: Blackwell; 1993.

Table 14.3.8   Life stage energy requirements for dogs

Life stage—canine	Energy requirement
Postweaning	$2 \times$ adult MER
40% adult weight	$1.6 \times$ adult MER
80% adult weight	$1.2 \times$ adult MER
Late gestation	1.25–$1.5 \times$ adult MER
Lactation	$3 \times$ adult MER
Prolonged physical work	2–$4 \times$ adult MER
Decreased environmental temperature	1.2–$1.8 \times$ adult MER

Source: Gross KL, Jewell DE, Yamka RM, et al. Macronutrients. In: *Small Animal Clinical Nutrition*, 5th edition, eds. MS Hand, CD Thatcher, RL Remillard, et al., pp. 50–88. Marceline, MO: Walsworth Publishing; 2010.

Table 14.3.9   Life stage energy requirements for cats

Life stage—feline	Energy requirement
Postweaned	250 kcal/kg BW
20 weeks	130 kcal/kg BW
Late gestation	$1.25 \times$ adult MER
Lactation	3–$4 \times$ adult MER

Source: Gross KL, Jewell DE, Yamka RM, et al. Macronutrients. In: *Small Animal Clinical Nutrition*, 5th edition, eds. MS Hand, CD Thatcher, RL Remillard, et al., pp. 50–88. Marceline, MO: Walsworth Publishing; 2010.

Using these equations and the energy density of the food, the amount of food to be fed to the individual animal can be calculated[12] (Tables 14.3.8 and 14.3.9).

Water requirements can be expressed in one of two ways, either two to three times the dry matter intake of the food, expressed in grams or by using the MER kilocalories per day estimates to also calculate water requirements.[12] The best recommendation is to have plenty of clean, fresh water available at all times, regardless of the animal's physiological state, caloric intake, or dry matter intake.

Weight gain

Assuming that there are no physiological reasons decreasing nutrient absorption or utilization, creating weight gain is simply a matter of increasing energy intake. When dealing with physiological problems affecting nutrient absorption (e.g., inflammatory bowel disease, lymphangiectasia, pancreatic exocrine insufficiency, and diabetes mellitus), weight gain will usually not occur without addressing the underlying disease. Fats are more calorically dense than are proteins or carbohydrates. Knowing this, increasing the amount of fat in a diet will increase the caloric density and will increase the number of calorics consumed if the amount eaten remains the same. For animals that are unable or unwilling to consume enough calories, the use of a feeding tube can help to ensure adequate nutrition is received to help with recovery.[12]

Weight loss

Conversely, weight loss is simply a matter of decreasing the calories consumed and increasing the calories used. This can be done by restricting the volume of food fed, by changing the nutrient distribution to decrease the caloric density, and by increasing the activity the animal receives every day. Usually, this is much easier said than done.

Muscle atrophy

Muscle atrophy can be caused either by decreased use of the muscle or through increased catabolism. Atrophy is a secondary affect, and the underlying problem must be addressed. Physical therapy and increased exercise can help with muscle disuse as long as the underlying issue is also addressed (e.g., pain with movement and neurological disorders). Muscle catabolism is usually caused through a disease process that either increases the body's protein requirements (e.g., some cancers) or through decreased protein intake in the food, causing secondary protein malnutrition. The underlying problem must first be treated in order to affect the secondary problem of muscle atrophy.[14,18]

Conclusion

Without the presence of an underlying disease, weight gain and weight loss is simply a matter of balance, energy in versus energy out. The presence of highly palatable and calorically dense foods, as well as decreased activity level, has tipped the balance and predisposed many of our pets to obesity.

A disease process can significantly affect the nutrient availability and therefore the amount of energy accessible to an animal. To successfully treat weight loss due to a disease process, the disease process itself must first be addressed.

Common measurements of energy

Basal Energy Requirement (BER). The energy requirement for a normal animal in a thermoneutral environment, awake but resting in a fasting state. This is also known as basal metabolic rate (BMR) or basal energy expenditure (BEE).

RER. The energy requirement for a normal animal at rest in a thermoneutral environment, awake but not fasted. RER accounts for the energy used for digestion, absorption, and metabolism of nutrients and for recovery from physical activity. Also known as resting metabolic requirement (RMR) or resting energy expenditure (REE).

Maintenance Energy Requirement (MER). The energy requirement for a moderately active adult animal in a thermoneutral environment. MER accounts for energy used for obtaining, digesting, and absorbing nutrients in an amount to maintain body weight, as well as energy used for spontaneous activity. This is also known as metabolic energy expenditure (MEE).

DER. The energy required for the average daily activity of any animal, dependent on lifestyle and activity. DER includes energy necessary for work, gestation, lactation, and growth, as well as energy needed to maintain normal body temperature.

Gross Energy (GE). The total amount of heat produced by burning a food in a bomb calorimeter.

Digestible Energy (DE). The energy in a food that is remaining after accounting for fecal losses, this amount is subtracted from GE.

Metabolizable Energy (ME). The energy in a food available to the animal after losses from feces, urine, and combustible gases; this amount is subtracted from GE.

Kilocalorie (kcal). The energy needed to raise the temperature of 1 g of water from 14.5 to 15.5°C. 1 kcal = 1000 cal.

3500 Kcal. The amount of energy required to lose or gain 1 lb.[14,15]

Refeeding syndrome

A phenomenon has been noted in historical records in humans describing epidemics of death when starving people gained access to food. When allowed to engorge themselves, they became severely ill and died. Those people that did not engorge themselves but consumed small amounts of food did not suffer the same fate.[19] In human medicine, this metabolic derangement is still seen in patients with severe anorexia nervosa or diabetic ketoacidosis, in chronic alcoholics, or in those individuals having gone on hunger strikes.[19,20]

More importantly to us in veterinary medicine, this metabolic derangement can also be seen in our patients. Typically, these patients present with a prolonged history of anorexia or other metabolic condition such as diabetic ketoacidosis or hepatic lipidosis.[19,21]

Physiology of starvation

When a body goes into a starvation situation, a complex set of changes or adaptations occur. By understanding these changes, we are better able to understand what happens when we start to "refeed."[20] Initially, the metabolic rate slows down decreasing the energy necessary to run the basic needs of the body; in addition, a reduction in the functional reserve of most if not all the organ systems occurs. Significant reductions occur in cardiac output and hemoglobin levels, therefore affecting the oxygen carrying capacity. Renal concentrating capacity, GI villous atrophy, and a slowing of GI motility also occurs.[20] These reductions in functional reserves are not severe enough to cause failure of any one organ system during starvation.

Physiology of refeeding

In humans, potential complications of refeeding include generalized muscle weakness, tetany, myocardial dysfunction, cardiac arrhythmias, seizures, excessive sodium and water retention, hemolytic anemia, and death from cardiac and respiratory failure.[20,22] While complications from refeeding are seen rarely in veterinary medicine, it is seen most often in those patients receiving enteral or parenteral nutritional support.[22]

When reintroducing food several areas need to be monitored closely to prevent the "refeeding syndrome." During recovery, excessively rapid refeeding (or hyperalimentation) can overwhelm the patient's already limited functional reserves.[20]

Refeeding causes a shift in the body from a catabolic state, where protein is the primary energy source, to an anabolic state, where carbohydrates are the preferred energy source.[20,23] Administration of enteral or parenteral nutrition stimulates the release of insulin; this causes dramatic shifts in serum electrolytes from the extracellular space to the intracellular space, primarily phosphorus, potassium, and, to a lesser degree, magnesium.[20,23,24] Insulin also promotes intracellular uptake of glucose and phosphorus for glycolysis.[23] Insulin acts like a doorknob into the cell; when the door is open, glucose can flow into the cell where it is converted into energy through the formation of adenosine triphosphate (ATP). Since glucose is not the only substance that passes in through this door, all of the intracellular electrolytes, as well as some metabolites, can also enter the cell. When exogenous insulin is supplied (injections) or endogenous insulin is produced (pancreatic release for glucose transport), shifts can also occur in these other substances. Increased insulin presence (exogenous or endogenous) drives intracellular electrolytes (phosphorus, potassium, magnesium) into the cells out of the bloodstream regardless of the amounts present in the bloodstream. In the case of refeeding syndrome, this can cause a sudden and dramatic decrease in the plasma levels of these electrolytes.

Prior to reintroducing food, the serum electrolyte levels are usually within normal ranges and may even be elevated.[20,22,23] During catabolism, as body cell mass shrinks, the intracellular ions (phosphorus, potassium, and magnesium) move in to the extracellular space.[20] From there, they are excreted through the kidneys as they reach the renal threshold. This loss through the kidneys will continue to happen even with continued depletion.[20]

During refeeding, these ions move back into the reexpanding intracellular space, and the serum levels can fall dangerously low within 24–72 h.[20,23] Treatment of uncontrolled diabetes with insulin can lead to identical electrolyte shifts.[20]

In addition to electrolyte abnormalities, another potential problem is fluid overload. Because of the decrease in functional reserve in the heart and kidneys, death from congestive heart failure is a possibility. If carbohydrates are reintroduced too quickly, the resulting fluid retention can overwhelm the patient's limited cardiac reserve causing heart failure.[20] Carbohydrate intake stimulates the release of insulin; one of the actions of insulin in addition to regulating glucose is to reduce sodium and water excretion.[20,24] Dextrose containing intravenous fluids can also cause the same problems without having food being given due to the rise in serum insulin levels driving the dextrose into the cells.

Risk assessment

Those patients most "at risk" for developing refeeding syndrome are the following:

Cats with hepatic lipidosis—the more severe, the more at risk

Diabetic ketoacidotics

Severe malnutrition/starvation

Hyperadrenocorticism (Cushing's disease)[21]

Phosphorus

Phosphorus in the form of phosphate is the most abundant intracellular anion.[21] Most intracellular phosphorus exists as organic compounds, such as creatine phosphate, adenosine monophosphate (AMP), and ATP.[19] Organic phosphate is also present in many compounds in the body such as phospholipids, phosphoproteins, nucleic acids, enzymes, cofactors, and biochemical intermediaries.[21] Phosphorus is involved in cell membrane integrity (the phospholipid layer), muscle and neurological function, carbohydrate, fat and protein metabolism, oxygen delivery from the RBC to the tissue, and the acid–base buffering system.[25] Phosphorus also aids in the transfer of energy to cells through the formation of ATP and is an essential component of bones and teeth.[25]

Most extracellular phosphorus is in the form of inorganic phosphorus; approximately 12–15% of this is protein bound, and the remaining 85–88% exists unbound as either monohydrogen phosphate or dihydrogen phosphate.[21] Only inorganic phosphate ions are measured when serum is analyzed for the presence of phosphorus.[21] Serum should be separated from cells within 1 h of sample collection; leakage of cellular organic phosphate into the serum may increase the inorganic phosphate concentration. Hemolysis can have the same effect.[21]

As with any ion found predominately in the intracellular space, serum concentrations do not represent total body stores.[21] Phosphorus normally shifts freely between the extracellular, intracellular, and bony compartments.[21] Hypophosphatemia does not imply that phosphorus depletion exists, just that it has shifted out of the measurable extracellular space.

Phosphorus moves into the cells with refeeding to support the increased production of phosphorylated intermediary components of energy metabolism. Severe hypophosphatemia, hemolytic anemia, and death can occur within 12–72 h of refeeding.

Because of the phosphorus requirements for the formation of ATP, signs of hypophosphatemia are often related to decreased energy stores and may include muscle weakness, anorexia, dysphagia, and respiratory failure caused by decreased diaphragmatic contractility and decreased cardiac output. Decreased oxygen delivery to cells, depleted cell energy stores, seizures, and coma may result.[25]

Severe hypophosphatemia may impair heart function by reducing the energy generating ability of the left ventricle. This is thought to be the result of depleted intracellular ATP stores and/or impaired calcium metabolism.[21] Approximately 20% of human patients show cardiac arrhythmias even when underlying heart disease was not present. After repletion of phosphorus, the severity of the arrhythmias improved.[19,21]

The RBC is the only tissue in the body that produces 2,3-diphosphoglycerate (2,3-DPG). 2,3-DPG is bound to hemoglobin and helps to enhance dissociation of oxygen from the hemoglobin molecule. A deficiency of RBC 2,3-DPG impairs the release of oxygen from the hemoglobin molecule, causing tissue hypoxia. A deficiency of phosphorus within the RBC affects not only its ability to function, but also the body tissues' ability to obtain oxygen.[19,21] This depletion also affects the phospholipid layer that helps maintain the cell integrity. This double hit causes RBC death and a secondary anemia.

Muscle contraction also requires ATP as an energy source; low concentrations of intracellular phosphorus results in depletion of these energy stores, causing muscular weakness and respiratory failure.[21]

ATP depletion is also the proposed mechanism by which hypophosphatemia may cause hemolysis. ATP is needed to maintain RBC membrane integrity, cell shape, and deformability. Glycolysis is the only means by which RBCs generate ATP. Decreased concentrations of inorganic phosphate therefore limit ATP production. ATP depletion may cause malfunction of the sodium–potassium pump, which causes decreased cell deformability and osmotic lysis. This can lead to severe hemolytic anemia.[23]

Phosphorus depletion can occur in the absence of hypophosphatemia in diabetic ketoacidosis. This is due to the effects of insulin on extracellular phosphorus and potassium and not necessarily due to the effects of "refeeding." Supplementation should be done in animals that have low normal or moderate hypophosphatemia prior to starting insulin therapy. Monitoring of serum phosphate is critical during the first 12–24 h after starting insulin and fluid therapy.[19,21]

Cats have low levels of hepatic glucokinase, the enzyme that phosphorylates glucose for hepatic use. This deficiency makes cats particularly susceptible to hyperglycemia when either feeding diets high in glucose or receiving fluids containing glucose.[23] This elevated serum glucose further stimulates the production of insulin, which causes an increased shift of phosphorus from the extracellular space into the intracellular space. Enteral diets high in simple carbohydrates can have the same effect.[21]

Potassium

Potassium is the primary intracellular cation, with at least 90% of the total body stores located in the intracellular space. Since potassium, like phosphorus, is located primarily intracellularly, serum levels often do not accurately represent the extent or severity of potassium deficiency, especially in cases of chronic disease. Potassium has a direct impact on cell, nerve, and muscle function by maintaining the cell's electrical neutrality and osmolality, aiding in neuromuscular transmissions, assisting skeletal and cardiac muscle contractility, and affecting the acid–base balance.[25]

Since potassium is an integral part of the sodium–potassium pump, hypokalemia usually results in muscle weakness and decreased GI motility.[25] An ECG will show prolonged repolarization (the period of time in which the Na^+–K^+ pump moves the potassium back into the cell and the sodium out), this causes a prolonged PR, QRS, and QT intervals, a decreased ST segment, and a flattened inverted T wave. When the plasma deficiency is severe, sinus bradycardia and heart block with atrioventricular dissociation can be seen.[25]

Insulin also pulls potassium along with phosphorus into the intracellular space with resumption of carbohydrate metabolism.[20,22] When potassium and glucose move into the cells with insulin, the Na^+–K^+ pump and glycogen synthesis is stimulated.

This further depletes the body of potassium since 0.33 mEq of potassium is required for each gram of glycogen produced.[22]

Magnesium

Magnesium is the second most abundant cation in the intracellular space. Approximately 60% of the body's magnesium can be found in the bones and teeth, 39% in the intracellular space, and less than 1% in the extracellular space. As with phosphorus and potassium, serum magnesium levels do not accurately reflect actual body stores because of the relatively small amounts found in the serum. Approximately 30% of the magnesium in the serum is protein bound; therefore, reduced albumin levels may falsely decrease the serum reading even if actual levels are within normal limits.[25]

Magnesium promotes enzymatic reactions within cells during carbohydrate metabolism and helps the body produce and use ATP. Signs of hypomagnesemia are similar to those seen with hypokalemia, respiratory muscle paralysis, complete heart block, and coma. Hypomagnesemia also causes an inappropriately high excretion of potassium through the urine, thus making worse any existing hypokalemia. This occurs because sodium–potassium ATPase, which is required for the reabsorption of potassium, is magnesium dependent. This also prevents correction of the hypokalemia even with high doses of potassium supplements until the hypomagnesemia is corrected.[20,22,25]

Hypomagnesemia can also cause a secondary hypocalcemia, which remains resistant to supplementation until magnesium is corrected.[20,22] This happens because with magnesium depletion, parathyroid hormone (PTH) is unable to elicit calcium release from the bone. Even though the body initially continues to secrete increased levels of parathyroid hormone to stimulate calcium release, the continued hypomagnesemia will eventually inhibit PTH secretion.[20,25] A patient with hypocalcemia due to hypomagnesemia may have a high, normal, or low PTH level. Animals with hypocalcemia can show signs of restlessness, muscle fasciculations, tetany, and convulsions.

Reintroduction of food

Current recommendations assert that no animal should go longer than 5 days without food.[26] As many of the animals that develop refeeding syndrome have already far exceeded this time frame, reintroducing food quickly is essential. It is important to keep in mind that the 5-day time frame is total days without food, not just hospital days.

It is essential that before starting nutritional support, rehydration, electrolyte, and acid–base status be addressed. We want to provide the best chance of a favorable outcome to our patients, and ensuring that everything starts off in the correct balance is essential to this.

When discussing nutritional support, the first consideration is how much food to feed. Using conservative energy estimates, as is now the current recommendation, the most accepted formulas would be RER = 70 × (body weight in kg)$^{0.75}$ or RER = 70 + (30 × body weight in kg). This formula can be used for animals weighing between 2 and 30 kg.[26] For cats, some recommend the alternate formula of RER = 40 × body weight in kg.

The ultimate goal would be to have the animal receiving 100% of their RER either through a feeding tube or orally soon after discharge from the hospital. Usually by this time, the animal is metabolically stable, tolerating the food well, off fluids and feeling better. Further nursing care can continue at home.

Recommendations for avoiding the refeeding syndrome

1. Anticipate the problem whenever a patient is at risk and refeed with formulations known to contain adequate levels of phosphorus, potassium, and magnesium.

2. Use initial nutritional refeeding rates not to exceed the patient's RER (30 × weight in kilograms) + 70. Consider refeeding a high fat, low carbohydrate diet to patients who have not eaten in more than 5 days, if their condition would not contraindicate such a diet.

3. Do not add extra energy to the caloric requirements by using an illness energy requirement adjustment to the RER.

4. Monitor phosphorus, potassium, magnesium, and PCV/TS at least daily, more often if indicated. Monitoring should start within 12 h of refeeding.

5. Supplement electrolytes as needed, either intravenous (IV) or with the food.

6. Monitor closely for signs of fluid overload and congestive heart failure.[20,22]

Conclusion

The take-home message here is to be aware, to monitor, and, when feeding, to "go slow, go low." Start feedings at 25–30% of RER with continuous rate infusion with a syringe pump works well for the first day. Some diarrhea is not unexpected in patients that have undergone prolonged starvation due to GI villous atrophy.

SECTION 4 DIAGNOSTIC PROCEDURES

Cystocentesis

Cystocentesis is performed to obtain a urine sample that is free of bacterial contamination from the distal urinary tract for urinalysis and/or culture, and in select emergent cases, to decrease the volume of urine in patients with a urethral obstruction. When properly performed, cystocentesis is a safe procedure. However, there are rare, serious, and even life-threatening complications that are seen more often with inappropriate techniques.

The relative contraindications of cystocentesis include uncooperative (unsedated) patients, ascites, coagulopathies, peritonitis,[1] insufficient urine volume, and the presence of a bladder mass within the bladder lumen. In addition, some authors suggest cystocentesis should not be performed in the presence of transitional cell carcinoma of the urinary bladder due to the increased risk of transfer of cancer cells along the cystocentesis needle track.[2]

The potential complications of cystocentesis include puncture of the abdominal aorta, vena cava, or an intra-abdominal organ (besides the urinary bladder); laceration of the bladder wall, leaking of urine into the abdomen from the cystocentesis site, transient hematuria, or bacterial contamination of the sample by inadvertent puncture of the small intestines or the colon.[3] Also, within 5–20 min postcentesis, transient clinical signs, unique to cats, have been reported characterized by collapse, respiratory distress, salivation, urination, and/or defecation. Although not proven, it is felt by some to be associated with vagal stimulation.[4,5]

Obtaining a diagnostic urine sample by cystocentesis

First, gently palpate the abdomen to assess the urinary bladder size and location. Insertion of a needle into the abdomen in the region of the urinary bladder without bladder palpation is not recommended as it increases the risk of complications. If the urinary bladder is not palpable or is too small to safely obtain a sample, the patient may be housed with access to water. A second attempt can be made in a few hours. In felines, do not allow access to a litter box during this time to avoid voiding of urine.

Cystocentesis may be performed in standing, lateral, or dorsal recumbency. The position chosen will depend on the operator's preference and patient comfort; for example, a patient with spinal or hip pain may resist being in dorsal recumbency.

Proper needle gauge, length, and insertion angle, as well as good restraint, will decrease the chance of complications. Although cystocentesis is generally well tolerated, sedation should be considered in uncooperative patients where movement during the procedure is a concern. To lessen the risk and amount of urine leakage postcentesis, the smallest gauge needle possible should be used. Some authors also suggest that reducing the volume of urine in the urinary bladder will decrease the risk of postcentesis urine leakage. The use of the shortest length of needle needed to reach the urinary bladder lumen reduces the risk of passing through the urinary bladder and the inadvertent puncture of the caudal vena cava and aorta. Historically, clipping hair and preparing the skin was not deemed necessary unless the patient was obviously dirty. In fact, a small study, conducted on 22 felines, revealed no bacterial contamination of samples when the hair was not shaved or the skin disinfected.[6] However, since the standards of care in veterinary medicine continue to rise, the study was very small and only cats were included; it is now the recommended practice to clip hair if needed and to disinfect the skin prior to insertion of the needle.

Palpate and immobilize the urinary bladder with the non-dominate hand so that it is either cranial or caudal to the operator's thumb; the location will depend on the bladder size and the operator's preference. Typically, a sterile 5- or 6-mL syringe with a 22- to 25-ga. 1.5-in. needle attached is chosen and is held in

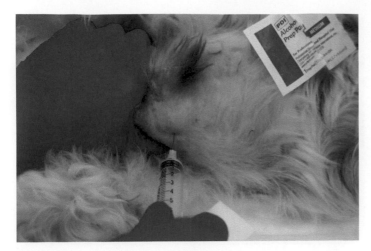

Figure 14.4.1 Hand position for cystocentesis.

the dominate hand, while the bladder is stabilized. The syringe should be held in a manner that will not require hand repositioning once the needle is in the bladder and aspiration begins. Place the needle cranial or caudal to the thumb (dependant on bladder location), through the skin in the ventral or ventrolateral abdomen, and into the urinary bladder. This approach reduces the risk of inadvertent puncture of the ureters and blood vessels that run dorsolaterally along the urinary bladder wall (Figure 14.4.1).

Pull back on the syringe plunger and aspirate 3–5 mL of urine. After releasing all negative pressure on the syringe, quickly remove the needle and syringe from the urinary bladder and abdomen. Releasing vacuum on the syringe prior to removal from the urinary bladder will help to prevent sample contamination by aspiration of intra-abdominal contents such as fat and intestinal bacteria.

To avoid laceration or injury of the urinary bladder or any internal structures, negative suction on the syringe should be immediately released and the needle removed quickly if there is any patient movement or blood obtained. Also, never blindly redirect the needle within the abdomen.

A new needle and syringe should be used for each centesis attempt to prevent contamination of the sample and to prevent spreading any bacteria that may be on the needle from the previous attempt.[7]

Ultrasound-guided cystocentesis

If ultrasound is available, it can be utilized to visualize small bladders and difficult to palpate bladders as seen in obese patients or in patients with tense abdomens. The procedure for an ultrasound-guided cystocentesis is the same as noted above except, instead of palpating the urinary bladder, the ultrasound machine is used to locate it. Avoid the use of ultrasound gel as a conduction medium since it may be inadvertently introduced into the abdomen during needle insertion; alcohol or water should be used.

Using the appropriate probe and settings on the ultrasound machine, the urinary bladder is visualized ultrasonographically.

Hold the probe in the nondominate hand with the notch (cranial marker) oriented toward the head of the patient in order to visualize a sagittal image of the urinary bladder. Optimize the settings on the machine (gain) to have a well-balanced image. The image of the urinary bladder should be adjusted (depth) to take up the entire screen. Once the distance to the far wall is determined, the appropriate needle length can be selected. This will decrease the chance of inserting the needle through the urinary bladder and into the colon or blood vessels. The needle is introduced into the bladder in the same orientation (parallel) as the ultrasound probe, along the notch on the front the probe, so that the needle can be visualized on the screen. Once in the urinary bladder, the syringe is then aspirated, observing the screen during the process to ensure the tip of the needle remains in the middle of the urinary bladder lumen during collection.

Therapeutic cystocentesis

This procedure may be performed in cases of urethral obstruction if the urinary bladder is overly distended and a urinary catheter cannot be readily passed. Therapeutic cystocentesis removes most of the urine from the urinary bladder, thereby relieving the excessive pressure within the urinary bladder lumen and temporarily addressing the obstructive effects on the urinary system (e.g., hydronephrosis and bladder wall necrosis[8]) and allowing time to relieve the urinary obstruction.

Abdominocentesis

Abdominocentesis is performed to confirm the presence of effusion, to obtain a diagnostic sample, and for therapeutic purposes. Therapeutic abdominocentesis will be discussed later in this section.

Blind abdominocentesis is a quick and simple procedure that may assist in the evaluation of a patient with abdominal disease or trauma. Limitations include inability to diagnose disease in the retroperitoneal space[9] and the potential for false positives and negatives (e.g., a false positive for peritonitis or hemoabdomen can occur from inadvertent sampling caused by a needle puncture of the intestine or spleen, respectively,[10] and small volumes or compartmentalized fluid can result in a false negative). It has been shown that at least 5–6 mL/kg of fluid must be present for a successful blind needle centesis.[11]

Complications from blind needle centesis include the development of a hemoabdomen from laceration of a blood vessel or organ (e.g., liver or spleen), peritonitis due to laceration of the intestine or other hollow viscus (internal organ), iatrogenic introduction of infection, or spread of a compartmentalized infection such as an abscess.

If blood is obtained during centesis, the needle should be immediately removed. The sample should be checked for clotting by injecting the sample into a blood tube without anticoagulants to rule out a traumatic centesis versus a hemoabdomen. Blood from a traumatic centesis will clot, whereas blood from within the peritoneal space (hemoabdomen) will defibrinate quickly and will not clot unless there is overwhelming ongoing hemorrhage.[12]

Ultrasound is a useful tool that can be utilized to guide aspiration of focal areas of fluid accumulation or compartments; however, it is not required to obtain a diagnostic sample. Additional procedures that may be performed include blind single- or four-quadrant centesis and diagnostic peritoneal lavage (DPL).

Contraindications for blind abdominocentesis include patients with coagulopathies, suspected abscess, large masses, pyometra, or other enlarged hollow viscera.[13]

As air may be introduced into the abdomen during centesis, abdominal radiographs should be obtained prior to centesis to avoid confusion when interpreting the radiographs. Iatrogenic free air in the abdomen may be misinterpreted as traumatic injury to a hollow viscus.

Laboratory samples collected should include EDTA tube for fluid analysis, slides prepared for cytology, culture media, and nonadditive red top tubes (RTTs) for possible chemistries. Which tests performed will depend on the suspected disease process. For example, if pancreatitis is suspected, an amylase may be performed on the abdominal fluid from the RTT and the results compared with those of a peripheral blood sample. If the abdominal fluid results are higher than the peripheral blood, it is a strong indicator for pancreatitis.[14]

Techniques

Blind abdominocentesis

When performing blind abdominocentesis, an over-the-needle IV catheter with or without additional fenestrations, or a 18- to 22-ga. 1.0- to 1.5-in. hypodermic needle may be used. Additional fenestrations in an IV catheter decrease the chance of occlusion, thus increasing the potential for a positive yield. Care must be taken when preparing and using the catheter. If the additional fenestrations are too large or close together, it will weaken the catheter, increasing the potential for a piece to break off within the abdominal cavity. To help maintain catheter integrity when aseptically adding additional fenestrations on the sides of a 14- to 18-ga. over-the-needle catheter, make sure they are smooth, never more than one-third the circumference of the catheter, and are spaced evenly apart (Figure 14.4.2).

Patient preparation should include emptying distended urinary bladders through voiding, expression, or catheterization to avoid inadvertent cystocentesis and a false positive for an uroabdomen. Left lateral recumbency is the preferred positioning, which will help avoid inadvertent splenic sampling. However, if due to a large quantity of effusion this position compromises the patient's comfort or ability to breathe, then standing may be the better option. Clip and aseptically prepare a large area of the ventral abdomen, from the xyphoid to the pubis. Preparing a large area in advance decreases the preparation time if a four-quadrant centesis is necessary. Local anesthesia is not required for needle centesis; however, it may be required when using a large-bore IV catheter. It is important to sedate uncooperative patients as any movement during the procedure increases the

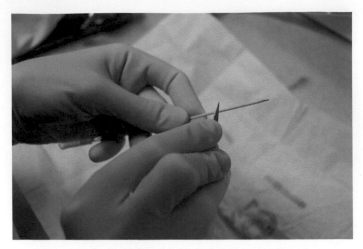

Figure 14.4.2 Demonstration of the technique to add fenestrations to an intravenous catheter.

risk of damage to internal structures; proper restraint is imperative for patient safety.

For a single-needle centesis with the patient properly restrained, after donning sterile surgical gloves, slowly insert a 22- to 18-ga. 1.0- to 1.5-in. needle or a fenestrated over-the-needle IV catheter into the abdomen, approximately 2 cm caudal and to the right lateral of the umbilicus. This approach will help avoid the spleen and also any falciform fat, which may interfere with sample collection.

Once the needle is in the abdomen, it may be gently rotated and the placement of a second needle approximately 2 cm caudal to the first may help to stimulate flow by altering intra-abdominal pressure. Any needle within the abdomen should never be blindly redirected. If using an IV catheter, once the catheter, and additional fenestrations if applicable, are within the peritoneum, the catheter is fed off the stylet and the stylet is removed.

Initially, a syringe should be left off to see if fluid flows by gravity alone. By allowing to free drip or to flow freely, you lessen the chance of occlusion by aspirating abdominal contents against the needle or catheter. If this method is successful, collect samples aseptically by allowing them to drip into previously mentioned specimen collection tubes. If fluid is not free flowing, carefully attach a 3-mL syringe and apply gentle suction. If the centesis is still negative at this point, remove the needle or catheter and perform a four-quadrant centesis (Figure 14.4.3).

Four-quadrant centesis

The four-quadrant centesis technique is similar in technique to single-needle centesis; however, rather than attempting to sample one area, needles will be consecutively placed in all four quadrants of the abdomen.

Visualize the four quadrants by dividing the abdomen into right and left cranial quadrants and into right and left caudal quadrants by crossing the lina alba and umbilicus, remaining medial to the mammary chain (Figure 14.4.4).

Aseptically place the needles in each quadrant, checking for a productive centesis at each site. Continue to place the needles in

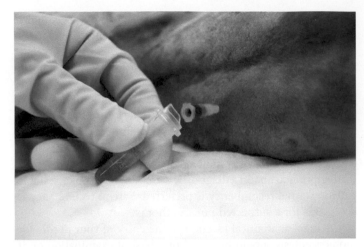

Figure 14.4.3 Image demonstrating abdominal fluid free dripping into a collection tube.

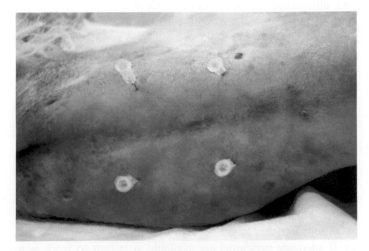

Figure 14.4.4 Needle position for a four-quadrant centesis.

each quadrant, leaving the previously placed needles in place to help stimulate flow. Continue until a positive result is obtained or until centesis has been performed on all four quadrants. Fenestrated catheters may also be used in lieu of a needle to help increase the chance of a positive sampling. If a diagnostic sample is not obtained, a diagnostic peritoneal lavage (DPL) may be performed.

Diagnostic peritoneal lavage

DPL is useful when small amounts of fluid are present as it can detect amounts as small as 1–5 mL/kg of fluid.[15]

In addition to the contraindications already listed, DPL on patients with potential trauma to the diaphragm should be excluded.

As described earlier, the patient should be properly restrained in left lateral or dorsal recumbency and the abdomen surgically prepared. Selection of catheter size will be dependent upon the size of the patient and thus the amount of fluid needed to be quickly infused. In smaller patients, an 18- to 20-ga. catheter

may be adequate. The location of catheter placement is the same as previously described.

If a large-bore catheter is to be used, aseptically instill lidocaine approximately two centimeters cranial and to the right of the umbilicus; include both the skin and body wall in the block. After waiting the appropriate time, a small skin stab incision is made usually with a number 11 scalpel blade. Introduce the 14- to 16-ga. over-the-needle IV catheter through the stab incision into the peritoneal cavity. Once the catheter is in place, remove the stylet and attempt to obtain fluid from this site. If the centesis is not productive, instill 22 mL/kg of warmed sterile saline into the abdomen by attaching an IV fluid bag and venoset or syringe and extension set to the catheter and quickly infuse the saline.

Gently rock the patient to distribute the fluid within the abdomen, taking care not to dislodge the catheter. Next, gently and slowly attempt to aspirate the fluid; place the sample in the appropriate containers as previously mentioned. The specimen will be diluted, and this must be taken into consideration when results are interpreted. As much of the instilled fluid as possible should be removed.

Therapeutic abdominocentesis

Excess effusion can cause the abdomen to become distended and tense, causing patient discomfort, and of greater concern, pressure on the diaphragm resulting in respiratory distress. There are many disease processes that may cause ascites, including, but not limited to, liver disease, cardiac disease, and neoplasia.

Currently, there is no consensus in veterinary medicine for the appropriate amount of fluid to be removed. Some recommend caution and to only remove enough fluid to relieve the respiratory distress and to increase patient comfort. However, others are concerned with the risks of frequent repeated centesis and recommend removing as much fluid as possible. Concerns with the removal of abdominal effusion include protein loss, volume depletion, stimulation of the formation of additional fluid, and infection.[16]

For therapeutic fluid removal, clip and aseptically prepare a wide area that is centered on, caudal to, and to the right of the umbilicus. The technique used to collect the effusion and the amount removed will be directed by clinician preference. Any of the techniques discussed previously may be used, for example, a hypodermic needle, over-the-needle IV catheters, or a fenestrated catheter attached to IV extension tubing and a three-way stop cock. Ideally, three people are available to assist with the procedure: one for restraint, one to insert and position the needle/catheter, and one to aspirate the fluid. The length and dimension of the catheter or needle selected will depend on the size of the patient and the volume of fluid to be removed. For example, a large-bore catheter up to 14 ga. by 3.5 in. can be used to efficiently remove large quantities of effusion in large breed patients. Obese patients may require longer catheters, and felines and small canines may do well with a butterfly catheter or a smaller-gauge IV catheter. Patients that have had chronic effusions may develop compartmentalized areas of fluid. If ultrasound guidance is available, it may prove helpful in identifying the best location for the most productive centesis.

The total volume of fluid removed should always be measured and recorded in the patient record. The patient should be reweighed after centesis to obtain an accurate weight.

Thoracocentesis

Thoracocentesis can be performed as a diagnostic procedure to collect a pleural effusion sample or as an emergent procedure to remove large volumes of pleural effusion or air. Complications of thoracocentesis include iatrogenic pneumothorax, lung laceration, hemothorax, and the introduction of infection. Relative contraindications include coagulopathy, thrombocytopenia, pulmonary bulla, as well as pleural space disorders not managed by thoracocentesis (e.g., pleural masses without effusions or pneumomediastinum without a pneumothorax).[17]

The pleural space is normally under negative pressure. It is occupied by a small volume of fluid that acts as a lubricant between the lungs, mediastinum, and diaphragm. In pleural space disorders, the normal flow of fluid, lymphatic drainage, hydrostatic pressure, or colloid osmotic pressure can be altered, resulting in a pleural effusion. Some causes of pleural effusions include blood from trauma or coagulopathy, chyle from cancers or idiopathic chylothorax, malignant effusion from cancers, modified transudate from heart failure, lung lobe torsion, or inflammatory process, or transudate from hypoalbuminemia.[18]

Normally, the mediastinum in dogs and cats is thin and semi-permeable to fluid. Some diseases can lead to inflammation, thickening, and a loss of this permeability, resulting in a unilateral pleural effusion.[19]

Air in the pleural space, pneumothorax, can be due to trauma, iatrogenic causes, or spontaneous. The causes of spontaneous pneumothorax include congenital abnormalities, ruptured lung abscesses, bulla, or advanced pulmonary disease. These patients are usually not known to have any history of pleural disease prior to presentation.[20]

A detailed history, thorough physical examination, and thoracic radiographs, when deemed safe to obtain, will help determine the cause of dyspnea in patients with pleural space disease. Thoracic auscultation often will reveal muffled heart sounds and lung sounds ventrally with effusion, either unilaterally or bilaterally, and dorsally with pneumothorax.

If the patient is not stable enough for radiographic conformation of a pneumothorax or pleural effusion, then thoracocentesis should be performed prior to any additional diagnostics tests and utilized as a diagnostic and lifesaving measure. If radiographs are deemed safe, a dorsoventral view can be less stressful; however, some patients may better tolerate a lateral view. Ideally, both radiographic views are recommended.

In all dyspnic patients, especially felines, stress should be kept to a minimum. Oxygen supplementation should begin upon presentation and continue during the patient's evaluation and treatment. Oxygen should be delivered via a method that is best tolerated by the patient (and therefore least stressful) and appropriate for the situation (e.g., flow-by or resting in an oxygen cage). Due to the fragile nature of dyspnic patients, you should always have the necessary equipment available for the possibility of respiratory arrest due to inadequate ventilation or patient fatigue due to increased respiratory effort. Fatigue may escalate into requiring general anesthesia and manual or mechanical ventilation.

When performing thoracocentesis, there are multiple options for patient positioning, and this will be determined by the stability of the patient and if effusion or pneumothorax is suspected. In emergent procedures, the patient should be allowed to assume a position of comfort as long as this allows appropriate access. If attempting to obtain a diagnostic sample of effusion on a stable patient, sternal recumbency is preferred. Lateral recumbency is acceptable for a suspected pneumothorax.

The exact anatomical location of the entry of your needle for thoracocentesis should be based on physical examination or, if available, radiographic findings. Another modality that can be helpful in collecting effusion is ultrasound. If only a small amount of effusion is present, or it has become compartmentalized, ultrasound guidance can be invaluable.

Most dyspnic patients will tolerate thoracocentesis with minimal restraint. Anesthesia and sedatives are avoided, if possible, but can be necessary in an uncooperative patient who will not safely permit thoracocentesis. If sedation is necessary, administration of a noncardiac or respiratory suppressive agent is recommended. See the respiratory anesthesia recommendations in Chapter 6.

There are several techniques used for thoracocentesis. A butterfly catheter, a hypodermic needle, and an IV over-the-needle catheter with an extension set, three-way stop cock, and syringe attached are all commonly used. The stop cock should always be turned off to the patient while the needle or catheter is being placed into the thoracic cavity. This will avoid an iatrogenic pneumothorax that might occur if the stop cock is open to the air. If adequate personnel are available, it is best to work as a team. One person works the stopcock and syringe, while the operator handles the needle, and a third and/or fourth person restrains the patient and provides flow by oxygen.

The technique used will be dependent on the patient, operator preference, and if fluid or air is expected. A 22- to 23-ga. butterfly catheter works well in nonobese felines and in small or thin canines. A hypodermic needle attached to a fluid extension set tubing can be used in larger patients. When determining the length and gauge of the needle or catheter to use, considerations include patient size, if effusion or air is to be removed, as well as type (e.g., a large-gauge needle is required for a pyothorax vs. a hydrothorax) and volume of effusion (e.g., in a large breed dog, a large bore, up to 14 ga. 3.5 in. through the needle catheter, will allow a large amount of chylous effusion to be removed efficiently; however, if air is being removed, an 18-ga. catheter may be more appropriate). The length must be able to adequately penetrate the thoracic cavity, and the smallest gauge should be used in order to avoid an iatrogenic pneumothorax due to a large needle tract.

One disadvantage of using a needle is the likely increased risk of creating a lung lobe laceration. The risk will increase as the air or fluid is removed, the lungs reexpand, and the lung margin is closer to the needle tip. The use of IV catheters has the advantage of a blunt atraumatic tip once the stylet is removed. Additional fenestrations may aseptically be added to the side of the catheter with a scalpel blade to assist in the removal of fluid (Figure 14.4.2). Make sure the fenestrations are smooth, not more than one-third of the circumference of the catheter, or spaced too closely to avoid structural weakening. The extra fenestrations lessen the chance of catheter occlusion if the effusion is flocculent. Disadvantages include kinking of the catheter or of a piece breaking off within the thorax. Prefenestrated centesis catheters are also commercially available.

Procedure

The patient should be clipped and a sterile surgical preparation performed prior to thoracocentesis. Initially, only one side of the chest may be clipped; this is true in unilateral effusions but also true if performing a diagnostic thoracocentesis. The hair should be clipped on both sides if a large bilateral effusion is present. The area to be prepped extends cranially from the 5th rib space caudally to the 10th rib space on the ventral one-half to two-thirds of the chest, although a much smaller area may be clipped for diagnostic thoracocentesis. The exception for a complete clip and surgical preparation is an emergent case, when it is acceptable to quickly clip a smaller area and wipe with an appropriate antiseptic.

The use of a local anesthetic is an operator preference. Arguments can be made for a local block (anesthesia to the area of centesis to improve comfort and cooperation) and against it (two needlesticks as opposed to one). If it is to be performed, a short-duration local anesthetic (i.e., lidocaine with or without sodium bicarbonate) is typically used.

After donning sterile gloves, the needle and the attached tubing are aseptically inserted between the sixth, seventh, or eighth rib, avoiding the vessels and nerves that run caudal to each rib. When air is suspected, the centesis should be directed toward the dorsal thorax; effusion will be ventral, near the level of the costochondral junction. Some feel it is easier to count spaces up from the last rib forward than it is to count down from the first rib backward.

Once the pleura has been punctured and therefore the needle tip is in the pleural space, the stop cock is opened to the patient and gentle aspiration on the syringe begins. This will assist in recognition of the appropriate needle depth as air or fluid is drawn into the needle or tubing. As the needle is advanced, the tip of the bevel should be directed toward the chest wall to avoid the bevel lacerating or puncturing the lungs during advancement. The needle may be redirected with a negative centesis, keeping the needle as parallel to the chest wall as possible. While the needle is being moved, continued gentle negative suction on the syringe will reveal a productive area. It is important to avoid the tendency to apply excessive suction on the syringe since this is likely associated with higher rates of lung trauma. If this fails, reposition the patient if tolerated; for example, roll the patient toward the side of the centesis or remove the needle and move to a different location within the parameters of the procedure. If this also produces a negative centesis, and there is a high suspicion of effusion, then centesis should be performed on the opposite side of the thorax, or if available, ultrasound guidance should be used. The addition of an extension set on the three-way stop cock allows the syringe to be emptied into your collection container with more ease and with less chance of splashing of the contents.

It is recommended with pleural effusions that centesis be performed on both sides of the thorax, even in the presence of a positive tap on the first side.

The technique for an IV catheter is similar; however, the exceptions are if a large-bore catheter is used, a local block and stab incision over the insertion site may be needed. Additionally, to avoid an iatrogenic pneumothorax due to the large needle tract, the overlying skin may be pulled 2 cm cranially prior to placement, thus allowing the skin to act as a seal once the needle is removed and the skin returns to its normal position. Once the catheter and, if applicable, added fenestrations are within the pleural space, the stylet is quickly removed, allowing the attachment of the extension tubing, three-way stop cock, and syringe.

If at any time during thoracocentesis the operator feels as if the lungs have come in contact with the needle or catheter, or frank blood is obtained, the needle or catheter should be withdrawn immediately. Blood may be indicative of a traumatic tap or a hemothorax. To differentiate between the two, check to see if the bloody effusion clots. Free fluid defibrinates and will not clot. If a hemothorax is diagnosed, only enough blood should be removed to relieve the respiratory distress as RBCs in the pleural space will be reabsorbed over several days.[21] Otherwise, when removing effusion or air, the largest amount possible should be removed. The site from which it was obtained, the measured total volume of fluid or air, the gross appearance of the fluid, and the postcentesis condition of the patient should be recorded in the patient's record. Additionally, if a large volume of fluid is removed, the patients should be reweighed to obtain an accurate and current body weight.

Any patient that has thoracocentesis performed should be monitored for several hours postcentesis for an iatrogenic pneumothorax due to a slow leaking puncture or laceration of the lung.

When fluid is collected, appropriate amounts should be saved in EDTA tubes for fluid analysis, sterile nonadditive RTTs for biochemical testing, aerobic and anaerobic culture swabs, and several slides should be prepared for cytology.

If negative pressure cannot be achieved or if multiple centesis are required to maintain negative pressure and normal respiratory rate and effort, then placement of an indwelling chest tube with a continuous suction device may need to be considered.

Numerous products are manufactured for use during centesis. One such device that is intended for use in place of a three-way stop cock and extension tubing is the Smart-Y* centesis device.[22] This device has tubing with two one-way valves and two locking injection ports attached to create a closed system. This allows for the appropriate direction of air or fluid movement during a procedure (Figure 14.4.5).

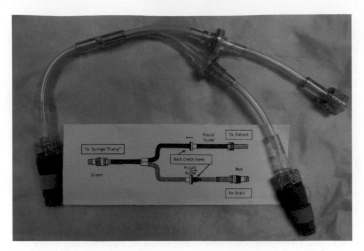

Figure 14.4.5   Example of a closed centesis device, the Smart-Y®.

Urinary catheters

Urethral catheterization is a common procedure performed in clinical practice and is often utilized for diagnostic as well as therapeutic purposes. Urinary catheterization may be needed to obtain a urine sample for diagnostic purposes (e.g., urine analysis, urine culture, urine cytology) when cystocentesis is contraindicated (i.e., bladder tumor present). Catheterization of the urethra may be utilized as a diagnostic aid to identify urethral obstruction or stricture. Documentation of the obstruction or stricture by instilling contrast media for contrast radiography is facilitated with urinary catheterization. Also, catheterization may be necessary to document urine retention or to monitor urine output. Therapeutic catheterization with an indwelling urinary catheter is often necessary in postobstructive or postsurgical cases and can be an essential part of nursing care for recumbent patients. Installation of medications through a urinary catheter may also be needed in some patients.

Types of urinary catheter

The common catheter types used in veterinary patients include soft polyvinyl ("red rubber") catheters (Kendall Sovereign®, Kendall, Mansfield, MA), semirigid polypropylene catheters (Kendall Sovereign, Kendall), and Foley balloon-tipped catheters (latex, Kendall, or silicon, Smiths Medical PM, Waukesha, WI) (see Figure 14.4.6). A stainless steel rigid "bitch" catheter (Jorgensen Laboratories, Loveland, CO) may be used in female dogs to collect a urine sample. The selection of a catheter is based on the indication of catheterization, the size of the patient, and the species. A soft and flexible catheter (i.e., polyvinyl, latex, or silicon) is less likely to induce trauma and is preferred for single catheterization. A Foley catheter is ideal when an indwelling catheter is needed. In dogs, the smallest-sized catheter that can be used will result in less trauma and secondary hematuria. Generally, sizes 3.5–10.0 Fr are used in male dogs (1 Fr unit equals 0.33 mm). In female dogs, sizes 5–12 Fr are typically used. The semirigid polypropylene tomcat catheters are often used in cats. Tomcat catheters are 3.5-Fr rigid polypropylene catheters that have either an open end or a closed end with side holes. The open-end catheter is shorter than the closed-end catheter (11.4 and 14.0 cm, respectively) and may not be of adequate length to empty the bladder in some cats. The open-end catheter, which allows for directed flushing of fluids into the urethra, is often utilized in urinary obstruction patients. However, the closed-end catheter causes less trauma to the urethra. Some emergency veterinarians prefer the Slippery Sam® tomcat urethral catheter (Surgivet, Smiths Medical PM, Inc., Wailesja, WI). This polytetrafluoroethylene (PTFE) rigid 3.5-Fr open-end urethral catheter has variable lengths (11–18 cm) and can be ordered with side holes.

Catheterization techniques

It is important to gather the needed equipment for catheterization prior to the procedure (see Table 14.4.1). The area around the urethral opening (prepuce and penis in the male, vulva in the female) should be gently scrubbed using a nonirritating surgical cleanser. The prepuce or vestibule can be flushed with a diluted antimicrobial solution, further disinfecting the area. Clipping of the fur can assist in providing an aseptic area, but care must be taken not to cause irritation of the skin in this sensitive area.

Sterile technique is mandatory to minimize contamination to the urinary tract. Technicians should thoroughly wash their hands prior to the procedure and should wear sterile surgical gloves. Placing sterile drapes around the area can allow easier

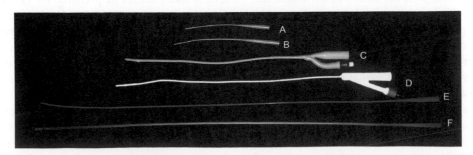

Figure 14.4.6   Common types of urinary catheters. A—open end tomcat catheter, B—closed end tomcat catheter, C—latex Foley catheter, D—silicone Foley catheter, E—polyvinyl "red rubber" catheter, F—polypropylene catheter.

Table 14.4.1 Equipment for urinary catheterization

Male dog or cat	Female dog or cat
Clippers	Clippers
Gauze sponges or cotton balls	Gauze sponges or cotton balls
Mild disinfectant	Mild disinfectant
Syringe for flushing	Syringe for flushing
Sterile aqueous lubricant	Sterile aqueous lubricant
Sterile urinary catheter	Sterile urinary catheter
Scissors to cut finger tab	Scissors to cut finger tab
Sterile surgical gloves	Sterile surgical gloves
Drape or sterile wrap from gloves	Vaginal or otoscope speculum
Appropriate urinary catheter	Light source
Drugs for sedation or anesthesia	Drape or sterile wrap from gloves
Sterile syringe or container for sample	Appropriate urinary catheter
	Drugs for sedation or anesthesia
	Sterile syringe or container for sample

Additional items for indwelling urinary catheter	
Sutured in place	Foley
Tape (if no tabs)	Appropriately sized syringe for balloon
Suture material	Sterile saline
Needle holder	Needle (for saline bottle— do *not* use on catheter)
Thumb forceps	
Suture scissors	

manipulation of the catheter without contaminating it against the animal's fur. The largest diameter catheter that will comfortably fit into the urethra should be chosen to prevent leakage of urine around the catheter. Diameter is less important when catheter placement is only for sample collection, but a catheter that is too small may be more difficult to pass and is more likely to fold on itself within the urethra (which can become a serious complication). The catheter should be long enough to reach the bladder comfortably. The catheter length should be measured against the animal's anatomy (while still in the sterile packaging) from the urethral tip (or vulvalar opening) to the estimated location of the urinary bladder. Many catheters have measurements on them that help to facilitate the proper insertion length. A sterile urinary catheter should be used and a small amount of sterile lubricant should be applied to the catheter tip. Sterile lidocaine gel can be used as an alternative if available and may

offer the benefit of local anesthesia. A gentle and careful approach is necessary to prevent trauma during the procedure. The use of force may result in severe trauma, such as rupture of the urethra or bladder.

Catheterization of the male dog

The dog is placed in lateral recumbency. Select an appropriate catheter size and measure the length of the catheter needed to pass the end of the catheter to the neck of the bladder. This step is very important to prevent coiling or knotting of the catheter within the bladder (see Figure 14.4.7). Retract the prepuce to expose the tip of the penis. The prepuce should be retracted during the entire procedure to maintain sterile technique. The end of the penis is cleaned with a mild disinfectant. Lubricate the end of the catheter with sterile aqueous lubricant. The packaging of the catheter can be cut to establish a "finger tab" to facilitate passage of the catheter into the urethral orifice and maintain sterile technique (see Figure 14.4.8). Insert the catheter into the external urethral orifice and advance the catheter gently to the premeasured length. Resistance may be encountered in the perineal region or in the area of the ischial arch. If there is difficulty passing the catheter in these areas, external palpation in the perineal region or rectal palpation may assist the passage of the catheter. When the catheter is advanced into the bladder (should be approximately to the premeasured length), urine should begin to flow through the catheter. The urine sample may be collected in a sterile container or withdrawn gently via a syringe.

Catheterization of the female dog

The patient is placed in sternal recumbency, some prefer the hind legs hanging off the end of the table. Excessive perivulvar hair is clipped and the area is cleaned and disinfected. A vaginal or sterile otoscope speculum can be used to directly visualize the urethral orifice (see Figure 14.4.9). Lubricate the end of the

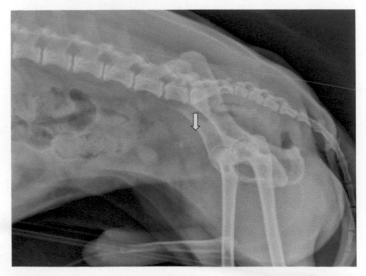

Figure 14.4.7 The urinary catheter is coiled within the urinary bladder (see arrow) of a dog due to improper measurement of the urinary catheter.

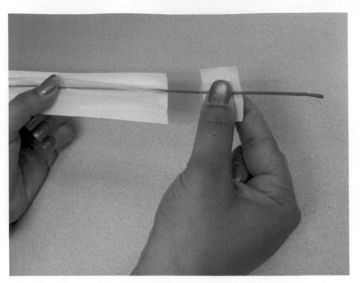

Figure 14.4.8   Urinary catheterization using the "finger tab" technique in a male dog.

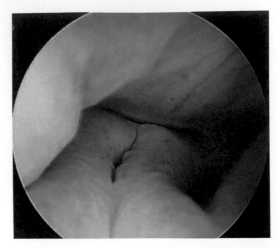

Figure 14.4.10   Endoscopic view of the urethral orifice of the dog.

obtained. Alternatively, a lubricated index finger can be inserted into the vaginal area and the urethral papilla can sometimes be palpated on the ventral floor. The catheter can be inserted ventral to the inserted finger, and fed into the urethral opening. The urine sample may be collected in a sterile container or withdrawn gently via a syringe.

Catheterization of the male cat

Most cats will require some degree of sedation or general anesthesia to facilitate gentle catheterization. Tomcat catheters are most commonly used to unblock male cats; however, red rubber or small Foley catheters are recommended for indwelling urinary catheters. It is important to premeasure the indwelling red rubber catheter length to prevent catheter folding or becoming knotted within the bladder. The cat is placed in lateral recumbency and the tail is held out of the way or in dorsal recumbency. The prepuce is disinfected and the penis is extruded and pushed dorsally to straighten the normal curvature. The catheter is lubricated and advanced into the urethral orifice until urine is obtained.

Catheterization of the female cat

As in the male cat, most female cats will require sedation or anesthesia. The cat is positioned in dorsal recumbency. The small cone of the otoscope can be used to visualize the urethral orifice. The catheter tip is lubricated and passed into the urethral orifice and advanced until urine is obtained. The feline urethra can be catheterized using the blind technique by directing the lubricated catheter slightly dorsal along the ventral floor of the vestibule. The catheter is advanced until urine is produced.

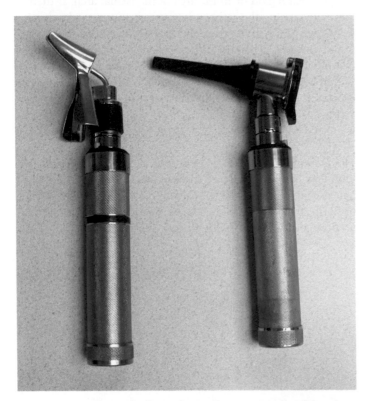

Figure 14.4.9   The vaginal speculum and otoscope are useful tools to catheterize a female dog.

catheter and insert the end into the urethral orifice (see Figure 14.4.10). Advance the catheter until urine is seen flowing from the catheter.

The blind catheterization technique may be performed when the urethral orifice is not easily visualized or in small patients. The catheter is inserted above the clitoral fossa and advanced in a cranioventral direction along the ventral midline until urine is

Indwelling urinary catheters

Indications for the use of indwelling urinary catheters include postobstruction diuresis, posturethral or bladder surgery, mechanism to measure urine output, decompressing a neurogenic bladder, or as a method to instill medication into the bladder.

When securing urethral catheters in place, thought should be taken to ensure maximum comfort for the patient. Poorly secured urinary catheters can cause discomfort and irritation to the skin and ureteral membranes. Urinary catheters without a balloon cuff must be sutured in place to prevent withdrawal during patient movement. Some catheters have anchor holes for suturing in place. If not, a piece of waterproof tape can be attached around the catheter in a butterfly pattern near the prepuce or vulva, and the tape can be attached to the skin with sutures. Placement of the tape too close to the penis or vulva and overtightening of the sutures in the patient can create dermal irritation and patient discomfort. Another method to secure the urinary catheter is tying a Chinese finger trap knot onto the soft catheters (i.e., red rubber or silicone urinary catheters).

Catheter care is important to prevent secondary urinary tract infections (UTIs). Flushing the vagina or prepuce with a mild disinfectant (e.g., 0.05% chlorhexidine solution) five times prior to placement is recommended. Catheter placement using sterile technique is mandatory. Maintaining a close collection system by attaching the urinary catheter to a sterile line and collection bag is important to help prevent secondary infections. A closed system uses an infection control urine drainage bag (Bard® Infection Control Urine Drainage Bag, Bard Medical Division, Covington, GA) and allows drainage without disconnection of the bag. In veterinary medicine, empty, recycled sterile IV fluid bags are attached to IV administration lines (macrodrips without backcheck valves) and connected to the urethral catheter. Barrett and Campbell performed aerobic cultures on stored used IV bags and demonstrated no bacterial growth in 95 bags when stored for ≤17 days. To empty the urine from the bag, the bag is disconnected and replaced with another empty IV bag. This system is considered open due to potential contamination between the bag and line. Technicians should wash hands and wear examination gloves when handling the urinary catheter, line and urine collection bag. Minimum nursing care of the patient with an indwelling urinary catheter involves regular visual inspection of the insertion site (for irritation), collection line (to ensure patency), and collection bag (to record volume and changes in urine color). The connections (catheter to line, line to collection bag) should be wiped with a disinfectant such as 0.05% chlorhexidine every 6–8 h. Urine collection bags should be changed every 6 h. Avoid having the catheter line and urine collection bag touching the floor by placing the bag on a clean blue pad (Chux, NorthShore Care Supply, Northbrook, IL) or cardboard tray (see Figure 14.4.11). Table 14.4.2 provides tips for troubleshooting problems of indwelling catheters.

Complications of urinary catheters

The major complications of urinary catheterization are trauma to the lower urinary tract and infection of the urinary tract. Trauma can be avoided by using smooth, soft and flexible catheters, and good technique. Hematuria, urethral spasms, or tearing of the urethral mucosa or bladder neck area can occur with poor technique or excessive force.

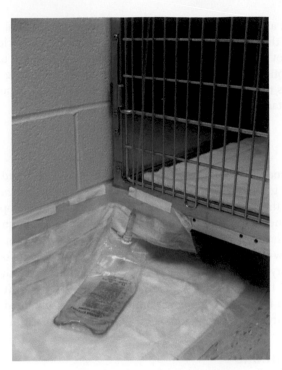

Figure 14.4.11   Example of a urine collection IV bag on a clean blue pad.

Table 14.4.2   Troubleshooting indwelling catheter and collection system

Problem	Solution
Urine not flowing into collection bag	
Line clamped off	Remove clamp
Catheter or line kinked or stuck in cage door	Tape lines to the side of the cage
Catheter is no longer in the urethra	Replace the urinary catheter
Collection line disconnected	Reconnect lines and tape
Urine not flowing from urethral catheter	
Clot or debris in the urinary catheter	Aspirate and/or flush catheter
Urinary catheter is kinked, coiled, or knotted in the bladder	Radiograph bladder, reposition or replace urinary catheter
Bladder is empty	
	Bladder or urethral rupture leading to uroabdomen

The normal flora of the distal urethra, prepuce, and vagina can be introduced into the bladder during catheterization. UTIs associated with indwelling urinary catheter have been reported in 10–59% of patients. Bubenik et al. found the odds of developing a UTI increased by 27% for each day the catheter was in place. Smarick et al. reported a low risk of UTI during the first

3 days after catheter placement. A study by Sullivan et al. suggested that the type of urinary collection system (open vs. closed) was not associated with the development of UTIs. The use of antibiotics to prevent infection in patients with indwelling catheters is not recommended due to the potential development of a resistant bacterial infection.

Bone marrow collection

Bone marrow biopsy or aspiration is a relatively quick and easy biopsy technique. The diagnostic procedure provides a means to access the cells of the bone marrow and, if indicated, a biopsy of the bone itself. In some practices, this technique is infrequently used; the clinician must be familiar with the techniques of bone marrow collection and handling of the sample in order to obtain a quality sample. Conversely, with proper training and if the law allows, this is a skill a veterinary technician can perform on a routine basis. Bone marrow samples should be submitted concurrently with a peripheral blood sample for comparison.

Indications

The indications for performing bone marrow sampling includes diagnosis of peripheral blood abnormalities of the RBC, white blood cell (WBC), or platelet cell lines, staging of neoplastic conditions, or as a test to further diagnose the causes of hypercalcemia, hyperproteinemia, or fever of unknown origin. Bone biopsy is indicated to evaluate lytic bone lesions.

Limitations

It is contraindicated in cases where sedation, anesthesia, or restraint is not possible, or in patients with a significant coagulopathy. However, it can be safely performed even in patients with severe thrombocytopenia with minimal hemorrhage. Bone marrow biopsy may miss limited or focal disease.

Advantages and disadvantages

If the clinician is comfortable with the procedure, bone marrow biopsy is relatively easy to perform, produces minimal trauma, and has a fast turnaround time.

The disadvantage is that specific equipment is required (must use a bone marrow needle), and depending on case load, may not be performed often enough to become proficient.

Potential complications

Complications with bone marrow aspiration are rare and include a minimal chance for infection or hemorrhage, even in thrombocytopenic patients. When using the most cranial aspect of the humerus with the needle direction toward the elbow, there is a slight chance of needle slippage into the joint capsule. If this occurs, the needle should be repositioned. If joint fluid is aspirated, a new needle should be chosen and redirected. When using the femur collection site, there is a slight chance for damage to the sciatic nerve should the needle slip off the periosteum; however, this is a rarely reported complication.

Contraindications

Sedation and local anesthesia to full anesthesia is required; restraint may be needed.

Patient preparation

If sedation or anesthesia is to be used, the patient should be fasted for 8–12 h prior to the procedure. Most patients tolerate this procedure with moderate sedation and local anesthesia. However, the aspiration portion of the procedure is painful; therefore, general anesthesia may be indicated; this is especially true in cases where the patient is difficult to restrain due to its size or behavior. General sedation with a benzodiazepine/opioid combination, propofol CRI, general anesthesia with induction and inhalant (isoflurane/sevoflurane), or local anesthesia with manual restraint are all commonly used protocols. The aspirate site is then shaved with approximately 2- to 3-in. margins around the desired entrance of the needle. Nonsterile localization of anatomy may be helpful in determining the area to be prepped. Once the area is shaved, a surgical scrub should be performed. Once the scrub is performed, aseptic technique should be followed. Using a gloved hand, sterile location of landmarks should be performed. If desired, a local anesthetic may be used at this time by injecting 0.25–0.5 mL from the periosteum to the surrounding tissues. Either 2% lidocaine or 0.5% bupivacaine is used. Lidocaine has a 5- to 10-min onset of action and a 1- to 2-h duration, where bupivacaine has a 20-min onset of action but typically lasts for up to 4–6 h. When using a local anesthetic and restraint or minimal sedation, it is important to be aware of the onset of action and duration of action for local anesthetics. Starting the procedure late or prematurely can cause unnecessary pain/distress to the animal and can greatly affect the ability to obtain a quality sample. It is also important to note that local anesthetic will not provide any relief for the actual aspiration portion of the procedure, which is the most painful. However, the use of local anesthetic can often provide significant postprocedure analgesia. Depending on the location selected, the animal may be in right or left lateral recumbency or in sternal recumbency. For aspiration of the femur or humerus, right/left lateral recumbency is chosen (based on dominant hand). When the iliac crest is chosen, the animal should be placed in sternal recumbency.

Patient monitoring

Anesthesia and sedation should be monitored as usual. Monitor the skin site postbiopsy for hemorrhage. Monitor patients postbiopsy for signs of hemorrhage (e.g., increasing heart or respiratory rate, pale mucus membranes, or decreasing blood pressure). Firm pressure may be applied to the biopsy site for 5 min postprocedure to facilitate clotting. Following either bone marrow aspiration or bone marrow core/biopsy, the patient should be monitored for pain. Pain levels can vary between patients and most may benefit from mild analgesia for 1–2 days postprocedure.

Techniques

The materials needed are as follows:

1. Bone marrow needle of choice

2. Sterile gloves

3. #11 scalpel

4. Sterile surgical drape (optional)

5. 10- to 12-mL syringe

6. Suture/surgical glue (optional)

7. Slides

8. Anticoagulant (EDTA or acid citrate dextrose [ACD])—optional

9. Plain PCV tubes (optional)

Personal preference and the patient size and condition will dictate the selection of the site for harvesting the bone marrow. The most common sites for the collection of bone marrow are the proximal humerus, the trochanteric fossa of the femur, and the iliac crest of the hip. The greater tubercle on the proximal humerus is often chosen for its large, flat surface area and small amount of surrounding tissue. When using this area, the bone marrow needle is inserted perpendicular to the greater tubercle.

Each location has its own advantages and disadvantages, including accessibility, overlying tissue thickness, and the size of the area for needle placement. The greater tubercle can be difficult to access in large dogs due to the general thickness of the periosteum; however, if the humerus is still the desired location, the most cranial aspect may be used by inserting the needle parallel to the length of the bone in the direction of the elbow. The trochanteric fossa of the proximal femur is often chosen for cats and small dogs. The needle is inserted into the trochanteric fossa parallel to the long axis of the femur. The iliac crest can be difficult in large, muscular, or obese patients as there is often a large amount of tissue covering the area. The widest, most dorsal portion of the wing is used and the needle is positioned perpendicular to the widest, most dorsal aspect. The sternum and rib have also been used for bone marrow collection but is typically not recommended due to the possibility of damage to vital structures should needle slippage occur.

The type of bone marrow needle selected is also clinician and patient driven. The most frequently used are the Illinois sternal, the Jamshidi*, and the Rosenthal. They come in a variety of gauges (15–18) and in a variety of lengths starting at 1 in. Jamshidi needles are typically reserved for bone marrow core or biopsy.

There are several anticoagulant options available for bone marrow aspiration including EDTA, ACD, or none. The choice of anticoagulant is based on personal choice, availability, and choice of slide preparation method. The most commonly used anticoagulant is EDTA. This can be difficult to find alone as an injectable; however, it can be compounded by capable pharmacies. If EDTA is desired and unable to be found, 0.5 mL of sterile saline may be added to a 7-mL EDTA blood tube to produce a solution for use. The other anticoagulant option is ACD solution from a blood collection bag, which is also available by the vial. With either anticoagulant, 0.5–1.0 mL is sterilely drawn into the syringe used to aspirate the sample and is allowed to coat the inside. The anticoagulant may then be flushed through the bone marrow needle to coat the inside, and either discarded, placed in a plain Vacutainer®, or into a Petri dish/cup/syringe cap for collection of individual spicules.

After sterile confirmation of landmarks, a #11 scalpel blade is used to make a small stab incision where the needle will be entering the tissue. This will allow for little resistance and easy seating of the needle on the periosteum. Use the nondominant hand to stabilize the limb. The bone marrow needle should be held with the dominant hand in a fashion similar to a pen, with the cap of the needle being braced by the palm or butt of the hand. It is important to ensure that the stylet is secured in place and completely occluding the lumen. Insert the needle through the stab incision and allow it to rest on the periosteum. Using rotating or clockwise–counterclockwise motion and gentle pressure, seat the bone marrow needle into the periosteum. Excessive pressure or movement can cause slippage. If this occurs, repositioning is required before further advancement of the needle should take place. Once the needle is seated well, continued gentle pressure and twisting should occur for several millimeters (varies depending on the size of the animal) until the needle has reached the marrow. When this occurs, the needle should be firmly planted into the bone and should move with the limb. A gentle tap of the end of the needle can also help determine if it is well seated.

Keeping a sterile field, the stylet is removed and a 10- to 12-mL syringe is quickly attached. Using 5–8 mL of negative pressure in two to three quick bursts of aspiration, 0.5–1.0 mL of bone marrow should be collected. If a sample is not obtained at this time, the stylet can be replaced and the needle advanced further and then aspirated a second time. If a sample is not obtained after further advancement of the needle, complete removal and repositioning should be considered. Once the sample is aspirated, the syringe should be quickly removed and slide preparation or bone marrow concentration should begin. Bone marrow will clot in less than 60 s and, once clotted, will be unusable as a diagnostic sample. Once the sample is placed either on slides or in the anticoagulant, the stylet should be replaced. At this time, microscopic evaluation should be performed to confirm that a diagnostic sample has been obtained (prior to removal of the bone marrow needle or recovery of the patient). Once the sample has been verified, the needle may be removed and direct pressure should be applied to the site. A small suture or surgical glue may be used if desired.

Bone marrow slide preparation

Slide preparation and verification of a diagnostic sample are imperative to bone marrow aspiration. As stated before, slide preparation can be dictated by the choice of anticoagulant. If no anticoagulant is used, brisk slide preparation at the time of aspiration should be performed as bone marrow will clot very quickly. A "drip" method can be performed by placing several slides upright and allowing a drop of bone marrow to fall down the slide. Once several slides have received a sample, a "spreader" slide may be used to smear the sample. Samples may also be placed on a slide laying on a flat surface prior to smearing. If an anticoagulant is used, the sample should go immediately into a storage container, either a plain Vacutainer or Petri dish. It is important to keep an approximate 1:1 ratio of bone marrow to anticoagulant to prevent clotting. Once the bone marrow is in the anticoagulant, slides should be prepared within 1 h.

A common practice in preparing bone marrow samples for cytology is a spicule collection or concentration method. With this procedure, approximately 1 mL of anticoagulant is placed in a plain Petri dish. If a Petri dish is unavailable, a paper/Styrofoam cup or a 35- to 60-mL syringe case cap may be used as well. Once the bone marrow sample has been aspirated, it is immediately placed into the dish containing the anticoagulant and gently swirled to mix. The dish is then tilted at a 45° angle allowing the sample to slide down, revealing the small spicules, which tend to stick to the surface of the dish. The spicules can be identified as small, irregular grains and can be collected with a plain PCV tube. The spicules may then be tapped or blown out onto a slide for squash preparation. This method has several benefits in that it allows the technician to make a large number of slides without the threat of coagulation, as well as provides a concentrated sample of bone marrow spicules to the pathologist.

Once the sample is on the slide, either via dripping, dotting, or a PCV tube, a second slide should be placed over the sample to create a "squash" prep, or compression smear, using a "slide over slide" technique. This may be done by placing the top, or spreader, slide either parallel or perpendicular to the slide containing the sample. If the spreader slide is placed perpendicular to the sample slide, the sample is allowed to spread for a few seconds, and then the spreader slide is gently pulled down the length of the sample slide with an even, steady motion. If the spreader slide is placed parallel to the sample slide, a small section of each slide should be left on either end for grip. Once the sample has spread for a few seconds, the slides are then steadily pulled down their lengths. With either method, it is important to place little to no downward pressure on the sample, which can lead to sample damage and nondiagnostic slides. When the samples are smeared out correctly, the bone marrow spicules can be seen grossly as a fine, granular material. In hemodilute but still diagnostic samples, this may not be grossly observed. Typically, a minimum of 4–5 unstained slides and a maximum of 10–15 unstained slides are submitted.

Verification of diagnostic sample

Verification of a diagnostic bone marrow aspiration is important to perform prior to the recovery of the animal from anesthesia or sedation. This step provides a second chance to obtain a diagnostic sample if needed, without additional stress or sedation/anesthesia to the animal. Once several slides have been prepared, one should be chosen and stained. In hospital, "diff-quick" stains are sufficient; however, it should be noted that due to the thickness of the bone marrow smear in contrast to a peripheral blood smear, increased staining time is recommended. Once the slide has been stained and air-dried, it should be microscopically evaluated. Evaluation should begin on the lowest objective (10×); this will help evaluate the quality of slide preparation as well as ensure that bone marrow collection occurred during the aspiration. Once slide quality is determined, a brief, high power examination (100×—oil immersion) can be performed to identify cells located within the bone marrow, ensuring a diagnostic sample. Once these RBC/WBC precursors are identified, adequate bone marrow aspiration has occurred and the patient may be recovered, and the remaining unstained slides may be submitted for pathology.

Most clinics do not have on-site pathologists, so shipment of unstained bone marrow slides is typical. It is always beneficial to reserve one to two unstained slides in the event that additional testing (immunofluorescent assay [IFA]/polymerase chain reaction [PCR]) is required. Once the slides have been allowed to air-dry, the samples should be packed in slide holders to prevent breakage. When shipping slides, it is important to ship them separate from formalin samples as the fumes can affect the staining performed by the pathologist and can lead to a nondiagnostic submission. In addition, a recent or concurrent complete blood count (CBC) and fresh peripheral blood smear should be provided to the pathologist, as well as a patient history, to assist in obtaining a diagnosis.

Bone biopsy

Under some circumstances, a bone marrow aspiration will be unable to provide a diagnostic sample, due to either inadequate collection technique or the patient's underlying disease state. In this circumstance, a bone marrow core may be obtained to provide better diagnostic information, although it is always recommended to attempt aspiration first as this is less invasive. Because there will be no hemodilution of the sample, bone marrow core samples can often provide a clearer picture of the cellularity and functionality of a patient's bone marrow. The sample site and preparation are similar to bone marrow aspiration; however, an anticoagulant is not used. The procedure is most commonly performed with a Jamshidi bone marrow needle due to its length and large diameter lumen. The Jamshidi also has a tapered end with a beveled cutting edge, which is used to excise a section of bone marrow. Alternately, a Goldenberg Snarecoil bone marrow needle will capture the sample, making breaking off the sample unnecessary. If a bone marrow aspiration has been performed, it is recommended to choose a different site for core collection. In addition, due to the pain associated with this procedure, general anesthesia is recommended.

Once the selected area has been surgically prepped and a local anesthetic applied, if desired, a stab incision is made as previously described for aspiration. The advancement of the needle is the same as with the aspiration technique; however, once the marrow is reached, the stylet is removed and the needle is rocked/rotated in approximately 1-in. circles to excise a small piece of bone marrow. The needle is then removed and a shepherd's hook tool provided with the Jamshidi needle is used retrograde to expel the sample through the proximal end of the needle. It is not recommended to force the sample back through the tapered end as damage can occur. Once the sample is removed from the needle, a small portion should be cut off using a scalpel. The largest portion should be placed in formalin for histopathology. The small section that was removed should be used to make slide samples by either rolling the sample down a slide or by making an impression smear. Making these extra slides will allow for additional testing, such as IFA or PCR, which cannot be performed once the sample is fixed in formalin.

To make a roll slide, the sample is gently rolled or pushed over a slide with a 20- to 22-ga. needle, creating tracts of bone marrow cells. An impression, or imprint smear, may also be made by holding the section of bone marrow core on the end of a needle, or with a small pair of forceps, and by repeatedly applying gentle pressure to the slide.

Once the core sample is obtained, direct pressure should be applied to the area and the patient should be monitored for hemorrhage and pain.

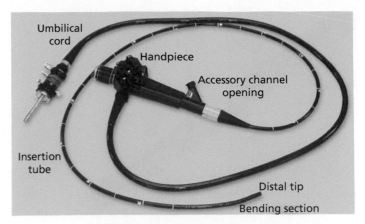

Figure 14.5.1 Olympus flexible fiberoptic endoscope XP20.
Source: http://www.endoscopy.com

SECTION 5 ENDOSCOPY

Endoscopy is a medical procedure that permits visualization of the interior of an organ (e.g., stomach with gastroscopy) or cavity (e.g., abdomen with laparoscopy) in a minimally invasive manner and, in many cases, simultaneously can be used to obtain a diagnostic sample (e.g., biopsy) or removal of a foreign body. Endoscopy is performed by utilizing either a flexible or a rigid endoscope, a light source, and a light-transmitting cable.[1] Although this is the minimal requirement to perform endoscopy, many accessory items (e.g., biopsy instrument) are frequently utilized when performing endoscopy. In many facilities, the veterinary technician is the main person responsible for the care of this very costly investment. This section will discuss flexible endoscopy and then rigid endoscopy.

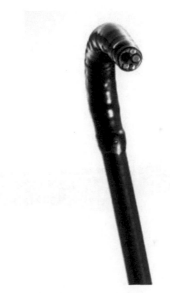

Figure 14.5.2 Insertion tube with a 2.8-mm channel—end-on view.
Source: http://www.endoscopy.com

Flexible endoscope

In order to understand how to handle, use, and clean a flexible endoscope, it is critically important to know the type of endoscope, the parts of the endoscope, and a number of endoscope safety precautions to prevent damage and costly repairs. The two basic types of flexible endoscopes are fiberoptic and videoendoscope. Fiberoptic endoscopes transfer images and light via optical glass fibers that are bundled together and surrounded by glass cladding. While with videoendoscopes, the image is transmitted electronically. The advantages of the fiberoptic endoscope include a less costly endoscope (compared to the videoendoscope), good image quality, and a wide range of endoscope diameters. Outer diameters range from as small as 2.3 mm to larger than 9.8 mm. The main advantage of the videoendoscope is an excellent image quality; however, these endoscopes are more costly and currently have limitations to the available diameters (which likely will not be an issue over time due to advances

in chip miniaturization).[1] The diameter size of the endoscope is the main limiting factor in the use of an endoscope.

There are three main sections of the fiberscope: the insertion tube, the handpiece, and the umbilical cord (see Figure 14.5.1). The *insertion tube* is a complex and fragile section that contains the many fiberoptic bundles to transmit images and light, multiple channels to permit suction, irrigation, and insufflation and an accessory channel to pass instruments, deflection cables (either two or four, depending on the type of endoscope, two- or four-way) and several layers of protective materials.[1] The bending section of the insertion tube is the last several centimeters, which are controlled via the deflection cables. Within the insertion tube, at the end of the fiberoptic bundles and the distal tip of the endoscope, is the objective lenses (see Figure 14.5.2), which serve to focus the image of the interior of the organ.

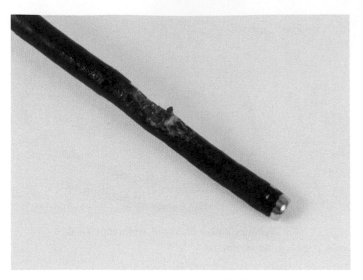

Figure 14.5.3   Damage to insertion tube of flexible endoscope.
Source: http://www.endoscopy.com

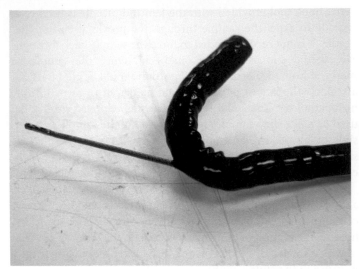

Figure 14.5.5   Hole in bending section of flexible endoscope.
Source: http://www.endoscopy.com

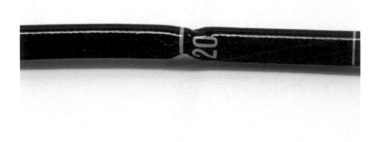

Figure 14.5.4   Bite damage to insertion tube of flexible endoscope.
Source: http://www.endoscopy.com

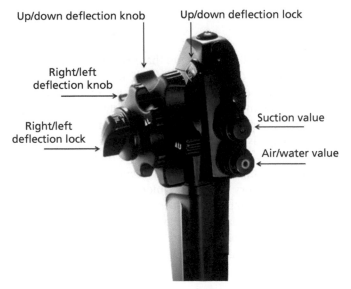

Figure 14.5.6   Video gastroscope GIF160 body close-up.
Source: http://www.endoscopy.com

The depth of field, which is determined with the ocular lenses in the eyepiece (see below) and the objective lenses, is from 3 to 100 mm in modern fiberscopes.[1] Due to the complexity of this section and the associated fragility of the parts, this section is the most costly to repair. Four very important tips on preventing damage to the insertion tube include the following[1]:

1. Avoid damage by preventing accidental striking of the insertion tube on hard surfaces (see Figure 14.5.3).

2. Ensure the endoscopist does not create a sharp bend, tight coiling, or twisting of the insertion tube.

3. Always use a mouth speculum when passing the tube through the oral cavity to protect the tube from inadvertent bite damage (see Figure 14.5.4).

4. Be very careful when passing items in the accessory canal and do not force equipment, especially if the insertion tube is being bent by the endoscopist (see Figure 14.5.5).

The *handpiece* (see Figure 14.5.6), designed to be held with the left hand, allows the endoscopist to control the tip of the insertion tube, to keep a clear image by the use of the suction, air, and water channels, and to visualize the interior of an organ and pass equipment in the accessory channel. It contains deflection control knobs and locks, suction and air/water valves, the eyepiece and diopter adjustment ring, and an opening to the accessory channel. The first valve on the handpiece (from the eyepiece) is the suction valve, which is activated by fully depressing the

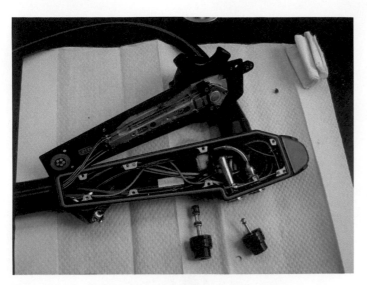

Figure 14.5.7   Storz endoscope handpiece with open cover.
Source: http://www.endoscopy.com

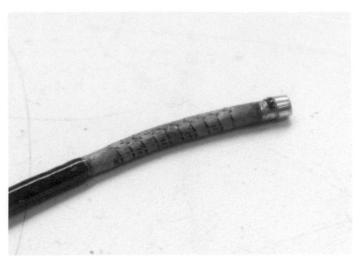

Figure 14.5.8   Corroded bending section of a flexible endoscope.
Source: http://www.endoscopy.com

valve. The second valve permits air insufflation by covering the hole in the valve with the fingertip, or water irrigation by fully depressing the valve (see Figure 14.5.7). For endoscopes with only a two-way deflection (e.g., bronchoscopy), the single up/down knob is controlled with the thumb of the left hand. For endoscopes with four-way deflection (e.g., gastroscopy), the larger knob is for up/down deflection and is controlled by the thumb of the left hand, and the smaller knob is for right/left deflection and is controlled by the right hand. A right/left deflection lock is attached to the smaller knob to allow a four-way deflection endoscope to work like a two-way endoscopy; it is important to set this to the unlock position when using the right/left deflection to avoid damaging the deflection cable. The right hand (or an endoscopist assistant) also controls the passage of the insertion tube through the mouth, applying rotational torque if needed, while avoiding excessive torque, and inserts equipment into the accessory channel.[1]

The *umbilical cord* is a very important section for the care of the flexible endoscope. This section is the portion that connects to the light source and has connectors for the air insufflation pump and water irrigation bottle (in four-way deflection endoscopes), suction pump, and a pressure compensation valve. As with other sections of the endoscope, it is important to carefully handle the umbilical cord to avoid damage to the light carrying fiber bundles passing through it. The pressure compensation valve prevents damage from external pressure changes (e.g., during ethylene oxide [EtO] sterilization or shipping by air). Also, the very important air leak tester attaches at this valve. The air leakage tester is critically important to detect internal leaks, and this should be used both before and after each use. After the manometer-type air leak tester is attached to the pressure compensation valve, the pressure bulb is compressed until the endoscope's manufacturer's specified desired pressure is reached, and then the needle of the pressure gauge is watched to ensure the

pressure remains stable.[1] This one step can allow early detection of leaks and can prevent costly water intrusion damage to the internal components of the fiberscope (see Figure 14.5.8), which is not always covered in warranty repairs.

Videoendoscope

The main sections and functions of the *videoendoscope* are similar to the fiberscope with one primary difference, the way the image is produced. Instead of fiberoptic bundles transferring an image, an electronic image is produced by a special device (CCD chip) in the distal tip of the endoscope and is transmitted along wires in the insertion tube to a processor. The processor can convert this electronic image into standard video signal, which can be viewed on a monitor, stored in an image storage system (e.g., computer or USB hard drive, CD, DVD, videocassette recorder), or transferred to a picture archiving and communication (PAC) system and printed.[1] An endoscopic video camera can be attached to the eyepiece of a fiberscope to accomplish indirect videoendoscopy; however, the videoendoscope provides a higher quality image than the fiberscope.[1]

Instrumentation

The accessory channel of both the fiberscope and videoendoscope is designed to accommodate a wide range of flexible instruments (see Figures 14.5.9–15). These instruments include biopsy and foreign body retrieval forceps, cytology brushes, injection/aspiration needles, polypectomy snares, aspiration tubing, mucous traps, scissors for cutting, and unipolar or bipolar coagulation. Instruments designed for use with a particular endoscope should be used whenever possible to avoid damaging the accessory channel. Other important techniques to avoid damaging the accessory channel include the following:

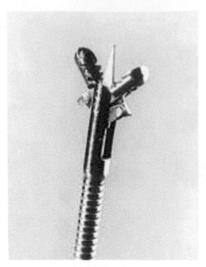

Figure 14.5.9   Serrated needle biopsy forceps—close-up.
Source: http://www.endoscopy.com

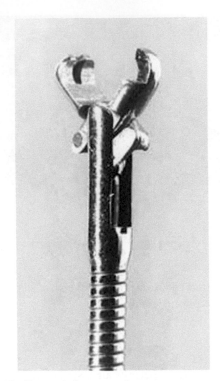

Figure 14.5.11   Rat tooth forceps—close-up.
Source: http://www.endoscopy.com

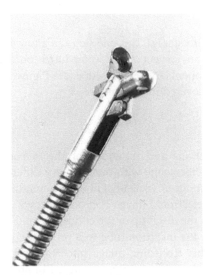

Figure 14.5.10   Oval cup forceps—close-up.
Source: http://www.endoscopy.com

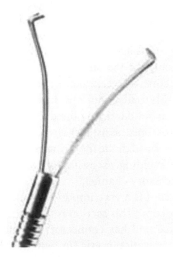

Figure 14.5.12   Forked jaw forceps—close-up.
Source: http://www.endoscopy.com

Only pass instruments with a diameter that does not exceed that recommended by the manufacturer; never force the instrument when resistance is met; follow the manufacturer's recommendations when passing instruments through a deflected tip; and do not remove foreign objects through the accessory channel; rather, with the foreign body firmly grasped pull the endoscope from the patient.[1]

Rigid endoscopes

In contrast to flexible endoscopes, rigid endoscopes do not have deflection cables or knobs, and as their names suggest, have a rigid tube, termed a telescope, which attaches to an eyepiece (see Figure 14.5.16). Rigid endoscopes are used when performing rhinoscopy, urethrocystoscopy, vaginoscopy, laparoscopy, and

thoracoscopy. The ranges of outer diameter sizes are 1.9–10.0 mm with 2.7, 4.0, 5.0, and 10.0 mm being the most common. Larger scopes produce a brighter and larger image; however, smaller scopes are less invasive and fit into smaller openings.[1] Also, in contrast to flexible endoscopes, rigid endoscopes are available with a range of viewing angles. The viewing angle is located at the distal tip of the telescope and includes 0° (forward viewing, same as a flexible endoscope) and 25° or 30° (which permits the endoscopist to view a larger area by rotating the endoscope).[1]

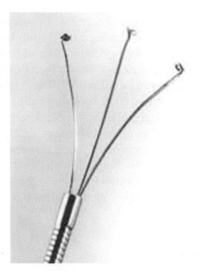

Figure 14.5.13   Tripod forceps—close-up.
Source: http://www.endoscopy.com

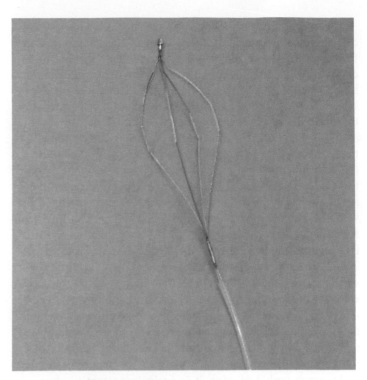

Figure 14.5.15   Basket forceps—close-up.
Source: http://www.endoscopy.com

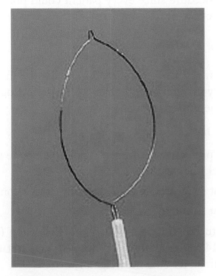

Figure 14.5.14   Small oval snare forceps—close-up.
Source: http://www.endoscopy.com

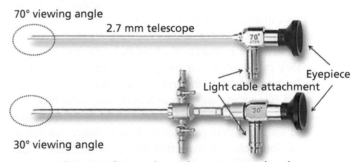

70° viewing angle
2.7 mm telescope
Eyepiece
Light cable attachment
30° viewing angle
2.7 mm telescope in urethrocystoscopy sheath

Figure 14.5.16   Rigid 2.7-mm telescope.
Source: http://www.endoscopy.com

Choosing the correct telescope size and viewing angle is an important part of setting up and performing rigid endoscopy. Due to the smaller available opening, rhinoscopy is often performed using a 2.7-mm telescope with either a 0°, 25°, or 30° viewing angle. Urethrocystoscopy and vaginoscopy are performed with either the 2.7-mm telescope (females weighing 5–45 lb) or the 4-mm telescope (females weighing greater than 15 lb), and often, a 25° or 30° viewing angle is utilized to maximize visualization. Urethrocystoscopy using a rigid endoscope in males or in females with larges scopes (>5 mm) can only be performed by a percutaneous approach. Laparoscopy and thoracoscopy can be performed with a wide range of diameter sizes; however, optimal image quality is obtained with the larger-scope diameters (5 and 10 mm). Laparoscopy can utilize the 0°, 25°, or 30° viewing angles; however, with thoracoscopy, the 25° or 30°

is more often used to permit optimal visualization. A last consideration when preparing for rigid endoscopy is if sterilization of the telescope will be required for the procedure. Some, but not all telescopes, are autoclavable. EtO sterilization is often an option, if available. It is important to check with the manufacturer of the telescope for recommended sterilization procedures. When considering sterilization, the sterility of the region being imaged is the deciding factor.[1] Rhinoscopy does not require sterilization since the nasal cavity is not sterile. However, urethrocystoscopy, laparoscopy, and thoracoscopy do require sterilization since these regions are sterile, in which introducing an infection needs to be avoided, even in the situation when a pathogenic infectious process is already occurring (e.g., pyothorax).

The light source for the flexible and rigid endoscopes is critically important to provide illumination during endoscopy. Many factors contribute to the brightness of the illumination during endoscopy, including the type and power of the light source, hours of use for certain light bulbs, the diameter of the endoscope, length, condition, capacity of the illumination chain, and the size of the cavity being imaged. In addition, two more easily adjustable factors that contribute to brightness are cleanliness of the lens at the distal tip of the endoscope and any other interface the light must pass through.[1] A xenon light source has become the standard in videoendoscopy since it offers excellent color reproduction and the 150–300 W of power recommended for veterinary endoscopy being videotaped. After 400–1000 h, a xenon lamp must be replaced.[1] Other types of light sources used in veterinary medicine include metal halide lamps, replaced after 200–250 h, and tungsten halogen lamps with a life span of approximately 100 h.[1] When choosing a light source for an endoscope, it is important to consider not only the type and power of the light source but also if the light source unit is compatible, or an adapter is available, with the type of endoscope being used.[1] For all rigid and some flexible endoscopes, light is transmitted via separate detachable cables rather than built into the endoscope's umbilical cord. It is again important to choose a compatible cable for the type of endoscope being used.[1]

As stated earlier, one of the advantages of a videoendoscope (or a fiberopic endoscope with an attached endoscopic video camera) is the ability to project an endoscopic image. The endoscopic video camera system needed to produce this image contains an endoscopic adapter, a camera head, a camera control unit (processor), and a monitor. Each of these parts plays a role in the quality of the projected image. The endoscopic adapter connects the camera head to the endoscope eyepiece and permits focusing and, depending on its focal length, magnification. The type of camera is based on the number of CCD chips. Although single-CCD chip cameras produce a slightly lower resolution and less accurate color reproduction image versus three-CCD chip cameras, the difference is minor and the three-CCD chip camera is more costly. The CCD chip converts an optical image to an electronic signal, which is transmitted via an attached cable to the processor. The processor is able to convert the information to a standard video signal, which can be distributed to a monitor or image storage system.[1] The standard video signals are sent to the monitor in one of three common formats: composite (the lowest cost but least detailed), S-video (recommended for single-chip cameras) and RGB (red-green-blue [recommended for three-chip cameras and the best detail]).[1] To maximize the image quality, the resolution of the monitor and any image storage system (e.g., VCR or printer) should be as close as possible or higher resolution than the camera.[1]

Reprocessing

A very important step in the care of any endoscope is cleaning, high level disinfecting, and with certain endoscopes, sterilization of the equipment. Collectively, this step is termed reprocessing. Reprocessing is critical to prevent cross contamination between patients and hospital-acquired infections. In veterinary medicine, most endoscopes are cleaned and disinfected by hand; however, in human medicine, a combination of hand cleaning and then a machine to disinfect the endoscopes (automated endoscope reprocessor) can be utilized.[2] Different types of detergents are used when cleaning endoscopes, including anionic (i.e., soap) and enzymatic detergents. Enzymatic detergents are low foaming detergents with enzymes capable of digesting organic material such as blood and mucous. Disinfection can be achieved with a chemical germicide (termed high level disinfectant [HLD]). EtO or steam autoclaving are used for sterilization.[2] High level disinfection destroys all vegetative microorganisms but not necessarily all bacterial spores.

Flexible endoscopes

The following is a list of steps that apply to most *flexible endoscopes*; however, always refer to the manufacturer's guidelines for each endoscope.[1] These steps should be followed after every endoscopy procedure since every patient could potentially be a source of infection.[2]

Precleaning

Precleaning an endoscope is started immediately after finishing the endoscopy procedure and prior to disconnecting the endoscope from the power source.

You will need the following:

a.   Personal protective equipment (gloves, eye/face protection, and impervious gown)

b.   Detergent solution (ideally enzymatic) and a container

c.   Sponge or soft, lint-free cloth

d.   Manufacturer's air and water channel cleaning (see Figure 14.5.17–14.5.19) adapters (if supplied, and not to be confused with an all-channel irrigator)

e.   Protective video caps if using video endoscopes

Precleaning Steps:

1.   Immediately after removing the endoscope from the patient, mechanically remove organic material from the endoscope by wiping the insertion tube with a wet cloth or sponge soaked in the detergent solution.

2.   Also at the patient side, alternate suctioning detergent and air, several times, through the biopsy/suction channel.

3.   Continuing to suction detergent until the solution is visibly clean and finish by suctioning air.

4.   Flush the water channel(s) and blow out the air channel per manufacturer's instructions.

5.   Detach the endoscope from the light source and suction pump.

6.   For videoscopes, place protective video cap.

7.   Transport the endoscope to the reprocessing area/room (Figures 14.5.17–14.5.19)

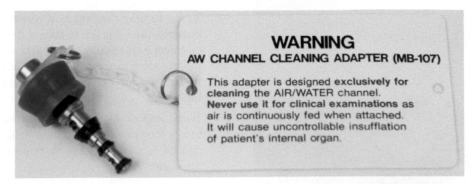

Figure 14.5.17 Olympus air water channel adapter.
Source: http://www.endoscopy.com

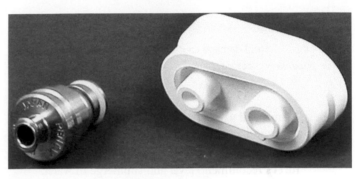

Figure 14.5.19 Pentax cleaning adapters.
Source: http://www.endoscopy.com

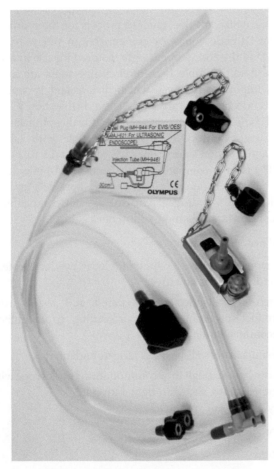

Figure 14.5.18 Olympus cleaning kit.
Source: http://www.endoscopy.com

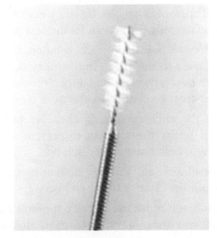

Figure 14.5.20 Channel brush.
Source: http://www.endoscopy.com

Cleaning

You will need the following:

a. Personal protective equipment (gloves, eye/face protection, and impervious gown)

b. Large sink or basin of detergent solution (ideally enzymatic)

c. Sponge or soft, lint-free cloth

d. Air leak tester

e. Manufacturer's all-channel irrigating cleaning adapters

f. Channel cleaning brushes (see Figure 14.5.20)

Cleaning Steps:

1. Air leak testing must always be done before immersion of an endoscope to detect damage to the interior or exterior of the endoscope. Always follow manufacturer's recommendations (see Figure 14.5.21):

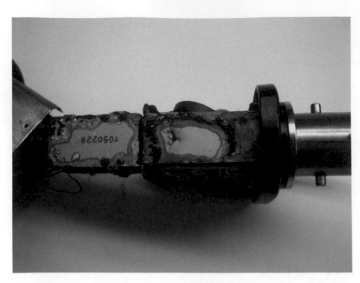

Figure 14.5.21   Fluid damage causing rusted connectors.
Source: http://www.endoscopy.com

   a.   Remove all valves (suction, air/water) and biopsy port cover and any other recommended detachable parts.

   b.   Attach the air leak tester; pressurize to the manufacturer's recommend level and submerge in water.

   c.   With only the pressurized insertion tube submerged, flex the distal tip in all directions and observe for bubbles. If none are noted, submerge the entire endoscope and observe all parts of the endoscope (i.e., universal cord, distal tip) for any bubbles. If a leak is detected, refer to the manufacturer's instructions for the next step.

2.   Fill a sink or basin with detergent solution. Ideally for each cleaning, use a freshly made, low foaming detergent so the device can be clearly visualized during the cleaning process and avoid cross contamination between cleanings.

3.   Immerse the endoscope and, whenever practical, leave immersed under the solution to prevent splashing and aerosolization of contaminated solution.

4.   Use a nonabrasive and lint-free cloth or sponge to wash all debris from the exterior of the endoscope.

5.   Use a small, soft brush to clean all removable parts, including inside and under all valves (suction, air/water), biopsy port cover, and openings.

6.   Pass the cleaning brush through the entire suction/biopsy channel including the insertion tube, umbilicus, and body or handpiece. There are brushes specific to the valve housing, biopsy port openings, and so on, and are dependent on manufacturer and model.

7.   Attach the manufacturer's air, water, suction, and biopsy channel cleaning adapters and flush the channels with the detergent solution to remove debris.

8.   If using an enzymatic detergent, soak the endoscope and its internal channels for the enzymatic detergent's recommended time period.

9.   If, due to time constraints, a complete reprocessing is not possible, then it is OK to stop at this step and to allow the endoscope to soak in a detergent solution until it can be thoroughly reprocessed. However, it is important to follow the manufacturer's recommendation for maximum soaking time.

10.   With clean or distilled water, depending on the manufacturer's recommendations, thoroughly rinse the endoscope and all removable parts to remove residual debris and detergent.

11.   Using forced air, purge water from all the channels.

Dry the exterior of the endoscope with a cloth.

High level disinfection

HLD is recognized as the standard process for the reprocessing of human GI endoscopes. By comparison, in veterinary medicine, HLD of the endoscope is only required for use in a sterile, operative field. Multiple high-level disinfectants are available and it is important to check which disinfectant is compatible with the endoscope you are performing disinfection. Glutaraldehyde (2%) (e.g., Cidex 7 or plus™) and ortho-phthalaldehyde (0.55%) (e.g., Cidex OPA™) are compatible with Olympus, Pentax, and Fujinon endoscopes.[3] Peracetic acid (0.2%) (e.g., Steris 20™) is only compatible with Pentax and Fujinon endoscopes.[3] Hydrogen peroxide (7.5%) (e.g., Sporox™) and 0.08% peracetic acid/1% hydrogen peroxide are not compatible with Olympus, Pentax, or Fujinon endoscopes.[3]

You will need the following:

   a.   Personal protective equipment (gloves, eye/face protection, and impervious gown)

   b.   High-level disinfectant (prepared and tested using a product-specific test strip, according to manufacturer recommendations)

   c.   Manufacturer's all-channel irrigator adapter(s)

   d.   Basin large enough to accommodate the endoscope without undue coiling and with tight-fitting lid

   e.   70% isopropyl alcohol

   f.   Soft, lint-free cloth

HLD Steps

1.   Completely immerse the endoscope and all removable parts in a basin with disinfectant.

2.   Inject disinfectant into all channels of the endoscope until a steady flow of disinfectant is observed exiting the opposite end. Ensure all channels are filled with the disinfectant and no air pockets are present.

3.   Soak the endoscope in a covered (to reduce exposure to chemical vapors) basin at the manufacturer-recommended temperature and duration. For 2% glutaraldehyde products, a 20-min soak at room temperature results in HLD.

4.   After completing the soak, purge the channels with air before removing the endoscope from the basin.

5. Using clean or distilled water, depending on the disinfectant's and endoscope's manufacturer recommendations, thoroughly rinse all surfaces and removable parts and flush all channels of the endoscope.

6. Using air, purge all channels until dry.

7. Flush all channels with 70% isopropyl alcohol until the alcohol can be seen exiting the opposite end of each channel.

8. Again, using air, purge all channels until dry.

9. Remove the manufacturer's all-channel cleaning adapters.

10. Dry the exterior of the endoscope with a soft cloth.

11. Thoroughly rinse and dry all removable parts.

Storage

1. During storage, do not attach removable parts to the endoscope.

2. Hang the endoscope vertically with the distal tip hanging. Do not store the endoscope in the carrying case.

Patient and equipment preparation

Since the vast majority of endoscopic procedures require anesthesia, patients should be fasted for a minimum of 12h prior to procedure time. Longer fasting periods are required for gastroscopy—12–24h, proctoscopy—1–3 days, and colonoscopy—2–3 days to permit adequate visualization of the mucosal surface. In addition to fasting, enemas and intestinal lavage solutions (e.g., GoLytely®) are essential for proctoscopy and colonoscopy, respectively.[4]

Prior to placing a patient under anesthesia for an endoscopic procedure, it is important to ensure all the equipment needed for a procedure is available, correctly set up, and functioning properly. Table 14.5.1 reviews a number of problems encountered during setup or a procedure with possible causes and corrections.[1]

Once a patient is placed under anesthesia, the next step is correctly positioning the patient on the table. The following will discuss standard starting positions; however, some endoscopists have alternative preferred positions.

Gastroduodenoscopy and colonoscopy is performed in left lateral recumbency to facilitate examination of the pylorus and ileocecal valve area.[4] By contrast, if a gastric feeding tube is being placed, the patient is positioned in right lateral recumbency to permit access to the gastric greater curvature. Esophagoscopy by itself can be performed in left lateral or sternal recumbency. Some endoscopists prefer sternal recumbency with esophageal foreign bodies to facilitate removal. Rhinoscopy, nasopharyngoscopy, and bronchoscopy are performed in sternal recumbency. Most endoscopists also perform vaginoscopy and cystoscopy in sternal recumbency; however, right lateral recumbency is preferred by some.

The author thanks Darlene Riel, RVT, VTS (SAIM), University of California, School of Veterinary Medicine, Davis, CA, for excellent manuscript review and additions.

SECTION 6 SELECTED NURSING CONSIDERATIONS OF INTERNAL MEDICINE PATIENTS

Thermoregulation

Normal thermoregulatory process

The anterior hypothalamus portion of the brain controls body temperature, hunger, thirst, fatigue, and circadian cycles. Thermoreceptors, both peripheral (cutaneous) receptors and central (deep) receptors, convey the external and internal temperature to the brain. Based on the normal set point of the body, the hypothalamus will instruct the body to increase or decrease the body temperature in response to this information, thereby achieving thermoregulation. In this process, heat generation is balanced with heat loss.

Each individual animal will have a set point that is considered "normal" for that animal in a healthy state. In addition, each animal will also exhibit a daily temperature swing based on its circadian cycle. In general, body temperature is lowest at about sunrise, increases slowly throughout the day, and peaks around sunset. It then slowly returns to its morning low overnight. In dogs, it has been shown that tiny dogs have a normal body temperature that is about 2°F higher than in large dogs.[1] For this reason, establishing a normal temperature for a specific patient when healthy can help to determine when or if the patient is hyperthermic or hypothermic.

When needed, the body can increase heat production through the effects of catecholamines and thyroxine and through the mechanical process of shivering. The body can also conserve heat by vasoconstriction, piloerection, postural changes, and heat-seeking behavior. Conversely, the body can dissipate heat by panting, vasodilation, postural changes, cool-seeking behavior, perspiration, and in cats also by grooming behaviors.

Fever or hyperthermia?

Fever is defined as a complex physiological response to disease mediated by pyrogenic cytokines and characterized by a rise in core temperature, generation of acute phase reactants, and activation of immunologic systems.[2] According to the *Textbook of Internal Medicine* the term fever is reserved for hyperthermic animals where the set point in the anterior hypothalamus has been "reset" to a higher temperature.[3] Pyrexia is another term that may be used, and it is synonymous with the term fever. Hyperpyrexia is an extremely high fever. Hyperthermia, in contrast, is defined as a therapeutically induced hyperpyrexia, but in actuality, it can mean any elevation in core body temperature above the accepted normal of that species without a change in the set point.

Pathophysiology of fever

Step 1. Exogenous pyrogens (fever-inducing agents produced outside the body) are the external stimuli that set this reaction

Table 14.5.1 Flexible endoscopy troubleshooting guide

Problem	Possible causes	Correction
Unclear or blurry image	Dirty objective lens	Press water valve to use water to clean lens; gently rub distal tip against mucosa.
	Dirty eyepiece, camera, or adaptor	Clean with alcohol-moistened cotton swab.
	Lens not focused for endoscopist	Focus image with diopter adjustment ring.
	Fluid damage inside distal end of eyepiece (see Figure 14.5.21)	Return endoscope to manufacturer for repair.
	Water on objective lens	Press air valve to use air to clear lens.
Image too dark or bright	Dirty light cable or distal tip	Clean light cable or distal tip with alcohol-moistened cotton swab.
	Improper light source settings	Adjust brightness control knob.
	Improperly installed or old lamp	Properly install or replace lamp.
	Broken (noncoherent) fiberoptic bundles	Replace/repair broken fiberoptic bundles
Absent/Decreased irrigation or Insufflation	Air or water channel (s) clogged	Soak distal tip in warm soapy water; pass water or enzymatic cleaner through channels.
	Air/water valve dirty	Clean and lubricate, with silicone oil, valve.
	Air pump not operating	Turn on switch on light source.
	Incompletely closed/loose water cap	Replace and tighten cap.
	Air/water channel damage/deformed	Return endoscope to manufacturer for repair.
	O-ring absent or displaced	Replace work or damaged O-ring.
	Straw missing or displaced	Reattach straw to water bottle cap.
Unable to irrigate	Water bottle empty or over filled	Fill two-thirds full.
Unable to suction	Suction channel obstructed	Clean suction channel in insertion tube and umbilical cord with cleaning brush.
	Dirty suction valve	Clean and lubricate, with silicone oil, valve.
	Absent, improperly attached, or leaky accessory channel valve	Ensure proper installation and function of valve.
	Suction pump problem	Ensure proper installation of pump tube, jar cap, valves, and suction settings.
Valve sticky	Dirty air/water or suction valve	Clean and lubricate, with silicone oil, valve.
Inappropriate water or air dispersed at distal tip	Worn or torn O-ring	Turn off air pump, remove air/water valve, and replace O-ring or entire valve, depending on manufacturer.
Resistance with turning deflection knobs	Deflection knob engaged	Turn lock to off position.
Forceps doesn't pass in channel smoothly	Bent or kinked forceps	Replace forceps.
	Broken jaws (often 1 "wing" of jaw has come apart at its weld	Repair or replace forceps.
Forceps will not open/ close	Dirty forceps cups	Place under running warm water, lubricate forceps, use enzymatic cleaner to help clean organic debris in wire-wrapped forceps, consider ultrasonographic cleaner.
	Bent or kinked forceps	Replace forceps.
Camera will not attach to fiberscope	Improperly positioned autofocus pin on fiberscope eyepiece	Reposition camera; refer to manufacturer's instructions.

Source: Adapted from Barlow DE. Fiberoptic instrument technology. In *Small Animal* Endoscopy, ed. TR Tam. St. Louis, MO: Mosby; 1990.

in motion. Pyrogens are numerous and include infectious agents such as bacteria or bacterial products like exotoxins and enterotoxins, fungi, virus, rickettsia, parasitic and protozoal agents. Pyrogens can also be nonmicrobial agents such as bile acids, some pharmacologicalal agents, tissue inflammation, and antigen-antibody complexes. These exogenous pyrogens stimulate the immune system to release endogenous pyrogens.

Step 2. Endogenous pyrogens (fever-inducing agents produced inside the body) are proteins, specifically fever-producing cytokines. These are produced and released by the immune system in response to stimulation. This reaction of the body is termed a "true fever." The part of the immune system that is stimulated to release these cytokines is primarily macrophages, but lymphocytes (B and T cells) and other leukocytes can be involved. Cytokines include some of the interleukins, interferons, tumor necrosis factors, and macrophage inflammatory proteins.

Step 3. Cytokines travel via the bloodstream to the anterior hypothalamus where they stimulate the anterior hypothalamus to release prostaglandin. The cytokines trigger the febrile response.

Step 4. Prostaglandins raise the set point of the anterior hypothalamus, which triggers heat conservation and heat production.

Causes of fever

The inability to adequately dispel body heat will result in a fever. High ambient temperatures, such as those produced in a car with inadequate ventilation, can overload the body and lead to heat stroke. Brachycephalic breeds and large breed dogs are more susceptible to heat stroke. This is when the term hyperthermia is utilized because the set point has not been altered.

Another form of inadequate heat dissipation is hyperpyrexic syndrome. This is typically seen in dogs that are jogging with an owner or hunting dogs that are working in a hot and humid environment.[3] These dogs will run or work beyond their normal limits, resulting in hyperthermia. The mechanism of this type of hyperthermia is a combination of two problems. In hot and humid environments, the body's ability to dissipate heat is less than in the equivalent temperature in a dry environment. This leads to faster net heat gain in the body. In addition, in response to extreme exercise, the cardiovascular system may give preferential blood flow to the skeletal muscles without allowing for the heat dissipation effects of vasodilation.

Hyperpyrexic syndrome differs from exercise-induced hyperthermia. Exercise-induced collapse (EIC) syndrome, also called exercise-induced hyperthermia, can occur with normal exercise but usually occurs during strenuous exercise. The clinical signs are a very elevated temperature (>107.6°F or >41.5°C), stiff gait, incoordination, rear leg collapse, and disorientation. Most dogs recover quickly with no residual effects. Genetic testing is available to identify the *DNM1* gene that is associated with this syndrome. EIC is an autosomal recessive trait found most commonly in Labrador retrievers, although other breeds can be affected.

Other causes of increased heat production are eclampsia (hypocalcemia) and seizure.

Pathological and pharmacological fevers

Fevers can also be pathological (resulting from disease) or pharmacological (resulting from pharmacological agents), although these types of fever are not frequently encountered. Brain lesions in the area of the anterior hypothalamus can interfere with the normal operation of the thermoregulatory center resulting in an inappropriate response to thermoreceptors. Hypermetabolic disorders, such as hyperthyroidism and pheochromocytoma, can cause an increase in heat production, an increase in heat conservation, or both effects. This results in a fever that is usually mild in nature.

Malignant hyperthermia (MH) is the result of a pharmacological or hypermetabolic myopathy. MH is an inherited disease effecting both dogs and cats with a breed predilection for some lines of greyhounds and Labrador retrievers. The increased muscular activity is caused by an inappropriate release of calcium by the muscle cells. Stress, exercise, and anesthetics (especially halothane) are the most common causative agents. The muscular activity is most often characterized as muscular rigidity, muscular fasciculations, and muscular rigor, resulting in increased heat production. The increased production leads to an increase in body temperature. This activity quickly depletes the ATP reserves that, in turn, coupled with tachypnea, create an acidotic state. This response may be quite pronounced and can quickly lead to a state of emergency. MH is also known as canine stress syndrome.

Fever of unknown origin

Fever of unknown origin (FUO) in human medicine is defined as an illness of more than 3 weeks' duration with a temperature higher than 101°F (38.4°C) on several occasions after 1 week of hospitalization and evaluation.[4] In veterinary medicine, FUO is also called fever of undetermined origin (FUD) since this term is applied rather loosely to any patient with an unexplained fever. Often, the causative agent has simply not been identified rather than being an unknown.

Diagnostics

Since the list of potential causes for fever is long, so is the list of diagnostics. The minimum database includes a CBC, chemistries, and urinalysis. Depending on the signalment and risk factors of the patient, additional laboratory diagnostic testing to consider are bacterial culture (blood and/or urine), fecal parasitology, infectious disease titers, coagulation testing, and radiographs. Advanced imaging such as CT or MRI, ultrasonography, and echocardiology, and advanced diagnostics such as needle biopsy, joint taps, bone marrow evaluation, and cerebrospinal (CSF) analysis may also be indicated in some cases.

Care of the febrile or hyperthermic patient

Nursing care for febrile patients includes frequent monitoring of the patient's temperature. The use of continuous temperature monitors may increase patient comfort by decreasing the need to disturb the patient with frequent rectal temperatures. Supportive care with fluid therapy to correct the accompanying dehydration is often prescribed. Strict asepsis during catheter placement and maintenance is indicated since the patient may already be septic. Medication protocols for febrile patients may be empirical or therapeutic in nature. These protocols may include antibiotics, corticosteroids, NSAIDs, phenothiazines, and antipyretics (e.g., dipyrone, acetylsalicylic acid). Close monitoring for a response to therapeutic treatment and/or response or side effects from empirical treatment is advised. Febrile patients are frequently anorexic, so their nutritional needs should be assessed and supported as indicated based on the RER and disease state calculations. These patients, while not usually overtly painful, generally exhibit malaise and may need additional care and comfort during the course of their hospital stay. Often, these patients are reluctant to utilize their bedding and elect to lie on cooler cages or run floors. Nursing attention to patient hygiene, opportunity to eliminate, and recumbent patient support of pressure-sensitive areas is essential.

Temperatures above 106°F (41°C) are considered emergent temperatures that require intervention. Temperatures above 107°F (41.6°C) can cause permanent organ damage, disseminated intravascular coagulopathy, or death. Total body cooling procedures can include cool water baths or rinses, wetting down and placing in front of a fan, administration of cool fluids, ice packs, gastric lavage, enemas, and treatment for shock. Too rapid or too slow of a cooling of the patient can have a deleterious effect on the survival of the emergent hyperthermic animal. An in-depth discussion of the emergency treatment of hyperthermia is not included in this text.

Conclusion

Even though this is the most basic vital sign, its importance should not be overlooked. Care of the febrile patient can be a short-term or a long-term process dependent on the causative agent and the patient response.

Hypothermia

Hypothermia is defined as a body temperature below normal for the species. The accepted normal temperature for dogs and cats varies by reference but is considered to be approximately 101.5°F (38.6°C). Hypothermia is typically classified as mild (96–99°F or 34–37°C), moderate (88–93°F or 31–34°C), and severe (<88°F or <31°C). The actual ranges used for these definitions may again vary based on the reference, but these values can serve as guidelines. In human medicine, profound hypothermia may also be included as a separate classification. Smaller, older, and sick or debilitated animals are more likely to become hypothermic as temperature control mechanisms may be impaired.[5]

Mechanisms of heat loss

The mechanisms by which the body can lose heat include radiation, convection, and conduction. The body radiates heat through the skin (primarily) and the lungs (to a lesser extent). Heat loss through liquids and the evaporative effects of heat loss are noted in convection. Direct contact with cold surfaces (e.g., stainless steel tables) leads to heat loss through conduction.

Causes of hypothermia

Hypothermia is further defined dependent on the causative reason, as accidental, pathological, or purposeful.

Accidental hypothermia

Accidental hypothermia is a decrease in core body temperature that is independent of the body's normal set point. This text, as it is not an emergency and critical care text, will not focus on the environmental exposure causes of hypothermia. Accidental hypothermia is also the type of hypothermia that can be seen in patients during an anesthesitic event. Anesthetics may cause vasodilation and can impair the function of the hypothalamus. These cooling effects coupled with exposure to cold tables, wet surgical preps, loss of hair, and so on, compound the heat loss and can lead to hypothermia. The resulting decreased metabolism will prolong recovery from the anesthetic drugs and can become a vicious circle of prolonged recovery.

Pathological hypothermia

Pathological hypothermia is the result of a disease or a disease process that decreases the metabolic rate or affects the thermoregulatory center. These include hypoglycemia, sepsis, shock, and major trauma. Endocrine diseases that can have this effect include hypothyroidism, hypopituitarism, and hypoadrenocorticism. These diseases usually produce a mild hypothermia. Brain lesions in the hypothalamus can have a direct effect on the set point of the body, causing either hypothermia or, as previously noted, hyperthermia. The treatment of pathological hypothermia includes treatment of the underlying disease or disease process in addition to the rewarming techniques described in this chapter.

Purposeful hypothermia

Purposeful hypothermia has been used in veterinary medicine during selected cardiac procedures to slow the metabolic rate. This decreases the oxygen consumption rate, which helps to preserve brain function in cases of surgically induced hypoxia. Purposeful hypothermia will not be discussed in this text, although treatment protocols are the same as for accidental hypothermia.

Pathophysiology of hypothermia

As discussed earlier, the body can generate heat through the mechanical process of shivering and can conserve heat through vasoconstriction, piloerection, postural changes, and heat-seeking behavior. In cases of mild hypothermia, the body will attempt to cope, exhibiting the above clinical responses. In addition, sympathetic nervous system excitation may result in hypertension, tachycardia, and tachypnea due to the increased oxygen demands from shivering.[6] Some degree of hepatic dysfunction may be noted and the sympathetic excitation can cause the release of glucose from the liver, resulting in hyperglycemia. Hyperglycemia may also be noted due to the decreased consumption of glucose by the cells and the decreased excretion of insulin.

Once the core temperature is below 94°F, the ability to generate heat through this process is lost or severely impaired. As core temperatures continue to drop, decreases in respiratory rate, heart rate, cardiac output, glomerular filtration rate, and blood pressure will be noted. Further decrease will result in loss of muscular control and a depression in consciousness. Hypothermia-induced cold diuresis is a common sequelae that may necessitate fluid therapy. This will be accompanied by a decrease in metabolic rate of most of the tissues of the body. Acidosis and electrolyte imbalances may be noted. Tachycardia and atrial fibrillation can occur. The end stages of hypothermia are unconsciousness and respiratory and cardiac arrest. In human medicine, paradoxical undressing may occur in that the patient removes clothing as the hypothermia worsens. Antidotal evidence of hypothermic animals climbing out of warm blankets and away from heat sources has been noted.

Diagnostics

An extended range thermometer that has the ability to read very low temperatures is needed in order to obtain an accurate core temperature. Monitoring of electrolytes, glucose levels, heart rate and rhythm, and acid–base status are indicated in moderate and severe cases of hypothermia.

Nursing care

There are three rewarming techniques: passive external, active external, and active internal. These techniques should be used according to the severity of the hypothermia. Frequent (e.g., every 15–30 min) turning or repositioning of the patient should occur to minimize the chance of thermal injury and to maximize rewarming efforts.

Passive external

Passive external rewarming techniques are aimed at preventing heat loss and allowing the body's natural heat conservation and heat-generating abilities to function. This is typically accomplished by providing clean, dry, warm bedding and assuring that the bladder is empty by providing an opportunity to void or mechanically emptying the bladder.

Active external

Active external rewarming techniques provide the patient with an external heat source in addition to the patient's natural abilities. External heat sources such as circulating water blankets, forced air blankets, heat lamps, and hot water or hot rice bags are some of the more typical external heat sources provided. Extreme care must be exercised whenever using an external heat source on a nonmobile patient in order to prevent thermal burns. This is particularly important when dealing with a vasoconstricted patient.

Active internal

Active internal rewarming techniques consist of warmed IV, peritoneal, gastric, and/or colonic lavage fluids. In addition, if the patient is under anesthesia or receiving oxygen, warming the inspired gas or gases can significantly help in the rewarming process.

Conclusion

Extreme care should be taken when rewarming the severely hypothermic patient. The emphasis in human medicine is to rewarm the patient's core while minimizing activity. This is to prevent the cool blood from the extremities from adversely affecting the core, particularly the heart, during the rewarming process. An in-depth discussion of the emergency protocol for the treatment of severe hypothermia can be found in an emergency text.

The sepsis syndrome

Sepsis is considered a malignant condition that occurs when there is an exaggerated and uncontrolled immune response to an infection that extends beyond the site of injury to normal tissue. The normal response to infection is a very intricate and complicated process that maintains a controlled response to the local affected area of injury. Sepsis occurs when regulation of the local response ceases and the inflammatory reaction spreads throughout the body. When the inflammation is no longer self-sustaining, toxins and cytokines are released, resulting in a condition called systemic inflammatory response syndrome, or "SIRS." As the SIRS process persists, another devastating chain of events can lead to organ failure and the development of multiple organ dysfunction syndrome, also known as "MODS." The sepsis syndrome proves to be a challenge with factors such as prevention, immediate clinical recognition, and implementing appropriate therapies influencing successful outcomes.

Sepsis occurs when a pathogen invades the body and ultimately enters the bloodstream, creating a systemic infection. Pathogens are primarily bacteria; however, viral and fungal infections can also cause sepsis. Although there are several conditions associated with the sepsis syndrome, essentially any condition resulting in hypoperfusion and subsequent hypoxia can lead to the sepsis syndrome. For the hospitalized patient, sources of infection include (but are not limited to) the GI system, the excretory system, and the respiratory system. It is important to note that the source of infection is not always identifiable. The pathogen responsible for the inflammatory process is not the direct cause of SIRS but rather the individual response to the pathogen (Table 14.6.1).

Pathophysiology

With normal tissue injury or infection, proinflammatory and anti-inflammatory elements are released simultaneously to

Table 14.6.1   Definition of infectious terms

Terms	Definition	Example
Infection	The presence or invasion of microorganisms to noninfected tissue resulting in an inflammatory response	Peritonitis, viremia
Bacteremia	The presence of bacteria in the blood steam	Endocarditis, nosocomial infections
Systemic inflammatory response syndrome (SIRS)	An immune response to a pathogen, which has resulted in systemic inflammatory state	Sepsis, septic shock, heat exhaustion
Acute sepsis	A systemic response to a pathogen, which is associated with organ dysfunction or failure	Oliguria, ischemic event, hypoperfusion
Septic shock	Sepsis or infection induced hypoperfusion, which results in organ dysfunction; refractory hypotension	Bacteremia, SIRS
Multiple organ dysfunction syndrome (MODS)	Organ dysfunction involving two or more organs, which requires medical intervention to maintain function	Hypoperfusion, tissue ischemia

balance tissue repair and healing. The endothelium is responsible for initiating the inflammatory process. The endothelium regulates blood vessel tone and vascular permeability and, in response to injury, will allow local vasodilation and therefore increased microvascular permeability, which results in localized edema. The endothelium also regulates WBC activity and attracts leukocytes to the local area of injury where phagocytosis can ensue. When macrophages invade bacteria, cytokines and proinflammatory mediators are activated and result in injury to the endothelial cell and the underlying tissue. Apoptosis and the formation of oxygen free radicals within the endothelial cell result in a localized removal of damaged and infected tissue. When cellular death occurs, creating gaps between cells, extravasation of protein-rich fluid and cellular material moves into interstitial spaces contributing to edema. In sepsis, the localized regulation becomes dysfunctional and the inflammatory process continues systemically as the endothelium covers a tremendous surface area (Table 14.6.2, Figure 14.6.1).

As the sepsis syndrome progresses, septic shock begins. Shock is defined as a disturbance of function. In veterinary medicine, shock is considered to be an imbalance between delivered oxygen and consumed oxygen where the former is deficient. For a basic review, the blood functions to deliver oxygen, nutrients, and hormones among other necessities to all the body's tissues. The blood also carries away waste products from those tissues and aids in the maintenance of the body's fluid balance. This delivery system is dependent on cardiac output, which is determined by heart rate and stroke volume consisting of cardiac preload. If cardiac function and perfusion is impaired, neurohormonal responses ensue and inflammatory mediators contribute to a vicious cycle as decompensation occurs (Tables 14.6.3 and 14.6.4).

During the initial stages of shock, cellular hypoxia causes an energy deficit as mitochrondia are no longer able to generate ATP. Anaerobic metabolism ensues, causing the pH to fall, leading to metabolic acidosis. An acute compensatory sympathetic response causes major arteries and veins to constrict. Initially, capillaries constrict, causing decreased perfusion to tissues; however, as anaerobic metabolism progresses, blood flow into the capillaries is increased as outflow is restricted, causing a volume shift of blood accumulating in the venules. This local "pooling" is responsible for the misdistribution of blood flow. Fluid and protein leak into the surrounding tissues, which effectively concentrates the blood and increases viscosity on a microvascular level. Prolonged vasoconstriction results in loss of blood flow to vital organs, which were previously protected by arterial shunting. The end result is catastrophic as some tissues are overperfused, while others suffer from ischemia. In the sepsis syndrome, hypovolemic shock, distributive shock, and cardiogenic shock are all responsible for the deterioration. To make matters worse, the pulmonary vascular blood flow become disrupted, leading to pulmonary edema and may progress to acute respiratory distress syndrome

The balance of coagulation systems is also regulated by the endothelium. Once inflammatory cytokines have affected the epithelium, a substance called tissue factor leads to the production of thrombin. Fibrin clots then develop in microvascular regions (capillary beds) and cannot be broken down naturally as interleukins and tissue necrosis factor (TNF) inhibit fibrinolysis. Antithrombin is unable to bind or inhibit thrombin due to prostaglandin production. As circulation continues with an increased cardiac effort, oxygen fails to be delivered to tissues due to the thrombi formation. Systemic vasodilation, poor perfusion, and subsequent oxygen demand and supply mismatch lead to tissue ischemia, resulting in organ dysfunction and failure (Figures 14.6.2 and 14.6.3).

Prevention, recognition, and management of the septic patient

There are many conditions that may lead to the sepsis syndrome; therefore, prevention and anticipation of sepsis are essential. It is imperative that veterinary nursing staff caring for patients not

Table 14.6.2   Pathophysiology of infection

Cytokines
Produced by tissue macrophages, monocytes, mast cells, platelets, and endothelial cells
Tissue necrosis factor (TNF) and interleukin (IL-1) are released, which initiate several cascades, including the production of other proinflammatory cytokines
TNF and IL-1 are responsible for the release of norepinephrine, vasopressin, activation of the renin–angiotensin–aldosterone system and fever
IL-1 and TNF cause fibrinolysis impairment
IL-6C stimulates release of reactive protein C and procalcitonin

Primary proinflammatory mediators	
Bacterial endotoxin	TNF
Leukotrienes	Prostaglandins
Interleukin-1	Interleukin-6
Interleukin-8	Nitric oxide
Interferon-gamma	Platelet-activating factor (PAF)
IL-6, IL-8, and interferon gamma	
Activate the coagulation cascade, complement cascade	
Release of nitric oxide, platelet-activating factor (PAF), prostaglandins, and leukotrienes	
Prostaglandins and leukotrienes contribute to endothelial damage	
Tissue factor initiates the production of thrombin and coagulation	
Disruption of naturally occurring anti-inflammatory mediators antithrombin and activated protein C	
Proinflammatory polypeptides contribute to the release of additional cytokines and cause vasodilatation, increasing vascular permeability	

Anti-inflammatory mediators	
Interleukin-4	Interleukin-6
Interleukin-10	Interleukin-12
Lipoxins	Granulocyte-macrophage colony-stimulating factor (GM-CSF)
Transforming growth factor (TGF)	Protein C
IL-1RA	PGE2
IL-4 and IL-10 decrease the production of TNF, IL-1, IL-6, and IL-8; antagonists to TNF and IL-1 receptors are produced	
Protease inhibitors	
Antioxidants	

only understand the anatomy, physiology, and pathophysiology of their patients' condition but also recognize changes and prepare for (and hopefully prevent) the next step of the disease process. Proactive nursing care involves critical thinking skills, preventing a patient from deteriorating, and ultimately improving the health and well-being of the patient.

Clinical recognition, beyond identification of at-risk patients, includes astute monitoring of vital signs and possible sources of infection such as urinary catheters, IV catheters, and surgical sites. The patient should be monitored for cardiovascular func-

tion, respiratory function, and thermoregulation, and evaluated for signs of pain and level of consciousness. Additionally, anticipation of GI bacterial translocation, kidney dysfunction, immunosuppression, and coagulation abnormalities should influence monitoring parameters. Laboratory findings may reveal an increase in lactate levels, abnormal coagulation parameters, acid–base status changes, hypoproteinemia, hypoglycemia, and abnormal CBC findings. In recent years, biomarkers have become available for procalcitonin, protein C, endotoxins, and TNF.

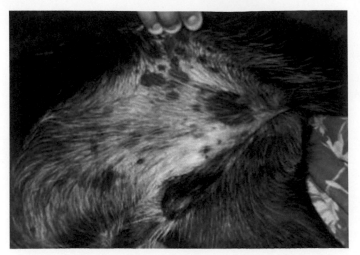

Figure 14.6.1 Sepsis patient in the coagulation cascade: anemia, thrombocytopenia, petechiae, ecchymosis (shown here), epistaxis, and hematuria present.

Table 14.6.3 Stages of sepsis

Stages	Description
1. SIRS	Fever + leukocytosis
2. Sepsis	SIRS + infection
3. Acute sepsis	Sepsis + MODS
4. Septic shock	Acute sepsis + refractory hypotension
5. MODS	Final end pathway

Table 14.6.4 Stages of MODS

First stage	Hypoglycemia, oliguria, mild respiratory alkalosis
Second stage	Moderate liver dysfunction, tachypnea, hypoxemia, hypocapnia
Third stage	Shock, azotemia, acid–base disorder, coagulopathy
Fourth stage	Lactic acidosis, ischemia, oliguria/anuria

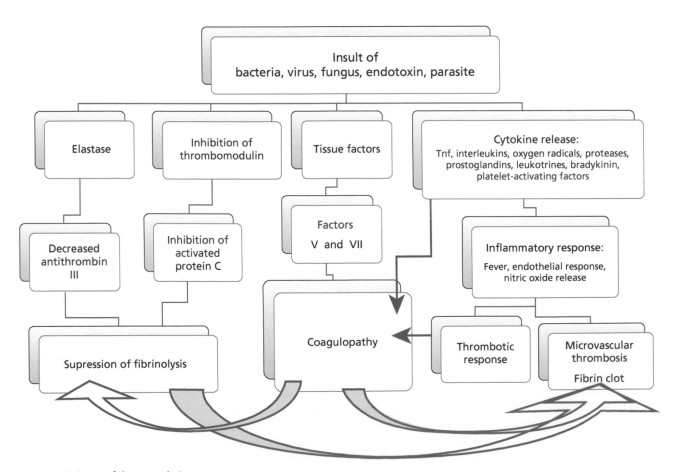

Figure 14.6.2 Balance of the coagulation system.

Nursing management of the septic patient includes supportive care, primarily with the goal of preventing progression of the disease state. Fluid balances should be assessed frequently in debilitated patients, particularly those suffering from renal disease or hypotension. Urine production generally reflects overall tissue perfusion. With each cardiac cycle, the kidneys receive 25% of cardiac output. Normal urine output is 1–2 mL/kg/h; by quantitating urine output, a rough assessment of tissue perfusion can be obtained. Additionally, other excretory means such as diarrhea, emesis, or even pleural fluid from a chest tube should be calculated in the fluid balancing. Critical patients at risk of third-spacing fluid shifts should be weighed up to every 2–4 h as part of the fluid balancing procedure. Fluid balancing is imperative in recognizing underhydration, overhydration and organ function (Figure 14.6.4).

Nutritional considerations of veterinary patients can largely influence healing and recovery. Patients should be assessed individually and a nutritional plan instituted based on the underlying disease and specific needs of the patient. In essence, nutrition should be applied as an addition to medical therapeutics, helping to harmonize the dynamics of veterinary care. Ill or injured patients require higher calories to sustain an increase in metabolic rate or catabolism will ensue. When nutrition is inadequate, the patient is at risk for a longer hospital stay, delayed wound healing, immunosuppression, muscle weakness, low serum albumin levels, and in cases where bacterial translocation occurs, sepsis, organ failure, and death.

Although there are many useful machines and monitoring units readily available in most veterinary settings, the most important one is the veterinary nursing staff. With that being said, utilizing the available instrumentation will help in better assessment and perhaps verification of clinical findings. The most commonly used devices are blood pressure monitors, pulse oximetry machines, electrocardiographs, and capnographs. These machines are useful in monitoring the ill or injured patient as hypotension, cardiac arrhythmias, hypoxemia due to V/Q mismatch, and so on.

Physical therapy enhances the natural healing process and improves surgery or injury recovery time. Physical therapy also increases blood flow, allows for better lymph drainage, prevents or reduces muscle atrophy, and reduces pain. In the recumbent patient, thoracic physical therapy helps improve breathing, thus increasing oxygen in systemic circulation. In addition, physical therapy is a noninvasive treatment, is generally low cost, and has psychological benefits for the patient. The main forethought in performing physical therapy is having an accurate understanding of the nature of the injury and the mechanism(s) involved in recovery. The use of physical therapy in the critical patient can help prevent secondary conditions from arising. Critical or recumbent patients often suffer from secondary illnesses such as atelectasis, pneumonia, thrombosis, and muscle atrophy.

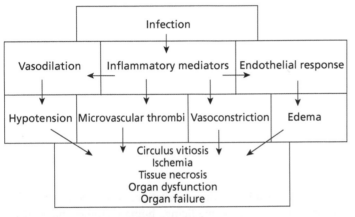

Figure 14.6.3 Stages of the sepsis syndrome.

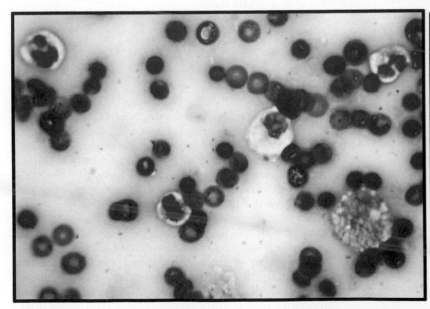
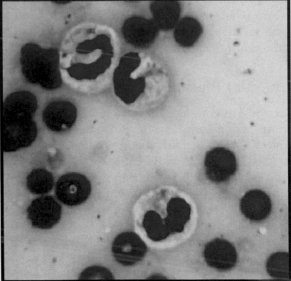

Figure 14.6.4 Peritoneal fluid cytology of a patient suffering septic peritonitis post-foreign body obstruction.

Techniques that are useful to the patient include massage, active and passive range of motion (PROM), thermal agents, positioning, postural drainage, percussion, vibration, and low level lasers. Physical therapy can be performed every 4–8h depending on the patients' needs. Massage and ROM exercises will help circulation, reducing the risk for thrombosis. ROM exercises will help prevent or reduce muscle atrophy. Thermal agents include the application of heat and/or ice. While heat dilates the capillaries and allows for better blood flow to the region, ice will cause vasoconstriction, reducing swelling and inflammation. Furthermore, both of these thermal agents contribute to pain management. Positional changes help prevent decubital ulcers, atelectasis, and peripheral edema. Postural drainage, percussion, and vibration should be implemented in the patient due to the inability to productively cough. Activity stimulates coughing; therefore, the recumbent, obtunded, or comatose patient may accumulate respiratory secretions and may suffer from conditions such as pneumonia as a sequelae.

Recognizing signs of pain and advocating pain management is a paramount element of patient care. It is well recognized that patients, both veterinary and human, suffer from longer hospital stays, greater complications, and increased mortality when pain is not controlled. It is assumed that any condition that may cause pain to humans would indeed cause pain to animals as well.

Sources for hospital-acquired infections include (but are not limited to) venous access sites, urinary catheter sites, and surgical sites or wounds. Maintenance and handling of access sites is an essential part of veterinary patient nursing when it comes to prevention of nosocomial infection. The single most effective way to prevent a nosocomial infection is hand washing. Veterinary personnel who do not wash hands between patients virtually become fomites and transfer microorganisms from one patient to another. When these microorganisms are transferred to an ill or injured patient, the effects can be devastating due to the compromised immune system of the patient. Patients undergoing surgical procedure are at risk for developing nosocomial infections; therefore, proper perioperative nursing is imperative to help reduce the risks of infection. Patients with wounds or bandages should be monitored to ensure perfusion, cleanliness, and comfort (Table 14.6.5).

Potential therapeutics for the future

Currently, in both human and veterinary medicine, successful treatment of the sepsis syndrome continues to be a major focus. Protein C is an antithrombotic, anti-inflammatory, and profibrinolytic agent that has been used for the treatment of sepsis in humans. A recombinant human activated protein C was approved by the FDA in 2001 for the treatment of sepsis and has decreased mortality rates. Other experimental therapies currently in development include focus on the ability to block cytokines, TNF, nitric oxide, endotoxins, and the clotting cascade. In human medicine, studies using drag-reducing polysaccharides, intracellular antioxidant solution, Ringer's ethyl pyruvate, and liposome-encapsulated nicotinamide adenine dinucleotide solution are showing hemodynamic improvement as well as

Table 14.6.5 Sepsis resuscitation

Steps for resuscitation	Example
Control infection source	Replace catheters (venous, urinary, etc.)
	Clean and debride wounds
Laboratory interventions	Blood culture: prior to antibiotics administration
	Maintain euglycemia
	Monitor serum lactate level
	Identify and monitor blood dyscrasias
Hemodynamic monitoring	Fluid therapy: crystalloids and colloids
	Vasopressors, positive inotropes
	Normalize cellular metabolism
	Ensure tissue perfusion
	Anticipate DIC
Organ support	Implement mechanical ventilation
	Prevent pulmonary edema
	Prevent renal hypoperfusion
	Level of consciousness
Miscellaneous	Nutritional support
	Supplemental oxygen

improved survival in shock resuscitation. Although not readily accessible in veterinary medicine, human studies have also shown that continual renal replacement therapy (CRRT), or hemodialysis, is effective in critically ill patients with renal failure and may in the future prove beneficial to the removal of cytokines seen in septic shock.

Bibliography

Section 1

1. Workers Compensation Board of BC. Joint Occupational Health and Safety Committee workbook. 2000, p. 5.
2. Washington State Department of Labor and Industries. [n.d., online] Veterinary hazards. http://www.lni.wa.gov/Safety/Topics/AtoZ/HazardsVeterinary/default.asp (accessed January 21, 2011).
3. Canadian Centre for Health and Safety. [December 12, 2005, online] Work-related musculoskeletal disorders. http://www.ccohs.ca/oshanswers/diseases/rmirsi.html#tphp (accessed January 14, 2011).
4. OSHA. 1974. Ionizing Radiation, Toxic and Hazardous Substances Part Number 1910, Subpart Z. Standard number 1910.1096.
5. U.S Department of Labor, Occupational Health and Safety Division. [May 18, 2000, online]. Anesthetic gases: Guidelines for workplace exposures; halogenated agents: section C, part 2. http://www.osha.gov/dts/osta/anestheticgases/index.html (accessed January 27, 2011).

6. United States Department of Labor. [September 25, 2008, online]. Latex allergy. http://www.osha.gov/SLTC/latexallergy/index.html (accessed March 6, 2011).

7. WorkSafe BC. [June 2005] Dealing with "Latex Allergies" at work. http://www.worksafebc.com/publications/health_and_safety/by_topic/assets/pdf/latex_allergies.pdf (accessed March 6, 2011).

8. Centers for Disease Control and Prevention. [1998, online]. Latex allergy a prevention guide. http://www.cdc.gov/niosh/docs/98-113/ (accessed March 6, 2011).

9. Canada West Veterinary Specialists. Infection control and Isolation Protocols Manual, 2009.

10. W.B Saunders. *Dorland's Pocket Medical Dictionary*, 24th edition, Philadelphia, PA: W.B Saunders Co; 1957.

11. Schlesinger DP, Joffee DJ. Raw food diets in companion animals, a critical review. *The Canadian Veterinary Journal* 2011;52: 50–54.

12. Centers for Disease Control and Prevention. [September 27 2010, online]. Salmonella. http://www.cdc.gov/salmonella/general/technical.html (accessed January 25, 2011).

13. Centers for Disease Control and Prevention, Healthcare-Associated Infections. [January 25 2011, online]. *Clostridium difficile* infection. http://www.cdc.gov/HAI/organisms/cdiff/Cdiff_infect.html (accessed January 31, 2011).

14. Henry CJ, Higginbotham ML, Royer NS. *Cancer Management in Small Animal Practice*, pp. 107–113. St. Louis, MO: Saunders Elsevier; 2010.

15. Withrow/Vail. *Small Animal Clinical Oncology*, 4th edition, pp. 167–169. St. Louis, MO: W.B. Saunders; 2007.

16. Withrow/MacEwan. *Small Animal Clinical Oncology*, 3rd edition, p. 95. Philadelphia, PA: W.B. Saunders; 2001.

Section 2

1. Trepanier LA. Top ten potential drug interactions, ACVIM Forum, Anaheim, CA 2010.

2. Plumb DC. *Plumbs Veterinary Drug Handbook*, 7th edition. Ames, IA: Blackwell Publishing; 2011.

3. Silverstein D, Hopper K. *Small Animal Critical Care Medicine*. St. Louis, MO: Elsevier Saunders; 2009.

4. Bonagura JD, Twedt DC. *Kirk's Current Veterinary Therapy XIV*. St. Louis, MO: Saunders Elsevier; 2009.

5. Mealey KL. MDR1 testing for prevention of chemotherapeutic adverse effects, ACVIM Forum, Anaheim, CA 2010.

6. Trpanier LA. Drug dose adjustments for disease. Proceedings from the CVC, April 7–12, 2010, Baltimore, MD.

7. Ettinger SJ, Feldman EC. *Textbook of Veterinary Internal Medicine*, 6th edition. St. Louis, MO: Elsevier Saunders; 2000.

8. Macintire DK, Drobatz KJ, Haskins SC, Saxon WD. *Manual of Small Animal Emergency and Critical Care Medicine*. Ames, IA: Blackwell Publishing; 2006.

9. Nelson RW, Couto CG, *Small Animal Internal Medicine*, 4th edition. St. Louis, MO: Elsevier Mosby; 2009.

10. Mathews KA *Veterinary Emergency and Critical Care Manual*, 2nd edition. Guelph, Ontario: Lifelarn; 2006.

11. Kirk RW. *Kirk's Current Veterinary Therapy VII*. St. Louis, MO: Saunders; 1980.

Section 3

1. Buffington CA, Hollaway C, Abood SK (eds.). Clinical dietetics. In: *Manual of Veterinary Dietetics*, pp. 54–60. St. Louis, MO: Elsevier; 2004.

2. Saker KE, Remillard R. Critical care nutrition and enteral-assisted feeding. In: *Small Animal Clinical Nutrition*, 5th edition, eds. MS Hand, CD Thatcher, RL Remillard, P Roudebush, BBJ Novotny, pp. 439–471. Marceline, MO: Walsworth Publishing; 2010.

3. Donaghue S. Nutritional support of hospitalized patients. *Veterinary Clinics of North America Small Animal Practice* 1989;19(3): 475–493.

4. Abood SK. Nutritional assessment of the critical care patient. In: Purina Nutrition Forum, pp. 16–19. St. Louis, MO: Ralston Purina; 1997.

5. Wingfield WE. The essentials of life in critically ill animals. In: Purina Nutrition Forum, pp. 2–15. St. Louis, MO: Ralston Purina; 1997.

6. Chan DL. 2005. In-hospital starvation: Inadequate nutritional support. In *11th International Veterinary Emergency & Critical Care Symposium proceedings*, pp. 515–518.

7. Torrance AG. Intensive care nutritional support. In: *Manual of Companion Animal Nutrition and Feeding*, ed. NC Kelly, JM Wills, pp. 171–180. Ames, IA: Iowa State University Press; 1996.

8. Hill RC. Critical care nutrition. In: *The Waltham Book of Clinical Nutrition of the Dog and Cat*, eds. JM Wills, KW Simpson, pp. 39–57. Tarrytown, NY: Pergamon Press; 1994.

9. Remillard RL, Saker KE. Parenteral-assisted feeding. In: *Small Animal Clinical Nutrition*, 5th edition, eds. MS Hand, CD Thatcher, RL Remillard, P Roudebush, BBJ Novotny, pp. 477–492. Marceline, MO: Walsworth Publishing; 2010.

10. Tennant B. Feeding the sick animal. In: *Manual of Companion Animal Nutrition and Feeding*, eds. NC Kelly, JM Wills, pp. 171–180. Ames, IA: Iowa State University Press; 1996.

11. Davenport D, Remillard R, Jenkins C. Gastric motility and emptying disorders. In: *Small Animal Clinical Nutrition*, 5th edition, eds. MS Hand, CD Thatcher, RL Remillard, P Roudebush, BJ Novotomy, p. 1044. Topeka, KS: Mark Morris Institute; 2011.

12. Case LP, Carey DP, Hirakawa DA, Daristotle L (eds.). Energy balance. In: *Canine and Feline Nutrition*, 2nd edition, pp. 75–88. St. Louis, MO: Mosby; 2000.

13. Will JM. Basic principles of nutrition and feeding. In: *Manual of Companion Animal Nutrition and Feeding*, eds. N Kelly, J Wills, pp. 19–21. Ames, IA: Iowa State Press; 1996.

14. Gross KL, Jewell DE, Yamka RM, et al. Macronutrients. In: *Small Animal Clinical Nutrition*, 5th edition, eds. MS Hand, CD Thatcher, RL Remillard, et al., pp. 50–88. Marceline, MO: Walsworth Publishing; 2010.

15. Burger IH. A basic guide to nutrient requirements. In: *The Waltham Book of Companion animal Nutrition*, eds. JM Wills, KW Simpson, pp. 6–10. Tarrytown, NY: Pergamon; 1993.

16. Xia L, Weihua L, Hong W, et al. July 2005. Pseudogenization of a sweet-receptor gene accounts for cats indifference toward sugar a http://www.plosgenetics.org, 1(1):27–35.

17. Crane SW, Cowell CS, Moser EA, et al. Commercial pet foods. In: *Small Animal Clinical Nutrition*, 5th edition, eds. MS Hand, CD Thatcher, RI Remillard, P Roudebush, B Novotny, p. 161. Marceline, MO: Walsworth Publishing; 2010.

18. Donoghue S. The underweight patient. In: *Manual of Companion Animal Nutrition and Feeding*, eds. N Kelly, J Wills, p. 103. Ames, IA: Iowa State Press; 1996.

19. Knochel JP. Phosphorus. In: *Modern Nutrition in Health and Disease*, 9th edition, eds. ME Shils, JA Olson, S Moshe, AC Ross, pp. 157–166. Philadelphia, PA: Lipponcott, Williams & Wilkins; 1999.

20. Hamaoui E, Kodsi R. Complications of enteral feeding and their prevention. In: *Clinical Nutrition, Enteral and Tube Feeding*, 3rd

edition, eds. JL Rombeau, RH Rolandelli, pp. 566–568. Philadelphia, PA: W.B. Saunders; 1997.

21. Forrester SD, Moreland KJ. Hypophosphatemia. *Journal of Veterinary Internal Medicine* 1989;1989(3):149–159.

22. Remillard RL, Armstrong PJ, Davenport DJ. Assisted feeding in hospitalized patients: enteral and parenteral nutrition. In: *Small Animal Clinical Nutrition*, 4th edition, eds. T Hand, R Remillard, p. 364. Marceline, MO: Walsworth Publishing; 2000.

23. Justin RB, Hosenhaus AE. Hypophosphatemia associated with enteral alimentation in cats. *Journal of Veterinary Internal Medicine* 1995;9:228–233.

24. Driscoll DF, Adolph A, Bistrian BR. Lipid emulsions in parenteral nutrition. In: *Clinical Nutrition, Parenteral Nutrition*, 3rd edition, eds. JL Rombeau, RH Rolandelli, p. 42. Philadelphia, PA: W.B. Saunders; 2001.

25. Wortinger A. Electrolytes, fluids and the acid-base balance. *Veterinary Technician Magazine* February 2001;22(2): 80–87; 2001.

26. Chan DL. Controversies in clinical nutrition therapy. In *IVECCS 2006 Proceedings*, San Antonio, TX, pp. 499–502; 2006.

Section 4

1. Cote E. *Clinical Veterinary Advisor Dogs and Cats*, pp. 1213–1214. St. Louis, MO: Mosby Elsevier; 2007.

2. Brown C. Diagnostic cystocentesis: technique and considerations. *Laboratory Animals* 2006;35(4):21–23.

3. Buckley GJ, Aktay SA, Raozanski EA. Massive transfusion and surgical management of iatrogenic aortic laceration associated with cystocentesis in a dog. *Journal of the American Veterinary Medical Association* 2009;235(3):288–291.

4. Lulich J. How I Get a Decent Urine Sample, British Small Animal Congress, 2007.

5. Caney SMA. Collecting Urine Samples From Cats: British Small animal Veterinary Congress, 2009.

6. Fry DR, Holloway SA. Comparison of normal urine samples collected by cystocentesis with or without prior skin disinfection. *Australian Veterinary Practice* 2004;24:2–5.

7. Macintire DK, Drobatz KJ, Haskins SC (eds.). Urologic emergencies. In: *Manual of Small Animal Emergency and Critical Care Medicine*, 1st edition, pp. 226–231. Philadelphia, PA: Lippincott Williams & Wilkins; 2005.

8. Kruger JM, Osborne CA, Ulrich LK. Cystocentesis, diagnostic and therapeutic considerations. *Veterinary Clinics of North America: Small Animal Practice* 1996;26(2):353–361.

9. Crowe DT. Diagnostic abdominal paracentesis techniques: clinical evaluation in 129 dogs and cats. *Journal of the American Animal Hospital Association* 1984;20:223–230.

10. Walters JM. Abdominal paracentesis and diagnostic peritoneal lavage. *Clinical Techniques in Small Animal Practice* 2003;18(1): 32–38.

11. Jandrey KE. Abdominocentesis. In: *Small Animal Critical Care Medicine*, Chapter 155, pp. 671–673. St. Louis, MO: Saunders Elsevier; 2009.

12. Mazzaferro EM. Abominocentesis and DPL; International Veterinary Emergency and Critical Care Symposium; 2006.

13. Smeak DD. Abdominocentesis; NAVC Clinicians Brief, September 2006.

14. Lee JA. Abdominal trauma: Evaluation and stabilization. International Veterinary and Critical Care Symposium; 2005.

15. Powell LL. The acute abdomen. Western Veterinary Conference; 2008.

16. Connolly DJ. The Ascitic Dog: British Small Animal Congress; 2006.

17. Blok B. Thoracocentesis. In: *Clinical procedures in Emergency Medicine*. Philadelphia, PA: Saunders; 2004.

18. Doelken P, Sahn SA. *Thoracocentesis Textbook of Critical Care*. Philadelphia, PA: Saunders; 2006.

19. Fossum TW. *Surgery If the Lower Respiratory System: Pleural Cavity and Diaphragm*, pp. 896–929. Philadelphia, PA: Mosby; 2007.

20. Battaglia A. *Small Animal Emergency and Critical Care A Manual for the Veterinary Technician*. Philadelphia, PA: Saunders; 2001.

21. Sauve' V. Pleural space disease. In: *Small Animal Critical Care Medicine*, pp. 125–130. Philadelphia, PA: Saunders; 2009.

22. I.C.U. Medical Inc. Smart-Y Centesis Device. http://www.icumedical.com

23. Chew DJ, Dibartola SP, Schenck PA. *Canine and Feline Nephrology and Urology*, 2nd edition, pp. 2–5. St. Louis, MO: Elsevier Saunders; 2011.

24. Wingfield WE. *Veterinary Emergency Medicine Secrets*, 2nd edition, pp. 449–455. Philadelphia, PA: Hanley & Belfus; 2001.

25. Bassert JM, McCurnin DM. *McCurnin's Clinical Textbook for Veterinary Technicians*, 4th edition, pp. 591–593. St. Louis, MO: Saunders Elsevier; 1998.

26. Barrett M, Campbell VL. Aerobic bacterial culture of used intravenous fluid bags intended for use as urine collection reservoirs. *Journal of the American Animal Hospital Association* 2008;44: 2–4.

27. Barsanti JA, Shotts EB, Crowell WA, Finco DR, Brown J. Effect of therapy on susceptibility to urinary tract infections in male cats with indwelling urethral catheters. *Journal of Veterinary Internal Medicine* 1992;6:64–70.

28. Barsanti JA, Blue J, Edmunds J. Urinary tract infection due to indwelling bladder catheters in dogs and cats. *Journal of the American Veterinary Medical Association* 1985;187:384–388.

29. Smarick SD, Haskins SC, Aldrich J, et al. Incidence of catheter-associated urinary tract infection among dogs in a small animal intensive care unit. *Journal of the American Veterinary Medical Association* 2004;224:1936–1940.

30. Ogeer-Gyles J, Mathews K, Weese JS, et al. Evaluation of catheter-associated urinary tract infections and multi-drug-resistant Escherichia coli isolates from the urine of dogs with indwelling urinary catheters. *Journal of the American Veterinary Medical Association* 2006;229:1584–1590.

31. Bubenik LJ, Hosgood GL, Waldron DR, Snow LA. Frequency of urinary tract infection in catheterized dogs and comparison of bacterial culture and susceptibility testing results for catheterized and noncatheterized dogs with urinary tract infections. *Journal of the American Veterinary Medical Association* 2007;231:893–899.

32. Bubenik J, Hosgood G, Hosgood G. Urinary tract infection in dogs with thoracolumbar intervertebral disc herniation and urinary bladder dysfunction managed by manual expression, indwelling catheterization or intermittent catheterization. *Veterinary Surgery: VS: the Official Journal of the American College of Veterinary Surgeons* 2008;37:791–800.

33. Sullivan LA, Campbell VL, Onuma SC. Evaluation of open versus closed urine collection systems and development of nosocomial bacteria in dogs. *Journal of the American Veterinary Medical Association* 2010;237:187–190.

34. McSherry LJ.. Techniques for bone marrow aspiration and biopsy. *Textbook of Veterinary Internal Medicine*, 7th edition, eds. SJ Ettinger, EC Feldman, pp. 383–385. St. Louis, MO: Saunders; 2010.

35. Hendrix CM. *Laboratory Procedure for Veterinary Technicians*, 5th edition, pp. 60–70, 290–301. St. Louis, MO: Mosby Elsevier; 2007.

36. Price A. Aspirating the answer: bone marrow aspirate basics, ACVIM 2010 Proceedings; 2010.

Section 5

1. Chamness CJ. Endoscopic instrumentation. In: *Small Animal Endoscopy*, 2nd edition, ed. TR Tams, pp. 3–27. St. Louis, MO: Mosby; 1999.

2. Committee SP. Standards of Infection Control in Reprocessing of Flexible Gastrointestinal Endoscopes. Society of Gastroenterology Nurses and Associates, Inc. (SGNA); 2007.

3. Committee SP. Guideline for Use of High Level Disinfectants & Sterilants for Reprocessing Flexible Gastrointestinal Endoscopes. Society of Gastroenterology Nurses and Associates, Inc. (SGNA); 2007.

4. Guilford WG, Center SA, Strombeck DR, Williams DA, Meyer DJ. *Strombeck's Small Animal Gastroenterology*, 3rd edition. Philadelphia PA: WB Saunders; 1996.

Section 6

1. Refinetti R. Big dogs cooler than small dogs. *Veterinary Forum* 2009;26(3):24.

2. Dirckx JH (ed.). *Stedman's Concise Medical Dictionary for the Health Professions*, 4th edition, Baltimore, MD: Lippincott, Williams, Wilkins; 2001.

3. Miller J. *Textbook of Veterinary Internal Medicine*, Ettinger & Feldman, 7th edition, Vols. 1 and 2, p. 41. St. Louis, MO: W.B. Elsevier Saunders; 2010.

4. Pachtinger G, King LG. Fever of unknown origin. *Clinician's Brief* 2010;8(3):29–31.

5. Taylor P. *Textbook of Veterinary Internal Medicine*, Ettinger & Feldman, 7th edition, Vols. 1 and 2, p. 46. St. Louis, MO: W.B. Elsevier Saunders; 2010.

6. Jack CM, Watson PM. *Veterinary Technician's Daily Reference Guide*, 2nd edition, p. 346. Ames, IA: Blackwell; 2008.

7. Laforcade AM. Mitochondrial Energetics in Sepsis. International Veterinary Emergency and Critical Care Symposium; 2003.

8. Laforcade AM. Postoperative Care of the Septic Patient. International Veterinary Emergency and Critical Care Symposium; 2003.

9. Silverstein D. Clinical Markers and Prevention of Sepsis. International Veterinary Emergency and Critical Care Symposium; 2003.

10. Rivera A. MODS and SIRS. International Veterinary Emergency and Critical Care Symposium; 2003.

11. Proulx J. Systemic Inflammatory Response Syndrome. American Animal Hospital Association Scientific Program; 2003.

12. Schaer M. Clinical Pearls in Intensive and Critical Care I and II. Western Veterinary Conference; 2003.

13. Otto C. Biomarkers of Sepsis. International Veterinary Emergency and Critical Care Symposium; 2006.

14. Rozanski A. Cytokines: Who's who and should I care? International Veterinary Emergency and Critical Care Symposium; 2006.

15. Schaffran N. Pain in critically Ill small animals: ethical aspects. *Veterinary Technician the Complete Journal for the Veterinary Hospital Staff* 1998;19(5):349–353.

16. Womack B. Providing nutritional support to critical care patients. *Veterinary Technician the Complete Journal for the Veterinary Hospital Staff* 2003;24(6):376–386.

17. Mott J. Ethical decision making: dealing with dilemmas and improving patient care. *Veterinary Technician the Complete Journal for the Veterinary Hospital Staff* 2004;25(2):126–131.

18. Limon L. Nosocomial infections. *The National Association of Veterinary Technicians in America Journal* 2006;(Winter):29.

19. Wilson JH. Avoiding nosocomial infections. *The National Association of Veterinary Technicians in America Journal* 2007;(Summer): 64–68.

20. Otto CM. Sepsis in veterinary patients: what do we know and where can we go? *Journal of Veterinary Emergency and Critical Care* 2007;17(4):329–331.

21. DeClue C. Acute respiratory distress syndrome in dogs and cats: a review of clinical findings and pathophysiology. *Journal of Veterinary Emergency and Critical Care* 2007;17(4):340–347.

22. Otto CM. Clinical trials in spontaneous disease in dogs: a new paradigm for investigation of sepsis. *Journal of Veterinary Emergency and Critical Care* 2007;17(4):359–367.

23. Nemzek JA, Agrodnia MA, Hauptman JG Breed specific pro-inflammatory cytokine production as a predisposing factor for susceptibility to sepsis in the dog. *Journal of Veterinary Emergency and Critical Care* 2007;17(4):368–372.

24. Fransson BA, Lagerstedt AS, Bergstrom A, et al. C-reactive protein, tumor necrosis factor a, and interleukin-6 in dogs with pyometra and SIRS. *Journal of Veterinary Emergency and Critical Care* 2007;17(4):373–381.

25. Wuestenberg K. Clinical recognition and treatment of shock. International Veterinary Emergency and Critical Care Symposium; 2008.

26. Hackett T. Fluid therapy. *The National Association of Veterinary Technicians in America Journal* 2008;(Summer)58–63.

27. Wortinger A. The benefits of using nutrition in the management of critical care cases. *Veterinary Technician the Complete Journal for the Veterinary Hospital Staff* 2009;30(3):26–28.

28. Wuestenberg K. Physical therapy interventions in the ICU. American College of Veterinary Internal Medicine Forum; 2009.

Appendix Accredited State Veterinary Diagnostic Laboratories

Arizona	Arizona Veterinary Diagnostic Lab 2831 N. Freeway Tucson, AZ 85705	Phone: 520-621-2356 Fax: 520-626-8696 http://cals.arizona.edu/vdl/
Arkansas	Veterinary Diagnostic Laboratory Arkansas Livestock and Poultry Commission Shipping Address: One Natural Resources Drive Little Rock, AR 72205 Mailing Address: PO Box 8505 Little Rock, AR 72215	Phone: 501-907-2430 Fax: 501-907-2410 http://alpc.arkansas.gov/Pages/default.aspx
California	CA Animal Health & Food Safety Lab System University of California, Davis Shipping Address: West Health Science Drive Davis, CA 95616 Mailing Address: PO Box 1770 Davis, CA 95617-1770	Phone: 530-752-8709 Fax: 530-752-5680 http://cahfs.ucdavis.edu
Colorado	Colorado State University Veterinary Diagnostic Lab Shipping Address: Fort Collins, CO 80523 Mailing Address: CSU DLab Fort Collins, CO 80523	Phone: 970-297-1281 Fax: 970-297-0320 http://www.dlab.colostate.edu

Small Animal Internal Medicine for Veterinary Technicians and Nurses, First Edition. Edited by Linda Merrill.
© 2012 John Wiley & Sons, Inc. Published 2012 by John Wiley & Sons, Inc.

Connecticut	Connecticut Veterinary Medical Diagnostic Laboratory Department of Pathobiology & Veterinary Science University of Connecticut Shipping Address: 61 N. Eagleville Road, Unit-3089 Storrs, CT 06269-3089 Mailing Address: 61 N. Eagleville Road, Unit-3089 Storrs, CT 06269-3089	Phone: 860-486-4000 Fax: 860-486-2794 http://www.patho.uconn.edu
Florida	Kissimmee Animal Disease Diagnostic Laboratory Florida Dept. of Agriculture & Consumer Services Shipping Address: 2700 N. John Young Parkway Kissimmee, FL 34741 Mailing Address: PO Box 458006 Kissimmee, FL 34745	Phone: 321-697-1400 Fax: 321-697-1467 http://www.freshfromflorida.com/ai/index.shtml
Georgia	Athens Veterinary Diagnostic Laboratory College of Veterinary Medicine University of Georgia Athens, GA 30602-7383	Phone: 706-542-5568 Fax: 706-542-5977 http://www.vet.uga.edu/dlab
	Veterinary Diagnostic and Investigational Laboratory University of Georgia Shipping Address: 43 Brighton Road Tifton, GA 31793 Mailing Address: PO Box 1389 Tifton, GA 31793	Phone: 229-386-3340 Fax: 229-386-7128 http://www.vet.uga.edu/dlab
Illinois	College of Veterinary Medicine Veterinary Diagnostic Laboratory Shipping Address: PO Box U Urbana, IL 61802 Mailing Address: 2001 South Lincoln Ave. Rm 1224 Urbana, IL 61802	Phone: 217-333-1620 Fax: 217-244-2439 http://www.cvm.uiuc.edu/vdl/
Indiana	Animal Disease Diagnostic Lab Purdue University 406 South University St. West Lafayette, IN 47907	Phone: 765-494-7440 Fax: 765-494-9181 http://www.addl.purdue.edu
Iowa	ISU- College of Vet Med Vet Diagnostic Lab 1600 S. 16th Street Ames, IA 50011	Phone: 515-294-1950 Fax: 515-294-3564 http://www.vdpam.iastate.edu
Kansas	Kansas State Veterinary Diagnostic Laboratory Kansas State University 1800 Denison Ave., Moiser Hall Manhattan, KS 66506	Phone: 785-532-5650 Fax: 785-532-4481 http://www.vet.k-state.edu/depts/dmp/

Kentucky	Murray State University	Phone: 270-886-3959

Kentucky
Murray State University
Breathitt Veterinary Center
Shipping Address:
715 North Drive
Hopkinsville, KY 42240
Mailing Address:
PO Box 2000
Hopkinsville, KY 42241-2000

Phone: 270-886-3959
Fax: 270-886-4295
http://breathitt.murraystate.edu/bvc

Livestock Disease Diagnostic Center
Shipping Address:
1490 Bull Lea Rd.
Lexington, KY 40511
Mailing Address:
PO Box 14125
Lexington, KY 40512

Phone: 859-253-0571
Fax: 859-255-1624
http://www.lddc.uky.edu/

Louisiana
LA Animal Disease Diagnostic Laboratory
Shipping Address:
1909 Skip Bertman Dr. Rm. 1519
Baton Rouge, LA 70803
Mailing Address:
PO Box 25070
Baton Rouge, LA 70894

Phone: 225-578-9777
Fax: 225-578-9784
http://laddl.lsu.edu

Michigan
Diagnostic Center for Population and Animal Health
Michigan State University
Shipping Address:
4125 Beaumont Road, Room 122
Lansing, MI 48910-8104
Mailing Address:
PO Box 30076
Lansing, MI 48909-7576

Phone: 517-353-0635
Fax: 517-353-5096
http://www.animalhealth.msu.edu

Minnesota
Veterinary Diagnostic Laboratory
University of Minnesota
1333 Gortner Avenue
St. Paul, MN 55108-1098

Phone: 612-625-8787
Fax: 612-624-8707
http://www.vdl.umn.edu

Mississippi
Mississippi Veterinary Research and Diagnostic
Laboratory System
Mississippi State University
Shipping Address:
3137 Highway 468 West
Pearl, MS 39208
Mailing Address:
P.O. Box 97813
Pearl, MS 39288

Phone: 601-420-4700
Fax: 601-420-4719
http://www.cvm.msstate.edu/diagnostic_labs/index.html

Missouri
Veterinary Medical Diagnostic Lab
University of Missouri
Shipping Address:
1600 East Rollins Road
Columbia, MO 65211
Mailing Address:
PO Box 6023
Columbia, MO 65205

Phone: 573-882-6811
Fax: 573-882-1411
http://www.vmdl.missouri.edu

Montana	Montana Department of Livestock Montana Veterinary Diagnostic Laboratory Shipping Address: South 19th and Lincoln Bozeman, MT 59718 Mailing Address: PO Box 997 Bozeman, MT 59771	Phone: 406-994-4885 Fax: 406-994-6344 http://www.liv.mt.gov/default.mcpx
Nebraska	Veterinary Diagnostic Center Fair Street, E. Campus Loop Shipping Address: PO Box 82646 Lincoln, NE 68501-2646 Mailing Address: PO Box 830907 Lincoln, NE 68583-0907	Phone: 402-472-1434 Fax: 402-472-3094 http://vbms.unl.edu/nvdls
New York	Animal Health Diagnostic Center College of Veterinary Medicine Cornell University Shipping Address: Upper Tower Road Ithaca, NY 14853 Mailing Address: PO Box 5786 Ithaca, NY 14852	Phone: 607-253-3900 Fax: 607-253-3943 http://ahdc.vet.cornell.edu/
North Carolina	North Carolina Department of Agriculture & Consumer Services Rollins Laboratory Shipping Address: 2101 Blue Ridge Road Raleigh, NC 27607 Mailing Address: 1031 Mail Service Center Raleigh, NC 27699-1031	Phone: 919-733-3986 Fax: 919-733-0454 http://www.ncagr.gov/vet/ncvdl/
North Dakota	Department of Veterinary Diagnostic Services North Dakota State University Shipping Address: 1523 Centennial Blvd., Van Es Hall Fargo, ND 58105 Mailing Address: PO Box 5406 Fargo, ND 58105	Phone: 701-231-8307 Fax: 701-231-7514 http://www.vdl.ndsu.edu/
Ohio	Animal Disease Diagnostic Lab 8995 E. Main Street, Building 6 Reynoldsburg, OH 43068	Phone: 614-728-6220 Fax: 614-728-6310 http://www.agri.ohio.gov/addl/
Oklahoma	Oklahoma Animal Disease Diagnostic Laboratory Oklahoma State University Shipping Address: Center for Veterinary Health Sciences Farm and Ridge Road Stillwater, OK 74078 Mailing Address: PO Box 7001 Stillwater, OK 74076-7001	Phone: 405-744-6623 Fax: 405-744-8612 http://www.cvm.okstate.edu

Oregon	Veterinary Diagnostic Laboratory Oregon State University Magruder Hall, Room 134 Shipping Address: 30th and Washington Way Corvallis, OR 97331 Mailing Address: PO Box 429 Corvallis, OR 97339-0429	Phone: 541-737-3261 Fax: 541-737-6817 http://oregonstate.edu/vetmed/diagnostic
Pennsylvania	Department of Agriculture Pennsylvania Veterinary Laboratory 2305 N. Cameron Street Harrisburg, PA 17110-9408	Phone: 717-787-8808 Fax: 717-772-3895 http://www.padls.org
	Pennsylvania State University PADLS—Penn State Animal Diagnostic Laboratory Orchard Road University Park, PA 16802-1110	Phone: 814-863-0837 Fax: 814-865-3907 http://www.padls.org
	University of Pennsylvania PADLS—New Bolton Center 382 West Street Road Kennett Square, PA 19348	Phone: 610-444-5800 Fax: 610-925-8106 http://www.padls.org
South Carolina	Clemson Veterinary Diagnostic Center Shipping Address: 500 Clemson Road Columbia, SC 29229 Mailing Address: PO Box 102406 Columbia, SC 29224-2406	Phone: 803-788-2260 Fax: 803-699-8910 http://www.clemson.edu/public/lph/lab/
South Dakota	Animal Disease Research and Diagnostic Laboratory South Dakota State University Shipping Address: Animal Disease Research Building, North Campus Drive Brookings, SD 57007-1396 Mailing Address: Box 2175, North Campus Drive Brookings, SD 57007-1396	Phone: 605-688-5171 Fax: 605-688-6003 http://www.sdstate.edu/vs/mission/index.cfm
Tennessee	CE Kord Animal Disease Diagnostic Laboratory Ellington Agricultural Center Shipping Address: 440 Hogan Rd., Porter Building Nashville, TN 37220 Mailing Address: PO Box 40627 Nashville, TN 37204	Phone: 615-837-5125 Fax: 615-837-5250 http://www.tn.gov/agriculture/regulatory/kord.shtml
Texas	Texas Veterinary Medical Diagnostic Laboratory (TVMDL) TVMDL-College Station Shipping Address: 1 Sippel Road College Station, Texas 77843 Mailing Address: P.O. Box 3040 College Station, Texas 77841-3040	Phone: 979-845-3414 Fax: 979-845-1794 http://tvmdl.tamu.edu/

	TVMDL—Amarillo Shipping Address: 6610 Amarillo Blvd., West Amarillo, Texas 79106 Mailing Address: P.O. Box 3200 Amarillo, Texas 79116-3200	Dr. Robert Sprowls Phone: 806-353-7478 Fax: 806-359-0636 http://tvmdl.tamu.edu/
	TVMDL—Gonzales Shipping Address: 1812 Water Street Gonzales, Texas 78629 Mailing Address: P. O. Box 84 Gonzales, Texas 78629	Phone: 830-672-2834 Fax: 830-672-2835 http://tvmdl.tamu.edu/
	TVMDL—Center Shipping/Mailing Address: 635 Malone Drive Center, Texas 79535	Phone: 936-598-4451 Fax: 936-598-2741 http://tvmdl.tamu.edu/
Utah	Utah Veterinary Diagnostic Laboratory Shipping and Mailing Address: 950 East 1400 North Logan, UT. 84341	Phone: 435-797-1895 Fax: 435-797-2805 http://www.usu.edu/uvdl/
Washington	Washington Animal Disease Diagnostic Laboratory Washington State University Shipping Address: 155N Bustad Hall Pullman, WA 99164-7034 Mailing Address: PO Box 647034 Pullman, WA 99164-7034	Phone: 509-335-9696 Fax: 509-335-7424 http://www.vetmed.wsu.edu/depts_waddl
Wisconsin	Wisconsin Veterinary Diagnostic Laboratory University of Wisconsin 445 Easterday Lane Madison, WI 53706	Phone: 608-262-5432 Fax: 847-574-8085 http://www.wvdl.wisc.edu
Wyoming	Wyoming State Veterinary Laboratory 1174 Snowy Range Road Laramie, WY 82070	Phone: 307-742-6638 Fax: 307-721-2051 http://wyovet.uwyo.edu/
Canada	Animal Health Laboratory University of Guelph Shipping Address: Door P2, Building 49, McIntosh Lane Guelph, Ontario N1G 2W1 Mailing Address: PO Box 3612 Guelph, Ontario N1H 6R8 CANADA	Phone: 519-824-4120 ext. 54502 Fax: 519-821-8072 http://www.guelphlabservices.com/AHL/
	Animal Health Branch 1767 Angus Campbell Road Abbotsford, BC V3G 2M3 CANADA	Phone: 604-556-3003 Fax: 604-556-3010 http://www.agf.gov.bc.ca/ahc/

Abbreviations

Abbr	Word/term
^{123}I	Iodine-123
^{131}I	Iodine-131
^{99m}TcO4-	Technetium-99m as pertechnetate
2-ME	2-Mercaptoethanol
α	Alpha
$α_1$-PI	Alpha$_1$-protease inhibitor
β	Beta
ω	Omega
AAFCO	American Association of Feed Control Officials
AAFP	Association of Feline Practitioners
AAHA	American Animal Hospital Association
AANAT	Serotonin N-acetyltransferase
AAROM	Active-assisted range of motion
ABG	Arterial blood gas
ACD	Acid citrate dextrose
ACE	Angiotensin-converting enzyme
ACEi, ACEI	Angiotensin-converting enzyme inhibitor
AChR	Acetylcholine receptor
ACL	Anterior cruciate ligament
ACT	Activated clotting time
ACTH	Adrenocorticotrophic hormone
ADH	Antidiuretic hormone
ADHF	Acutely decompensated heart failure
AD-MSC	Adipose-derived mesenchymal stem cell
ADP	Adenosine diphosphate
Ag	Antigen
AGID	Agar gel immunodiffusion
AIDS	Acquired immune deficiency syndrome
ALP	Alkaline phosphatase
ALT	Alanine aminotransferase
AMP	Adenosine monophosphate
ANA	Antinuclear antibodies
ANP	Atrial natriuretic peptides
APC	Activated protein C
aPTT, APTT	Activated partial thromboplastin time
APUDoma	Amine precursor uptake and decarboxylation tumor
ARDS	Acute respiratory distress syndrome
ARF	Acute renal failure
AROM	Active range of motion
AST	Aspartate aminotransferase
AT	Antithrombin
ATE	Arterial thromboembolism
ATP	Adenosine triphosphate
AV	Atrioventricular valves
AVMA	American Veterinary Medical Association
AVP	Arginine vasopressin
BAL	Bronchoalveolar lavage
BCS	Body condition score
BER	Basal energy requirement
BFU-E	Burst-forming unit-erythroid
BGC	Blood glucose concentration
BID	Bis in die (twice a day)
BIPS	Barium-impregnated polyethylene spheres
BMBT	Buccal mucosal bleeding time

Small Animal Internal Medicine for Veterinary Technicians and Nurses, First Edition. Edited by Linda Merrill.
© 2012 John Wiley & Sons, Inc. Published 2012 by John Wiley & Sons, Inc.

BNP	Brain natriuretic peptide		CRTZ	Chemoreceptor trigger zone
BP	Blood pressure		CRYOPP	Cryoprecipitate poor plasma
BPH	Benign prostatic hyperplasia		CSA	Chondrosarcoma
BSA	Body surface area		CSD	Cat scratch disease
BUN	Blood urea nitrogen		CSF	Cerebral spinal fluid
C	Celsius		CT	Computed tomography
C3	Complement 3		CUPS	Chronic ulcerative paradental stomatitis
Ca^{2+}	Calcium		CVP	Central venous pressure
CACH	Copper-associated chronic hepatitis		D5W	Dextrose 5% in water
CaO_2	Changes in arterial oxygen concentration		DABP	Direct arterial blood pressure
CATE	Canine arterial thromboembolism		DCM	Dilated cardiomyopathy
CAV2	Canine adenovirus 2		DDAVP	Deamino-8-d-arginine vasopressin
CBC	Complete blood count		DE	Digestable energy
CCD	Charge-coupled device		DEA	Dog erythrocyte antigen
CCK	Cholecystokinin		DER	Daily energy requirements
CCK-2	Cholecystokinin 2		DES	Diethylstilbestrol
CD	Cluster of differentiation/designation		DHA	Docosahexaenoic acid
CD	Compact disk		DI	Diabetes insipidus
CDV	Canine distemper virus		DIC	Disseminated intravascular coagulation
CE	Client education		DJD	Degenerative joint disease
CF	Complement fixation		DKA	Diabetic ketoacidosis
CFU-E	Colony-forming unit-erythroid		dL	Deciliter
CGE	Canine granulocytic ehrlichiosis		DM	Diabetes mellitus
CGMS	Continuous glucose monitoring system		DM	Dry matter
CHF	Congestive heart failure		DMSO	Dimethyl sulfoxide
CHOP	Cyclophosphamide, hydroxydoxorubicin (doxorubicin), Oncovin˙ (vincristine), prednisone		DNA	Deoxyribonucleic acid
			DNM	Dynamin
			DPG	Diphosphoglycerate
CHV	Canine herpesvirus		DPL	Diagnostic peritoneal lavage
CIBDAI	Canine IBD Activity Index		DV	Dorsoventral
CIRDC	Canine infectious respiratory disease complex		DVD	Digital versatile disk
CIV	Canine influenza virus		Dx	Diagnosis
CK	Creatine kinase		EB	Eosinophilic bronchopneumopathy (formerly known as PIE)
CKCS	Cavalier King Charles spaniel			
CKD	Chronic kidney disease		ECF	Extracellular fluid
CLAD	Canine leukocyte adhesion deficiency		ECG	Electrocardiogram
cm, cm^3	Centimeter, cubic centimeter		ECM	Erythema chronicum migrans
CME	Canine monocytic ehrlichiosis		EDTA	Ethylenediaminetetraacetic acid
CNP	C-type natriuretic peptide		EE	Eosinophilic enteritis
CNP	Circulating neutrophil pool		EFA	Essential fatty acid
CNS	Central nervous system		EGE	Eosinophilic gastroenteritis
CO_2	Carbon dioxide		EHBO	Extrahepatic biliary obstruction
COPD	Chronic obstructive pulmonary disease		EHEC	Enterohemorrhagic *Escherichia coli*
COPV	Canine oral papillomavirus		EIA	Enzyme immunoassay
COX	Cyclooxygenase		EIC	Exercise-induced collapse
CPiV	Canine parainfluenza virus		ELISA	Enzyme-linked immunosorbent assay
CPK	Creatine phosphokinase		EMG	Electromyogram
cPLI	Canine pancreatic lipase		EPA	Eicosapentaenoic acid
CPV	Canine parvovirus		EPI	Exocrine pancreatic insufficiency
CRF	Chronic renal failure		EPO	Erythropoietin
CRH	Corticotropin-releasing hormone		EpoR	Erythropoietin receptor
CRI	Continuous/Constant Rate Infusion		ERD	Early renal damage
CRI	Chronic renal insufficiency		EtO	Ethylene oxide
CRRT	Continuous renal replacement therapy		E-tube	Esophagostomy tube
CRT	Capillary refill time		F	Fahrenheit

FA	Fluorescent antibody	GS	Gingivostomatitis
FAO	Food and Agriculture Organization	GSPC	Gingivitis–stomatitis–pharyngitis complex
FAT	Functional adrenal tumor	GT	Glanzmann's thrombastenia
FATE	Feline arterial thromboembolism	G-tube	Gastrostomy tube
Fc	Fragment, crystallizable	Gy	Gray
FCV	Feline corona virus	h	Hour
FDA	Food and Drug Administration	H^+	Hydrogen
FDP	Fibrin degradation products	H_2	Histamine 2
FEGC	Feline eosinophilic granuloma complex	H_2O	Water
FeLV	Feline leukemia virus	HA (H)	Hemagglutinin
FFP	Fresh frozen plasma	HAC	Hyperadrenocorticism
FHV	Feline herpesvirus	Hb, Hgb	Hemoglobin
FIBDAI	Feline IBD Activity Index	HCM	Hypertrophic cardiomyopathy
FIC	Feline idiopathic cystitis	HCO_3-	Bicarbonate
FiO_2	Fractional concentration of oxygen	HCS	Hepatocutaneous syndrome
FIP	Feline infectious peritonitis	HCT	Hematocrit
FIV	Feline immunodeficiency virus	HDDST	High dose dexamethasone suppression test
FLUTD	Feline lower urinary tract disease	HE	Hepatic encephalopathy
FNA	Fine needle aspirate/aspiration	Hg	Mercury
FOS	Fructooligosaccharides	hIVIG	Human intravenous immunoglobulin
FP	Frozen plasma	HLD	High level disinfectant
FPn	Feline pneumonitis	HMWK	High molecular weight kininogen
FPV	Feline panleukopenia virus	HPAA	Hypothalmic–pituitary–adrenal axis
FPV	Feline parvovirus	hpf	High power field
FR	French	HSA	Hemangiosarcoma
FSA	Fibrosarcoma	HT	Hydroxytryptamine
FSH	Follicle-stimulating hormone	HUS	Hemolytic uremic syndrome
fT4 (ED)	Free T4 by equilibrium dialysis	IBD	Inflammatory bowel disease
FUD	Fever of undetermined origin	ICH	Infectious canine hepatitis
FUO	Fever of unknown origin	ICU	Intensive care unit
FUS	Feline urologic syndrome	IDDM	Insulin-dependent diabetes mellitus
FWB	Fresh whole blood	IFA	Immunofluorescent assay
g	Gram	IFN-α	Interferon alpha
ga.	Gauge	Ig	Immunoglobulin
GAG	Glycosaminoglycans	IGF	Insulin-like growth factor
gag	Group-specific antigens	IL	Interleukin
GALT	Gastrointestinal (gut)-associated lymphoid tissue	IM	Intramuscular
		IMHA	Immune-mediated hemolytic anemia
GBM	Gallbladder mucocoele	IMPA	Immune-mediated polyarthropathy
G-CSF	Granulocyte colony-stimulating factor	IMT	Immune-mediated thrombocytopenia
GDV	Gastric dilatation–volvulus	IPF	Idiopathic pulmonary fibrosis
GE	Gross energy	IRIS	International Renal Interest Society
GFR	Glomerular filtration rate	ISF	Interstitial fluid
GGT	Gamma-glutamyl transferase	IU	International units
GGT	Gamma-glutamyl transpeptidase	IV	Intravenous
GH	Growth hormone	IVD(D)	Intervertebral disk (disease)
GHIH	Growth hormone release-inhibiting	K^+	Potassium
GHLO	Gastric *Helicobacter*-like organism	kcal	Kilocalorie
GI	Gastrointestinal	KCl	Potassium chloride
GIP	Gastric inhibitory polypeptide	KCS	Keratoconjunctivitis sicca
GIT	Gastrointestinal tract	kg	Kilogram
GM	Granulocyte-macrophage	kJ	Kilojoules
GMC	Giant migrating contractions	KKK	Kininogen–Kallikrein–Kinin system
GnRH	Gonadotropin-releasing hormone	K-time	Clot formation time
GP	Glycoprotein	L	Lumbar

L	Liter		NAC	N-acetylcysteine
LADA	Latent autoimmune diabetes of adults		NaCl	Saline
lbs	Pounds		NADPQI	N-acetyl-p-benzoquinoneimine
LD	Loading dose		NE	Nasoesophageal
LDDST	Low dose dexamethasone suppression test		ng	Nanogram
LMWH	Low molecular weight heparin		NIDDM	Non-insulin-dependent diabetes mellitus
LPC	Lymphocytic plasmacytic colitis		NK	Natural killer
LPE	Lymphocytic plasmacytic enteritis		NMDA	N-methyl-D-aspartate
lpf	Low power field		NME	Necrolytic migratory erythema
LPGS	Lymphoplasmacytic gingivitis-stomatitis		nmol	Nanomole
LRS	Lactated Ringer's solution		NormR	Normosol-R
LS-CHF	Left-sided congestive heart failure		NPH	Neutral protamine Hagedorn
LYST	Lysosomal trafficking gene		nRBC	Nucleated red blood cells
m	Meter		NSAID	Non-steroidal anti-inflammatory drug
MA	Maximum convergence		NT-proANP	N-terminal prohormone of atrial natriuretic peptide
MAP	Mean arterial pressure			
MAT	Microscopic agglutination test		NT-proBNP	N-terminal prohormone of brain natriuretic peptide
MC	Mast cell			
mcg, μg	Microgram		O_2	Oxygen
MCHC	Mean corpuscular hemoglobin concentration		OA	Osteoarthritis
mcL, μL	Microliter		ORSA	Oxacillin-resistant *Staphylococcus aureus*
mcm, μm	Micron		OSA	Osteosarcoma
MCT	Medium chain triglycerides		OSHA	Occupational health and safety
MCV	Mean corpuscular volume		Osp	Outer surface protein
MDR	Multidrug resistance		OSPT	One-Step prothrombin time
ME	Metabolizable energy		PAC	Picture archiving and communication
MEE	Metabolic energy expenditure		$PaCO_2$	Partial pressure of carbon dioxide
mEq	Milliequivalent		pANCA	Perinuclear antineutrophilic cytoplasmic antibodies
MER	Maintenance energy requirements			
mg	Milligram		PaO_2	Partial pressure of oxygen
MH	Malignant hyperthermia		PCD	Primary ciliary dyskinesia
MIC	Minimum inhibitory concentration		PCR	Polymerase chain reaction
mL	Milliliter		PCV	Packed cell volume
MLK	Morphine–lidocaine–ketamine		PD	Polydipsia
MLV	Modified live virus		PDH	Pituitary-dependent hyperadrenocorticism
mm	Millimeter		PEEP	Positive end-expiratory pressure
mmHg	Millimeter of mercury		PEG	Percutaneous endoscopic (placed) gastrostomy
MMF	Mycophenolate mofetil			
MMM	Masticatory muscle myositis		PET	Positron emission tomography
mmol	millimole		P-gp	P-glycoprotein
MNP	Marginal neutrophil pool		pH	Potential hydrogen
MODS	Multi (multiple) organ dysfunction syndrome		PH	Pulmonary hypertension
mOsm	milliosmol		PIE	Pulmonary infiltrates with eosinophils (now known as eosinophilic bronchopneumopathy)
MRI	Magnetic resonance imaging			
mRNA	messenger RNA		PIV	Parainfluenza virus
MRSA	Methicillin-resistant *Staphylococcus aureus*		PIVKA	Protein induced by vitamin K antagonism
MRSA-CA	Community-associated MRSA		PK	Pyruvate kinase
MRSA-HA	Hospital or Health-Care-Associated MRSA		PLE	Protein-losing enteropathy
MRSA-LA	Livestock-associated MRSA		PLN	Protein-losing nephropathy
MSDS	Material safety data sheet		PO	Per os (by mouth)
MCT	Mast cell tumor		PP	Pancreatic polypeptide
MST	Median survival time		PPE	Personal protection/protective equipment
n-3	Omega-3		PPI	Proton pump inhibitors
NA	Noradrenaline		PPN	Partial parenteral nutrition
NA (N)	Neuraminidase		PR	Pulmonic regurgitation
Na^+	Sodium		PRA	Plasma renin activity

PRAA	Persistent right aortic arch	SCF	Stem cell factor
pRBC	Packed red blood cell	SCFA	Short-chain fatty acids
PRN	Pro re nata (as needed/as required)	SI	Small intestine
PROM	Passive range of motion	SIBO	Small intestinal bacterial overgrowth
PRP	Platelet-rich plasma	SID	Semel in die (once a day)
PSIg	Platelet surface-associated immunoglobulin	SIRS	Systemic inflammatory response syndrome
PSS	Portosystemic shunt	SLE	Systemic lupus erythematosus
PT	Prothrombin time	SND	Superficial necrolytic dermatitis
PTE	Pulmonary (arterial) thromboembolism	SpO$_2$	Saturation of peripheral oxygen
PTFE	Polytetrafluoroethylene	spp.	Species
PTH	Parathyroid hormone	SRIF	Somatotropin release-inhibiting factor
PTT	Partial thromboplastin time	SST	Somatostatin
PU	Polyuria	SSTR	Somatastatin receptor
PUFA	Polyunsaturated fatty acids	SWB	Stored whole blood
PVC	Polyvinylchloride	T$_3$	Triiodothyronine
PZI	Protamine zinc insulin	T$_4$	Thyroxine
q	Quaque (every)	TCC	Transitional cell carcinoma
Q	Cardiac output	TCO$_2$	Total carbon dioxide
RA	Rheumatoid arthritis	TEG	Thromboelastography
RAAS	Renin–angiotensin–aldosterone system	TENS	Transcutaneous electrical neuromuscular stimulation
RAST	Radioallergosorbent testing		
RBC	Red blood cell	TF	Tissue factor
RCCT	Randomized controlled clinical trials	THM	Tamm–Horsfall mucoprotein
RCM	Restrictive cardiomyopathy	TID	Ter in die (three times a day)
RDVM	Referring DVM	TIVA	Total intravenous anesthesia
RER	Resting energy requirement	TL	Thoracolumbar
RF, RhF	Rheumatoid factor	TLI	Trypsin-like immunoassay
rhG-CSF	Recombinant granulocytic colony-stimulating factor	TNF (-α)	Tumor necrosis factor (-alpha)
		TNM	Tumor node metastasis
rHuEPO	Recombinant human EPO	TPA, tPA	Tissue plasminogen activator
RIA	Radioimmunoassay	TPH	Tryptophan hydroxylase
RMSF	Rocky Mountain spotted fever	TPN	Total parenteral nutrition
RNA	Ribonucleic acid	TR	Tricuspid regurgitation
ROM	Range of motion	TRH	Thyrotropin-releasing hormone
RSA	Rhabdomyosarcoma	TS	Total solids
RSAT	Rapid slide agglutination test	TSH	Thyroid-stimulating hormone
RS-CHF	Right-sided congestive heart failure	TT	Thrombin time
RT	Radiation therapy	TT4	Total T4
RT, RT-PCR	Reverse transcriptase	TTW	Transtracheal wash
R-time	Reaction time	Tx	Treatment
RTT	Red top tube	U	Units
RVOT	Right ventricular outflow tract	UC:CR	Urine cortisol:creatinine ratio
S	Sacral	UDCA	Ursodeoxycholate
SOAP	Subjective, objective, assessment plan	UP:C	Urine protein-to-creatinine ratio
S1	First heart sound	uPA	Urokinase plasminogen activator
S2	Second heart sound	USB	Universal serial bus
S3	Third heart sound	USG	Urine specific gravity
S4	Fourth heart sound	USMI	Urethral sphincter mechanism incompetence
SA	Sinoatrial	UTI	Urinary tract infection
SAA	Sulfasalicylic acid	UV	Ultraviolet
SAMe	S-adenosylmethionine	VAC	Vincristine adriamycin cyclophosphamide
SaO$_2$	Saturation of oxygen	VAS	Visual analogue scale
SAP	Serum alkaline phosphatase	VBTA	Veterinary bladder antigen test
SBP	Systemic blood pressure	VCR	Video cassette recorder
SBS	Short bowel syndrome	VD	Ventrodorsal
SC, SQ	Subcutaneous	VIP	Vasoactive intestinal peptide

VIP	Vasoactive intestinal protein		WBC	White blood cell
VIPoma	Vasoactive intestinal peptide secreting tumor		WHO	World Health Organization
VPCs	Ventricular premature contractions		WMSD	Work-related musculoskeletal disorder
VSD	Ventricular septal defect		XSCID	X-linked severe combined immunodeficiency
VS-FCV	Virulent systemic feline calicivirus		ZF	Zona fasciculata
vWD	von Willebrand disease		ZG	Zona glomerulosa
vWF	von Willebrand factor		ZR	Zona reticularis

Index

Note: Page numbers in *italics* refer to figures; those in **bold** to tables.

Small Animal Internal Medicine for Veterinary Technicians and Nurses, First Edition. Edited by Linda Merrill.
© 2012 John Wiley & Sons, Inc. Published 2012 by John Wiley & Sons, Inc.